Transcultural Nursing
ASSESSMENT & INTERVENTION

Seventh Edition

Transcultural Nursing

ASSESSMENT & INTERVENTION

Joyce Newman Giger, EdD, APRN, BC, FAAN
Professor Emerita
School of Nursing
University of California at Los Angeles
Los Angeles, California

ELSEVIER

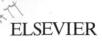
ELSEVIER

3251 Riverport Lane
St. Louis, Missouri 63043

Notices

Knowledge and best practice in this field are constantly changing. As new research and experience broaden our understanding, changes in research methods, professional practices, or medical treatment may become necessary.

Practitioners and researchers must always rely on their own experience and knowledge in evaluating and using any information, methods, compounds, or experiments described herein. In using such information or methods they should be mindful of their own safety and the safety of others, including parties for whom they have a professional responsibility.

With respect to any drug or pharmaceutical products identified, readers are advised to check the most current information provided (i) on procedures featured or (ii) by the manufacturer of each product to be administered, to verify the recommended dose or formula, the method and duration of administration, and contraindications. It is the responsibility of practitioners, relying on their own experience and knowledge of their patients, to make diagnoses, to determine dosages and the best treatment for each individual patient, and to take all appropriate safety precautions.

To the fullest extent of the law, neither the Publisher nor the authors, contributors, or editors, assume any liability for any injury and/or damage to persons or property as a matter of products liability, negligence or otherwise, or from any use or operation of any methods, products, instructions, or ideas contained in the material herein.

Cover image credits: Blend Images, Jon Feingersh/the Agency Collection/Getty Images, Comstock Images/Getty Images, Image Source/Getty Images, Medioimages/Photodisc/Getty Images, UpperCut Images/Tim Dolan Photography/Getty Images.
Previous editions copyrighted 2013, 2008, 2004, 1999, 1995, 1991

Library of Congress Cataloging-in-Publication Data
Names: Giger, Joyce Newman, editor.
Title: Transcultural nursing : assessment & intervention / [edited by] Joyce Newman Giger.
Other titles: Transcultural nursing (Giger)
Description: Seventh edition. | St. Louis, Missouri : Elsevier, [2017] | Includes bibliographical references and index.
Identifiers: LCCN 2015049612| ISBN 9780323399920 (pbk. : alk. paper) | ISBN 9780323400046 (eISBN)
Subjects: | MESH: Transcultural Nursing | Nursing Assessment | Culturally Competent Care | United States
Classification: LCC RT86.54 | NLM WY 107 | DDC 610.73–dc23 LC record available at http://lccn.loc.gov/2015049612

Content Strategist: Tamara Myers
Content Development Manager: Billie Sharp
Content Development Specialist: Charlene Ketchum
Project Manager: Srividhya Vidhyashankar
Design Direction: Maggie Reid

Printed in the United States of America

Last digit is the print number: 9   8   7   6   5   4   3   2

Working together to grow libraries in developing countries

www.elsevier.com • www.bookaid.org

To My Mother
The late Ionia Holmes Newman

To My Husband
Argusta Giger Jr.

To My Mentors
Richmond Calvin, EdD; the late Frances P. Dixon, BS

To My Children
D'artagnan, Carolyn, Taye

*To the students of Bethel College, past, present, and future,
and all the nurses and students who seek a better way to render culturally appropriate care*

CONTRIBUTORS

Susan J. Appel, PhD, ACNP-BC, FNP-BC, CCRN, FAHA
Professor
School of Nursing
University of Alabama at Tuscaloosa
Tuscaloosa, Alabama

Najood G. Azar, PhD, RN
Assistant Professor
School of Nursing
Azusa Pacific University
Azusa, California

Chyi-Kong (Karen) Chang, RN, MSN, PhD
Associate Professor
School of Nursing
Purdue University
West Lafayette, Indiana

Anita Renau Bralock, PhD, CNM
President & CEO
Bralock and Associates Consultancy
Los Angeles, California

Brenda Cherry, MSN, RN, FNP
Associate Professor
Professor Emerita
Georgia Perimeter College

Yoshiko Yamashita Colclough, PhD, RN
Assistant Professor
College of Nursing
Montana State University
Bozeman, Montana

Tina D. DeLapp, EdD, RN FAAN
Emeritus Professor
Carmen Mason School of Nursing
University of Alaska—Anchorage
Anchorage, Alaska

Dawn Liam Doutrich, PhD, RN, CNS
Associate Professor of Nursing
Founder and Director, Linfield Transcultural Nursing
    Program
Washington State University
Vancouver, Washington

Jai Bun K. Earp, PhD, ARNP, FNP-BC, CNE
UAB Gerontology Scholar
Professor & Associate Dean
Graduate Program
School of Nursing
Florida A&M University

Christina R. Esperat, RN, PhD, ARNP, BC, FAAN
Professor and Assistant Dean for Practice and Research
School of Nursing
Texas Tech University, Health Sciences Center
Lubbock, Texas

Miguel A. Franco, PhD
Staff Psychologist, Student Affairs
Assistant Professor of Psychology
Notre Dame University
Notre Dame, Indiana

Deborah R. Gillum, RN, MSN, PhD, ANP, FNP
Dean, School of Nursing
Assistant Professor
Bethel College
Mishawaka, Indiana

Elizabeth W. Gonzalez, PhD, APRN-BC
Associate Professor
College of Nursing & Health Professions
Drexel University
Philadelphia, Pennsylvania

Linda G. Haddad, RN, PhD, FAAN
Associate Dean
Academic Affairs
College of Nursing
University of Florida
Gainesville, Florida

Catherine E. Hanley, RN, BSN, MPH, FAAN, FACHE
Hospital and Health Care Consultant
Flagstaff, Arizona

Anita Hunter, PhD, MSN, RN
Associate Director of Nursing Programs, College of Nursing
Washington State University—Vancouver Campus
Vancouver, Washington

Razia Askaryar Iqbal, PsyD
Clinical Psychologist and Program Director
Jewish Family and Children Services, East Bay
Walnut Creek, California

Kira Ann Lass, MSN, RN, CNS, CCRN
Interventional Radiology
Eden Medical Center
Castro Valley, California

Henry Lewis, III, PharmD
President & CEO
Lewis and Associates
Tallahassee, Florida

Juliene G. Lipson, PhD MA, RN, FAAN
Professor Emerita
Community Health Systems
University of California—San Francisco
San Francisco, California

Cheryl M. Martin, RNC, WHNP, PhD
Associate Professor
School of Nursing
University of Indianapolis
Indianapolis, Indiana

Scott Wilson Miller, RN, MS
Clinical Coordinator, Surgical Services
Ambulatory Surgery Unit, Olson Pavilion
Northwestern Memorial Hospital
Chicago, Illinois

Sherrica Miller, PhD(c), PNP
Doctoral Student
University of California at Los Angeles
Los Angeles, California

Linda McMurry, DNP, RN, NEA-BC
Executive Director
Larry Combest Community Health and Wellness Center
Lubbock, Texas

Cordelia Chinwe Nnedu, PhD, RNc, WHCNP
Professor, Department of Nursing
School of Nursing & Allied Health
Tuskegee University
Tuskegee, Alabama

Cheryl Smythe Padgham, DNP, RN, WHNP,-BC
President & CEO
Padgham & Associates
Newport Beach, California

Donna C. Owen, PhD, RN, CNE
Professor
School of Nursing
Texas Tech University Health Sciences Center
Lubbock, Texas

Mary Reidy, RN, BN, MSC, PhD
Associate Professor Emerita
School of Nursing
University of Montreal
Quebec, Canada

Cynthia C. Small, DNP, MSN, RN, APRN, BC, FNP
Instructor Emerita
Lake Michigan College
Lakeland Regional Health Systems
Benton Harbor, Michigan

Linda S. Smith, PhD, MS, RN, CLNC
Affiliate Faculty
Idaho State University
Vice President for Research
Data Design, Inc.
Horseshoe Bend, Arkansas

Ora L. Strickland, PhD, RN, FAAN
Dean and Professor
College of Nursing and Health Sciences
Florida International University
Miami, Florida

Huaxin Song, PhD
Sr. Research Associate
Texas Tech University Health Sciences Center
Lubbock, Texas

Marilyn Oreta Uvero, PhD(c), Ed.D, MSN, RN
Uvero & Associates Consultancy
Long Beach, California

Mary Grace Umlauf, PhD, RN
Professor Emerita
Capstone College of Nursing
University of Alabama at Tuscaloosa
Tuscaloosa, Alabama

Thad Wilson, PhD, RN, FAAN
Executive Associate Dean
The University of Iowa
College of Nursing
Iowa City, Iowa

FOREWORD

Angela Barron McBride, PhD, RN, FAAN
Distinguished Professor–University Dean Emerita
Indiana University School of Nursing, Indianapolis, IN

Because minorities tend to receive a lower quality of health care even when their access to services is similar to non-minorities and because the diversity—ethnic, racial, age, lifestyle, economic, sexual preferences, and so forth—of the U.S. population is growing, the Institute of Medicine (2003) has advocated cross-cultural education in the health professions as a key strategy in ending such disparities. Nursing has long focused on both personal and population-based caregiving issues (American Nurses' Association, 1980) and has a proud tradition of cross-cultural assessment and intervention dating back to the pioneering work of Leininger (1977). Indeed, one of the first issues of the *Annual Review of Nursing Research* contained a chapter on cross-cultural nursing research (Tripp-Reimer & Dougherty, 1985).

Building on this proud tradition and mindful that there is an urgency all providers must demonstrate in addressing these disparities, Joyce Newman Giger has prepared a new and expanded edition of this award-winning book on transcultural nursing, though with a sense of sadness because her collaborator heretofore, Ruth Davidhizar, died much too young in 2008. Their jointly developed Transcultural Assessment Model, which has been used extensively to develop effective educational and clinical interventions in the past, continues to provide a needed framework for this edition. It focuses on the six cultural phenomena believed to shape care—communication, space, social organization, time, environmental control, and biological variations. Many of the chapters specify how a particular racial/ethnic group (e.g., African-Americans or Appalachians) may vary in these six areas and how these variations must be taken into account in planning care.

While it has become commonplace for nurses to urge culturally appropriate care, what that really means is not always clear, other than some general admonition to be aware that not all patients with the same medical diagnosis are likely to have the same background and experience. The notion that patients and their families make choices based on the unique meaning they assign to their experience is often discounted on a day-to-day basis when the prevailing emphasis seems to be more on the importance of procedures and coverage than on providing tailored interventions. That is why this volume can be so useful to students and seasoned clinicians alike, because it provides many examples of how individual experience is likely to vary in ways that go well beyond the patterning of medical symptoms: Is this man one who responds well to frequent touching? Does this woman need considerable personal space? Will an effective intervention necessarily have to involve the patient's extended family? Is this person likely to make eye contact with a provider? What are this couple's beliefs about the nature of illness? What does well-oxygenated skin color look like when the infant being rated on the Apgar scale is dark skinned? Will the observation of certain rituals ease the anguish parents feel at their child's death?

This edition, which draws on the clinical experience of many individuals, speaks to the needs of our pluralistic society by providing a wealth of insights about how cultural assessment is integral to understanding the meaning of behaviors that, if not understood within the context of ethnic values, might be regarded as puzzling or even negative. All of the disease incidence and prevalence rates cited build on the 2010 Census, and there is up-to-date information on how genetics confounds our understandings of who is vulnerable and what will be helpful. This edition provides details that will make us sensitive to the concerns of specific population groups, while all the while providing us with a framework with broad generic applicability.

On September 27, 2010, the Institute on Minority Health and Health Disparities was created within the National Institutes of Health. The purpose of that agency is to increase understanding of how the incidence, prevalence, mortality, and burden of disease vary among specific population groups. This volume is an important resource in this journey as caregivers move away from paternalistically thinking that one approach or one treatment applies to all and, instead, wisely customize their approach, bearing in mind patients' predispositions and situations. Ruth Davidhizar, who grew up in an isolated Alaskan enclave, learned to do this, and now the rest of us must learn to follow her example.

REFERENCES

American Nurses' Association (1980). *Nursing: a social policy statement.* Kansas City, MO: ANA.

Inst B. D. Smedley, A. Y. Stith, & A. R. Nelson (Eds.), *Unequal treatment. Confronting racial and ethnic disparities in health care.* Washington, DC: The National Academies Press.

Leininger, M. (1977). *Transcultural care of infants and children: proceedings from the first transcultural conference.* Salt Lake City: University of Utah.

Tripp-Reimer, T., & Dougherty, M. C. (1985). Cross-cultural nursing research. *Annual Review of Nursing Research* (Vol. 3, pp. 77–104). New York: Springer.

PREFACE

After writing this book for nearly three decades, it is still true that the concept of transcultural nursing is relatively new to the nursing literature. In fact, it has been only in the past four decades that nurses have begun to develop an appreciation for the need to incorporate culturally appropriate clinical approaches into the daily routine of client care. Although nurses have begun to recognize the need for culturally appropriate clinical approaches, the literature on the subject is either scanty or does not provide a systematic method for comprehensive assessment and intervention. However, a good foundation in transcultural nursing is essential for the nurse because it can provide a conceptual framework for holistic client care in a variety of clinical settings and assist the nurse throughout a nursing career.

When the late Dr. Ruth Davidhizar and I were challenged nearly 30 years ago by the nursing students at Bethel College to develop a systematic approach to client assessment for use with individuals from diverse cultural backgrounds, we had no idea how profoundly important this topic would become for all health care providers. The United States is rapidly becoming a multicultural, heterogeneous, pluralistic society. With changing demographics, it is imperative that nurses develop not only sensitivity but also cultural competence to render safe, effective care to all clients.

Dr. Davidhizar and I discovered that the students had difficulty finding adequate literature to assist in planning for clients from diverse cultural backgrounds. Like our students, each of us had identified a similar need by virtue of our own diverse cultural backgrounds: One of us is African-American and was raised in the South, and the other was White and was raised in an Eskimo setting in Alaska. Thus, in response to both a personal interest and the need identified by our students, Dr. Davidhizar and I set about to synthesize a body of literature that would assist students in developing the theoretical knowledge necessary to provide culturally appropriate care. Although the literature has vastly improved since the initial release of this text, there is still much work to be done in this area.

This text, like the six previous editions, is divided into two parts. The first part, which focuses on theory, includes an introduction and six chapters describing the six cultural phenomena that make up our transcultural conceptual theory of assessment. The six cultural phenomena that we identified as being evidenced in all cultural groups are (1) communication, (2) space, (3) social organization, (4) time, (5) environmental control, and (6) biological variations. The chapters in Part One describe how these phenomena vary with application and utilization across cultures.

Part Two contains chapters by contributing authors in which the six cultural phenomena are systematically applied to the assessment and care of individuals in specific cultures. The cultures selected for inclusion represent those most likely to be encountered by a nurse practicing in the United States.

In the seventh edition, I have once again selected contributing authors with expertise and clinical backgrounds in the care of selected cultural groups. While we have lost, through death, some of the contributors who were with this work from the beginning, we are carrying on in their memories. Many of our chapters were written by contributing authors who actually represent, by ethnic heritage, the cultural group described. Not only are unique and diverse cultures represented, but also the contributing authors span the North American continent with representation truly from coast to coast and from California to Alaska and Hawaii. Thus the assessment model is applied to persons in diverse cultural settings by nurses who have expertise and sensitivity in the cultural group and in the unique care strategies that a nurse should use in providing culturally appropriate and competent care.

Because the first edition was translated into French, we perceived a need to incorporate some of the cultural uniqueness of our neighbors to the north (the people of Québec in Canada). This perceived need led to a book, *Canadian Transcultural Nursing,* published in 1998. In this seventh edition I have tried to select cultural groups who by virtual numbers reflect the greater percentage of our current population. As always, I recognize and value the diversity of all the cultural groups found in the United States, but because of space and fiscal considerations, we have selected the most populous groups.

Since publication of the first edition, Dr. Davidhizar and I developed a quick reference, user-friendly assessment tool for use with clients in diverse clinical settings. The Giger and Davidhizar model has been cited, excerpted, or modified for inclusion in more than 1000 new nursing, medical, and allied health textbooks. Our model has shown great applicability across clinical disciplines. As such, the text was included in the library of the Education Testing Service (ETS) for many years as the only text of its kind to validate test items developed for the former RN-NCLEX© and the current RN-CAT. I have added clear and more concise definitions of health disparities and disabilities as a culture. For the first time, we have included a colleague from Pharmacy, Henry Lewis, III, PharmD, so that we can further understand ethnopharmacology.

This book was written primarily for all nurses and nursing students who are interested in developing knowledge of transcultural concepts to apply to client-centered care. However, we believe this new edition will also be applicable across other disciplines, such as psychology, sociology, medicine, and anthropology, because it provides not only a nursing perspective but also a historical and biotechnological approach to transcultural health care.

In my commitment to transcultural nursing, I have once again made every effort, through extensive research, to be as culturally sensitive as possible and not offend readers or specific racial, cultural, ethnic, or religious groups. Despite careful attention to detail to prevent this from happening, I realize that the presentation of literature and research findings is often interpreted differently by individuals. I apologize for any content that readers may find insensitive and assure our readers that as a nurse researcher, clinician, and academician, I have as my only intent the presentation of factual information.

ACKNOWLEDGMENTS

On behalf of the late **DR. RUTH ELAINE DAVIDHI-ZAR,** I would like to acknowledge and thank our former editors: Linda Duncan, whose vision of the future allowed this project to come to fruition; Loren Wilson, who continued to challenge us to provide the best referenced text on this subject; Michael Ledbetter, who worked diligently on past editions of this text; Robin Carter, who also served as a past editor; Jean Sims Fornango, who took up the challenge; and finally, Tamara Myers, who worked diligently to bring this present project to completion.

A special recognition goes to the people who, by their religious affiliation, proved to be invaluable content experts in providing advice, counsel, and information on special religious groups. These individuals include Judy Mason, a former member of the staff at the University of Alabama at Birmingham, School of Nursing, whose expert advice on Jehovah's Witnesses proved to be invaluable. Similarly, we would like to thank Tamara Walters, a former baccalaureate nursing student at the University of Tulsa in Tulsa, Oklahoma, who read our first edition and graciously provided in-depth insight into the Church of Jesus Christ of Latter Day Saints (Mormons); Dr. Mary Grace Umlauf, who through her extensive travels to Jordan not only contributed to that chapter but also helped us through her extensive ties to the Muslim world to understand Islam as a world religion; Dr. Joan Earle Hahn, who developed the disability cultural schematic model based on Giger and Davidhizar; and Dr. Henry Lewis III, PharmD, who contributed significantly to broaden and enhance ethnopharmacology. I wish to thank April Clements for invaluable contributions in securing data, interpreting data, and other tasks.

I wish to thank the many persons who took the photos and provided them for use in this textbook and all the individuals who posed for these pictures. Special thanks go to Dottie Kauffman, the photographer, who labored on this project for some 20 years. I wish to thank the chapter contributors who believed in this project. Each of you has made invaluable contributions. Finally, I would like to acknowledge the friendship and respect that grew over 25 years between me and the late Dr. Ruth E. Davidhizar. Without a doubt, the diversity of our heritages and our ability to complement each other were testimonials to the achievement of racial, ethnic, and cultural harmony across the United States, Canada, and countries throughout the world. Well into the second decade of the new millennium, I am hopeful that all health care providers will continue to strive to achieve cultural competence.

SPECIAL ACKNOWLEDGMENT

Many of you know that I lost my good friend, fellow transcultural scholar, and writing partner in 2008. It was my pleasure to have traveled the road to discovery that has led to more culturally competent care with such a wonderful friend as Ruth Davidhizar. We began this odyssey more than 30 years ago. Unlike most writing partners, I think we began as friends, and our relationship grew steadily over the decades. Since we lost Ruth, there is not a day that I do not think of her and remember her very quiet, unassuming manner. Every time I take up the task of revising this book, I am reminded that I truly MISS YOU My Buddy! My Friend!

Joyce Newman Giger

CONTENTS

PART ONE

Framework for Cultural Assessment and Intervention Techniques

1

Introduction to Transcultural Nursing

Theories of transcultural nursing with established clinical approaches to clients from varying cultures are relatively new. According to Madeleine Leininger (1977, 1991), who founded the field of transcultural nursing in the mid-1960s, the education of nursing students in this field is only now beginning to yield significant results. Today, nurses with a deeper appreciation of human life and values are developing cultural sensitivity for appropriate, individualized clinical approaches. Transcultural nursing concepts are being incorporated into the curricula for student nurses in the United States and Canada.

The Transcultural Nursing Society, founded in 1974, is promoting interest in transcultural concepts and the education of transcultural nurses at the graduate level (Giger & Davidhizar, 2002; Wenger, 1989). Since its inception, the society has promoted such efforts at annual transcultural nursing conferences in different worldwide locations. The society also implemented the first certification plan in transcultural nursing. Through the efforts of the society, a number of U.S. and Canadian nurses have received certification. Other international conferences, such as that supported by the Rockefeller Foundation in October 1988 in Bellagio, Italy, have sought to promote international health care management. The society also publishes the *Transcultural Nursing Society Newsletter* and the *Journal of Transcultural Nursing*. In addition, other transcultural publications include the *International Journal of Nursing Studies* and the *International Nursing Review*. Although the literature on patient approaches in culturally diverse situations is mushrooming and nurses are beginning to perform transcultural research studies, up to now relatively few theories on transcultural nursing have provided a systematic method for comprehensive nursing assessment (Brink, 2001a, 2001b; Leininger, 1985a, 1985b, 1991;

Spector, 1996; Tripp-Reimer, 1984a, 1984b; Tripp-Reimer & Dougherty, 1985; Tripp-Reimer & Friedl, 1977).

CULTURE DEFINED

Culture is a patterned behavioral response that develops over time as a result of imprinting the mind through social and religious structures and intellectual and artistic manifestations. Culture is also the result of acquired mechanisms that may have innate influences but are primarily affected by internal and external environmental stimuli. Culture is shaped by values, beliefs, norms, and practices that are shared by members of the same cultural group. Culture guides our thinking, doing, and being and becomes patterned expressions of who we are. These patterned expressions are passed down from one generation to the next. Other definitions of culture have been offered by Leininger (1985a, 1985b, 1991), Leininger and McFarland (2006), Spector (2008), and Andrews and Boyle (2008). According to Leininger (1985a, 1985b, 1991) and Leininger and McFarland (2006), culture is the values, beliefs, norms, and practices of a particular group that are learned and shared and that guide thinking, decisions, and actions in a patterned way. Spector (2008) contends that culture is a metacommunication system based on nonphysical traits such as values, beliefs, attitudes, customs, language, and behaviors that are shared by a group of people and are passed down from one generation to the next. According to Andrews and Boyle (2008), culture represents a unique way of perceiving, behaving, and evaluating the external environment and as such provides a blueprint for determining values, beliefs, and practices. Regardless of the definition chosen, the term *culture* implies a dynamic, ever-changing, active, or passive process.

Cultural values are unique expressions of a particular culture that have been accepted as appropriate over time. They guide actions and decision making that facilitate self-worth and self-esteem. Leininger (1985a, 1991) postulates that cultural values develop as a direct result of an individual's desirable or preferred way of acting or knowing something that is often sustained by a culture over time and that governs actions or decisions.

THE NEED FOR TRANSCULTURAL NURSING KNOWLEDGE

It is believed that demography is destiny, demographic change is reality, and demographic sensitivity is imperative. The United States is rapidly becoming a multicultural, pluralistic society. In 2010, 72.4% of the population in the United States was White of European descent; 14%, African-American; 17.3%, Hispanic-American; 4.8%, Asian American; and 0.9%, American Indian (U.S. Department of Commerce, Bureau of Census, 2010 Census Briefs, 2011). It is projected that by the year 2020, only 53% of the U.S. population will be White of European descent. It is further projected that by the year 2021, the number of Asian Americans and Hispanic-Americans will triple, and the number of African-Americans will double (U.S. Department of Commerce, Bureau of the Census, American Community Survey, 2009).

If the 2010 census data on fertility, birth, and mortality are correct, conceivably it will be almost impossible to isolate and identify a "pure" race of Whites of European descent by the year 2070 (U.S. Department of Commerce, Bureau of Census, 2010 Census Brief, 2011). In light of these statistical data, it is imperative that the nursing workforce rapidly adapt itself to a changing, heterogeneous society.

Providing culturally appropriate and thus competent care in the twenty-first century will be a complex and difficult task for many nurses. In many professional health career programs, such as nursing, medicine, and respiratory therapy, students are rarely taught culturally appropriate and competent care techniques. Thus, when these individuals encounter clients from culturally diverse backgrounds in the clinical setting, they are often unable to accurately assess and provide the kinds of interventions that are culturally appropriate.

The burden of teaching nurses culturally competent care techniques will rest not only with the individual programs of practice development but also with the health care agency itself. Regardless of who is responsible for this task, nurses must develop an understanding about culture and its relevance to competent care.

A nurse who does not recognize the value and importance of culturally appropriate care cannot possibly be an effective care agent in this changing demographic society. If nurses do not recognize that the intervention strategies planned for an African-American client with diabetes are uniquely different from those planned for a Vietnamese American, an Italian American, and so forth, they cannot possibly hope to change health-seeking behaviors or actively encourage the wellness behaviors of this client or any client. When nurses consider race, ethnicity, culture, and cultural heritage, they become more sensitive to clients. This is not to suggest that there is a cookbook approach to delivering care to clients by virtue of race, ethnicity, or culture. There is as much variation within certain races, cultures, or ethnic groups as there is across cultural groups. When the informed nurse considers the significance of culture, clients are approached with a more informed perspective.

The time to learn differing perspectives about culture is at hand. As professional health care providers, nurses will be asked to step forward to provide the leadership to ensure that all people have equal access to high-quality, culturally appropriate, and culturally competent health care. This task can be accomplished only through culturally diverse nursing care.

CULTURAL ASSESSMENT

Using Non-nursing Models

In a pluralistic society, nurse practitioners need to be prepared to provide culturally appropriate nursing care for each client, regardless of that client's cultural background. To provide culturally appropriate nursing care, nurses must understand specific factors that influence individual health and illness behaviors (Tripp-Reimer, Brink, & Saunders, 1984). According to Affonso (1979), cultural assessment can give meaning to behaviors that might otherwise be judged negatively. If cultural behaviors are not appropriately identified, their significance will be confusing to the nurse.

Although transcultural nursing theories have appeared in the literature (Affonso, 1979; Leininger, 1991), adequate nursing assessment methods to accompany these theories have not been provided consistently. One of the most comprehensive tools used for nursing cultural assessment is the *Outline of Cultural Materials* by Murdock et al. (2004); however, this tool was developed primarily for anthropologists who were concerned with ethnographic descriptions of cultural groups. Although the tool is well developed and contains 88 major categories, it was not designed for nurse practitioners and thus does not provide for systematic use of the nursing process. Another assessment tool is in

Brownlee's (1978) *Community, Culture, and Care: A Cross-Cultural Guide for Health Workers.* Brownlee's work is devoted to the process of practical assessment of a community, with specific attention given to health areas. The work deals with three aspects of assessment: what to find out, why it is important, and how to do it. Brownlee's assessment tool has been criticized as being too comprehensive, too difficult, and too detailed for use with individual clients. Although this tool was developed for use by health care practitioners, it is not exclusively a nursing assessment tool.

Using Nursing-Specific Models

Transcultural nursing is defined by Leininger (1991; Leininger & McFarland, 2006) as a "humanistic and scientific area of formal study and practice which is focused upon differences and similarities among cultures with respect to human care, health (or well-being), and illness based upon the people's cultural values, beliefs, and practices." According to Leininger (1991), the ultimate goal of transcultural nursing is use of relevant knowledge to provide culturally specific and culturally congruent nursing care to people. From this theoretical perspective, Leininger (1985a, 1985b; Leininger & McFarland, 2006) provides a comprehensive transcultural theory and assessment model. For more than 30 years, this model has helped nurses discover and understand what health care means to various cultures. Leininger's sunrise model symbolizes the rising of the sun (care). The model depicts a full sun with four levels of foci. Within the circle in the upper portion of the model are components of the social structure and worldview factors that influence care and health through language and environment. These factors influence the folk, professional, and nursing systems or subsystems located in the lower half of the model. Also included in the model are levels of abstraction and analysis from which care can be studied at each level. Various cultural phenomena are studied from the micro, middle, and macro perspectives (Leininger, 1985a, 1985b). Leininger's model has served as the prototype for the development of other culturally specific nursing models and tools (Bloch, 1983; Branch & Paxton, 1976; Orque, 1983; Rund & Krause, 1978).

An Analysis of Culturally Specific Models and Tools

Tripp-Reimer et al. (1984), in one of the first studies of its kind, analyzed selected culturally appropriate models and tools to determine whether the models significantly differed. They concluded that most cultural assessment guides are similar because they all seek to identify major

cultural domains that are important variables if culturally appropriate care is to be rendered. Nine culturally appropriate models or guides were analyzed: Aamodt (1978), Bloch (1983), Branch and Paxton (1976), Brownlee (1978), Kay (1978), Leininger (1977), Orque (1983), Rund and Krause (1978), and Tripp-Reimer (1984b). In analyzing the models, Tripp-Reimer et al. (1984) concluded that the same two limitations existed in each guide. The first limitation was the tendency to include too much cultural content, ultimately negating the "heart of the matter," which is the process itself. The second limitation was that it is often impossible to separate client-specific data from normative data.

Using Nursing Diagnoses

The relative significance of culturally appropriate health care cannot be understood if the nurse does not understand the value of culturally relevant nursing diagnoses. Geissler (1991) reported a study to determine the applicability of the North American Nursing Diagnosis Association (NANDA) taxonomy as a culturally appropriate assessment tool for use with diverse populations. In the study, three nursing diagnoses were analyzed to validate their cultural appropriateness: (1) impaired verbal communication, (2) social isolation, and (3) noncompliance in culturally diverse situations. Participants in the study ($n = 245$ nurses) were experts in the field of transcultural nursing and were members of either the Transcultural Nursing Society or the American Nurses Association Council on Cultural Diversity (Geissler, 1991). Findings from this study also indicate that nursing diagnoses tend to (1) focus on the client rather than the provider and therefore do not acknowledge the existence of other culturally relevant viewpoints (such as those expressed by the provider); (2) be generalized and, as a result, increase the likelihood, when applied in diverse cultural settings, for stereotyping and victimization because so-called non-Western medical models are believed to be "abnormal" and thus require necessary interventions; and (3) involve mislabeling phenomena, which in actuality arise as expressions of cultural dissonance rather than expressions of political, social, psychological, or economic factors.

In a classic, but relevant, study reported by Geissler (1991), the NANDA nursing diagnosis of "impaired communication, verbal, related to cultural differences" is an excellent example of a client-oriented diagnosis that does not recognize linguistic cultural differences. The study concludes that the NANDA diagnosis of "impaired verbal communication" connotes that the client's verbal communication and ability to understand and use language are impaired in some way. This diagnosis does not consider the causative factors creating the impairment (Giger, Davidhizar, Evers, & Ingram, 1994). It is apparent that individuals who speak a language different from that used by health care providers or nurses may be very capable of both use and comprehension of a specific language when interacting with persons fluent in that language (Giger et al., 1994). According to Geissler (1991), if the client in this situation is "verbally impaired," the nurse is equally impaired. Geissler also concludes that the NANDA diagnosis of "impaired verbal communication" does not adequately address the issue of nonverbal communication, which was identified in the earlier nursing literature as an essential assessment factor (Giger & Davidhizar, 1990, 1994).

According to Geissler (1991), nursing diagnoses related to social isolation and noncompliance need further defining characteristics for use with culturally diverse populations. Rather than use the term *noncompliance,* Geissler (1991) suggests that the term *nonadherence* may be more appropriate because this term may more accurately reflect behavior resulting from cultural dissonance. At the same time, the use of *nonadherence* may remove the stigma of guilt experienced by the health care recipient who is inappropriately labeled noncompliant.

GIGER AND DAVIDHIZAR'S TRANSCULTURAL ASSESSMENT MODEL

In response to the need for a practical assessment tool for evaluating cultural variables and their effects on health and illness behaviors, a transcultural assessment model is offered that greatly minimizes the time needed to conduct a comprehensive assessment in an effort to provide culturally competent care. The metaparadigm for the Giger and Davidhizar Transcultural Assessment Model includes (1) transcultural nursing and culturally diverse nursing, (2) culturally competent care, (3) culturally unique individuals, (4) culturally sensitive environments, and (5) health and health status based on culturally specific illness and wellness behaviors.

Transcultural Nursing Defined

In the context of Giger and Davidhizar's Transcultural Assessment Model (1990, 2002), transcultural nursing is viewed as a culturally competent practice field that is client centered and research focused. Although transcultural nursing is viewed as client centered, it is important for nurses to remember that culture can and does influence how clients are viewed and the care that is rendered.

Every individual is culturally unique, and nurses are no exception to this premise. Nonetheless, nurses must use caution to avoid projecting on the client their own cultural uniqueness and worldviews if culturally appropriate care is to be provided. Nurses must carefully discern personal cultural beliefs and values to separate them from the client's beliefs and values. To deliver culturally sensitive care, the nurse must remember that each individual is unique and a product of experiences, beliefs, and values that have been learned and passed down from one generation to the next.

According to Stokes (1991), nursing as a profession is not "culturally free" but rather is "culturally determined." Nurses must recognize and understand this fact to avoid becoming grossly ethnocentric (Stokes, 1991). Because there is a contingent relationship between cultural determination and the delivery of culturally sensitive care, the transcultural nurse must be guided by acquired knowledge in the assessment, diagnosis, planning, implementation, and evaluation of the client's needs based on culturally relevant information. This ideology does not presuppose that all individuals within a specific cultural group will think and behave in a similar manner with relative predictability. The astute nurse must remember that there is as much diversity within a cultural group as there is across cultural groups. Nonetheless, the goal of transcultural nursing is the discovery of culturally relevant facts about the client to provide culturally appropriate and competent care.

Although transcultural nursing is becoming a highly specialized field of specially educated individuals, every nurse, regardless of academic or experiential background, must use transcultural knowledge to facilitate culturally appropriate care. Regardless of preparation in the field of transcultural nursing, every nurse who is entrusted with care of clients must make every effort to deliver culturally sensitive care that is free of inherent biases based on gender, race, or religion.

Culturally Diverse Nursing Care

Culturally diverse nursing care refers to the variability in nursing approaches needed to provide culturally appropriate and competent care. Nurses need to use transcultural knowledge in a skillful and artful manner to render culturally appropriate and competent care to a rapidly changing, heterogeneous client population. Culturally diverse nursing care must take into account six cultural phenomena that vary with application and use, yet are evident in all cultural groups: (1) communication, (2) space, (3) social organization, (4) time, (5) environmental control, and (6) biological variations (Figs. 1-1 and 1-2).

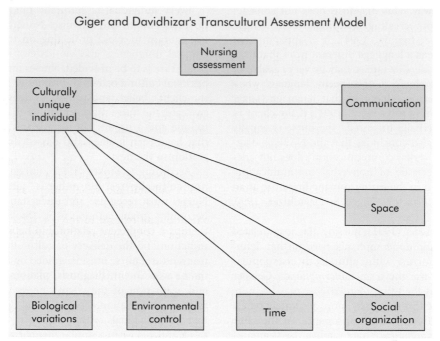

FIG 1-1 Application of cultural phenomena to nursing care and nursing practice.

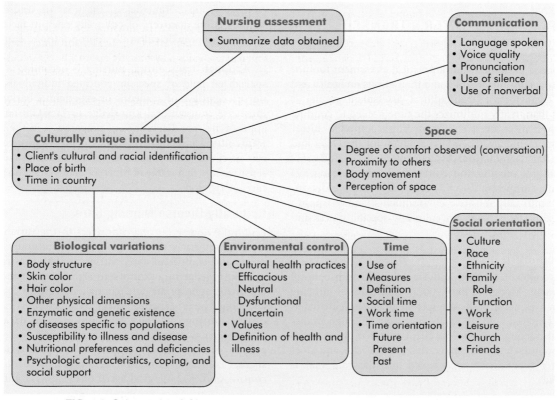

FIG 1-2 Schematic of Giger and Davidhizar's Transcultural Assessment Model.

Culturally Competent Care Defined

As a heightened awareness of transcultural health care has been espoused, so too has the widened use of the term *cultural competence*. There are as many varying definitions for this term as there are for the term *culture*. Purnell and Paulanka (2008) note that *cultural competence* is the act whereby a health care professional develops an awareness of one's existence, sensations, thoughts, and environment without letting these factors have an undue effect on those for whom care is provided. Further, they conclude that cultural competence is the adaptation of care in a manner that is congruent with the client's culture. In this sense, cultural competence is a conscious process and as such cannot be necessarily viewed as linear (Purnell & Paulanka, 2008).

According to Smith (1998b), cultural competence is a continuous process of awareness, knowledge, skill, interaction, and sensitivity that is demonstrated among those who render care and the services they provide. Smith concludes that cultural competence requires continuous seeking of skills, practices, and attitudes that enable nurses to transform interventions into positive health outcomes, such as improved client morbidity and mortality, as well as augmenting client and professional levels of satisfaction.

Cultural competence is a dynamic, fluid, continuous process whereby an individual, system, or health care agency finds meaningful and useful care-delivery strategies based on knowledge of the cultural heritage, beliefs, attitudes, and behaviors of those to whom they render care. To develop cultural competence, it is essential for the health care professional to use knowledge gained from conceptual and theoretical models of culturally appropriate care. In addition, cultural competence connotes a higher, more sophisticated level of refinement of cognitive and psychomotor skills, attitudes, and personal beliefs. Attainment of cultural competence can assist the astute nurse in devising meaningful interventions to promote optimal health among individuals, regardless of race, ethnicity, gender identity, sexual identity, or cultural heritage. It is interesting to note that in searching for an adequate definition for *cultural competence*, Cohall and Bannister (2001), writing in a seminal text by Braithwaite and Taylor (2001), used the *cultural competency* definition proposed by Giger and Davidhizar.

Giger and Davidhizar took a major lead along with colleagues from the American Academy of Nursing's Expert Panel on Cultural Competence (2007) to develop an important consensus paper that addressed ways to eliminate health disparities using culturally competent care techniques. This Expert Panel made 12 consensus recommendations to assist health care professionals in the endeavor to not only eliminate health disparities across racial/cultural groups but to do so using culturally competent care techniques appropriate to that particular group.

Culturally Unique Individuals

To provide culturally appropriate and competent care, it is important to remember that each individual is culturally unique and as such is a product of experiences, cultural beliefs, and cultural norms. Cultural expressions become patterned responses and give each individual a unique identity (see Fig. 1-2). Although there is as much diversity within cultural and racial groups as there is across and among cultural and racial groups, knowledge of general baseline data relative to the specific cultural group is an excellent starting point to provide culturally appropriate care.

Culturally Sensitive Environments

Culturally diverse health care can and should be rendered in a variety of clinical settings. Regardless of the level of care—primary, secondary, or tertiary—knowledge of culturally relevant information will assist the nurse in planning and implementing a treatment regimen that is unique for each client.

In response to the apparent lack of practical assessment tools available in nursing for evaluating cultural variables and their effects on health and illness behaviors, this text provides a systematic approach to evaluating the six essential cultural phenomena to assist the nurse in providing culturally appropriate nursing care. Although the six cultural phenomena are evident in all cultural groups, they vary in application across cultures. Thus, an individualized assessment of these areas is necessary when working with clients from diverse cultural groups (Fig. 1-3).

DEVELOPMENT AND REFINEMENT OF GIGER AND DAVIDHIZAR'S TRANSCULTURAL ASSESSMENT MODEL

Clinical and Educational Application

Since its introduction in 1991, Giger and Davidhizar's Transcultural Assessment Model has been applied to the care of clients in a variety of clinical specialties, including the maternity client (Giger, Davidhizar, & Wieczorek, 1993), the operating room client (Bowen & Davidhizar, 1991), the psychiatric client (Giger et al., 1994), and others.

In 1993, Spector illustrated the model's utility by combining it with the Cultural Heritage Model. The

GIGER AND DAVIDHIZAR'S TRANSCULTURAL ASSESSMENT MODEL

CULTURALLY UNIQUE INDIVIDUAL

1. Place of birth
2. Cultural definition
   What is . . .
3. Race
   What is . . .
4. Length of time in country (if appropriate)

COMMUNICATION

1. Voice quality
   A. Strong, resonant
   B. Soft
   C. Average
   D. Shrill
2. Pronunciation and enunciation
   A. Clear
   B. Slurred
   C. Dialect (geographical)
3. Use of silence
   A. Infrequent
   B. Often
   C. Length
      (1) Brief
      (2) Moderate
      (3) Long
      (4) Not observed
4. Use of nonverbal
   A. Hand movement
   B. Eye movement
   C. Entire body movement
   D. Kinesics (gestures, expression, or stances)
5. Touch
   A. Startles or withdraws when touched
   B. Accepts touch without difficulty
   C. Touches others without difficulty
6. Ask these and similar questions:
   A. How do you get your point across to others?
   B. Do you like communicating with friends, family, and acquaintances?
   C. When asked a question, do you usually respond (in words or body movement, or both)?

D. If you have something important to discuss with your family, how would you approach them?

SPACE

1. Degree of comfort
   A. Moves when space invaded
   B. Does not move when space invaded
2. Distance in conversations
   A. 0 to 18 inches
   B. 18 inches to 3 feet
   C. 3 feet or more
3. Definition of space
   A. Describe degree of comfort with closeness when talking with or standing near others
   B. How do objects (e.g., furniture) in the environment affect your sense of space?
4. Ask these and similar questions:
   A. When you talk with family members, how close do you stand?
   B. When you communicate with coworkers and other acquaintances, how close do you stand?
   C. If a stranger touches you, how do you react or feel?
   D. If a loved one touches you, how do you react or feel?
   E. Are you comfortable with the distance between us now?

SOCIAL ORGANIZATION

1. Normal state of health
   A. Poor
   B. Fair
   C. Good
   D. Excellent
2. Marital status
3. Number of children
4. Parents living or deceased?
5. Ask these and similar questions:
   A. How do you define social activities?
   B. What are some activities that you enjoy?
   C. What are your hobbies, or what do you do when you have free time?

FIG 1-3 Giger and Davidhizar's Transcultural Assessment Model.

GIGER AND DAVIDHIZAR'S TRANSCULTURAL ASSESSMENT MODEL–cont'd

D. Do you believe in a Supreme Being?

E. How do you worship that Supreme Being?

F. What is your function (what do you do) in your family unit/system?

G. What is your role in your family unit/system (father, mother, child, advisor)?

H. When you were a child, what or who influenced you most?

I. What is/was your relationship with your siblings and parents?

J. What does work mean to you?

K. Describe your past, present, and future jobs.

L. What are your political views?

M. How have your political views influenced your attitude toward health and illness?

TIME

1. Orientation to time
   A. Past-oriented
   B. Present-oriented
   C. Future-oriented
2. View of time
   A. Social time
   B. Clock-oriented
3. Physiochemical reaction to time
   A. Sleeps at least 8 hours a night
   B. Goes to sleep and wakes on a consistent schedule
   C. Understands the importance of taking medication and other treatments on schedule
4. Ask these and similar questions:
   A. What kind of timepiece do you wear daily?
   B. If you have an appointment at 2 PM, what time is acceptable to arrive?
   C. If a nurse tells you that you will receive a medication in "about a half hour," realistically, how much time will you allow before calling the nurses' station?

ENVIRONMENTAL CONTROL

1. Locus-of-control
   A. Internal locus-of-control (believes that the power to affect change lies within)

   B. External locus-of-control (believes that fate, luck, and chance have a great deal to do with how things turn out)
2. Value orientation
   A. Believes in supernatural forces
   B. Relies on magic, witchcraft, and prayer to effect change
   C. Does not believe in supernatural forces
   D. Does not rely on magic, witchcraft, or prayer to affect change
3. Ask these and similar questions:
   A. How often do you have visitors at your home?
   B. Is it acceptable to you for visitors to drop in unexpectedly?
   C. Name some ways your parents or other persons treated your illnesses when you were a child.
   D. Have you or someone else in your immediate surroundings ever used a home remedy that made you sick?
   E. What home remedies have you used that worked? Will you use them in the future?
   F. What is your definition of "good health"?
   G. What is your definition of illness or "poor health"?

BIOLOGICAL VARIATIONS

1. Conduct a complete physical assessment noting:
   A. Body structure (small, medium, or large frame)
   B. Skin color
   C. Unusual skin discolorations
   D. Hair color and distribution
   E. Other visible physical characteristics (e.g., keloids, chloasma)
   F. Weight
   G. Height
   H. Check lab work for variances in hemoglobin, hematocrit, and sickle cell phenomena if Black or Mediterranean
2. Ask these and similar questions:
   A. What diseases or illnesses are common in your family?

FIG 1-3, cont'd *Continued*

GIGER AND DAVIDHIZAR'S TRANSCULTURAL ASSESSMENT MODEL–cont'd

B. Has anyone in your family been told that there is a possible genetic susceptibility for a particular disease?

C. Describe your family's typical behavior when a family member is ill.

D. How do you respond when you are angry?

E. Who (or what) usually helps you to cope during a difficult time?

F. What foods do you and your family like to eat?

G. Have you ever had any unusual cravings for:
(1) White or red clay dirt?
(2) Laundry starch?

H. When you were a child what types of foods did you eat?

I. What foods are family favorites or are considered traditional?

NURSING ASSESSMENT

1. Note whether the client has become culturally assimilated or observes own cultural practices.

2. Incorporate data into plan of nursing care:
   A. Encourage the client to discuss cultural differences; people from diverse cultures who hold different world views can enlighten nurses.
   B. Make efforts to accept and understand methods of communication.
   C. Respect the individual's personal need for space.
   D. Respect the rights of clients to honor and worship the Supreme Being of their choice.

E. Identify a clerical or spiritual person to contact.

F. Determine whether spiritual practices have implications for health, life, and well-being (e.g., Jehovah's Witnesses may refuse blood and blood derivatives; an Orthodox Jew may eat only kosher food high in sodium and may not drink milk when meat is served).

G. Identify hobbies, especially when devising interventions for a short or extended convalescence or for rehabilitation.

H. Honor time and value orientations and differences in these areas. Allay anxiety and apprehension if adherence to time is necessary.

I. Provide privacy according to personal need and health status of the client (NOTE: the perception of and reaction to pain may be culturally related).

J. Note cultural health practices.
(1) Identify and encourage efficacious practices.
(2) Identify and discourage dysfunctional practices.
(3) Identify and determine whether neutral practices will have a long-term ill effect.

K. Note food preferences.
(1) Make as many adjustments in diet as health status and long-term benefits will allow and that dietary department can provide.
(2) Note dietary practices that may have serious implications for the client.

FIG 1-3, cont'd

combination of these two models (Fig. 1-4), which appears in Potter and Perry's *Fundamentals of Nursing* textbook, is unique because it provides a holistic method of providing culturally competent care. In addition, using Giger and Davidhizar's six cultural phenomena, although in a different hierarchical arrangement, Spector (1996) created a unique quick-reference guide for cultural assessment

of people from a variety of racial and cultural groups (Table 1-1).

In 1994, Kozier, Erb, Blaise, Johnson, and Smith-Temple used the model to provide a mechanism by which cultural behaviors relevant to health assessment could easily be identified across cultural groups. Their work relative to Giger and Davidhizar's Transcultural Assessment Model

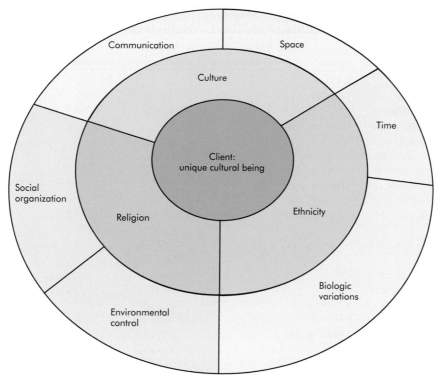

FIG 1-4 Model of the client within a culturally unique heritage and the cultural phenomena that have a profound effect on nursing care. (Compiled from Spector, R. [1996]. *Cultural diversity in health and illness* [3rd ed.]. Norwalk, CT: Appleton & Lange; Spector, R. [2000]. *Cultural diversity in health and illness* [5th ed.]. Englewood Cliffs, NJ: Prentice Hall Health; and Giger, J., & Davidhizar, R. [1995]. *Transcultural nursing* [2nd ed.]. St. Louis: Mosby.)

compiles basic culturally relevant information (Table 1-2). This work was further used in 1995 by Kozier, Erb, Blaise, and Wilkinson. In addition, in 1992, the editors at Editions Lamarre translated the model into French for use by French and French-Canadian nurses. In 1998, Giger and Davidhizar's work was further expanded on the international horizon to include a method for assessing select cultural groups in Canada.

In 1993, the National League for Nursing published *Nursing Management Skills: A Modular Self-Assessment Series, Module IV, Transcultural Nursing* (Sheridan & Zimbler, 1993). Included in this publication are numerous articles on the application of the model in a variety of clinical situations to be used by nurses to learn and refine managerial skills. In 1994, the Nashville-based production company Envision, Inc., produced a half-inch VHS-format video titled "Cultural Diversity in Healthcare: A Different Point of View" that used Giger and Davidhizar's Transcultural Assessment Model as its overarching framework.

In 1994, the fourth edition of *Mosby's Medical, Nursing, and Allied Health Dictionary* was published. Included in the new edition is "Guidelines for Relating to Patients from Different Cultures," which was excerpted from the work of Giger and Davidhizar.

In 1995, Burk, Wieser, and Keegan proposed a method for analyzing the cultural beliefs and health behaviors of pregnant Mexican-American women using the Giger and Davidhizar Transcultural Assessment Model as an underpinning for assessment.

In 2004, the Office of Minority Health (U.S. Department of Health and Human Services, Office of Minority Health, 2004) used the Giger and Davidhizar Transcultural Assessment Model as one of the overarching models for rendering culturally competent care. In their review, they note that on balance, health care organizations reported using the Giger and Davidhizar Transcultural Assessment Model more frequently than university programs. This statement might be debatable because a great number of schools have reported using the Giger and Davidhizar

TABLE 1-1   Cross-Cultural Examples of Cultural Phenomena Impacting Nursing Care

Nations of Origin	Communication	Space	Time Orientation	Social Organization	Environmental Control	Biological Variation
Asia China Hawaii Philippines Korea Japan Southeast Asia (Laos, Cambodia, Vietnam)	National language preference Dialects, written characters Use of silence Nonverbal and contextual cuing	Noncontact people	Present	Family: hierarchical structure, loyalty Devotion to tradition Many religions including Taoism, Buddhism, Islam, and Christianity Community social organizations	Traditional health and illness beliefs Use of traditional medicines Traditional practitioners: Chinese doctors and herbalists	Liver cancer Stomach cancer Coccidioidomycosis Hypertension Lactose intolerance
Africa West Coast (as slaves) Many African countries West Indian Islands Dominican Republic Haiti Jamaica	National languages Dialect: pidgin, Creole, Spanish, and French	Close personal space	Present over future	Family: many female, single-parent Large, extended family networks Strong church affiliation within community Community social organizations	Traditional health and illness beliefs Folk medicine tradition Traditional healer: root-worker	Sickle cell anemia Hypertension Cancer of the esophagus Stomach cancer Coccidioidomycosis Lactose intolerance
Europe Germany England Italy Ireland Other European countries	National languages Many learn English immediately	Noncontact people Aloof Distant Southern countries: closer contact and touch	Future over present	Nuclear families Extended families Judeo-Christian religions Community social organizations	Primary reliance on modern health care system Traditional health and illness beliefs Some remaining folk medicine traditions	Breast cancer Heart disease Cirrhosis of the liver Diabetes mellitus
American Indian 500 American Indian tribes Aleuts Eskimos	Tribal languages Use of silence and body language	Space very important and has no boundaries	Present	Extremely family oriented Biological and extended families	Traditional health and illness beliefs Folk medicine tradition	Accidents Heart disease Cirrhosis of the liver Diabetes mellitus

TABLE 1-1 Cross-Cultural Examples of Cultural Phenomena Impacting Nursing Care—cont'd

Nations of Origin	Communication	Space	Time Orientation	Social Organization	Environmental Control	Biological Variation
				Children taught to respect traditions Community social organizations	Traditional healer: medicine man	
Hispanic countries Spain Cuba Mexico Central and South America	Spanish or Portuguese primary languages	Tactile relationships Touch Handshakes Embracing Value physical presence	Present	Nuclear family Extended families *Compadrazgo*: godparents Community social organizations	Traditional health and illness beliefs Folk medicine traditions Traditional healers: *curandero, espiritista, partera, señora*	Diabetes mellitus Parasites Coccidioidomycosis Lactose intolerance

Compiled by Rachel Spector, RN, PhD. In Potter, P. A., Perry, A. G. (1997). *Fundamentals of nursing: concepts, process, and practice* (4th ed.). St. Louis: Mosby.

Transcultural Model in their curriculum (Lipson & Desantis, 2007). Kaplow and Hardin (2007), using the Giger and Davidhizar Transcultural Model, developed a streamlined version of the model for use with critical care patients. These authors suggested that instead of the normal 45-minute time frame required to complete the Giger and Davidhizar Transcultural Assessment Model, the Critical Care Cultural Assessment (modified from Giger and Davidhizar) could be completed in a staggered time frame. Similarly, in 2008, the Royal College of Nursing, London, England, used the Giger and Davidhizar Transcultural Assessment Model as one of the overarching conceptual and theoretical models to provide care globally to a changing, heterogeneous, culturally diverse society.

In 2003, the Emergency Nurses Association used the Giger and Davidhizar Transcultural Assessment Model to guide the development of its position statement on Diversity in Emergency Care. Similarly, in 2010 and in the update in 2011, the American Association of Colleges of Nursing used the Giger and Davidhizar Transcultural Assessment Model as one of the overarching theoretical frameworks to not only develop an undergraduate but a graduate toolkit to assist in developing cultural competence (American Association of Colleges of Nursing, 2008, 2011). In 2010, Felemban, from Melbourne, Australia, used the Giger and

Davidhizar Transcultural Assessment Model as one of the overarching models to create strategies for educators around the world to teach transcultural health and nursing concepts to their students. The Giger and Davidhizar Transcultural Assessment Model has been widely incorporated into schools of nursing throughout the United States (Lipson & Desantis, 2007).

Application to Other Disciplines

The model is broad enough in scope to be recognized for applicability by many other health care professions (e.g., medical imaging, dentistry, education and training departments, and hospital administration) (Dowd, Giger, & Davidhizar, 1998). This model has had numerous applications in medical imaging: a description of its use in dealing with diversity in radiology departments (Davidhizar, Dowd, & Giger, 1997a), a proposal for its use in the theory base of the profession of radiography (Davidhizar, Dowd, & Giger, 1997b), and a method for how to deal with cultural differences affecting pain response (Davidhizar, Dowd, & Giger, 1997c). Dental hygienists are also involved with clients from diverse cultures. "Transcultural Patient Assessment: A Method of Advancing Dental Care," published in *Dental Assistant* (Davidhizar & Giger, 1998a, 1998b), illuminates how awareness of the behavior of clients in the dental office

TABLE 1-2   Cultural Behaviors Relevant to Health Assessment

Cultural Group	Cultural Variations (Common Beliefs/Practices)	Nursing Implications
African-Americans	Dialect and slang terms require careful communication to prevent error (e.g., "bad" may mean "good").	Question the client's meaning or intent.
Mexican Americans	Eye behavior is important. An individual who looks at and admires a child without touching the child has given the child the "evil eye."	Always touch the child you are examining or admiring.
American Indian	Eye contact is considered a sign of disrespect and is to be avoided.	Recognize that the client may be attentive and interested even though eye contact is avoided.
Appalachians	Eye contact is considered impolite or a sign of hostility. Verbal patter may be confusing.	Clarify statements.
American Eskimos	Body language is very important. The individual seldom disagrees publicly with others. Client may nod yes to be polite, even if not in agreement.	Monitor own body language closely as well as client's to detect meaning.
Jewish Americans	Orthodox Jews consider touching, particularly from members of the opposite sex, offensive.	Establish whether client is an Orthodox Jew and, if so, avoid excessive touch.
Chinese Americans	Individual may nod head to indicate yes or shake head to indicate no. Excessive eye contact indicates rudeness. Excessive touch is offensive.	Ask questions carefully and clarify responses. Avoid excessive eye contact and touch.
Filipino Americans	Offending people is to be avoided at all cost. Nonverbal behavior is very important.	Monitor nonverbal behaviors of self and client, being sensitive to physical and emotional discomfort or concerns of client.
Haitian Americans	Touch is used in conversation. Direct eye contact is used to gain attention and respect during communication.	Use direct eye contact when communicating.
East Indian Hindu Americans	Be aware that men may view eye contact by women as offensive. Avoid eye contact.	Women avoid eye contact as a sign of respect.
Vietnamese Americans	Avoidance of eye contact is a sign of respect. The head is considered sacred; it is not polite to pat the head. An upturned palm is offensive in communication.	Limit eye contact. Touch the head only when mandated and explain clearly before proceeding to do so. Avoid hand gesturing.

From Giger, J., & Davidhizar, R. (1995). *Transcultural nursing* (2nd ed.). St. Louis: Mosby; also appears in Kozier, B., Erb, G., Blaise, K., Johnson, J. Y., & Smith-Temple, J. (1993). *Techniques in clinical nursing* (2nd ed.). Reading, MA: Addison-Wesley.

is often culturally motivated. The model is also described in journals that cross health care professions, such as *Hospital Topics* (Davidhizar & Giger, 1996), *Community Health: Education and Promotion Manual* (Giger, Davidhizar, Johnson, & Poole, 1996), and *Health Care Traveler* (Giger, Davidhizar, Johnson, & Poole, 1997). Application of Giger and Davidhizar's model to diverse clinical settings is quickly producing a way for staff across disciplines to understand

cultural diversity and learn techniques of culturally competent care. In addition, Giger and Davidhizar's Transcultural Assessment Model has been shown to be applicable to the analysis of current trends in multiculturalism in health care (Smith, 1998a). In 2010, Singh and Duggal, while writing for the Light on Ayurveda Foundation, used the Giger and Davidhizar Transcultural Assessment Model as the overarching framework to explain the synergistic relationship between ethnopharmacology and traditional medicine. While using the model as the framework, these authors offered challenges and opportunities for ethnopharmacology and traditional medicine and cultural relativism.

Refinement through Research

Refinement of Giger and Davidhizar's Transcultural Assessment Model is also being enhanced through the research efforts of various individuals. For example, in 1992, a graduate student from the University of Kansas completed a master's thesis titled *Utilizing Giger and Davidhizar's Transcultural Assessment Model for the Cultural Assessment of Farm Families* (Daugherty, 1992). In 1993, a graduate student at Georgia Southern University at Statesboro conducted a research study on the health beliefs and self-care practices of hypertensive African-American women by using Giger and Davidhizar's Transcultural Assessment Model as a theoretical framework to guide and evaluate research findings (Walthour, 1993). In addition to these master's theses, several doctoral dissertations have been completed using the model. In 1995, a group of interdisciplinary researchers (nursing, behavioral medicine, lipoprotein research, human genetics, preventive medicine, nutrition, biostatistics) at the University of Alabama at Birmingham and at Emory University received $750,000 from the Uniformed Health Sciences, University of the Health Sciences, Tri-Services Nursing Military Research Group, and Department of Defense to identify behavioral risk-reduction strategies and chronic indicators for premenopausal African-American women with coronary heart disease or associated risk factors. The model served as the overarching theoretical framework to test its usefulness as an educational tool to enhance and promote compliance. The study is titled "Behavioral Risk Reduction Strategies for Chronic Indicators and High Risk Factors for Premenopausal African-American Women (25–45) with Coronary Heart Disease" (Giger & Strickland, 1995).

In 1988, Linda Smith, a doctoral student at the University of Alabama at Birmingham, completed a pilot study guided by Giger and Davidhizar's Transcultural Assessment Model as the overarching theoretical framework. The primary purpose of this descriptive correlational study was to describe the relationship among scores and subscores on scales measuring concepts of cultural competence. A secondary purpose of this study was to develop reliability and validity data on each of three cultural scales for a population ($n = 51$) of hospital-based registered nurses. These three scales were (1) the Cultural Attitude Scale (CAS), originally developed by Bonaparte (1977, 1979) and modified by Rooda (1990, 1992); (2) the Cultural Self-Efficacy Scale (CSES), developed by Bernal and Froman (1987); and

(3) knowledge base questions (Rooda, 1990). Each of the scales had previously reported reliability and validity data but was administered to populations potentially different from hospital-employed registered nurses. Giger and Davidhizar's Transcultural Assessment Model served as the theoretical foundation, and the CSES, the CAS, and the knowledge base questions were the chosen instruments. Analysis of the data indicates that, for this study population, the reliability analysis scale (alpha) was 0.9778 for the 58-item CSES, 0.6412 for the 40-item CAS, and 0.6038 for the 22 knowledge base questions. Canonical correlation analysis was performed between a set of attitude variables and a set of self-efficacy variables. Both sets of variables demonstrated statistically significant relationships (at an *a priori* alpha of 0.05) to each other (with an approximate eta-squared value for practical significance of 0.365), providing sufficient evidence to reject the non-relationship null hypothesis. For this sample and for these data, cultural self-efficacy toward Asian, African-American, and Hispanic clients and self-efficacy regarding nursing skills when caring for diverse clients related to cultural attitudes and cultural self-efficacy. Nursing care, cultural health beliefs, and cultural health attitudes are related to attitudes toward care of diverse clients. Both sets of variables relate to each other as qualities of culturally competent nursing care (Smith, 1998b).

In 1998, Sharon S. Mullen and Carla G. Phillips at Ohio University School of Nursing also used Giger and Davidhizar's Transcultural Assessment Model as the overarching theoretical framework to explore the cultural beliefs of Appalachians from southeastern Ohio (Mullen & Phillips, 1998). The primary purpose of the qualitative ethnographic study was to identify cultural beliefs as a means of providing culturally competent nursing care. Giger and Davidhizar's Transcultural Assessment Model was used to identify cultural beliefs from six phenomena of interest: (1) communication, (2) space, (3) social organization, (4) time, (5) environmental control, and (6) biological variations. The participants were 14 adults who were native to southeastern Ohio and who had resided in the area their entire lives. Giger and Davidhizar's Transcultural Assessment Model, which also included interview questions and observational guidelines, was used for structured interviews. Findings from this study suggest that these individuals were more socially inclined, communicated more openly, had more of an internal locus of control, had fewer personal space needs, were more future oriented, used no significant home remedies, were more conscientious about getting to appointments on time, and were more likely to follow medical protocols than Appalachians in general. However, findings also suggest that these individuals still resembled the mainstream Appalachian population in that they tended to have a strong character, tended to be stoic and nonassertive, and also tended to have a strong belief in a Supreme Being.

In 2006, Eggenberger, Grassley, and Restrepo used the Giger and Davidhizar model to provide an overarching theory to develop an understanding of Mexican-American women's health care views. From the Giger and Davidhizar model, these researchers conceptualized and developed an interview guide, which was based on social organization and environmental control. Findings from this study suggested that the thematic analysis of interviews with six Mexican-American women indicated the importance of the family, religion, and locus of control in the health beliefs, attitudes, and lifestyle practices of this culture. These researchers concluded that using the voices of Mexican-American women was an excellent starting point for health care practitioners to promote understanding of the Mexican-American culture as a guide for nursing care.

The Giger and Davidhizar Transcultural Assessment Model has also enjoyed tremendous interest and appeal to those striving to conduct culturally competent research. For example, Tanrıverdi, Bayat, Sevig, and Birkök (2011) used the Giger and Davidhizar Transcultural Assessment Model in an effort to discern what cultural factors, if any, existed when clients decided to accept health care services in Eastern Turkey. These researchers postulated that such knowledge was paramount to elevating the quality of services so that clients would accept and use such services. The primary purpose of this qualitative study was to evaluate the effect of cultural characteristics on use of health care services using Giger and Davidhizar's Transcultural Assessment Model. The sample in this study consisted of 31 ($n = 31$) individuals who volunteered to participate in the study and who lived in rural Eastern Turkey. Findings from this study suggested that the limitations and obstacles as stated by these participants included the widespread gender differences of the subjects, use of traditional treatment methods, a high level of environmental control, and a fatalistic attitude about health. One primary conclusion was that for these participants, and given their country of residence, one of the most important limitations or obstacles to appropriate utilization of available health care services was being a woman.

For more than 20 years, the Giger and Davidhizar Transcultural Assessment Model has served to inform all health care practitioners in the art and science of the delivery of culturally competent and appropriate health care. In recognition of this stellar body of work, the American Academy of Nursing recognized the model as one of its Edge Runners for that year. To date, it is the only transcultural model to be so honored by this distinguished body of scholars.

ORGANIZATION OF THE TEXT

In this book, the six cultural phenomena (communication, space, social organization, time, environmental control, and biological variations) are presented in individual chapters with areas that must be assessed when working with clients from multicultural populations. In addition, these six phenomena are applied to the care and management of clients in 16 subcultural groups found in the United States and throughout the world. The Web site used in the fourth and fifth editions has been further refined to assist in the clinical application of Giger and Davidhizar's Transcultural Assessment Model, which has been applied to six additional ethnic and cultural groups. At the end of each chapter, test questions based on the National Council Licensure Examination–Registered Nurse (NCLEX-RN®) review format are found. In addition, http://evolve.elsevier .com/Giger/ provides a user-friendly cultural competency test based on the NCLEX-RN test format with supporting key for faculty use. This tool is based on Giger and Davidhizar's Transcultural Assessment Model. The NCLEX-RN test bank was originally developed by Kenneth Farr, Doris Bartlett, Joyce Newman Giger, and Ruth Davidhizar and revised in this edition by Joyce Newman Giger. Concept analyses of individual items were provided by the developers, and the concepts were found to be valid. Ambiguous or difficult concepts were discarded or reworded after concept analyses. To date, 108 nursing faculty have taken the test as a pre- and post-test to establish reliability. Reliability of this instrument ranged from 0.82 to 0.91 on the pre-test and 0.91 to 0.94 on the post-test. In the future, reliability and validity of the test will be further assessed. It is important to remember that a comprehensive nursing assessment is necessary for both the nurse practitioner and the researcher to provide culturally appropriate nursing care.

REFERENCES

Aamodt, A. M. (1978). The care component in a health and healing system. In E. Bauwens (Ed.), *The anthropology of health*. St. Louis: Mosby.

Affonso, D. (1979). Framework for cultural assessment. In A. L. Clark (Ed.), *Childbearing: a nursing perspective* (2nd ed., pp. 107–119). Philadelphia: F. A. Davis.

American Association of Colleges of Nursing. (2008). *Tool kit of resources for cultural competent education for baccalaureate nurses*. Available at <http://www.aacn .nche.edu/education/pdf/toolkit.pdf> Retrieved March 30, 2011.

American Association of Colleges of Nursing. (2011). *Tool Kit for Cultural Competence in Master's and Doctoral Education*. Available at <http://www.aacn.nche.edu/education/pdf/

Cultural_Competency_Toolkit_Grad.pdf> Retrieved on
March 30, 2011.

Andrews, M., & Boyle, J. (2008). *Transcultural concepts in nursing care* (5th ed.). Philadelphia: Lippincott Williams & Wilkins.

Bernal, H., & Froman, R. (1987). The confidence of community health nurses in caring for ethnically diverse populations. *Image: Journal of Nursing Scholarship, 19*(4), 201–203.

Bloch, B. (1983). Bloch's assessment guide for ethnic/cultural variations. In M. S. Orque, B. Bloch, & L. S. A. Monrroy (Eds.), *Ethnic nursing care: a multicultural approach* (pp. 49–75). St. Louis: Mosby.

Bonaparte, B. H. G. (1977). *An investigation of the relation between ego defensiveness and open-closed mindedness of female registered professional nurses and their attitude toward culturally different patients.* New York: New York University.

Bonaparte, B. H. G. (1979). Ego defensiveness, open-closed mindedness, and nurses' attitude toward culturally different patients. *Nursing Research, 28*(3), 166–172.

Bowen, M., & Davidhizar, R. (1991). Communication with the client in the OR. *Today's OR Nurse, 1*, 11–14.

Braithwaite, R., & Taylor, S. (2001). *Health issues in the black community* (2nd ed.). San Francisco: Jossey-Bass.

Branch, M. F., & Paxton, P. P. (Eds.) (1976). *Providing safe nursing care for ethnic people of color.* Englewood Cliffs, NJ: Prentice-Hall.

Brink, P. J. (2001a). *Transcultural nursing: a book of readings.* Long Grove, IL: Waveland Press.

Brink, P. J. (2001b). Cultural diversity in nursing: how much can we tolerate. In J. McCloskey & H. Grace (Eds.), *Current issues in nursing* (6th ed.). St. Louis: Mosby.

Brownlee, A. T. (1978). *Community, culture, and care: a cross-cultural guide for health workers.* St. Louis: Mosby.

Burk, M., Wieser, P., & Keegan, L. (1995). Cultural beliefs and health behaviors of pregnant Mexican-American women: implications for primary care. *Advances in Nursing Science, 17*(4), 37–52.

Cohall, A., & Bannister, H. (2001). The health status of children and adolescents. In R. Braithwaite & S. Taylor (Eds.), *Health issues in the black community* (pp. 13–43). San Francisco: Jossey-Bass.

Daugherty, B. (1992). *Utilizing Giger and Davidhizar's transcultural assessment model for the cultural assessment of farm families* (Unpublished master's thesis). Lawrence, KS: University of Kansas.

Davidhizar, R., Dowd, S., & Giger, J. (1997a). Managing a multicultural radiology staff. *Radiology Management, 19*(1), 50–55.

Davidhizar, R., Dowd, S., & Giger, J. (1997b). Model for cultural diversity in the radiology department. *Radiologic Technology, 68*(3), 233–238.

Davidhizar, R., Dowd, S., & Giger, J. (1997c). Cultural differences in pain management. *Radiologic Technology, 68*(4), 345–348.

Davidhizar, R., & Giger, J. (1996). Reflections on the minority elderly in health care. *Hospital Topics, 74*(3), 20–24.

Davidhizar, R., & Giger, J. (1998a). Caring for the patient from another culture. *Journal of the Canadian Dental Association, 39*(1), 24–27.

Davidhizar, R., & Giger, J. (1998b). Transcultural patient assessment: a method of advancing dental care. *The Dental Assistant, 39*(1), 40–43.

Dowd, S., Giger, J., & Davidhizar, R. (1998). Use of the Giger and Davidhizar Model by other health professions: contributions of nursing science. *International Nursing Review, 45*(4), 119–203.

Eggenberger, S., Grassley, J., & Restrepo, E. (2006). Culturally competent nursing care for families: listening to the voices of Mexican-American women. *OJIN: The Online Journal of Issues in Nursing, 11*(3).

Emergency Nurses Association. (2003). *Emergency Nurses Association Position Statement.* Available at <http://www.ena.org/SiteCollectionDocuments/Position%20Statements/Diversity_in_Emergency_Care_-_ENA_PS.pdf> Retrieved June 25, 2011.

Felemban, E. (2010). Transcultural competency in the curricula of nursing. *Middle East Journal of Nursing, 4*(2), 23–30.

Geissler, E. M. (1991). Transcultural nursing and nursing diagnosis. *Nursing and Health Care, 12*(4), 190–203.

Giger, J., & Davidhizar, R. (1990). Transcultural nursing assessment: a method for advancing practice. *International Nursing Review, 37*(1), 199–203.

Giger, J., & Davidhizar, R. (1994). Transcultural nursing: have we gone too far or not far enough? In O. Strickland & D. Fishman (Eds.), *Nursing issues in the 1990s* (pp. 491–504). New York: Delmar.

Giger, J., & Davidhizar, R. (1998). *Canadian transcultural nursing, assessment, and intervention.* St. Louis: Mosby.

Giger, J., Davidhizar, R., Evers, S., & Ingram, C. (1994). Cultural factors influencing mental health and mental illness. In C. M. Taylor (Ed.), *Mereness' essentials of psychiatric nursing* (14th ed., pp. 217–236). St. Louis: Mosby.

Giger, J., Davidhizar, R. E., Johnson, J., & Poole, V. (1996). Health promotion in minority populations. In C. S. Schust (Ed.), *Community health: education and promotion manual.* Gaithersburg, MD: Aspen.

Giger, J., Davidhizar, R. E., Johnson, J., & Poole, V. (1997). The changing faces of America: using cultural phenomena to improve care. *The Health Care Traveler, 4*(4), 10–40.

Giger, J., Davidhizar, R., & Wieczorek, S. (1993). Culture and ethnicity. In I. Bobak & M. Jensen (Eds.), *Maternity and gynecological care* (5th ed., pp. 43–67). St. Louis: Mosby.

Giger, J. N., & Davidhizar, R. (2002). The Giger and Davidhizar Transcultural Assessment Model. *Journal of Transcultural Nursing, 13*, 185–188.

Giger, J., & Strickland, O. (1995). *Behavioral risk reduction strategies for chronic indicators and high risk factors for premenopausal African-American women (25–45) with coronary heart disease.* Grant Number N95–019, Department of Defense, Uniformed Health Services. Bethesda, MD: University of the Health Sciences, Tri-Service Nursing Research.

Giger, J. N., et al. (2007). American Academy of Nursing Expert Panel Report: Developing cultural competence to eliminate health disparities and other vulnerable populations. *Journal of Transcultural Nursing, 18*(2), 95–102.

Kaplow, R., & Hardin, S. (2007). *Critical care nursing: synergy for optimal outcomes.* Boston, MA: Jones and Bartlett.

Kay, M. (1978). Clinical anthropology. In E. E. Bauwens (Ed.), *The anthropology of health* (pp. 3–11). St. Louis: Mosby.

Kozier, B., Erb, G., Blaise, K., Johnson, J., & Smith-Temple, J. (1995). *Techniques in clinical nursing* (2nd ed.). Reading, MA: Addison-Wesley.

Leininger, M. (1977). Transcultural nursing and a proposed conceptual framework. In M. Leininger (Ed.), *Transcultural nursing care of infants and children: proceedings from the first transcultural conference.* Salt Lake City: University of Utah.

Leininger, M. (1985a). *Qualitative research methods in nursing.* Orlando, FL: Grune & Stratton.

Leininger, M. (1985b). Transcultural care, diversity and universality: a theory of nursing. *Nursing and Health Care, 6*(4), 209–212.

Leininger, M. (1991). Transcultural nursing: the study and practice field. *Imprint, 38*(2), 55–66.

Leininger, M., & McFarland, M. (2006). *Culture care diversity and universality: a worldwide nursing theory* (2nd ed.). Sudbury, MA: Jones and Bartlett.

Lipson, J., & Desantis, L. (2007). Current approaches to integrating elements of cultural competence in nursing education. *Journal of Transcultural Nursing, 18,* 10S–20S.

Mullen, S., & Phillips, C. (1998). *Cultural beliefs of southeastern Ohio Appalachians. Proceedings of the Fourth International and Interdisciplinary Health Research Symposium 1998 Health Care and Culture School of Nursing.* Morgantown, VA: West Virginia University.

Murdock, G. P., et al. (2004). *Outline of cultural materials* (5th ed.). New Haven, CT: Human Relations Area Files.

Orque, M. S. (1983). Orque's ethnic/cultural system: a framework for ethnic nursing care. In M. S. Orque, B. Bloch, & L. S. A. Monrroy (Eds.), *Ethnic nursing care: a multi-cultural approach* (pp. 5–48). St. Louis: Mosby.

Purnell, L. D., & Paulanka, B. J. (Eds.) (2008). *Transcultural health care* (2nd ed.). Philadelphia: F. A. Davis.

Rooda, L. (1990). *Knowledge and attitudes of nurses toward culturally diverse patients* (Unpublished doctoral dissertation). West Lafayette, IN: Purdue University.

Rooda, L. (1992). Attitudes of nurses toward culturally diverse patients: an examination of the social contact theory. *Journal of the National Black Nurses Association, 6*(1), 48–56.

Royal College of Nursing. (2008). *Transcultural health care practice: foundation module section three: models of transcultural care.* Available at <http://www.rcn.org.uk/development/learning/transcultural_health/foundation/sectionthree> Retrieved March 15, 2011.

Rund, N., & Krause, L. (1978). Health attitudes and your health programs. In E. E. Bauwens (Ed.), *The anthropology of health* (pp. 73–78). St. Louis: Mosby.

Sheridan, D., & Zimbler, E. (1993). *Nursing management skills: a modular self-assessment series, module IV, transcultural nursing.* New York: National League for Nursing.

Singh, A., & Duggal, S. (2010). Ethnopharmacology and traditional medicine—exploring challenges and opportunities. *The Light of Ayurveda Foundation.* Available at <http://www.loaj.com/ayurvedic_herbology.html> Retrieved March 30, 2011.

Smith, L. (1998a). Trends in multiculturalism in health care. *Hospital Material Management Quarterly, 20*(1), 61–69.

Smith, L. (1998b). Concept analysis: culture competence. *Journal of Cultural Diversity, 5*(1), 4–10.

Spector, R. (1996). *Cultural diversity in health and illness* (3rd ed.). Norwalk, CT: Appleton & Lange.

Spector, R. (2008). *Cultural diversity in health and illness* (8th ed.). Upper Saddle River, NJ: Pearson Prentice Hall.

Stokes, G. (1991). A transcultural nurse is about. *Senior Nurse, 11*(1), 40–42.

Tanriverdi, G., Bayat, M., Sevig, U., & Birkök, C. (2011). Evaluation of the effect of cultural characteristics on use of health care services. Using the Giger and Davidhizar's Transcultural Assessment Model: a sample from a village in eastern Turkey. *Use of Health Care Services, 4*(1), 19–24.

Tripp-Reimer, T. (1984a). Research in cultural diversity. *Western Journal of Nursing Research, 6*(3), 353–355.

Tripp-Reimer, T. (1984b). Cultural assessment. In J. P. Bellack & P. A. Bamford (Eds.), *Nursing assessment: a multidimensional approach* (pp. 226–246). Monterey, CA: Wadsworth.

Tripp-Reimer, T., Brink, P., & Saunders, J. (1984). Cultural assessment: content and process. *Nursing Outlook, 32*(2), 78–82.

Tripp-Reimer, T., & Dougherty, M. C. (1985). Cross-cultural nursing research. *Annual Review of Nursing Research, 3,* 77–104.

Tripp-Reimer, T., & Friedl, M. (1977). Appalachians: a neglected minority. *Nursing Clinics of North America, 12*(1), 41–54.

U.S. Department of Commerce, Bureau of the Census. (2009). *American Community Survey, 2009.* Washington, DC: U.S. Government Printing Office. Internet update.

U.S. Department of Commerce, Bureau of Census. (2011). *2010 Census Briefs.* Washington, DC: U.S. Government Printing Office.

U.S. Department of Health and Human Services, Office of Minority Health. (2004). *Cultural competency and nursing: a review of current concepts, policies, and practices.* Contract Number: 233-02-0082, Task Order #1, Task 2: Curriculum Synthesis Report. Washington, DC: U.S. Government Printing Office.

Walthour, E. (1993). *Health beliefs and self-care practices of hypertensive African-Americans* (Unpublished master's thesis). Statesboro, GA: Georgia Southern University.

Wenger, F. (1989). President's address. *Transcultural Nursing Society Newsletter, 9*(1), 3.

2

Communication

BEHAVIORAL OBJECTIVES

After reading this chapter, the nurse will be able to:

1. Describe the importance of communication as it relates to transcultural nursing assessment.
2. Delineate barriers to communication that hinder the development of a nurse–client relationship in transcultural settings.
3. Understand the importance of dialect, style, volume, use of touch, context of speech and kinesics and their relationship to transcultural nursing assessment and care.
4. Describe appropriate nursing intervention techniques to develop positive communication in the nurse–client relationship.

5. Understand the significance of nonverbal communication and the use of silence, and their relationship to transcultural nursing assessment and care.
6. Explain the significance of the structure and format of names in various cultural groups.
7. Explain the significance of variations in word meanings across and within various cultural and ethnic groups.

The word *communication* comes from the Latin verb *communicāre*, "to make common, share, participate, or impart" (Guralnik, 1989; Tuleja & O'Rourke, 2009). Communication, however, goes further than this definition implies and embraces the entire realm of human interaction and behavior. All behavior, whether verbal or nonverbal, in the presence of another individual is communication (Potter & Perry, 2005; Tuleja & O'Rourke, 2009; Watzlawich, Beavin, & Jackson, 1967).

As the matrix of all thought and relationships among people, communication provides the means by which people connect. It establishes a sense of commonality with others and permits the sharing of information, signals, or messages in the form of ideas and feelings. Communication is a continuous process by which one person may affect another through written or oral language, gestures, facial expressions, body language, space, or other symbols.

Nurses have long recognized the importance of communication to health. Effective communication of health care information motivates individuals to work with their health care providers to manage their health. Giorgianni

(2000) notes that individuals who have had effective health care communication are better informed and more confident in pursuing health care. Communication received increased visibility nationally with the inclusion of an entire chapter on health communication in *Healthy People 2010,* and this trend continues in the new *Healthy People 2020* (U.S. Department of Health and Human Services, 2000, 2011). In *Healthy People 2010,* among the six national objectives were increased access to the Internet from home, increased satisfaction by individuals in the communication skills of their health care providers, and increased research on health communication. Effective communication of health care information is critical if individuals are to take action on behalf of their own health, the strategic goal of *Healthy People 2010.* For *Healthy People 2020,* the communication objective is centered on health communication and health information technology (U.S. Department of Health and Human Services, 2011).

Communication is the core of most nursing curricula. However, if effective communication is to occur in today's multicultural setting, nursing curricula not only need to provide skills in communication but also must teach diversity as a value (Cook & Cullen, 2000). To accomplish this, nursing curricula are increasingly reflecting integration of culture as a central concept (Davidhizar & Eshleman, 2006; Davidhizar & Giger, 2001; Wood, 2001). Furthermore, to promote effective communication, health care settings are modifying the climate of units and organizations to accommodate multiculturalism (Buerhaus & Auerbach, 1999; Byrne, 2002; Davidhizar, Dowd, & Giger, 1998; Davidhizar & Shearer, 2005; Davidhizar, Shearer, & Giger, 2002).

Nevertheless, communication frequently presents barriers between nurses and clients, especially when the nurses and the clients are from different cultural backgrounds. If the nurse and the client do not speak the same language or if communication styles and patterns differ, both the nurse and the client can feel alienated and helpless. When communication is impaired, the physical healing process may be impaired. Nurses may also feel angry and helpless if their communication is not understood or if they cannot understand the client. With ineffective communication, certain physiological problems such as pain may not be controlled (Davidhizar & Hart, 2005). Nurses need to have not only a working knowledge of communication with clients of the same culture but also a thorough awareness of racial, cultural, and social factors that may affect communication with persons from other cultures. Communication with family members is also crucial to client and family satisfaction. When Shields and King (2001) interviewed family members in four countries, all the respondents identified the importance of communication with family members in the provision of care.

Nurses must have an awareness of how an individual, although speaking the same language as the nurse, may differ in communication patterns and understandings as a result of cultural orientation. Nurses must also have communication skills in relating to individuals who do not speak a familiar language (Davidhizar & Brownson, 2000; Ericksen, 2002; Sieh & Brentin, 1997). Nurses generally assume that their perceptions and assessment of the client's health status are accurate and congruent with those of the client. However, there is evidence that discrepancies in perceptions persist and may interfere with the provision of care to special populations with higher-than-average risk of developing health problems (Crump, Bartman, Walker, & Mitchell, 2000). Many factors obstruct high-quality client care, including cost, fear, poor communication, noncompliance with the treatment regimen, inadequate or unnecessary treatment, and ethical problems. All these factors combine to create discrepancies in perceptions between nurse and client (Andrews & Boyle, 2003; Crump et al., 2000; Giger, Davidhizar, Johnson, & Poole, 1997; Lester, 1998).

COMMUNICATION AND CULTURE

Communication and culture are closely intertwined. Communication is the means by which culture is transmitted and preserved (Delgado, 1983; Orlando & Nickoloff, 2007; Tohidian & Tabatabaie, 2010). Culture influences how feelings are expressed and what verbal and nonverbal expressions are appropriate. Americans may be more likely to conceal feelings, and the United States is generally considered a low-touch culture, whereas a member of an Eastern culture may be open and loud with expressions of grief, anger, or joy and may use touch more (Davidhizar & Giger, 2002; Giger & Davidhizar, 2002; Hall, 1966; Thayer, 1988). Other cultural variables, such as the perception of time, bodily contact, and territorial rights, also influence communication. The cultural differences in contact can be quite dramatic. In a classic study, Sidney Jourard (1972) reported that when touch between pairs of people in coffee shops around the world was studied, touch occurred more in certain cities. For example, touch occurred as frequently as 180 times an hour between couples in San Juan, Puerto Rico, and 110 times an hour in Paris, France. In other cities there was less touch; specifically, touch occurred twice an hour between couples in Gainesville, Florida, and zero times an hour in London, England.

Cultural patterns of communication are embedded early, typically by age 5, and are found in child-rearing practices (Anderson, 2003; Capirci, Iverson, Pizzuto, & Volterra, 1996). In a classic study, Gibson (1984) studied the playgrounds and beaches of Greece, the Soviet Union, and the United States, and compared the frequency and nature of touch between caregivers and children ranging from 2 to 5 years of age. The analysis of data indicates that although rates of touching for retrieving or punishing the children were similar, rates of touching for soothing, holding, and playing were dissimilar. American children were less likely to be touched than children from other cultures. The communication practices of persons in different cultural groups affect the expression of ideas and feelings, decision making, and communication strategies. The communication of an individual reflects, determines, and consequently molds the culture (Hedlund, 1993; Krech, Crutchfield, & Ballachey, 1962). In other words, a culture may be limited and molded by its communication practices. As early as 1929, Sapir proposed that individuals are at the mercy of the particular language that has become the medium of expression of their society. Experiences are determined by language habits that predispose the individual to certain conceptions of the world and choices of interpretation. Kayser (1996) noted that educational programming that is provided to children of different cultural and linguistic backgrounds is critical for the successful implementation of language interventions. Focusing on English-language development while minimizing learning opportunities limits children who do not speak English as their first language from the development of higher-level cognitive skills.

Variations in communication may be limited to specific meanings for a few individuals in a small group, such as a family. On the other hand, unique communication patterns are frequently found among persons from the same ethnic and cultural group, such as the Gypsies or the Amish (Banks & Banks, 1995; Beachy, Hershberger, Davidhizar, & Giger, 1997). Some persons consider the deaf a cultural group. In any case, persons who are deaf have a unique language and communication patterns that require nurses to use special communication approaches (McLeod & Bently, 1996). However, the nurse must be cautious about assuming that a certain communication pattern can be generalized to all persons in a designated cultural group because communication patterns are often unique. In assessing the client, the nurse should keep in mind common cultural patterns and approach the client as an individual who should not be categorized because of cultural heritage.

LINGUISTICS

Because communication is a broad concept and encompasses all human behavior, it has been conceptualized in many ways. One way is to consider the structure of communication, as in linguistics. Linguistics is the area within anthropology concerned with the study of the structure of language. Linguistic patterns represent more than the use of grammatically nonequivalent words; these patterns can create real disparity in social treatment. The major focus on the structure of communication has been developed within the fields of ethnomethodology in sociology and of linguistics in anthropology. Structure may be perceived as a form of language and the use of words and behaviors to construct messages. The role of ethnomethodologists is to consider the structure and effects of communication and to look at rules of communication and the consequences of breaking these rules. Ethnomethodologists not only have emphasized the study of the structure and rules of language but also have studied the structure and rules of nonverbal communication (Garfinkel, 2002; Sudnow, 1967).

FUNCTIONS OF COMMUNICATION

Another way to think about communication is to consider what it achieves or accomplishes in human interaction. Consideration of the functions of communication refers to examining what the communication accomplishes rather than how the communication is structured. A relationship exists between communication structure and communication function in the sense that structure does affect function.

As a part of human interaction, communication discloses information or provides a specific message. Messages can be sent with no expectation of a response. Included in the disclosure of information may be an element of self-disclosure. Communication may or may not be intended as a method of self-disclosure or a means to provide information about the self or the individual's perception of self (Hedlund, 1993; Luft & Ingham, 1984; Myers, 2007). Perceptions of self include acts that describe the self and estimations of self-worth. In some situations self-awareness may be achieved through communication; this function of communication involves interaction with people (Davidhizar & Dowd, 2005). Through communication with others, an individual may become more aware of personal feelings. Communication can also serve the important interpersonal functions of conveying respect and giving or taking away power (Beutter & Davidhizar, 1999; Davidhizar & Dowd, 2004; Miller & Davidhizar, 2001).

PROCESS OF COMMUNICATION

Communication may be conceptualized as a process that includes a sender, a transmitting device, signals, a receiver, and feedback (Varcarolis, 2006). A sender attempts to relay a message, an idea, or information to another person or group through the use of signals or symbols. Many factors influence how the message is given and how it is received. For example, physical health, emotional well-being, the situation being discussed and the meaning it has, other distractions, knowledge of the matter being discussed, skill at communicating, and attitudes toward the other person and the subject being discussed may all affect the communication that takes place (Box 2-1). In addition, personal needs and interests; background, including cultural, social, and philosophical values; the senses and their functional ability; a personal tendency to make judgments and be judgmental of others; the environment in which the communication takes place; and experiences that relate or are related to the present situation may all affect the message that is received. The receiver then interprets the message. Feedback is given to the sender about the message, and more communication may occur. If no feedback is given, there may be no reciprocal interaction. Cultures such as the mainstream U.S. culture may be low context whereas the Asian cultures are high context; that is, very little of the message is the coded, explicit, transmitted part of the message. Members of individualistic cultures have a tendency to communicate in a more direct manner that has

BOX 2-1   Factors Influencing Communication

1. Physical health and emotional well-being
2. The situation being discussed and its meaning
3. Distractions to the communication process
4. Knowledge of the matter being discussed
5. Skill at communicating
6. Attitudes toward the other person and toward the subject being discussed
7. Personal needs and interests
8. Background, including cultural, social, and philosophical values
9. The senses involved and their functional ability
10. Personal tendency to make judgments and be judgmental of others
11. The environment in which the communication occurs
12. Experiences that relate to the current situation

TABLE 2-1   Languages Other Than English Spoken by Persons Residing in the United States

Language Spoken at Home for Persons Over 18 Years of Age	Number
Spanish or Spanish Creole	34,560,000
Chinese	2,466,000
French (including patois, Cajun)	1,979,000
Tagalog	1,488,000
Vietnamese	1,225,000
German	1,122,000
Korean	1,052,000
African languages	742,000
Japanese	440,000
Miao, Hmong	190,000
Mon-Khmer, Cambodian	183,000
Navajo	171,000
Laotian	147,000

Adapted from the U.S. Bureau of the Census. (2011). *Statistical Abstracts of the United States* (13th ed.). Washington, D.C.: The National Data Book, U.S. Government Printing Office.

relatively low dependence on context, whereas members of collectivistic cultures use high-context messages in a more indirect fashion (Xu & Davidhizar, 2005).

Although the process of communication is universal, nurses should be aware that styles and types of feedback may be unique to certain cultural groups. For example, before the assimilation of the Alaskan Eskimo into the American culture, the Alaskan Eskimo would indicate that a message was received by blinking rather than by making a verbal response (Davidhizar & Giger, 2000). Nonverbal responses are also found in the Vietnamese. Vietnamese persons may smile, but the smile may not indicate understanding. A Vietnamese person may say *yes* simply to avoid confrontation or out of a desire to please. A smile may cover up disturbed feelings. Nodding, which nurses commonly interpret as understanding and compliance, may, for a Vietnamese individual, simply indicate respect for the person talking (Hoang & Erickson, 1982; Lindsay, Narayan, & Rea, 1998). The nurse may be surprised later when the Vietnamese client who smiled and nodded does not follow through with the instructions given.

In today's health care system, optimal communication includes use of technology. E-mail, cell phones, voice mail, and PDAs have greatly improved timeliness in communication (Davidhizar & Dowd, 2006). E-mail messages can be printed to provide hard copy for documentation purposes. Notebook computers with cell phone modem connections to access clinical information can be used in a client's home in a rural setting to give clients more efficient service. Past health records can be accessed via the computer to be viewed by health professionals. Nurses can use the Internet and search Web sites to keep up-to-date on health care information and to print health education material for clients. Clients can be assisted to find age- and language-appropriate TV programs as well as Web sites for health information (Jones, 2000). Health promotion strategies can include CD-ROMs, health consumer e-journals, toll-free telephone numbers, and DVDs.

Linguistic Isolation in the United States

In the United States, some 43 million adults are linguistically isolated, do not speak English well, or speak a language other than English at home (U.S. Department of Commerce, Bureau of the Census, American Community Survey Briefs, 2010a). Table 2-1 shows some of the languages spoken in the United States.

VERBAL AND NONVERBAL COMMUNICATION

Another way to conceptualize communication is in terms of verbal and nonverbal behavior (Box 2-2). Communication first of all involves language or verbal communication, including vocabulary or a repertoire of words and grammatical structure (Barkauskas, 1994; Halliday & Webster, 2006).

BOX 2-2 Verbal and Nonverbal Communication

Language or Verbal Communication
Vocabulary
Grammatical structure
Voice qualities
Intonation
Rhythm
Speed
Pronunciation
Silence

Nonverbal Communication
Touch
Facial expression
Eye movement
Body posture

Communications That Combine Verbal and Nonverbal Elements
Warmth
Humor

Although foreign-born persons need to demonstrate English proficiency to obtain U.S. citizenship, the nurse may encounter many persons in the United States who are not fluent in English. In 2009, 38.5 million members of the U.S. population were foreign born, representing 12.5% of the total U.S. population. It is interesting to note that between 2000 and 2009, the foreign-born population increased by 11.3 million people. This figure represents a percentage of change of 23.5% and a share of change of 28.6%. Among the foreign-born in 2009, 53.7% were born in Latin America, 28% were born in Asia, 13.1% were born in Europe, 2.2% were born in other regions of North America, and 4.3% were born in Africa and other regions of the world. In fact, among the foreign-born, the top four countries representing the greatest number were Mexico (11.5 million; 29.8%), China (2 million; 5.2%), the Philippines (1 million; 4.5%), and India (1 million; 4.3%). As previously indicated, of the total number of foreign-born, 43.7% are U.S. citizens, and 17.9% live in poverty (*Time Almanac,* 2011; U.S. Department of Commerce, Bureau of the Census, American Community Survey Briefs, 2010a). In fact, in 2009, of the number of foreign-born, 56.2% were not U.S. citizens and only 43.7% had obtained citizenship through naturalization (U.S. Department of Commerce, Bureau of the Census, American Community Survey Briefs 2010b).

Among the foreign-born, four of every five speak a language other than English at home. This translates roughly to 83% of the foreign-born older than 5 years of age who speak a language other than English at home. This figure includes 52.3% who speak Spanish, 21.9% who speak other Indo-European languages, and 21.6% who speak Asian or Pacific Island languages. In 2008, of the number of foreign-born who spoke a language other than English at home, only 38.5% spoke English "very well," whereas 12.2% of the foreign-born did not speak English at all. Among the foreign-born who speak Spanish at home, only 48% speak English very well (*Time Almanac,* 2011; U.S. Department of Commerce, Bureau of the Census, American Community Survey Reports, 2010a; U.S. Department of Commerce, Bureau of the Census, 2010). In 2008, 283,150,000 persons older than 5 years of age spoke English at home; 34,560,000 spoke Spanish; 1,979,000, French; 782,000, Italian; 2,466,000, Chinese; 1,488,000, Tagalog; and 620,000, Polish. Vietnamese was spoken by 1,225,000, Portuguese by 661,000, Japanese by 440,000, Greek by 337,000, Arabic by 786,000, and Hindi by 560,000. Russian, Yiddish, Thai, Persian, French Creole, Armenian, Navajo, Hungarian, Hebrew, Dutch, Khmer (Cambodian), and Gujarati were all spoken by at least 100,000 people (U.S. Department of Commerce, Bureau of the Census, 2011). In addition to these persons registered as living in households, many other non–English-speaking persons are in the United States as visitors, on temporary visas, or illegally. Approximately one sixth (31,845,000) of the population reported that they spoke another language besides English in the home, yet only a small minority of caregivers speak a language other than English (U.S. Department of Commerce, Bureau of the Census, 2011).

It is important to appreciate that along with language, significant communication cues are received from voice quality, intonation, rhythm, and speed, as well as from the pronunciation used. Dialect may differ significantly among persons both across and within cultures. Silence during communication may itself be a significant part of the message.

Communication involves nonverbal messages, which include touch, facial expressions, eye behavior, body posture, and the use of space (Giger & Davidhizar, 1990a). Spatial behavior also affects communication and encompasses a variety of behaviors, including movement and proximity to others and to objects in the environment (see Chapter 3). Although nonverbal communication is powerful and honest, its importance and meaning vary among and within cultures; therefore, it is essential that the nurse have an awareness and appreciation of the role that body language may have in the communication process. In addition, some communications combine nonverbal and verbal components in the message that is sent. Two examples of combination messages are warmth and humor.

Language, or Verbal Communication

Language is basic to communication. Without language, the higher order cognitive processes of thinking, reasoning, and generalizing cannot be attained. Words are tools or symbols used to express ideas and feelings or to identify or describe objects. Words shape experiences and influence cultural perceptions. Words convey interpretations and influence relationships (Pirandello, 1970; Talbot, 1996; Varcarolis, 2006). Although words provide a special way of looking at the world, the same words often have different meanings for different individuals within cultural groups. In addition, word meanings change over time and in different situations. It is important to ascertain that the message is received and understood as the sender intended. As early as 1954, Sullivan emphasized the importance of ongoing validation in a therapeutic relationship to verify interpretations made on the behavior and words of another. Even today, this validation remains relevant in a nurse–client relationship in which many experiential, educational, and cultural differences are present. Smith and Cantrell (1988) reported a study comparing the effect of personal questions and physical distance on anxiety rates. Pulse rates were higher when the investigator asked personal questions, regardless of the physical distance from subjects. Although the data from this study indicate that the most important part of a message may be verbal, the opposite has also been found to be true. Thus, both verbal and nonverbal communication must be considered before a conclusion about the true meaning of a message can be determined.

To provide culturally appropriate nursing care, nurses must separate values based on their own cultural background from the values of the clients to whom care is given. Transcultural communication and understanding break down when caregivers project their own culturally specific values and behaviors onto the client. Thiederman (1986) has suggested that projection of values as well as hindering care may actually contribute to noncompliance.

Vocabulary. Even though people may speak the same language, establishing communication is often difficult because word meanings for both the sender and the receiver vary according to past experiences and learning. Words have both denotative and connotative meanings. A denotative meaning is one that is in general use by most persons who share a common language. A connotative meaning usually arises from a person's personal experience. For example, although all Americans are likely to share the same general denotative meaning for the word *pig*,

depending on the occupation and cultural perception of the person, the connotation may be entirely different and precipitate completely different reactions. The word *pig* will invoke either negative or positive reactions from certain people on the basis of occupation and culture. For example, an Orthodox Jew's reactions will differ from those of a pig farmer. For an Orthodox Jew, the word *pig* is synonymous with the word *unclean* or *unholy* and thus should be avoided. On the other hand, for a pig farmer the word *pig* implies a clean, wholesome means of making a living. Numerous conflicts resulting from differences in word meaning among various ethnic and racial groups are reported in the literature. Among her many famous cultural studies, Margaret Mead (1947) reported on the different meanings that the word *compromise* carries for an Englishman and an American:

> In Britain, the word compromise *is a good word, and one may speak approvingly of any arrangement that has been a compromise, very often including one in which the other side has gained more than 50% of the points at issue. Whereas, in Britain, to compromise means to work out a good solution, in America it usually means to work out a bad one, a solution in which all the points of importance are lost.*

Often people who have learned a language have learned the meaning for the word in only one context. For example, Díaz-Duque (1982) reported that a Hispanic person who was told he was going "to be discharged tomorrow" somehow interpreted this to mean that he was going to develop "a discharge from below." Díaz-Duque also indicated that for Hispanics, problems arise with cognates such as *constipation* because for Hispanics this term generally refers to nasal congestion rather than intestinal constipation. Lunsford (2006) recounts the story of Xial Ming Li, now a college teacher, who came to the United States from China where she had been a good writer. However, in college in the United States she struggled to understand what faculty expected of her writing. Although she used appropriate words and sentence grammar, she needed tutors to assist her to write in the "U.S.A. style" that was expected.

Although barriers exist when people speak the same language, more profound barriers are present when different languages are spoken. Each language has a whole set of unconscious assumptions about the world and life. Understanding differences in the meaning of words can provide insight into people of different cultures. For example, many English-speaking Americans are puzzled by what seems to be a different time orientation among Hispanic peoples. An understanding of the meaning of the word *time* helps provide insight into this different orientation. In Spanish, time is defined as "passing"—a clock "passes time" or "moves," whereas in English a clock "runs." If time is moving rapidly, as English usage declares, we must hurry. On the other hand, the Spanish definition allows for a more leisurely attitude (Randall-David, 1989). Such cultural understandings can provide insight into the reasons why Spanish individuals are often late for health care appointments.

Language reflects the dominant concerns and interests of a people, which can be noted in the number of words for certain things. Some classic studies have reported that certain cultures use many words to describe a particular object of importance. For example, Eskimos have 20 or so words for snow depending on consistency and texture (Tohidian & Tabatabaie, 2010). The language of a people is a key that unlocks their culture. A nurse who is familiar with the language of clients will have the best chance of gaining insight into their culture.

Names. Names have a special psychological and cultural significance. All people have names, and in every culture naming a newborn is considered important. The considerations that go into the naming process vary greatly from culture to culture. For example, in Roman tradition there is a given name for boys; a family name, which is second; and a third name that specifies an extended family unit. The name *Caius Julius Caesar* illustrates the importance of tribal connections as well as male chauvinism (Clemmens, 1988). In Roman times, girls had only one name, the female version of the family name; for example, Caesar's sister was Julia, as were his father's sister and other relatives. During the early Roman times, women lacked individuality and thus in Roman society were not worth being named.

The Hebrew tradition has a patrilineal way of looking at names—that is, a given name plus "son of." Mothers' names are not included. A spiritual and traditional continuity is evidenced in this system of naming. The Hebrew tradition can be seen today in Iceland, where all males have their given names, followed by their father's given name, ending in "son." In contemporary Western society as well, there are systems of naming. The most common one in the dominant culture in the United States is a patrilineal succession plus one or more given names. In the United States, the middle name is often one that relates to the family, such as the mother's maiden name.

The Russian system of naming provides a clue to the significance placed on relating son and father, as well as daughter and father. The mother is left out, with Russians habitually addressing each other by the individual's given name together with the patronymic. The family name is omitted. Spaniards and Latin Americans include women more than other cultures, with children carrying their father's name first and their mother's name second. The mother's name usually appears only on documents and for formal occasions because the addition of the mother's name makes the name quite long. Another variation is seen in the Dutch, who have the option of using both the husband's and the wife's family names jointly. Among the various cultures, the most common theme of naming is pride in lineage (Clemmens, 1985, 1988).

Grammatical Structure. Cultural differences are reflected in grammatical structure and the use and meaning of phrases. "That's all right" is a phrase frequently used by African-Americans when they actually mean "I have some plans, but I am not telling you what they are" (Mitchell, 1978). In another example, for some Hispanic-American women, having a stillborn baby or a miscarriage does not equate with a pregnancy—rather, pregnancy is equated only with a successful live birth (Haffner, 1992). It is important for nurses to keep in mind that there is little validity in generalizations about the meaning of phrases by persons in varying cultures.

Length of sentence and speech forms may vary not only with culture but also with social class. For example, Argyle (1992) noted that persons from the lower class commonly use short, simple sentences and are more direct than are persons with more education. Word choice, grammatical structure, speech fluency, and articulation provide cues to social status and class. Jargon is also a speech variation that may prove to be a barrier to communication. Nurses frequently have difficulty expressing things in simple, jargon-free language (without medical terms) that clients can understand. On the other hand, a nurse who does not know the jargon used by the clients served may have a difficult time relating to them.

For some cultures, patterns of social amenities can create communication problems. Small talk, social chit-chat, and discussion of mundane topics that may appear to "kill time" are sometimes necessary as preliminaries for more purposeful discussion. Yet the busy nurse seeking short, succinct answers to questions may be annoyed by the amount of anecdotal information that a Hispanic-American client, for example, gives. Many clients tend to add irrelevant material because it lessens embarrassment. They may be more comfortable if attention is not focused on their medical problems, and so they may intersperse actual symptoms with other biographical data. Cultural factors may also play a role in what seems to be verbal rambling. Patients who are used to folk healers believe that information on the weather, the environment, and eating habits are really important pieces of information for the health professional.

Voice Qualities. *Paralinguistics,* or *paralanguage,* refers to something beyond the words themselves. Voice quality, which includes pitch and range, can add an important element to communication. The commonly used phrase "Don't speak to me in that tone of voice" indicates the significance of this aspect of the communication message.

The softer volume of Asian-American or American-Indian speech may be interpreted by the nurse as shyness. On the other hand, the nurse's behavior may be viewed as loud and boisterous if the volume is loud and if there is a deliberate attempt to accent particular words. Sometimes people who speak softly, slowly, and without emphasis on particular words are viewed as wishy-washy. When the nurse cannot hear what the client is saying, there is a tendency for the nurse to speak louder. It is important to remember that amplifying the volume does not necessarily equate with being understood or understanding. Nurses must remember when they are assessing the client that paralinguistic behavior is an important cultural consideration. The nurse can recognize this behavior by listening to tone of voice, quality of voice, and nonword vocalizations, such as sobbing, laughing, and grunting.

Intonation. Intonation is an important aspect of the communication message. When people say they feel "fine," they may mean they genuinely do or they may mean they do not feel fine but do not wish to discuss it. If said sarcastically, it may also mean they feel just the opposite of fine. There is often a latent or hidden meaning in what a person is saying, and intonation frequently provides the clue that is needed to interpret the true message.

Techniques of intonation vary among cultures. For example, Americans put commands in the form of suggestions and often as questions, whereas Arabic speech contains much emphasis and exaggeration (Argyle, 1992). Some cultures value indirectness and subtlety in speech and may be alienated by the frankness of Western health care professionals. Asian clients, for example, may interpret this method of communication as rude, immature, and lacking finesse. On the other hand, health care professionals may label Asian clients as evasive, fearful, and unable to confront problems (Sue & Sue, 1999).

Rhythm. Rhythm also varies from culture to culture; some people have a melodic rhythm to their verbal communication, whereas others appear to lack rhythm. Rhythm may also vary among persons within a culture. For example, some African-American ministers use a singsong rhythm to deliver fiery sermons.

Speed. The rate and volume of speech frequently provide a clue to an individual's mood. A depressed person will tend to talk slowly and quietly, whereas an aggressive, dominating person is more apt to talk rapidly and loudly.

Pronunciation. Persons from some cultural groups may be identified by their dialect, such as Black dialect or Black English, Irish brogue, or a Brooklyn accent. Black English includes words and expressions not commonly found in Standard English and is sometimes spoken by African-Americans. It ranges on a continuum from being more to less Africanized, with the mild end of the continuum being much like Standard English (Taylor, 1976). However, even persons with dialects at the mild end of the continuum may have a "Black sound" that identifies them as African-American. A person may hear a boil called a "raisin" or difficult breathing called "the smothers" (Snow, 1976); dentures may be called "racks" (Dillard, 1973). Some African-Americans speak in dialect when they do not want others to understand what is being said. One function of the Black dialect may be to enhance the in-group solidarity of African-Americans (Taylor, 1976).

Utterances of "ahs," "ers," and grunts also provide important dimensions to communication. Although hesitations may indicate a person who is unsure and slow to make a commitment, for some cultures this can have the opposite meaning.

Silence. The meaning of silence varies among cultural groups. Silences may be thoughtful, or they may be blank and empty when the individual has nothing to say. A silence in a conversation may also indicate stubbornness and resistance, apprehension, or discomfort. Silence may be viewed by some cultural groups as extremely uncomfortable; therefore, attempts may be made to fill every gap with conversation. Persons in other cultural groups value silence and see it as essential to understanding a person's needs. Many American Indians have this latter view of silence, as do some traditional Chinese and Japanese persons. Therefore, when one of these persons is speaking and suddenly stops, what may be implied is that the person wants the nurse to consider the content of what has been said before continuing. Other cultures may use silence in yet other ways. For example, English and Arabic persons use silence for privacy, whereas Russian, French, and Spanish persons may use silence to indicate agreement between parties. Some persons in Asian cultures may view silence as a sign of respect, particularly toward an elder. Mexicans may use silence when instructions are given by a person in authority rather than showing the disrespect of disagreement (Quarnero, 2005).

Nurses need to be aware of possible meanings of silence so that personal anxiety does not promote the silence to be interrupted prematurely or to be nontherapeutic. A nurse who understands the therapeutic value of silence can use this understanding to enhance the care of clients from other cultures.

Nonverbal Communication

Hall (1966) suggested that 65% of the message received in communication is nonverbal. Through body language or motions (kinetic behavior), the person conveys what cannot or may not be said in words. For a message to be accurately interpreted, not only must words be translated but also the meaning held by nuances, intonation patterns, and facial expressions. Just as verbal behavior may undo nonverbal behavior, nonverbal behavior may repeat, clarify, contradict, modify, emphasize, or regulate the flow of communication. Nonverbal behavior is less significant as an isolated behavior, but it does add to the whole communication message. To understand the client, the nurse may wish to validate impressions with other health team members, since different people often interpret nonverbal behavior differently. It is important for the nurse to be aware not only of the client's nonverbal behavior but also of personal nonverbal behavior that may add to, undo, or contradict verbal communication (Reusch, 1961).

Touch. Touch, or tactile sensation, is a powerful form of communication that can be used to bridge distances between nurse and client (Bronstein, 1996; Davidhizar & Giger, 1988; Giger, Davidhizar, & Wieczorek, 1993). Touch has many meanings (Box 2-3). It can connect people, provide affirmation, be reassuring, decrease loneliness, share warmth, provide stimulation, and increase self-concept. Being touched can be highly valued and sought after. On the other hand, touch can also communicate frustration, anger, aggression, and punishment; invade personal space and privacy; and convey a negative (such as a subservient) type of relationship. In certain situations touch can be disconcerting because it signals power. In a study reported by Thayer (1988), higher status individuals were found to enjoy more liberties concerning touch than their lower status associates. It is generally considered improper for individuals to put their hands on superiors.

Touching or lack of touch has cultural significance and symbolism and is a learned behavior. Cultural uses of touch vary. Each culture trains its children to develop different kinds of thresholds to tactile contacts and stimulation so that their organic, constitutional, and temperamental characteristics are accentuated or reduced. Some cultures are characterized by a "do not touch me" way of life. These persons may view fondling and kissing as embarrassing. Some cultures include every possible variation on the theme of tactility. In the United States, the dominant culture generally tolerates hugs and embraces among

---

BOX 2-3   Meanings of Touch

Touch may:
1. Connect one individual with another, both literally and figuratively, by indicating availability.
2. Provide affirmation and approval.
3. Be reassuring by providing empathy, interest, encouragement, nurturance, caring, trust, concern, gentleness, and protection.
4. Decrease loneliness by indicating a relationship with another.
5. Share warmth, rapport, love, intimacy, excitement, and happiness.
6. Provide stimulation by being a mode of sensation, perception, and experience.
7. Increase self-concept.
8. Communicate frustration, anger, aggression, or punishment.
9. Invade personal space and privacy by physical and psychological assault or intrusion.
10. Convey a negative type of relationship with another.
11. Cause sexual arousal.
12. Allow a person to perform a functional or professional role, such as a physician, barber, or tailor, and be devoid of personal message.
13. Reflect cordiality, such as a handshake by business associates and among strangers and acquaintances.

---

intimates and a pat on the shoulder as a gesture of camaraderie. The firm, hearty handshake is symbolic of good character and a sign of strength. In some American-Indian groups, however, the hand is offered in some interpersonal interactions, but the expectation is different. Rather than a firm handshake, there is a light touch or grasp or even just a passing of hands. Some American Indians interpret vigorous handshaking as an aggressive action and are offended by a firm, lengthy handshake (Montagu, 1986).

Americans often give a lingering touch a sexual connotation. For some Americans, even casual touching is considered taboo and may be a result of residual Victorian sexual prudence (DeThomaso, 1971). Other cultures also consider touching taboo; the English and Germans carry untouchability further than Americans do. On the other hand, highly tactile cultures do exist, such as the Spanish, Italians, French, Jews, and South Americans (Montagu, 1986). However, generalizations about diverse national or ethnic groups in the area of touch can be problematic. For example, Shuter (1976) reported on studies of touch in Costa Rica, Colombia, and Panama. Findings from this study indicate that Latin Americans are commonly oriented toward high contact. Thayer (1988) also compared couples in Costa Rica, Colombia, and Panama and found that partners in Costa Rica were touched and held more often than partners in the other two countries.

Most cultures give touch different rules and meanings depending on the sex of the persons involved. Whitcher and Fisher (1979) reported that women in a hospital study had a strikingly positive reaction to being touched, with subsequent lowered blood pressure and anxiety before surgery, whereas men found the same experience upsetting, with a subsequent increase in blood pressure and anxiety. Thayer (1988) reported on a study at the Kansas City International Airport that found women greeted women and men more physically, with lip kisses, embraces, and more kinds of touch and holding and for longer periods than did men. For men, a more common greeting was to shake hands. Regardless of sex, some research has shown that people who are most uncomfortable with touch are also uncomfortable with communicating through other means and have lower self-esteem (Thayer, 1988). Other studies have shown that people who touch more are less afraid and suspicious of other people's motives and intentions and have less anxiety and tension in their everyday lives. In some cultures, leaning back, showing the palm of the hand, and fussing with the other person's collar may be perceived as possible courting behaviors because they may convey an invitation for closeness or affiliation. Touching behaviors such as reaching out during conversation to poke the other person in the chest may be viewed as domineering behavior. However, laughing while being poked may be a way to submit to and at the same time trivialize or eliminate the other person's aggressive intent (Scheflen & Scheflen, 1972).

In some cultures touch is considered magical and healing (Mackey, 1995). For example, some Mexican Americans and American Indians view touch as symbolic of "undoing" an evil spell, as a means for prevention of harm, or as a means for healing (Montagu, 1986). On the other hand, Vietnamese Americans may find touching shoulders with another to be anxiety producing, since they believe that the soul can leave the body on physical contact and that health problems may result (Rocereto, 1981). The Vietnamese regard the human head as the seat of life and therefore highly personal. Procedures that invade the surface or any orifice of the head can frighten the Vietnamese, who fear that these procedures could provide an escape for the essence of life (Stauffer, 2005).

Nurses must be alert to the rules of touch for individuals encountered in the work role. Lane (1989) found that nurses perceive male clients as being less receptive to touch and closeness than their female counterparts, which could be attributed to the fact that males generally have a larger personal space than females. Thus it is believed that people generally maintain a greater distance from males (Insel & Lindgren, 1978; Sommer, 1959). Lane (1989) concluded that there may be a double standard concerning touch because of societal norms and expectations: male clients may be more receptive to touch than are female nurses, but female nurses are perhaps more comfortable with the closeness and touch of female clients.

Although the rules of touch may be unspoken and unwritten, they are usually visible to the observer. A nurse should stay within the rules of touch that are culturally prescribed. It is essential that the nurse uses touch judiciously and avoids forcing touch on anyone. Nurses must keep in mind that the message conveyed through touch depends on the attitude of the other person involved and on the meaning of touch both to the person touching and to the person being touched. Generally, the need for intimacy and touch is so strong that the satisfaction of that need is a greater influence on behavior than fears about its inappropriateness (Johnson, 1965). A momentary and seemingly incidental touch can establish a positive, temporary bond between strangers, making them more compliant, helpful, positive, and giving. In all cases, touch needs to be applied deliberately, with empathy, and with close attention to the person's particular needs. All cultural groups have rules, often unspoken, about who touches whom, when, and where. To avoid being perceived as intrusive, the astute nurse must be mindful of the client's reaction to touch.

Facial Expression. Facial expression is commonly used as a guide to a person's feelings. Research shows that generally, in Americans, facial expression is used as a part of the communication message. A constant stare with immobile facial muscles indicates coldness. During fear, the eyes open wide, the eyebrows rise, and the mouth becomes tense with the lips drawn back. When a person is angry, the eyes become fixed in a hard stare with the upper lids lowered and the eyebrows drawn down. An angry person's lips are often tightly compressed. Eyes rolled upward may be related to tiredness or may show disapproval. Narrowed eyes, a curled upper lip, and a moving nose commonly signal disgust. A person who is embarrassed or self-conscious may turn the eyes away or down; have a flushed face; pretend to smile; rub the eyes, nose, or face; or twitch the hair, beard, or mustache. A direct gaze with raised eyebrows shows surprise (Ekman & Friesen, 1975; Polhemus, 1978).

Facial expression also varies with culture. Italian, Jewish, African-American, and Hispanic persons smile readily and use many facial expressions, along with gestures and words, to communicate feelings of happiness, pain, or displeasure. Irish, English, and northern European persons tend to have less facial expression and are generally less responsive, especially to strangers. Facial expression can also be used to convey an opposite meaning of the one that is felt; for example, in Asia negative emotions may be concealed with a smile (Sue & Sue, 2003).

Eye Movement. Research on eye movement has vastly increased as a result of the development of computer-based data collection and analysis routines. Recording techniques for eye movements provide a vast array of data to the researcher (Grainger, 1992; Rayner, 1992; Shapiro, 1991).

Eye movement is an important aspect of interpersonal communication. Generally, during social interaction, most people look each other in the eye for short periods (Argyle & Dean, 1965; Davidhizar, 1988a). People use more eye contact while they are listening and may use glances of about 3 to 10 seconds. When glances are longer than this, anxiety is aroused.

Eye contact is an important tool in transcultural nursing assessment and is used both for observation and to initiate interaction. In the United States, those of the dominant culture (predominantly Whites) value eye contact as symbolic of a positive self-concept, openness, interest in others, attentiveness, and honesty. Eye contact can communicate warmth and bridge interpersonal gaps between people. A nurse who wears glasses and wants to make a point may increase the intensity of eye contact by taking off the glasses. The removal of glasses has also been cited as a technique that can humanize an individual's face, since barriers to eye contact are removed (Giger & Davidhizar, 1990b).

Lack of eye contact may be interpreted as a sign of shyness, lack of interest, subordination, humility, guilt, embarrassment, low self-esteem, rudeness, thoughtfulness, or dishonesty. In social interaction the speaker glances away from the listener to indicate collecting of thoughts or planning of what is to be said. If contact is not resumed, lack of interest may be interpreted. Pupil dilation and constriction can also be a clue to anxiety level and positive response (Hess, 1965, 1975).

Most Mexican-American and African-American clients are comfortable with eye contact (Guruge & Donner, 1996; Murray & Huelskoetter, 1991). In contrast to this view, others have suggested that through a process of socialization in a "minority status" of relative powerlessness, some African-Americans have learned to deliberately avoid eye contact with others (Giger, Davidhizar, Evers, & Ingram, 1994). In fact, in the United States avoidance of eye contact is sometimes considered rude, an indication of lack of attention, or a sign of mental illness (Bigham, 1964; Paynich, 1964). On the other hand, McKenzie and Chrisman (1977) reported that, for some Filipinos, eye contact that turns away is associated with the possibility of being a

witch. Other groups who find eye contact difficult include some Asian people and some American Indians, who relate eye contact to impoliteness and an invasion of privacy. Many American Indians regard eye contact as disrespectful because it is believed that "looking in an individual's eyes" is "looking into an individual's soul" (Galanti, 2003; Giger & Davidhizar, 2001; Henderson & Primeaux, 1981; Poole, Davidhizar, & Giger, 2003).

Persons in certain Indian cultures avoid eye contact with persons of a higher or lower socioeconomic class. The Vietnamese generally practice less eye contact (Rocereto, 1981), and prolonged eye contact is also avoided by some African-Americans (Giger & Davidhizar, 1990b). In some Indian cultures eye contact is given a special sexual significance. Some Orthodox Jews also attribute a sexual significance to eye contact by an elderly man with a woman other than his wife (Sue & Sue, 1999). Some Appalachian people tend to avert their eyes because for them eye contact is related to hostility and aggressiveness (Tripp-Reimer & Friedl, 1977). Certain cultures place more focus on the eyes than others; for example, in India and Greece the use of the eyes is all important (Eibl-Eibesfelt, 1972).

Body Posture. Communication is also affected by body posture. A nurse can bridge distance in an interaction by placing the forearms on the table, palms up. In Western culture, palms up can send a message of acquiescence even while disagreeing. However, the nurse should also recognize that palms up in other cultures may have a sexual implication. Therefore, the decision to use this gesture should be weighed carefully.

Body posture can provide important messages about receptivity. In some Western cultures, such as among Whites in the United States, the closer a listener's overall posturing matches the posture of the speaker, the higher the likelihood of receptivity. If the individuals' unconscious gestures differ, probably their perspective on the matter at hand is also different. Matching body movements to those of another person can communicate a sense of solidarity, even if solidarity is not present. Body posture can also communicate attitude toward a person. For example, within the dominant culture of Whites in the United States, an attentive posture is indicated by leaning toward a person. Attentive posture is used toward people of higher stature and toward people who are liked (Mehrabian, 1968, 1981). An American man may indicate sexual attraction by placing his arms in front of his body with his legs closed. An American woman, on the other hand, indicates attraction by a more open posture, that is, arms down at the side (Hall, 1966). Physical pain is communicated by rigid muscles, flexed body, and cautious movements. Argyle, Salter, Nicholson, Williams, and Burgess (1970) reported that in England dominance is communicated when the dominant person stands or sits more erectly than the compliant or submissive person. Knowledge of sociocultural heritage is essential in interpreting body language, since various body parts are used differently in different cultures.

Communications That Combine Verbal and Nonverbal Elements

Many interpersonal communications combine both verbal and nonverbal elements. Warmth and humor are two of these.

Warmth. Warmth is a quality or state that promotes feelings of friendship, well-being, or pleasure. Warmth can be communicated verbally ("You really lay still during the procedure, and that helped us to do it as quickly as possible") and may also be communicated nonverbally, as by a pat on the shoulder or a gentle smile.

Although warmth is also a matter of perception, communication that focuses on human needs is more likely to be related to warmth in the speaker. Statements that show respect, address the human need to be needed, and promote self-acceptance will usually be interpreted positively and can increase motivation, morale, and cooperation. Personal recognition and concern also communicate warmth. Verbal recognition (for example, a hello on meeting) or a statement of genuine concern (for example, "How are you feeling?") can convey interest and may facilitate a positive relationship between client and family and the nurse (Davidhizar, 1989).

The nurse's communication of warmth is an important and dynamic aspect of a therapeutic nurse–client relationship. If the client is from another culture and is having difficulty with understanding communication, the nurse's warmth may be vital to promoting a positive relationship. Graham-Dickerson (1996) suggests that the healing process is promoted by the interrelation between the nurse and the client and that without this relationship the client from another culture may not be engaged in the healing process.

Humor. Humor is a powerful component of verbal and nonverbal communication. Humor can create a bond of shared pleasure between people, decrease anxiety and tension, build relationships, promote problem solving and learning, provide motivation, and enable personal survival. As a healthy and constructive coping mechanism, humor can provide a discharge for aggressive feelings in a more or less acceptable way and can enable management of stressful situations (Davidhizar, 1988b). Humor that is therapeutic does not ridicule and rarely uses cynicism (Huckaby, 1987). Personality, culture, background, and levels of stress and pain may influence reactions to humor. When people are

from a different culture, humor must be used in a limited and deliberate manner since humor can be an obstacle to a relationship if it is misunderstood. The nurse must carefully assess the individual client and the situation to decide if humor is appropriate. Humor not only can improve communication when used appropriately but may also affect the immune system by promoting the body's ability to combat such problems as cancer and diseases of the connective tissue, such as arthritis and lupus (Simonton, Simonton, & Creighton, 1978).

When the individual spoken with does not have a full grasp of the language and the nuances and puns that are often involved in humor, jokes and statements meant humorously may not be understood or may be misinterpreted. It is also important for an individual who tries to speak in another language to be prepared to precipitate laughter. A statement meant to be serious may be perceived as comical. The ability to laugh at oneself and with others can ease the anxiety that may be present in an intercultural situation.

IMPLICATIONS FOR NURSING CARE

Guidelines for Relating to Patients from Different Cultures

Nurses commonly relate to clients in an interview setting. The nurse may also relate during the process of client care or at a more informal level on the hospital unit or in the clinic. Although cultural issues may cause the client to interpret the nurse's behavior from a unique perspective, adherence to the following guidelines will increase the likelihood that the nurse–client relationship will be positive (Box 2-4).

1. Assess Personal Beliefs of Persons from Different Cultures. Awareness of the nurse's personal beliefs is vital in relating to clients from diverse cultural backgrounds (Boone, 2005). A nurse working with a client from another background should carefully review personal beliefs and experiences to determine conscious and unconscious attitudes. It is important for the nurse to set aside personal values, biases, ideas, and attitudes that are judgmental and may negatively affect care. The nurse can learn to control personal reactions by a broadened understanding of others' beliefs and behaviors (Winans-Orr & McIntosh, 1996). Leininger and McFarland (2006) contend that there is a major crisis in nursing in that most nurses are unprepared to function effectively with migrants and cultural strangers. Understanding of other cultures can be enhanced through immersion in another culture. In addition, use of cultural assessment tools provides a method to assess personal attitude (Anthony, 1997).

BOX 2-4 Guidelines for Relating to Patients from Different Cultures

1. Assess your personal beliefs surrounding persons from different cultures. Review your personal beliefs and experiences.
   - Set aside any values, biases, ideas, and attitudes that are judgmental and may negatively affect care.
2. Assess communication variables from a cultural perspective. Determine the ethnic identity of the patient, including generations in the United States.
   - Use the patient as a source of information when possible.
   - Assess cultural factors that may affect your relationship with the patient and respond appropriately.
3. Plan care according to the communicated needs and cultural background. Learn as much as possible about the patient's cultural customs and beliefs.
   - Encourage the patient to reveal cultural interpretation of health, illness, and health care.
   - Be sensitive to the uniqueness of the patient.
   - Identify sources of discrepancy between the patient's and your own concepts of health and illness.
   - Communicate at the patient's personal level of functioning.
   - Evaluate effectiveness of nursing actions and modify nursing care plan when necessary.
4. Modify communication approaches to meet cultural needs. Be attentive to signs of fear, anxiety, and confusion in the patient.
   - Respond in a reassuring manner in keeping with the patient's cultural orientation.
   - Be aware that in some cultural groups discussion with others concerning the patient may be offensive and impede the nursing process.
5. Understand that respect for the patient and communicated needs is central to the therapeutic relationship. Communicate respect by using a kind and attentive approach.
   - Learn how listening is communicated in the patient's culture.
   - Use appropriate active listening techniques.
   - Adopt an attitude of flexibility, respect, and interest to help bridge barriers imposed by culture.
6. Communicate in a nonthreatening manner. Conduct the interview in an unhurried manner.
   - Follow acceptable social and cultural amenities.
   - Ask general questions during the information-gathering stage.
   - Be patient with a respondent who gives information that may seem unrelated to the patient's health problem.
   - Develop a trusting relationship by listening carefully, allowing time, and giving the patient your full attention.
7. Use validating techniques in communication. Be alert for feedback that the patient is not understanding.
   - Do not assume meaning is interpreted without distortion.
8. Be considerate of reluctance to talk when the subject involves sexual matters. Be aware that in some cultures sexual matters are not discussed freely with members of the opposite sex.
9. Adopt special approaches when the patient speaks a different language. Use a caring tone of voice and facial expression to help alleviate the patient's fears.
   - Speak slowly and distinctly but not loudly.
   - Use gestures, pictures, and play acting to help the patient understand.
   - Repeat the message in different ways if necessary.
   - Be alert to words the patient seems to understand and use them frequently.
   - Keep messages simple and repeat them frequently.
   - Avoid using medical terms and abbreviations that the patient may not understand.
   - Use an appropriate language dictionary.
10. Use interpreters to improve communication. Ask the interpreter to translate the message, not just the individual words.
   - Obtain feedback to confirm understanding.
   - Use an interpreter who is culturally sensitive.

2. Assess Communication Variables from a Cultural Perspective. To communicate with a client from another culture, it is essential to assess each client from a cultural perspective. Oxendine (2000) reports a health education project in which Zuni, Pueblo, Hopi, and Navajo women showed no interest in breast cancer brochures with pictures of breasts on the cover. The women said they found the pictures of breasts unsuitable and wanted the term *breast health* rather than *breast cancer* used. When a contest was held to pick new cover art for the brochure, 120 American-Indian artists entered. Carneiro (2000) describes a health education program for a Hispanic Latino community in which a video featured a slim, blond, blue-eyed model who did not look at all Latino. The educators did not appreciate that in the Latino communities, being chubby is viewed by some as being healthier and that some Latino parents still associate a skinny baby with not having enough money to feed the child. The nurse must also assess whether the individual is from a culture in which priority is given to context versus content since this will influence communication style (Goldman & Schmalz, 2005; Xu & Davidhizar, 2005). The cultural phenomenon of communication cannot be minimized when providing culturally appropriate nursing care. The nurse who understands differences in communication variables can attempt to transcend communication barriers to provide high-quality client care.

It is important to realize that cultural assessment does not require information on every aspect of a specific culture. However, data should elicit ethnic identity, including generation in the United States (that is, first or second generation); the beliefs of a first-generation immigrant, regardless of ethnic heritage, may differ from those of a second-generation person. Whenever possible, the client should be used as the primary informant, since others, even though close to the client, may have different ideas and beliefs.

After a careful assessment of cultural factors that may enter into a relationship, the nurse must respond appropriately. For example, for African-Americans and Mexican Americans who tend to value eye contact, it is important for the nurse to use this practice (Kendall, 1996). On the other hand, when relating to Filipino Americans who are afraid of eye contact, the nurse should avoid eye contact. When relating to Southeast Asians, it is important to remember that persons from this cultural background usually are very formal in their language. It is essential that courtesy be shown by use of the family name or a title until one is given permission to address the client by a given name. Asians also use an indirect approach to obtaining information, so direct questions are not received well; such questions are considered rude, and the interviewer is not likely to receive the information sought (Hagen, 1988; Mattson, 1995). If communication is to be effective in today's multicultural society, relating in a culturally sensitive manner is essential (Campinha-Bacote, 1995).

3. Plan Care Based on the Communicated Needs and Cultural Background.
Care for persons from other cultures must be consistent with the client's lifestyle and unique needs that have been communicated by the client to the nurse and mutually agreed on (Geissler, 1991; Grossman, 1996). To establish an appropriate plan, it is essential to improve personal knowledge about the customs and beliefs of the culture of the clients receiving care. The

nurse should encourage the client to communicate interpretations of health, illness, and health care since culture influences what are considered appropriate approaches to health, wellness, illness, and death (Sieh & Brentin, 1997). A client's perception of illness will affect not only communication but also the care that is planned. Sensitivity to the uniqueness of each client is required if the nurse is to work effectively, particularly with clients from different cultures. This sensitivity can be gained only through appropriate communication techniques. In addition, nurses who cannot communicate and correctly interpret cultural behavior will feel inadequate and helpless and quickly experience stress and burnout (Scholz, 1990). It is important to remember that the best teacher in learning about culture is people themselves. Individuals must be communicated with at their personal level of functioning. Values and beliefs of persons from different cultures may affect the way care is delivered. Many cultures have similar idiosyncrasies that must be considered. Finally, it is important to evaluate the effectiveness of nursing actions with clients from diverse culture groups. It may be necessary to modify the plan of care to provide an effective intervention based on communicated needs.

4. Modify Communication Approaches to Meet Cultural Needs.
A factor that commonly interferes with care delivery to a person from another culture is confusion and fear about the treatment process. The nurse must be attentive to signs of anxiety and respond in a reassuring manner in keeping with the client's cultural orientation. When English is the client's second language, the nurse should be alert to the fact that meanings of words and how facts are presented may vary according to the family and culture of origin (Davidhizar & Brownson, 2000).

Some cultures are primarily oral and do not rely on a written form of communication. In such a society, the spoken word holds greater meaning and power. For example, Hmong are considered an oral cultural group. For these individuals, the formation of and acceptance in a social group is primarily dependent on the spoken word (Shadick, 1993). When interacting with individuals from an oral culture, the nurse must remember that if the teaching–learning process is to be effective, instruction must be oral.

Some Muslim sects do not believe in prevention and thus are unwilling to perform the most basic health intervention and promotion activities. Taking active measures to prevent disease is thought to go against the wishes of Allah (Carneiro, 2000; Davidhizar & Giger, 2002). The nurse must appreciate the impact of this cultural belief on health behavior in order to think of communication strategies to respond to health needs.

5. Understand That Respect for the Client and Communicated Needs Is Central to the Therapeutic Relationship.
The need to communicate respect for the client is a nursing concept that crosses all cultural boundaries and conserves use of resources (Purnell, 2001). Regardless of the language spoken or the cultural orientation, the nurse whose approach focuses on individuals and their emotional and physical needs increases communication and reduces interpersonal distance. Communication of respect is central to a focus on emotional needs. Respect for clients is communicated by a kind and attentive approach in which the client is heard. Active listening techniques are used, such as encouraging clients to share thoughts and feelings by reflecting back what has been heard. The nurse should be attentive to how listening is communicated in the client's culture. For example, for some persons, listening may be indicated by eye contact, whereas for others listening may mean having the listener turn a listening "ear." Predictions about what the client is trying to express may be made to encourage elaboration. At the heart of the task of hearing is the art of listening (Martin, 1995). Listening communicates genuine interest and caring. The feeling of being heard is powerful, reducing distance and drawing people together into positive interpersonal interactions. An attitude of flexibility, respect, and interest can bridge the artificial barriers of distance imposed by culture and role.

6. Communicate in a Nonthreatening Manner.
The interview should be started in an unhurried manner, with adherence to acceptable social and cultural amenities. It is usually wise to start with general social topics and to make some connection with the individual before asking questions (Wissing, 2000). Being aware of and using cultural information provides a valuable base from which to proceed (Sieh & Brentin, 1997). During the information-gathering stage, general rather than specific questions should be asked. The interviewer should allow time for the respondent to give what appears to be unrelated information. For many persons a direct approach appears rude and uncaring. For example, persons of European background and Hispanic individuals often value "small talk" and will not relate optimally to the nurse who talks only about illness-related matters. Many persons, specifically Asian and Spanish-speaking persons, respond better to a nondirective approach with open-ended questions than to direct questions (Giger & Davidhizar, 1990b). Storytelling (Evans & Severtsen, 2001), photography (Killion, 2001), and literature (Barton & Richardson, 1998; Studer, 2002) can provide important information to assist in understanding individuals and their cultural orientation.

7. Use Strategies to Develop Trust.
When personal matters are discussed, it is important to allow time for the development of a relationship. In a significant book on cultural perspective, *The Spirit Catches You and You Fall Down,* Fadiman (1997) provides an example of a health care worker visiting a pregnant Hmong woman with tuberculosis who was refusing her medication. The interpreter stopped the caregiver from starting on this topic but rather started the conversation by wishing the patient's family well and initiating conversation with the husband. Once friendly contact had been established, the social worker inquired as to why the wife was not taking medications and was told that they feared that the baby would be born without arms and legs. When this misunderstanding was corrected, she took her medication. It is essential to first communicate a positive attitude in order to promote trust and confidence if collaboration about health care needs is to occur (Jenkins & Fallowfield, 2000). The appearances of being too busy, of not having time to listen, of not giving sufficient time for an answer, and of not really wanting to hear are equally effective in cutting off the client. Research has demonstrated that racial and ethnic minorities have lower levels of trust in health care providers than do White Americans (Satcher & Pamies, 2006). For example, LaVeist, Nickerson, and Bowie (2000) reported that African-Americans were more likely to perceive racism in the health care system and report distrust.

When working with persons from diverse cultural backgrounds, the astute nurse must recognize that the communication process may be impeded by hesitancy to speak to Westerners about health concerns. Some American Indians are becoming more confident and willing to speak out about their personal needs. Hagey and Buller (1983) noted that the Ojibway people traditionally avoided direct oral questioning by health care workers and viewed it as a violation of dignity and thus inappropriate. Such questions could be met with complete silence and meaningless answers (in response to a question, it would be entirely acceptable for an answer to be given in a few days or weeks). It is critical that the nurse serve as a client advocate to provide culturally sensitive care. It is also essential that the nurse learn to appreciate a value held by some Ojibway that espouses deep-rooted ideals of noninterference, which may be found among some Native and ethnic groups (Grypma, 1993; Reimer & Redskye, 1998). Regardless of cultural background, listening is one of the most effective therapeutic techniques (Potter & Perry, 2005).

8. Use Validating Techniques in Communication.
Although validating techniques are always important, they are especially important when the client is from a different culture. The nurse should be alert for feedback that the

client is not understanding and should use restating and validating techniques, such as "Did I hear and understand you correctly?" When the nurse has difficulty understanding, it may help to find out precisely what the topic is, such as "Are you telling me where you're having pain?" By determining the topic, the number of words can be decreased. If the message is not understood—people usually know when they are understood—it may be helpful to have the client try to convey the message in another way, such as through pointing or imitation. The nurse should never pretend to understand a message; in doing so, the nurse conveys that the message is not really important (Pore, 1995).

9. Be Considerate of Reluctance to Talk When the Subject Involves Sexual Matters.
Hispanic and Indian clients, who tend to be hesitant to talk about sexually related matters, may talk more freely to a nurse of the same sex. When talking about sexual matters with a male child from certain cultures (such as Spanish, Pakistani, or Arabic), it is important to have the father rather than the mother present.

10. Adopt Special Approaches When the Client Speaks a Different Language.
A client who enters the health care system without being able to speak the dominant language of the caregivers enters a frightening and frustrating world. This may also be true for clients whose first language differs from that of the nurse (Davidhizar et al., 2002). The nurse should keep in mind that for clients who cannot speak the language of the professionals encountered, basic procedures such as registering at the emergency desk or for a diagnostic procedure may be very anxiety producing. Clients who do not understand are more likely to be hostile and belligerent, to be uncooperative, or to withdraw (Spector, 2004).

The nurse should be alert for the client who pretends to understand to please the caregiver and gain acceptance. This patient will usually say yes to all questions. Without the availability of words, the nurse must relate to a client at an affective level. A tone and facial expression of caring can be vital in alleviating a client's fear.

If an interpreter is not available and the client seems to have some understanding of the language, speaking slowly and distinctly, using a lot of gestures, acting out, using pictures, and repeating the message several times in different ways may enable the client to understand what is being said. The nurse should be alert for words that the client seems to understand so that these words can be used more frequently. Messages should be kept simple and stated sentence by sentence, not paragraph by paragraph. Clients who appear to be having difficulty understanding should be asked to provide feedback on what they have heard to provide an opportunity for further clarification.

It is especially necessary to avoid using medical terms and jargon when speaking to a client with only a partial understanding of the language. Abbreviations such as *TPR* and *BP* should be avoided. An individual usually first understands standard words and picks up slang expressions and professional terms at a much later stage of language acquisition.

The nurse should select a dictionary that has both the language the nurse speaks and the language the client speaks, such as a Spanish–English, English–Spanish dictionary. In addition, standard nursing references, such as *Taber's Cyclopedic Medical Dictionary* (Venes, 2009) and *Mosby's Dictionary of Medicine, Nursing, and Health Professions* (2012), have sections that give common medical statements and questions in several languages. Nursing textbooks are increasingly adding sections related to speaking to non–English-speaking clients. In addition to assessing how much English a client knows, it is important to assess whether the client can read English or is literate in the language spoken so that appropriate printed information on the agency, consent forms, and health information can be obtained. With online technology, multilingual and even age-specific communication can automatically occur, making health care and prescription drug information available in whatever language is selected (Giorgianni, 2000). However, as Mika, Kelly, Price, Franquiz, and Villarreal (2005) note, a significant portion of the U.S. population has serious problems with both literacy and understanding how to effectively use health-related information. An adult literacy survey found that 45% of the adult population in the United States had limited literacy skills (Kirsch, Jungeblut, Jenkins, & Kolstad, 1993). A more recent survey of adult literacy skills suggested that while the number of those considered to have limited literacy skills had dropped dramatically to approximately 23% of the adult U.S. population, even this percentage represented a higher number of adults with limited literacy for a highly technological society like the United States (Guy, 2005). The cultural orientation of the client also affects such factors as assignment of caregivers. For example, for conservative Arab, Afghan, or other Muslim clients, females giving instructions to males may not be effective (Davidhizar & Giger, 2002). If a male nurse is providing services to a female Arab client, strict rules require that a family member always be present. Older Arab clients may not comply with direct instructions given by a young staff member; with these clients, indirect requests and suggestions are the desired methods (Nellum-Davis, 2002; Wilson, 1996).

11. Use Interpreters to Improve Communication.
When the client and nurse do not speak the same language, an interpreter must be obtained. When a medical interpreter

is not available, a family member may be used. However, use of a child should be avoided since a child may not adequately understand or explain technical information (Davidhizar & Brownson, 2000). The nurse should evaluate whether having a family member interpret is satisfactory to the client because some clients may not be willing to confide certain information to a family member (Clark, 1995). Hallenbeck (2004) notes that if a family member serves as translator, family values such as not talking openly about cancer or death may affect the translation. The interpreter should be able to translate not only the literal meaning of the words but also the nonverbal messages that accompany the communication. Interpreters who act out their message through intonation, facial expression, or gestures are more likely to be effective in getting the message across. Even when every effort is made to ensure effective interpretation, neither the nurse nor the interpreter can be completely sure that accurate communication has been accomplished; therefore, obtaining feedback remains essential. Communication through a third party compounds the problem of sending a message clearly. Interpreters often face the difficulty of interpreting versus translating. Although a message may be translated into another language, helping another understand is much more complex and involves interpreting the message into understandable terms. An interpreter must have transcultural sensitivity, understand how to impart knowledge, and understand how to be a client advocate to represent the client's needs to the nurse. Interpreting with cultural sensitivity is much more complex than simply putting the words into another language (Díaz-Duque, 1982; Wolfson, 1996). Monolingualism in multicultural practices frequently presents ethical dilemmas. If the nurse, the interpreter, and the client's views on the ethical principles regarding care differ, problems can be compounded (Kaufert & Putsch, 1997). Boston (1993) conducted a study of Italian immigrant families in Montreal to determine whether they felt frustration with their caregivers because of language barriers. Findings from this study indicated that respondents expressed fear and helplessness about their treatment because of the language barriers. Even when an interpreter was provided, family members believed that their own deeper concerns and fears were not adequately communicated. Communication extends beyond conveying information and must include methods of conveying emotional and social support (Papadopoulos & Lees, 2004). England, Doughty, Genc, and Putkeli (2003) also reported that even when interpreters are provided, staff should be concerned that communication problems related to other social issues may remain unaddressed.

When the health professional can speak the language of the client, cultural barriers will be lowered. Even if the nurse knows only key words or phrases, this can significantly affect communication and satisfaction with care (Burnard & Naiyapatana, 2004).

CASE STUDY

A 37-year-old Black woman who was recently diagnosed as having hypertension is admitted for a medical work-up examination. Her history reveals that she has recently moved from New Orleans to New York. The nurse is having difficulty communicating with the client because she not only speaks in Black English but also has a heavy Southern drawl and tends to speak in pidgin English. Another factor complicating the development of the nurse–client relationship is that not only does the client not understand the hospital jargon and medical terms, but also word meanings for the nurse and the client vary. For example, when the nurse asks if the client likes her physician, she responds, "He's bad." Only later does the nurse discover that the client was speaking in an argot that is a special linguistic code for some Blacks. The client appears very fearful and anxious about being in the hospital. When questioning the client, the nurse finds that the fear and anxiety are related to the connotative and denotative meanings of the word "hospital." In this case, the client believes that hospitals are associated with death and that she may not leave the hospital alive. When the nurse communicates with the client, she speaks very loudly and repeats the same words again and again.

CLINICAL DECISION MAKING

1. Describe at least two problems encountered by the nurse when giving nursing care to persons who do not speak English as their primary language.
2. Describe four communication approaches that the nurse can use to give culturally appropriate care.
3. Describe approaches the nurse can use when relating to a client whose primary language is not English.
4. Describe at least two nonverbal indicators of anxiety the nurse may encounter when dealing with a client who does not speak English.
5. List at least two problems encountered by the nurse who assumes that speaking louder will improve communication.

REVIEW QUESTIONS

1. While assessing a client who does not speak English, the nurse is aware of nonverbal indications of anxiety that include which of the following?
   a. Being uncooperative and withdrawn.
   b. Looking directly at the nurse and nodding yes.
   c. Looking at the blood and nodding no.
   d. Being cooperative and outgoing.
2. When analyzing the assessment data on the admissions of a client with limited English skills, the nurse realizes the client has answered yes or nodded the head indicating yes to all questions. The nurse interprets this as indicating which of the following?
   a. The client intended to answer all questions as yes.
   b. The client nodded the head and responded yes to indicate cooperation.
   c. The nurse should repeat the questions more loudly so the client will hear.
   d. The nurse should get an interpreter to assist with the assessment.
3. The nurse plans to use an interpreter when teaching a Spanish-speaking client about diabetes mellitus. The best interpreter for the nurse to select is which of the following?
   a. A family member who lives with the client.
   b. One who translates not only the words but the nonverbal messages too.
   c. One who can translate the words into Spanish.
   d. One who can translate the words into oral and written format.

REFERENCES

Anderson, M. (2003). Transcultural perspectives in the nursing care of children. In M. Andrews & J. Boyle (Eds.), *Transcultural concepts in nursing care*. Philadelphia: Lippincott Williams & Wilkins.

Andrews, M. M., & Boyle, J. S. (2003). *Transcultural concepts in nursing care* (4th ed.). Philadelphia: Lippincott Williams & Wilkins.

Anthony, M. (1997). A cultural values assessment tool. *Journal of Cultural Diversity*, 4(2), 49–52.

Argyle, M. (1992). *The social psychology of everyday life*. New York: Routledge.

Argyle, M., & Dean, J. (1965). Eye-contact, distance, and affiliation. *Sociometry*, 28, 289–304.

Argyle, M., Salter, H., Nicholson, N., Williams, M., & Burgess, P. (1970). The communication of inferior and superior attitudes by verbal and nonverbal signals. *British Journal of Social and Clinical Psychology*, 9, 221–231.

Banks, A., & Banks, S. (1995). Cultural identity, resistance, and "good theory": implications for intercultural communication theory from Gypsy culture. *Howard Journal of Communication*, 6(3), 146–163.

Barkauskas, P. (1994). *Quick reference to cultural assessment*. St. Louis: Mosby.

Barton, G., & Richardson, L. (1998). Using literature to create cultural competence. *Image: Journal of Nursing Scholarship*, 30(1), 75–79.

Beachy, A., Hershberger, E., Davidhizar, R., & Giger, J. (1997). Cultural implications for nursing care of the Amish. *Journal of Cultural Diversity*, 4(4), 118–128.

Beutter, B., & Davidhizar, R. (1999). A home care provider's challenge: caring for the Hispanic client in the home. *Journal of Practical Nursing*, 49(3), 26–36.

Bigham, C. (1964). To communicate with Negro patients. *American Journal of Nursing*, 64(9), 113–115.

Boone, S. (2005). Talk directly to patients about beliefs, practices. *Hospital Care Management*, 13(6), 95–96.

Boston, P. (1993). Culture and cancer: the relevance of cultural orientation within cancer education programmes. *European Journal of Cancer Care*, 2, 72–76.

Bronstein, M. (1996). Healing hands. *The Canadian Nurse*, 92(1), 32–34.

Buerhaus, P., & Auerbach, D. (1999). Slow growth in the United States of the number of minorities in the RN workforce. *Image: Journal of Nursing Scholarship*, 31(2), 179–183.

Burnard, P., & Naiyapatana, W. (2004). Culture and communication in Thai nursing: a report of an ethnographic study. *The International Journal of Nursing Studies*, 41(7), 755–765.

Byrne, M. (2002). Diversity and the subculture of healthcare. *Healthcare Traveler*, 9(6), 14–16, 59, 60.

Campinha-Bacote, J. (1995). The quest for cultural competence in nursing care. *Nursing Forum*, 30(4), 19–24.

Capirci, O., Iverson, J., Pizzuto, E., & Volterra, V. (1996). Gestures and words during the transition in two-word speech. *Journal of Child Language*, 23, 645–673.

Carneiro, J. (2000). Know the audience. *The Pfizer Journal: Innovations in Communication*, 4(3), 19–27.

Clark, C. (1995). Enhancing communication with families. *Health Traveler*, 3(2), 34.

Clemmens, E. (1985). An analyst looks at languages, cultures, and translations. *American Journal of Psychoanalysis*, 45(4), 310–321.

Clemmens, E. (1988). Some psychological functions of language. *American Journal of Psychoanalysis*, 43(4), 294–304.

Cook, P., & Cullen, J. (2000). Diversity as a value in undergraduate education. *Nursing and Health Care Education*, 21(4), 178–183.

Crump, R., Bartman, B., Walker, D., & Mitchell, J. (2000). Special populations: who are they and what makes them so special? *Community Health Forum*, 2(2), 35–37.

Davidhizar, R. (1988a). Distance in managerial encounters. *Today's OR Nurse*, 10(10), 23–29.

Davidhizar, R. (1988b). Humor—no nurse should be without it. *Today's OR Nurse*, 10(1), 18–20.

Davidhizar, R. (1989). Developing managerial warmth. *Dimensions of Critical Care*, 8(1), 28–34.

Davidhizar, R., & Brownson, K. (2000). Literacy, cultural diversity, and client education. *Home Health Care Management Practice, 12*(2), 38–44.

Davidhizar, R., & Dowd, S. (2004). When your boss is evil. *RT, 17*(40), 4–7.

Davidhizar, R., & Dowd, S. (2005). The trick about leadership is to make it look easy. *Healthcare Traveler, 13*(2), 2631.

Davidhizar, R., & Dowd, S. (2006). Taking criticism. *Journal of Practical Nursing, 56*(2), 21–24.

Davidhizar, R., Dowd, S., & Giger, J. (1998). Prepare now to work with diverse staff. *Case Management Advisor, 9*(9), 149–151.

Davidhizar, R., & Eshleman, J. (2006). Strategies for developing cultural competency in an RN-BSN program. *Journal of Transcultural Nursing, 17*(2), 179–183.

Davidhizar, R., & Giger, J. (1988). Managerial touch. *Today's OR Nurse, 10*(7), 18–23.

Davidhizar, R., & Giger, J. (2000). Culture and care: profiling Alaskan Eskimos. *Healthcare Traveler, 7*(4), 43–47.

Davidhizar, R., & Giger, J. (2001). Teaching culture within the nursing curriculum using the Giger-Davidhizar model of transcultural nursing assessment. *Journal of Nursing Education, 40*(6), 282–284.

Davidhizar, R., & Giger, J. (2002). Cultural issues: using a transcultural assessment model to understand Afghanis and Islamic culture and religion. *Advances for Nurses,* 37–38.

Davidhizar, R., & Hart, A. (2005). Pain management. *Healthcare Traveler, 13*(6), 3–41.

Davidhizar, R., & Shearer, R. (2005). When your nursing student is culturally diverse. *Health Care Manager, 24*(4), 356–363.

Davidhizar, R., Shearer, R., & Giger, J. (2002). The challenges of cross-cultural communication. *RT Image, 15*(11), 18–23.

Delgado, M. (1983). Hispanics and psychotherapeutic groups. *International Journal of Psychotherapy, 33*(4), 507–520.

DeThomaso, M. (1971). Touch power and the screen of loneliness. *Perspectives in Psychiatric Care, 9*(3), 112–117.

Díaz-Duque, O. F. (1982). Overcoming the language barrier: advice from an interpreter. *American Journal of Nursing, 82*(9), 1380–1382.

Dillard, J. (1973). *Black English: its history and usage in the United States.* New York: Vintage Books.

Eibl-Eibesfelt, I. (1972). Similarities and differences between cultures in expressive movements. In R. A. Hinde (Ed.), *Nonverbal communication* (pp. 297–312). Cambridge, England: Cambridge University Press.

Ekman, P., & Friesen, W. (1975). *Unmasking the face: a guide to recognizing emotions from facial clues.* Englewood Cliffs, NJ: Prentice Hall.

England, R., Doughty, K., Genc, S., & Putkeli, Z. (2003). Working with refugees: health education and communication issues in a child health clinic. *Health Education Journal, 62*(4), 359–368.

Ericksen, A. (2002). Culturally speaking. *Healthcare Traveler, 9*(6), 8–12, 59–60.

Evans, B., & Severtsen, B. (2001). Storytelling as cultural assessment. *Nursing and Health Perspectives, 22*(4), 180–183.

Fadiman, A. (1997). *The spirit catches you and you fall down: Hmong child, her American doctors, and the collision of two cultures.* New York: Noonday Press.

Galanti, G. (2003). *Caring for patients from different cultures: case studies from American hospitals* (3rd ed., pp. 26–27). Philadelphia: University of Pennsylvania Press.

Garfinkel, H. (2002). *Ethnomethodology's program.* New York: Rowman and Littlefield.

Geissler, E. (1991). Transcultural nursing and nursing diagnosis. *Nursing and Health Care, 12*(4), 190–192.

Gibson, J. (1984). As they grow: 1 year olds. *Parents,* 128.

Giger, J., & Davidhizar, R. (1990a). Culture and space. *Advancing Clinical Care, 6*(6), 8–10.

Giger, J., & Davidhizar, R. (1990b). Transcultural nursing assessment: a method for advancing nursing practice. *International Nursing Review, 37*(1), 199–202.

Giger, J., & Davidhizar, R. (2001). Diversity in caring. In P. Potter & A. Perry (Eds.), *Fundamentals of nursing* (5th ed.). St. Louis: Mosby.

Giger, J., & Davidhizar, R. (2002). Culturally competent care: emphasis on understanding the people of Afghanistan, Afghanistan Americans, and Islamic culture and religion. *International Nursing Review, 49,* 79–86.

Giger, J., Davidhizar, R., Evers, S., & Ingram, C. (1994). Cultural factors influencing mental health and mental illness. In C. Taylor (Ed.), *Mereness' essentials of psychiatric nursing* (pp. 214–238). St. Louis: Mosby.

Giger, J., Davidhizar, R., Johnson, J., & Poole, V. (1997). Health promotion among ethnic minorities: the importance of cultural phenomena. *Rehabilitation Nursing, 22*(6), 303–307, 310, 336.

Giger, J., Davidhizar, R., & Wieczorek, S. (1993). Culture and ethnicity. In I. M. Bobak & M. Jensen (Eds.), *Maternity and gynecological care* (5th ed., pp. 43–67). St. Louis: Mosby.

Giorgianni, S. (2000). Activating the health consumer. *The Pfizer Journal: Innovations in Communication, 4*(3), 4–36.

Goldman, K., & Schmalz, K. (2005). E = MC^2: Effective multiple competence. *Health Promotion Practice, 6*(3), 237–239.

Graham-Dickerson, P. (1996). Healing through discourse for culturally diverse people within the health care system. *The Journal of Multicultural Nursing and Health, 2*(3), 33–37.

Grainger, R. (1992). Eye movements: a new psychotherapeutic tool. *American Journal of Nursing, 92*(5), 18.

Grossman, D. (1996). Cultural dimensions in home health care nursing. *American Journal of Nursing, 96*(7), 33–36.

Grypma, S. (1993). Culture shock. *The Canadian Nurse, 89*(8), 33–36.

Guralnik, D. (Ed.), (1989). *Webster's new world dictionary: student edition* (3rd ed.). New York: Prentice Hall.

Guruge, S., & Donner, G. (1996). Transcultural nursing in Canada. *The Canadian Nurse, 92/8*(36–40), 34–39.

Guy, T. (2005). *The adult literacy education system in the United States. Background paper prepared for the Education for All Global Monitoring Report 2006.* Athens, GA: University of Georgia. Available at: <http://unesdoc.unesco.org/images/0014/001462/146281e.pdf> Retrieved July 24, 2011.

Haffner, L. (1992). Translation is not enough: interpreting in a medical setting. *Western Journal of Medicine, 157*(3), 248–254.

Hagen, E. (1988). *Southeast Asians in the United States: an overview of belief systems, and the refugee experience.* Long Beach, CA: St. Mary Medical Center. Paper presented at the seminar: Working with the Southeast Asian Health Consumer.

Hagey, R., & Buller, E. (1983). Drumming and dancing: a new rhythm in nursing care. *The Canadian Nurse, 79*(4), 28–31.

Hall, E. T. (1966). *The silent language.* New York: Anchor Books.

Hallenbeck, J. (2004). Communication across cultures. *Journal of Palliative Medicine, 7*(3), 477–480.

Halliday, M., & Webster, J. (2006). *On language and linguistics.* London: Continuum International Publishing.

Hedlund, N. (1993). Communication. In R. P. Rawlins, S. Williams, & C. K. Beck (Eds.), *Mental health–psychiatric nursing: a holistic life approach* (3rd ed.). St. Louis: Mosby.

Henderson, G., & Primeaux, M. (1981). *Transcultural health care.* Menlo Park, CA: Addison-Wesley.

Hess, E. H. (1965). Attitude and pupil size. *Scientific American, 212*, 46–54.

Hess, E. H. (1975). The role of pupil size in communication. *Scientific American, 233*(5), 110–119.

Hoang, G., & Erickson, R. (1982). Guidelines for providing medical care to Southeast Asian refugees. *Journal of the American Medical Association, 248*(6), 710–714.

Huckaby, D. (1987). Take time to laugh. *Nursing, 87*(17), 81.

Insel, P. M., & Lindgren, H. C. (1978). *Too close for comfort: the psychology of crowding.* Englewood Cliffs, NJ: Prentice Hall.

Jenkins, V., & Fallowfield, L. (2000). Reasons for accepting or declining to participate in randomized clinical trials for cancer therapy. *British Journal of Cancer, 82*, 1782–1788.

Johnson, B. (1965). The meaning of touch in nursing. *Nursing Outlook, 13*(2), 59–60.

Jones, R. (2000). Developments in consumer health informatics in the next decade. *Health Libraries Review, 17*(1), 26–31.

Jourard, S. (1972). *The transparent self: self disclosure and well-being* (2nd ed.). New York: Van Nostrand-Reinhold.

Kaufert, J., & Putsch, R. (1997). Communication through interpreters in healthcare: ethical dilemmas arising from differences in class, culture, language, and power. *The Journal of Clinical Ethics, 8*(1), 71–87.

Kayser, H. (1996). Cultural/linguistic variations in the United States and its implications for assessment and intervention in speech-language pathology: an epilogue. *Language, Speech, and Hearing Services in Schools, 27*(4), 385–387.

Kendall, J. (1996). Creating a culturally responsive psychotherapeutic environment for African-American youths: a critical analysis. *Advances in Nursing Science, 18*(4), 11–28.

Killion, C. (2001). Understanding cultural aspects of health through photography. *Nursing Outlook, 49*(1), 50–54.

Kirsch, I., Jungeblut, A., Jenkins, L., & Kolstad, A. (1993). *Adult literacy in America: a first look at the results of the National Adult Literacy Survey.* Washington, DC: National Center for Education Statistics, U.S. Dept. of Education.

Krech, D., Crutchfield, R., & Ballachey, E. (1962). *Individual in society: a textbook of social psychology.* New York: McGraw-Hill.

Lane, P. (1989). Nurse–client perceptions: the double standard of touch. *Issues in Mental Health Nursing, 10*, 1–13.

LaVeist, T., Nickerson, K., & Bowie, J. (2000). Attitudes about racism, medical mistrust, and satisfaction with care among African American and white cardiac patients. *Medical Care Research Review, 57*(Suppl. 1), 146–161.

Leininger, M., & McFarland, M. (2006). *Culture care diversity and universality* (2nd ed.). Sudbury, MA: Jones and Bartlett.

Lester, N. (1998). Cultural competence: a nursing dialogue. *American Journal of Nursing, 98*(8), 26–33.

Lindsay, J., Narayan, M., & Rea, K. (1998). Nursing across cultures: the Vietnamese client. *Home Healthcare Nurse, 16*(10), 693–700.

Luft, J., & Ingham, H. (1984). The Johari window: a graphic model of awareness in interpersonal relations. In J. Luft (Ed.), *Group processes: an introduction to group dynamics* (3rd ed.). Palo Alto, CA: Mayfield.

Lunsford, A. (2006). *Easy writer: a pocket reference* (3rd ed.). Boston: Bedford/St. Martin's.

Mackey, R. (1995). Discover the health power of therapeutic touch. *American Journal of Nursing, 95*, 27–32.

Martin, B. (1995). The difficult art of listening. *Gospel Herald, 88*(48), 1–2.

Mattson, S. (1995). Culturally sensitive perinatal care for Southeast Asians. *Journal of Obstetric and Gynecological Neonatal Nursing, 24*(4), 335–341.

McKenzie, J., & Chrisman, N. (1977). Healing herbs, gods, and magic folk health beliefs among Filipino-Americans. *Nursing Outlook, 25*(5), 326.

McLeod, R., & Bently, C. (1996). Understanding deafness as a culture with a unique language. *Advanced Practice Nursing Quarterly, 2*(2), 50–58.

Mead, M. (1947). The application of anthropological technique to cross-national communication. *Transcultural New York Academy of Science, Series II, 9*, 4.

Mehrabian, A. (1968). The influence of attitudes from the posture, orientation, and distance of a communicator. *Journal of Consulting Clinical Psychology, 32*, 296–308.

Mehrabian, A. (1981). *Silent messages: implicit communication of emotions and attitudes.* Belmont, CA: Wadsworth.

Mika, V., Kelly, P., Price, M., Franquiz, M., & Villarreal, R. (2005). The ABCs of health literacy. *Family Community Health, 28*(4), 351–357.

Miller, S., & Davidhizar, R. (2001). Sociocultural aspects of adherence to medical regimens for Mexican Americans. *Journal of Care Management, 7*(3), 44–48.

Mitchell, A. (1978). Barriers to therapeutic communication with Black clients. *Nursing Outlook, 26*, 109–112.

Montagu, A. (1986). *Touching: the human significance of the skin* (3rd ed.). New York: Columbia University Press.

Mosby's dictionary of medicine, nursing, and health professions (2012). (9th revised ed.). St. Louis: Mosby.

Murray, R., & Huelskoetter, N. (1991). *Psychiatric/mental health nursing: giving emotional care* (3rd ed.). Norwalk, CT: Appleton & Lange.

Myers, A. (2007). *A study on the differences between appropriate interpersonal self-disclosure in a work environment.* Wichita, KS: Wichita State University.

Nellum-Davis, P. (2002). Clinical practice issues. In D. E. Battle (Ed.), *Communication disorders in multicultural populations* (3rd ed.). Boston: Andover Medical Publishers.

Orlando, O., & Nickoloff, J. (2007). *An introductory dictionary of theology and religious studies.* Collegeville, MN: A Micheal Glazier Book/Liturgical Press.

Oxendine, J. (2000). Creating culturally-sensitive health materials for American Indians. In *Closing the Gap: A Newsletter* (p. 12).

Papadopoulos, I., & Lees, S. (2004). Cancer and communications: similarities and differences of men with cancer from six different ethnic groups. *European Journal of Cancer Care, 16,* 154–162.

Paynich, M. (1964). Cultural barriers to nurse communication. *American Journal of Nursing, 64*(2), 87–90.

Pirandello, L. (1970). Language and thought. *Perspectives in Psychiatric Care, 8*(5), 230.

Polhemus, T. (Ed.), (1978). *The body reader: social aspects of the human body.* New York: Pantheon Books.

Poole, V., Davidhizar, R., & Giger, J. (2003). Cultural aspects of psychiatric nursing. In N. Keltner, L. Schwecke, & C. Bostrom (Eds.), *Psychiatric nursing* (4th ed.). St. Louis: Mosby.

Pore, S. (1995). I can't understand what my patient is saying. *Advance for Nurse Practitioners, 3,* 47–48.

Potter, P., & Perry, A. (2005). *Fundamentals of nursing* (6th ed.). St. Louis: Mosby.

Purnell, L. (2001). Guatemalans' practices for health promotion and the meaning of respect afforded them by health care providers. *Journal of Transcultural Nursing, 12*(1), 40–47.

Quarnero, P. (2005). Mexicans. In J. Lipson & S. Dibble (Eds.), *Culture and clinical care.* San Francisco: UCSF Nursing Press: School of Nursing, University of California.

Randall-David, E. (1989). *Strategies for working with culturally diverse communities and clients* [Brochure]. Washington, DC: Association for the Care of Children's Health.

Rayner, K. (1992). *Eye movements and visual cognition: scene perception and reading.* New York: Springer-Verlag.

Reimer, J., & Redskye, C. (1998). The Canadian Ojibwa. In R. Davidhizar & J. Giger (Eds.), *Canadian transcultural nursing: assessment and intervention.* St. Louis: Mosby.

Reusch, J. (1961). *Therapeutic communication.* New York: W. W. Norton.

Rocereto, L. (1981). Selected health beliefs of Vietnamese refugees. *Journal of School Health, 51*(1), 63–64.

Sapir, E. (1929). The status of linguistics as a science. *Language, 5,* 207–214.

Satcher, D., & Pamies, R. (2006). *Multicultural medicine and health disparities.* New York: McGraw-Hill.

Scheflen, A., & Scheflen, A. (1972). *Body language and social order.* Englewood Cliffs, NJ: Prentice Hall.

Scholz, J. (1990). Cultural expressions affecting patient care. *Dimensions in Oncology Nursing, 4*(1), 16–20.

Shadick, K. (1993). Development of a transcultural health education program for the Hmong. *Clinical Nurse Specialist, 7*(2), 48–53.

Shapiro, F. (1991). Eye movement desensitization and reprocessing procedure: from EMD to EMD/R—a new treatment model for anxiety and related traumata. *The Behavioral Therapist, 14,* 133–135.

Shields, L., & King, S. (2001). International pediatric nursing: qualitative analysis of the care of children in hospital in four countries. *Journal of Pediatric Nursing: Nursing Care of Children and Families, 16*(3), 206–213.

Shuter, R. (1976). Proxemics and tactility in Latin America. *Journal of Communication, 26*(3), 46–52.

Sieh, A., & Brentin, L. (1997). *The nurse communicates.* Philadelphia: Saunders.

Simonton, O. C., Simonton, S., & Creighton, J. (1978). *Getting well again: a step-by-step, self-help guide to overcoming cancer for patients and their families.* New York: Bantam Books.

Smith, B., & Cantrell, P. (1988). Distance in nurse-patient encounters. *Journal of Psychosocial Nursing, 26*(2), 22–26.

Snow, L. (1976). "High blood" is not "high blood pressure." *Urban Health, 5*(3), 54–55.

Sommer, R. (1959). Studies in personal space. *Sociometry, 22,* 247–260.

Spector, R. (2004). *Cultural diversity in health and illness* (6th ed.). Upper Saddle River, NJ: Pearson Prentice Hall.

Stauffer, R. (2005). *Personal communication.* Harrisburg, VA.

Studer, C. (2002). Reflections: body language—melting pain into song. *American Journal of Nursing, 102*(1), 45.

Sudnow, D. (1967). *Passing on: the social organization of dying.* Englewood Cliffs, NJ: Prentice Hall.

Sullivan, H. (1954). *The interpersonal theory of psychiatry.* New York: W. W. Norton.

Sue, D. W., & Sue, D. (1999). *Counseling the culturally different: theory and practice* (3rd ed.). New York: John Wiley & Son.

Sue, D. W., & Sue, D. (2003). *Counseling the culturally diverse: theory and practice* (4th ed.). New York: John Wiley.

Talbot, L. R. (1996). The power of words. *Canadian Journal of Nursing Research, 28*(1), 9–15.

Taylor, C. (1976). Soul talk: a key to Black cultural attitudes. In D. Luckroft (Ed.), *Black awareness: implications for Black patient care.* New York: American Journal of Nursing.

Thayer, S. (1988). Close encounters. *Psychology Today, 10*(1), 31–36.

Thiederman, S. (1986). Ethnocentrism: a barrier to effective health care. *Nurse Practitioner, 11*(8), 52–59.

Time Almanac. (2011). Chicago: Encyclopedia Britannica.

Tohidian, I., & Tabatabaie, S. (2010). Considering the relationship between language, culture and cognition to scrutinize the lexical influences on cognition. *Current Psychology, 29,* 52–70.

Tripp-Reimer, T., & Friedl, M. (1977). Appalachians: a neglected minority. *Nursing Outlook, 32*(2), 41–45.

Tuleja, E., & O'Rourke, J. (2009). *Intercultural communication for business.* Mason, OH: South-Western, Cengage Learning.

U.S. Department of Commerce: Bureau of the Census. American Community Survey Briefs. (2010a). *The foreign-born population in the United States: current populations reports* (pp. 20–534). Washington, DC: U.S. Census Bureau.

U.S. Department of Commerce, Bureau of the Census, American Community Survey Briefs. (2010b). *Nativity status and citizenship in the United States: 2009.* Washington, DC: U.S. Government Printing Office.

U.S. Department of Commerce, Bureau of the Census, American Community Survey Briefs. (2010c). *Place of birth of the foreign-born population: 2009.* Washington, DC: U.S. Government Printing Office.

U.S. Department of Commerce, Bureau of the Census. (2011). *Statistical Abstracts of the United States. The national data book* (130th ed.). Washington, DC: U.S. Government Printing Office.

U.S. Department of Health and Human Services. (2000). *Healthy people 2010.* Washington, DC: U.S. Government Printing Office.

U.S. Department of Health and Human Services. (2011). *Healthy people 2020.* Available at <http://www .healthypeople.gov/2020/TopicsObjectives2020/pdfs/ HP2020_brochure.pdf> Retrieved July 24, 2011.

Varcarolis, E. (2006). *The clinical interview and communication skills. Foundations of psychiatric mental health nursing* (5th ed.). Philadelphia: Saunders.

Venes, D. (2009). *Taber's cyclopedic medical dictionary* (20th ed.). Philadelphia: F. A. Davis.

Watzlawich, P., Beavin, J., & Jackson, D. (1967). *Pragmatics of human communication: a study of interactional patterns, pathologies, & paradoxes.* New York: W. W. Norton.

Whitcher, S. J., & Fisher, J. D. (1979). Multidimensional reaction to therapeutic touch in hospital setting. *Journal of Personality, Sociology, and Psychology, 37*(1), 87–96.

Wilson, M. (1996). Arabic speakers: language and culture, here and abroad. *Topics in Language Disorders, 18*(4), 65–80.

Winans-Orr, P., & McIntosh, M. (1996). Putting control theory to work. *The Canadian Nurse,* 51–52.

Wissing, D. (2000). Respect is key to great people pictures. *Journey,* 12.

Wolfson, L. (1996). Breaking the language barrier. *Hemispheres (Paris, France),* 37–38.

Wood, D. (2001). Learning about difference. *Minority Nurse Spring,* 45–50.

Xu, Y., & Davidhizar, R. (2005). Intercultural communication in nursing education: when Asian students and American faculty converge. *Journal of Nursing Education, 44*(5), 209–215.

Space

After reading this chapter, the nurse will be able to:

1. Discuss factors related to distance and immediate receptors that influence spatial behavior.
2. Define the term *personal space,* and relate its significance to care plan development for clients from varying cultures.
3. Explain how actions of the nurse may contribute to feelings of anxiety and loss of control for clients from transcultural backgrounds.
4. List actions the nurse can take to promote feelings of autonomy and self-worth when caring for clients from transcultural backgrounds.
5. Delineate the difference between tactile space and visual space, and show their relationship to transcultural nursing care.

Personal space is the area that surrounds a person's body; it includes the space and the objects within the space. *Personal space* can also describe inner space that filters the incoming stimuli that a person receives (Scott & Dumas, 1995). Scott (1988) defines *inner personal space* as dynamic, invisible lines of demarcation that can be divided into four concentric areas of space: (1) the inner spirit core, (2) an area of thoughts and feelings perceived as unacceptable, (3) an area of thoughts and feelings perceived as acceptable, and (4) an area of superficial public image. An individual's comfort level is related to both inner and outer personal space; discomfort is experienced when personal space is invaded. Although personal space is an individual matter and varies with the situation, dimensions of the personal space comfort zone also vary from culture to culture (Davidhizar, Shearer, & Giger, 2002).

Traditionally, nursing research paid little attention to geographical approaches and the dynamics of nursing and space. However, change is occurring and research is beginning on the relationships among nursing, space, and place as an emerging geography of nursing and a health geography subdiscipline (Andrews, 2003; Halford & Leonard, 2003). Andrews postulates that from a disciplinary perspective, studying the geography of nursing can explain the relationship between health geography and mainstream health service and medical concerns in a place-sensitive, patient-sensitive, and qualitative form (Andrews, 2002; Andrews & Andrews, 2003; Andrews & Phillips, 2002). Nevertheless, nurses have long drawn from the social science disciplines and appreciated that spatial behavior is an important consideration in measuring distance in relationships. Since spatial behavior is usually judged to be spontaneous and unintentional, individuals are typically more likely to trust the accuracy of actions rather than words as a reflection of true feelings. Although a large percentage of spatial behaviors are spontaneous and unintentional, communication in this domain can be managed to promote favorable and desired impressions. For example, a nurse may choose to stand when greeting a client to show respect.

To understand human behavior, one must understand something of the nature of our receptor systems and how the information received by these systems is modified by culture. Because spatial behavior is a response to sensory stimulation in the internal and the external environment, the phenomenon of space can be understood only as an integral part of the sensory systems—that is, sight, sound, touch, and smell. Spatial behavior encompasses a variety of behaviors, including proximity to others, objects in the environment, and movement.

PERCEPTION OF SPACE

Sensory apparatuses fall into two categories:

1. *Distance receptors* are concerned with the examination of distant objects. The sensory receptors for distance include the eyes, ears, and nose.
2. *Immediate receptors* are used to examine the world up close. Sensory receptors used to examine the world up close include touch, which is the sensation received from the skin membranes (Hall, 1969, 1977).

These two classifications can be broken down even further to facilitate the nurse's understanding of the phenomenon of space. For example, the skin is the chief organ of touch and is sensitive to heat gain and heat loss; both radiant and conducted heat are detected by the skin. Therefore, the skin must be perceived as both an immediate receptor and a distance receptor. In general, there is a relationship between the evolutionary age of the receptor system and the amount and quality of information it can convey to the central nervous system. Many psychologists estimate that the touch system is as old as life itself (Hall, 1966). Because the ability to respond to stimuli is based on touch, the response to touch is one of the basic criteria for the maintenance of life. In comparison, sight is believed to be the last and most specialized sense to develop in humans. From an anthropological view, vision became more important than olfactory response when our ancestors left the ground and took to trees in search of food and safety. Stereoscopic vision became essential for primitive humans because without it, jumping from branch to branch was difficult and dangerous.

Distance Receptors

Distance receptors include sensory apparatuses for visual, auditory, and olfactory perception. It is essential that the nurse understand the relationship between sight, touch, and smell and how the reaction to these stimuli can be modified by culture.

Visual and Auditory Perception. As indicated earlier, vision was the last of the senses to evolve. However, it is by far the most complex. Seemingly, more data are fed to the nervous system through the eyes at a much greater rate than through the senses of touch or hearing. For example, the information a blind person can gather outdoors is limited to a circle of 20 to 100 feet because a blind person can perceive by way of auditory or olfactory stimuli only what is immediately surrounding him or her. However, with sight a person can see the stars at night. Even very talented blind persons are limited to an average speed of perception of 2 to 3 miles an hour over familiar territory. In contrast, with sight a person has to fly faster than sound

before additional visual aids are needed to avoid bumping into things. The amount of information that can be gathered by the eyes in contrast to the ears cannot be calculated precisely. Such a calculation would require not only a translation process but also the knowledge of precisely what to count. A general notion held by most scientists is that the relative complexities of the two systems, visual and auditory, can be obtained by comparison of the size of the nerves connecting the eyes and the ears to the centers of the brain (Brown, Leavitt, & Graham, 1977; O'Shea, Roeber, & Bach, 2010).

The optic nerve contains roughly 18 times as many neurons as the cochlear nerve; therefore, one might assume that it transmits at least that much more information. The eyes may act as a defense mechanism because they normally alert us to danger; the eyes may be as much as a thousand times more effective than the ears in gathering information to protect us from harmful stimuli. The area that the unaided ear can effectively cover in the course of daily living is quite limited. The ear is very efficient but only up to a distance of 20 feet. At about 100 feet, one-way vocal communication is possible but at a somewhat slower rate than at a conversational distance. Although two-way conversation is also possible at this distance, it is considerably altered. Beyond this distance the auditory cues begin to break down rapidly. The unaided eye, on the other hand, can gather an extraordinary amount of information within a 100-yard radius and is efficient for human interaction at up to a mile (Hall, 1969).

The impulses that activate the eyes and the ears differ in speed and quality. For example, at a temperature of $0°C$ ($32°F$) at sea level, sound waves can travel 1100 feet per second and be heard in frequencies of 50 to 1500 cycles per second (Hertz). On the other hand, light rays can travel 186,000 miles (300,000 km) per second and thus are visible at a maximal frequency of 500 trillion at yellow-green (Hall, 1969).

Many complex and remarkable instruments have been invented to extend the eyes and ears. Radio, television, and the Internet have revolutionized the perception of space and shortened distances among people worldwide. During World War II, radio was relied on quite extensively to bring news from the occupied countries to parts of the free world. Perhaps one of the most famous broadcasts of this period was done by Tokyo Rose, whose broadcasts, which were reported to be untrue, influenced many people in the listening audience about the nature and direction of World War II. However, radio lacked the visual stimuli offered later by television, which filled in perception gaps left by radio. Television came of age in the 1960s, when for the first time, brighter, clearer, and bolder pictures were offered to viewers. The addition of color filled another perception gap and enhanced our receptor fields. For the first time in history, from their living rooms, the people of the United States could view their president doing the ordinary, the extraordinary, and the unusual. For example, the people of the United States were informed about the Cuban missile crisis by U.S. President Kennedy on television. They were also able to see this president playing with his children in the Oval Office. In 1963, when President Kennedy was assassinated, little was left to the imagination of the people of the United States, who were mesmerized by complete television coverage from assassination to burial. Because of television, the nation and the world at large experienced grief that is still present today and mourned collectively.

The development of cyberspace technology has added another visual dimension to space. On September 11, 2001, the nation and the world collectively experienced shock as terrorists crashed airplanes into the World Trade Center and the Pentagon. Not only did many view the disasters as they happened on television and on the Internet, but also horrific images and reports of the September 11 terrorist attacks were broadcast for weeks. Technology also allowed the world to see the emotional reactions of others to the disaster and in turn precipitated responses of condolence. Immediately, e-mail messages offering sympathy to grieving Americans poured in from friends around the world. Cyberspace technology united the world in grief as memorials on each continent were displayed on the Internet. The visual impressions provided by technology enabled persons who did not directly experience the disaster to be profoundly disturbed by it (Davidhizar & Shearer, 2002). In 2005, the nation experienced a similar phenomenon with the devastation of Hurricane Katrina that became a part of the lived experience of persons who had access to television or the Internet (Thomas, 2006). The Internet and multimedia technologies provided a range of quasi-public spaces that encouraged debate and active citizenship to assess the reaction of the government and the nation to this event (Thomas, 2006). More recently, natural disasters such as the massive earthquake in Haiti in 2010, which killed approximately 250,000 people, and the earthquake and tsunami in Japan in 2011 that killed thousands and caused a nuclear disaster have all been widely covered not only on television but through other social networks such as Twitter, Facebook, and YouTube.

In summary, visual space has an entirely different character from that of auditory space. The overriding quality that differentiates visual space from auditory space is that visual information tends to be less ambiguous and more focused than auditory information. Therefore, visual information is less subject to external manipulation than is auditory information. One major exception to this rule is the blind person who has learned to understand selectively the higher audio frequencies, which can assist him or her in locating objects within a familiar or unfamiliar room. For example, a blind person may know where the door is in a room by the relationship of the sound that comes from that direction.

Even today it is not known what effects the incongruities between auditory and visual space have on individuals. Some data indicate that auditory space is a factor in performance. J. W. Black, a phonetician, demonstrated that the size and reverberation (vibrations of external sounds) of a room can affect an individual's reading rate. In a classic study, Black (1950) found that people read more slowly in larger rooms, where the reverberation time, or circulation of sound, is slower than that in smaller rooms. Hall (1966, 1969) interviewed subjects in regard to the slowing of reverberation time in a larger room. Among the interviewees was a gifted English architect who improved the performance of a malfunctioning committee by simply blending the auditory and visual worlds of the conference chamber where the committee met. The complaint the architect had received was that the chairman was inadequate and was about to be replaced. However, the architect had reason to believe that the difficulties this committee encountered were caused by more in the environment than just the chairman. In this situation the meeting room was next to a busy street, and traffic noises were intensified by reverberations from the hard walls and rugless floors inside the building and particularly in the meeting room. The architect was able to adjust the room by adding an acoustic ceiling, carpet, and soundproof walls. Once interferences were reduced, the chairman was able to conduct the meeting without undue strain, and complaints about the chairman ceased.

People who are brought up in different cultures learn unknowingly to screen out various bits of information and to sort information into relevant or irrelevant categories; once set, these perceptual patterns remain stable throughout life. For example, Japanese individuals tend to give meaning to spaces that a Westerner may classify as empty (Gregg, 1996). Japanese readers expect to be presented with the parts first and then the whole rather than getting the "big picture" and then a breakdown of material into its component parts (Davidhizar, Dowd, & Bowen, 1998; Simply Stated, 1985). In addition, Japanese people screen visually in a variety of ways and are more perceptive to visual stimuli. Japanese people are therefore perfectly content with paper walls as acoustic screens. A Westerner who finds himself in a Japanese inn where a party is going on next door may be in for a new sensory experience since only paper-thin walls separate each room. In contrast, German and Dutch people depend on double doors and thick walls to screen out sound and may have difficulty if they must rely on their own powers of concentration to do so. If two rooms are the same size and one screens out sound and the other does not, a sensitive German or Dutch person who is trying to concentrate will feel less intruded on in the former and thus less crowded (Hall, 1966, 1969). Cultural patterning of space can also be seen in the arrangements of urban space in different cultures. For example, U.S. cities are usually laid out along a grid with the axis north–south and east–west. In Paris, main streets are laid out radiating from centers with no grid system (Gregg, 1996). The layout of French cities is only one aspect of the theme of centralization that characterizes French culture. In French offices, the most important person has the desk in the middle of the office.

Yet another aspect of cultural patterning of space is function of space. For example, space in India is sometimes related to concepts of superiority and inferiority. In Indian cities, villages, and even homes, spaces may be designated as inferior or polluted. Spaces in India are divided so that high and low castes, secular and sacred activities, and male and female can be kept segregated (Gregg, 1996).

Olfactory Perception. Some cultures place more importance on olfactory perceptions than do others. For example, Americans are culturally underdeveloped in the use of their olfactory apparatuses (Hall, 1966, 1969). Hall (1966) contended that the deprivations of the olfactory stimulus are a result of the extensive use of deodorants and the suppression of odors in public places, which has resulted in a land of olfactory blandness and sameness that is difficult to duplicate anywhere else in the world.

People in the United States are continuously bombarded with commercials for room deodorizers, antiperspirants, mouthwashes, carpet deodorizers, and so on. All of these factors result in bland, undifferentiated spaces and deprive many people in the United States of the richness and variety of life. For example, if one is cooking with garlic, a room deodorizer may be used during the cooking process, causing the garlic smell to be eliminated. It is this type of behavior on the part of people of the United States that obscures memories. It is believed that smells evoke much deeper memories than either vision or sound; when the sound or the sight of what has happened has passed, the memory of the smell lingers on. Even today many U.S. citizens equate certain holidays, such as Christmas, with certain smells. For example, because Christmas is traditionally equated with the smell of baked goods, holly, pine, and fruit, today many people in the United States try to reproduce these smells at Christmas. An individual who has an artificial Christmas tree may buy a pine-scented spray to create the effects of a fresh tree. Another old-fashioned scent for many U.S. citizens is country potpourri,

which has now been simulated in aerosol cans for easy dispensing. A new car odor can be simulated by a car spray that smells like new leather. Soap may be purchased to re-create a desired feeling; for example, the soap Mother used at home may create a feeling of hominess. Smells may also create a negative reaction; for example, an individual who washes with lye soap may be thought to have body odor because the smell is unusually strong and medicinal. A medicinal smell is perceived by most individuals in the United States to be appropriate for a hospital room but not elsewhere.

Odor is perhaps one of the most basic methods of communication. It is primarily chemical in nature and is therefore referred to in a chemical sense. The olfactory sense has diverse functions and not only differentiates individuals but also makes it possible to identify the emotional state of others. Even an infant can learn to identify his or her parents through the sense of smell. Although the young infant has not learned to see and discriminate patterns well, the infant can distinguish identity through the olfactory sense.

In a hospital setting an employee who has an unpleasant odor creates a real management dilemma. The supervisor may counsel and even reprimand the employee for poor hygiene. Employees who have the smell of alcohol may be sent home. It is important that the nurse appreciate that odors may be caused by pathological conditions, as in certain diabetic states, or the result of certain mouthwashes or soaps. If a client has an unpleasant odor, the nurse should first assess whether some pathological condition is present, such as an inflammatory process. In a psychiatric hospital, a client's odor could be associated with a condition such as schizophrenia, and although there is some thought that such an odor may be pathological, it is more likely to be related to a lack of motivation for self-care skills.

Immediate Receptors

Immediate receptors are those that examine the world up close, such as tactile stimuli received by way of the skin membranes. It is important that the nurse appreciate the effect culture may have on an individual's reaction to these stimuli and how these stimuli can be modified by cultural influences.

Skin Membranes. Human beings receive a tremendous amount of information from the distance receptors, which include the eyes, ears, and nose. Because of the vast amount of information that is received from the distance receptors, few people think of the skin as a major sense organ. However, if we humans lacked the ability to perceive heat and cold, we would soon perish. Without the ability to perceive heat and cold and to react appropriately to these stimuli, we would freeze in the winter and become overheated in the summer. The skin, as a major sense organ, is so grossly overlooked that even some of its subtle sensing and communicating qualities go unnoticed. Nerves called *proprioceptors* keep us informed as to exactly what is happening as we work our muscles. These nerves provide the feedback that enables us to move our bodies smoothly; thus, they occupy a key position in kinesthetic space perception. The body also has another set of nerves called *exteroceptors,* which are located in the skin and convey the sensations of heat, cold, touch, and pain to the central nervous system. In light of the fact that two different systems of nerves are used in the perception of space, kinesthetic space is considered qualitatively different from thermal space. However, nurses must remember that these two systems work together and are mutually reinforcing most of the time.

It has been only in modern scientific times that some remarkable thermal characteristics of the skin have been discovered. The capacity of the skin for emitting and detecting radiant or infrared heat is extraordinarily high. One might assume that is so because it was important to survival in the past and most certainly had a significant function in early human beings. Although the discovery of the thermal characteristics of the skin has been only within recent times, the nurse should not overlook the importance of the skin as an immediate receptor.

Humans are well equipped to send and receive messages concerning emotional states based on changes in skin temperature. Skin temperature can give very important clues to the emotional state of the individual. A common indicator of embarrassment or anger in fair-skinned individuals is blushing. However, dark-skinned people also blush. Therefore, blushing cannot be perceived as simply a matter of change in skin coloration. The nurse must carefully observe dark-skinned persons when looking for changes in emotional state, such as embarrassment or anger, by noting a swelling of regions of the forehead. The additional blood to these areas will raise the temperature, and these areas will appear flushed. Therefore, even if there is no significant change in color to these areas in dark-skinned individuals, these areas will feel warm to the touch.

Many novel instruments have been developed to study heat emission. These instruments should make it possible to study the thermal details of interpersonal communication, an area not previously accessible to direct observation. Thermographic devices (infrared-detection devices and cameras) that were originally developed for satellites and homing missiles have been used for recording subvisual phenomena. Photographs taken in the dark using the radiant heat of the human body have shown that an inflamed area of the body actually emits more heat than the surrounding areas. Diagnosis of cancer is also possible with thermographic devices that measure blocked circulation of blood. Thermographic devices have been useful in health care delivery because skin color does not affect the amount of heat delivered; dark skin does not emit more or less heat than light skin. Thus, the observable phenomenon in all individuals regarding heat emission is the blood supply in a given area of the body.

Increased heat on the surface is detected in three ways:
1. Thermal detectors in the skin, particularly if two individuals are close enough to each other.
2. Intensified olfactory interactions, which are augmented when skin temperature rises. Perfumes and lotions may be smelled at a greater distance when the body temperature is increased.
3. Visual examination, which can give clues to an increase or decrease in body temperature. For example, an individual who is pale may have a decrease in body temperature, whereas a person who appears flushed may have an increase in body temperature.

Certain individuals or racial groups are more aware of subtle changes in skin temperature. In addition, some persons accentuate or take advantage of this medium of communication. For example, an individual knowledgeable about variations in skin temperature according to location may apply perfume to certain parts of the body. The phenomenon of crowding is a chain reaction set in motion when there is not enough space to dissipate the heat within a crowd and the heat intensifies. A hot crowd will require more room than a cool crowd if they are to maintain the same degree of comfort and lack of involvement. It is important for the nurse to remember that when thermal spaces overlap and people can smell each other, they become more involved and may even be under the chemical influences of each other's emotions. Some individuals by virtue of cultural heritage have trouble with the phenomenon of crowding. These individuals are more likely to be unable to sit in a chair soon after someone else has vacated it. An example of this phenomenon is often given by sailors on submarines who are forced to participate in "hot bunking," the practice of sharing a bunk as soon as someone gets out of it. It is not understood why one's own heat is not objectionable whereas a stranger's may be. It may be attributable in part to the fact that humans have a great sensitivity to small differences; therefore, individuals respond negatively to a heat pattern that is not familiar (Hall, 1966, 1969).

Body-heat regulation lies deep in the brain and is controlled by the hypothalamus. Culture affects attitudes in regard to the perception of skin temperature changes.

Human beings exert little or no conscious control over the heat system of the body. Many cultural groups tend to stress phenomena that can be controlled and deny those that cannot. In other words, because some individuals by virtue of their cultural heritage have been taught to ignore certain uncontrollable stimuli, they experience body heat as a highly personal stimulus. Body heat is therefore linked to intimacy as well as to the experiences of childhood. An adult who as a child was used to close personal contact with parents and other loved ones may have a pleasant association when in a crowded environment where heat and warmth are radiated. On the other hand, an adult who was subjected to discomfort in close relationships or who was not exposed to closeness as a child may experience a great deal of difficulty and anxiety when in a close environment, such as an overcrowded bus.

A person born in a heavily populated country where closeness was necessitated by overcrowding may experience conscious discomfort in moving to another locality where closeness is not the norm. On the other hand, persons born in thinly populated countries may have a conscious feeling of overcrowding in a country where closeness is the norm. For example, a tourist from the United States visiting a country such as Jamaica or China or a city such as Hong Kong, all of which are extremely overpopulated, may quickly react to the experience of closeness and associate the country or this particular city with unpleasantness. This experience is not limited to different cultures but may also be noted when a rural person visits an urban setting, such as a person from rural Mississippi visiting New York City.

The English language is full of expressions that relate to skin sensation and body temperature changes. For example, it is not uncommon in the United States to hear individuals say that another person made them hot under the collar, gave them a cold stare, involved them in a heated argument, or warmed them up. These expressions may be more than just a figure of speech; they may be a way of recognizing the changes in body temperature that occur both personally and in other people. Thus, these common experiences have been incorporated into language in the United States.

Relationship between Tactile Space and Visual Space

Touch and visual spatial experiences are so interwoven that they cannot be easily separated. Young children and infants learn to reach, grasp, fondle, and mouth everything in the environment. Teaching children the relationship between tactile and visual space is a difficult task that requires many years of training for children to subordinate the world of touch to the visual world. Visual and tactile space can be distinguished by the fact that tactile space separates the viewer from the object, whereas visual space separates objects from each other. As early as 1945, Michael Baliant described two different perceptual worlds: sight oriented and touch oriented. According to Baliant, the touch-oriented world is both immediate and friendlier than the sight-oriented world, in which space is friendly but filled with dangerous and unpredictable objects—namely, people. Using Baliant's definition of tactile space, it is difficult to conceive that designers and engineers have failed to grasp in all of their scientific research the deep significance of touch, particularly active touch (actually contacting others or objects). Individuals incorporate both tactile and visual stimuli in relating to the world. For example, although automakers tend to rely heavily on visual perception when designing a particular car, they are also concerned with tactile perception, as evidenced by their attention to such things as luxury upholstery, automatic windows, doors, gas-cap locks, ornate trimmings, and carpeting. In response to such stimuli, prospective buyers touch both the car's interior and exterior before making a purchase.

Some objects in the environment are appraised and appreciated almost entirely by touch, even when these objects are visually presented, such as objects made from wood, cloth, or ceramics. The Japanese are very conscious of the significance of texture. Emphasis is placed on the smoothness of the item being crafted. It may be perceived that it requires more time to make a smooth-textured item than a rough-textured item and that the time spent on the crafted item is related to the care and concern of the craftsman. The objects that are produced by Japanese people may be perceived as being made by caring craftsmen.

Touch is the most personal of all the sensations. Touch is sometimes described as the most important sense because it confirms the reality perceived through the other senses (Montagu, 1986). As discussed in Chapter 2, touch is central to the human communication process and is often used to communicate messages. Touch is a part of most intimate relationships, which are increasingly recognized as integral to health. Although relationships can exist without touch, distance creates loneliness, which has been related to lack of health (Cacioppo et al., 2000). James Lynch, author of *The Broken Heart: The Medical Consequences of Loneliness,* noted that there is a cardioprotective nature of community life and loving relationships (Lynch, 1998). In fact, studies have found that loneliness at the time of surgery is a contributor to death at both 30 days and 5 years following coronary artery bypass grafting and that the recurrent cardiac event rate at 6 months after initial myocardial infarction was significantly higher among those who lived alone (Case, Moss, Case, McDermott, & Eberly, 1992; Herlitz et al., 1998). Positive intimate relationships increase longevity, lower morbidity, and increase personal happiness (Giorgianni, 2000).

In contrast to tactile space is the phenomenon of visual space. To understand visual space, the nurse must understand that people do not see exactly the same thing when actively using their eyes in a natural situation; people do not relate to the world around them in exactly the same way. For example, different persons will visually notice different objects because of perceptual differences (Davidhizar, Dowd, & Giger, 1997). It is important for the nurse to recognize these differences and at the same time be able to translate from one perceptual world to another. The distance between the perceptual worlds of two persons of the same culture may be considerably less than the distance between the perceptual worlds of two persons of different cultures. There is significant evidence that people brought up in different cultures live in different perceptual worlds. North Americans tend to have a more linear perceptual field. This difference is demonstrated in art and architectural design. American artists prefer designs that are linear, whereas Chinese and Japanese artists prefer depth and maintaining constancy in a design.

SPATIAL BEHAVIOR

Spatial behavior is often described in nursing literature in relation to the universal need for territoriality (Allekian, 1973; Brant, 1983; Davidhizar, 1988; Davidhizar & Giger, 1998; Oland, 1978). People by nature are territorial. *Territoriality* refers to a state characterized by possessiveness, control, and authority over an area of physical space. If the need for territoriality is to be met, the person must be in control of some space and must be able to establish rules for that space. The need for territoriality cannot be fully met unless individuals can defend their space against invasion or misuse by others (Roberts, 1978). Hayter (1981) has suggested three important aspects of territoriality to consider when planning nursing care: a physical space of one's own, a personal space, and the territory of expertise or role. One can also relate territoriality needs to spatial behaviors of or proximity to others, to objects in the environment, and to body movement or position. Territoriality serves to achieve diverse functions for individuals, including meeting needs for security, privacy, autonomy, and self-identity. Group rights must also be considered in relation to space. In cultures where priority is given to the group over the individual (Asian cultures, many Latino and Mediterranean cultures, most Arab cultures, and cultures of Africa and the Middle East), group rights and shared space are important considerations. In cultures where priority is given to the individual rather than the group (United States, Canada, cultures of North and West Europe,

Australia, and New Zealand), privacy is more likely to be valued (Goldman & Schmalz, 2005). In a culture where priority is given to the individual, a person may choose to be alone when feeling ill or in pain (Davidhizar & Hart, 2005). Palos, a multicultural researcher at the Department of Symptom Research at the University of Texas M. D. Anderson Cancer Center and School of Public Health in Houston, states that finding 20 relatives at the bedside arises out of the concept of collectivity rather than polarity and may be a strange concept to health care professionals oriented to the biomedical model based on autonomy (Kaegi, 2004). It is important for the nurse to understand the effect such variables may have on spatial behavior and the ethical implications (Piaschenko, 1997).

Proximity to Others

Proxemics is the term for the study of human use and perception of social and personal space (Hall, 1974). Individuals tend to divide surrounding space into regions of front, back, right, and left (Franklin, Henkel, & Zangas, 1995). The front region is considered the most important, is the largest, is recalled with the greatest precision, and is described with the greatest detail. Proxemics has been shown to allow one to predict self-esteem and self-evaluative moods, even after controlling for the contribution of the personality dimensions of neuroticism, extroversion, and agreeableness (Hart, Field, Garfinkle, & Singer, 1997). Physical distancing from others varies with setting and is culturally learned (Murray & Huelskoetter, 1991). Generally, in Western culture there are three primary dimensions of space: the intimate zone (0 to 18 inches), the personal zone (18 inches to 3 feet), and the social or public zone (3 to 6 feet) (Hall, 1966). The intimate zone may be used for comforting, protecting, and counseling and is reserved for people who feel close. The personal zone usually is maintained with friends or in some counseling interactions. Touch can occur in the intimate and personal zones. The social zone is usually used when impersonal business is conducted or with people who are working together. Sensory involvement and communication are often less intense in the social zone. Wide variations to these general dimensions do occur and are often influenced by cultural background (Giger & Davidhizar, 1990). Montagu (1986) has suggested that childrearing practices affecting sleep behavior may have an effect on the use of space, especially as it determines acceptable interaction distance. He reported on varying cultural approaches apparently related to family group sleeping arrangements and the Western middle-class practice of separating the child from parents for sleep. According to Oland (1978), the Western practice of putting small children in a room of their own, which separates them from other family members, may enculturate children to desire isolation and separation and cause or facilitate a desire for more extensive territory.

Among the Eskimos and Northern Indians of Canada, the practice of separate bedrooms varies dramatically because living quarters are often small, with all persons sleeping in the same room (Burke, Maloney, Pothaar, & Baumgart, 1988; Giger & Davidhizar, 1998; Young, 1988). For these individuals, proximity to others in small living quarters is often a necessity for survival since staying inside and near the body heat of others may be necessary to avoid freezing in the frigid arctic temperatures. The need for space also varies for many Southeast Asian immigrants who have come to the United States as refugees. These individuals are also accustomed to living in crowded living situations. Therefore, for some Southeast Asian Americans, spacious living accommodations may cause discomfort (Van Esterik, 1980). Sinha and Mukherjee (1996) investigated college students at Dayalbagh, India, and noted that more roommates led to larger space requirements, decreased tolerance for crowding, and a more negative attitude toward room environment. However, high cooperation among roommates moderated the effects of crowding. Walkey and Gilmour (1984) noted that a preferred interpersonal distance score in inmates was effective in predicting prison fighting behavior with a 71% degree of success.

Spatial needs and the desire for a certain proximity to certain people continue through life and have been studied in the elderly. In nursing homes, elderly clients may have certain chairs identified as theirs and become upset when a stranger sits in that chair or in the seat nearby that is reserved for a special friend. Moving from household to household to stay with adult children on a rotating basis, rather than being viewed as a pleasant variation, is also likely to be upsetting to older people. Since the elderly are more likely to experience separation from others through the death of a spouse and the moving away of offspring, their spatial needs may appear to change; that is, they may withdraw or may reach out more for others (Ittelson, Proshansky, Rivlin, & Winkel, 1974).

Interpersonal messages are communicated not only by body proximity but also by the location and availability of the nurse during the day. A client who knows that the nurse will answer when the call bell is pressed feels differently from the client who does not understand how the call bell works or feels that it is an imposition to ask for help and waits for the nurse to ask what can be done (Schuster & Ashburn, 1992).

Individuals have different requirements for sensory stimulation. Either overstimulation, as by crowding, or understimulation, as by isolation, may cause an untoward reaction. For example, in times of disaster, overstimulation induced by crowding can be so extreme that it can result in insanity or death. In this example, a person is perceived as being in a little black figure and unable to move about freely, which causes the person to jostle, push, and shove. How the individual responds to jostling and therefore to the enclosed space depends on how he or she feels about being touched by strangers. This constant touching and being touched may result in widespread panic and "freezing" in disaster situations (Hall, 1966).

An enclosed space requirement can also be overstimulating. For example, a client who must remain in a hospital room in bed and in isolation for a lengthy period can be overstimulated because of the spatial limits presented by the boundaries, including bed rest and the four walls of the room. Nursing interventions for this client include opening curtains, frequently calling by intercom to check on the client, and stopping by to see the client as often as possible. A client in isolation can suffer from understimulation in regard to tactile stimulation. The few people who do enter the room may hesitate to touch the client out of fear of contracting the illness. One of the greatest problems expressed by clients with acquired immunodeficiency syndrome (AIDS) is the isolation they experience because of physical distance from others. Family members afraid of catching AIDS may hesitate to touch, hug, or kiss the AIDS victim. Caregivers also may show their fear by standing a greater distance from the client, wearing gloves, and having less frequent encounters with the client (Zook & Davidhizar, 1989). How individuals perceive and interact with human immunodeficiency virus (HIV) risk varies by a myriad of social, contextual, and setting-related issues (Brown & Maycock, 2005). The strong link between curing, the major focus of health care, and caring by health care practitioners has been emphasized by Leininger and McFarland (2006), who cite touch as one of the special constructs of the caring process. As a therapeutic element of human interaction, touch can help the nurse to show caring. Marx, Wener, and Cohen-Mansfield (1989) noted a divergent response to touch among elderly in a nursing home. For some, touching was interpreted as a violation of personal space, while at other times touching was perceived as a comforting form of communication.

The image of the nurse as someone standing close to the bedside and having physical proximity is changing. Within the wider discourse of fiscal restraint on health care spending, professional nurses need not be in physical proximity for meanings to be generated, to be acted upon, and to have effects in the present. Modern technology is redefining the need for physical proximity. The needs of modern health care are redefining where the nurse's presence needs to be to accomplish the needs of professional nursing (Purkis, 1996).

Cultural Implications

Watson (1980) noted that although there are variations in spatial requirements from person to person, individuals in the same cultural group tend to act similarly. For example, nomads do not seem to desire a permanent territory but are content with establishing a temporary territory and then moving on. Because individuals are usually not consciously aware of their personal space requirements, they frequently have difficulty understanding a different cultural pattern. What may be considered an act of friendliness by one person (such as standing close to another person) may be perceived by the other as a threatening invasion of personal space. A person who wishes to maintain distance will indicate this by body language. Clients who step back, do not face the nurse directly, or pull their chair back from the nurse are sending messages indicating additional space requirements. The nurse's responsiveness to the client's spatial requirements is an important factor in the client's emotional comfort. It is important that the nurse be cognizant of the effects of culture on the client's spatial needs and use sensitivity in responding to the client's need for personal territory. Subtle cultural variations in the use of nonverbal signals often lead to misunderstanding; thus, to meet the client's needs, it is essential that the nurse have knowledge of cultural variations in spatial requirements.

Nurses and clients from the population groups of American Indians, Appalachians, Japanese Americans, and Mexican Americans often find a comfortable position between the personal and social distance (Tripp-Reimer & Lively, 1993). Watson (1980) studied cultural differences in the use of personal space. He compiled a range of space by nationality and found that persons in the United States, Canadians, and the British require the most personal space, whereas Latin American, Japanese, and Arabic persons need the least. These latter groups seemingly have a much higher tolerance for crowding in public spaces than some other cultural groups, such as North Americans and northern Europeans, but they also appear to be more concerned about their own requirements for the space they live in. In particular, the Japanese tend to devote more time and attention to the proper organization of their living space for perception by all the senses (Hall, 1966). Asians are generally more sensitive to personal space and are more likely to feel comfortable conversing from a distance of 5 or 6 feet. Maintaining distance for some Asian Americans is an indication of respect. Therefore, it is important to remember to avoid invading the personal space of these individuals. Some West Indians maintain little space between friends when communicating, but for some West Indians, an outsider is expected to maintain some distance when interacting (Carson, 2000). Arab Americans value

modesty and privacy, particularly with strangers. Comfort and personal disclosure are increased if the care provider is of the same sex (Davidhizar & Giger, 2002; Giger, Davidhizar, & Wieczorek, 1993; Meleis, 2006).

A White American female nurse from a nontactile culture may experience discomfort when a male client from a tactile culture, such as the Latin American, African-American, or Indonesian cultures, stands in the intimate zone while describing symptoms (Rawlins, Williams, & Beck, 1993; Tripp-Reimer & Friedl, 1977). Touching between persons of the same sex, including men, is more common among Arabs than it is among Americans. However, among some Asian cultures, touch between women is less common. For example, in some Asian cultures women do not shake hands with each other or with men (Randall-David, 1989). In the United States the kind of familiarity common among Arabs may be considered a homosexual pass (Hall, 1966). Hall and Whyte (1990) note that a handshake in Latin America, particularly between two men, is seen as cold and impersonal. For some Latins, the *doble abrazo,* in which two men embrace by placing their arms around each other's shoulders, is the accepted form of greeting. On the other hand, touching the shoulders of a Japanese man is seen as a humiliation and an unpardonable breach of traditional etiquette. Argyle and Dean (1965) reported that members of some societies in Africa and Indonesia also came closer and maintained body contact during conversation.

Abuse and violence involve intrusion on the physical, personal, or cognitive space (verbal functioning or mental strategizing) of another. However, violence is interpreted in a cultural context and according to cultural norms (Burlae, 2004). Wife beatings may not be considered abuse in some cultures. Violence can be subtler. A contemptuous boss may give a female employee an office in the basement or a desk in a public area while male employees have private offices near the employer. This invasion of space carries with it an innuendo that can lead to violence (Burlae, 2004).

In the Thai and Vietnamese cultures, the head is sacred, and patting the head of a small child is considered offensive. For these individuals the head is considered to be the "seat of life." When the head is touched, it is believed that the spirit leaves through this channel. Therefore, when the head needs to be touched for medical reasons, it is important to explain the reason and to ask permission of the adults (Carson, 2000; Randall-David, 1989).

In the United States, a person who stands at a slight angle to another person indicates a body position of readiness to communicate. A desire to exclude a third person can be shown by two persons who face each other directly and have ongoing eye contact. Rejection is also communicated by a person who stands at a right angle to another (Scheflen & Scheflen, 1972). The position of the toes can create distance by communicating rank. A person who feels subordinate will usually stand with the toes inward, whereas a person who feels superior will stand with the toes facing out (*Personal Report,* 1987). A comparison of the movie shown in the United States, *Three Men and a Baby,* and the French comedy on which it was based, *Three Men and a Cradle,* illustrates the differences in responses in the two cultures. In the French version, when the natural father returns to the two bachelors who have been inconvenienced by the care of the baby, icy silence occurs. The two men sit stiffly in their chairs and refuse to answer their friend's questions or even acknowledge his presence. In the version seen in the United States, when the natural father returns, he is pummeled and a loud scene occurs (Grosvenor, 1989).

Territoriality influences relationships between people. Some German people tend to need a larger space and are less flexible in their spatial behavior than some American, French, and Arab people. Differences in spatial patterns between persons in different cultures apply not only to their body proximity but also to such behavior as changing geographic location. For example, Germans often live in the same house their entire lives, whereas Americans tend to change houses approximately every 5 years, and nomads are content with temporary territories rather than permanent ones. According to Evans and Howard (1973), some Puerto Ricans and African-Americans may have different perspectives about space. Some African-Americans have more eye contact when they speak, have greater body activity, and have a closer personal space (Sue & Sue, 2003). However, as indicated in Chapter 2, some African-Americans have been socialized through a long history of hostile, punitive interactions with Whites to avoid direct eye contact. This behavior may also influence personal space zones (Giger, Davidhizar, Evers, & Ingram, 1994).

OBJECTS IN THE ENVIRONMENT

Objects in the environment offer additional dimensions to communication and can provide both positive and negative qualifiers to verbal communication. Easily movable chairs in a waiting room or office can be pulled together to provide physical closeness or separated to provide distance. Positioning chairs at a 90-degree angle can communicate a cooperative stance, whereas a side-by-side arrangement of chairs can decrease communication. Discomfort and, consequently, emotional distance can be created by uncomfortable furniture. The nurse's position during the conversation (such as sitting behind a desk or leaning against the corner of the desk while looking down on the client seated at a lower level) can also promote the perception of psychological distance. Health care icons, such as stethoscope, name tag, uniform, nurse's cap, or lab coat, are also objects that can convey a message to the client about the nurse's authority (Bechtel & Davidhizar, 1998). However, all icons can have positive and negative associations for different individuals—for example, a stethoscope can be associated with a person who cares for a patient, or it may be associated with a stranger who invades personal space (Andrews, 2003). The nurse must be aware of the effect culture may play on the client's reaction to objects in the environment and should respond in a way that increases client comfort. The nurse dealing with Eskimos should appreciate the value Eskimos place on objects they possess. These individuals tend to highly value generosity and a sense of sharing, as in "What is mine is here for all." For some of these people, only what is needed for the present is taken and used. This can be a problem for the Eskimo who is diabetic because if food is available, it will be shared with anyone, regardless of the special health needs (Davidhizar & Giger, 2000).

Cleanliness in the environment may also be a significant factor in creating a healthy and comfortable milieu. This is particularly true in surgical areas, where space is used in designing a physical layout that will allow for maintaining aseptic technique (Fox, 1997). Comfortable air conditioning in a client waiting room on a hot day can facilitate a client's ease and decrease anxiety. On the other hand, when the air conditioning is absent or malfunctioning on a hospital ward on a hot day, client and staff anxiety can escalate.

Structural Boundaries

The term *personal boundaries* is sometimes used to describe the use of structural boundaries in the environment. A boundary separates a person from others and also helps define a person's space. Fences, doors, curtains, walls, desks, chairs, and other objects may create boundaries between persons (Scott, 1988). The purpose of a boundary is to facilitate individuation or separation from the environment. Developmentally, this concept begins at approximately 6 months of age. Mahler, Pine, and Bergman (1975) described an infant's first attempts at separation or individuation as behaviors such as pulling at the parent's hair, ears, or nose and pushing the body away from the parent to get a better look at him or her. At 7 to 8 months of age the infant begins to differentiate self from the parent. The child may examine the parent's jewelry or glasses and is anxious around others. These crucial developmental steps are indicative of the child's beginning formation of boundary, which continues through the toddler stage. By 3 years of age the toddler has a fairly stable sense of identity and self-boundaries.

Doors, walls, glass panels, and waist-high partitions serve as structural boundaries for nurses' territories in health care settings. Doors, curtains, and furniture arrangements may define client territories. Structural boundaries can help the individual adapt to both internal and external stresses. On the other hand, when structural boundaries are violated, anxiety may increase. The nurse needs to assess whether the client has rigid or flexible boundaries. If a client has open boundaries, less anxiety will be encountered in interactions with health professionals that may violate personal boundaries. If the client has rigid boundaries, the nurse should guard against approaches that may be perceived as threatening.

The use of restraints with agitated clients involves physical invasion of both intimate space and body boundaries. This personal invasion may cause patients to resist restraints and become aggressive and combative.

Just as individuals can be described by personal boundaries that determine comfort levels in relation to others, territoriality also describes an interpersonal phenomenon in the environment. As indicated earlier, territoriality is a state characterized by possessiveness, control, and authority over an area of physical space (Hayter, 1981). For the need for territoriality to be met fully, the person must be in control of some space, be able to establish rules for that space, and be able to defend it against invasion or misuse by others. In addition, the person's right to do things in the space must be acknowledged by others (Roberts, 1978). For example, a hospitalized client needs not only a personal sleeping area but also a place to put and arrange personal belongings without fear that they will be disturbed by others. The nurse should respect patient privacy and knock before entering the room (Stuart, 2005).

Nurses also have professional territorial imperatives. Nurses' stations and lounges may be designated as staff territory. When a psychiatric unit is renovated and the staff are asked by the administration to change from a locked-nursing station to an open-nursing station so that clients may come to an open half-wall to interact openly with staff who may be inside, the staff may find this very intrusive of "their" territory and object to this invasion of their space. Nursing staff may also fear personal assault (Croker & Cummings, 1995; Roberts, 1989, 1991). McMahon (1994) noted that, for psychiatric staff, space in the ward office serves several significant functions, including the opportunity for informal contact between nurses and a place to have a liaison with visiting professionals, to store possessions, to provide a "patient-free" zone, and to serve as a communication center. Staff needs for territory must be considered when unit staff and clients' areas are designed. Restricting certain staff from certain hospital areas (such as the mailroom or the copy machine room) may be seen as punitive and dehumanizing. Thus, it is essential that explanations given for this restriction be clearly understood to avoid paranoid interpretations of this action.

Cultural Implications

Color is a phenomenon with cultural implications. In many North American cultures, warm colors such as yellow, red, and orange tend to stimulate creative and happy responses. In some Asian countries, white is associated with a funeral. In many African countries, red symbolizes witchcraft and death (Carson, 2000). In the dominant culture in the United States, good mental health is often associated with the ability to coordinate the color of one's wardrobe (Ramírez, 1991). In contrast, in some countries, including those in Africa, the Caribbean, and the South Pacific, bright, multiple colors are the accepted norm of dress (Carson, 2000). Leff and Isaacs (1996) noted that a scarf tied around the forehead may not indicate "royalty" or schizophrenia but the cultural response by a West Indian to a headache. In Western culture, cool colors such as blue, green, and gray tend to encourage meditation and deliberation and thus may have a dampening effect on communication. The nurse should plan color in the environment to be therapeutic in an effort to enhance communication (Bartholet, 1968; Mufford, 1992).

For clients who have a chronic disability with difficulty in moving, it is important that space in the living environment be arranged to maximize power and use of resources (Moss, 1997). Access and ability to negotiate space in the living environment can be critical to quality of life and maximum independence (Useh, Moyo, & Munyonga, 2001). Space can also be used to promote health. Andersen, Franckowiak, Snyder, Bartlett, and Fontaine (1998) reported that signs promoting the health and weight-control benefits of stair use as a community intervention significantly increased the physical activity of 17,901 persons in a shopping mall. However, more lean persons as compared with overweight persons, and more Whites than Blacks, changed their behavior as a result of the sign intervention.

BODY MOVEMENT OR POSITION

Body movement or position can also communicate a message to others. This concept has been well documented by the pioneering work of Efron (1941), Birdwhitstell (1970), Scheflen and Scheflen (1972), Ekman and Friesen (1975), and Ekman (2001) and by other reviews of the state of the art in this field (Bull, 1983; Davis, 1975; Davis & Skupien, 1982; Hickson & Stacks, 2002; Leathers, 1997; Wolfgang, 1984). This information has also been applied to counseling and psychotherapeutic techniques through the work of Moreno (1946), Gendlin (1969), Steere (1982),

Marcus (1985), and Perls, Hefferline, and Goodman (1983), all of whom made body movement and awareness central aspects of their therapeutic approach. Thus, a broad body of knowledge supports the premise that through body movement, a person may convey what is not verbalized.

It is well known that body movements may be of particular importance during periods of stress. Expressions of self through movement are learned before speech; therefore, when stress is experienced, a person may revert to a form of expression used at an earlier level. Attention to body movement can facilitate understanding of a person experiencing stress. There are endless expressions of body movement, such as finger pointing, head nodding, smiles, slaps on the back, head and general body movements, and even body sounds, including belching, knuckle cracking, and laughing. A seemingly insignificant act, such as how a doorbell is rung, may bear the stamp of an individual's personality as well as an emotional state. For example, the doorbell may be rung loudly, impatiently, repetitively, tentatively, feebly, or aggressively (Bendich, 1988).

The nurse must also consider the effect of slow versus fast movements (Newman, 1976). In an emergency, rapid movements are essential. On the other hand, a young child in the hospital for the first time may be frightened by a health professional who enters the room quickly, approaches the child rapidly, and immediately picks up the child. In another situation, an agitated psychiatric client who is approached slowly and with a quiet voice may be calmed by the slow movements of the nurse, which are seen as reassuring.

Nurses are also exploring movement as a therapeutic medium, such as movement therapy for the aged (Goldberg & Fitzpatrick, 1980; Stevenson, 1989), movement therapy after inactivity or infection (Folta, 1989; Kasper, 1989), dance and movement therapy, and exercise to music. It has been thought that movement therapy can provide a way to communicate when the ability to communicate feelings is limited. Movement therapy has also been used for relaxation and to provide relief of blocked emotion.

Body motions, or kinetic behaviors, can be categorized as follows (Knapp & Hall, 1992):

1. *Emblems.* Nonverbal actions that have a verbal translation into a word, phrase, or symbol. They include sign language used in the operating room or the gesture of thumb and forefinger to form a circle to say "A-OK" in the United States or to indicate an obscenity in Brazil.
2. *Affect displays.* Facial expressions, such as a frown, a smile, or lips pulled down at the corners.
3. *Illustrations.* Nonverbal acts accompanying speech. Examples include an upturned thumb to indicate that a ride is desired or pointing a finger to indicate a direction.
4. *Adapters.* Nonverbal behavior that modifies or adds to what is being said. For example, folded arms may indicate disgust or that a person is feeling closed to others; a wave may be used as a friendly greeting; leg swinging and finger tapping may indicate anxiety.
5. *Regulators.* Movements that maintain interaction and provide feedback. Head nods or changing gaze can indicate that it is the other person's turn to talk. A head nod can also indicate listening.

Cultural Implications

Body movement is also related to culture. For example, in the United States head nodding is common, whereas in Africa the torso is frequently moved (Eibl-Eibesfeldt, 1972). Gestures are used by Americans and the British to denote activity and by Italian or Jewish persons to emphasize words (Bigham, 1964). In some cultures, certain actions are not considered proper with strangers, such as touching, standing close to, or looking directly at the individual. Some cultures give certain body movements a sexual interpretation. In the Western culture, stroking the hair, adjusting the clothes, or changing position to accent maleness or femaleness may have or be given a sexual connotation (Scheflen & Scheflen, 1972). Although a kiss is often given a sexual connotation in the United States, the Japanese kiss to show deference to superiors (Sue & Sue, 2003). When Brazilian clients were compared with American clients for space and motion discomfort in relation to anxiety disorders, a country bias was noted. Brazilian clients were more likely than American clients to endorse symptoms, thus showing a transcultural bias (Romas, Jacob, & Lilienfeld, 1997).

IMPLICATIONS FOR NURSING CARE

Nurses can create a healing environment by influencing a client's inner personal space as well as by creating a therapeutic outer space for the client to occupy (Birx, 2002). It is important for the nurse to remember that the need for space serves four functions: security, privacy, autonomy, and self-identity (Oland, 1978). The nurse needs an understanding of cultural diversity and culturally appropriate behaviors in relation to these functions. Security includes actual safety from harm and giving the person a feeling of being safe. The nurse must also remember that if a client is in a place where a feeling of control is experienced, the client will feel safer, less threatened, and less anxious (Sheeshka et al., 2001). People generally tend to feel safer in their own territory because it is arranged and equipped in a familiar manner. In addition, most people believe there is a degree of predictability associated with being in one's own personal space and that this degree of predictability is hard to achieve elsewhere. Nurses must also remember that the anxiety level of a client is increased when the client is hospitalized. However, the same client may experience a decrease in anxiety if the client is allowed to return home, even if still sick. Some terminally ill clients request to go home because of the feeling of security experienced in one's own personal space.

In addition to security, personal space provides privacy and at the same time protected communication. Most people believe it is not necessary to be on guard or to keep up pretenses—not be themselves—in the security of one's personal space. The fulfillment of the desire to be oneself contributes to feelings of decreased anxiety and promotes relaxation. Many people may complain of feeling tense and tired after a long day at work but may experience relaxation and ease of tension as soon as they get home. Contributing to these feelings are the facts that activities at home are different from those at work and that people experience more relaxation in their personal space (Hayter, 1981). In some instances, hospital staff members tend to treat elevators as private space and make inappropriate comments while riding back and forth on them. Hospital employees need to be very careful to consider certain hospital locations, such as elevators, as public spaces and to guard against violation of client privacy (Ubel et al., 1995). If it becomes necessary to transfer a client from one room to another or from one floor to another, the nurse should remember that the client may experience increased anxiety because of the loss of security and privacy of the room to which the client has become accustomed (Smith, 1976). This feeling of loss of security and privacy can also be related to nursing practice. For example, a nurse manager who returns from vacation to find office furniture rearranged may feel unsettled until the furniture is returned to a familiar arrangement. The nurse should remember that clients may already be experiencing feelings of anxiety that are related to the reasons for seeking health care. Additional anxiety invoked by issues involving territoriality can be minimized by the nurse who develops an understanding of culture and its implications for territoriality or interpersonal space.

Another important aspect of territoriality for nurses is the function of autonomy. Autonomy is the means by which a person controls what happens. In personal territory a person may feel free to ask questions, resist suggested actions, hold out for those things that are most important personally, and share personal feelings. A client, on the other hand, is out of personal territory and lacks control. Therefore, it is important for the nurse to determine if the client has an adequate understanding of the treatment regimen and is not submitting to treatment merely because of a lack of control of territory. Statements to the client that maximize feelings of control, such as "How do you want to

CASE STUDY

Mr. Bernhard Wolfgang, a 56-year-old German immigrant who works as an engineer, is admitted with chest pain and shortness of breath. Mr. Wolfgang is admitted to the coronary care unit to rule out myocardial infarction. Immediately after admission, Mr. Wolfgang's wife comes to the coronary care unit with personal items such as family portraits, some roses from the client's garden, and some personal clothing. However, since the coronary care unit is restricted in space, personal items are not allowed and the wife is instructed to take the items home. On admission, Mr. Wolfgang's vital signs are stable and his color is good. He reports that the chest pain is not debilitating and is more or less an occasional dull ache. After 2 days, the diagnosis of myocardial infarction is confirmed, and Mr. Wolfgang remains restricted to bed but is transferred to a semi-private room in the coronary care step-down unit. After admission to the coronary care step-down unit, the nurse observes that Mr. Wolfgang is anxious, somewhat withdrawn, and unable to express his needs and feelings.

arrange the room?" or "Are you concerned about your treatment? We can walk down the hall to the visiting room, where it is private, to discuss your feelings," should promote feelings of security and autonomy for the client. Feelings of autonomy are also evidenced in nursing practice. For example, when a nurse manager needs to counsel an employee, the manager's control will be maximized if the counseling occurs in the manager's office. On the other hand, a manager who is viewed as too controlling may intentionally select a more neutral territory for the counseling, such as a conference room.

It is essential to remember that having personal space promotes self-identity by affording opportunities for self-expression and that personal well-being is often related to the critical distance a person keeps from others (Giger & Davidhizar, 2001; Giger, Davidhizar, Johnson, & Poole, 1997; Wilson & Kneisl, 1995). Another way to define self-identity in relation to personal space is to view self-identity as a mode of individuality. The personal space over which a person has jurisdiction often becomes a personal extension of self and a reflection of characteristics, personality, and interest. A nurse may communicate warmth and reduce feelings of anxiety by moving close to a client. On the other hand, rapidly moving toward an anxious client may dramatically increase the client's anxiety. People have a need to organize and arrange personal space so that it maximizes functioning and at the same time meets needs. For example, when a person purchases a new home, it becomes essential for that home to take on the person's identity. This is evidenced by the desire of the new occupants to change such items as the wallpaper, colors of the walls, carpet, lighting fixtures, and draperies. Regardless of whether these items are new, each person has a need for self-expression or individuality. When clients set out personal pictures of their family and other personal items from home and wear their own sleepwear, self-identity is enhanced. Therefore, changing items to reflect this individuality becomes an essential aspect of personal security and autonomy. Self-identity is also created by the nurse when he or she is negotiating symbolic space.

CLINICAL DECISION MAKING

1. When assessing Mr. Wolfgang, the nurse should realize that some German people have specific needs that are related to territoriality and space. Name at least two factors that affect some Germans and their spatial behavior.
2. List ways the nurse could enable Mr. Wolfgang to meet his needs for privacy and autonomy while in a semiprivate room.
3. Identify markers that would indicate Mr. Wolfgang's need for the establishment of a temporary territorial space.
4. Identify ways in which illness and hospitalization could threaten Mr. Wolfgang's personal sense of territoriality.
5. Identify factors present in a coronary care unit that could negatively affect spatial behavior.
6. List two factors related to perceptual and visual stimuli that adversely affect some German clients.
7. List ways the nurse could control perceptual and verbal stimuli that may affect Mr. Wolfgang.

REVIEW QUESTIONS

1. Encouraging clients to set out personal items and wear their own sleepwear is a means of promoting which of the following?
   a. Personal space
   b. Self-identity
   c. Visual space
   d. Autonomy
2. Because touching the head has specific meaning in the Vietnamese culture, before measuring the head circumference of a child, the nurse should:
   a. Explain the procedure and ask permission of the parent.

b. Play a game with the child.
c. Provide privacy by pulling the curtains.
d. Sit the child on the parent's lap.
3. When assessing an Asian client, the best way to obtain information is to:
   a. Use an interest approach to get information.
   b. Ask questions through an interpreter.
   c. Ask family members to answer questions.
   d. Ask short-answer questions.

REFERENCES

Allekian, C. E. (1973). Intrusions of territory and personal space. *Nursing Research, 22,* 236–241.

Andersen, R., Franckowiak, S., Snyder, J., Bartlett, S., & Fontaine, K. (1998). Can inexpensive signs encourage the use of stairs? Results from a community intervention. *Annals of Internal Medicine, 129,* 363–369.

Andrews, G. (2002). Towards a more place-sensitive nursing research: an invitation to medical and health geography. *Nursing Inquiry, 9*(4), 221–238.

Andrews, G. (2003). Locating a geography of nursing: space, place and the progress of geographical thought. *Nursing Philosophy, 4*(3), 231–248.

Andrews, G. J., & Phillips, D. (2002). Changing local geographies of private residential care for older people 1983–1999: lessons for social policy in England and Wales. *Social Science and Medicine, 55,* 63–78.

Andrews, G. J. P., & Andrews, G. J. (2003). Life in a secure unit: the rehabilitation of young people through the use of sport. *Social Science and Medicine, 56,* 531–550.

Argyle, M., & Dean, J. (1965). Eye-contact, distance, and affiliation. *Sociometry, 28,* 289–304.

Baliant, M. (1945). *Individual differences of behavior in early infancy.* London: Dissertation for Master of Science in Psychology.

Bartholet, M. (1968). Effects of color on dynamics of patient care. *Nursing Outlook, 6*(10), 51–53.

Bechtel, G., & Davidhizar, R. (1998). *Culture, personal space, and health. Competence matters.* Birmingham, AL: University of Alabama at Birmingham.

Bendich, S. (1988). Appreciating bodily phenomena in verbally oriented psychotherapy sessions. *Issues in Mental Health Nursing, 9,* 1–7.

Bigham, C. (1964). To communicate with Negro patients. *American Journal of Nursing, 64*(9), 113–115.

Birdwhitstell, R. (1970). *Kinesics and context: essays on body motion communication.* Philadelphia: University of Pennsylvania Press.

Birx, E. (2002). *Healing Zen.* Ontario, Canada: Viking Compass.

Black, J. W. (1950). The effect of room characteristics on vocalizations and rate. *Journal of Acoustical Society in America, 22,* 174–176.

Brant, C. (1983). *Native ethics and rules of behavior.* London, Ontario: University of Western Ontario.

Brown, G., & Maycock, B. (2005). Different spaces, same faces: Perth gay men's experiences of sexuality, risk and HIV. *Culture, Health and Sexuality, 7*(1), 59–72.

Brown, J. W., Leavitt, L., & Graham, F. (1977). Response to auditory stimuli in six- and nine-week-old infants. *Developmental Psychobiology, 10*, 255–266.

Bull, P. (1983). *Body movement and interpersonal communication.* New York: John Wiley & Sons.

Burke, S., Maloney, R., Pothaar, D., & Baumgart, A. (1988). *Four views of childbearing and child health care: northern Indians, urban natives, urban Euro-Canadians and nurses.* A report for the National Health Research Development Program, Health and Welfare Canada.

Burlae, K. (2004). The theory of mindful space. *Identifying, Understanding, and Preventing Violence, 19*(1), 85–98.

Cacioppo, J., et al. (2000). Lonely traits and concomitant physiological process: the MacArthur social neuroscience studies. *International Journal of Psychophysiology, 35*, 143–154.

Carson, V. (2000). *Mental health nursing: the nurse-patient journey* (2nd ed.). Philadelphia: Saunders.

Case, R., Moss, A., Case, N., McDermott, M., & Eberly, S. (1992). Living alone after myocardial infarction. *Journal of the American Medical Association, 267s*, 515–519.

Croker, K., & Cummings, A. (1995). Nurses' reactions to physical assault by their patients. *Canadian Journal of Nursing Research, 27*(2), 81–93.

Davidhizar, R. (1988). Distance in managerial encounters. *Today's OR Nurse, 10*(10), 23–30.

Davidhizar, R., Dowd, S., & Bowen, M. (1998). The educational role of the surgical nurse with the multicultural patient and family. *Today's Surgical Nurse, 20*(4), 20–22.

Davidhizar, R., Dowd, S., & Giger, J. (1997). Model for cultural diversity in the radiology department. *Radiology Technology, 68*(3), 233–240.

Davidhizar, R., & Giger, J. (1998). *Canadian transcultural nursing: assessment and intervention.* St. Louis: Mosby.

Davidhizar, R., & Giger, J. (2000). Culture and care: profiling Alaskan Eskimos. *Health Traveler: The Magazine for Healthcare Travel Professionals, 7*(4), 43–47.

Davidhizar, R., & Giger, J. (2002). Cultural issues. *Advances for Nurses*, 37–38.

Davidhizar, R., & Hart, A. (2005). Pain management. *Healthcare Traveler, 13*(6), 3–41.

Davidhizar, R., & Shearer, R. (2002). Helping children cope with public disasters. *American Journal of Nursing, 102*(3), 26–32.

Davidhizar, R., Shearer, R., & Giger, J. (2002). The challenges of cross-cultural communication. *RT Image, 15*(11), 18–20.

Davis, M. (1975). *Towards understanding the intrinsic in body movement.* New York: Ayer.

Davis, M., & Skupien, J. (1982). *Body movement and nonverbal communication: an annotated bibliography, 1971–1981.* Bloomington: Indiana University Press.

Efron, D. (1941). *Gesture and environment: a tentative study of the spatio-temporal and "linguistic" aspects of the gestural behavior of Eastern Jews and Southern Italians in New York City living in similar as well as different environmental conditions.* New York: King's Crown Press.

Eibl-Eibesfeldt, I. (1972). Similarities and differences between cultures in expressive movements. In R. A. Hinde (Ed.), *Nonverbal communication* (pp. 297–312). Cambridge, England: Cambridge University Press.

Ekman, P. (2001). *Telling lies: clues to deceit in the marketplace, politics, and marriage.* New York: W. W. Norton.

Ekman, P., & Friesen, W. (1975). *Unmasking the face: a guide to recognizing emotions from facial clues.* Englewood Cliffs, NJ: Prentice Hall.

Evans, G. W., & Howard, R. B. (1973). Personal space. *Psychological Bulletin, 80*, 335–344.

Folta, A. (1989, April 3). *Exercise and functional capacity after myocardial infarction.* Paper presented at the 13th annual Midwest Nursing Research Society Conference, Cincinnati, Ohio.

Fox, N. J. (1997). Space, sterility, and surgery: circuits of hygiene in the operating theater. *Social Science & Medicine, 45*(5), 649–657.

Franklin, N., Henkel, L., & Zangas, T. (1995). Parsing surrounding space into regions. *Memory and Cognition, 23*(4), 397–407.

Gendlin, E. T. (1969). Focusing. *American Journal of Psychotherapy, 1*, 1–18.

Giger, J., & Davidhizar, R. (1990). Culture and space. *Advancing Critical Care, 5*(8), 8–11.

Giger, J., & Davidhizar, R. (1998). *Canadian transcultural nursing, assessment, and intervention.* St. Louis: Mosby.

Giger, J., & Davidhizar, R. (2001). Diversity in caring. In P. Potter & A. Perry (Eds.), *Fundamentals in nursing* (5th ed.). St. Louis: Mosby.

Giger, J., Davidhizar, R., Evers, S., & Ingram, C. (1994). Cultural factors influencing mental health and mental illness. In C. Taylor (Ed.), *Mereness' essentials of psychiatric nursing* (14th ed., pp. 215–238). St. Louis: Mosby.

Giger, J., Davidhizar, R., Johnson, J., & Poole, V. (1997). The changing face of America. *Health Care Traveler, 4*(4), 11–17.

Giger, J., Davidhizar, R., & Wieczorek, S. (1993). Culture and ethnicity. In I. Bobak, M. Jensen, & D. Lowdermilk (Eds.), *Maternity and gynecologic care: the nurse and the family* (5th ed.). St. Louis: Mosby.

Giorgianni, S. (2000). *Intimate relationships: a vital component of health.* New York: Pfizer.

Goldberg, W., & Fitzpatrick, J. (1980). Movement therapy with the aged. *Nursing Research, 29*, 339–346.

Goldman, K., & Schmalz, K. (2005). E = MC^2: effective multicultural communication. *Health Promotion Practice, 6*(3), 237–239.

Gregg, J. (1996). *Communication and culture: a reading and writing text* (4th ed.). Boston: Heinle.

Grosvenor, G. M. (1989). Viva la différence [President's editorial]. *National Geographic, 15.*

Halford, S., & Leonard, P. (2003). Space and place in the construction and performance of gendered nursing identities. *Journal of Advanced Nursing, 42*(2), 201–208.

Hall, E. T. (1966). *The silent language.* New York: Anchor Books.

Hall, E. T. (1969). *The hidden dimension*. New York: Anchor Books.

Hall, E. T. (1974). Proxemics. In S. Weitz (Ed.), *Nonverbal communication* (2nd ed.). New York: Oxford University Press.

Hall, E. T. (1977). *Beyond culture*. New York: Anchor Books.

Hall, E., & Whyte, W. (1990). Interpersonal communication: a guide to men of action. In P. J. Brink (Ed.), *Transcultural nursing: a book of readings*. Prospect Heights, IL: Waveland Press.

Hart, D., Field, N., Garfinkle, J., & Singer, J. (1997). Representations of self and others: a semantic space model. *Journal of Personality*, 65(1), 77–105.

Hayter, J. (1981). Territoriality as a universal need. *Journal of Advanced Nursing*, 6, 79–85.

Herlitz, J., et al. (1998). The feeling of loneliness prior to coronary artery bypass grafting might be a predictor of short- and long-term postoperative morbidity. *European Journal of Vascular and Endovascular Surgery*, 16, 120–125.

Hickson, M. L., & Stacks, D. W. (2002). *Nonverbal communication: studies and applications* (4th ed.). Los Angeles: Roxbury.

Ittelson, W., Proshansky, H., Rivlin, I., & Winkel, H. (1974). *An introduction to environmental psychology*. New York: Holt, Rinehart, & Winston.

Kaegi, L. (2004 Summer). What color is your pain? *Minority Nurse*, 28–35.

Kasper, C. (1989). *Exercise-induced degeneration of skeletal muscle following inactivity*. Paper presented at the 13th annual Midwest Nursing Research Society Conference. Cincinnati, OH.

Knapp, M., & Hall, J. (1992). *Nonverbal communication in human interaction* (3rd ed.). New York: Holt, Rinehart, & Winston.

Leathers, D. B. (1997). *Successful nonverbal communication: principles and applications* (3rd ed.). Boston: Allyn & Bacon.

Leff, J., & Isaacs, A. (1996). *Psychiatric examination in clinical practice* (3rd ed.). Boston: Blackwell Scientific.

Leininger, M., & McFarland, M. (2006). *Cultural care diversity and universality* (2nd ed.). Sudbury, MA: Jones and Bartlett.

Lynch, J. J. (1998). Decoding the language of the heart: developing a physiology of inclusion. *Integrative Physiological and Behavioral Science*, 33, 130–136.

Mahler, M., Pine, F., & Bergman, A. (1975). *The psychological birth of the human infant: symbiosis and individuation*. New York: Basic Books.

Marcus, N. (1985). Utilization of nonverbal expressive behavior in cognitive therapy. *American Journal of Psychotherapy*, 39(4), 467–478.

Marx, M., Wener, P., & Cohen-Mansfield, J. (1989). Agitation and touch in the nursing home. *Psychological Reports*, 64(3 Pt. 2), 1019–1026.

McMahon, B. (1994). The functions of space. *Journal of Advanced Nursing*, 19, 362–366.

Meleis, A. (2006). Arabs. In J. Lipson & S. Dibble (Eds.), *Culture and clinical care*. San Francisco: UCSF Nursing Press.

Montagu, A. (1986). *Touching: the human significance of the skin*. New York: Harper & Row.

Moreno, J. L. (1946). *Psychodrama* (Vol. 1). New York: Beacon House.

Moss, P. (1997). Negotiating spaces in home environments: older women living with arthritis. *Social Science Medicine*, 45(1), 23–33.

Mufford, C. (1992). A cure of many colors. *The New Physician*, 14–19.

Murray, R., & Huelskoetter, M. (1991). *Psychiatric-mental health nursing: giving emotional care* (3rd ed.). Norwalk, CT: Appleton & Lange.

Newman, M. (1976). Movement therapy and the experience of time. *Nursing Research*, 25, 273–279.

Oland, L. (1978). The need for territoriality. In H. Yura & M. B. Walsh (Eds.), *Human needs and the nursing process*. Norwalk, CT: Appleton-Century-Crofts.

O'Shea, R. P., Roeber, U., & Bach, M. (2010). Evoked potentials: vision. In E. B. Goldstein (Ed.), *Encyclopedia of perception* (pp. 399–400). Los Angeles: Sage.

Perls, F. S., Hefferline, R., & Goodman, P. (1983). *Gestalt therapy*. New York: Dell.

Personal Report for the Executive. (1987). New York: National Institute of Business Management.

Piaschenko, J. (1997). Ethics and the geography of the nurse-patient relationship: spatial vulnerable and gendered space. *Scholarly Inquiry of Nursing Practice*, 11(1), 45–59.

Purkis, M. E. (1996). Nursing in quality space. *Nursing Inquiry*, 3(2), 101–111.

Ramírez, M. (1991). *Psychotherapy and counseling with minorities*. New York: Pergamon Press.

Randall-David, E. (1989). *Strategies for working with culturally diverse communities and clients* [Brochure]. Washington, DC: U.S. Department of Health and Human Services.

Rawlins, R., Williams, S., & Beck, C. (1993). *Mental health-psychiatric nursing: a holistic life cycle approach* (3rd ed.). St. Louis: Mosby.

Roberts, S. (1989). *The effects of assault on nurses who have been physically assaulted by their clients*. Toronto, Ontario: University of Toronto.

Roberts, S. (1991). Nurse abuse: a taboo topic. *The Canadian Nurse*, 87(3), 23–25.

Roberts, S. L. (1978). *Behavioral concepts and nursing throughout the life span*. Englewood Cliffs, NJ: Prentice Hall.

Romas, R. T., Jacob, R. G., & Lilienfeld, S. O. (1997). Space and motion discomfort in Brazilian versus American patients with anxiety disorders. *Journal of Anxiety Disorders*, 11(2), 131–139.

Scheflen, A., & Scheflen, A. (1972). *Body language and social order: communication as behavioral control*. Englewood Cliffs, NJ: Prentice Hall.

Schuster, C., & Ashburn, S. (1992). *The process of human development: a holistic lifespan approach* (3rd ed.). New York: Lippincott.

Scott, A. (1988). Human interaction and personal boundaries. *Journal of Psychosocial Nursing*, 26(8), 23–28.

Scott, A., & Dumas, R. (1995). Personal space boundaries: clinical applications in psychiatric mental health nursing. *Perspectives in Psychiatric Care, 31*(3), 14–19.

Sheeshka, J., Potter, B., Norrie, E., Valaitis, R., Adams, G., & Kuczynski, L. (2001). Women's experiences breastfeeding in public places. *Journal of Human Lactation, 17*(1), 81–88.

Simply Stated (1985). *Writing user manuals for Japanese readers*, No. 57.

Sinha, S., & Mukherjee, N. (1996). The effect of perceived cooperation on personal space. *Journal of Social Psychology, 136*(5), 655–657.

Smith, M. (1976). Patient responses to being transferred during hospitalization. *Nursing Research, 25*, 192–196.

Steere, D. A. (1982). *Bodily expressions in psychotherapy*. New York: Brunner/Mazel.

Stevenson, J. (1989). *Exercise in frail elders: findings and methodological issues*. Paper presented at the 13th annual Midwest Nursing Research Society Conference. Cincinnati, OH.

Stuart, G. (2005). Therapeutic nurse patient relationship. In G. Stuart & M. Larai (Eds.), *Principles and practice of psychiatric nursing* (8th ed.). St. Louis: Elsevier.

Sue, D. W., & Sue, D. (2003). *Counseling the culturally diverse: theory and a holistic life cycle approach* (4th ed.). New York: John Wiley.

Thomas, E. (2006). Taken by storm. *Newsweek*, 46–66.

Tripp-Reimer, T., & Friedl, M. (1977). Appalachians: a neglected minority. *Nursing Clinics of North America, 12*(41), 41–54.

Tripp-Reimer, T., & Lively, S. (1993). Cultural considerations in mental health-psychiatric nursing. In R. Rawlins, S. Williams, & C. Beck (Eds.), *Mental health-psychiatric nursing* (3rd ed.). St. Louis: Mosby.

Ubel, P., Zell, M., Miller, D., Fischer, G. S., Peters-Stefani, D., & Arnold, R. M. (1995). Elevator talk: observational study of inappropriate comments in a public space. *American Journal of Medicine, 99*(2), 190–194.

Useh, U., Moyo, A., & Munyonga, E. (2001). Wheelchair accessibility of public buildings in the central business district of Harare, Zimbabwe. *Disability and Rehabilitation, 23*(11), 490–496.

Van Esterik, P. (1980). Cultural factors affecting adjustment of Southeast Asian refugees. In E. Tepper (Ed.), *Southeast Asian exodus: from tradition to resettlement* (pp. 151–172). Ottawa, Ontario: The Canadian Asian Studies Association.

Walkey, F., & Gilmour, R. (1984). The relationship between interpersonal distance and violence in imprisoned offenders. *Criminal Justice and Behavior, 11*(3), 331–340.

Watson, O. M. (1980). *Proxemic behavior: a cross-cultural study*. The Hague, the Netherlands: Mouton.

Wilson, H., & Kneisl, C. (1995). *Psychiatric nursing* (5th ed.). Reading, MA: Addison-Wesley.

Wolfgang, A. (Ed.). (1984). *Nonverbal behavior: perspectives, applications, and intercultural insights*. Lewiston, New York: C. J. Hogrete.

Young, T. (1988). *Health care and cultural change: the Indian experience in the central subarctic*. Toronto: University of Toronto Press.

Zook, R., & Davidhizar, R. (1989). Caring for the psychiatric inpatient with AIDS. *Perspectives in Psychiatric Nursing Care, 25*(2), 3–8.

4

Social Organization

After reading this chapter, the nurse will be able to:

1. Describe how cultural behavior is acquired in a social setting.
2. Define selected terms unique to the concept of social organization, such as *culture-bound, ethnocentrism, homogeneity, bicultural, biracial, ethnicity, race, ethnic people of color, minority,* and *stereotyping.*
3. Describe significant social organization groups.
4. Define family groups, including *nuclear, nuclear dyad, extended, alternative, blended, single parent,* and special forms of family groups.
5. List at least two primary goals inherent in the American culture in regard to the family as a unit.
6. Describe the significant influence that religion may have on the way individuals relate to health care practitioners.

Cultural behavior, or how one acts in certain situations, is socially acquired, not genetically inherited. Patterns of cultural behavior are learned through a process called *enculturation* (also referred to as *socialization*), which involves acquiring knowledge and internalizing values. Most people achieve competence in their own culture through enculturation. Children learn to behave culturally by watching adults and making inferences about the rules for behavior (Kalish & Shiverick, 2004; Nolt, 1992). Patterns of cultural behavior are important to the nurse because they provide explanations for behavior related to life events. Life events that are significant transculturally include birth, death, puberty, childbearing, childrearing, illness, and disease. Children learn certain beliefs, values, and attitudes about these life events, and the learned behavior that results persists throughout the entire life span unless necessity or forced adaptation compels them to learn different ways. Patterns of cultural behavior are also apparent in rituals. Some commonly observed rituals include weddings, funerals, and special holiday meals (Bonder, Martin, & Miracle, 2002). It is important for the nurse to recognize the value of social organizations and their relationship to physiological and psychological growth and maturation.

CULTURE AS A TOTALITY

Most anthropologists believe that to understand culture and the meaning assigned to culture-specific behavior, one must view culture in the total social context. The concept of holism requires that human behavior not be isolated from the context in which it occurs. Therefore, culture must be viewed and analyzed as a totality—a functional, integrated whole whose parts are interrelated and yet interdependent. The components of culture, such as politics, economics, religion, kinship, and health systems, perform separate functions but nevertheless mesh to form an operating whole. Culture is more than the sum of its parts (Goldsby, 1977; Henderson & Primeaux, 1981).

Culture-Bound

As children grow and learn a specific culture, they are to some extent imprisoned without knowing it. Some anthropologists have referred to this existence as "culture-bound." In this context the term *culture-bound* describes a person living within a certain reality that is considered "the reality." Most people have learned ways to interpret their world based on enculturation. Thus, although certain interpretations are understandable and persuasive to persons brought up to share the same frame of reference, other people may not share these interpretations and therefore may make little sense out of the context. Shipler (1997), who has traveled extensively around the United States, notes that connecting across racial lines is among the most difficult things on earth. In a perceptive work, *A Country of Strangers,* he notes, "Even as we look upon each other like strangers from afar, we are trapped in each other's imaginations." In *Liberal Racism,* Sleeper (1997) suggests that rather than trying to overcome racism and create a color-blind world, individuals should fight for equality on nonracial terms. In fact, in polls most Americans agree that people should be judged for themselves, not for their race (Sniderman & Carmines, 1997).

Nurses are also culturally bound within the profession because they are likely to bring a unique scientific approach—the nursing process—to determining and resolving health problems. Many nurses are likely to consider the nursing process the best and only means of meeting the needs of all clients, regardless of their cultural heritage. However, clients may view this modern scientific approach differently, believing that the nursing process meets their needs in some ways but not in others. The nursing process may not consider alternative health services, such as folk remedies, holistic health care, and spiritual interventions. In these cultures, medicine is often practiced in unscientific ways, according to the Western viewpoint. Therefore, desirable outcomes for treatment may occur independently of medical and health care interventions.

Traditionally, American nurses have been socialized to believe that modern Western medicine is the answer to all humanity's health needs. Most illnesses have been attributed to a biological cause (Grypma, 1993). More recently, Americans have been moving toward a more harmonious relationship with nature in which there is a growing sensitivity to the environment. Traditional attitudes toward disease are being reassessed. Today, more attention is given to the concept of the individual as an organic whole. Nurses are beginning to study and assess options outside of Western medicine that have been used by other cultures, such as Zen meditation, a Buddhist practice (Birx, 2002), or tai chi, an exercise treatment used in China for hundreds of years to reduce chronic pain in older adults (Adler, Good, Roberts, & Snyder, 2000). Many nursing leaders in America are calling for a change in nursing paradigms from scientific to holistic (Davidhizar, King, Bechtel, & Giger, 1998; Guruge & Donner, 1996; Thomas, 2001).

Culture-Bound Syndromes

The nurse should appreciate that some illnesses are uniquely found in a given cultural group. *Culture-bound syndromes* is a term that refers to "diseases" that seem to be specific to a single culture or a group of related cultures. Culture-bound syndromes are generally limited to specific societies or culture areas and are localized, folk, diagnostic categories that frame coherent meanings for a pattern of sets of experiences (American Psychiatric Association [APA], 2000). In some cases the "illness" may be linked to a category in the *Diagnostic and Statistical Manual of Mental Disorders* (APA, 2014) but have symptoms, a course, and social responses that are influenced by local cultural factors. Examples are *amok,* a mental or emotional affliction known in the Philippines that causes one to become a killer, and *susto,* an ailment widely associated with Spanish-speaking groups in which the soul is believed to leave the body as a result of a frightening event (Bonder et al., 2002).

Ethnocentrism

For the most part, people look at the world from their own particular cultural viewpoint. *Ethnocentrism* is the perception that one's own way is best. Even in the nursing profession, there is a tendency to lean toward ethnocentrism. Nurses must remain cognizant of the fact that their ways are not necessarily the best and that other people's ideas are not "ignorant" or "inferior." Nurses must remember that the ideas of laypersons may be valid for them and, more importantly, will influence their health care behavior and consequently their health status. In contrast to the term *ethnocentrism* is the word *ethnic,* which relates to large groups of people classed according to common traits or customs. In populations throughout the world, people are bound by common ties, elements, life patterns, and basic beliefs germane to their particular country of origin.

In general, the medical paradigm used in Western culture views health, illness, and dying as biophysical realities. However, the meaning a nurse places on life can affect relationships with clients. For example, a nurse's belief that there is no relationship between illness and evil may conflict with a client's belief that illness is a punishment from God or the work of spirits (Gregory, 1992; Grypma, 1993; Zola, 1972). On one hand, some Puerto Ricans believe that sickness and suffering are a result of one's evil deeds; on the other hand, many Ugandans believe that an infant's illness or death is the result of a neighbor's curse (Grypma, 1993).

It is also important for the nurse to be aware of treatment practices clients may present that do not appear in Western medicine and may seem shocking. For example, female genital cutting, which may range from a ceremonial pricking of the genitalia to the removal of the clitoris, occurs in 28 African countries with prevalence rates estimated at 50% (Natinsky, 2001). Yet another concept that the nurse should appreciate is that moral definitions of an illness may arise from particular historical, social, or medical circumstances that are different in each society. For example, in some societies leprosy is common and considered just another debilitating illness, which many families tolerate. In other societies leprosy has been stigmatized, and lepers are quickly divorced, are pushed out of their homes, and end up as beggars (Wexler, 1981).

Homogeneity

It is difficult to find a homogeneous culture in the United States. If a homogeneous culture did exist, all individuals would share the same attitudes, interests, and goals—a phenomenon referred to as *ethnic collectivity*. People who are reared in ethnic collectivity share a bond that includes common origins, a sense of identity, and a shared standard for behavior. These values are often acquired from experiences that are perceived to be cultural norms and determine the thoughts and behaviors of individual members (Harwood, 1981; Saunders, 1954). The ultimate consequences of enculturation are carried over to health care and become an important influence on activities relative to health and illness behaviors. In the American culture there is a tendency to speak of culture as if it included a set of values shared by everyone. However, even within an ethnic collectivity, intraethnic variations occur and are obvious in health behaviors. For example, intraethnic variations are seen in the concept of mental illness (Berry, 1988; Guttmacher & Elinson, 1972; Sands & Berry, 1993), in cultural definitions of health and illness, in skepticism about medical care and consequently the use or lack of use of health care services (Berkanovic & Reeder, 1973; Spector, 2008), and in the willingness of the individual to assume a dependent role when ill (Suchman, 1964). Since there may not be obvious clues (e.g., language, physical appearance, clothing) to alert the nurse to intraethnic variations, it is essential to be alert to the presence of differences and to be sensitive in interactions with the client when nurse–client variations become evident (Bonder et al., 2002).

Bicultural

The term *bicultural* is used to describe a person who crosses two cultures, lifestyles, and sets of values. Some children of African-American, Hispanic, Asian, and American Indian heritage are socialized to be bicultural—that is, to acquire skills to function in both a minority and a majority culture (Andrews & Boyle, 2008; Zayas & Solari, 1994).

Ethnicity

Ethnicity is frequently and perhaps erroneously used to mean "race," but the term *ethnicity* includes more than the biological identification. *Ethnicity* in its broadest sense refers to groups whose members share a common social and cultural heritage passed on to each successive generation. The most important characteristic of ethnicity is that members of an ethnic group feel a sense of identity.

Race

Efforts to precisely delineate the term *race* have been made by many scientists (American Association of Physical Anthropologists [AAPA], 1996). The AAPA suggests that race, in a pure sense of genetically homogeneous populations, does not exist in any human species today. Freeman (1998) also proposes that the biological concept previously held to be the "one drop rule" is dated and as such is no longer tenable in today's society. Nonetheless, many biological scientists suggest that while socioeconomic status may have a more profound effect on health status, *race* is a viable term that merits attention. Thus, in contrast to the term *ethnicity* is the term *race,* which is related to biology. Members of a particular race share distinguishing physical features, such as skin color, bone structure, or blood group. Ethnic and racial groups can and do overlap because in many cases the biological and cultural similarities reinforce one another (Bullough & Bullough, 1982). A more precise definition of race is a breeding population that primarily mates within itself (Giger, Davidhizar, & Wieczorek, 1994). There are very few races that still mate largely within the group, but some pure-blooded lineages are found in certain parts of the world, such as some of the descendants of West Africans who live along the Georgia and South Carolina seacoasts in the United States. These people have protected their lineage because they have refused to intermarry. These individuals are known as the *Gullah people;* they have not only their own lineage but also their own distinct dialect of English (Wolfram & Clark, 1971). It is important for the nurse to remember that regardless of race, all people have a cultural heritage that makes them ethnic. It is also important to appreciate that race has an interrelational effect with family structure and income that can influence health and academic and professional achievement (Blum, Buehring, & Rinehart, 2000).

As views of racial and ethnic identities have changed over time, so have official categories and measurement procedures. The U.S. government weighed in on the question of race as far back as 1790, beginning the arduous process of classifying people into racial categories. Nonetheless, the categories and the method of measuring race or ethnicity have changed dramatically in the intervening decades since the first census was taken in concert with the political and economic forces that have evolutionarily defined this nation. With early censuses, the census takers simply answered the race question based on their perception of the individual. These early censuses were at the very least racially insensitive in that slave status was used as a proxy for a racial category. Even so, at that time, the only race options available for selection include "free White persons," "slaves," or all other "free persons" (Sandefur, Martin, Eggerling-Boeck, Mannon, & Meier, 2001; U.S. Department of Commerce, Bureau of the Census, American Community Survey, 2015. As the census continued to evolve, the necessity for more specificity in racial categories became clear for those of mixed African-American and White descent, such as *mulatto, quadroon,* and *octoroon.* Beginning in the late 1800s, Asian groups were listed on the census for the first time. Those groups included Chinese, Japanese, and Filipinos (Hirschman, Alba, & Farley, 2000). In 1870, other Asian groups were added and included Korean, Vietnamese, and Asian Indian. Likewise, in 1870, American Indians for the first time were included as a separate group. Similarly, counting and measuring the Hispanic population has varied over time. Census takers began by identifying who was Hispanic by looking for a Spanish surname, the use of the Spanish language in the home, and the birthplace of the respondent or parents to indicate Hispanic ethnicity (Hirschman et al., 2000). Over time, this crude way of measurement and counting any racial or ethnic group would prove to be obsolete.

By 1970, racial classification on the census changed from the census taker's identification to self-identification. Yet, while this was a fairly significant change, it had a relatively minor impact on the count of racial and ethnic groups in the 1970 census compared with the 1960 census. Nonetheless, this change was the catalyst that would spur even greater changes in the census count in subsequent years (Hirschman et al., 2000). The Office on Management and Budget (OMB) announced new standards for federal data on race and ethnicity in 1997 (OMB, 2000). The Census Bureau, taking its cues from the OMB standards, recategorized racial categories to include, for the first time in 2000, five suggested categories, including White, Black/African-American, American Indian/Alaska Native, Asian, and Native Hawaiian/other Pacific Islander. The Census Bureau also added a sixth category, "some other race." The Native Hawaiian/other Pacific Islander category was separated from the Asian category for the first time. A significant change—another first since the census started—allowed respondents to choose more than one racial category.

Biracial

When an individual crosses two racial and cultural groups, the individual is considered "biracial." To be both biracial and bicultural often creates an almost insurmountable dilemma for an individual. Physical attributes such as color, shape of eyes, or hair may have a profound influence on others' acceptance of the "biracial" individual. One problem associated with biracialism is the inability of the individual to identify or find acceptance in any one of the biologically related racial groups (Giger, Davidhizar, Evers, & Ingram, 1994). It is the total exclusion and the sense of not belonging to either of the racial or cultural groups that often create the dilemma. For example, an African-American who is an "octoroon," a person with one eighth African-American blood, may have difficulty being accepted as African-American because of the lightness of the skin. Conversely, this same individual might be ostracized by some Whites because of the "blackness of the blood lineage." Although interracial marriages are on the rise, issues of discrimination still occur. Golf champion Tiger Woods revealed in 1997 that in spite of his national stature, his mixed-race origin of White, Black, Indian, and Asian was sometimes met with hostility (Cose, 2000). This probably is also true for Barack Obama, the first Black president elected in the United States in 2008, who is also of mixed racial heritage. Cose suggests that even in the emerging U.S. mestizo future, if the Latin American experience is a guide, people who are whiter will still have the advantage. Even in Brazil, where racial mixing is sometimes celebrated, status and privilege are still related to lighter skin. For some people of color, there is a perception that White America believes that color is the difference that makes the differences (Giger, Johnson, Davidhizar, & Fishman, 1993).

Minority

A minority can consist of a particular racial, religious, or occupational group that constitutes less than a numerical majority of the population. With use of this definition for the term *minority,* it is obvious that all types of people can belong to various kinds of minorities (Bullough & Bullough, 1982). Often a group is designated *minority* because of its lack of power, assumed inferior traits, or supposedly undesirable characteristics. In any society, cultural groups can be arranged in a hierarchical power structure. Dominant groups are considered to be powerful, whereas those in minority groups are considered inferior and lacking in power.

The term *minority* is not synonymous with numbers. In the United States, people of color (African-Americans, Latin Americans, Asian Americans) are considered minorities. However, when the population of the world is considered in its aggregate, it is obvious that people of color are in the majority.

Gender is another example of how the term *minority* is used erroneously. Females in the United States are a larger numerical percentage (50.9%) than males (49.1%) but are considered to be in the minority because of their under-representation in high-level managerial positions in the workplace (U.S. Department of Commerce, Bureau of the Census, Asian American Community Survey, 2012).

The significance of the term *minority* cannot be over-emphasized. The central defining characteristic of any minority group, according to Adams (1995, p. 6), is its "experience with various disadvantages at the hands of another social group."

Ethnic Minority

The term *ethnic minority* is often used because it is less offensive to people of color than other terms. Supposedly it takes into account ethnicity, race, and the relative status of the groups of persons included in the category. Were it not for the use of the word *minority,* perhaps this terminology would be less culturally offensive to some groups of people (that is, ethnic people of color). According to Gary (1991), use of the term *people of color* might be the preferable option, particularly in situations where sensitivity to racial preferences needs to be heightened. It is estimated that by the year 2050 about half of the total American population will be nonwhite, thus eliminating the meaning of the term *ethnic minority* (Kunen, 1996; U.S. Department of Commerce, Bureau of the Census, Asian American Community Survey, 2012).

Stereotyping

Stereotyping is the assumption that all people in a similar cultural, racial, or ethnic group are alike and share the same values and beliefs. For example, stereotyping occurs when an African-American nurse is assigned to care for an African-American client simply because of ethnicity and race. It is stereotypical when the assumption is made that all African-Americans are alike and therefore the African-American nurse is more likely to be more sensitive to the needs of the African-American client. Race and ethnicity do not, in and of themselves, make persons "resident experts" on the belief and value systems of other persons. Whether stereotyping is engaged in as a result of scientifically proved, research-based data or because of past associations and experiences, stereotyping can ultimately lead to faulty data gathering and wrong interpretations.

Role of Gender and Cultural Significance

In traditional Chinese society, women have held subordinate roles to men, a belief that dates back to the first millennium B.C. (Mo, 1992). Traditional Chinese believe that the universe developed from two complementary opposites: *yin* (Cantonese, *yam*), the female, and *yang* (Cantonese, *yeung*), the male. For some traditional Chinese Americans, the *yin* represents the dark, cold, wet, passive, weak, feminine aspect of humankind. In stark contrast, the *yang* represents the bright, hot, dry, active, strong,

masculine aspect of humankind (Mo, 1992). In traditional societies, there are written and unwritten roles that dictate the behavior of girls and women (Strickland & Giger, 1994). Although some countries in North America are highly evolved technologically, traditional beliefs about the role of women in society still persist throughout many regions of America. Peitchinis (1989) noted that discrimination exists for women in the workplace because women are viewed as having a higher absentee rate than their male counterparts. For many women, discrimination creates a barrier to entrance into the workplace and, even more important, places a "glass ceiling" on advancement that their male counterparts need not overcome (Misener, Sowell, Phillips, & Harris, 1997).

According to a U.S. General Accountability Office study in 2000 (Associated Press, 2000; General Accountability Office, 2010), salaries of women and men in managerial jobs were even farther apart in 2000 than in 1995 in 7 of the 10 industries that employ the most women in the United States. By 2008, this disparity apparently had not ended. For example, in 2008, women who were full-time wage and salary workers had median weekly earnings of $638, or about 80% of the $798 median for their male counterparts (U.S. Department of Labor Statistics, Bureau of Labor Statistics, 2015).

In 1995, female managers in entertainment earned 83 cents for every dollar earned by a male manager; by 2000, female managers in the industry earned only 62 cents. By 2008, the range of pay in the category now called *Leisure and Hospitality* ranged from the lower limits to 78 cents to 83 cents of their male counterparts (General Accountability Office, 2010). Although women have tended to be an oppressed group in the workplace, numerous studies have indicated efforts by industries to implement policies and procedures to prevent discrimination on the basis of sex. For example, women may have access to benefits such as child care leave, alternative working arrangements, child care arrangements, special brief leaves to deal with family problems, and free prenatal classes (Danyliw, 1997). Because breastfeeding reduces the incidence and severity of diarrhea, ear infections, allergies, and sudden infant death syndrome and lessens the risk of ovarian and breast cancer in mothers, programs that allow mothers to do so can result in significant savings for companies in medical claims (Danyliw, 1997).

In some cultures, nursing is a low-status occupation. For example, in Saudi Arabia and Kuwait, care for the sick is carried out by health care providers hired from abroad for the purpose of caring for the bodily needs of the sick (Andrews & Boyle, 2008). Clients or physicians from a culture where nurses are in the lower class may have difficulty accepting the nurse as being in a role of authority and as having expertise. In many parts of the world, female purity and modesty are major values, and disregard of these values can cause distress. For example, female purity is especially important in the Middle East and Muslim countries. In some cultures it is preferable to assign nurses of the same gender as care providers (Habel, 2001). If the nurse is female and the client is male and is from a cultural group where touch is permitted only between members of the same sex and where direct eye contact is avoided, special modifications in care may be needed (Kulwicki, 2003; Meleis, 2006).

Role of Disability and Culture

Today, almost exclusively, more attention has been directed toward a definition of *culture* that includes groups of people by such characteristics of race/ethnicity, religion, and cultural heritage. In addition, the same is true for the term *health disparities*. Statistical data now suggest that other population data, not just race and ethnicity, should now be used to define cultures of people, including those living with health disparities. Disabled people, for example, can now be considered a cultural group that lives with a number of health disparities. A person with a long-lasting condition or disability can be described as suffering from a health disparity. In 2009, 41.2 million individuals in the United States had disabilities (U.S. Department of Commerce, Bureau of the Census, Disability Census Briefs, 2012). Kinne, Patrick, and Doyle (2004) reported a two to three times greater likelihood that individuals with disabilities would suffer from each of 16 secondary conditions, including falls or other injuries, respiratory infections, asthma, sleep problems, chronic pain, and periods of depression. Individuals with disabilities are also at higher risk for preventable physical, mental, or social disorders that may result from the initial disabling condition. Individuals with disabilities are more likely to report that their health is poor or fair (44.8%) than are individuals without disabilities (9.4%) (U.S. Department of Health and Human Services, 2002). These individuals are less likely to be involved in physical activity and more likely to smoke and be overweight (U.S. Department of Health and Human Services, 2002, 2011). Negative social and economic circumstances are also more likely among individuals with disabilities, including decreased participation in social relationships, decreased employment, and decreased income for those employed (U.S. Department of Health and Human Services, 2002, 2011). Thus, it is important to assess the individual with a disability by using the six phenomena of the Giger and Davidhizar model to determine the specific difficulties that this culturally unique individual may experience (Hahn, 2006) (Figure 4-1).

SOCIAL ORGANIZATION GROUPS AS SYSTEMS

Social organizations are structured in a variety of groups, including family, religious, ethnic, racial, tribal, kinship, clan, and other special interest groups. Groups are dependent on particular persons and are more affected by changes in members than are other systems. In most groups, except for racial and ethnic groups, members may come and go. Thus, the formation and the disintegration of groups are more likely to occur during the members' lifetimes than are the formation and the disintegration of other systems.

According to general systems theory, social organization groups are characterized by a steady state and a sense of balance or equilibrium that is maintained even as the group changes. Most groups form, grow, and reach a state of maturity. Social organization groups begin with a variety of elements that include individuals with unique personalities, needs, ideas, potentials, and limits. In the course of development of the group, a pattern of behavior and a set of norms, beliefs, and values evolve. As the group strives toward maturity, parts become differentiated, and each member assumes special functions.

Family Groups

One group of paramount concern for the nurse when working transculturally is the family. In fact, as the family goes, so goes the health care system. Nevertheless, a consensus about the definition of the word *family* does not exist. *Merriam-Webster's Dictionary* (2003 online edition) offers 21 definitions of *family*. In terms of the U.S. Census, the term *family households* is defined as "people who occupy a housing unit" (U.S. Department of Commerce, Bureau of the Census, American Community Survey, 2012). It is estimated that in 2010, there were 77,538,296 family households and 39,177,996 nonfamily households, representing 66.4% and 33.6% of all U.S. households, respectively. Married couples maintained 48.4% of all families, whereas women with no husband maintained 13.1% (U.S. Department of Commerce, Bureau of the Census, American Community Survey, 2012).

Regardless of cultural background or the nature of the family, the family is the basic unit of society in the United States. From a sociological perspective, *family* may be defined as a social unit that interacts with a larger society. The discipline of economics may define *family* in terms of how it works together to meet material needs. From a psychological perspective, *family* may be defined as a basic unit for personality development and the development of subgroup relationships, such as parent–child relationships. Still another definition is offered from a biological

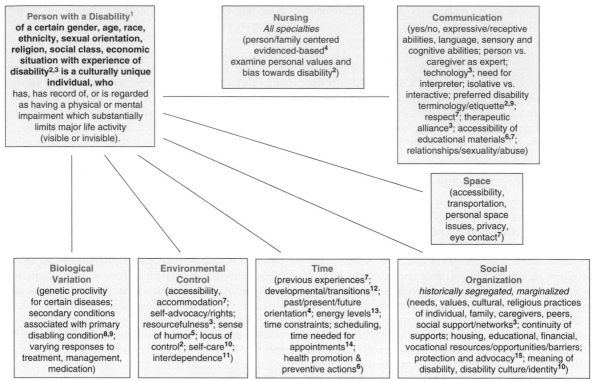

FIG 4-1 Hahn's Culture and Disability Assessment Model. (Adapted from Giger, J. N., Davidhizar, R. (2004). *Transcultural nursing assessment and intervention,* St. Louis: Mosby.)

perspective, which conceptualizes the family as a unit with the biological function of perpetuating the species. However, even while families deliver most health care and at one time being in a family was expected, today not being in a family is both common and accepted and has profound implications for health care delivery (Giorgianni, 2003).

Types of Family Structures

Traditional Nuclear Family. According to Virginia Satir (1983), the traditional nuclear family consists of one man and one woman of the same race, religion, and age who are of sound mind and body and who marry during their early or middle twenties, are faithful to the other for life, have and raise their own children, retire, and finally die. This definition appears narrow; however, it has maintained popularity over the years and is still seen by many persons as the most desirable family form. Today a more current definition of the nuclear family allows for more variation: a family of two generations formed by a married woman and man with their children by birth or adoption (Jones, 2003). Within this particular family form, as within all

identified family forms, the assigned roles and functions performed by each member vary. One common family structure has the father working outside the home and the mother working at home taking care of the children and household tasks. However, today the traditional nuclear family often finds both mother and father working outside the home. Thus, childrearing and childcare may be shared by both parents as well as by others outside the family, such as a day care center.

The most common type of household, married-couple families, changed from 55% to 51.65% of all households from 1990 to 2012. In the United States in 2010, there were 120,768,000 married-couple families with the spouse present, representing 43% of all families in all races, with an additional 4% of households headed by males and 12% of households headed by females with no spouse present (*World Almanac,* 2015; U.S. Department of Commerce, Bureau of the Census, American Community Survey, 2015). The number of married-couple households varies by state, with the highest number in Utah and Idaho and in the west-central section of the country, which corresponds with the 2010 census (*World Almanac,* 2015). A total of 44% of married-couple families have children under age 18 in their home. The average size of the nation's households declined from 2.63 persons in 1990 to 2.57 persons in 2012. In 2004, first marriage occurred at age 25.8 years for women and 27.4 years for men. An increasing and less stigmatized trend today is for adult children to live at home. In 2004, 2.72 million males and 1.56 million females between the ages of 25 and 34 were still living at home. This is approximately double the number in 1970 (Jayson, 2006). Certain ethnic groups, including Asians, African-Americans, and Hispanics, are more likely to stay home longer and are less likely to move far away.

The median age of the U.S. population in 2012 was 37.2 years, the highest it has ever been, up from 32.9 years in 1990. As the median age rose, so did the age of first marriage. The average age at first marriage in 2010 was 26.8 for men and 25.1 for women, and it has been creeping upward (U.S. Department of Commerce, Bureau of the Census, American Community Survey, 2015). As the population continues to age, relatively fewer families will have children—a projected 39% in 2012, down from 50% in 1994. Among families with children, a lower proportion includes two married parents—49.3%, significantly down from 74% in 1994. It is estimated that fewer than 14% of American children living today are growing up in two-parent nuclear families (U.S. Department of Commerce, Bureau of the Census, American Community Survey, 2015). While the number of children in a family is decreasing, increasing numbers of married and unmarried Americans are seeking children to adopt. In 1998, a survey of American women found just 200,000 considering adoption; in 2000, by contrast, 500,000 wanted to adopt a child. Because fewer children are available in the United States, there has been a concomitant sharp increase in foreign adoptions, with 18,441 in 2000 (Clark & Shute, 2001).

Interestingly, although the nuclear family is on the decline, immigration laws still lean toward "family preference." In the interest of keeping families together, U.S. policy allows an unlimited number of visas to certain relatives of U.S. citizens and of permanent resident aliens. Thus, an illiterate laborer with no skills but with a parent in the United States has a better chance of immigration than a graduate school–educated foreigner with no family or employer in the United States. In 1995, about 68% of immigrants came to the United States through the family preference, and about 10% of them came as adult siblings. People born in Mexico, which sends more legal immigrants—18%—to the United States than does any other country, have responded to family preference in particularly high numbers, and they are more likely to use ties to extended family members than any other group. The result is a family-based immigrant population that, for Mexicans and Central Americans at least, is skewed toward unskilled labor (Headden, 1998).

The second most common type of household, consisting of people living alone, rose from 28.15% in 2000 to 30% of all households in 2012 (U.S. Department of Commerce, Bureau of the Census, American Community Survey, 2015).

Nuclear Dyad Family. The nuclear dyad family consists of one generation and is made up of a married couple without children. In the United States, 56.5 million people (19.4% of the population) report that they live in a household with only a spouse (U.S. Department of Commerce, Bureau of the Census, American Community Survey, 2015). There are numerous reasons why a family may remain childless: the family may have chosen not to have children, they may not be able to have children or to adopt them, or the children may have died. Unlike their parents, couples who married in the United States in 2002 were more likely to delay having children (Orecklin, 2002). In some cultures this family form is considered a beginning point for the formation of the family. However, in other cultures the nuclear dyad family is considered a part of the mainstream of the social organization of the family.

Extended Family. The extended family is multigenerational and includes all relatives by birth, marriage, or adoption. The family group includes grandparents, aunts, uncles, nieces, nephews, cousins, brothers, sisters, and in-laws. In today's society there is a tendency for children to leave the homes and communities of their parents, which has resulted in a separation of the nuclear family from the extended family. As longevity in America increases, increasing numbers of people are elderly. In 2010, 22.9% of Americans were over age 65 (U.S. Department of Commerce, Bureau of the Census, 2010 Census Brief, 2015). Concomitantly, the number of multigenerational or extended family households is increasing. In 2019, more than 24 million (23.4%) households included individuals 65 years of age and older. The elderly are increasingly living alone. More than 9 million (9.2%) persons 65 years of age and older were in nonfamily households (U.S. Department of Commerce, Bureau of the Census, American Community Survey, 2015).

Skip-Generation Family. Grandparents who are taking care of grandchildren are a growing family group. With increasing numbers of parents dying of acquired immunodeficiency syndrome (AIDS) and single parents who are not interested in child care, grandparents are finding themselves in the role of primary caregiver (McMahon, 1997). An estimated 7.8 million of America's children live with at least one grandparent; this figure represents a 64% increase since 1991 when only 4.7 million children reportedly lived with a grandparent. Among children living with a grandparent, 76% also were living with at least one parent in 2009, which was not statistically different from the 77% who lived with at least one parent in 1991 (U.S. Department of Commerce, Bureau of the Census, American Community Survey, 2015).

Alternative Family. The alternative family consists of adults of a single generation or a combination of adults and children who live together without the social sanction of marriage. The alternative family is often either a communal arrangement—composed of roommates who might be either homosexual or heterosexual—or a love relationship between a man and a woman. Unmarried partners form 5.5 million households in the United States, including 5 million of the opposite sex and 600,000 of the same sex. These unmarried-partner households made up 8.9% of all households in 2010, an increase from 4% in 1990 and 2% in 1980 (*World Almanac*, 2015).

Single-Parent Family. The single-parent family consists of two generations and is made up of a mother or a father and children by birth or adoption. The reasons for a single-parent family include electing to be a single parent, divorce, death, separation, or abandonment. The prevalence of the single-parent family is increasing because of such factors as divorce and the acceptability of being a single parent. In 2010, families maintained by women with no husband present edged up to 13.1%, for a total of 15.2 million. Among female-headed households, 15,250,349 or 13.1% of all households had children under age 18 years (U.S. Department of Commerce, Bureau of the Census, American Community Survey, 2015). Between 2005 and 2013, 44.3 children per 1000 were born to unmarried women 15 to 44 years of age, compared with 3.8% in 1940 (U.S. Department of Health and Human Services, Health United States, 2013). This is a 7% increase in these births; however, the median age of the unmarried mothers is in the late twenties, they may be divorced or never married, and 40% are living with a man who may be the father of one or more of the children (U.S. Department of Commerce, Bureau of the Census, American Community Survey, 2015). More than half of the youngsters born in the 1990s are predicted to spend at least part of their childhood in a single-parent home. Single fathers account for 2.7 million households, representing little variation since 1994 (U.S. Department of Commerce, Bureau of the Census, American Community Survey, 2015).

Reconstituted or Blended Family. The reconstituted or blended family is formed by "put-together parts" of previously existing families with the intention of forming a new nuclear family (Satir, 1983). The blended family, like the traditional nuclear family, is two-generational. However, the blended family differs in form and may consist of a single person who marries a person with children or of a man and a woman, both of whom have children, who marry. This family form may also yield biological children; thus, there may be children who are "yours," "mine," and "ours" in the family. The blended family can become very complicated because of the composition of family members, which may include stepbrothers, stepsisters, stepparents, and stepgrandparents. Unipolar blended and bipolar blended describe whether one or both parents bring stepchildren to a marriage. If one parent's children do not live with the family, the family is a secondary-step, bipolar family. If one parent brings children from two previous marriages, the term *double-step family* is used (Rosemond, 1994). Nearly 25% of all minor children live in a stepfamily (Jones, 2003).

Special Forms of Families: Communal Families and Gay Families. In some cultures, an even wider array of family forms occurs, particularly if ideas about marriage and the requirement that the nuclear family is essential to family definition are disregarded. These groups function as families and therefore must be recognized. These special forms of families may be either unigenerational or multigenerational. Two or more adults constitute these special family forms, and they may or may not be of the same sex.

A commune is a group of people that intertwines husband–wife, parent–child, and brother–sister types of relationships of individuals who have elected to live together in one household or in closely adjoining structures. Family members in a commune must express a feeling of commitment to others in the group. Assigned family roles as well as responsibilities are divided among the members of the group. Generally there are specific rules and expectations for each member of the group. A commune may be formed when people have a common goal, such as a religious, philosophical, or political goal, or a common need, such as an economic, social, or physical need. Examples of communes include Israeli kibbutzim, religious cults, retirement homes for the elderly, and households where couples share resources.

Some gay households consist of two persons and generally function as a nuclear dyad. Other gay households may consist of more members, such as a commune. Today, perhaps as a result of the gay rights movement, homosexual couples have openly taken up residence together. In 1999, many members of society rejected this particular family form, as indicated in a survey by the *Washington Post,* Harvard University, and the Kaiser Family Foundation (1999) in which 53% of respondents stated they believed sexual relationships between two adults of the same sex were always wrong. By 2015, this prevailing attitude had switched occurring to data from a Pew Poll whereas now 55% of Americans) support same-sex marriage, compared with 39% who oppose it.

To combat discrimination against gays and lesbians, legislation regarding the workplace, marriage, and adoption is increasingly being enacted at the state and federal level. In 1996, Congress passed a bill dubbed the "Defense of Marriage Act," which prohibited federal benefits for spouses in same-sex marriages and guaranteed that no state shall be required to legally recognize same-sex unions. In June of 2015, the Supreme Court of the United States, writing in a decision in the case of *Obergefell v. Hodges,* upheld the principle *that marriage is a fundamental right* that all couples are entitled to under the Fourteenth Amendment of the Constitution, which provides for equal protection to all citizens under the law (Supreme Court of the United States, 2015). In 1997, a New Jersey gay couple was allowed to jointly adopt a child, as New Jersey became the first state to explicitly allow lesbian and gay couples to adopt children jointly, just as married couples do. As gay and lesbian baby boomers enter their golden years, the estimated current number of 1 to 3 million gay and lesbian seniors is expected to skyrocket. Gay retirement communities are being developed from Boston to Palm Springs to offer retirees the opportunity to be part of a like-minded community that stands against discrimination (Rosenberg, 2001). Young gays are disclosing their sexual orientation earlier. Whereas in 1997 there were approximately 100 gay–straight alliances (clubs for gays and gay-friendly kids) on U.S. high school campuses, today there are nearly 3000 (Cloud, 2005). The nursing literature is increasingly addressing variations in sexual orientation and encouraging nurses to come to terms with their own feelings about homosexuality and to practice unconditional acceptance of the individual regardless of sexual orientation (Townsend, 2006).

Characteristics of a Family System

According to general systems theory, a system is a group of interrelated parts or units that form a whole. When general systems theory is applied to the family, the individual family members are those units that make up the identifiable family system. These parts or units act as one or more subsystems within the larger system. Within the family system, the *subsystems* refer to the ways in which the members align themselves with one another. For example, in the family system, the parents may be one subsystem and

the children another subsystem. At the same time, males and females of the family system may be two other subsystems. A subsystem may consist of any number of members who are linked by some common factor. Within the family system, membership in a particular subsystem may be determined by generational considerations, sexual identity, areas of interest, or a specifically designated function. Individual family members may belong to several different subsystems. Family members also belong to external systems, such as the community system, the school system, and career systems. Subsystems may be constructed to ensure that important functions within the family system are carried out to maintain the overall family structure.

Fawcett (1975) studied the family as a living open system and thus viewed family nursing as an emerging conceptual framework for nursing care. Nurses have cared for families for years; however, it is only recently that nurses have begun to study the family as a whole (Finkleman, 2000; Kearney, York, & Deatrick, 2000).

Family as a Behavioral System. The family is conceptualized as a behavioral system with unique properties inherent to the system. A close interrelationship exists between the psychosocial functioning of the family as a group and the emotional adaptation of individual family members. A distinguishable link exists between disorders of family living and disorders of family members. This link can best be understood in the context of systems theory. Systems theory is an orientation whereby people are recognized and defined by who they are in the context of their relationship with family, friends, and the society in which they live. Family systems theories were developed in the 1950s on both the East and West coasts of the United States. On the West Coast, a group of people that included Jackson, Haley, and their associates in Palo Alto, California, explored the notions of communication theory and homeostasis applied to the family with a schizophrenic member (Bateson, Jackson, Haley, & Weakland, 1968; Satir, 1983). On the East Coast, in Washington, DC, Bowen (1985) conceptualized a family systems theory based on a biological systems model. In Philadelphia, Minuchin (1974) used a systems model in his research with families with psychosomatic disorders.

Lewis, Beavers, Gossett, and Phillips (1976) and Caplan (1976) explored both disturbed families and healthy families from a systems perspective. A system is a whole that consists of more than the sum of its parts; a system can be divided into subsystems, but the subsystems are not representative pieces of the whole. To study the family from a cultural perspective, one must understand the basic characteristics of a family system and of a living system. Today in nursing, the family nursing process is the same whether the focus is on the family as the client or the family as the environment. Therefore, the nursing process used in family nursing is the same as that used with individuals, that is, assessment, nursing diagnosis, planning, intervention, and evaluation. According to Friedman (1986), the only distinguishable difference is that both the individual and the family receive care simultaneously. There are some inherent underlying assumptions germane to the family approach to the nursing process, including the beliefs that all individuals must be viewed within their family context, that families have an effect on individuals, and that individuals have an effect on families. As nursing becomes more involved in the delivery of care in the community, it is imperative to strengthen nursing expertise in the delivery of care to the entire family (Hitchcock, 2003).

Independent Units. All systems have basic units that make functioning possible. Within the structure of the family system, the basic interdependent units are the individual family members. As in any open system, change within one family member affects the entire family system. For example, when one family member becomes physically or emotionally ill, the entire family system is changed in some way. Additional alterations in the family system occur because of the changing composition of family membership as a result of events such as birth, divorce, death, hospitalization, leaving home for college, or marriage. All these variables, whether positive or negative, may bring about disruption and disequilibrium in the family system. All family systems have dynamic characteristics that must be used when disruption or disequilibrium occurs if the family system is to be permitted to return to equilibrium as matter, energy, and information are exchanged (Lewis, 1979).

The number of adults who are unmarried (never married, widowed, or divorced) is dramatically increasing in the United States. Between 2000 and 2009, the number of young adults between 25 and 34 years who were married dropped precipitously by 10% from 55% to 45%. It is interesting to note that during that same period, the percent of adults in the same cohort who were never married dramatically increased from 34% to 46%. These data indicate a dramatic reversal between individuals who have been married and those who have not and for the first time those who have not exceed those who have (U.S. Department of Commerce, Bureau of the Census, American Community Survey, 2015; *World Almanac,* 2015). In 2012, widowed persons represented 13.8 million (2.3% of males and 10.3% of females) of the population while divorced individuals represented 21.5 million (8.8% of males and 11.5% of females) of the population (*World Almanac,* 2015).

Environment. As with all open systems, an internal and external environment controls the direction of growth of the family system. The internal environment involves the social and physical factors within the family boundaries, the quality of which is reflected by such factors as (1) marital relationship, (2) location of power, (3) closeness of family members, (4) communication, (5) problem-solving abilities, (6) free expression of feelings, (7) ability to deal with loss, (8) family values, (9) degree of intimacy, and (10) autonomy of family members. Within the family system, the external environment is the social and physical world outside the family, such as church, neighbors, extended family, school, friends, work, health care system, political system, and recreation.

Boundaries. Within the family system, the "boundary" is the imaginary line or area of demarcation that keeps the family system separate and unique from its external environment. As with all open systems, energy, in the form of information, material goods, and feeling states, passes among family members and the external environment. Openness and closeness in a family system are governed by the degree of information or energy that is exchanged and the nature of the boundaries. Information coming into the family system provides the family with information about the environment and about family functioning. If the family accepts the information, it may be used to formulate and respond to the environment, assist the family in coping with disequilibrium, or rejuvenate the family. Energy coming into the family can also be stored until needed. Finally, energy or information coming into the family can be rejected or ignored (Satir, 1983).

As with all open systems, the amount of energy or information that enters and leaves the system must be balanced within certain limits to maintain a steady state of functioning or homeostasis if proper adaptation of the system is to occur. Any system can become dysfunctional if the system is allowed to become too open or too closed. No truly closed systems exist, except in a theoretical sense. On the other hand, if a family system were totally open, the family system would probably lose its identity as a system separate from other systems to which family members belong. Therefore, the family members might suffer from alienation, rootlessness, and a lack of belonging. The opposite extreme, a theoretically closed family system, would have very rigid boundaries, and family members would become enmeshed, fixed, and unable to move out, grow, or change.

Communication within the Family System

The verbal and nonverbal interaction among family members is communication. Factors that contribute to the family members' patterns of communication include (1) the pattern of members in acknowledging each other's verbal and nonverbal messages, (2) the degree of responsibility each member takes for expressing individual feelings, thoughts, and reactions in a constructive way, (3) the extent to which the family encourages a clear exchange of words, (4) the extent to which family members are allowed to talk for themselves, and (5) the patterns of spontaneous talking. Bonding among family members results from the forms of communication patterns that exist.

Roles in the Family

Family member roles are patterns of wants, goals, beliefs, feelings, attitudes, and actions that family members have for themselves and others in the family. Roles are both assigned and acquired, and they specify what individuals do in the family. Although they are usually dependent on social class and cultural norms, roles are dynamic and change in response to factors both within the family and without. Roles are reciprocal and complement roles taken by other family members. Family equilibrium is dependent on how well roles in the family are balanced and reciprocated (Duvall & Miller, 1985; Friedman, 1986).

The way in which a family member assumes a particular role is influenced by various factors, including temperament, height, weight, gender, birth order, age, and health status. Certain roles, however, depend solely on the sex of the family member. Females can be sister, daughter, wife, mother, or girlfriend, whereas males can be brother, son, father, husband, or boyfriend. Other roles, such as breadwinner, childrearer, homemaker, cook, handyman, and gardener, are performance roles and depend on the person's ability to perform a certain task. In contrast to performance roles are emotional roles, such as leader, nurturer, scapegoat, caretaker, jester, arbitrator, or martyr, which may be adopted at certain times as a means of adjusting to the demands of a family system, to an extended family crisis such as a long-term family illness, or to long-term family conflict. The functions of emotional roles are to reduce conflict among family members and to promote temporary adaptation among family members. However, consistent use of emotional roles may impair adaptation, thus hindering the growth of the family. An example is when one family member, perhaps the oldest child, assumes the role of family caretaker, supporting other members and arbitrating disputes. The role may take on negative characteristics in this instance because the family caretaker may appear outwardly strong and capable but inwardly have unrealistic feelings, such as "I can't fail" or "I can't be weak." In this emotional role, this person may function under pressure to be perfect but at the same time have feelings of self-doubt and fear. It is important for the nurse to remember that roles have a significant effect on individual

adjustment. Role function is influenced by the values of social groups to which the individual belongs. For example, in an international study by Vehvilainen (1998), Finnish Lutheran women placed less value on bearing and rearing children than other groups studied (American Mormons and Canadian Orthodox Jews).

Family Organization

To understand family organization, the nurse must remember that structuring of both functions and goals must be addressed. It is also important for the nurse to remember that most families are dynamic, endlessly adaptable, and continuously evolving in both structure and function. The functional ability of a family depends in part on the individual needs and wants of the members. If the nurse is unable to assist family members in meeting needs within the family structure, pain may be felt and confusion may exist. The nurse must keep in mind that, in the American culture, families are expected to be self-perpetuating and at the same time be the primary system for the transfer of social values and norms.

In the American culture, two primary goals are inherent in the family: (1) the encouragement and nurturance of each individual and (2) the production of autonomous, healthy children (O'Brien, 1992). Marital partners are expected to be supportive and protective of each other. Both the husband and the wife are expected to share a sense of meaning and emotional closeness within the boundaries of their relationship, thus fostering the goal of personality development. In families in which supportive relationships do not exist, the achievement of the first goal (the encouragement and nurturance of each individual) is not attainable. The second goal of the family includes encouraging children to develop their own identity and individuality by allowing them to develop ideals, feelings, and life directions. At the same time, children are encouraged to sense both similarities to and differences from others and to be able to initiate activities based on this information (Lewis, 1979). Factors that must be addressed to determine the degree to which the family will accomplish these two primary goals include the patterns of relationships and adaptive mechanisms that are present. There are many reasons why some families fail to accomplish these two primary goals, including psychiatric disturbance of family members, incomplete maturation of children, and disintegration of the family system. When the family uses adaptive mechanisms, internal equilibrium may result. These adaptive mechanisms are dependent on (1) the level of communication skills within the family, (2) the individual contributions of each family member to the family welfare, (3) the mutual respect and love within the family, (4) the types, kinds, and amounts of stressors encountered, (5) the response pattern to stressors encountered in the internal and external environment, and (6) the support or resources available and the opportunity to participate in support systems (Ackerman, 1984; Black, 2001). For example, a family that has an alcoholic father may not be able to accomplish goals because this problem may result in psychiatric disturbances in the wife and children, and ultimately the family system may disintegrate. The reasons for the disintegration of this family include not only the individual psychiatric disturbances but also accompanying difficulties, such as incomplete maturation of children and adult members, financial instability, inability to adapt successfully to stressors, and, more important, the inability of each family member to perceive the family unit as caring and loving (Brown, 1986).

Levels of Functioning. Four levels of family functioning that have been identified form a continuum in increasingly abstract levels (Box 4-1): (1) family functions and activi-

ties, (2) intrafamilial interactions, (3) interpersonal relationships, and (4) the family system (Averaswald, 1983).

To understand the family from a cultural perspective, it is essential that the nurse recognize that family relationships are stronger among some ethnic or cultural groups than among others. However, the importance of socioeconomic class cannot be overlooked. According to Casavantes (1976), a pattern of strong family relationships exists, particularly among poor people who have few resources and must rely on the support of the family kinship network to meet physical and emotional needs. Middle- or upper-class people often have resources that extend beyond the extended family and are therefore able to avail themselves of physical and emotional support within the community. It is often believed that when people do not have money or other available resources for recreation and social activities in the community, they tend to spend more time together and depend on the family group for recreational and social outlets.

BOX 4-1   Levels of Family Functioning

Least Abstract
Level I: Family functions and activities
Level II: Intrafamilial interactions
Level III: Interpersonal relationships

Most Abstract
Level IV: The family system

Level I deals with family affairs and functions. Included in this level are tangible, pragmatic activities that are observable or easily identified; more important, these are things that family members are most comfortable discussing. Four categories of family functioning have been identified in Level I:

1. **Activities of family living.** Families are expected to provide physical safety and economic resources. Included in this category is the ability of family members to obtain such necessities as food, clothing, shelter, and health care.
2. **Ability of the family members to assist one another.** Included in this category is the family's ability to assist other members in developing emotionally and intellectually and at the same time attaining a personal as well as a family identity.
3. **Reproduction, socialization, and release of children.** Included in this category are functioning goals that allow the family to become closely aligned,

thereby allowing the transmission of subcultural roles and values.

4. **Integration between the family, its culture, and society.** Included in this category is the ability of the family to use external environmental resources for support and feedback.

Level II deals with communication and various interactions between family members, including what is said, how it is said, patterns of communication over time, the ability of each family member to communicate, and the quality of communication skills. Also included in this level is the transfer of information from family member to family member.

Level III deals with the way family members interact in relationships that occur within the family constellation. The dimensions of closeness and power and the degree of empathy, support, and commitment among family members are important. How the family functions in regard to decision making and problem solving is included in this level.

Level IV deals with the concepts of the family system, as well as how the family functions as a system. Level IV is the most abstract level of family functioning. It encompasses the concepts of wholeness, openness or closedness, homeostasis, and rules.

Data obtained from Schneider, R. (1980, June). *Conceptual scheme of family organization and function.* Paper presented at St. Louis University Medical Center conference, St. Louis, MO.

Regardless of socioeconomic class, families must organize and structure themselves. *Structure* refers to the organization of the family and includes the type of family, such as nuclear or extended. The value system of the family dictates the roles assigned in the family, communication patterns within the family, and power distribution within the family (Friedman, 1986; Schneflen, 1972). The basic beliefs about humankind, nature, the supernatural (fate), time, and family relationships constitute a family's value system. Value systems are often clustered by socioeconomic status or ethnic groups. For example, families from lower socioeconomic groups tend to have a present-time orientation and view themselves as being subjugated by the environment or the supernatural (fate). Often the family relationships are disrupted by desertion of a spouse or by the early emancipation of the children because of severe economic difficulties. These families have been able to survive and adapt by taking in children of other extended family members; for example, a grandmother may provide direct assistance by raising her son's or daughter's children. In these families, power is usually authoritarian or not exerted at all.

Middle- and upper-class families in the United States for the most part espouse the Protestant work ethic values, which dictate the importance of working and planning for the future. These values encompass the belief that although humanity is somewhat evil, behavior is changeable by hard work. In the middle- and upper-class family structure, financial stability and success are viewed as rewards for hard work. Within these classes, family relationships center on the nuclear family, socialization occurs with work-related or neighborhood friends, and power may be more egalitarian than in the lower-class family. Power tends to become more male dominated as the economic level of a family rises. Middle- and upper-class families often see themselves as able to control or have mastery over their environment (O'Brien, 1992).

When typical White American families are compared with Asian American families, some differences can generally be noted. The typical White American family defines itself by the present generation, is fiscally independent, has the core relationship as husband–wife, emphasizes happiness of the individual, and is more feeling oriented. In contrast, the Asian family is defined by past, present, and future generations; feels economic obligations to kin; has parent–child as the core relationship; emphasizes the welfare of the family; and is more task oriented (Hsu, 1985). The Asian client's explanatory model of illness is greatly influenced by the family (Smart, 1991), and the discussion of illness is related to a sense of obligation to the family (Nilchaikovit, Hill, & Holland, 1993).

The nurse must keep in mind that these statements on structure and organization of a family by class are broad generalizations of social class values and in themselves cannot account for cultural differences. For example, many ethnic groups, such as the Newfoundland Inuit family, regardless of socioeconomic status, place great importance on extended family relationships rather than on the individualism valued by White, Protestant, middle-class Americans. A family with a good income but with a time orientation in the present, such as that commonly found among persons in the lower socioeconomic class, may fail to recognize the importance of saving money and thus may always struggle financially. To understand whether a family system organizes itself around a family unit, such as the extended family, or tends to be a more individualistic system, such as the nuclear family, the nurse must assess the family as a group. The American family is composed of diverse multicultural populations and is defined by three criteria: kinship, function, and location.

Kinship

In the first criterion, kinship, there are three dyads that imply the existence of or location for the individual within the family structure: husband–father, wife–mother, or child–sibling. There are several conventional forms of family structures that are composed of these positions, including the nuclear family and the stem family. The nuclear family, which was discussed earlier, may consist of a husband, a wife, and their nonadult children and is based on all three dyads, with their marital, parental, and sibling elements. Whereas the nuclear family is restricted to a depth of two generations, the stem family encompasses three generations: grandparents, parents, and children.

Function

The second criterion, function, describes the purpose, goals, and philosophy of the family organization. *Family function* is defined as the expected action of an individual in a given role. In a description of family organization, the term *function* is used to depict family roles and the assigned tasks for those roles. Every family has unit functions that must be performed to maintain the integrity of the family unit and to meet the needs of the family. If individual family members' needs and societal expectations are to be met, the functioning role of the family must be clearly delineated. In family systems with two or more individuals, the family members have unit functional responsibilities related to their social positions. Depending on position within the family structure, an individual may function in a variety of roles, such as companion, decision maker, health motivator, or sexual partner. It is important for the nurse to remember that the maintenance of the family system is dependent on these various roles. Some cultural groups function in traditional ways in which the family is viewed as a holistic functioning unit. Other cultural groups may function as a disaggregate unit, meaning that the family does not function as a unit but that members function independently.

When the nurse is providing care, it is particularly important to assess who has the decision-making function in the family. For example, a decision about consent to treatment, receiving care or teaching, or whether to follow instructions may need to be made individually (Haddad, 2001). On the other hand, a client may not feel comfortable in making a health care decision without the spouse or family. In some situations the client may defer to the spouse for decision making (Dowd, Davidhizar, & Giger, 2007). In still other situations, another individual or group, such as a deacon or a church, may need to be involved. In a traditional Mexican family, the man is the decision maker. When a decision regarding health care is needed, a woman may defer any decision until her husband can arrive (Bechtel & Davidhizar, 1998). Consideration for families' decision-making style is included in the recent additions to the standards of the Joint Commission for the Accreditation of Healthcare Organizations (JCAHO), which acknowledge the autonomy of the client and/or of the family in the health care decision-making process (JCAHO, 2000). Decisions about who makes decisions regarding the end of life may also be culturally determined, although it can never be assumed that all members of the group will act the same or share the same beliefs. For example, among Asian and Pacific Island cultures, the interaction of Buddhism, Confucianism, and Christianity generally supports filial piety. While the family assumes the decision-making role, terminating treatment for a parent can influence the fate of the living and be equated with ancestor murder. Thus, many families will want to provide artificial feedings and hydration to the terminally ill and to demented patients not taking food and fluids orally since they feel that only God decides when it is time to die (Mitty, 2001).

Another family function that the nurse needs to examine is in relation to the family's physical, affectional, and social properties (Murray, Meili, & Zentner, 1993). Physical functions include providing food, clothing, and shelter; protecting against danger; and providing health care. Affectional functions include meeting emotional needs. Social functions include providing social togetherness, fostering self-esteem, and supporting creativity and initiative. Another approach to examining family functions views the family from a task-oriented perspective (Sussman, 1971). Tasks include socialization of children, strengthening competency of family members in relation to their adjustments within organizations, appropriate use of social

organizations, providing an environment that fosters the development of identities and affectional behavior, and creating a satisfying, emotionally healthy environment essential to the family's well-being. Adaptation is essential to the family's ability to carry out functions and tasks and to meet the changing needs of society and other social systems, such as political and health–illness systems.

One of the most significant dimensions affecting child-rearing practices in America today is managing children's time with computers, TV, and video games. It is estimated that the average American child in 2002 spent an average of 4.5 hours a day at home in front of a screen, an increase of 30 minutes from the previous year. In 1999, the average American child grew up in a home with two TVs, two VCRs, three audiotape players, two CD players, one video-game player, and one computer, according to a Kaiser Family Foundation study; children had an increasingly sedentary lifestyle and increased exposure to violent and sexual images (Kaiser Family Foundation, 1999). Parents are challenged to protect their children online using software packages such as Cyber Patrol, Net Nanny, and Cybersitter, but nothing is promoted as perfect, and children remain vulnerable to pornography and sex predators on the Internet (Dunnewind, 2001; Nordland & Bartholet, 2001).

Location

Family location is also a significant criterion for understanding the family. Martin (1978) and Leininger (1995) discussed the variations that occurred among values of African-American families when families were evaluated in urban versus rural settings. Martin found that when families moved from rural to urban settings, there was an erosion of values emphasizing "mutual aid" and a contrasting increase in individualism, materialism, and secularism. When urban African-Americans are compared with their rural counterparts, it appears that urban African-Americans may view their counterparts as lacking the toughness and sophistication needed to make headway in a dominant urban culture. Despite the variations that occur with location changes, geographical separation does not mean a severing of kinship ties, according to Martin; rather, geographical separation may strengthen the emotional bonds among relatives. Today there is a tendency among African-Americans, whether urban or rural, toward a migration back home and getting back to their people. For some African-Americans there has been an increasing awareness that the urban centers have not met their hopes and aspirations. From the 1940s to the 1970s, there was a migration by some African-Americans away from the rural South. In the 1980s there was a trend toward migration of some African-Americans away from the urban North back to the urban South. For example, significant numbers of urban Northern African-Americans have migrated to such cities as Atlanta, Dallas, and Houston (Kunen, 1996).

Religious Groups

According to many sociologists, religion is a social phenomenon (Carroll, Johnson, & Marty, 1979). Religious practices, therefore, are usually rooted in culture, and each culture typically has a set of beliefs that define health and the behaviors that prevent or treat illness (Davidhizar, Bechtel, & Cosey, 2000). However, many persons, particularly those with religious convictions, tend to think of religion in an entirely different way. For some people religion is seen in the context of a person's communion with the supernatural, and religious experiences fall outside ordinary experiences, whereas other people view religion as an expression of an instinctual reaction to cosmic forces (Johnstone, 2007). Another worldview of religion depicts it as an explicit set of messages from a deity. For the most part, all these beliefs tend to de-emphasize, ignore, and perhaps even reject the sociological dimensions of religion. Nevertheless, whether it is being considered in general, in regard to a particular religious family such as Christianity or Buddhism, or in regard to a very specific religious group, such as Baptists, religion is believed to interact with other social institutions and forces in society and to follow and illustrate sociological principles and laws. In other words, regardless of what religion is or is not, it is a social phenomenon and as such is in a continual reciprocal, interactive relationship with other social phenomena.

Regardless of its definition, be it theological or sociological, many different kinds of groups are based on religion. Generally, religious structures fall into two basic types: the church type and the withdrawal-group type. The church type of structure is broadly based and represents the normative spiritual values of a society that most people adhere to by virtue of their membership in the society, such as Hinduism in India or Catholicism in Spain. For the most part, membership in certain societies dictates the faith that the person should belong to if that person has not made a conscious, deliberate choice to adhere to something else. The church type of structure is generally a comprehensive system that allows for individual variations and in practice does not make extremely rigorous demands on its members. In the United States, the church type of structure is encompassed within numerous major denominations. This denominational structure is in sharp contrast with the church type of structure in other countries, such as India or Spain, where most of the people belong to one faith and one church. In some countries, particularly the United States, individual churches are often closely identified with an ethnic group rather than with a social class, and churches

thrive, more or less, as a means of asserting ethnic identity. For example, the Black church, regardless of denominational faith, has become synonymous with the Black life experience. The Amish people, on the other hand, subscribe to one denominational belief; however, the belief is synonymous with the Amish life experience.

The second type of religious structure is the withdrawal group, which expresses the beliefs of those for whom personal commitment and experience are more important than the family and the community functions of religion (Ellwood, 2005). Withdrawal groups meet the needs of those who believe that the majority's faith or lack of faith is not for them. Persons involved in withdrawal groups define themselves by making a separate choice. These groups include the Amish or Jehovah's Witnesses, which tend to represent a more intense or unbending commitment than that held by the average person adhering to a religion. These groups may be called *sects*. Groups that combine separation with syncretism and new ideas and that emphasize mystical experience are often referred to as *cults*. However, the word *cult* is often used in Western society with caution because it has acquired a negative connotation. In some religious groups, such as the Church of Jesus Christ of Latter-Day Saints (Mormons), Muslims, Jehovah's Witnesses, Seventh-Day Adventists, Buddhists, or Hindus, as well as that of the Gypsy culture, the extended social organization of the religion is considered more important than membership in the individual family. It is essential to remember that while this view is held by some theological scholars (Ellwood, 2005), many members of these religious groups do not necessarily share this belief. For example, in the Church of Jesus Christ of Latter-Day Saints (the Mormon Church), children are taught at a very young age that families are eternal. In this sense, the family is viewed as a stable, cohesive group bonded by love and as such is one of the most important units on earth today (Sheler, 2000).

As persons from different religions increasingly intermarry, it is becoming more common for parents not to share the same faith. The proportion of Jews who married Gentiles, around 10% for the first half of the century, according to the American Jewish Committee, doubled in 1960, doubled again by the early 1970s, and in the 1990s leveled off at just over 50%. Approximately one of three American Jews lives in an interfaith household (Wingert, Springen, Stone, et al., 1997). Comparable figures are 21% for Catholics, 30% for Mormons, and 40% for Muslims. Thus, a new form of religious identification in America is developing that is analogous to a "mixed race." However, although diversity is increasingly acceptable among American religions, observances inevitably involve some sectarianism. Even though raising children in two faiths promotes diversity, it is sometimes confusing for the children, who may feel that they are not as good as their all-Jewish or all-Christian cousins. Although attitudes toward intermarriage are becoming more liberal, for some it creates confusion over which holidays to celebrate and which church children should attend. On the other hand, intermarriage is not completely accepted in the United States. There are conservative sects, such as Old Colony Mennonites and Missouri Synod Lutherans, who are less tolerant of intermarriage and insist on born-again spouses (Wingert, Springen, Stone, et al., 1997).

There are 215 distinct church traditions represented in the United States. Many of these groups represent the process of dividing and reuniting that has been a characteristic of religious life in America (Kosmin & Keysar, 2009; Lindner, 2004). Data from the American Religious Identification Survey indicated that there were 228,182,000 persons in the United States in 2008 who considered themselves members of a church; this is up from 2000, when more than 152 million claimed membership (Kosmin & Keysar, 2009). The denomination with the largest membership is the Catholic Church, with 57,199,000 members, comprising 24% of the U.S. population; the Southern Baptist Convention has 16.2 million (all Baptists, including Southern Baptists, total 36,148,000), the United Methodist Church has 11,366,000, and the Church of God in Christ has 6.4 million. The Church of Jesus Christ of Latter-Day Saints ranks fifth, with a membership of 3,158,000, but is noted to have had a very brisk increase in membership since its origin in 1830. The Church of God in Christ, which has historically been the largest Black Pentecostal church, is now among the five largest denominations, indicative of the growth of Pentecostal churches (Lindner, 2004) (Tables 4-1 and 4-2).

Worldwide, the vitality of Christianity is fading in the West, especially in Europe, where Christians often do not go to church. The center of Christianity is shifting to the developing world, as persons in Nigeria and India embrace the faith (Woodward, 2001). Christianity's identification with the poor is drawing the impoverished and the downtrodden. Christianity in the United States is attracting many young believers with an entertainment explosion. Alternative rock is just one part of the entertainment-led revolution that spans from the popular *Left Behind* novels, which have sold 65 million copies, which is up from $28 million in 2001, to live festivals with Grammy-winning singers (Ali, 2001; *Left Behind* series, 2011). Some 79% of Americans describe themselves as "spiritual"; 64% say they are "religious" (Underwood, 2005). 67% believe that when they die their souls will go to heaven or hell; 24% do not believe that heaven or hell exists. Beliefnet.com, a religious Web site, sends out more than 8 million daily

TABLE 4-1   Largest Denominational Families in the United States

Denomination	2008 Estimated Adult Population
Roman Catholic Church	78,000,000
Baptist	39,299,000
Methodist/Wesleyan	14,174,000
Lutheran	9,110,000
United Church of Christ	6,448,000
Church of Jesus Christ of Latter-Day Saints	3,158,000
Presbyterian	5,187,000
Assemblies of God	810,000
Episcopal	2,405,000
Churches of Christ	1,921,000
Congregational/United Church of Christ	736,000
Jehovah's Witnesses	1,914,000
Seventh-Day Adventist	938,000
Orthodox Church in America	900,000
Christian Churches (Unspecified)	786,000

Data reported via self-identification in the American Religious Identification Survey (2009).

TABLE 4-2   Largest Organized Religions in the United States

Religion	2008 Estimated Adult Population	% of U.S. Population, 2008
Christianity	159,030,000	76.7
Judaism	2,680,000	1.2
Islam	1,349,000	0.6
Buddhism	1,189,000	0.5
Hinduism	766,000	0.4
Unitarian Universalist	629,000	0.3
Wiccan/Pagan/Druid	307,000	0.1
Spiritualist	116,000	*
American Indian Religion	103,000	*
Baha'i	84,000	*

*Less than 0.05%.

Data reported via self-identification in the American Religious Identification Survey (2009). Nonreligious, Atheist, and Agnostic categories have been dropped from this list.

e-mails of spiritual wisdom in various flavors to more than 5 million subscribers. Generic "inspiration" is the most popular type of e-mail (2.4 million), followed by the Bible (1.6 million), but there are 460,000 subscribers to the Buddhist thought for the day, 313,000 Torah devotees, 268,000 subscribers to Daily Muslim Wisdom, and 236,000 who get the Spiritual Weight Loss message. Islam is the fastest growing religion in the world, with more than 7 million American believers (Ali, 2005). Campo-Flores (2004) describes the increasing number of Christian nightclubs that are proliferating in Dallas, Nashville, and Tamarac, Florida, along with the "Get your praise on" Christian movement.

Over the past decades, there has been a trend within nursing theory to separate religion from spirituality and to make spirituality the legitimate focus of nursing care (Kirkham, Pesut, Meyerhoff, & Sawatzky, 2004). A priority in spiritual care is end-of-life care. Interest in transcultural nursing toward dying, death, and bereavement has dramatically increased in recent years (Fordham, Giger, & Davidhizar, 2006). Of particular interest are the disadvantaged dying: those who are older and are dying with other long-term degenerative and ultimately fatal illnesses; these patients are unlikely to be given the label of "terminally ill" or to be aware of their prognosis (Exley, 2004).

JEHOVAH'S WITNESSES

Although each group has unique practices that should be considered by the nurse, two groups with particular significance for the nurse are Jehovah's Witnesses and Seventh-Day Adventists.

The founder of the Watchtower Bible and Tract Society, which is the legal corporation now used by Jehovah's Witnesses, was Charles Taze Russell. The name "Jehovah's Witnesses" was taken in Columbus, Ohio, in 1931 in an attempt to differentiate between the Watchtower Tract Society and the true followers of Russell, who were represented by the Dawn Bible Students and the Layman's Home Missionary Movement. From 1876 to 1879, Russell served as pastor of a Bible class he organized in Pittsburgh, Pennsylvania, and was also the assistant editor of a small monthly magazine in Rochester, New York. However, he resigned from the editorial position in 1879 when controversy arose over his counterarguments on the atonement of Christ. In 1879 he founded the magazine *Herald of the Morning*, which developed into the magazine that is distributed today as *The Watchtower Announcing Jehovah's Kingdom*. This magazine has grown from a circulation of 6000 to 39 million per month and is published in 188 languages and is considered to be the most widely circulated publication in the world. Today there is another Watchtower periodical titled *Awake*;

it has a circulation of 38 million issues twice a month and is published in 88 languages (Jehovah's Witnesses official Web site, 2014).

In 1884, Russell incorporated Zion's Watchtower Tract Society, in Pittsburgh, which published a series of seven books. Russell himself wrote six of these books. The seventh volume, *The Finished Mystery*, caused a split in the group that culminated in a clean division. The larger portion of the group followed Joseph Franklin Rutherford, whereas the smaller portion subsequently became known as the Dawn Bible Students Association. Under Rutherford's leadership, the Watchtower Bible Society began to attack the doctrines of organized religion. This group eventually became known as the present-day Jehovah's Witnesses and has branches in 233 countries with 5.9 million members. According to 2008 statistics, there are 1,914,000 Jehovah's Witnesses in the United States (Kosmin & Keysar 2009). The U.S. headquarters is located in Brooklyn, New York (Lindner, 2004).

Modern-day Jehovah's Witnesses still await the millennium. They regard Christ as a creature who will come to destroy the forces of evil at Armageddon, and they teach that sinners who are not saved will perish, whereas the faithful will enter into the Kingdom of Joy and Happiness. Because they believe in the Second Coming of the Kingdom, they undertake no military service. They also hold the belief that the institutions of government are under the control of Satan. It is this belief that has been the basis for some of the persecution they have undergone over the years. One view of this group is that Jehovah's Witnesses are peaceful but somewhat fanatical and that they know their Bible backward and forward (Smart, 1991). Some theologians believe that this religion appeals to persons of very modest education (Smart, 1991). The Jehovah's Witness faith is based on the doctrines presented in Box 4-2.

Implications for Nursing Care

There are many implications for the nurse who provides culturally appropriate nursing care to a Jehovah's Witness. The paramount concern for the nurse is that Jehovah's Witnesses are opposed, on the basis of scripture and Christian history, to homologous (amologous) blood transfusions (blood obtained from a blood bank or through donations). Blood that is precollected from the client for future use and stored as either whole blood or as packed cells is also not acceptable (Watchtower, 1989). Jehovah's Witnesses hold the view that "God's determination is that blood represents life and thus is sacred" (Watchtower, 1989). They believe that it is God's commandment that no human should sustain life by taking blood. Jehovah's Witnesses believe that if blood is taken from a creature and not

BOX 4-2   Beliefs of Jehovah's Witnesses

1. Jehovah's Witnesses believe that there is one solitary Being from all eternity and that that Being is Jehovah, God, the creator and preserver of the universe in all things that are visible and invisible.

2. Jehovah's Witnesses do not believe in the Holy Trinity of three Gods in one—God the Father, God the Son, and God the Holy Ghost—who are equal in power, substance, and eternity (Watchtower Bible & Tract Society, 1953). Rather, they believe that Satan is the originator of the Trinity doctrine and that this doctrine is just another of Satan's attempts to keep people from learning the truth about Jehovah and his Son, Christ Jesus, which is that there is no Trinity (Watchtower Bible & Tract Society, 1953).

3. Jehovah's Witnesses believe that there is only one God and that he is greater than his Son. They believe that the Son, the firstborn and only begotten, was sent by God but is not God himself and is not equal with God.

4. On the subject of the virgin birth, Jehovah's Witnesses believe that Jehovah God took the perfect life of his only begotten Son and transferred it from heaven to the womb of the unmarried virgin, Mary. They believe that Jesus' birth was not an incarnation but that he was emptied of all things heavenly and spiritual. This was a miracle in the sense that Jesus was born a man (and was flesh) instead of a spirit–human hybrid (Martin, 2003).

5. Jehovah's Witnesses believe that the human life that Jesus Christ laid down in sacrifice must be viewed as exactly equal to the life that Adam forfeited for all of his offspring. Thus, Jesus' life must be viewed as a perfect human life, no more and no less (Watchtower Bible & Tract Society, 1955).

6. Jehovah's Witnesses believe that immortality is a reward for faithfulness and that it does not come automatically to a human at birth (Watchtower Bible & Tract Society, 1953).

7. On the subject of the resurrection of Christ, Jehovah's Witnesses believe that Christ was raised from the dead, not as a human creature, but as a spirit (Watchtower Bible & Tract Society, 1953).

8. Jehovah's Witnesses believe that Christ Jesus will return again, not as a human but as a glorious spirit. National flags or symbols of the sovereign power of a nation are forbidden by Exodus 20:2–6. Thus, those who believe and ascribe salvation only to God may not salute a national emblem without violating Jehovah's commandments against idolatry (Watchtower Bible & Tract Society, 1953).

9. Jehovah's Witnesses believe that the hell mentioned in the Bible is mankind's common grave and that even an honest child can understand it. Thus, the doctrine of a burning hell where the wicked are tortured after death cannot be true.

10. Jehovah's Witnesses believe that man is a combination of two things: dust of the ground and breath of life. The combining of these two things produces a living soul, or a creature called man.

11. Jehovah's Witnesses believe that the undefeatable purpose of Jehovah God is to establish a righteous kingdom in these last days and that this purpose has already been fulfilled.

12. Jehovah's Witnesses believe that the Levitical commandments given by God to Moses included the commandment that no one in the House of David should eat blood or he would be cut off from people.

---

used for sacrifice, it should be disposed of and covered with dust. People who subscribe to this belief are likely to refuse any surgical or medical interventions that will require homologous blood transfusion. Even in the face of ominous danger and with the impending threat of loss of life, a Jehovah's Witness will refuse treatment for self and family members if a homologous transfusion is the only plausible blood replacement option available. However, many but not all Jehovah's Witnesses will submit to certain types of autologous blood transfusions (autotransfusion). Whether autologous blood transfusions will be accepted by a Jehovah's Witness depends on the type of autologous transfusion—one type that might be acceptable is blood retrieved through induced hemodilution at the start of surgery (blood that is directed to storage bags outside the client's body while plasma expanders [perfluorocarbons] are given to maintain blood volume). The blood is then reinfused toward the end of surgery or during the postoperative period. Although this type of autologous transfusion might be acceptable, other types, such as use of blood collected from a wound by aspiration, pumped through a filter or a centrifuge to remove debris and clots, and then returned to the client, would not be an acceptable alternative (Watchtower, 1989). Many Jehovah's Witnesses carry a card stating that they refuse blood in all circumstances and the type of blood expander that is acceptable. The caregivers should ask the client for this extremely important card or, if the client is unconscious, examine the client's personal belongings to find it. When autologous blood transfusions or blood volume expanders are not plausible alternatives, many physicians look to alternatives during major surgery that are acceptable to Jehovah Witnesses, including colloids or colloid replacement fluids, electrocautery, hypotensive anesthesia, or hypothermia. Researchers continue to seek a red blood cell substitute that is practical and safe, but the products that have been tried have not been pronounced successful. Many legal battles have been waged in the courts with regard to parents' refusal to allow surgical or medical interventions in their minor children. The consensus of the court in some countries, such as the Supreme Court in the United States, has been that a person of adult majority age has the right to refuse treatment but cannot withhold treatment from a minor child.

A second concern for the nurse is the refusal of Jehovah's Witnesses to eat certain foods to which blood has been added, such as some sausages and lunch meats. The nurse must take extra care to ensure that blood has not been added to foods that are served to Jehovah's Witnesses. Because Jehovah's Witnesses are pacifists and conscientious objectors, the nurse must also take extra care to avoid raising such issues during interactions. In general, topics related to politics, government rule, and the like should be avoided. Because Jehovah's Witnesses do not observe any national holidays or ceremonies, including Christmas, the nurse should avoid any attempts to involve the client in preparations for such celebrations.

SEVENTH-DAY ADVENTISTS

The Seventh-Day Adventist religion sprang from the "Great Second Advent Awakening" that shocked the religious world just before the middle of the nineteenth century. During this period, reemphasis on the second advent of Jesus Christ was rampant in England and in Europe. It was not long before many of the Old World views and prophetic interpretations crossed the Atlantic and began to penetrate American theological circles (Martin, 2003). The American Seventh-Day Adventist group began in upper New York (Ellwood, 2005).

The first leader of the Seventh-Day Adventists was William Miller, a Baptist minister from Lower Hampton, New York. The Seventh-Day Adventist religion is based largely on the apocalyptic books of Daniel and Revelation. Many of the early students of the Seventh-Day Adventist religion, following the chronology of Archbishop Ussher, interpreted the 2300 days of Daniel as 2300 years, and thus they concluded that Christ would come back in about the year 1843. In 1818 Miller taught many of his followers that in about 25 years (1843), Jesus Christ would come again. Miller and his associates pinpointed October 22, 1843, as the specific final date on which Jesus Christ would return for his saints, visit judgment on sin, and establish the Kingdom of God on earth. Many theologians disagreed with Miller's contentions because they believed that Miller was teaching in contradiction to the Word of God. According to biblical scripture, "the day and hour knoweth no man, no, not the angels of heaven but God alone" (Matthew 24:36). Because of Miller's early teaching, the first group of Seventh-Day Adventists were called Millerites. However, the mistake of setting an exact date for Christ's Second Coming led to failure for the first Seventh-Day Adventist movement in the United States.

The modern Seventh-Day Adventist movement is based on the prophecy of Ellen G. White. White made an early assertion about Miller's prophecy that supported it and gave a date that she considered to be correct: October 22, 1844. Despite this failure in prediction, the group has grown and been active in evangelism. Today Seventh-Day Adventists believe that Christ will return again very soon and that Christians have an obligation to keep some of the laws of Moses, including worship on Saturday, the old Sabbath. Thirteen issues on doctrine that give direction for living and that are upheld by the Seventh-Day Adventist Church are presented in Box 4-3.

There were 914,106 members of the Seventh-Day Adventist Church in North America in 2012. The Seventh-Day Adventist Church is one of the fastest growing churches in the world today, passing the 18-million mark in 1998 (General Conference of the Seventh-Day Adventists, 2014). The worldwide Seventh-Day Adventist Church headquarters are located in Washington, DC.

Implications for Nursing Care

The religious doctrines of Seventh-Day Adventists teach that the body is a temple of God and thus should be kept healthy. Persons who subscribe to this faith may avoid such items as seafood, meat, caffeine, alcohol, drugs, and tobacco in all forms. To provide culturally appropriate nursing care to a Seventh-Day Adventist, the nurse must know and understand the religious doctrines of the Seventh-Day Adventist Church. A Seventh-Day Adventist may refuse surgical intervention on a Friday evening or Saturday morning or afternoon because the client may interpret such an intervention as being in direct conflict with religious doctrines. This same client may also refuse other medical interventions that might normally take place at these times, such as respiratory or physical therapy.

The religious doctrine regarding unclean foods may cause some clients to refuse to eat certain foods with shells,

BOX 4-3   Beliefs of Seventh-Day Adventists

1. **Inspiration and authority of the scriptures.** Seventh-Day Adventists believe that the scriptures of both the Old Testament and the New Testament were inspired by God and constitute the very Word of God. They hold the Protestant position that the Bible is the sole root of the faith and practice of Christians.

2. **The nature of Christ.** Christ, called the Second Adam, is pure and holy, connected with God, and beloved by God. Seventh-Day Adventists believe that Christ is God and that he has existed with God for all eternity (Martin, 2003).

3. **The Atonement.** Seventh-Day Adventists do not believe that Christ made partial or incomplete sacrificial atonement on the cross. The all-sufficient sacrifice of Jesus was completed on the cross at Calvary.

4. **The Resurrection.** Seventh-Day Adventists believe that Jesus rose from the grave, ascended literally and bodily into heaven, and serves before God. They believe that there will be a resurrection of both the just and the unjust. For the just, this resurrection will take place at the Second Coming of Christ, whereas the resurrection of the unjust will take place 1000 years later, at the close of the millennium (Revelations 20:5–10).

5. **The Second Coming.** Seventh-Day Adventists believe that Jesus Christ will assuredly come the second time and that his second advent will be visible, audible, and personal.

6. **The plan of salvation.** Seventh-Day Adventists believe that one must be born again and fully accepted by the Lord. They believe that there is nothing an individual can ever do that will merit the salvation of God. Salvation is by grace (Romans 3:20).

7. **The spiritual nature of man.** Seventh-Day Adventists believe that man rests in the tomb until the resurrection of the just, when the righteous will be called

forth by Christ (Revelations 20:4–5). It is at this point that the just will enter into everlasting life in their eternal home in the Kingdom of Glory.

8. **Punishment of the wicked.** Seventh-Day Adventists reject the doctrine of eternal torment because everlasting life is a gift from God (Romans 6:23). The wicked do not possess this and therefore shall not have eternal life (John 3:36).

9. **Sanctuary and investigative judgment.** Seventh-Day Adventists believe that the acceptance of Christ at conversion does not seal a person's destiny; rather, it determines his life's work after conversion. Man's record is closed when he comes to the end of his days; he is responsible for his influences during life and is likewise responsible for his evil influences after he is dead.

10. **Scapegoat teaching.** Seventh-Day Adventists repudiate the idea that Satan is the sin bearer.

11. **The Sabbath and the Mark of the Beast.** This doctrine is based on the Bible as interpreted by Seventh-Day Adventists and not according to Ellen White's writings. Seventh-Day Adventists do not believe that keeping the Sabbath is a means of keeping salvation or willing merit before God. They believe that man is saved only by grace.

12. **The question of unclean food.** Seventh-Day Adventists refrain from eating certain foods, not because of the laws of Moses but because it is a Christian duty to preserve the body in the best of health for the service and glory of God (1 Corinthians 3:16).

13. **The "remnant church."** Seventh-Day Adventists believe God has a precious remnant, a multitude of earnest and sincere individuals, in every church. The majority of God's children are scattered throughout the world and may practice their religion on Sunday.

such as lobster or crab; scavenger fish, such as catfish; or certain meats. This refusal to eat some foods high in iodine or protein may cause these clients to have iodine and protein deficiencies; thus, it is important for the nurse to teach these clients that iodine and protein substitutes are necessary in the diet. Some specialty shops that have a Seventh-Day Adventist clientele stock a variety of protein substitutes for meats. These substitutes are often made from vegetables such as soybeans and may take the place of meats such as ground beef. These substitutes should be

encouraged, particularly when they appear to be free of preservatives.

The nurse and the nurse manager should also be aware that a colleague who is a Seventh-Day Adventist may refuse to accept assignments on Friday evenings or Saturday during the day, since the Sabbath begins on Friday at dusk and extends to Saturday at dusk. It is important for the nurse who is a Seventh-Day Adventist to ascertain at the time of employment whether working on Friday evenings or Saturday during the day is a requirement of the job. On the other hand, it is also important for the nurse manager to include staff in making nondiscriminatory policies in this regard. Inclusion of staff in policy making may minimize implementation difficulties.

ISLAM: THE RELIGION*

According to a study of mosques (Bagby, Perl, & Froehle, 2001), Islam is the fastest growing religion in the United States. Between 1994 and 2000, the number of mosques increased from 962 to 1209, an increase of 25%. Much of the growth in these congregations occurred in less than 20 years; about one third of mosques were established in the 1980s and another third in the 1990s. The ethnic distribution of members of the average mosque is 25% Arab, 33% South Asian, and 30% African-American. Most organizations are involved in some outreach activities: 70% provide some type of assistance for the needy, and 20% have full-time schools for children. Based on the 2 million persons associated with a mosque in this study, the total U.S. Muslim population is estimated at 6 to 7 million persons and growing. Part of this increase in numbers is attributed to conversion to Islam, which has been estimated at 17% to 30% of membership.

The three major monotheistic religions of the world—Judaism, Christianity, and Islam—share common cultural roots and history. All three originated in the Middle East, and each developed and dispersed globally in response to cultural influences and world politics. The Arabic word *Islam* means "peace, submission, and obedience." Islam is a monotheistic religion that recognizes Muhammad as the last of the great prophets, following in the footsteps of Noah, Abraham, Moses, and Jesus. The life and writings of Muhammad, the Qur'an, serve as a template for Muslims to worship, pray, raise their families, and conduct daily life. The tenets of Islamic life are described as the "Five Pillars of Islam." Although religious groups often become well known by the actions of their extremist members, Islam is not typically practiced as a fundamentalist religion. The practice of Islam is less well known because Muslims are a religious minority primarily represented by immigrant populations. This demographic is changing with the increase in membership by African-Americans.

The Five Pillars of Islam

1. The declaration of faith: The first article of faith in Islam is to recognize the existence of one Supreme Being. Muslims bear witness that there is none worthy of worship except Allah and that Muhammad is his messenger to all humanity until the day of judgment. The prophethood of Muhammad obliges Muslims to follow his exemplary life as a model.
2. Daily prayers: Muslims offer prayers five times a day as part of their religious duty to remain focused on spiritual connectedness. These prayers are scheduled throughout the day at designated times and are observed at work, in school, and at home. The result is a rhythm of daily life that is punctuated with communal religious devotion.
3. Fasting during Ramadan: Islam uses both solar and lunar calendars, and the observance of daytime fasting occurs during the ninth lunar month, Ramadan. During this 28-day period Muslim adults abstain from food and drink from dawn to sunset. The purpose of this communal fast, known as *sawm,* is to develop restraint, self-control, self-discipline, and self-obedience. Pregnant or lactating women, children, the sick, and the elderly are excused from fasting, but those who can afford it may be expected to provide a meal to a poor person for each day they cannot fast.
4. Giving alms to the poor: *Zakat* is an annual payment or tithe of a percentage of income given to the poor or needy. All Muslims are bound by this religious duty, although the amount is based on the individual's ability to pay.
5. Pilgrimage to Mecca: Each Muslim is obligated to perform *hajj,* a pilgrimage to the holy city of Mecca in Saudi Arabia. Hajj is required once during a lifetime, provided that the individual Muslim is physically and financially able.

Common Muslim Phrases

"God willing" or "If God wills it" (pronounced *in sha'allah*) is a common phrase used regarding future events to acknowledge the limited control of humans and the supremacy of Allah in daily life. For example, one person asks, "When will you return?" The respondent will often say something like "God willing, I will come again tomorrow."

"Thanks be to God" (pronounced *hamdu'allah*) is a phrase commonly used to acknowledge the hand of God in all things good. For example, when common greetings are exchanged, such as "How are you today?" the response is often "I am doing well. Thanks be to God." (Also see Box 4-4 for common Islamic terms.)

Social Differences in Islamic Culture

Apart from religious adherence, Islamic culture manifests itself in many ways that are similar to other cultural groups in the United States. The importance of the extended

---

*The section on Islam (Muslims) was written by Mary Grace Umlauf, PhD, RN, FAAN.

BOX 4-4   Common Islamic Terms

Allah: The Supreme Being, the one and only God, the same God as that worshiped by Jews and Christians.

Azan: The call for daily prayers, broadcast five times a day in Arabic over a loudspeaker in the minaret, or tower, of the mosque.

Eid: A religious festival. There are two main celebrations in Islam. The Eid Al Fitr marks the end of Ramadan, a month of fasting. The Eid Al-Adhha is the Feast of Sacrifice in memory of when the prophet Abraham was asked to sacrifice his son Ishmael.

Hadith: A collection of sayings and traditions of the prophet Muhammad that are used to guide daily life, dietary practices, and social interactions.

Halal: A term meaning "lawful," which refers to compliance with the Qur'an and the Hadith. In Muslim communities, grocery stores advertise halal meat for sale. Like the Jewish Kosher tradition, these vendors have followed the Islamic practices required in the preparation and killing of animals.

Haram: The converse of halal, unlawful according to the tenets of the Qur'an and the Hadith. Eating pork is considered haram for Muslims. Sex outside of marriage is also haram or forbidden.

Imam: A religious leader who leads congregational prayers at the mosque. This person is not viewed as infallible. The imam is not ordained or assigned to a particular mosque by any higher religious authority.

Jihad: An Arabic word derived from the word *jahada,* which means to strive for a better way of life or endeavor, strain, exertion, effort, diligence, or fighting to defend one's life, land, and religious freedom. Extremists may use this concept as justification for violence, whereas most Muslims understand this concept to mean the intrapersonal struggle to overcome evil and to live a just and good life.

Masjid: The Arabic word for "mosque." The three holiest mosques are located in the Middle East. Al-Masjid Al-Haram and Al-Masjid Al-Nabawi are located in Mecca and Madinah, Saudi Arabia, where Islam originated. The third is Al-Masjid Al-Aqsa in Jerusalem.

Muhammad: The last and final prophet who established the monotheistic religion of Islam in the midst of a climate of political polytheism. He was born in 570 and died in 632 A.D. He was a husband, father, religious leader, political leader, and reformer. The contents of the Qur'an were revealed to him at the age of 40 through the angel Gabriel.

Muslim (or Moslem): A believer in Islam. The term "Muhammadan" is viewed as incorrect and inappropriate to Muslims because it implies that they worship Muhammad in the way Christians worship Christ. Moslems assert, as a primary article of faith, that they believe in Allah and do not deify Muhammad.

Qur'an (or Koran): The holy scripture of Islam revealed by Allah to Muhammad over a period of 23 years. The Qur'an is maintained in Arabic and studied in its original form. Translation of the text is said to dilute or reinterpret the original meaning of the text.

Zakah: Giving alms, one of the five pillars of Islam. The money collected is to be used for the welfare of society in the following categories: the poor, the needy, the sympathizers, the captives, the debtors, the cause of Allah, the wayfarers, and those who collect it. The amount collected ranges from 2.5% to 10%, depending upon the resources of the individual.

---

family unit is a pervasive theme among Muslims and other persons who come from countries that are historically Islamic. Social customs, such as styles of women's clothing, are distinct, but the theme of modest clothing for women is common to many other faiths and communities, such as the Amish and Orthodox Jews. Likewise, the prohibition against eating pork is also held in common with Judaism.

Emphasis on Family

In the context of Islamic culture, the value of the family group supersedes the importance of the individual. Individuals draw their identity and strength from their families. Family can be counted upon to provide nurturing, social support, economic assistance, and caregiving. Children are highly valued and lavished with affection by all members of the family. Children are more often cared for by family members and are seldom cared for by unrelated persons. Adolescents and young people develop strong bonds with other members of the family of the same sex, who provide career guidance and mentoring. Primary allegiance is deferred to parents, who make important decisions such as advanced schooling or career selection on behalf of the child, even into adulthood. This is not to say that the child has no input in decision making or that personal skill or ability is not considered. Typically, the parent and child discuss the pros and cons of a given course of action. The parent ultimately confirms or negates a decision, and the child is usually persuaded to accept the outcome. After marriage, this pattern of decision making is more consultative in nature. Marriage partners confer with each other, while also taking input from the other family members into account.

Social Support

Because family members prefer to live in close proximity and typically spend a lot of time together, the extended family can provide a great deal of support if there are problems in the nuclear family. For example, if a married couple is experiencing problems, it is usually apparent or known to some degree. Individually, the husband or wife will often confer with a trusted family member about the problem. Regardless of the nature of the problem, the family mobilizes to problem-solve or to reconcile differences between the partners. Although divorce is permitted in Islam, divorce is not preferable when children are involved. In general, problems of an individual or an individual nuclear family are also the concerns of the family group.

The Crisis of Infertility

Among families that are newly emigrated from Islamic countries, fertility problems are viewed as particularly disastrous for married partners. Because of the high value placed on children in the family, infertility may be an acceptable justification for divorce in an immigrant's country of origin. Some Islamic countries recognize polygamy as a social tradition that can remedy this problem for the male partner who is fertile. In those countries he can retain an infertile wife and marry another wife who is likely to be fertile. However, polygamy is not permitted in the United States. Thus, an infertile Muslim woman may be at risk for an unwanted divorce because she now lives in the United States. An infertile man is also at risk of being rejected by his wife, who is likely to have full support of her family for this action. Medical interventions for infertility that involve sperm or egg donation are unacceptable under Islamic law because they violate the primary recognition of family membership. Each child must carry the name of his father and family. Anonymous donation of genetic material violates this essential directive. Adoption outside the family unit is not an attractive option for infertile couples for the same reason. Conversely, adoption of orphaned family members is viewed as a family obligation and right.

Covered Women

One of the most noticeable differences about practicing Muslims is the way some of the women dress. As Muslim girls are growing up, they are taught the importance of *hijab,* or modesty. Modesty, particularly the covering of the hair and arms when in public, is meant to avoid pride or showiness in outward appearance, much like the practice of Amish women or religious orders of Catholic women. As a matter of religious preference, when a girl reaches puberty, she can choose to cover herself when in public by wearing a headscarf and long-sleeved clothing. Typically, Muslim women also wear longer skirts or long pants. At home and in the presence of family members or groups of women only, these same women do not cover. Even though a woman may be dressed in a scarf and a somber-colored full-length dress in public, underneath she may be wearing the latest fashion and the brightest colors. Although the practice of *hijab* is viewed as a form of modesty and religiosity, becoming covered also marks a rite of passage and evolving membership for young women in the family and social group. Thus, very young girls make a very demur debut as young women in the Muslim community when they begin to cover.

Women who practice *hijab* are also likely to avoid situations where they must touch or be in very close proximity to men. These women may avoid shaking hands with men and will avoid sitting next to a man on public transportation, such as a bus or plane. Male health care providers may not be able to perform physical assessments or provide personal care to these women because of their commitment to modesty. A female nurse may have to perform breast or pelvic examinations in lieu of a male physician or male nurse.

Sex and Marriage

Along with the emphasis on family and on modesty among women, sex outside of marriage is highly discouraged. Young people are encouraged to maintain strong social ties with others of the same sex. Activities sponsored by mosques and related organizations will congregate men with men and women with women. Only infrequently will there be activities that include a mixed group. Even wedding celebrations will provide separate but adjoining halls or ballrooms for men and women to congregate separately, and the children often migrate between rooms at will. In the more traditional families, dating does not begin unless there is an interest in marriage and the woman's family has approved beginning a relationship. The selection of a marriage partner is a planned activity, and the extended family may be called upon to identify well-qualified marriage partners. Families try to identify potential marriage partners with a good family background, a good education, a good job, and a compatible temperament who are also Muslim. In general, Muslim families will accept a marriage with a non-Muslim, but Christian families from an Islamic background will not accept a marriage with a Muslim.

Families do not arrange marriages per se, but there is an active interest in making sure that the wrong type of person is not considered. Because this is an acceptable practice in Islamic cultures, there is less pressure for dating and pre-marital sex among young people. Concurrently, there is greater communal support for having a good reputation, an education, and a good job, as well as a good family background.

Stereotypes about Muslims

1. All Arabs are Muslims, all Muslims are Arabs: Arabs may be of any faith, and many are Orthodox Christians. Muslims may be from any ethnic group. Many U.S. converts to Islam are African-Americans. However, converts must learn Arabic to study the Qur'an.
2. Most Muslims are from the Middle East: There are more Muslims in Indonesia than in all Arab countries combined. Many Muslims also come from Asia and sub-Saharan Africa, or they may be American residents who have recently converted to Islam.
3. Islam promotes violence, or Muslims are violent people: Most Muslim immigrants come from developing countries with unstable political and economic systems. Many come to the United States to avoid the strife of war and to live peaceful lives with their families.
4. Muslims do not recognize the rights of women to go to school or to have jobs: Social custom or political oppression should not be confused with religious and cultural practices. Although there have been recent examples of the oppression of women in a few Islamic countries, the Qur'an does not deny women the freedom to learn, to be productive, or to own property.
5. Family violence is common among Muslims: Family violence can occur in any household regardless of religious background or economic status. Although no data are available, marital conflicts may occur more often among new immigrant families because they lack the economic and social support offered by extended families in their home countries. In response to this need, many mosques have initiated programs to address this problem. For example, the Islamic community in Oakland, California, has developed an outreach program called "Muslims against Family Violence" that includes public education, a toll-free number for assistance, and a Web site that describes their prevention program.

ETHNIC GROUPS IN RELATION TO FAMILY IN THE UNITED STATES

The 2010 census reveals some interesting trends in both population growth and changes in the geographic location of the population. For example, according to the 2010 census data, the state with the fastest population growth was Nevada (by 35.1%), followed by Arizona (by 24.6%), Utah (by 23.7%), Idaho (by 21.3%), and finally Texas (20.6%). The slowest growing states were Rhode Island, Louisiana, and Ohio. The only state with a reported decline was Michigan, losing 0.6% of its population (U.S. Department of Commerce, Bureau of the Census, 2010 Census Briefs, Distribution and Change, 2013). According to the 2010 census, there were an estimated 320,786,413 people living in the United States (U.S. Department of Commerce, Bureau of the Census, 2010 Census Brief, Race, 2013). Of these, 45,003,665 (14.0%) were Black, 2,932,319 (0.9%) were American Indian/Eskimo-Aleut, 14,674,252 (5.6%) were Asian, and 378,782 (0.3%) were Pacific Islander. In addition, 50,477,594 (17%) were Hispanic, representing a 43% change since the 2000 census. Some 223,553,265 (72.4%) of the total population classified themselves as non-Hispanic White (U.S. Department of Commerce, Bureau of the Census, 2010 Census Brief, Race, 2013). It is estimated that by 2050, the United States will have 393.9 million people, 40% more than the population today. It is also estimated that the population will be more diverse. The non-Hispanic White share of the population is projected to fall from the current 70.38% to 53% by 2050. Meanwhile, persons of Hispanic origin will increase from 16.3% to 24% of the population. Asians and Pacific Islanders will see their population climb from 5.60% to 9%. Increases are expected to be smaller for American Indian, Eskimo, and Aleut populations, from slightly under 1%, and for African-Americans, from 12.6% to 16% (U.S. Department of Commerce, Bureau of the Census, American Community Survey, 2013). Two ethnic groups will be discussed in relation to family as follows.

American Indians

According to the 2010 census, there are 2,932,248 American Indians living in the United States (U.S. Department of Commerce, Bureau of the Census, 2010 Census Brief, Race, 2013). Because there are more than 565 different federally recognized tribes of American Indians and an additional 200 who do not benefit from federal recognition, it is difficult to predict patterns of residency unless one is dealing with specific tribes (Palacios, Butterfly, & Strickland, 2006). In 2010, the 10 states with the largest American Indian populations, in order, were California, Oklahoma, Arizona, Texas, New Mexico, New York, Washington, North Carolina, Michigan, and Alaska. Florida was the only other state with more than 100,000 American Indians. These 11 states are home to 62% of the total U.S. American Indian population (U.S. Department of Commerce, Bureau of the Census, American Community

Survey, 2013). In the United States, Indian reservations are places where very slow and very rapid changes are occurring simultaneously. It is estimated that 72% of Navajo homes still do not have a telephone and that many homes lack plumbing. On the other hand, among American Indians type 2 diabetes mellitus and obesity have suddenly appeared with the highest incidence in the world (Reid, 2000). Providing culturally appropriate nursing care is complicated because each nation or tribe of American Indians has its own language and religion, and belief system practices differ significantly among groups as well as among members of the same tribe (Palacios et al., 2006).

The American Indian family is frequently composed of extended family members who may encompass several households. Through various religious ceremonies, other individuals can become the same as a parent in the family network. In some American Indian tribes, grandparents are viewed as the family leaders, and respect for individuals increases with their age. In some tribes, the family is viewed as important, particularly in periods of crisis, when family members are expected to serve as sources of support and security. It is important for the nurse to remember that because some American Indian tribes tend to place great emphasis on the extended family as a unit, the opinions and ideas of the family members should be solicited in order to give culturally appropriate nursing care. Even though physicians and hospitals may be available to American Indians, some families may still hold traditional healing ceremonies in high regard, and it may be important to incorporate old ways to treat illnesses for a treatment plan to be effective.

The Hmong

The Hmong are of Asian descent and are an ethnic–cultural group of people who originally lived in the rural highlands of Laos (Johnson & Hang, 2006; Lester, 2006). Many of the Hmong living in the United States today were displaced from their homeland because of their alignment with the United States during the Vietnam War (Johnson & Hang, 2006). There are 260,073 Hmong residing in the United States (U.S. Department of Commerce, Bureau of the Census, Asian Census Brief, 2013). The mean age for the rest of the general United States was 37.2; for Asian Americans it was 33 years; in contrast, in 2010, the median age of Hmong who made the United States their home was 19.1 years. Hmong, by median age, are still reported to be the youngest ethnic cultural group in the United States (U.S. Department of Commerce, Bureau of the Census, American Community Survey, Asian Briefs, The Hmongs, 2013). Not only are Hmong one of the youngest cultural groups residing in this country, but they also tend to have larger families (6.5 persons) than other Asian Americans (2.59

persons) and the general U.S. population (3.2 persons) (U.S. Department of Commerce, Bureau of the Census, Asian Brief, The Hmongs, 2013; U.S. Bureau of the Census, American Community Survey, 2013). Of the Hmong residing in the United States who are 25 years of age or older, 6.2% were less than a high school graduate, 81.1% were high school graduates, 16.8% had some college experience, and 13.4% held a Bachelor's degree or higher (U.S. Bureau of the Census, American Community Survey, 2013; U.S. Department of Commerce, Bureau of the Census, The Hmongs, Brief, 2013). Of the Hmong in the United States, 96.9% speak an Asian or Pacific Island language at home, 58.6% do not speak English well, and 43.9% are reported to be linguistically isolated (U.S. Bureau of the Census, American Community Survey, 2013; U.S. Department of Commerce, Bureau of the Census, Asian Brief, 2012).

The Hmong are primarily an oral cultural group, a statement implying that some Hmong have never learned to read Hmong or any other language (Shadick, 1993). In the 1950s, French missionaries introduced to the Hmong a form of written Hmong, which is based on the Roman alphabet (Shadick, 1993). There are two major dialectal variations in the oral Hmong language, Hmoo Daw (White Hmong) and Hmoo Ntsua (Blue Hmong) (Dunnigan, 1986). According to Catlin (1982), Hmong is spoken by using one of eight tones. For some Hmong, the oral word holds greater meaning and power than does the written word (Shadick, 1993). Some Hmong consider the spoken word to be the primary tool and mechanism for passing on traditions, rituals, and information to future generations (Shadick, 1993). It is important for the nurse to remember this when interacting with Hmong clients. Because they tend to be primarily an oral cultural group, culturally appropriate care is hindered when treatment plans and protocols are given to the client in a written form (even when the client does speak English). Hmong shamen are influential individuals within their community and often serve as resources for health information (Hensel, Mochel, & Bauer, 2005).

Special Interest Groups

Special interest groups are a significant part of the social structure of the United States. Individuals may join a group for many reasons, including support and self-help. Support groups provide the opportunity to increase the participant's social network, share solutions to common problems, and reshape perceptions of self and the environment. Examples of support groups include quality-of-life groups, caregiver support groups, and bereavement support groups (McMahon & Presswalla, 1997). Self-help groups are attractive to members because they promote well-being. Self-help groups are usually focused on particular clinical states, such as chronic mental illness; a particular social state, such as divorce; or special psychosocial issues, such as chemical dependency. Examples include Alcoholics Anonymous (AA), Narcotics Anonymous (NA), and Overeaters Anonymous (OA). Support groups may replace or augment the family or formal health care system and generally aim to link health behaviors with everyday existence. Self-help groups foster self-reliance and are a form of healing (McMahon & Presswalla, 1997). A network of friends, relatives, and neighbors can be crucial to psychological well-being and can relieve social isolation, promote mental health, facilitate coping, alleviate problems by preventive problem solving, and assist persons in preparing for stressful events in life (Brown, 1990).

Implications for Nursing Care

When nurses provide care to clients from a sociocultural background other than their own, they must have an awareness of and a sensitivity to the clients' sociocultural background, including knowledge of family structure and organization, religious values and beliefs, and how ethnicity and culture relate to role and role assignment within group settings. Friedman (1986) contends that nursing care must be directed to the family as a whole as well as to the individual family member. The nurse must therefore view the family as having two separate entities, the first being the family as an environment and the second being the family as the client. Both approaches to client care can be useful when the nurse attempts to provide culturally appropriate nursing care.

If the family is viewed as an environment, the primary focus of nursing care is the health and development of individual family members within a very specific environment. In this context it is important for the nurse to assess the extent to which the family provides the individual basic needs of each person. It is also essential that the nurse remember that individual needs vary, depending on developmental level and the current situation. The nurse should recognize that families provide more than just the physical necessities; the ability of the family to help the client meet psychosociological needs is paramount.

When families are viewed as an environment, it is extremely important for the nurse to recognize that other family members may also need intervention. For example, when a child is hospitalized, the parents may feel anxiety and stress; therefore, intervention with them is just as important as intervention with the hospitalized child (Davidhizar, Havens, & Bechtel, 1999; Sydnor-Greenberg & Dokken, 2000).

When families are viewed as clients, it is important to assess crucial factors that are germane to family structure and organization. For example, if a hypertensive client is

admitted to a hospital unit, it is crucial that the nurse assess several factors related to the family, including the following:

1. The family's current dietary patterns
2. The family's desire, as well as resources, for changing the dietary patterns
3. The family's knowledge about hypertension and its effects on the body
4. The family's ability to support a hypertensive family member
5. The family's ability to cope with and manage stress and anxiety

Whether the family is viewed as an environment or as the client, it is essential to incorporate cultural concepts when the nursing plan of care is being developed. The nursing process is used regardless of whether the family is viewed as an environment or as the client. The delineations or differences that occur in the nursing process are the result of cultural variables and beliefs that are germane to a particular ethnic or cultural group. Therefore, it is essential that the nurse incorporate cultural beliefs and concerns shared by family members into the plan of care.

CASE STUDY

Susie Chung, a 24-year-old Chinese American, is admitted with right lower-quadrant abdominal pain. Within a few hours Miss Chung is taken to surgery for an appendectomy. When she returns to the floor, her vital signs remain stable. The nurse notes that even though Miss Chung is rapidly recovering, her immediate and extended family appear to hover about her. The nurse also notes that it is very difficult to administer nursing care because of the number of family members who are keeping a constant vigil.

CLINICAL DECISION MAKING

1. List at least three social organization factors that influence the interactions between members of the same ethnic group or members of varying ethnic groups.
2. List at least two social organization factors that contribute to the development of cultural behavior.
3. Explain the role that religion may play for Susie Chung with regard to sociopsychological adaptation to her illness.
4. List at least three nursing interventions that minimize the confusion caused by the large number of family

members who are keeping constant vigil in Susie Chung's room.

5. List at least two reasons why the family members of Susie Chung have congregated in the hospital room.

6. List at least three factors that would support Susie Chung's family being defined as a behavioral system.

7. List at least two imaginary and two real boundaries that would be found within Susie Chung's family structure.

8. List at least two roles that Susie Chung may take on in a social context within her family structure.

REVIEW QUESTIONS

1. When planning to teach an Islamic client, the nurse needs to be aware of which of the following?
   a. Decision making tends to be male dominated.
   b. Decision making tends to be female dominated.
   c. Decision making tends to be generally consultative between spouses.
   d. Decision making tends to be consultative with the entire family.

2. When planning care for the patient who is a Jehovah's Witness and may need blood in an upcoming surgery, the nurse should be aware of which of the following?
   a. The patient will not accept whole blood.
   b. The patient will not accept predeposited autologous blood.
   c. The patient may accept autologous blood through induced hemodilution.
   d. The patient will accept wound-aspirated blood that has been filtered.

3. In developing a culturally sensitive care plan for a Hmong (Asian-American) psychiatric patient, which of the following would be inappropriate?
   a. Including the family in the plan of care.
   b. Showing respect by avoiding eye contact.
   c. Avoiding touching the head.
   d. Communicating all instructions in a written form.

REFERENCES

Ackerman, N. (1984). *The theory of family systems.* New York: Gardner Press.

Adams, D. (1995). Cultural diversity and institutional inequity. In D. L. Adams (Ed.), *Health issues for women of color.* Thousand Oaks, CA: Sage.

Adler, P., Good, M., Roberts, B., & Snyder, S. (2000). Fourth Quarter). The effects of Tai Chi on older adults with chronic arthritis pain. *Journal of Nursing Scholarship, 32*(4), 377–378.

Ali, L. (2001). The glorious rise of Christian pop. *Newsweek,* 38–41.

Ali, L. (2005). New welcoming spirit of the Mosque. *Newsweek,* 52.

American Association of Physical Anthropologists (AAPA). (1996). AAPA statement on biological aspects of race. *American Journal of Physical Anthropology, 101,* 569–570.

American Psychiatric Association (APA). (2000). *Diagnostic and statistical manual of mental disorders,* Text Revision (4th ed.). Washington, DC: American Psychiatric Association.

Andrews, M., & Boyle, J. (2008). *Transcultural concepts in nursing care* (5th ed.). Philadelphia: Lippincott.

Associated Press. (2000). Study: earnings gap between genders growing. *USA Today,* 1.

Averaswald, E. (1983). Families, change and the ecological perspective. In A. Ferber (Ed.), *The book of family therapy.* New York: J. Aronson.

Bagby, I., Perl, P. M., & Froehle, B. T. (2001). *The mosque in America: a national portrait.* Washington, DC: Council on American-Islamic Relations.

Bateson, G., Jackson, D., Haley, J., & Weakland, J. (1968). Toward a theory of schizophrenia. In D. D. Jackson (Ed.), *Communication, family and marriage.* Palo Alto, CA: Science & Behavior Books.

Bechtel, G., & Davidhizar, R. (1998). Mexicans in the psychiatric care setting. *Psychosocial Nursing and Mental Health Services, 36*(11), 20–27.

Berkanovic, E., & Reeder, L. G. (1973). Ethnic, economic and social psychological factors in the source of medical care. *Social Problems, 21,* 246–259.

Berry, J. (1988). Acculturation and psychological adaptation: a conceptual overview. In J. W. Berry & R. C. Annis (Eds.), *Ethnic psychology: research and practice with immigrants, refugees, native peoples, ethnic groups and sojourners.* Amsterdam: Swets & Zeitlinger.

Birx, E. (2002). *Healing Zen.* Ontario, Canada: Viking Compass.

Black, C. (2001). *It will never happen to me* (2nd ed.). Center City, MN: Hazelden.

Blum, R., Buehring, T., & Rinehart, P. (2000). *Protecting teens: beyond race, income, and family structure.* Minneapolis, MN: Center for Adolescent Health, University of Minnesota.

Bonder, B., Martin, L., & Miracle, A. (2002). *Culture in clinical care.* Thorofare, NJ: Slack.

Bowen, M. (1985). *Family therapy in clinical practice.* Northvale, NJ: Jason Aronson.

Brown, S. (1986). Children with an alcoholic parent. In N. Estes & M. Heinemann (Eds.), *Alcoholism: development, consequences, and interventions* (3rd ed., pp. 207–220). St. Louis: Mosby.

Brown, R. (1990). Self-help and therapy groups. *The Marshall Cavendish encyclopedia of personal relationships: human behavior.* New York: Marshall Cavendish.

Bullough, V. L., & Bullough, B. (1982). *Health care for the other Americans.* East Norwalk, CN: Appleton-Century-Crofts.

Campo-Flores, A. (2004). Get your praise on. *Newsweek,* 56.

Caplan, G. (1976). The family as a support system. In G. Caplan & M. Killilea (Eds.), *Support systems and mutual help: multidisciplinary exploration.* New York: Grune & Stratton.

Carroll, J., Johnson, D., & Marty, M. (1979). *Religion in America: 1950 to present.* New York: Harper & Row.

Casavantes, E. (1976). Pride and prejudice: a Mexican American dilemma. In C. A. Hernandez, M. J. Haug, & N. N. Wagner (Eds.), *Chicanos: social and psychological perspectives* (2nd ed., pp. 9–14). St. Louis: Mosby.

Catlin, A. R. (1982). Speech surrogate systems of the Hmong: from singing voices to talking reeds. In B. T. Downing & D. P. Olney (Eds.), *The Hmong in the West* (pp. 170–197). Minneapolis, MN: Center for Urban and Regional Affairs, University of Minnesota.

Clark, K., & Shute, N. (2001). The adoption maze. *U.S. News, 130*(10), 60–64.

Cloud, J. (2005). The battle over gay teens. *Time,* 43–51.

Cose, E. (2000). Our new look: the colors of race. *Newsweek,* 28.

Danyliw, N. (1997). Got mother's milk? *U.S. News and World Report, 123*(23), 79.

Davidhizar, R., Bechtel, G., & Cosey, E. (2000). Hospital extra: the spiritual needs of hospitalized patients. *American Journal of Nursing, 25,* 282–289.

Davidhizar, R., Havens, R., & Bechtel, G. (1999). Assessing culturally diverse pediatric clients. *Pediatric Nursing, 25*(4), 371–376, 393–394.

Davidhizar, R., King, V., Bechtel, G., & Giger, J. (1998). Nursing clients of Greek ethnicity at home. *Home Healthcare Nurse, 16*(9), 618–623.

Dowd, S., Davidhizar, R., & Giger, J. N. (2007). The mystery of altruism and transcultural nursing. *The Health Care Manager, 26*(1), 64–67.

Dunnewind, S. (2001). Saturated. *Pittsburgh Post-Gazette AP from the Seattle Times,* E-2.

Dunnigan, T. (1986). Process of identity maintenance in Hmong society. In G. L. Hendricks, B. T. Downing, & S. Deinard (Eds.), *The Hmong in transition* (pp. 41–53). Staten Island, NY: Center for Migration Studies.

Duvall, E., & Miller, B. (1985). *Marriage and family development* (6th ed.). New York: Harper & Row.

Ellwood, R. (2005). *Many peoples, many faiths* (8th ed.). Upper Saddle River, NJ: Pearson Prentice Hall.

Exley, C. (2004). Review article: the sociology of dying, death, and bereavement. *Sociology of Health and Illness, 26*(1), 110–122.

Fawcett, J. (1975). The family as a living open system: an emerging conceptual framework for nursing. *International Nursing Review, 22,* 113.

Finkleman, A. (2000). Psychiatric patients and families: moving from catastrophic event to long-term coping. *Home Care Providers, 5*(4), 142–147.

Fordham, P., Giger, J., & Davidhizar, R. (2006). Multi-cultural and multi-ethnic considerations and advanced directives: developing cultural competency. *Journal of Cultural Diversity, 13*(1), 3–9.

Freeman, H. P. (1998). The meaning of race in science—considerations for cancer research: concerns of special populations in the National Cancer Program. *Cancer, 82,* 219–225.

Friedman, M. M. (1986). *Family nursing: theory and assessment* (2nd ed.). East Norwalk, CT: Appleton-Century-Crofts.

Gary, F. (1991). Sociocultural diversity and mental health nursing. In F. Gary & C. Kavanaugh (Eds.), *Psychiatric nursing* (pp. 138–163). Philadelphia: J. B. Lippincott.

General Accountability Office. 2010. Washington, DC: Author.

General Conference of the Seventh Day Adventists. (2014). *Facts and figures.* Available at <http://www.adventist.org/>. Retrieved May 16, 2002.

Giger, J., Davidhizar, R., Evers, S., & Ingram, C. (1994). Cultural factors influencing mental health and mental illness. In C. Taylor (Ed.), *Mereness' essentials of psychiatric nursing* (14th ed., pp. 215–238). St. Louis: Mosby.

Giger, J., Davidhizar, R., & Wieczorek, S. (1994). Transcultural nursing: have we gone too far or not far enough? In D. Strickland & D. Fishman (Eds.), *Nursing in a diverse society.* Albany, NY: Delmar.

Giger, J., Johnson, J., Davidhizar, R., & Fishman, D. (1993). Strategies for building a supportive faculty. *Nursing and Health Care, 14*(3), 144–159.

Giorgianni, S. (2003). How families matter in health. *The Pfizer Journal, 7*(1), 1.

Goldsby, R. A. (1977). *Race and races* (2nd ed.). New York: Macmillan.

Gregory, D. (1992). Nursing practice in native communities. In A. Baumgart & J. Larson (Eds.), *Canadian nursing faces the future* (2nd ed.). St. Louis: Mosby.

Grypma, S. (1993). Culture shock. *The Canadian Nurse, 89*(8), 33–36.

Guruge, S., & Donner, G. (1996). Transcultural nursing in Canada. *The Canadian Nurse, 92*(8), 36–40.

Guttmacher, S., & Elinson, J. (1972). Ethno-religious variation in perception of illness: the use of illness as an explanation for deviant behavior. *Social Science Medicine, 5*(2), 117–125.

Habel, M. (2001). Caring for people of many cultures. *Nurse Week,* 20–22.

Haddad, A. (2001). Ethics in action (competent, elderly Chinese woman … can't give consent because she must wait for her family to arrive to give approval. *RN, 64*(3), 21–22, 24.

Hahn, J. (2006). Hahn's culture and disability assessment model (unpublished). Adapted from J. Giger & R. Davidhizar. (2004). In *Transcultural nursing assessment and intervention.* St. Louis: Mosby.

Harwood, A. (1981). *Ethnicity and medical care.* Cambridge, MA: Harvard University Press.

Headden, S. (1998). Favor aliens with job skills. *U.S. News and World Report, 123*(25), 83–85.

Henderson, G., & Primeaux, M. (1981). *Transcultural health care.* Reading, MA: Addison-Wesley.

Hensel, D., Mochel, M., & Bauer, R. (2005). Chronic illness and Hmong shaman. *Journal of Transcultural Nursing, 16*(2), 150–154.

Hirschman, C., Alba, R., & Farley, R. (2000). The meaning and measurement of race in the U.S. census: glimpses into the future. *Demography, 3*(37), 281–393.

Hitchcock, J. (2003). Framework for assessing families. In J. Hitchcock, P. Schubert, & S. Thomas (Eds.), *Community health nursing caring in action* (2nd ed.). San Francisco: Delmar.

Hsu, J. (1985). Asian family interaction patterns and their therapeutic implications. In P. Picot, P. Berner, R. Wolf, & K. Thau (Eds.), *Psychiatry: the state of art* (Vol. 8, pp. 599–606). New York: Plenum Press.

Jayson, S. (2006). Is "failure to launch" really a failure? *USA Today*, D1.

Jehovah's Witnesses Official Website. (2014). Retrieved from <http://www.jw-media.org/aboutjw/article43.htm#Publishing>.

Johnson, S., & Hang, A. (2006). Hmong. In J. Lipson & S. Dibble (Eds.), *Culture and clinical care*. San Francisco: UCSF Nursing Press.

Johnstone, R. (2007). *Religion in society* (7th ed.). Upper Saddle River, NJ: Pearson Prentice Hall.

Joint Commission of Accreditation of Healthcare Organizations (JCAHO). (2000). *Accreditation manual for hospitals*. Oakbrook Terrace, IL: Joint Commission of Accreditation of Healthcare Organizations.

Jones, A. (2003). Reconstructing the stepfamily: old myths, new stories. *Social Work*, *48*(2), 228–234.

Kaiser Family Foundation. (1999). *Kids and media at the new millennium: a comprehensive national analysis of children's media use*. Menlo Park, CA: The Henry J. Kaiser Family Foundation.

Kalish, C., & Shiverick, S. (2004). Children's reasoning about norms and traits as motives for behavior. *Cognitive Development*, *19*, 401–416.

Kearney, M., York, R., & Deatrick, J. (2000). Fourth Quarter). Effects of home visits to vulnerable young families. *Journal of Nursing Scholarship*, *32*(4), 309–314.

Kinne, S., Patrick, D. L., & Doyle, D. L. (2004). Prevalence of secondary conditions among people with disabilities. *American Journal of Public Health*, *94*(3), 443–445.

Kirkham, S., Pesut, B., Meyerhoff, H., & Sawatzky, R. (2004). Spiritual caregiving at the juncture of religion, culture, and state. *Canadian Journal of Nursing Research*, *36*(4), 148–169.

Kosmin, B., & Keysar, B. (2009). *American religious identification survey (ARIS)*. Hartford, CT: Trinity College.

Kulwicki, A. P. (2003). People of Arab heritage. In L. Purnell & B. Paulanka (Eds.), *Transcultural health care: a culturally competent approach* (2nd ed.). Philadelphia: F. A. Davis.

Kunen, J. (1996). The end of integration. *Time*, 39–44.

Left Behind Series. Leftbehind.com. Official Web site of the book series. Retrieved July 20, 2011.

Leininger, M. (1995). *Transcultural nursing: concepts, theories, research, and practices*. New York: McGraw-Hill.

Lester, M. (2006). MCC workers help preserve Hmong culture. *Mennonite Weekly Review*, 6.

Lewis, H. (1979). *How's your family?* New York: Brunner/Mazel.

Lewis, J. M., Beavers, W. R., Gossett, J. T., & Phillips, V. A. (1976). *No single thread: psychological health in family systems*. New York: Brunner/Mazel.

Lindner, E. (2004). *Yearbook of American and Canadian churches*. Nashville: Abingdon Press.

Martin, E. P. (1978). *The Black extended family*. Chicago: University of Chicago Press.

Martin, W. (2003). *The kingdom of the cults* (revised ed.). Minneapolis: Bethany House.

McMahon, A. (1997). Working with families. In J. Haber, D. Krainovich-Miller, A. McMahon, & P. Price-Hoskins (Eds.), *Comprehensive psychiatric nursing*. St. Louis: Mosby.

McMahon, A., & Presswalla, J. L. (1997). Working with groups. In J. Jaber, B. Krainovich-Miller, A. McMahon, & P. Price-Hoskins (Eds.), *Comprehensive psychiatric nursing* (4th ed.). St. Louis: Mosby.

Meleis, A. I. (2006). Arabs. In J. Lipson & S. Dibble (Eds.), *Culture and health care*. San Francisco: UCSF Nursing Press.

Merriam-Webster's Collegiate Dictionary (11th ed.). <http://www.merriam-webstercollegiate.com>.

Minuchin, S. (1974). *Families and family therapy*. Cambridge, MA: Harvard University Press.

Misener, T., Sowell, R., Phillips, K., & Harris, C. (1997). Sexual orientation: a cultural diversity issue in nursing. *Nursing Outlook*, *45*(4), 178–182.

Mitty, E. (2001, First Quarter). Ethnicity and end of life decision making. *Reflections on Nursing Leadership*, *46*, 28–31.

Mo, B. (1992). Modesty, sexuality, and breast health in Chinese American women. *Western Journal of Medicine*, *157*, 260–264.

Murray, R., Meili, P., & Zentner, J. (1993). The family—basic unit for the developing person. In R. Murray & J. Zentner (Eds.), *Nursing concepts for health promotion* (5th ed.). Englewood Cliffs, NJ: Prentice Hall.

Natinsky, P. (2001). Female genital cutting: why are women mutilated? *Community Health Forum*, *2*(5), 41–43.

Nilchaikovit, T., Hill, J. M., & Holland, J. C. (1993). The effects of culture on illness behavior and medical care: Asian and American differences. *General Hospital Psychiatry*, *15*(1), 41–50.

Nolt, S. (1992). *A history of the Amish*. Intercourse, PA: Good Books.

Nordland, R., & Bartholet, J. (2001). The web's dark secret. *Newsweek*, 44–50.

O'Brien, S. (1992). Fall). Gender bias in family benefit provision. *Canadian Journal of Community Mental Health*, *11*(2), 163–186.

Office of Management and Budget. (2000). *Provisional guidance on the implementation of the 1997 standards for federal data on race and ethnicity*. Available at <http://www.ofm.wa.gov/pop/race/omb.pdf>. Accessed February 2, 2011.

Orecklin, M. (2002). If at first you don't succeed. *Time*, 14.

Palacios, J., Butterfly, C., & Strickland, C. (2006). American Indians. In J. Lipson, S. Dibble, & P. Minarik (Eds.), *Culture and clinical care*. San Francisco: UCSF Nursing Press.

Peitchinis, S. (1989). *Employment standards handbook*. Toronto: McClelland Stewart.

Reid, R. (2000). American Indian health. *Medicine of the Americas*, *1*(1), 53.

Rosemond, J. (1994). Stepfamilies: a family by any other name. *Hemispheres (Paris, France)*, 93.

Rosenberg, D. (2001). A place of their own. *Newsweek*, 54–56.

Sandefur, G. D., Martin, M. A., Eggerling-Boeck, J., Mannon, S., & Meier, A. (2001). An overview of racial and ethnic demographic trends. In N. J. Smelser, W. J. Wilson, & F. Mitchell (Eds.), *America becoming: racial trends and their consequences*. Washington, DC: National Academy Press.

Sands, E., & Berry, J. (1993). Acculturation and mental health among Greek-Canadians in Toronto. *Canadian Journal of Community Mental Health, 12*(2), 117–124.

Satir, V. (1983). *Conjoint family therapy* (3rd ed.). Palo Alto, CA: Science & Behavior Books.

Saunders, L. (1954). *Cultural differences and medical care*. New York: Russell Sage Foundation.

Schneflen, A. (1972). *Body language in social order*. Englewood Cliffs, NJ: Prentice Hall.

Schneider, R. (1980). *Conceptual scheme of family organization and function*. Paper presented at St. Louis University Medical Center Conference, St. Louis, MO.

Shadick, K. (1993). Development of a transcultural health education program for the Hmong. *Clinical Nurse Specialist, 7*(2), 48–53.

Sheler, J. (2000). The Church of Latter-Day Saints grows by leaps and bounds. *U.S. News and World Report, 129*(19), 59–65.

Shipler, D. (1997). *A country of strangers*. New York: Alfred A. Knopf.

Sleeper, J. (1997). *Liberal racism*. New York: Viking Press.

Smart, N. (1991). *The religious experience of mankind* (4th ed.). New York: Macmillan.

Sniderman, P. M., & Carmines, E. G. (1997). *Reaching beyond race*. Cambridge, MA: Harvard University Press.

Spector, R. (2008). *Cultural diversity in health and illness* (7th ed.). Upper Saddle River, NJ: Pearson Prentice Hall.

Strickland, O., & Giger, J. (1994). Women's health in the decade of the woman. In O. Strickland & D. Fishman (Eds.), *Nursing issues and ethics* (pp. 362–399). Albany, NY: Delmar.

Suchman, E. A. (1964). Sociomedical variations among ethnic groups. *American Journal of Sociology, 70*, 319–331.

Supreme Court of the United States. (2015). Syllabus Obergefell et al. *v*. Hodges, Director, Ohio Department of Health, et al. Certiorari to the United States Court of Appeals for the Sixth Circuit. no. 14–556. Argued April 28, 2015—Decided June 26, 2015.

Sussman, M. B. (1971). Family systems in the 1970s: analysis, politics, and programs. *Annals of American Academy of Political Social Science, 396*, 40–56.

Sydnor-Greenberg, N., & Dokken, D. (2000). Family focus. Communicating information at diagnosis: helping families and children manage asthma. *Journal of Child and Family Nursing, 3*(4), 290–295.

Thomas, N. (2001). The importance of culture throughout all of life and beyond. *Holistic Nursing Practice, 15*(2), 40–46.

Townsend, M. (2006). *Psychiatric mental health nursing concepts of care* (5th ed.). Philadelphia: F. A. Davis.

Underwood, A. (2005). Spirituality in America. *Newsweek*, 45–64.

U.S. Department of Commerce, Bureau of the Census. (2004). *We the American Asians*. Washington, DC: U.S. Government Printing Office.

U.S. Department of Commerce, Bureau of the Census. (2012). *The Asian American Community Survey 2012*. Washington, DC: U.S. Government Printing Office.

U.S. Department of Commerce Economics and Statistics Administration. (2012). *U.S. Census Bureau*. (2012) Disability brief. Washington, DC: US Government Printing Office.

U.S. Department of Commerce, Bureau of the Census. (2013). *Asian Census Brief, 2013*. Washington, DC: U.S. Government Printing Office.

U.S. Department of Health and Human Services. (2013). *Health United States, 2013*. Hyatttsville, MD: U.S. Government Printing Office.

U.S. Department of Commerce, Bureau of the Census. (2013). Population Distribution and Change: 2000 to 2010: *2010 Census Briefs*. Washington, DC: U.S. Government Printing Office.

U.S. Department of Commerce, Bureau of the Census. (2013). American Community Survey, *Asian Briefs, The Hmongs*. U.S. Government Printing Office, 2013.

U.S. Department of Commerce, Bureau of the Census. (2015). *American Community Survey 2015*. Washington, DC: U.S. Government Printing Office.

U.S. Department of Health and Human Services. (2011). *National Center for Health Statistics (2010)*. Health United States 2010 with Special Feature on Death and Dying. Hyattsville, MD: U.S. Government Printing Office.

U.S. Department of Health and Human Services. (2002). *Healthy People 2010: Understanding and improving health* (2nd ed.). Washington, DC: U.S. Government Printing Office.

U.S. Department of Labor Statistics. (2015). Employment Situation Summary. Bureau of Labor Statistics, 2015.

Vehvilainen, K. (1998, Second Quarter). Wake up to Finnish nursing. *Reflections in Nursing Leadership*, 28–29.

Watchtower. (1989). Questions from readers. *Watchtower*, 30–31.

Watchtower Bible & Tract Society (1953). *Let God be true* (revised ed.). New York: Author.

Watchtower Bible & Tract Society (1955). *You may survive Armageddon into God's new world*. New York: Author.

Wexler, N. E. (1981). Learning to be a leper. In E. G. Mishler, L. R. AmaraSingham, S. T. Hauser, R. Liem, & S. D. Osherson (Eds.), *Social context of health, illness and patient care*. Cambridge, England: Cambridge University Press.

Wingert, P., et al. (1997). A matter of faith. *Newsweek*, 49–53.

Wolfram, W. A., & Clark, H. (1971). *Black–White speech relationships*. Washington, DC: Center for Applied Linguistics.

Woodward, K. (2001). The changing face of the church. *Newsweek*, 45–50.

World Almanac. (2015). New York: World Almanac Books.

Zayas, L., & Solari, F. (1994). Early childhood socialization in Hispanic families: context, culture, and practice implications. *Professional Psychology, Research and Practice, 25*(3), 2100–2206.

Zola, I. (1972). The concept of trouble and sources of medical assistance to whom one can turn with that. *Social Science and Medicine, 6*, 673–679.

Time

BEHAVIORAL OBJECTIVES

After reading this chapter, the nurse will be able to:

1. Postulate an adequate definition for the term *time* in relation to transcultural nursing care.
2. Understand the significant role that culture plays in the understanding and perception of time.
3. Understand the significant role that the developmental process plays in the understanding and perception of time.
4. Understand the significance of the measurement of time and the relationship to transcultural nursing care.
5. Differentiate the terms *social time* and *clock time.*
6. Describe the worldview of clock time and social time.
7. Define the three broad areas of the structure of social time: temporal patterns, temporal orientation, and temporal perspectives.

Since the beginning of life on earth, time has been the greatest mystery of all. The mystery of time becomes evident as soon as thought is given to the concept. Our experience with time continuously leads us into puzzles and paradoxes. According to the classic work of Wessman and Gorman (1977), it is through an awareness and conception of time that the products of the human mind— that is, time itself—seem to possess an existence apart from time's passage, which is perceived as personal and inexorable. We measure time, and time measures us. It is this intimate and personal yet aloof and detached character that constitutes the paradox of human time.

CONCEPT OF TIME

The concept of the passage of time is very familiar to most people regardless of cultural heritage. The days and nights come and go, and with each passing day and night humankind grows older. In today's highly mechanized world, there are numerous clocks and watches that ceaselessly tick away time and determine the schedules by which hundreds of millions of people live. Thus, it would seem that the concept of the passage of time should be second nature to humankind and thoroughly understood by all people (Spector, 2004).

However, developing an awareness of the concept of time is not a simple phenomenon but a gradual process (Hymovich & Chamberlin, 1980). Most people, regardless

of cultural heritage, remember a time when their perception of the passage of time was altered. Such occasions might have been during times of boredom or of highly emotional and stressful events. During these events time might have seemed to have passed very slowly, or it might have seemed to have passed all too quickly. It must be remembered that a sense of time is not innate but is developed early as a result of everyday experiences that are common to all people. Thus, a sense of time results from learning. It becomes a part of human nature before one is conscious of its presence. Even infants perceive the essence of time. Infants are fed on demand or according to a strict timetable and experience the succession of day by night. Infants are thereby exposed to regular rhythmic changes that are reflected in rhythmic changes in bodily conditions, including being sated, awake, or asleep. Thus, one phenomenon of time is its association with rhythm and change.

Infants grow, develop, and begin to move through crawling. The speed with which crawling occurs determines the time it takes to get from one place to another. Thus, even this simple task makes individuals aware that time is associated with speed and velocity, which is the second phenomenon of time. As individuals grow older, they learn speech as they listen to stories that begin with "once upon a time." It is through these storytelling sessions that children learn that things did happen before they were born; thus, time is associated with history and goes backward as well as forward with the succession of events. As the growth and development of the child continue, an awareness of punctuality is developed. Children may be punished for being slow or late, and regardless of their reaction to it, the punishment contributes to the formation of character and the development of the understanding of time. Therefore, the third phenomenon of time is its association with social behavior (Sideleau, 1992).

The child begins to become conscious of time and asks questions such as "Where was I before I was born?" and "What did God do before He created the world?" and "What will happen to me after I die?" Such questions lead to an understanding that time is associated with philosophy and religion. Children are taught to read time on a clock, and as they grow to adulthood, they learn that the clock is ubiquitous and that life is governed by the clock. Thus, there is an erroneous identification of time with the clock. Through questioning, individuals begin to contemplate existence on earth and to develop an understanding that time is associated with something external over which there is no control and that appears absolute (Elton, 1975; Sideleau, 1992).

Developing an understanding of the definition of time by looking at the developmental process is clearly too simple. The development of the awareness of time is directly influenced by earlier ideas and prejudices that are mostly unconscious. However, because it is the nature of humankind to have a questioning frame of mind, ideas and prejudices may become conscious.

Other considerations concerning time include the question of whether time is concrete or abstract. Time is perceived as real in the sense of being concrete and having direct effects, or it is regarded as not real in the sense of being abstract. The mathematical and physical sciences adopt the view that time is an abstract dimension with only a locational or reference function (McGrath & Kelly, 1986). On the other hand, the biological sciences adopt the view that time is an essential ingredient in many life and behavioral processes, such as gestation, healing, and metamorphosis. This difference in conceptualization of time may be related to an obvious difference between the physical and biological sciences and how each treats the concept of entropy. For the physical sciences, entropy, or randomness, continuously increases over time, whereas the biological sciences see organization, structure, and information residing within the organism and in the organism's relation to its environment as increasing over time.

MEASUREMENT OF TIME

Time has two distinct, although related, meanings. The first meaning is that of duration, which is an interval of time.

The second meaning is that of specified instances, or points in time. These two meanings are related because a point in time is identified as being the end of a time interval that starts at an arbitrary or fixed reference point, such as the founding of Rome or the birth of Christ. Thus, if one asks the question "What is the time?" and the answer given is "It is 10:00 a.m.," this answer refers to a point in time. At the same time, the answer refers to a time interval, since it indicates the time from a certain reference point, which in this case is midnight the previous night (Elton, 1975; Sideleau, 1992). The two meanings are quite different and must not be confused with each other. Measuring devices are meant to determine intervals of time, and clocks and watches are designed to read direct points in time. Clocks and watches therefore have to be standardized against a standard clock. The purpose of a standard clock is to measure accurately the time interval up to the present time. This phenomenon goes back to one universal standard clock against which all standard clocks are calibrated.

The purpose of a universal standard clock is to define operational time in terms of both time interval and point in time (Landes, 2000). The purpose of measuring devices is to define time; however, people need to have intuitive ideas about time to specify the properties of the instrument. Measuring devices of a phenomenon such as time are more accurate than measuring devices of some other phenomena. For example, if a person wanted to measure the weight of another person, this weight could be defined operationally as a point or reading on a scale. Thus a good scale would give accurate weight, just as any good clock would give accurate time. On the other hand, if an individual wanted to define a person's intelligence quotient (IQ) as the score obtained on an intelligence test but there was no general agreement about what constituted intelligence and what constituted a good intelligence test, the scores would not be so relevant or so meaningful as the weight or time measures.

Throughout the history of humankind, there have been two obvious standards of time: the day and the year. The day is a remarkably easy period of time to recognize because of the experience of daylight and darkness, which result from the earth's spinning on its axis. The year is also easy to recognize because of the passage of the seasons, which are caused by the tilting of the earth's axis. Thus, a day is the period of time required for one complete revolution of the earth about its axis, whereas a year is the time taken for the earth to move one complete revolution around the sun, which takes just under 365.25 days. Therefore, it is completely natural that we choose to mark the passage of time by first marking the days and then marking the years. Time measurement during the day has been divided into hours, and the hours in turn have been divided by 60 to give minutes. The minutes have been divided by 60 to give seconds.

Very early in the history of civilization, the middle of each day was determined as the point when the sun was at its highest point during the day. This point was defined as noon, and clocks were made to read 12 when it occurred. Thus, if it is noon in one place, it is midnight at the opposite side of the earth and different times at other places on the earth. To understand how time varies, the earth must be viewed as a circle that passes through both the North Pole and the South Pole.

Traditionally in science, Greenwich, the observatory in London, has been taken to have 0 degrees of longitude; the longitudes of all other places on Earth are given as so many degrees east or west of Greenwich. Therefore, one half of the earth's surface has a longitude of up to 180 degrees east of Greenwich, whereas the other half has a longitude of up to 180 degrees west of Greenwich. The times of all places east of Greenwich are ahead of that of Greenwich, and the times of all places west of Greenwich lag behind that of Greenwich. For example, if a person started from Greenwich and traveled eastward to a longitude of 45 degrees, the time would be 3 hours ahead of Greenwich time. The converse is that if a person started at Greenwich and traveled westward to a longitude of 180 degrees, the time would be 12 hours behind that of Greenwich. In simpler terms, if it is 2 a.m. on Sunday morning at Greenwich, it is 2 p.m. on Sunday at a longitude 180 degrees east of Greenwich and 2 p.m. on Saturday at a longitude 180 degrees west of Greenwich (Elton, 1975).

This phenomenon of time presents some interesting effects on persons who travel great distances. For example, it is possible for an international traveler to have two birthdays (birthday anniversaries); that is, if a person crosses the international date line traveling eastward at 2 a.m. Sunday morning, at which point it suddenly becomes 2 a.m. Saturday, that person has Saturday all over again and thus is able to celebrate the birthday again. If this same international traveler who is about to celebrate a birthday on Saturday leaves from the point of origin at 2 a.m. on Saturday but crosses the international date line westward, the traveler suddenly finds that it is 2 a.m. Sunday morning, and apparently almost the entire day of Saturday and the birthday have been missed (Elton, 1975).

Clocks

According to historians and philosophers, the earliest clocks were undoubtedly sundials of various kinds, which were probably followed by devices that used the regular flow of a substance such as water, oil, or sand, or the steady combustion of oil or candles. The earliest clocks have been dated back to 1600 B.C. in Egypt, and clocks were used throughout classical times and the Middle Ages.

The thirteenth century saw the invention of a rhythmic motion clock, which was a sawtoothed crown wheel. However, the most important development in clock construction occurred with the introduction of the pendulum, which was discovered by Galileo in 1581. Galileo found that a swinging pendulum would readily tick away a unit of time by a specific number of swings and that even if the swings gradually died, the unit of time would remain relatively unaffected. Thus, for the first time in history, time was measured more accurately.

Tropical Years

An important distinction that scientists have made is the difference between a calendar year and a tropical year. According to scientists, a calendar year consists of 365 days, whereas a tropical year consists of 365.242199 solar days. (The word *tropical* in this instance has nothing to do with a hot climate.) The difference between these two numbers (tropical year and calendar year) is the reason for the necessity of leap years. Time that is based on the length of a tropical year is called *ephemeris time*. One tropical year is defined in terms of having 31,556,925.9747 seconds. Today, atomic clocks have replaced the old, outdated pendulum and weight- and gravity-driven clocks. Atomic clocks are so accurate that in due course scientists speculate that the difference between atomic time and ephemeris time will become very apparent. In fact, atomic clocks are said to be 10 million times more accurate than any other clock on earth and are never more than 1 billionth of a second off. Atomic clocks are considered to be so accurate that the exact second of an event can be obtained at the time of the event.

Solar Time

Solar time is perhaps the earliest way that time was measured (Dossey, 1993). Solar time considers a focal point, 12:00 noon, which is precisely the point at which the sun passes directly overhead (vertically above the meridian). The time between successive crossings of the sun directly over the same meridian is called a *solar day*. However, this measurement of time is not without its problems. When days are measured in this way, they turn out to be not exactly constant. A solar day varies slightly in length throughout the year because of the orbiting of the earth around the sun.

The concept of solar time has many implications for nurses who work at extreme southern or northern points of the earth—for example, at the North or South Pole. A nurse working in the northernmost part of Canada may find Indians operating on "Indian time" because the sun remains up during most of the summer and down during much of the winter. Activities requiring daylight can therefore be done anytime during a 24-hour period. Staying up much of the night and sleeping in the daytime is consistent with an orientation to do what feels right at the present time. On the other hand, "White man's time" is more future oriented and adheres to clocks and schedules rather than to the sun (England, 1986; Wuest, 1992; Young & Hayne, 1988). Generally, Whites who have not grown up in the northernmost part of Canada but have relocated to this area tend to work during familiar working hours and to sleep during familiar sleeping hours. However, this pattern may not necessarily correlate with the same time orientation for others who are native to the northernmost part of Canada.

Calendar

Inventing a simple yet efficient calendar has presented difficulties since the invention of the first calendar. Scientists believe that these difficulties lie in the fact that the three obvious periods are due to the rotation of the earth about the sun. These three revolutional periods are not simply related one to the other. In fact, they have obvious differences. For example, 1 tropical year equals 365.224 solar days, and 1 month is considered to be the observed time between one full moon and the next, or 29.5306 solar days.

Throughout history we have measured time by counting the months and the calendar years and combining the two. However, this combination of months and years has proved to be most confusing. Even if we ignored the moon, there would still be the problem of the solar year not being a whole number of days, although this problem has conceivably been dealt with by the system of leap years. With so many different civilizations contributing to the development of the calendar, it is no wonder that we are left with a complicated system that children and even adults, regardless of ethnic or cultural heritage, find difficult to remember or understand. Many of the significant events linked with the calendar can be traced to specific persons in history, such as Julius Caesar, who decreed that months should alternately have 30 and 31 days with the exception of February (which at that time was the last month of the Roman calendar). Historians believe that all would have been well with the calendar if Julius Caesar had not decided to call the fifth month Julius in his honor. The problem began when Augustus followed Julius Caesar and also wanted a month. He promptly chose the month that followed Julius and named it "Augustus." However, he very soon realized that his month was shorter than Julius Caesar's month and promptly took a day from February, added it to his month, and readjusted the rest of the year. The result was that there were three long months in succession,

that is, June, July, and August. Even today, because of the vanity of Emperor Augustus, children continue to chant, "Thirty days hath September."

According to the earlier decree by Julius Caesar, September would have been an alternate month with 31 days if August had been given 30 days as originally planned (Elton, 1975). Although there have been attempts over the past 50 years to standardize the calendar by international agreement through the United Nations, these attempts have uniformly failed. For example, the day that is considered the beginning of the New Year in the United States is January 1, but the beginning of the New Year is different in many countries.

SOCIAL TIME VERSUS CLOCK TIME

The word *time* immediately presents an image of a clock or calendar. However, the term *social time* is not equivalent with *clock time*. *Social time* refers to patterns and orientations that relate to social processes and to the conceptualization and ordering of social life. For centuries, many of the great thinkers have argued that social time must be distinguished from clock time. As early as 1910, Henri Bergson insisted that the homogeneous time of Newtonian physics was not the time that revealed the essence of humankind. On the other hand, Phillip Bock (1964), an anthropologist, showed that an Indian wake could be meaningfully analyzed in terms of "gathering time," "prayer time," "singing time," "intermission time," and "meal time." None of these times has a particular relationship to clock time. They all simply imply the passage of the mourner from one time to another by consensual feelings rather than by the clock.

According to some sociologists, certain kinds of psychological disorders may be viewed in terms of the individual living wholly in the present, the implication being that the past and the future are completely severed from consciousness. The difference, therefore, between social time and clock time is that the former is a more inclusive concept whereas the latter may or may not be. Hoppe and Heller (1974) conducted a study on Mexican Americans and proposed that Mexican Americans have a present-time orientation that may account for the tendency to be late for appointments. It is believed that present-time orientation, particularly in high-risk settings such as mental health facilities, may result in a crisis approach rather than a preventive one. For example, a client who has an immediate need at home may be late for appointments at the clinic or hospital or may miss them altogether. The nurse should also keep in mind that clients with a present-time orientation may be reluctant to leave an appointment simply because the time is up.

This same lack of correlation between social time and clock time can be seen in mystical beliefs. According to mystical thought, magic can be used to negate the temporal order that infers causality. For example, an Indian warrior who is wounded by an arrow may attend to his pain by hanging the arrow up where it is cool or by applying ointment to the arrow. What the Indian warrior is attempting to do is to reverse the clock time—that is, wrench the present back into the past to alter the course of events. For people who have mystical beliefs, temporal intervals are not simple, homogeneous series; rather, they contain an inherent quality and meaning or an essence and efficacy of their own (Cassirer, 1992). Therefore, the objectivity represented by clock time is unknown to a person with mystical beliefs.

Many sociologists believe that people who lack or minimize clock time also lack regularity or temporal measurement. The natural and social phenomena may dictate regularity and measurement. Ariotti (1995) provides several examples of natural events that have been used to time human activities: (1) the arrival of the cranes in ancient Greece marked the time for planting; (2) the return of the swallow marked the time for the end of pruning; (3) the South African Bushmen note the rising of Sirius and Canopus and are able to depict the progress of winter by the movement of these celestial bodies across the night sky.

Archaeologists have been able to piece together the history of humankind by measuring the passage of time, using the method of geologists. This measure of time is based on rates of deposits to and erosion of natural early elements. An example of this kind of measurement is tree-ring chronology (Weyer, 1961).

WORLDVIEW OF SOCIAL TIME VERSUS CLOCK TIME

People throughout the world view social time and clock time differently (Davidhizar, Dowd, & Giger, 1997). For example, Sorokin (1964) noted that the division of time by weeks reflects social conditions rather than mechanical Newtonian divisions. Most societies have some kind of week, but the weeks vary in length from 3 to 16 or more days. In most cases, weeks reflect the cycle of market activities. The Khasi people have an 8-day week because they hold market every eighth day, and they have named the days of the week after the places where the principal markets occur (Sorokin, 1964).

Some cultural groups exhibit a social time that not only is different from clock time but also is actually scornful of clock time. For example, there are peasants in Algeria who live with a total indifference to the passage of clock time and who despise haste in human affairs. They have no

notion of exact appointment times, they lack exact times for eating meals, and they have labeled the clock as the "devil's mill" (Thompson, 1967). Some Amish keep "slow time." When those around them adjust their time to go from daylight savings time to standard time, the Amish set clocks a half-hour ahead (Gingerich, 1972; Nolt, 1992; Randall-David, 1989; Wenger, 2006). This has important implications for the nurse who is trying to emphasize the importance of keeping medical appointments.

Despite the way people in various cultures view clock time as opposed to social time, the nurse must remember that clock time should not be regarded as unimportant or irrelevant. Although for some people in some cultural groups there is no necessary correlation of clock time and social time, clock time does not take on paramount importance in a social context such as the modern Western world, where the watch or the clock can become something of a tyrant. In Jonathan Swift's *Gulliver's Travels*, Gulliver never did anything without looking at his watch, which he called his "oracle." He said that his watch pointed out the time for every action of his life. Because of Gulliver's obsession with his watch, the Lilliputians concluded that the watch was Gulliver's god.

Aside from literature, many actual examples of human obsessive behavior in regard to clock time can be found. Lebhar (1958) wrote that he was exactly 43 years old and had probably only 227,760 hours to live, and he proceeded to detail how he would maximize the use of those remaining hours of his life. He concluded that if he reduced his sleep time from 8 hours to 6 hours, the 2 hours a day saved from sleeping would amount to 18,980 hours over a period of 26 years. If this savings were converted into 18-hour days, which is the equivalent of about 2 years and 11 months, he could virtually lengthen his remaining time alive by 2 years and 11 months. This example illustrates how human life can be turned into a lengthy succession of minutes and hours, with the individual's existence reduced to a compulsive and frantic effort to avoid waste.

Gilles and Faulkner (1978) conducted a study of the role of time in television news work. They found that time is a major factor in the production of unscheduled "hard" news. The definition for "hard" news refers to events such as fires, homicides, and accidents, which have a certain urgency to them. They summarized the findings of their research in three propositions. In the first proposition they concluded that the news value of an event is directly proportional to the time invested in covering it. An event may turn out to be relatively minor in the sense of not involving the trauma or shock value that was anticipated, but this factor is not considered when a news crew has invested time in the event, and the story is likely to be used in the evening news program anyway. They found in the second proposition that what is considered news by the news crew depends on when it happens and how long it lasts. Although viewers tend to believe that what they see on the evening news is a compilation of the universal news events for that particular day, what is telecast each evening is actually a compilation of news events that the news crew was able to learn about, get a story line on, capture on film, and then process and edit on film. The researchers found in the third proposition that bias in the news reflects occupational assumptions and temporal constraints more than it does the political or social views of the news crew. More important than political and social biases are the assumptions that the news crew makes about what will make good news on television and the severe time constraints on those persons assigned to locate film and write about events in time for the evening news program. The researchers concluded that because of deadline pressures, it is inevitable that events are reduced to surface actions and that the visuals seen each evening are of only the most dramatic events.

In today's modern technological society, clock time is of paramount importance. However, we must remember that even in a modern society the clock may be a relatively peripheral part of social life. Not all people in a modern technological society function under the inevitable tyranny of the clock. In a survey of a representative sample of the French population, approximately 21% of the respondents indicated a belief that there was no urgency about being punctual and also stated that they had not experienced the feeling of wasting time (Stoetzel, 1953). It is the perception of some people in some cultural groups that there is little correlation between being punctual and wasting time (Hein, 1980). Hein further postulated that assumptions and definitions in regard to time are determined by culture and cultural variables and are reflected in interactions with others, personal views concerning punctuality, use or waste of time, and value and respect for time or a lack thereof. Waiting is a cultural counterpart to time because a particular behavior, person, or event is anticipated within a particular time frame. Waiting may have a meaning similar to that of time for some African-American clients. The nurse may schedule an appointment for an African-American client and wait for the client to arrive for the appointment. However, the client may not arrive for several hours, or perhaps even a few days, because of other important issues that in the client's mind took precedence over the appointment. Although the nurse viewed this time as waiting and therefore wasting time, the client for whom the appointment was made was not wasting time (Randall-David, 1989).

In some cultures, for example, among some persons of Asian origin, time is viewed as flexible, and so there is no need to hurry or be punctual except in extremely important cases. Asians may spend hours getting to know people and view predetermined abrupt endings as rude (Stauffer, 1995). Nonetheless, the nurse should emphasize the importance of keeping scheduled appointments. Hispanics or Latinos as well often have difficulty with scheduled appointments and are sometimes said to be on "Latin time." However, this is sometimes explained by Hispanics as the result of consideration for others who were not ready to leave for the appointment (Hoppe & Heller, 1974; Ruiz, 2003; Ruiz & Padella, 1977).

In the American nursing profession, many nurses have related professionalism and success in their careers to a sense of precision about clock time. For example, in many health care facilities, a medication error is considered to occur when a medication is not given within 30 minutes of the prescribed time, even when the medication is given daily and is not a time-released medication. Thus the nurse must complete a medication error form for not giving a routine daily medication such as a vitamin or laxative, which is neither time released nor urgent.

Most agencies relate medication errors to disciplinary action and dismissal. In some facilities the nurse is expected to complete all morning or evening care in a precise time frame, even though many clients may not operate in the same time sphere as the facility schedule for client care. For example, a client may become upset when the night nurse refuses to help the client to shower at 3 a.m. because showering is a stated day-shift activity. In this case the client may be used to starting the day at 3 a.m. and unwilling to wait until 7 a.m. to do so. Another example is early-morning vital signs, which may be taken by the night nurse to facilitate a timely assessment of the client's condition for the physician who makes early morning rounds. The client may be annoyed at being awakened for such a brief procedure and then instructed by the nurse to return to sleep.

According to Zerubavel's (1979) analysis of the temporal order of the hospital, any unit of clock time is equal to any other unit, whether one is talking about minutes, hours, days, or weeks. However, Zerubavel concluded that different days mean quite different things to different people. Because people perceive days differently, it is important to remember that some days are more or less desirable for some people. For example, some health care personnel may perceive the fact of working two weekends in succession as unfair. Similarly, evening or night duty is usually considered less desirable than day duty. Thus it is important for hospital administrators to understand the necessity for fairness in scheduling. Some hospitals have a policy that all personnel are expected to work their share of the less desirable times. In other hospitals the staff are paid differentials for working what are perceived as the less desirable times—that is, evenings, nights, weekends, and holidays.

STRUCTURE OF SOCIAL TIME

The structure of social time is a complex phenomenon. To understand it, three broad areas of social time must be analyzed: temporal pattern, temporal orientation, and temporal perspective.

Temporal Pattern

Hawley (1986) identified the temporal pattern of social time as one of the most important aspects of ecological organization. He concluded that there are five basic elements in the temporal pattern of any social phenomenon: periodicity, tempo, timing, duration, and sequence.

Periodicity. *Periodicity* refers to the various rhythms of social life and is characterized by activities related to both the needs and the activities of people. For example, every community has a functional routine that is supposedly peculiar to that community, such as the search for food, shelter, and mates, which occurs more or less with regular periodicity. People also have transcendental needs that are pursued with regular periodicity. For example, people may attend church weekly in pursuit of satisfying transcendental needs. Even physical functions of the body occur in a periodic manner. There are cyclical variations in physiological functions of the body, such as body temperature, blood pressure, and pulse.

In a classic study, Nelkin (1970) studied the behavior patterns of migrant workers and found several daily, weekly, and seasonal rhythms that were germane to their existence. Nelkin concluded that these migrant workers seemed to alternate between compact and diffuse time. Migrant time was seen to be very present-oriented, irrational, and highly personal. Nelkin concluded that migrant time was in sharp contrast to the typical time perception, which was future-oriented, rational, and impersonal. Findings from the study indicate that social time for the migrants differed because it was a series of disconnected periods rather than a continuous and predictable process, which in part accounted for maladaptive behaviors such as excessive drinking, gambling, volatile social relationships, and apathy.

Periodicity is also considered important at the managerial level. An important aspect of managerial life concerns the periodicity of meetings. For example, it is inappropriate for managers of a volunteer organization to plan frequent meetings for the membership. It is believed that a volunteer organization can engage in systematic self-destruction and ensure itself of a high turnover of membership if the group seeks to gather its members too often. These organizations must justify their demands on the members' time and at the same time create the novelty necessary to maintain the interest of the membership. In contrast to this are nonvoluntary groups, such as those that are part of a job assignment. For example, in nursing administration, regular meetings are necessary as part of the required management structure and are not usually planned with the intent of being novel and interesting. Because the management structure requires regular meetings, the meetings are planned regardless of specific agenda items.

Periodicities are also noted at the individual level. It is believed that when people are able to control their own work patterns (periodicity), satisfaction and productivity are maximized (Strauss, 1963). Some individuals spontaneously choose to alternate bouts of intense work with periods of idleness.

It is important for the manager to realize that productivity is cyclic and that equal periods of productivity cannot always be maintained. For example, after a period in which a nursing care unit experiences high client acuity, necessitating an extremely heavy work load for staff, employees will need to recover with a period of less intense pressure. It is unwise to follow a period of high acuity with another assignment that requires major time on the task. However, some work environments by their very nature cannot provide for individual periodicity. For example, industrial workers often must work at a continuous rhythmic pace, such as that seen on an automobile assembly line.

To understand periodicity, the nurse must remember that it is an important aspect of human life and the first aspect of the temporal pattern. Periodicity therefore refers to the recurrence of a social phenomenon with some kind of regularity that can be measured by clock time or by comparison of the social phenomenon with other social phenomena.

Tempo. Tempo is the second aspect of the temporal pattern and refers to rate (Morgenstern, 1960; Wang, Lui, & Ahalt, 1996). *Tempo* may refer to the frequency of activities in some unit of social time or to the rate of change of some phenomenon. An example is the industrialization of the United States, which differs from that of Russia and China because of different rates (Gioscia, 1971; Wang, Lui, & Ahalt, 1996). In a study done by the Southern Illinois University Foundation (Veterans World Project, 1972), it was suggested that one major problem among Vietnam veterans resulted from the rapidity with which they were brought home. The study concluded that the sudden transition from combat back to the United States by way of jet flights required a psychological adjustment that was often quite traumatic for these veterans.

Tempo also includes perceived rapidity of time and experience and the rapidity of various modes of social life, such as urban versus rural and work versus leisure. For example, the tempo of life in a large city such as Chicago or New York is much different from the tempo of life in a small, rural Midwestern town. Thus a person who relocates may have difficulty adjusting to the different tempo.

Tempo has several important consequences at the individual level because control of the tempo of one's work seems to be important for a healthful self-concept (Kohn, 1977). The tempo of change in social order appears to be related to emotional health; thus, the more rapid the change, the greater the stress of the individual. This thought became the theme of Alvin Toffler (1970), who coined the term *future shock*—the psychological disruptions that result from experiencing too much change in too short a time. An example of this is noted with Japanese people, who traditionally have had to change their culture and society at a very rapid pace. The very rapid tempo of the deliberate transformation of the Meiji era in Japan produced considerable stress for the Japanese people. Some historians have concluded that the 1878 revolution in Japan did save Japan from Western domination, but the generations that followed experienced the brunt of the hectic rate of change and suffered extraordinary mental agonies as a result of these forced changes (Pyle, 1969).

Timing. Timing is the third element in the temporal pattern and is referred to as *synchronization*. Timing involves the adjustment of various social units and processes with each other. The necessity for synchronization has led to the emphasis on clock time in modern society. Timing can be a crucial factor in the initiation of planned social changes and is of obvious importance in numerous social contexts, such as industrial processes, military campaigns, and political campaigns. A presidential candidate who supports a particular view that is not popular or timely may lose an election but win at a later time when the view becomes popular or another view emerges. For example, Richard Nixon ran for president of the United States in 1960 and lost. Eight years later he ran for president again at the height of the Vietnam War, and because the issue of the war was a timely one, he campaigned on this issue and won. Success is related to being at the right place at the right time with popular ideas.

Another example of the importance of timing is provided by research data on institutionalized disturbed children. These children, because of their psychological limitations, can be permitted to engage in activities such as competitive sports for only limited amounts of time. The restrictions on time are necessary because the process of the game and the psychological processes can mesh for only limited periods of time before the two processes begin to conflict and lead to destructive behavior (Doob, 1971).

Some researchers have concluded that one of the most serious problems of the modern American family is the difficulty of synchronizing family life because of the diverse activities in which each member is engaged. Another difficulty that has emerged over the years lies in the efforts of rural immigrants to adjust to the stringent demands of industrial life. Some researchers have suggested that habitual functioning of these rural immigrants must be synchronized with the industrial process and that such synchronization disallows the individual's self-actualization.

Duration. Duration is the fourth element of the temporal pattern. It has been the concern of psychologists more than it has been the concern of sociologists. The psychological concern about duration is related to the duration of which the individual is conscious, or to what has been referred to as the "spacious present." According to the classic early work of James (1990), one of the early writers in the field of social psychology, longer or shorter periods are conceived symbolically by adding to or dividing the vaguely bound unit that is the spacious present.

Duration has significance beyond the psychological level, however. Some noted sociologists have set forth a number of laws that relate to duration and behavior in organizations (Parkinson, 1970). Parkinson developed the laws of triviality and delay. The law of triviality states that the amount of time spent on any item in the agenda of an organizational meeting is inversely proportional to the money involved with that item. People may quibble far more about an item costing $50 than about an item costing $10,000. For example, in professional staff meetings at a state psychiatric hospital, an inordinate amount of time was spent discussing the purchase of a 75-cent plastic receptacle for holding clients' personal items such as toothbrushes and soap. A year later, when some plastic lids were missing, several meetings were devoted to developing a strategic nursing procedure for safeguarding these "valuable plastic receptacles." The policy developed to safeguard these receptacles mandated that the staff send a written requisition to the director of nursing, who in turn was required to write a written justification for replacement of the receptacle or the lid. The law of delay asserts that delay is the deadliest form of denial. In addition, duration is perceived as a useful variable.

Researchers continue to investigate the effects of various phenomena such as perceived importance of time, anxiety, and boredom on the perception of time. For example, researchers have concluded that workers' morale may be improved if time is subjectively made to pass more quickly and if there are several methods whereby the apparent length of a period of time can be manipulated (Meade, 1960).

Sequence. Sequence is the fifth element of the temporal pattern and is derived from the fact that there are activities requiring order. An obvious evidence of the utility of sequence is the measuring of values. For example, work before play is an ordering of activities that reflects a valuing hierarchy. In a classic 1972 study, Freedman and colleagues measured values relating to physical activities, theoretical–scientific interests, and aesthetic interests, and found that study participants made similar choices on both time and money scales. Friedman concluded that when cost and time are equalized, similar preferential orderings are made for various activities.

In modern American society, time is indeed money. It is conceivable, however, that the sequential ordering of activities may reflect necessity rather than values as an industrial process. Conflict may also arise over whether the sequence actually does represent necessity rather than values. Generally, this kind of conflict is more common in organizational settings in which disputes arise over the necessity of sequential orderings that are demanded by bureaucratic rules.

Finally, sequential ordering may reflect habit. Rituals of primitive societies are ordered in accordance with custom. Modern rituals also fall in this category, even though some are more appropriately viewed as reflections of values. For example, the ritual of a man removing his hat before entering a room or elevator is a habitual sequence. However, the ritual of the same man removing his hat before the national anthem is played is a sequence demanded by values.

Temporal Orientation

Temporal orientation refers to the ordering of past, present, and future and to the fact that individuals and groups may be differentiated according to whether behavior is primarily related to the past, present, or future. Psychologists and sociologists, however, have raised objections to this particular ordering. One objection is that past, present, and future are perceived to make up an organic whole that cannot be separated (Cassirer, 1992; Sideleau, 1992). A second objection involves variations in the ordering of past, present, and future among various groups. For example, the argument is made that an actor's orientation to a situation always contains an "expectancy aspect," which implies that all orientations are to a future state of a situation as well as to the present. However, this may be true only in a limited sense because actors generally do not anticipate their demise in the situation. It is also untrue that orientation to the future is a universal and inherent aspect of all social action.

Future orientation refers to the fact that the future is a dominant factor in present behavior, and as such this kind of orientation is by no means universal. For example, the Navajo Indians' view of time does not include the expectancy aspect. In years past, efforts to get the Navajo Indians to engage in range control and soil conservation programs were extremely frustrating for government employees because the Navajos simply do not have a view of temporality that would lead them to act on the basis of an expected future (Hall & William, 1960). For the Navajo people the only real time, like the only real space, is that which is here and now (Iverson, 1990). For some Navajo Indians there is little reality of the future; thus the promise of future benefits is not worth thinking about (Hall & William, 1960). It is important for the nurse to remember that the way in which a society, group, or individual orders past, present, or future will be consequential for behavior.

Kluckhohn and Strodtbeck (1973) argued in their classic work that the knowledge of rank ordering of these three modes can tell much about a social unit and the direction of change for that unit. Some Americans have typically placed a dominant emphasis on the future, which does not imply that they ignore either the past or the present. Although there are some undesirable connotations for the label "old fashioned," few Americans express total contentment with the present state of affairs. According to Kluckhohn and Strodtbeck, American values change easily as long as the change does not contradict what is perceived as the American way of life. There is a direct relationship between the extended future orientation and the amount of change. However, the change perceived is not expected to be the kind that threatens the existing order.

Generally speaking, resistance to change should be expected where there is a past orientation. Thus it should be expected that serious problems would arise in efforts to industrialize a society that lacks a future orientation. For example, in a classic 1953 study, Ritzenhaler found that among the Chippewa Indians, who traditionally lack any concern for the future, there were serious problems when attempts were made to industrialize their work. Ritzenhaler also noted that the Chippewa Indians quit work as soon as they had sufficient money for immediate needs.

Temporal orientations are not immutable; they can change, and along with change come various behavioral changes. Therefore, a shift of orientation to the present may have significant consequences in several contexts (Ketchum, 1951). For example, in a crowd situation the orientation may be drawn to the present, wherein some of the typical behaviors of crowds may manifest themselves as overreacting behaviors, such as struggling at a department store sale, racing to the exit doors in a fire, or panicking in an airplane during turbulence. Similarly, in a marriage or relationship where the partners perceive the relationship to be of uncertain duration, they may begin to act in accordance with feelings rather than stable values. For example, one of the partners may transfer joint banking accounts and charge card accounts to individual status. In other words, when situations are structured so that people function in a present orientation that lacks future and past orientations, a variety of self-destructive and self-limiting behaviors may result.

Whenever a change is anticipated, individuals or groups may resist orientation to the change, and serious consequences generally follow. The intermingling of traditional orientation, which is somewhat past-oriented, with the pressures manifested by modernization, which may be somewhat present- or future-oriented, may cause societal agony. For example, many problems arose in a factory in Cantal, Guatemala, because the management refused to be sensitive to market variations or to the problem of obsolete equipment (Nash, 1967). Worse situations occurred in Iran, which is a past-oriented society. In past-oriented societies, the past is of primary importance and the future of minimal significance. In Iran, businessmen invested considerable sums of money in factories without any real plan for how to use these factories (Hall & William, 1960).

Temporal orientation is an important variable in societal behavior and is also significant at the societal level. Some psychological studies indicate that temporal orientation may be directly related to various kinds of emotional disorders, such as alcoholism, and to certain kinds of deviant behaviors, such as juvenile delinquency.

Temporal Perspective

Temporal perspective refers to the image of past, present, and future that prevails in a society, a social group, or individuals. The rank ordering of past, present, and future is of significance, yet it is insignificant in gaining an adequate understanding of social time. For example, if a particular group is future-oriented—that is, it ranks the future highest in its hierarchy of values—its behavior will depend largely on the way it perceives the future. If people in a society perceive that they may be extinct in the future, efforts may be made to ensure survival. The converse of this is that if people in a society perceive that they do not have a future (e.g., they will be eradicated in a nuclear holocaust), they may adopt a present orientation, desiring to live life now to its fullest. An excellent example of this is found with the dying client's perception of time. For the dying client, living in the present is very important; however, the nurse should recognize other realms of time perception. The nurse should ascertain precisely how the client views the past, present, and future because these views may assist the nurse in helping the client cope with

death and the challenges faced in the process (Maguire, 1984). An image of the future functions to direct present behavior in accordance with specific values, and some sociologists view a society as being magnetically pulled toward a future fulfillment of its own image of the future as well as being pushed from behind by its past (Polick, 1973).

A future orientation to illness, disease, and health care is essential to preventive medicine. Actions are taken in the present to safeguard the future, particularly regarding certain disease conditions, such as using condoms to prevent acquired immunodeficiency syndrome (AIDS), practicing safe sex, adhering to a diet to prevent elevated cholesterol or blood glucose levels, not driving while under the influence of alcohol, and using seat belts.

TIME AND HUMAN INTERACTION

Up to this point, an effort has been made to create an awareness that social time arises out of interaction. Regardless of the cultural heritage of an individual or group, there is no kind of time that is natural to humans. Instead, time is a result of the structuring and functioning of social order. When a particular temporality emerges, it tends to persist and to influence subsequent interaction. Various cultural groups construct systems of time that have diverse meanings and therefore diverse consequences on social interactions. The most fundamental differences in the meaning of time occur when cultural groups measure time predominantly by either social events or the clock.

Cultural groups that measure time predominantly by social events construct time according to the activities of the group. Conversely, cultural groups that measure time by the clock schedule activities according to the clock. In this regard, time is perceived basically as qualitative for those who measure time by social life and activities and as quantitative for those who measure time by the clock. When measured by social activities, time has significance only in terms of the activities that are occurring. When time is measured by the clock, it has significance only in terms of money, which is perceived to be a scarce commodity, and all activities that take place do so in the shadow of the clock.

Few cultural groups or societies could be characterized as bound exclusively by the clock or as wholly independent of any constraints of temporality. How a group perceives time, nevertheless, has implications for interactions. For example, the Balinese people have a detemporalizing concept of time (Geertz, 1975). For these people, social time includes a calendar with a complex system of periodicities. According to Geertz, this is called a "premutational calendar" because it contains 10 different cycles of days ranging in length from 1 to 10 days. Although this is a complex system, it nevertheless serves various religious and practical purposes; it identifies nearly all the holidays and temple celebrations and at the same time guides the individual in daily activities. According to Geertz, the structure of this complex system allows and disallows certain activities on certain days. For example, certain days are good or bad for building a house, starting a business enterprise, moving from one location to another, going on a trip, and harvesting and planting crops.

In contrast to the belief of the Balinese people is the belief held by some Americans that time is money and therefore a scarce commodity. Thus human interactions are controlled in accordance with some notion of the appropriate amount of time for a particular situation. For example, some Americans distinguish the amount of time that can rightfully be consumed by strangers from that which can be given to friends and relatives. Weigert (1981) concluded that interaction time is a measure of the meaning of the relationship between two persons. In the event that two casual acquaintances meet somewhere, it is unlikely that they will take more than a few minutes to express recognition or perhaps exchange a pleasantry or two; therefore, the interaction time for such a meeting is limited. The converse of this is that if two good friends meet and one of the friends attempts to limit the interaction, the other friend may feel rejected. Therefore, the violator is expected to account for the behavior, and if this accounting is not forthcoming, the friendship may be severely strained. A single logical conclusion is that interaction can be evaluated in terms of time consumption.

In the United States, methods to save time or to use time more effectively are in high demand. Numerous books, articles, workshops, tapes, and seminars imply that most Americans value time but at the same time do not think they use it wisely. Many busy professionals feel torn between wise use of time and taking time for interpersonal relationships with fellow workers or friends. For example, a dilemma may arise when a person is busy and a coworker drops in and asks, "Do you have a minute?" If time is considered money, a minute is costly. Because this worker values time, a reply of "yes" may be viewed as costly and thus unjustifiable. On the other hand, "no" may be perceived by the other person as a lack of sensitivity, coldness, and a lack of interest. Therefore, much of the advice given by time-efficiency experts can do much to depersonalize human interactions. A person who follows the advice of these experts to the letter may have far more hours in which to accomplish tasks but at the same time may have fewer friends and fewer intimate relationships.

Drucker (1993) called the executive a captive because everyone can move in on an executive's time, and, generally speaking, everybody does. An executive's time is often preempted by matters that are important to other people; therefore, the executive has little or no time for self. A nurse manager who is responsive to others may find there is little time to do paperwork in the office and thus may take a lot of work home. A nurse manager's personal priorities are often modified when employees present "more urgent" problems.

CULTURAL PERCEPTIONS OF TIME

Appreciating cultural differences regarding time is important for the nurse in relating to both peers and clients. When people of different cultures interact, as is frequently the case in health care settings, there is a great potential for misunderstanding. If nurses are to avoid misreading issues that involve time perceptions, they must understand how other persons in different cultures view time (Tripp-Reimer & Lively, 1993).

Campinha-Bacote (1997) compared time orientation among certain groups in relation to future-time and present-time orientation:

- Dominant American: future over present
- African Black: present over future
- Puerto Rican American: present over future
- Mexican American: present
- Chinese American: past over present
- American Indian: present

Individuals with Future-Oriented Perceptions

Most middle-class Americans, regardless of ethnic or cultural heritage, tend to be future oriented (Tripp-Reimer & Lively, 1993). For example, some middle-class Americans tend to defer gratification of personal pleasure until some future objective has been met, such as advanced education. Thus they delay starting families, purchasing homes, buying an expensive car, or investing money until they have prepared for a profession through advanced education. Another noted difference among members of the dominant American culture is that these individuals tend to structure time rigidly. For these people, adhering to a time-structured schedule is a way of life, regardless of whether the schedule involves work or leisure. For the nurse who works with future-oriented individuals, it is important to talk about events in relation to the future and to adhere to the schedule for planned events in a timely and precise manner.

Individuals with Present-Oriented Perceptions

Present-oriented individuals do not necessarily adhere strictly to a time-structured schedule. The present takes precedence over the future and the past for these individuals. More specifically, whatever is occurring at a precise moment may be more important than a future appointment. It is important for the nurse to avoid labeling such individuals as lazy, disrespectful, or lacking interest. Hoppe and Heller (1974) concluded that present-time orientation may be a reason why some Hispanic clients are late for appointments. Carter (1979) noted that it is important to gain an awareness of differences in values for African-Americans from low socioeconomic groups and proposed that instead of labeling tardiness as a blatant disregard for time, problems related to health, economics, and transportation should be considered with these individuals. Another explanation of individuals with present-time orientation is that they tend to react to time in a linear fashion. Because they perceive time as being on a straight plane, they believe that a present moment spent on a particular task or with a particular individual cannot be regained: "We will never have this moment again" or "We must do it now because we'll pass this way only once." This idea is in contrast to the thoughts held by persons with circular-time orientation, who say, "I'll get back with you" or "We can do it later." The implication of these latter statements is that both persons will be around and the essence of the moment can be relived. In relation to health care, present-oriented individuals are not likely to be involved in preventive care; however, they will seek out emergency care in acute care facilities (Grypma, 1993; Guruge & Donner, 1996). Grypma (1993) notes that after setting up a prenatal class for some American Indian women residing on a reservation, although these individuals had preregistered for the class and confirmed their appointments, they did not keep the appointment. The reason given by these women for not attending the class was a sudden weather shift and the low tide, which provided optimal conditions for picking abalone at islands nearby. For these women, the present-oriented need for food took precedence over planning for the future event of having a baby (Thompson & McDonald, 1989).

A common belief shared by some African-Americans and Mexican Americans is that time is flexible and events will begin when they arrive. For African-Americans this belief has been translated through the years as a perception of time wherein lateness of 30 to 60 minutes is acceptable. Mbiti (1990) traced this perception of time back to West Africa, where the concept of time was elastic and encompassed events that had already taken place, as well as those that would occur immediately.

Many American Indians and Inuits believe that only what is needed for the day should be used and that nature will continue to provide for future needs (McRae, 1994). Atcheson (1987) noted that health, and therefore life, is a spiritual experience for Indians, and the gifts of the Great Spirit should never be abused. Some American Indians and Inuits believe that the person who gives the most to others should be respected. This is also in keeping with the notion of being present-oriented. Many American Indians and Inuits have been taught to live in the present and not be concerned with the future. Therefore, they share what they have today (Hagey & Buller, 1983; McRae, 1994; Young, Ingram, & Swartz, 1990).

It is important for the nurse to remember that time perception may also be related to socioeconomic status. For example, although some African-Americans and Mexican Americans can be characterized as present-oriented individuals, others have been assimilated into the dominant culture, are very time-conscious, and take pride in punctuality. These African-Americans and Mexican Americans are more likely to be future-oriented and therefore are more likely to save and plan for important events. They are also likely to be well educated and to hold professional positions. This may not always be the case, since some individuals may not be well educated or hold professional positions yet may value time and have future hopes for themselves and their children. According to Pouissant and Atkinson (1970), these individuals are more likely to encourage their children to seek higher education and to begin saving for the future.

Time perception may also be related to religious orientation. Some American Indians, Mexican Americans, and African-Americans hold strong religious beliefs, and their concept of time is therefore very future-oriented. These individuals, who may come from all socioeconomic and educational levels, have in common the belief that life on earth, with all of its pain and suffering, is bearable only because of the chance for future happiness after death. Such individuals, according to Smith (1976), may plan future activities related to their deaths; for example, they may plan their funeral, including their eulogy; purchase a grave plot; make a will; and otherwise prepare to die. Such individuals may also threaten heirs with disinheritance and talk about what the heirs will do with their hard-earned money.

Levine and Wolff (1985), with the assistance of colleagues Laurie West and Harry Reis, compared the time sense of male and female students in Niterói, Brazil, with similar students at California State University at Fresno. A total of 91 Brazilian students and 107 students from California were surveyed. The universities selected in Brazil and California were similar in academic quality and size, and the cities in which they were located were secondary metropolitan centers with populations of approximately 350,000. The researchers asked students about their perception of time in several situations, including what they considered late or early for a hypothetical lunch appointment with a friend. According to the data, the average

Brazilian student defined lateness for the hypothetical lunch as 33 minutes after the scheduled lunchtime, whereas the Fresno students defined lateness for the hypothetical lunch as 19 minutes after the scheduled lunchtime. The Brazilian students allowed an average of 54 minutes before they considered someone early for an appointment, whereas the Fresno students drew the line for earliness at 24 minutes. When the Brazilian students were asked to give typical reasons for lateness, they were less likely to attribute it to a lack of caring than their North American counterparts were. Instead, the Brazilian students pointed to unforeseen circumstances that an individual could not control without prior knowledge. In addition, the Brazilian students appeared less inclined to feel personally responsible for their own lateness. The question that comes to mind for the nurse is "Are Brazilians more flexible in their concepts of time and punctuality?" Another question for the nurse to consider is "If Brazilians are more flexible in their concepts of time and punctuality, how does this relate to the stereotypical picture of the fatalistic and irresponsible temperament associated with Latins?" This example illustrates the need for nurses to guard against formulating stereotyped images of persons from other cultures. Instead, the nurse must have an understanding of cultural variables that differ among cultures, such as the variation in viewing time.

Levine and Wolff (1985) found similar differences in how students from North America and Brazil characterize people who are late for appointments. In the survey, the Brazilian students indicated that a person who is consistently late is probably a person who is more successful than one who is consistently on time. These students seemed to accept the premise that someone of great stature is expected to arrive late; therefore, a lack of punctuality is a badge of success. In contrast, according to the North American students, persons who arrive late for scheduled appointments, rush in late to meetings, turn in assignments late, or fail to notify others when they find that they are going to be late are generally unorganized, have trouble with priorities, are inconsiderate, and thus will fail to advance professionally and will be less successful. Popular literature in the United States on creating a successful business and professional image espouses the need for continued punctuality.

PHYSIOCHEMICAL INFLUENCES IN RELATION TO TIME

Research on biological rhythms has found that internal body rhythms fluctuate within a 24-hour period. Biological capacities for some individuals are at a low ebb in the daytime, whereas for others, they are at a high level during the day (Biological Rhythms, 1970; Yogman, Lester, & Hoffman, 1983; Ziac, 1984). Research has shown that the time of day in which medication is given influences its effectiveness and its side effects; drugs may be more potent when biological capacities are at a low ebb. However, it is important for the nurse to remember that although drugs might be more potent with low biological capacities, the treatment may be less therapeutic. Health care professionals often fail to take into account the client's biological rhythms when scheduling surgical procedures and diagnostic tests. For example, surgical interventions should be avoided when a client's biological capacities are low. Persons who are at a low ebb of biological functioning may be at greater risk for an exaggerated response to anesthesia or may be less able to respond to blood loss (Bremner, Vitiello, & Prinz, 1983; Sideleau, 1992). Evidence also exists that diagnostic tests and treatments may be tolerated better by certain clients when they are timed according to biological rhythms. Hormones and other homeostatic physiological mechanisms fluctuate in the body in a rhythmic way. The timing of the collection of blood and urine samples is important and influences the interpretation of the information obtained.

Physiochemical levels are also related to age. Children have a higher metabolic rate, which tends to make time appear to move more slowly for children. On the other hand, older individuals have a slower metabolic rate, which results in time appearing to move more quickly.

Body rhythms may influence waking at a preselected time. Waking, however, is also a conditioned response. Body systems, including the nervous and endocrine systems, are the result not only of internal biological rhythms but also of psychological phenomena, such as the time or date of previous traumatic events.

Psychological phenomena can greatly affect the client's time perception. For example, according to Sideleau (1992), persons with psychiatric problems can manifest several types of time impairments, including the following:

1. Perception as related to rate and flow of time; that is, a sense that time passes too quickly or too slowly.
2. Failure to recognize finite division of time, which is manifested by confusion related to the inability to distinguish night from day.
3. Attention or inattention to time; that is, adhering too rigidly to schedules or the complete disregard for the value of time constraints or schedules.

It is important for the nurse to carefully discern whether the client's time perception is attributable to cultural phenomena or to some biochemical or psychological manifestation. For example, drug abusers tend to have an altered sense of time. If a hallucinogenic or excitatory drug is being used, the individual may experience temporal contraction and spatial expansion. For these persons, the distortion in time is so profound that they often arrive early for appointments (Sideleau, 1992). In stark contrast, individuals who are influenced by the effects of tranquilizers experience time expansion and space contraction. These individuals are more likely to arrive late for an appointment. Although all these phenomena can be experienced by clients who have a biochemical imbalance or a psychological disorder, the nurse must carefully determine if the faulty perception is caused by the disorder or by a cultural phenomenon (Giger, Davidhizar, Evers, & Ingram, 1994; Giger, Davidhizar, Johnson, & Poole, 1997).

IMPLICATIONS FOR NURSING CARE

The nurse who gains an understanding of time as a cultural variable with a significant effect on clients and ultimately on client care must also gain an understanding of how time is managed to give high-quality client care. A general attitude shared by health care professionals is that time is irreplaceable and irreversible and that to waste time is to waste life. Moreover, there is no such thing as a lack of time; regardless of the way individuals spend time, it goes at the same pace (Salmond, 1986). That is, each individual has 168 hours to live per week, no more and no less. As health care needs have changed over the years, so have the demands that are placed on nurses. Nurses are constantly being challenged to work in a more time-efficient manner, causing high levels of stress. Some nurses maintain that they are losing control and lack personal satisfaction and thus are becoming burned out. However, it is important for the nurse to remember that one way to remain in control and to have personal satisfaction as opposed to burnout is to adopt an efficient system of time management. Getting organized and precisely articulating priorities are related to job satisfaction (Feldman, Monicken, & Crowley, 1983; MacStavic, 1978; McNiff, 1984). Nurses have long known the importance of working smarter rather than longer or harder (Barros, 1983).

Conflicts between nurses and physicians are sometimes complicated by differences in time perception. Nurses tend to operate on an hourly time sense with adherence to rigid schedules to complete client care assignments. Physicians tend to measure time with the client not in actual time spent with the client, which often is quite brief, but in the duration of the illness or its treatment. Physicians are less likely to schedule time strictly and often appear not to appreciate the nurse's sense of time (Sheard, 1980; Young & Hayne, 1988).

For the nurse, time-management issues involve how to manage both personal time and time at work to meet professional goals. In addition, as cost-containment issues are gaining increased attention in nursing, time-management concerns also necessitate precise assessment of client care needs to plan the hours of nursing time required to meet these needs and to manage the time of staff who are supervised in the delivery of care (Vestal, 1987). In the 1970s, the concern with cost-effectiveness of client care and the realization that census may not be an adequate determinant of the demand for care prompted the development of client classification systems. These classification systems were used initially in general hospitals to determine needs for nursing resources by grouping clients into categories that reflected the magnitude of nursing care time. By 1979, over 1000 hospitals reported using some method of classifying levels of care and the time required (Schroder, Washington, Deering, & Coyne, 1986). In 1983 the development of client classification systems received a significant impetus when the Joint Commission on Accreditation for Hospitals and the American Hospital Association Standards recommended client classification systems in all hospitals. As psychiatric hospitals began to seek accreditation under the American Hospital Association Standards, increasing attention was given to client classification systems in psychiatric hospital settings.

Appropriate grouping of clients in a hospital (such as having a unit for colostomy clients) can contribute to effective use of staff time. In addition, grouping client activities into a logical sequence (such as changing the client's bed after the colostomy irrigation is finished) can save the nurse time.

Organization of supplies and tasks is important when activities are grouped together. Organizing items prevents multiple interruptions during a procedure to collect things that were forgotten. A nurse who must leave a procedure to get items that are needed but were forgotten not only wastes time but also appears incompetent.

Nursing efforts to reduce hospitalization time are a serious concern as health care costs spiral (Midgley & Osterhage, 1973). Yet another dimension of time management for nurses today involves appropriately timed data collection to determine client needs and to collect data about the nursing process (Felton, 1970; Polit & Hungler, 2004). If assessment of client and nursing needs is inadequately timed, inaccurate solutions may be planned. The nurse who is aware of the importance of time must also consider the time constraints of data collection. Although a 24-page nursing assessment may provide optimal client data, if the time taken to collect these data would result in other client care being neglected, time constraints will by necessity influence the length of the assessment. Time constraints also influence data collection for research purposes in a health care setting. If financial restraints prohibit additional staff for research purposes, a decision must be made about the priority of the research versus the priority of other nursing staff duties (Monette, Sullivan, & Dejong, 2008).

As change agents, nurses are also concerned with time in relation to change. According to organizational change theory, if change merely involves knowledge, change can be achieved in a short time with little difficulty. If attitudes are involved, somewhat longer periods of time are needed. If the behavior of an individual is involved, a moderate amount of time is required, and moderate difficulty may be encountered. If the behavior of a group is involved, a large amount of time may be required and a high level of difficulty may be encountered (Hersey & Blanchard, 2001).

Lest the nurse stereotype all persons in the United States as valuing timeliness, it must be emphasized that time and punctuality vary considerably from place to place and region to region. Each region and even each city has its own rhythm and rules. Words such as *now* and *later* can convey vastly different meanings. *Now* and *later* may also be interpreted differently by persons from different ethnic or cultural groups. For some African-Americans, *now* may not really imply "immediately"; rather, *now* may mean "soon," so that it could be hours before an action is taken. For the same African-American, later may not really imply "within a few hours," but "when you get around to it" (Mbiti, 1990). In contrast, for some future-oriented Americans, *now* means "immediately," and thus action is expected at once. For these same persons, *later* means "within a few hours."

For Americans who travel abroad, major differences encountered, surpassed only by language problems, are the contrasting paces of life and the punctuality differences of people from other countries. These differences can also be noted in the United States when one travels from region to region. For example, in the South, regardless of whether the area is rural or urban, the general pace of life is slow and laid back, and punctuality is not of paramount importance; thus people from this region may be stereotyped as "country." In contrast, in a large metropolitan area such as New York City, the pace of life is associated with more rapid activity, such as walking fast, talking fast, and making decisions quickly. Time differences are also seen in various agencies and among various health professionals. For example, the nurse may find that a more rapid pace is required in a particular hospital setting. The pace may also vary in different clinical disciplines. Duties may differ, and the pace may be more accelerated in high-risk areas such as the intensive care unit, coronary care unit, emergency department, operating room, and psychiatric unit. On the other hand, these areas also experience "slow time" or "down time" when the census is low.

When caring for clients who may have present-oriented time perceptions, such as some African-Americans, some

Americans from Puerto Rico, some American Indians, some Mexican Americans, and some Chinese Americans, the nurse must remember that it is necessary to avoid adhering to time as a fixed resource. (An example would be rigid schedules for nursing care procedures such as baths, medications, and meals.) In this case the nurse may find that the standards of the institution regarding time and the time orientation of the client may be in conflict. Again, it is important for the nurse to remember that such persons may perceive time as flexible and that what is happening now is more important than what is going to happen in the future. Therefore, the nurse must be able to adapt client care within a range in time rather than according to fixed hours. It is important for the nurse to recognize that time is perceived differently by some individuals from diverse ethnic, cultural, age, and socioeconomic groups (Gaglione, 1988). Accepting that there are different ways of perceiving time is the first step to increasing tolerance for time-related cultural behaviors. The nurse should appreciate the breadth of factors that affect perception of time. For example, Carter, Green, Green, and Dufour (1994) noted that homeless individuals are very present-oriented. This can significantly affect follow-up care and adherence to treatment recommendations. On the other hand, certain illnesses may affect time perception. Individuals with schizophrenia tend to be present-oriented and have a limited ability to focus on the future. This can significantly affect adjustment to the hospital and community living situations (Suto & Frank, 1994). Chronic illness may affect perception of time for the future. For some persons, hope is important for an orientation to the future (Alberto, 1990).

CASE STUDY

Miss Susie Jones is a 37-year-old African American client who has been coming to the hospital's outpatient clinic because she has brittle diabetes. Miss Jones's diabetes was diagnosed 6 months previously; however, the diabetes remains uncontrolled by insulin. The client was put on a regimen of 40 units of Lente insulin with 5 units of regular insulin at 7 a.m. and at 4 p.m. When Miss Jones comes to the clinic today, she relates to the nurse that she had an episode of "blacking out" or an "insulin reaction," because she forgot to eat after taking her morning insulin. This morning, as frequently in the past, Miss Jones is at least 1 hour late for her scheduled appointment. The following questions relate to variable time and its significance in relation to Susie Jones.

CLINICAL DECISION MAKING

1. List at least two things in relation to the perception of time and culture that may be contributing factors in Susie Jones's tardiness for appointments.
2. List at least two things that the nurse could suggest to Susie Jones that would assist her in being on time for future clinic appointments.
3. List at least two factors about time that contribute to Susie Jones's nonadherence to the medical regimen.
4. Identify ways that the nurse could assist Susie Jones in developing an understanding about time and its relationship to important medications such as insulin.
5. Identify a contributing factor to the insulin reaction Susie Jones described to the nurse.

REVIEW QUESTIONS

1. In teaching a patient with present time orientation, the nurse should consider which of the following?
   a. Result in taking medication in a timely manner.
   b. Result in adherence to a preventive health regimen.
   c. Result in the patient's attending to other events that are happening rather than focusing on times medication is to be taken.
   d. Influence actions related to a future benefit.
2. A nurse doing discharge teaching with a Navajo diabetic patient should recognize that the patient may experience which of the following?
   a. May have trouble with keeping appointments.
   b. Will adhere to taking medication by associating it with mealtimes.
   c. Is future oriented and therefore motivated to be adherent.
   d. Is likely to perform illness prevention activities to be in harmony with nature.
3. When a nurse is discussing a medication home regimen with an Alaskan Eskimo patient, the nurse might expect which of the following?
   a. Focused on present events.
   b. Focused on the benefit of present events as they affect the future.
   c. Primarily concerned with past historic events.
   d. Unaffected by time orientation.

REFERENCES

Alberto, J. (1990). A test of a model of the relationships between time orientation, perception of threat, hope, and self-care behaviors of persons with chronic obstructive pulmonary disease (unpublished doctoral dissertation). Indiana University School of Nursing, Bloomington, IN.

Ariotti, P. E. (1995). The concept of time in Western antiquity. In J. T. Fraser & N. Lawrence (Eds.), *The study of time* (Vol. 3, pp. 69–80). New York: Springer-Verlag.

Atcheson, J. (1987). Traditional health beliefs and compliance in Native American tuberculosis patients (unpublished master's thesis). McMaster University, Hamilton, Ontario.

Barros, A. (1983). Time management: learn to work smarter, not longer. *Medical Laboratory Observer*, 107–111.

Biological rhythms in psychiatry and medicine. (1970). Chevy Chase, MD: U.S. Department of Health, Education, and Welfare, National Institute of Mental Health.

Bock, P. (1964). Social structure and language structure. *Southwestern Journal of Anthropology, 20*, 393–403.

Bremner, W. J., Vitiello, M. V., & Prinz, P. N. (1983). Loss of circadian rhythmicity in blood testosterone levels with aging in normal man. *Journal of Clinical Endocrinology and Metabolism, 56*(6), 1278–1281.

Campinha-Bacote, J. (1997). Understanding the influence of culture. In J. Haber, B. Krainovich-Miller, A. McMahon, & P. Hoskins (Eds.), *Comprehensive psychiatric nursing* (5th ed., pp. 76–90). St. Louis: Mosby.

Carter, J. (1979). Frequent mistakes made with Black clients in psychotherapy. *Journal of the National Medical Association, 71*(10), 56–64.

Carter, K., Green, R., Green, L., & Dufour, L. (1994). Health needs of homeless clients accessing nursing care at a free clinic. *Journal of Community Health Nursing, 11*(3), 139–147.

Cassirer, E. (1992). *An essay on man.* New Haven, CT: Yale University Press.

Davidhizar, R., Dowd, S., & Giger, J. (1997). Model for cultural diversity in the radiology department. *Radiology Technology, 68*(3), 233–240.

Doob, L. (1971). *Patterning of time.* New Haven, CT: Yale University Press.

Dossey, L. (1993). *Healing words.* San Francisco: Harper.

Drucker, P. (1993). *The effective executive.* New York: Harper Business.

Elton, L. (1975). *Time and man.* New York: Pergamon Press.

England, J. (1986). Cross-cultural health care. *Canada's Mental Health, 34*(4), 13–15.

Feldman, E., Monicken, L., & Crowley, M. (1983). The systems approach to prioritizing. *Nursing Administration Quarterly, 7*(2), 57–62.

Felton, J. S. (1970). Communicating in writing I and II. *Occupational Health Nursing, 18*(5), 13–19, *18*(6), 13–25.

Freedman, J. L., Levy, A., Buchanan, R., & Price, J. (1972). Crowding and human aggressiveness. *Journal of Experimental Social Psychology, 8*, 528–548.

Gaglione, B. (1988). *Cognitive orientations of three healthy retired American men* (unpublished doctoral dissertation). Rutgers–The State University of New Jersey, New Brunswick, NJ.

Geertz, C. (1975). *The interpretation of cultures.* London: Hutchinson.

Giger, J., Davidhizar, R., Evers, S., & Ingram, C. (1994). Cultural factors influencing mental health. In C. Taylor (Ed.),

Essentials of psychiatric nursing (14th ed., pp. 215–238). St. Louis: Mosby.

Giger, J., Davidhizar, R., Johnson, J., & Poole, V. (1997). The changing face of America. *Health Traveler, 4*(4), 11–17.

Gilles, R., & Faulkner, R. (1978). Time and television news work: task temporalization in the assembly of unscheduled events. *Sociological Quarterly, 19*, 89–102.

Gingerich, O. (1972). *The Amish of Canada.* Waterloo, Ontario, Canada: Council Press.

Gioscia, V. (1971). On social time. In H. Yaker, H. Osmond, & F. Cheek (Eds.), *The future of time* (pp. 73–141). Garden City, NY: Doubleday.

Grypma, S. (1993). Culture shock. *The Canadian Nurse, 89*(9), 33–37.

Guruge, S., & Donner, G. (1996). Transcultural nursing in Canada. *The Canadian Nurse, 92*(9), 34–39.

Hagey, R., & Buller, E. (1983). Drumming and dancing: a new rhythm in nursing care. *The Canadian Nurse, 79*(4), 28–31.

Hall, E., & William, F. (1960). Intercultural communication: a guide to men of action. *Human Organization, 19*, 7–9.

Hawley, A. (1986). *Human ecology.* Chicago: Chicago University Press.

Hein, E. C. (1980). *Communication in nursing practice* (2nd ed.). Boston: Little, Brown.

Hersey, P., & Blanchard, K. (2001). *Management of organizational behaviors* (8th ed.). Upper Saddle River, NJ: Prentice Hall.

Hoppe, S., & Heller, P. (1974). Alienation, familism, and the utilization of health services by Mexican Americans. *Journal of Health and Social Behavior, 15*, 304.

Hymovich, D. P., & Chamberlin, R. W. (1980). *Child and family development.* New York: McGraw-Hill.

Iverson, P. (1990). *The Navajos.* New York: Chelsea House Publishers.

James, W. (1990). *Principles of psychology* (2nd ed., Vol. 1). Chicago: Encyclopaedia Britannica.

Ketchum, J. D. (1951). Time, values, and social organization. *Canadian Journal of Psychology, 5*, 97–109.

Kluckhohn, F., & Strodtbeck, F. (1973). *Variations in value orientation.* Westport, CT: Greenwood Press.

Kohn, M. (1977). *Class and conformity* (2nd ed.). Chicago: University of Chicago Press.

Landes, D. (2000). *Revolution in time* (revised ed.). Cambridge, MA: Harvard University Press.

Lebhar, G. (1958). *The use of time* (3rd ed.). New York: Chain Store.

Levine, R., & Wolff, E. (1985). Social time: the heartbeat of culture. *Psychology Today*, 29–35.

MacStavic, R. E. (1978). Setting priorities in health planning: what does it mean? *Inquiry: A Journal of Medical Care Organization, Provision and Financing, 45*(1), 20–24.

Maguire, D. C. (1984). *Death by choice.* Garden City, NY: Image Books.

Mbiti, J. S. (1990). *African religions and philosophies* (2nd ed.). Portsmouth, NH: Heinemann.

McGrath, J., & Kelly, J. (1986). *Time and human interaction.* New York: Guilford Press.

McNiff, M. (1984). Getting organized—at last. *RN, 47*, 23–24.

McRae, L. (1994). Cultural sensitivity in rehabilitation related to native clients. *Canadian Journal of Rehabilitation, 7*(4), 251–256.

Meade, R. (1960). Time on their hands. *Personnel Journal, 39*, 130–132.

Midgley, J. W., & Osterhage, R. A. (1973). Effect of nursing instruction and length of hospitalization on postoperative complications in cholecystectomy patients. *Nursing Resident, 22*(1), 69–72.

Monette, F. C., Sullivan, T., & Dejong, C. (2008). *Applied social research* (7th ed.). Belmont, CA: Thomson Higher Education.

Morgenstern, I. (1960). *The dimensional structure of time.* New York: Philosophical Library.

Nash, M. (1967). *Machine age Maya.* Chicago: University of Chicago Press.

Nelkin, D. (1970). Unpredictability and life style in a migrant camp. *Social Problems, 17*, 472–487.

Nolt, S. (1992). *A history of the Amish.* Intercourse, PA: Harold Press.

Parkinson, C. (1970). *The law of delay.* London: John Murray.

Polick, F. (1973). *The image of the future* (Vol. 1–2). San Francisco: Jossey-Bass.

Polit, D., & Hungler, B. P. (2004). *Nursing research: principles and methods* (7th ed.). Philadelphia: Lippincott Williams & Wilkins.

Pouissant, A., & Atkinson, C. (1970). Black youth and motivation. *The Black Scholar, 1*, 43–51.

Pyle, K. (1969). *The new generation of Meiji Japan.* Stanford, CA: Stanford University Press.

Randall-David, E. (1989). *Strategies for working with culturally diverse communities and clients [Brochure].* Washington, DC: Department of Health and Human Services.

Ritzenthaler, R. E. (1953). The Impact of Small Industry on an Indian Community. *American Anthropologist, 55*(1), 143–148.

Ruiz, R. (2003). Cultural and historical perspectives in counseling Hispanics. In D. Sue (Ed.), *Counseling the culturally diverse: theory and practice* (4th ed.). New York: Wiley.

Ruiz, R. A., & Padella, A. M. (1977). Counseling Latinos. *The Personnel and Guidance Journal, 55*, 401–408.

Salmond, S. (1986). Time management: the time is now. *Orthopedic Nursing, 5*(3), 25–32.

Schroder, P. J., Washington, W. P., Deering, C. D., & Coyne, L. (1986). Testing validity and reliability in a psychiatric patient classification system. *Nursing Management, 17*(1), 49–54.

Sheard, T. (1980). The structure of conflict in nurse–physician relations. *Supervisor Nurse, 11*(8), 14–16.

Sideleau, B. (1992). Space and time. In J. Haber, A. Leach-McMahon, P. Price-Hoskins, & B. Sideleau (Eds.), *Comprehensive psychiatric nursing* (4th ed.). St. Louis: Mosby.

Smith, J. A. (1976). The role of the Black clergy as allied health care professionals in working with Black patients. In J. D. Luckraft (Ed.), *Black awareness: implications for Black care* (pp. 12–15). New York: American Journal of Nursing Company.

Sorokin, P. (1964). *Sociocultural causality, space, time.* New York: Russell & Russell.

Spector, R. (2004). *Cultural diversity in health and illness* (6th ed.). Upper Saddle River, NJ: Prentice Hall.

Stauffer, R. (1995). Personal communication. Harrisburg, VA.

Stoetzel, J. (1953). The contribution of public opinion research techniques to social anthropology. *International Social Science Bulletin, 5,* 494–503.

Strauss, G. (1963). Group dynamics and intergroup relations. In A. O. Lewis Jr. (Ed.), *Of men and machines* (pp. 321–327). New York: E. P. Dutton.

Suto, M., & Frank, G. (1994). Future time perspective and daily occupations of persons with chronic schizophrenia in a board and care home. *American Journal of Occupational Therapy, 48*(1), 7–18.

Thompson, E. (1967). Time, work-discipline, and industrial capitalism. *Past and Present, 38,* 58–59.

Thompson, P., & McDonald, J. (1989). Multicultural health education: responding to the challenge. *Health Promoting, 28*(2), 8–11.

Toffler, A. (1970). *Future shock.* New York: Random House.

Tripp-Reimer, T., & Lively, S. H. (1993). Cultural considerations in mental health–psychiatric nursing. In R. P. Rawlins, R. S. Williams, & C. K. Beck (Eds.), *Mental health–psychiatric nursing* (3rd ed., pp. 166–177). St. Louis: Mosby.

Vestal, K. (1987). *Management concepts for the new nurse.* Philadelphia: J. B. Lippincott.

Veterans World Project. (1972). *Wasted men: the reality of the Vietnam veteran.* Edwardsville, IL: Southern Illinois University.

Wang, D., Liu, X., & Ahalt, S. (1996). On temporal generalisation of simple recurrent networks. *Neural Networks, 9,* 1099–1118.

Weigert, A. (1981). *Sociology of everyday life.* New York: Longman.

Wenger, A. (2006). The culture care theory and the older order Amish. In M. Leininger (Ed.), *Cultural care diversity and universality: a theory of nursing* (2nd ed.). Sudbury, MA: Jones and Bartlett.

Wessman, A., & Gorman, B. (1977). The emergence of human awareness and concepts of time. In B. S. Gorman & A. E. Wessman (Eds.), *Personal experience of time* (p. 3). New York: Plenum Press.

Weyer, E. (1961). *Primitive peoples today.* Garden City, NY: Doubleday.

Wuest, J. (1992). Joining together: students and faculty learn about transcultural nursing. *Journal of Nursing Education, 31*(2), 90–92.

Yogman, M. W., Lester, B. M., & Hoffman, J. (1983). Behavioral rhythmicity and circadian rhythmicity during mother, father, stranger, infant social interaction. *Pediatric Research, 17*(11), 872–876.

Young, D. E., Ingram, C., & Swartz, L. (1990). *Cry of the eagle: encounters with a Cree healer.* Toronto: University of Toronto Press.

Young, L., & Hayne, A. (1988). *Nursing administration: from concepts to practice.* Philadelphia: Saunders.

Zerubavel, E. (1979). *Patterns of time in hospital life.* Chicago: University of Chicago Press.

Ziac, D. C. (1984). Menstrual synchrony in university women. *American Journal of Physical Anthropology, 63*(2), 237.

Environmental Control

BEHAVIORAL OBJECTIVES

After reading this chapter, the nurse will be able to:

1. Recognize relevant cultural factors that affect health-seeking behaviors related to environmental control.
2. Recognize relevant cultural factors that affect illness behaviors related to environmental control.
3. Identify various types of cultural folk health practices and the effect on health-seeking behaviors.
4. Recognize the relationship between external locus of control and fatalistic or health-seeking behaviors.
5. Recognize factors affecting external locus of control for persons in selected cultural groups.

Environmental control refers to the ability of an individual or persons from a particular cultural group to plan activities that control nature. Environmental control also refers to the individual's perception of ability to direct factors in the environment. This definition in itself implies that the concept of environment is broader than just the place where an individual resides or where treatment occurs. In the most practical sense, the term *environment* encompasses relevant systems and processes that affect individuals (Sideleau, 1997).

Systems are organized structures that may influence and be influenced by individuals. Processes may be viewed as organized, purposeful patterns of operation. Processes generally include the dynamics and interactions among families, groups, and the community at large. On the basis of these definitions, it is evident that the environment and humans have a reciprocal relationship in the sense that humans and the environment are constantly exchanging matter and energy. When this exchange has purpose and is goal directed, the interaction and exchange processes are considered functional and useful. However, when the exchange has no purpose and lacks goal direction, a dyssynchronous relationship occurs (Haber et al., 1997).

In the broadest sense, health may be viewed as a balance between the individual and the environment. Health practices such as eating nutritiously, subscribing to preventive health services available in the community, and installing hazard- and pollution-control devices are all believed to have a positive effect on the individual, who in turn can positively affect the environment (Spector, 2004).

Complex systems of health beliefs and practices exist across and within cultural groups. In addition, variations, whether extreme or modest, to cultural beliefs and practices are found across ethnic and social class boundaries and even within family groups. Today the most widely accepted approach to health care is the biomedical model. This model emphasizes biological concerns, which are considered by those who support this model as more "real" and significant than psychological and sociological issues (Kleinman, Eisenberg, & Good, 1978).

Today in modern Western society, health care practitioners remain primarily interested in abnormalities in the structure and function of body systems and in the treatment of disease. According to Kleinman et al. (1978), the biomedical approach is culture-specific, culture-bound, and value-laden. The biomedical model represents only one end of a continuum. At the opposite end of the continuum is the traditional model, which espouses popular beliefs and practices that diverge from medical science (Chrisman, 1977). Persons who subscribe to beliefs encompassed in the traditional model have varying health beliefs and practices, including folk beliefs and traditional beliefs that are also shaped by culture (Spector, 2004).

DISTINCTION BETWEEN ILLNESS AND DISEASE

During the past few decades, scientists and anthropologists began to make a distinction between the terms *illness* and *disease*. The individual experiences that relate to illnesses do not necessarily correlate with the biomedical interpretation of disease. *Illness* can be defined as an individual's perception of being sick. On the other hand, *disease* is diagnosed when the condition is a deviation from clearly established norms based on Western biomedical science (Fabrega, 1971; McGrattan, 2004). Illness can and does occur in the absence of disease; approximately 50% of visits to physicians are for complaints without a definite basis. According to Kleinman et al. (1978), illness is culturally shaped in the sense that it is individually perceived. In other words, how one experiences and copes with disease is based on the individual's explanation of sickness. Disease is described in detail in medical–surgical nursing textbooks. However, nurses need to remember to incorporate both personal and cultural reactions of the client to illness, disease, and discomfort to give culturally appropriate nursing care.

Just as culture influences health-related behavior, it also has a profound effect on the expectations and perceptions of sickness that shape the labeling of sickness and on how, when, and to whom communication of health problems occurs (Campinha-Bacote, 1997). The astute nurse must keep in mind the fact that perceptions of health and illness are shaped by cultural factors. As a direct result of cultural shaping, individuals vary in health care behaviors, health status, and health-seeking attitudes (Grypma, 1993; Guruge & Donner, 1996; McRae, 1994; Thompson, 1993).

The term *health care behavior* is defined as the social and biological activities of an individual that are based on maintaining an acceptable health status or manipulating and altering an unacceptable condition (Bauwens & Anderson, 1992). The term *health status,* on the other hand, is defined as the success with which an individual adapts to the internal and external environment (Bauwens & Anderson, 1992; Rumsfeld, 2002). Thus, health care behavior influences health status, which in turn influences health care behavior. Because health care behavior and health status are reciprocal in nature, they both can be affected by sociocultural forces, such as economics, politics, environmental influences, and the health care delivery system itself (Elling, 1977).

CULTURAL HEALTH PRACTICES VERSUS MEDICAL HEALTH PRACTICES

Cultural health practices are categorized as efficacious, neutral, dysfunctional (Pillsbury, 1982), or uncertain.

Efficacious Cultural Health Practices

According to Western medical standards, efficacious cultural health practices are beneficial to health status, although they can differ vastly from modern scientific practices. Because efficacious health practices can facilitate effective nursing care, nurses need to actively encourage these practices among and across cultural groups. Nurses must keep in mind that a treatment strategy that is consistent with the client's beliefs may have a better chance of being successful. For example, persons from cultural groups who subscribe to the theory of hot and cold, such as some Mexican Americans, may actually benefit from this particular belief. Individuals who subscribe to this theory may avoid hot foods in the presence of stomach ailments such as ulcers, a practice that is consistent with the bland diet used in a medical regimen for the treatment of ulcers. Thus scientific health care practices may be blended with efficacious cultural health practices.

Neutral Cultural Health Practices

Neutral cultural health practices have no effect on the health status of an individual. Although some health care practitioners may consider neutral health practices irrelevant, the nurse must remember that such practices may be extremely important because they might be linked to beliefs that are closely integrated with an individual's behavior (Pillsbury, 1982). In Greene's classic work (1981), several examples of neutral practices were cited, including "the ritual disposal of the placenta and cord," interpretation of signs in the cord, avoidance of sexual activity during various stages of pregnancy, certain hygiene practices, and avoidance of exposure to luminous rays of the moon during a lunar eclipse. Many Southeast Asian women believe that sitting in a door frame or on a step while they are pregnant will complicate labor and delivery. In waiting and examination rooms, these women avoid areas near doors. These women may also think that overeating or inactivity during pregnancy will cause a difficult delivery and that sleeping late or during the day will have the same effect. Hill tribeswomen (Hmong and Mien) avoid contact with scissors and knives because they fear sharp instruments may cause cleft lip or abortion. There is a general belief among these women that reaching overhead for something or working too hard may cause miscarriage or birth defects (Lew, 1989; Mattson, 1995). Although these practices require no planned nursing interventions, the astute nurse must recognize their significance and respect the client's right to subscribe to and practice such beliefs.

Dysfunctional Cultural Health Practices

Dysfunctional cultural health practices are harmful. An example of a dysfunctional health care practice found in the United States is the excessive use of such items as over-refined flour and sugar. The nurse must be aware of practices that are dysfunctional and should work to establish educational training programs that help individuals identify dysfunctional health practices and develop beneficial practices. A dysfunctional health care practice was noted among women of various racial, ethnic, and cultural groups in British Columbia in Canada (Hislop, Deschamps, Band, Smith, & Clarke, 1992). Findings from this study noted that implementation of a population-based cervical cytology screening program in British Columbia that began in 1955 decreased the mortality from invasive squamous cervical cancer by more than 70%. However, the mortality from cervical cancer, despite the implementation of this innovative program, remained high among the Canadian Native population (Inuits, Indians, Métis). In fact, the mortality was four times higher among Canadian Native women than among their non-Native counterparts (Threlfall, 1986). Although approximately 85% of the women in the general population complied with screening recommendations, the compliance by Canadian Native women was approximately 30% less. Whether this under-participation by Native woman resulted from beliefs and attitudes or from lack of availability of resources was not determined.

Uncertain Cultural Health Practices

In 1994, Williams, Baumslag, and Jelliffe developed a cultural assessment system that included a category of cultural health practices with unknown effects. Classified as uncertain, these practices included such things as swaddling a newborn infant to maintain body temperature and using an abdominal binder for mother and infant to prevent umbilical hernias.

The nurse must remember that in most instances health practices do not fit perfectly into one category or another. According to Greene (1981), health practices are subjectively evaluated as more or less beneficial or harmful when they are compared with the alternative practices available to the user.

VALUES AND THEIR RELATIONSHIP TO HEALTH CARE PRACTICES

Values may be viewed as individualized sets of rules by which people live and are governed. They serve as the cornerstone for beliefs, attitudes, and behaviors. Cultural values are often acquired unconsciously as an individual assimilates the culture throughout the process of growth and maturation. It is important for the nurse to recognize that because cultural values are believed to exist almost

solely on an unconscious level, they are the most difficult to alter. Cultural values therefore have a pervasive and profound influence on the individual (Giger, Davidhizar, Johnson, & Poole, 1997).

Value Orientations

Kluckhohn and Strodtbeck (1973) defined *value orientations* as "complex but definitely patterned principles which give order and direction to the ever-flowing stream of human acts and thoughts as they relate to the solution of common human problems." Kluckhohn and Strodtbeck also proposed that it is entirely possible for an individual to hold a value orientation different from the rest of the same cultural group. However, they concluded that despite differences in value orientation within a cultural group, dominant value orientations can be identified for most persons of a particular cultural group.

In their classic work, Kluckhohn and Strodtbeck (1973) compared the way people in different cultural groups organize their thinking about such things as time, personal activity, interpersonal relationships, and their relationship to nature and the supernatural. They developed an orientation framework that includes temporal, activity, relational, people-to-nature, and innate human nature orientations.

Temporal Orientation

Temporal orientation refers to the method by which persons from particular cultural groups divide time. Time is generally divided into three frames of reference: past, present, and future. According to Kluckhohn and Strodtbeck (1973) and Haber et al. (1997), most cultures combine all three orientations, but one is more likely to dominate than another.

Activity Orientation

Activity orientation refers to whether a cultural group is perceived as a "doing"-oriented culture, which is oriented toward achievement, or as a "being"-oriented culture, which values "being" and views people as an important link between generations. In other words, the "doing"-oriented culture values accomplishments, whereas the "being"-oriented culture values inherent existence.

Relational Orientation

Relational orientation from a cultural perspective distinguishes interpersonal patterns. More specifically, *relational orientation* refers to the way in which persons in a culture set goals for individual members. Relational orientations are found in three modes: lineal, individualistic, and collateral.

Lineal Mode. When the lineal mode is dominant within a particular cultural group, the goals and welfare of the group are viewed as major concerns. Other major concerns are the continuity of the group and the orderly succession of the group over time. Cultures that are perceived as subscribing to the lineal mode view kinship bonds as the basis for maintaining lineage.

Individualistic Mode. Cultures in which the dominant mode is individualistic value individual goals over group goals. Thus, each individual is responsible for personal behaviors and ultimately is held accountable for personal accomplishments.

Collateral Mode. When the collateral mode is dominant in a cultural group, the goals and welfare of lateral groups such as siblings or peers are of paramount importance. Examples are found in Russia and in Israel, where the goals of individuals are subordinate to those that affect the entire lateral group.

People-to-Nature Orientation

People-to-nature orientation implies that people dominate nature, live in harmony with nature, or are subjugated to nature. The conceptual framework of people dominating nature is based on the view that humans dominate nature and further indicates that humankind can master or control natural events. When people live in harmony with nature, there is an integration among them, nature, and the universe. When the view that humans are subjugated to nature is held, a philosophy of fatalism is adopted; that is, fate is considered inevitable, and individuals perceive themselves as having no control over nature or their future—they consider themselves powerless to guide personal destiny. An example is the belief held by some Appalachian people that "If I'm going to get cancer, I'm going to get it," so that taking preventive measures to avoid cancer would be of no benefit. This fatalistic attitude, however, is not completely consistent because most Appalachian people will go to a physician or hospital if they believe they are extremely ill.

Innate Human Nature Orientation

The innate human nature orientation distinguishes an individual's human nature as being good, evil, or neutral. Some cultural groups view human beings as having a basic nature that is either changeable or unchangeable. For example, an individual may be viewed as evil and unchangeable, evil but changeable, or neutral (subject to both good and negative influences).

LOCUS-OF-CONTROL CONSTRUCT AS A HEALTH CARE VALUE

The locus-of-control construct, which originated in social learning theory, is defined as follows:

> When a reinforcement is perceived as following some action but not being entirely contingent upon (personal) action then in our culture it is typically perceived as a result of luck, chance, and fate, as under the control of powerful others, or unpredictable because of the great complexity of the forces surrounding [the individual]. When the event is interpreted in this way by an individual, this is labelled as a belief in external control. If a person perceives that the event is contingent upon his own behavior or his own permanent characteristics, we have termed this a belief in internal control. (Rotter, 1966)

This definition presupposes that individuals who believe that a contingent relationship exists between actions and outcomes have internal feelings of control and thus act to influence future behaviors and situations. Individuals who believe that efforts and rewards are uncorrelated, and who thus have external feelings of control, view the future as the result of luck, chance, or fate, and are less likely to take action to change the future. The locus-of-control construct can be applied to a variety of phenomena, including the weather, preventive health, curative health actions, and feelings of well-being. For example, individuals who believe that a contingent relationship exists between compliance to preventive and treatment regimens and health have an internal locus of control and are likely to respond positively to affect the future and thus promote good health. On the other hand, individuals who believe that compliance behaviors and health are unrelated have an external locus of control and have little motivation to develop behaviors that could affect the future and enhance good health. Rotter (1975) concluded that the locus of control does not in itself represent a behavior trait and can be modified by interaction with others.

While the locus-of-control construct originates in social learning theory (Rotter, 1966, 1975, 1992), it is essential to note that Siegleman (1992) believed that locus of control is often too general and tends to collapse good and bad events. However, in contrast, Peterson and Stunkard (1992) noted that thousands of researchers have scientifically examined the locus-of-control construct. In fact, Phares (1978), in summarizing the multitude of investigations on the locus-of-control construct, noted that, compared with the external, the internal is often resistant to such factors as social pressure and is frequently dedicated to the pursuit of excellence. While Phares (1978) has been quick to add a disclaimer that internality is not necessarily good, the remainder of the research indicates that in a responsive environment, individuals who have an internal locus of control have been able to benefit from such beliefs (Peterson & Stunkard, 1992). Rotter (1992) noted that his 1966 monograph had been cited more than 4700 times in the literature, thereby giving credence for its validity as an applicable construct. Some cultural experts in nursing, such as Giger, Davidhizar, and Turner (1992), espouse the usefulness of the locus-of-control construct to understand individuals from diverse cultural backgrounds.

The astute nurse should recognize that persons who subscribe to an external locus of control tend to be more fatalistic about nature, health, illness, death, and disease. For example, some Hispanics, Appalachians, and Puerto Ricans are reported to have an external locus of control. Some American Indians, Chinese Americans, and Japanese Americans or Japanese Canadians are said to be more or less in harmony with nature; therefore, their cultural beliefs fall outside the locus-of-control construct. However, northern European Americans and African-Americans are reported to fall within both the internal and the external locus-of-control construct (Kluckhohn & Strodtbeck, 1973). The nurse can help the client modify behaviors that fall within the realm of the external locus-of-control construct by showing the effects of certain behaviors on illnesses, health, and disease and thus promote the development of an internal locus of control.

FOLK MEDICINE

Folk medicine, or what is commonly referred to as "Third World beliefs and practices," is often called "strange" or "weird" by nurses and other health professionals who are unfamiliar with folk medicine beliefs (Giger, Davidhizar, & Turner, 1992; Snow, 1981). In reality, whether or not something seems "strange or weird" depends on familiarity with the beliefs. In most instances folk medicine practices do not seem strange or weird once health care providers become familiar with them.

The astute nurse must distinguish between practices that are familiar and practices that are desirable, since becoming familiar with something does not imply acceptance. In this situation, tolerance becomes a two-way process: people who subscribe to folk medicine practices need not feel compelled to abandon these beliefs and practices when they become familiar with modern medicine, and health care practitioners should not feel compelled to abandon modern medical practices when they become familiar with folk medicine practices.

An individual's worldview largely determines beliefs about disease and the appropriate treatment interventions. For example, a belief in magic may lead to the assumption that a disease is a result of human behavior and that a cure can be achieved by magical techniques. A religious belief may lead to the assumption that the disease is a result of supernatural forces and that a cure can be achieved by appealing to supernatural forces. The scientific view may lead to the assumption that the disease is a result of the cause-and-effect relationship of natural phenomena and that a cure is achieved by scientific medicine (Henderson & Primeaux, 1981).

Folk Medicine Beliefs as a System

The folk medicine system classifies illnesses or diseases as natural or unnatural. This division of illnesses or diseases into natural and unnatural phenomena is common among Haitians, persons from Trinidad, Mexicans and Mexican Canadians, African Canadians, and some Southern White Americans (Snow, 1981).

Distinction between Natural and Unnatural Events

The simplest way to distinguish between natural and unnatural illnesses is that, according to this belief system, natural events have to do with the world as God made it and as God intended it to be. Thus, natural laws allow a measure of predictability for daily life. Unnatural events, on the other hand, imply the exact opposite because they upset the harmony of nature. Unnatural events can therefore be viewed as events that interrupt the plan intended by God and at their very worst represent the forces of evil and the machinations of the devil. Unnatural events are frightening because they have no predictability. They are outside the world of nature, and so when they do occur, they are beyond the control of ordinary mortals.

Germane to the tendency to view phenomena in terms of opposition, such as good versus evil and natural versus unnatural, is the belief held by some folk medicine systems that everything has an exact opposite. For example, some African Canadians who subscribe to a folk medicine system believe that for every birth there must be a death, for every marriage there must be a divorce, and for every person with good health there must be someone with bad health. This belief is so encompassing that such individuals believe that every illness has a cure, every poison has an antidote, every herb has a healing purpose, and so forth (Snow, 1981). Because of this belief, some cultural groups do not accept the chronicity of such diseases as acquired immunodeficiency syndrome (AIDS), herpes, or syphilis.

Herbal medicine continues to enjoy a "rebirth" (French, 1996). Eisenberg et al. (1993) noted that 34% of all U.S. citizens use herbal products in some way. In 1990, they spent $13.7 billion on "unconventional" therapy, with 75% of this cost being out-of-pocket. Canadians are also participating in this resurgence with an increased use of herbal medicines (Abarts, 1995).

In 2007, the number of what is now termed *natural medicines* in some circles had increased again dramatically. Natural medicines also include vitamins, dietary supplements, and alternative medicines. In fact, the use of dietary supplements and alternative medicines continues to gain popularity among health-seeking consumers. Today, more than 40% of all U.S. residents have tried some type of alternative medication, whereas 50% of U.S. residents 35 to 49 years of age have tried alternative medicines. It fact, it has been reported that in the United States:

- 106 million people use vitamins and minerals.
- 44.6 million people use herbal remedies.
- 24.2 million people use specialty dietary supplements (Institute for Safe Medication Practices, 2007).

Distinction between Natural and Unnatural Illnesses

Illnesses are generally classified as *natural* or *unnatural*, which affects the type of cure or practitioner sought. All illnesses can be viewed as representing disharmony and conflict in some particular area of life and thus tend to fall into two general categories: natural illnesses as environmental hazards and unnatural illnesses as divine punishment.

Natural Illnesses as Environmental Hazards. Natural illnesses in the folk medicine belief system occur because of dangerous agents, such as cold air or impurities in the air, food, and water. Natural illnesses are based on the belief that everything in nature is connected and that events can be both interpreted and directed by an understanding of these relationships. Sympathetic magic, the basis for popular folk medicine beliefs and practices, can be divided into two categories: contagious and imitative magic. At the root of contagious magic is the premise that the parts do represent the whole. Many witchcraft practices are based on contagious magic, including such practices as an evil-doer obtaining a lock of the victim's hair or shavings from the victim's skin to do harm. Imitative magic, on the other hand, is based on the premise that like will follow like. For example, a knife under the bed will cut labor pains. To assist the client in preventing natural illnesses, the nurse must comprehend the direct connections between the body and natural phenomena, such as the phases of the moon, the position of the planets, and the changing of the seasons. Because in this belief system good health is

contingent on these phenomena, it is imperative that one be able to read these signs if the body is to remain in harmony with nature.

Unnatural Illnesses as Divine Punishment. Unnatural illnesses are believed to occur because a person has become so grave a sinner that the Lord withdraws his favor. In fact, illnesses may be attributed to punishment for failure to abide by the proper behavior rules given to man by God (Gregory, 1992). The cause of unnatural illnesses, for those who subscribe to these beliefs, is based on the continual battle between the forces of good and evil as personified in God and the devil. Evil influences may be blamed for any unnatural illness, which may range from nightmares to tuberculosis to cancer (Boston, 1993). An example of a person subscribing to this belief is a diabetic African-American woman who consistently refuses to inject herself with insulin because she believes her illness is the direct result of punishment by the devil for her sinful youth. However, unnatural illnesses are also believed to result from witchcraft. Witchcraft is based on the belief that there are individuals who have the ability to mobilize unusual powers for good and evil.

Comparison of the Folk Medicine System and Other Medical Systems

To develop an understanding of folk medicine as a system, the system itself must be examined, along with the ecological model, the Western medical system, alternative therapies, and religious systems. Every medical system is based on the philosophy of survival of the human organism. According to the classic work of Thomas Weaver (1970), both folk practices and Western medical practices are social systems with interdependent parts or variables that include beliefs, attitudes, practices, and roles associated with the concepts of health and disease and with the patterns of diagnoses and treatments.

All medical systems have an adaptive nature. As such, the term *medical system* can be defined as the pattern of cultural tradition and social institutions that evolves from deliberate behavior to improve health status, regardless of the outcome of a particular behavior (Dunn, 1998).

To achieve good health, an individual must develop an idea of what constitutes disease, with its counterpart conditions of pain and suffering. Once an individual adopts a philosophy of health, various health roles are delineated. These health roles require specific health care practitioners who are duly initiated into the rites of practice. Practitioner status may be granted by medical societies or, in the case of folk medicine practices, by supernatural forces. The body is an integral part of each individual; therefore, all medical systems use body parts or excreta for diagnostic purposes. In addition, folk medicine practices, in most cases, prescribe medicine to rub into the skin, to irrigate the body, or to anoint the sick.

Ecological Model. The ecological model is closely related to the folk medicine system. Kay (1979) defined *ecology* as having three foci: (1) biological, or the branch of biology that deals with the relationship between organisms and the environment; (2) social, or the relationship between people and institutions and the interdependence between the two; and (3) cultural, or the relationship between culture and the environment, which also includes culture and societies in the environment. Ecological dimensions of health care can assist the nurse in providing plausible explanations as to why certain individuals contract specific diseases and why other individuals do not. Over the past decade, health care practitioners have become increasingly concerned with the ecological dimensions of race and ethnic minority group health problems such as AIDS and sickle cell anemia.

Western Medical System. In contrast to the folk medicine system, which attempts to explain illness in terms of balances between an individual and the physical, social, and spiritual worlds, is the Western medical system of diagnoses and scientific explanations for illness. Western medical practices focus on preventive and curative medicine, whereas folk medicine practices focus on personal rather than scientific behavior. In the folk medicine system, it may make all the sense in the world to burn incense and to avoid certain individuals, cold air, and the "evil eye." According to Kay (1979), one person's religion is another person's magic, witchcraft, or superstition. However, it is very difficult for health care professionals to see these entities as directly relevant to medical practice or to recognize that for some cultural groups, religion is the equivalent of a science.

Although many differences in focus can be seen when Western and folk medicine health practices are compared, some of these differences may not be that significant. For example, Western medical relationships are generally dyads, such as physician–client, physician–nurse, and nurse–client relationships, whereas folk medicine networks are generally multiperson health care networks that may consist of parents, other relatives, and nonrelatives as health caregivers. However, today multiperson health care networks are no longer dismissed by Western health care practitioners as irrelevant and thus dysfunctional. In fact, multiperson networks are slowly being incorporated into the Western medical system of health care.

Ethnic diets are an important aspect of human ecology, and health care providers are beginning to incorporate the use of ethnic diets into practice and to understand their significance. A person, regardless of ethnic group, must consume enough food to meet nutritional requirements for energy, fat, protein, vitamins, and minerals to keep the body functioning. Rittenbaugh (1992) noted that very little is known regarding the range of human variability both among and within human populations, particularly regarding common parameters such as nutritional requirements, physiological response to malnutrition, and digestive capabilities. It is perhaps this lack of knowledge that has in the past resulted in Western-oriented health care providers prescribing diets unacceptable to persons from diverse and multicultural backgrounds. In fact, some individuals from diverse cultural backgrounds may have physical incompatibility with certain Western foods. Therefore, the nurse must consider factors regarding ethnic diets and other such folk practices when developing care plans for culturally specific nursing care.

Alternative Therapies. In 1990, 36% of Americans, approximately 61 million people, used one or more nonmedical forms of therapy to treat illness. Most of these individuals used these alternative therapies without informing their health practitioner (Eisenberg et al., 1993). In contrast, William LaValley, founder of the Nova Scotia Medical Society's Complementary Medicine Section, estimates that 25% of the Canadian population sought health care from alternative practitioners (University of Calgary–Complementary Medicine Seminar, 1995). Other presenters at the University of Calgary–Complementary Medicine Seminar (1995) reported that 18% of patients seen at the Calgary human immunodeficiency virus (HIV)/AIDS clinic and 27% of those seen at the University of Calgary gastroenterology clinic had tried alternative therapies. Some 44% of physicians from Alberta indicated that they made referrals to practitioners of alternative therapies, even though only 10% considered themselves informed on the subject (Peterson, 1996). Although Western medicine tends to focus on illness care, alternative therapy addresses the whole patient (Peterson, 1996). In alternative therapy, symptoms are seen as the tip of the iceberg and the body's means for communicating to the mind that something needs to be changed, removed, or added to one's life (Peterson, 1996). In alternative therapy, the mind and the body are seen as a whole. Acupuncture, holistic healing, therapeutic touch, aromatic therapy, meditation, guided imagery, and a variety of other techniques prevail as feasible alternative therapies (Barnum, 1994). Practitioners of alternative therapies include therapeutic touch experts, homeopaths, naturopaths, massage therapists, and reflexologists (Cronsberry, 1996). According to Dossey (1993), scientists working in the new field of psychoneuroimmunology have demonstrated the existence of intimate links between parts of the brain concerned with thought and emotion and the neurological and immune systems. Based on these discoveries, Dossey (1993) concluded that thought can become biology. Although the scientific value of alternative, or complementary, therapies is yet to be proved, there is a psychological component that allows the client to have a sense of control. For this reason, nurses should be well informed about nontraditional methods (Cronsberry, 1996).

Over the past 20 years the use of complementary therapies increased from 36.3% in 1990 to 46.3% of the U.S. population by 1997 and remained stable from 1997 to 2002 (Tindle, Davis, Phillips, & Eisenberg, 2005). The increasing prevalence of Alzheimer's disease in an aging U.S. population with concomitant behavioral symptoms of dementia (BSD), coupled with the numerous side effects experienced when medications are used to ameliorate these symptoms, has resulted in the current recommendations for nonpharmacological treatments (NPTs) for BSD. Several of the therapies that demonstrate efficacy for alleviating BSD in Alzheimer's disease are complementary therapies such as aromatherapy (Ballard, O'Brien, Reichelt, & Perry, 2002) and calming interventions such as therapeutic touch (Woods, Beck, & Sinha, 2009; Woods, Craven & Whitney, 2005; Woods, Rapp, & Beck, 2004; Woods & Dimond, 2002). Research studies conducted by Woods et al. (2005, 2009) and reviewed by Jain and Mills (2010) show a moderate effect for therapeutic touch on BSD. In a randomized, double-blind, three-group experimental interrupted design, Woods et al. (2005) examined the effect of therapeutic touch on BSD nursing home residents with dementia. Fifty-seven residents 67 to 93 years of age who exhibited BSD were randomized to one of three groups (experimental, placebo, control) within each of three special care units within three long-term care facilities. Direct behavioral observation was completed every 20 minutes from 8:00 a.m. to 6:00 p.m. for 3 days preintervention and for 3 days postintervention by trained observers who were blind to group assignment. The intervention consisted of therapeutic touch given twice daily for 5 to 7 minutes for 3 days between 10:00 a.m. and 11:30 p.m. and between 3:00 p.m. and 4:30 p.m. The main outcome variable was overall BSD including six specific behaviors: restlessness, escape restraints, tapping, searching, pacing, and vocalization. Findings from this study using analysis of variance (ANOVA) (F = 3.331, P = 0.033) and Kruskal-Wallis (X^2 = 6.661, P = 0.036) indicated a significant difference in overall BSD, restlessness, and vocalization when the experimental group was compared with the placebo and control groups. Therapeutic touch significantly decreased restlessness and vocalization when the experimental group was compared with the control group, whereas the placebo group indicated a decreasing trend in BSD. In a similarly designed study, Woods et al. (2009) found that therapeutic touch decreased BSD in the experimental group compared

with the control group (P = 0.03), with a significant difference in morning cortisol (P = <0.001). At a time when cost containment is a consideration in health care, therapeutic touch is a complementary therapy that is noninvasive, readily learned, and able to provide an alternative for selected persons with BSD.

Religious Systems. Some religious groups have elaborate rules concerning health care behaviors, including such things as the giving and receiving of health care. Religious experiences are based on cultural beliefs and may include such things as blessings from spiritual leaders, apparitions of dead relatives, and even miracle cures. Healing power based on religion may also be found in animate as well as inanimate objects. Religion can and does dictate social, moral, and dietary practices that are designed to assist an individual in maintaining a healthy balance and, in addition, plays a vital role in illness prevention. Examples of religious health care practices include illness prevention through such acts as the burning of candles, rituals of redemption, and prayer. Religious practices such as the blessing of the throats on St. Blaine's feast day are performed to prevent illnesses such as sore throats and choking. Baptism may be seen as a ritual of cleansing and dedication, as well as a prevention against evil. In addition to its meaning as dedication to God's will and a preparation for death, anointing the sick is related by some religious and cultural groups to recovery and may be performed in the hope of a miracle. Circumcision is also a religious practice in that it may be viewed as having redemptive values that may prevent illness and harm (Morgenstern, 1966; Spector, 2004).

It is important for the nurse to learn to distinguish between a shaman and a priest. A shaman derives power from the supernatural, whereas a priest learns a codified body of rituals from other priests and from biblical laws. In traditional folk medicine systems, some of the most significant religious rituals are those that mediate between events in the here and now and events in the hereafter or "out there" in the netherworld (Morley & Wallis, 1978).

Another example of a religious system is the Amish movement. For the Amish, religion and custom are inseparable and blend into a way of life (Randall-David, 1989). Religious considerations determine hours of work, occupation, means, destination of travel, and choice of friends and mates. The Amish value the importance of working with the elements of nature rather than mastery over these elements. Closeness to soil, animals, plants, and weather is valued. Salvation is viewed as obedience to the community (Wenger, 2006). The Amish have the belief that the human body was created by God and should not be tampered with. Some Amish believe that although medication may help, it is God who heals (Randall-David, 1989).

Many Amish have been increasingly influenced by special health food interests, vitamins, and food supplement industries (Wenger, 1988). Folk medical practices and opposition to health care seem to be dominant in some family systems (Hostetler, 1980). Egeland (1967) hypothesized that there is a relationship between the concept of family culture and health behavior. Clusters of family cultures serve as basic socializers of health (Egeland, 1967). *Friendshaft*, a concept that crosses distinct church lines, produces distinct patterns of behavior and personality in the Amish community related to choice of type of physician. It also influences choice of curative diet therapy, folk remedies, and family coding of preference of treatment in reference to the presumed cause of symptoms (Brewer & Bonalumi, 1995; Wenger, 1995).

Death and Dying and End-of-Life Decision Making across Cultures

Some researchers have noted that grieving and death rituals vary across cultures and for the most part are often heavily influenced by religion (Chachkes & Jennings, 1994; Younoszai, 1993). It is essential to remember that how and to what extent rituals regarding death and dying are practiced will certainly vary and will depend on the country of origin and level of acculturation into the mainstream of U.S. society. Clements et al. (2003) also noted that the duration, frequency, and intensity of the grief process by various cultural groups is often also based on the manner in which death is experienced and on the family cultural beliefs (Clements et al., 2003).

Cultural Beliefs and Advanced Directives. The U.S. health care system is based on three values:

1. Life is sacred and should be preserved at all costs.
2. Autonomous decision making should be maintained at all times.
3. Above all, it is important that no individuals suffer needlessly (Kagawa-Singer, 1998).

It is interesting to note that findings from some studies suggest that there are cultural variations in attitude toward concepts such as truth telling, life-prolonging techniques, and decision-making styles at the end of life that are obvious between and across cultures (Giger, Davidhizar, & Fordham, 2006). Advanced directives are suggested for those who want to maintain some autonomy and decision making about their health care, yet some cultural groups have been slow to embrace this concept. For example, some African-Americans continue to distrust the health care system. This distrust is perhaps the result of such things as the Tuskegee Syphilis Study. While decision making for many African-Americans certainly varies by virtue of individual history, religiosity, and socioeconomic status, a great number of African-Americans may regard an advanced directive as a way to legalize neglect, perhaps deny treatment, and commit genocide of the race (DeSpelder & Strickland, 2005).

Autonomy in Decision Making and Truth Telling about Death and Dying. In the United States, the value of autonomous decision making is valued by many persons from diverse cultures (Giger et al., 2006). Blackhall, Murphy, Frank, Michel, and Azen (1995) found that when it comes to decision making in the case of the terminally ill, some Korean Americans and Mexican Americans subscribe to a family-centered model of decision making as opposed to a patient-centered model. For example, they noted that some Korean Americans may seek to avoid the unnecessary suffering of a loved one, particularly if they believe that more negative results would occur if a loved one were told of an unfavorable prognosis. In this case, the family serves as a group decision maker. Examples of other cultural groups that may subscribe to such beliefs include some Japanese Americans and Hispanic individuals (Giger et al., 2006; Kagawa-Singer, 1996, 1998).

Findings from one study suggested that Mexican Americans and Korean Americans are significantly less likely than Whites and African-Americans to believe that a family member should be told of a diagnosis, particularly a diagnosis such as metastatic cancer (Blackhall et al., 1995). In fact, Koreans (47%) and Mexican Americans (65%) were significantly less likely than Whites (87%) and African-Americans (88%) to believe that a loved one should be told of a diagnosis such as metastatic cancer. A surprising finding from this study (Blackhall et al., 1995) was that Korean Americans (28%) and Mexican Americans (41%) tended to hold an overriding belief that loved ones should not be allowed to make decisions about life-supporting measures as compared with 56% of Whites. In fact, some researchers suggest that among Mexican Americans there is a belief that the dying should be protected from knowing the prognosis. Yet when it comes to the decision of quality over quantity of life, some cultural groups also vary in this regard. For example, Blackhall et al. (1995) noted that some African-Americans are about only half as likely as their White counterparts to opt for pain medications that might improve the quality of their lives at the expense of the length of life, even if it means that the physiological pain might be constantly present. On the other hand, Whites are more likely to refuse such life-sustaining measures as intubation than their Hispanic or African-American counterparts (Giger et al., 2006).

The astute nurse who works with persons from diverse cultural backgrounds must be cognizant of the variations not only in the beliefs about death and dying but also about such keys issues as advanced directives, truth telling, and autonomy in decision making.

IMPLICATIONS FOR NURSING CARE

The nurse must keep in mind that regardless of whether a client believes in internal or external locus of control or whether the client uses a folk medicine system, religious system, or ecological system, there is still safety in harmony and balance, and there may be danger in anything that is done to the extreme. In other words, it is bad for the body to eat too much, drink too much, stay out too late, and so on. In a classic 1972 study in Harlem, it was reported that 90% of African-American adolescents surveyed believed that good health was largely a matter of looking after oneself. These adolescents concluded that the results of excess may not be immediately visible but sooner or later will affect the individual because the body has become weakened (Brunswick & Josephson, 1972).

There seemingly is a gender and age differential that is associated with strengths and weaknesses among individuals. Generally speaking, strength is correlated with a person's ability to withstand illness, whereas weakness is correlated with a person's heightened susceptibility. For example, strength has been related to the male of our species. In Canada, females are generally regarded as weaker than their male counterparts, and as a result women are generally perceived as being more prone to illness, primarily because of functional blood loss and anatomical differences. Certain age groups have also been related to individual strength and weakness. Infants and unborn fetuses are considered the weakest of all and are perceived to be at the mercy of the mother's behavior, including prenatal behavior. During pregnancy, harmony and moderation are the keys to a healthy baby; thus the pregnancy period carries the greatest taboos among most cultural groups. For example, some Mexican Americans, Amish, and Hutterites and Whites and African-Americans subscribe to the doctrine of maternal moderation in pregnancy (Bauer, 1969). It is even believed that the mother's emotional state during pregnancy may affect the baby, particularly in the case of pity, fear, mockery, or hate. For example, some southern African-Americans believe that feelings of hate for a particular individual may cause the baby to resemble that person or that a child could be subject to seizures if the mother saw someone having a seizure and felt pity. Some African-Americans, persons from the southern United States, and Mexican Americans also believe that when a pregnant woman makes fun of someone with a physical affliction, the baby may be born with the same affliction, thus punishing the mother for lack of charity (Snow, 1981).

Because some cultural groups believe in a direct connection between the body and the forces of nature, it is important for the nurse to recognize the relevance of natural phenomena such as phases of the moon, positions of the planets, and seasons of the year.

In the rural South in the United States, there is a dependence on natural signs to regulate behavior. Some of these people rely on the *Old Farmer's Almanac* to guide such events as planting crops, setting hens' eggs, destroying weeds, weaning babies, and fishing. The *Almanac* is consulted for many health needs, such as the best time to extract teeth or to have teeth filled. (According to the *Almanac,* the best time to have teeth extracted is during the moon's increase, and the best time to have teeth filled is during the moon's decrease.) The *Almanac* may also be used to determine the optimal time to undergo surgical procedures. The nurse must remember that the *Almanac* is used not only by rural southern people but also in northern urban areas, where many African-American pharmacists give copies of the *Almanac* as gifts to their customers for the New Year. Interestingly, the first *Old Farmer's Almanac* is reported to have been written by a physician in 1897.

It is also important for the nurse to remember that many people from diverse cultural groups use the zodiacal signs to manipulate health regimens but do not mention this practice to health professionals for fear of being ridiculed. Use of zodiacal signs illustrates how external forces are brought to bear on the individual; these signs are the basis for a lively practice of self-medication, dietary regulation, and behavior modifications. The nurse should remember that some of these practices are harmful, some are neutral, and some are beneficial. For example, it would be extremely detrimental for a client in need of a life-saving surgical procedure to wait for a full moon to have the procedure done. It is important for the nurse to devise training programs that will teach clients to manipulate behaviors and interpret zodiacal signs in a way that will maintain health and prevent illness and disease.

The nurse should also appreciate that dreams may have a role in health. Many Haitians believe that dreams are important events that allow the individual to communicate with inhabitants of the supernatural world. When dead relatives appear in a dream, they bring messages from the other world, which the Haitian individual is likely to see as reliable (Holcomb, Parsons, Giger, & Davidhizar, 1996; Randall-David, 1989).

In a study of the folk medicine system, it may become obvious that this system reflects a view of the world as a dangerous place, where the individual must be constantly on guard against nature, other persons, and possible punishment from God. This worldview teaches the individual that it is best to look out for oneself and that mistrust is wiser than trust. For example, Hispanics or Latinos may believe that illness has its roots in physical imbalances or supernatural forces that include God's will, magical powers, evil spirits, powerful human forces, or emotional upsets. For some Hispanics or Latinos, treatment comes primarily through a variety of healers that include the *curandero* (healer who uses prayer and artifacts), *yerbero* (herbalist), *espiritista* (practitioner of *espiritismo,* a religious cult concerned with communication with spirits and the purification of the soul through moral behavior), and *santero* (practitioner of *Santería,* a religious cult concerned with teaching people how to control or placate the supernatural) (Randall-David, 1989; Richardson, 1982; Ruiz, 1985; Wanderer & Rivera, 1986; Weclew, 1975). It may be necessary to involve spiritual healers and priests in crisis intervention therapy to treat the client.

The presence of an alternative medical (folk medicine) system that is different from and possibly in direct conflict with the Western medical system can complicate matters. Not only is it a matter of offering health care in the place of no health care or offering superior health care in lieu of inferior health care, but also the nurse must remember that persons from diverse cultural backgrounds have deeply ingrained beliefs about how to attain and maintain health. These beliefs, which may be linked to the natural and supernatural worlds, may adversely affect the physician–client and nurse–client relationships and thus influence the individual's decision to follow or not follow prescribed treatment regimens. For example, in certain cultures, the occurrence of cancer may be attributed to insufficient use of herbal medicine, an insult to an ancestor, or a perceived punishment. Thus, standard Western medical approaches may not always appear relevant to certain clients in multicultural populations (Boston, 1993).

The nurse might correctly assume that when a low-income African-American, southern White American, Puerto Rican, or Mexican American arrives for professional care, every home remedy known to the client has already been tried. It is important for the nurse to determine what the client has been doing to combat the illness. If the home remedy is harmless, it is best left in the treatment plan with the nurse's own suggestions added. However, harmful practices must be eliminated. One of the best ways for the nurse to eliminate harmful practices is to inquire whether the practice has worked. If the client assumes that it has not worked, the nurse can simply suggest that something else be tried. If the client perceives that a harmful practice is beneficial, the nurse must provide education that will illuminate the dangers of this harmful practice.

Nurses have begun to explore the relationship of person and environment in nursing research. A classic exploratory study by Pyles (1989) related Etzioni's compliance theory to satisfaction by nursing employees in a school of nursing. Data from the study indicated that a normative power structure in the school and the resultant moral involvement profile in the faculty were compatible for an organization such as a university, which displays cultural goals. In another classic study, Gould (1989) examined 112 elderly residents in three metropolitan nursing homes. The data indicated that life satisfaction is an indicator of well-being, which is useful as a measure of quality of care because of its linkage to health. The data also indicated that bonding develops between institutionalized elderly persons and their caregivers, which precludes the drive for self-determination. Thus, the data explained why lower income elderly persons demonstrated high levels of life satisfaction despite low levels of perceived influence over the institutional environment.

CASE STUDY

Martha Brown is a 27-year-old woman who lives in the hills of northern Kentucky in a small cabin that has no indoor plumbing. She lives with her husband and six small children. The public health nurse makes a home visit after three of the children have been diagnosed by the school nurse as having lice. While the nurse is explaining the use of Rid (lice treatment) to the mother, she notes that Mrs. Brown has a persistent cough that she states she has had for 2 years. The nurse notes that the cough is productive, that Mrs. Brown looks emaciated, and that her color is extremely ashen. She tires easily. Although health insurance is a benefit of her husband's job in a nearby mine, Mrs. Brown's children were born at home, and she has never had a complete physical. When asked why she has not gone to a nearby free health clinic, Mrs. Brown replies, "Sickness is God's will, and he will cure me if he wants to. Anyway, my family comes first, and I don't have the time. Besides, doctors can't be trusted. My Aunt Jane went to one once, and she died the next week."

CLINICAL DECISION MAKING

1. Based on the fact that Mrs. Brown is Appalachian and taking into consideration the fact that every individual is unique, decide whether Mrs. Brown is more likely to be "being" oriented or "doing" oriented in regard to activity orientation.

2. Decide what the relational orientation is for Mrs. Brown, based on her reply to the public health nurse about why she has not sought treatment.
3. Based on Mrs. Brown's reply to the public health nurse and the fact that she is Hispanic, what people-to-nature orientation is she likely to have?
4. Decide, on the basis of Mrs. Brown's comment and the fact that she is Hispanic, what view of human nature she is likely to hold.
5. List at least three reasons why Mrs. Brown might be apprehensive about seeking medical help.

REVIEW QUESTIONS

1. A nurse is teaching an Appalachian patient who says, "Whatever will be, will be." The nurse understands that which of the following is most accurate about this scenario?
   a. External feelings of control are related to compliance.
   b. Internal feelings of control are related to compliance.
   c. A fatalistic point of view is related to taking preventative health care actions.
   d. Feelings of internal control are not necessary for compliance.
2. When caring for the patient who believes there is a relationship between outcomes and internal feelings of control, the patient can be expected to do which of the following?
   a. Follow directions given for health care.
   b. View the future as a result of luck, chance, or fate.
   c. Believe compliance behaviors and health are unrelated.
   d. Adhere to beliefs of external control.
3. The nurse who is caring for a patient with an external locus of control can anticipate which of the following?
   a. The patient will be more likely to be fatalistic about nature and illness.
   b. The patient is more likely to feel in control of events that affect him or her.
   c. The patient will expect to be able to modify behaviors to reach health goals.
   d. The patient will desire help to control health and illness outcomes.

REFERENCES

Abarts, L. (1995). University of Calgary hosts complementary medicine society. *Holistic and Complementary Medical Society of Alberta Newsletter, 1*(1), 1.

Ballard, C. G., O'Brien, J. T., Reichelt, K., & Perry, E. K. (2002). Aromatherapy as a safe and effective treatment for the management of agitation in severe dementia: the results of a double-blind, placebo-controlled trial with Melissa. *Journal of Clinical Psychiatry, 63,* 553–558.

Barnum, B. S. (1994). *Nursing theory* (4th ed.). Philadelphia: J. B. Lippincott Co.

Bauer, W. W. (1969). *Potions, remedies, and old wives' tales.* Garden City, NY: Doubleday.

Bauwens, E., & Anderson, S. (1992). Social and cultural influences on health care. In M. Stanhope & J. Lancaster (Eds.), *Community health nursing: process and practice for promoting health* (3rd ed., pp. 89–108). St. Louis: Mosby–Year Book.

Blackhall, L. J., Murphy, S. T., Frank, G., Michel, V., & Azen, S. (1995). Ethnicity and attitudes towards patient autonomy. *Journal of the American Medical Association, 274,* 820–825.

Boston, P. (1993). Culture and cancer: the relevance of cultural orientation within cancer education programmes. *European Journal of Cancer Care, 2,* 72–76.

Brewer, J. A., & Bonalumi, N. M. (1995). Cultural diversity in the emergency department. *The Journal of Emergency Nursing, 2*(6), 494–497.

Brunswick, A. F., & Josephson, E. (1972). Adolescent health in Harlem. *American Journal of Public Health, 72*(Suppl.), 7–47.

Campinha-Bacote, J. (1997). Understanding the influence of culture. In J. Haber, B. Krainovich-Miller, A. McMahon, & P. Price-Hoskins (Eds.), *Comprehensive psychiatric nursing* (5th ed.). St. Louis: Mosby.

Chachkes, E., & Jennings, R. (1994). Latino communities: coping with death. In B. Dane & C. Levine (Eds.), *AIDS and the new orphans: coping with death* (pp. 77–100). Westport, CT: Greenwood Press.

Chrisman, N. J. (1977). The health seeking process. *Culture and Medicine in Psychiatry, 1,* 351–377.

Clements, P. T., et al. (2003). Cultural perspectives of death, grief, and bereavement. *Journal of Psychosocial Nursing, 41*(7), 18–26.

Cronsberry, T. (1996). Alternative cancer therapies. *The Canadian Nurse, 92*(4), 35–38.

DeSpelder, L., & Strickland, A. (2005). *The last dance: encountering death and dying* (7th ed.). Boston: McGraw-Hill.

Dossey, L. (1993). *Healing words.* San Francisco: Harper.

Dunn, F. L. (1998). Transcultural Asian medicine and cosmopolitan medicine as adaptive systems. In E. Leslie (Ed.), *Asian medical systems: a comparative study* (p. 135). Delhi: Motilal Banarsidass Publishers.

Egeland, J. (1967). *Belief and behavior as related to illness: a community case study of the old order Amish* (Doctoral dissertation, Yale University). Ann Arbor, MI: University Microfilms International: Dissertation Abstracts International, X.

Eisenberg, D., Kessler, R., Foster, C., Norlock, E. F., Calkins, D. R., & Delbanco, T. L. (1993). Unconventional medicine in the United States: prevalence, costs, and patterns of use. *New England Journal of Medicine, 328*(4), 246–252.

Elling, R. H. (1977). *Socio-cultural influences on health and health care*. New York: Springer Publishing.

Fabrega, H. (1971). Medical anthropology. In B. J. Siegel (Ed.), *Biennial review of anthropology*. Stanford, CA: Stanford University Press.

French, M. (1996). The power of plants. *Advances for Nurse Practitioners*, 16–18.

Giger, J. N., Davidhizar, E., & Fordham, P. (2006). Multicultural and multi-ethnic considerations and advanced directives: developing cultural competency. *Journal of Cultural Diversity*, 13(1), 3–9.

Giger, J., Davidhizar, R., Johnson, J., & Poole, V. (1997). The changing face of America. *Health Traveler*, 4(4), 11–17.

Giger, J., Davidhizar, R., & Turner, G. (1992). Black American folk medicine health care beliefs: implication for nursing plans of care. *The ABNF Journal*, 2(3), 42–46.

Gould, M. (1989). *The relationship of perceived social-environmental factors and functional health status to life satisfaction in the elderly*. Paper presented at Sigma Theta Tau International Conference, Indianapolis, IN.

Greene, L. (1981). *Social and biological predictors of nutritional status, physical growth, and neurological development*. New York: Academic Press.

Gregory, D. (1992). Nursing practice in native communities. In A. Baumgart & J. Larson (Eds.), *Canadian nursing faces the future* (2nd ed.). St. Louis: Mosby–Year Book.

Grypma, S. (1993). Culture shock. *The Canadian Nurse*, 89(8), 33–37.

Guruge, S., & Donner, G. (1996). Transcultural nursing in Canada. *The Canadian Nurse*, 92(8), 36–40.

Haber, J., Giuffra, M., Haber, J., Hoskins, P., Leach, A., & Sideleau, B. (1997). Sociocultural issues. In *Comprehensive psychiatric nursing* (5th ed.). St. Louis: Mosby.

Henderson, G., & Primeaux, M. (1981). *Transcultural health care*. Reading, MA: Addison-Wesley.

Hislop, T. G., Deschamps, M., Band, P. R., Smith, J. M., & Clarke, H. F. (1992). Participation in the British Columbia Cervical Cytology Screening Programme by Native Indian women. *Canadian Journal of Public Health*, 83(5), 344–345.

Holcomb, L. O., Parsons, L. C., Giger, J. N., & Davidhizar, R. (1996). Haitian Americans: implications for nursing care. *Journal of Community Health Nursing*, 13(4), 249–260.

Hostetler, J. (1980). *Amish society* (3rd ed.). Baltimore: Johns Hopkins University Press.

Institute for Safe Medication Practices. (2007). *A white paper on medication safety in the U.S. and the role of community pharmacists*. Institute for Safe Medication Practices: Huntingdon Valley. Available at: <http://www.ismp.org/pressroom/viewpoints/CommunityPharmacy.pdf>.

Jain, S., & Mills, P. J. (2010). Biofield therapies: helpful or full of hype? A best evidence synthesis. *International Journal of Behavioral Medicine*, 17, 1–16.

Kagawa-Singer, M. (1996). Cultural systems related to cancer. In R. McCorkle, M. Grant, M. Grant-Strong, & S. B. Brains (Eds.), *Cancer nursing* (2nd ed., pp. 38–52). Philadelphia: Saunders.

Kagawa-Singer, M. (1998). The cultural context of death rituals and mourning practices. *Oncology Nursing Forum*, 25(10), 1725–1756.

Kay, M. (1979). Clinical anthropology. In E. E. Bauwens (Ed.), *The anthropology of health* (pp. 3–11). St. Louis: Mosby.

Kleinman, A., Eisenberg, L., & Good, B. (1978). Culture, illness and care. *Annals of Internal Medicine*, 88, 251–258.

Kluckhohn, K., & Strodtbeck, F. (1973). *Variations in value orientations*. Westport, CT: Greenwood Press.

Lew, L. (1989). Southeast Asian Health Project: application for mother, children and infants demonstration grant (Unpublished grant proposal). Ottawa, Ontario.

Mattson, S. (1995). Culturally sensitive perinatal care for southeast Asians. *Journal of Obstetric and Gynecological Neonatal Nursing*, 24(4), 335–341.

McGrattan, M. (2004). *The social construction of disease: why homosexuality isn't like cancer*. Available at: <http://www.interdisciplinary.net/ptb/mso/hid/hid3/McGrattan%20paper>. Retrieved July 24, 2011.

McRae, L. (1994). Cultural sensitivity in rehabilitation related to native clients. *Canadian Journal of Rehabilitation*, 7(4), 251–256.

Morgenstern, J. (1966). *Rites of birth, marriage, death, and kindred occasions among the Semites*. Chicago: Quadrangle.

Morley, P., & Wallis, R. (1978). *Culture and caring*. London: Peter Owen.

Peterson, B. (1996). The mind-body connection. *The Canadian Nurse*, 92(1), 29–31.

Peterson, C., & Stunkard, A. (1992). Cognates of personal control: locus of control, self-efficacy, and explanatory style. *Applied & Preventive Psychology*, 1, 111–117.

Phares, E. (1978). Locus of control. In H. London & J. Exner (Eds.), *Dimensions of personality* (pp. 263–304). New York: Wiley.

Pillsbury, B. (1982). Doing the month: confinement and convalescence of Chinese women after childbirth. In M. Kay (Ed.), *Anthropology of human birth*. Philadelphia: F. A. Davis.

Pyles, C. (1989). *Power compatibility profile in a school of nursing*. Paper presented at the Sigma Theta Tau International Conference, Indianapolis, IN.

Randall-David, E. (1989). *Strategies for working with culturally diverse communities and clients* [Brochure]. Washington, DC: U.S. Department of Health and Human Services.

Richardson, L. (1982). Caring through understanding: part 2. Folk medicine in the Hispanic population. *Imprint*, 29(2), 21.

Rittenbaugh, C. (1992). Human foodways: a window on evolution. In E. E. Bauwens (Ed.), *The anthropology of health* (3rd ed.). St. Louis: Mosby–Year Book.

Rotter, J. B. (1966). Generalized expectancies for internal versus external control of reinforcement. *Psychological Monographs*, 80(1), 1–28.

Rotter, J. B. (1975). Some problems and misconceptions related to the construct of internal versus external control of reinforcement. *Journal of Consulting and Clinical Psychology*, 43, 56–67.

Rotter, J. B. (1992). Some comments on the "Cognates of personal control." *Applied & Preventive Psychology, 1,* 127–129.

Ruiz, P. (1985). Cultural barriers to effective medical care among Hispanic-American patients. *Annual Review of Medicine, 36,* 63–71.

Rumsfeld, J. S. (2002). Health status and clinical practice. *Circulation, 106,* 5–7.

Sideleau, B. (1997). Space and time. In J. Haber, A. McMahon, P. Price-Hoskins, & B. Sideleau (Eds.), *Comprehensive psychiatric nursing* (5th ed.). St. Louis: Mosby.

Siegleman, M. (1992). Power and powerlessness: comments on "Cognates of personal control." *Applied & Personal Psychology, 1,* 119–120.

Snow, L. F. (1981). Folk medical beliefs and their implications for the care of patients: a review based on studies among Black Americans. In G. Henderson & M. Primeaux (Eds.), *Transcultural health care.* Reading, MA: Addison-Wesley.

Spector, R. (2004). *Cultural diversity in health and illness* (6th ed.). Upper Saddle River, NJ: Pearson Prentice Hall.

Thompson, K. (1993). Self-governed health. *The Canadian Nurse, 89*(8), 29–32.

Tindle, H. A., Davis, R. B., Phillips, R. S., & Eisenberg, D. M. (2005). Trends in use of complementary and alternative medicine by US adults: 1997–2002. *Alternative Therapies in Health and Medicine, 11*(1), 42–49.

Threlfall, W. J. (1986). Cancer patterns in British Columbia Native Indians. *Medical Journal, 28,* 508–510.

University of Calgary Complementary Medicine Seminar (1995). Calgary, Alberta, Canada: University of Calgary.

Wanderer, J., & Rivera, G. (1986). Black magic beliefs and white magic practice: the common structures of intimacy, tradition and power. *Social Science Journal, 23*(4), 419.

Weaver, T. (1970). Use of hypothetical situations in a study of Spanish-American illness referral systems. *Human Organisms, 29,* 141.

Weclew, R. V. (1975). The nature, prevalence, and level of awareness of curanderismo and some of its implications for community mental health. *Community Mental Health Journal, 11*(2), 145–154.

Wenger, A. (1988). The phenomenon of care in a high context culture: the old order Amish (Unpublished doctoral dissertation). Detroit, MI: Wayne State University.

Wenger, A. (1995). Cultural context, health, and health care decision making. *Journal of Transcultural Nursing, 7*(1), 3–14.

Wenger, A. (2006). The culture care theory and the older order Amish. In M. Leininger (Ed.), *Cultural care diversity and universality: a theory of nursing* (2nd ed.). Sudbury, MA: Jones and Bartlett.

Williams, C. D., Baumslag, N., & Jelliffe, D. B. (1994). *Mother and child health: Delivering the services.* New York: Oxford University Press.

Woods, D. L., Beck, C., & Sinha, K. (2009). The effect of therapeutic touch on behavioral symptoms and cortisol in persons with dementia. *Forschende Komplementärmedizin/ Research in Complementary Medicine, 16,* 181–189.

Woods, D. L., Craven, R. F., & Whitney, J. (2005). The effect of therapeutic touch on behavioral symptoms of persons with dementia. *Alternative Therapies of Health and Medicine, 11,* 66–74.

Woods, D. L., & Dimond, M. (2002). The effect of therapeutic touch on agitated behavior and cortisol in persons with Alzheimer's disease. *Biologic Research for Nursing, 4,* 104–114.

Woods, D. L., Rapp, C. G., & Beck, C. (2004). Escalation/ deescalation patterns of behavioral symptoms of persons with dementia. *Aging and Mental Health, 8,* 126–132.

Younoszai, B. (1993). Mexican American perspectives related to death. In D. P. Irish, K. F. Lundquist, & V. J. Nelson (Eds.), *Ethic variations in dying, death, and grief.* Washington, DC: Taylor & Francis.

Biological Variations

BEHAVIORAL OBJECTIVES

After reading this chapter, the nurse will be able to:

1. Articulate biological differences among individuals in various racial groups.
2. Relate the importance of knowledge of biological differences that may exist among individuals in various racial groups to the provision of health care by the nurse.
3. Describe nursing implications that may arise when providing care for individuals in different cultural and racial groups.
4. Describe nutritional preferences and deficiencies that may exist among persons in different cultural groups.
5. Explain how psychological characteristics may vary from one culture to another.
6. Explain how susceptibility to disease may differ among individuals in different racial groups.

It is a well-known fact that people differ culturally. Cultural differences are evident in communication, spatial relationships and needs, social organizations (family, kinships, and tribes), time orientation, and ability or desire to control the environment. Less recognized and understood are the biological differences among people in various racial groups. It is becoming more evident to nurses that a body of scientific knowledge does exist about biological cultural differences. References to and information about biocultural differences are mushrooming in the literature and have resulted in a field of study known as *biocultural ecology* (Bandara, 2009), which focuses on human adaptation and homeostasis. The purpose of biocultural ecology is to transcend the fragmentation inherent in the separation of culture, human biology, and ecology and the environment. Biocultural ecology is an examination of diverse human populations by means of this three-way interaction system and focuses on specific, localized individuals and populations within a given environment. Data relative to all the variables significant to people within a racial group are essential for complete understanding of the people. Not only are no two persons alike, but also no two cultural or racial groups are alike, and all phenomena relative to both individuals and cultural or racial groups must be understood.

Although the significance of biocultural ecology concepts has been studied in other disciplines, such as sociology and medical anthropology, the nursing literature has only recently documented the importance of this field for nurses. A focus on transcultural issues that began in the mid-1960s with the impetus of nurses such as Madeleine Leininger (2007) has helped nurses to develop cultural insights and a deeper appreciation for human life and values from a cultural perspective. However, despite the introduction of transcultural nursing concepts, the nursing literature remains scanty on biological variations among people in various racial groups. The strongest argument for including concepts on biological variations in nursing education and subsequently nursing practice is that scientific facts about biological variations can aid the nurse in giving culturally appropriate health care. Nurses who care for people transculturally need to be cognizant of certain basic biological differences to give nonharmful and competent care.

Most nurses in the United States have been educated in a system of nursing practice based on biological baselines of the dominant White race. Because studies on biological baseline data in growth and development, nutrition, and other biological phenomena have been conducted with White subjects, standardized norms available to the nurse do not reflect biological variations among different racial groups. That people in various racial groups differ tremendously is evidenced externally and is related to biogenetic variations that have occurred internally. Therefore, values uniracially normed are inappropriate when applied across racial groups. In the United States, White-standardized values for factors related to growth and development, nutrition, and susceptibility to disease are often applied to African-Americans, Asians, and American Indians. Therefore, significant deviations from the norm that may be labeled "nonnormal" might be more appropriately labeled "non-White" (Overfield, 1995). In fact, biological variations among racial groups are so diverse that multiple dimensions are encompassed.

DIFFERENTIATION AMONG HEALTH DISPARITIES, HEALTH CARE DISPARITIES, HEALTH INEQUALITIES, AND HEALTH INEQUITIES

To understand the significance of biological variations, it is essential to understand other key terms, such as *health disparities, health care disparities, health inequities,* and *health inequalities.* These terms have augmented significance when health care professionals attempt to render culturally competent care to diverse, multicultural groups of people.

Health Disparity

A *health disparity* can be defined from a sociological, population-specific, or biopsychosocial perspective.

For example, from a sociological perspective, health disparity can be viewed as a chain of events signified by differences in (1) environment; (2) access to, utilization of, and quality of care; (3) health status; and (4) health outcome.

On the other hand, in its broadest sense, a *health disparity* can be defined as a "population-specific difference in not only disease, but health outcomes, or access to health care" (U.S. Department of Health and Human Services, 2011). In fact, the first National Institutes of Health (NIH) Working Group on Health Disparities succinctly narrowed the definition somewhat by defining health disparities as "differences in the incidence, prevalence, mortality, and burden of disease and other adverse health conditions that exist among specific population groups in the US" (Committee on Review and Assessment, 2006; NIH, 2003). It is essential to remember that because the impact of health care on health disparities is an important factor, a definition of racial and ethnic health care disparities was provided by the Institute of Medicine's Committee on Understanding and Eliminating Racial and Ethnic

Disparities in Health Care (Smedley, Stith, & Nelson, 2003). The committee unequivocally noted that a health disparity "more likely than not is a racial and ethnic difference in the quality of health care usually arising as a result of access-related factors or clinical needs, preferences and appropriateness of the intervention" (Smedley et al., 2003). In fact, the committee unequivocally noted that disparities in health care for the most part are consistent regardless of the nature of the illness or the time of services rendered (Smedley et al., 2003).

It is interesting to note that neither the sociological nor population-specific definitions allow for the inclusion of biological variations that may occur in groups of people regardless of race, ethnicity, socioeconomic status, and access to care issues. With this thought in mind, another approach to health disparity from a biopsychosocial perspective is offered that works in tandem with the concept of biological variations. From a *biopsychosocial* perspective, genes and biology, environment, and behavior all come together in a cataclysmic way to create a health disparity (Giger, 2011; Giger & Davidhizar). It is essential to note that socioeconomic status plays a major contributing factor in unequal treatment, particularly where ethnic minorities are concerned. Although this definition does take into account the issue of vulnerability or race and ethnicity, socioeconomic status, geographical location, and access to care issues (Appel, Giger, & Davidhizar, 2005), Braithwaite and Taylor (2001) noted that even if income levels were standardized and all impediments regarding access to care were eliminated, disparities in health outcomes might still exist. They contend that this argument gives credence to the need to eliminate cultural incompetence among health care providers. The biopsychosocial perspective does not negate the fact that certain groups, including specific racial and ethnic groups, persons residing in certain geographic locations, the poor and underserved, and the disabled, are more likely to suffer disproportionately from health disparities (Atrash & Hunter, 2001). It is also interesting to note that the term *disparity* is almost exclusively used in the United States, whereas the terms *health inequality* or *inequity* are more commonly used outside of the United States.

Health Care Inequality

Inequality, particularly when referring to health care, is a term used to refer to differences in age, rank, condition, lack of excellence in treatment, or dissimilitude (vast differences) in services available. *Inequity* is similarly defined as a condition of "being unequal" or "lack of opportunity, treatment or status." Yet another view of the term *health disparity* is that in the context of public health and the social sciences, the term has begun to take on a meaning of injustice (Atrash & Hunter, 2001). In fact, Atrash and

Hunter (2001) contend that in the United States, there is growing concern that even when there are equivalent levels of access to care, most racial and ethnic minorities continue to experience a lower quality of health services and are therefore less likely to receive needed routine medical procedures than their White counterparts. For example, African-Americans are less likely to receive peritoneal dialysis and kidney transplants for end-stage renal disease than their White counterparts (Barker-Cummings, McClellen, Soucie, & Krisher, 1995; Kasiske, 1998; National Healthcare Disparities Report, 2014). Similarly, some data suggest that African-American and Hispanic clients with long-bone fractures who are seen in the emergency department are far less likely than their White counterparts to receive necessary analgesics to suppress the pain (Todd, Deaton, D'Adamo, & Goe, 2000). Yet another example of health care disparities includes studies suggesting that African-American Medicare patients with congestive heart failure or pneumonia, for example, are more likely to receive a poorer quality of care than are their White counterparts (Vaccarino, et al., 2002; Wheeler, 2004).

DIMENSIONS OF BIOLOGICAL VARIATIONS

A direct relationship exists between race and body structure, skin color, other visible physical characteristics, enzymatic and genetic variations, electrocardiographic patterns, susceptibility to disease, nutritional preferences and deficiencies, and psychological characteristics. Differences among people in various racial groups in each of these areas are discussed in the following sections.

Body Structure

One category of difference between racial groups is body structure, which includes both body size and body shape. Newborn body proportions differ among racial groups. Although research on this topic remains scanty, it has been postulated that newborn body proportions appear to be genetically programmed to conform to the pelvic shape of the mother (Nold & Georgieff, 2004; Overfield, 1995).

Body structure as well as bone density also differs among adults. For example, the prevalence of osteoporosis and the incidence of vertebral fractures are both reported to be substantially lower in African-American women than in White American women (Aloia, 2008; Melton & Riggs, 2000; Wagner & Heyward, 2000). This finding is generally attributed to racial differences in adult bone mass (Aloia, 2008).

Among adults, bone density is greater in African-Americans than in White Americans of either sex (Shaffer et al., 2007). However, differences in adult bone density are not necessarily confined to these two racial groups. In fact, the bone density of adult Polynesians is reported to be greater than that of age-matched Whites (Shaffer et al., 2007). In contrast, Asian Americans generally have lower values for bone density than other racial groups (Shaffer et al., 2007). Biological markers that account for the variations in adult bone mass among racial groups are unknown. In addition, the time of life at which these differences are manifested is uncertain. According to Wagner and Heyward (2000), prepubertal African-American children tend to have higher values for bone density than do their White counterparts. Some researchers (Selemenda, Peacock, Hui, Zhou, & Johnston, 1997) have speculated that such findings indicate that racial differences in skeletal mass develop early in childhood and persist throughout life.

In regard to body structure and size, the face is perhaps one of the most fascinating areas of the body because it has many parts that combine to make the whole. The face tends to be the one prominent area that can visibly categorize people by race. For example, eyelids vary from racial group to racial group. In some racial groups the eyelids droop over the cartilage plate above the eye, and in other racial groups the eyelids do not droop. The epicanthic fold, another variation of the eyelids, is found predominantly in persons with Asian characteristics but may be present in other racial groups.

Ears are another fascinating part of the face because they have a variety of shapes. Earlobes can be free and floppy or attached close to the face as if the intent were to make sure the lobe stayed in place. Earlobes that are free and floppy are very handy for attaching earrings. When earlobes are attached, they are the least defined, and wearing objects such as earrings may be difficult.

Noses come in all sizes and shapes; however, nose size and shape correlate directly with one's racial ancestry. It has been postulated that small noses were an evolutionary result of living in cold climates, such as the classic Asian nose, and that noses with high bridges were a result of living in climates that were dry, such as the classic Iranian and American Indian noses. People who lived in moist, hot climates developed broad, flat noses, such as those found on Africans and African-Americans (Overfield, 1995).

Teeth offer another important variation in body size and shape. Tooth size, which is important because the teeth help shape the size of the lower face, varies among racial groups. For example, Australian aborigines have the largest teeth in the world, as well as four extra molars. Asian Americans and African-Americans have very large teeth, whereas White Americans have very small teeth. People with very large teeth tend to have their jaws projecting beyond the upper part of the face. This projection tends to be a normal variation and not an orthodontic problem. There is also a tendency among some racial groups for fewer teeth. For example, some racial groups do not have a third molar or maxillary lateral incisors. Peg teeth are sometimes a step in the evolutionary process that facilitates the presence or absence of a particular type of tooth (Johe, Steinhart, Sado, Greenberg, & Jing, 2010; Overfield, 1995).

As teeth vary among racial groups, so do tongues. The most common variances are scrotal tongues, which occur in 5% of the population in some racial groups; geographic tongues, which occur in 3% of the population in some racial groups; and fissured tongues, which occur in 5% to 40% of the population in some racial groups (Witkop & Barros, 1963).

The mandibular or palatine torus is also of concern to the nurse when inspecting the mouth. The torus is a bony protuberance, and the palatine torus occurs on the midline of the palate, whereas the mandibular torus occurs as a lump on the inner side of the mandible near the second molar. Tori are fairly common, with palatine tori occurring in up to 25% of the population in most racial groups studied. Mandibular tori occur in 7% of Whites, 2% of African-Americans, and 40% of Asians (White & Pharoah, 2009).

Another variation in body size and structure is attributable to muscle size and mass. In certain racial groups, specific muscles are absent altogether. The peroneus tertius muscle, which is found in the foot, and the palmaris longus muscle, which is found in the wrist, are absent in individuals in some racial groups. However, muscle absence in general does not appear to be more prevalent in any particular racial group, nor does absence of a particular muscle correspond with absence of another muscle.

Numerous studies have investigated inheritability of stature (Overfield, 1995; Silventoinen, 2003). In general, the studies conclude that people vary in height as a result of race and that in the United States, African-Americans and White Americans are the tallest, American Indians are either similar in height or a few inches shorter than Mexican Americans, and Asian Americans are the shortest. Individuals of higher socioeconomic status in all ethnic groups are taller (Overfield, 1995; Silventoinen, 2003). In regard to physical growth and developmental rates, African-Americans are generally advanced, whereas Asians are generally lower when these groups are compared with White norms.

Body Weight

Weight differs in individuals both by race and by gender. African-Americans and Whites are less similar in weight than they are in height. This is believed to occur because African-Americans have heavier bone and muscle mass than Whites (Khan, 2001; Wagner & Heyward, 2000). On the average, African-American men weigh less than their White counterparts (166.1 lb compared to 170.6 lb, respectively) (Greenberg, Dintiman, & Oakes, 2004). In stark contrast, African-American women are consistently heavier at every age group than their White American counterparts (149.6 lb compared to 137.0 lb, respectively). In addition, African-American women average about 20 lb heavier than their White American counterparts from 35 to 65 years of age (Greaves, Puhl, Baranowski, Gruben, & Seale, 1989). Similarly, Mexican American Whites, on the average, weigh more than non-Hispanic Whites as a result of truncal fat (Greaves et al., 1989). On average, obesity is more pronounced in the lower class, less pronounced in the middle class compared with their lower-class counterparts, and even less pronounced in the upper class compared with their middle-class counterparts (Winkleby, Robinson, Sundquist, & Kraemer, 1999).

If the health care statistics in *Healthy People 2010* and *2020* are dismal for African-American, Hispanic, and American Indian women and men, they are even worse for their children (U.S. Department of Health and Human Services, 2000). If being overweight is a common problem in the general U.S. population, it is said to be at epidemic proportions for children in this country (Strauss & Pollack, 2001). Data from the Department of Health and Human Services, Youth Risk Behavioral Surveillance 2013 survey (2014) indicated that the prevalence of overweight among children was higher among non-Hispanic Black (15.1%) and Hispanic children (15.1%) than non-Hispanic White children (10.3%) and higher among non-Hispanic Black female (11.1%) and Hispanic female (11.2%) than White female (6.2%) students (U.S. Department of Health and Human Services, Youth Risk Behavioral Surveillance [YRBS] 2013 survey, 2014; Ogden et al., 2006). In a comparison of obesity rates in male students, the highest rate was in Hispanic (21.3%) and non-Hispanic Blacks (18.2%) than in Whites (14.0%). Nonetheless, childhood obesity continues to increase steadily and rapidly among African-American children (Strauss & Pollack, 2001). Some researchers conclude that childhood obesity often serves as a primary marker for high-risk dietary and physical inactivity practices (Crawford, Story, Wang, Ritchie, & Sabry, 2001). Childhood obesity can also contribute to the development of metabolic syndrome (syndrome X), also referred to as *insulin resistance.*

The Development of Metabolic Syndrome (Syndrome X) from Childhood to Adolescence.* The metabolic syndrome (syndrome X) is a clustering of abnormalities characterized by the primary defect of compensatory insulin

---

*Portions of the section on childhood adiposity and metabolic syndrome (syndrome X) are excerpted with permission from a prior publication by Giger, J., Richardson, J., & Jones, D. (2002, July), African-American children: a precious commodity at risk. *Journal of the National Black Nurses Association* (editorial), *13*(1), vii–viii.

resistance, glucose intolerance, dyslipidemia, and centrally distributed obesity (Matthews et al., 1985; Ravean, 2011). Chen et al. (2000) conducted a study to examine the age-related patterns of cardiovascular risk factor clusters relative to metabolic syndrome (syndrome X) among African-American and White children. The clusters in this study for metabolic syndrome (syndrome X) included (1) insulin resistance index, (2) body mass index (BMI), (3) triglycerides/HDL cholesterol ratio, and (4) mean arterial pressure. Regardless of age, four mediating factors contribute to the development of coronary heart disease: hyperinsulinemia (metabolic syndrome [syndrome X]), hypercholesterolemia, hypertension, and obesity. A sedentary lifestyle, the large amount of fat consumed per day by some children (such as African-Americans), and the prevalence of obesity may all contribute to the development of metabolic syndrome (syndrome X). In other words, African-American, Hispanic, or American Indian children are not exempt because of their tender years from developing metabolic syndrome (syndrome X) and starting the downward spiral toward diabetes and ultimately coronary heart disease.

It is interesting to note that findings from the study of Chen et al. (2000)—follow-up findings to the Bogalusa Heart Study—suggest that overall, White children had a higher total of adverse clusters among the four indices measured (9.8; $P < 0.01$) than their African-American counterparts (7.4; $P < 0.01$). Previous and recent analyses of these data sets suggest that while predictability of childhood adiposity and insulin resistance syndrome is difficult to determine with certainty in children, the contributions of these adverse clusters can provide convincing evidence for the future development of metabolic syndrome (syndrome X), thereby leading to the development of coronary heart disease in adulthood (Srinivasan, Myers, & Berenson, 2002). As African-Americans age, the adverse clusters outrank those of their White counterparts, and this ultimately leads to the development of metabolic syndrome (syndrome X) and coronary heart disease in adulthood (Giger, Richardson, & Jones, 2002). Srinivasan et al. (2002) examined the contributions of childhood adiposity and insulin as weighted predictors to adulthood risk of developing metabolic syndrome (syndrome X) among African-American and White children with baseline ages of 8 to 17 years. Using a logistic regression model, these researchers noted that childhood BMI and insulin resistance served as significant predictors of adult clustering for metabolic syndrome (syndrome X). In this study, BMI was the strongest indicator, exhibiting a curvilinear relationship. Further findings from this study also suggest that childhood obesity often is a powerful predictor of the development of metabolic syndrome (syndrome X) later in

life. These findings suggest that children, and particularly ethnic minorities such as African-American children, can benefit tremendously from programs that underscore the importance of weight control and increased physical activity (Srinivasan et al., 2002). Nurses must rise to the challenge of helping these vulnerable families reduce the epidemic of childhood obesity among children.

Strategies to reduce childhood obesity appear obvious but often are ignored by parents and even health care practitioners. These strategies include increasing the physical activity of vulnerable children, reducing the amount of television watched each day, and restricting the amount of fat consumed, particularly in nonefficacious foods (Davis, Northington, & Kolar, 2000). In a classic study, Lindquist, Reynolds, and Goran (1999) found obvious sociocultural determinants of physical activity among children. Findings from this study suggest that although there is greater television viewing among children from single-parent homes, there is more vigorous exercise among these same children. This finding seems contradictory in terms of the amount of television watched. However, it is plausible to assume that in single-parent homes children are often responsible for themselves while the parent works. Although these children tend to watch more television, they also tend to engage in more outdoor activities because they do not have to seek permission to do so. Further findings from this study also suggest that there is less habitual physical activity among girls and less mandatory physical exercise among African-American children, particularly from single-parent homes (Lindquist et al., 1999). There appears to be no plausible explanation for why some ethnic minority children such as African-American children engage in less physical exercise as mandated in many school systems. Nurses must rise to the clarion call of assisting parents and their children in developing an understanding about the importance of physical activity, proper dietary intake, and methods to increase the amount of fiber and fruits consumed per day. In addition, it is essential for nurses to underscore to parents the importance of limiting harmful activities, such as extensive television viewing.

Skin Color

When working with people from diverse cultural backgrounds, the nurse should understand how different races evolved in relation to the environment. Biological differences noted in skin color may be attributable to the biological adjustments a person's ancestors made in the environment in which they lived. For example, it has been scientifically postulated that the original skin color of humans was black (Jablonski & Chaplin, 2000; Overfield, 1995) and that white skin was the result of mutation and environmental pressures exerted on persons living in cold, cloudy northern Europe. The mutation is believed to have occurred because light skin was better able to synthesize vitamin D, particularly on cloudy days. It is believed that black skin became a neutral trait in climates where protection from the sun and heat of the tropics was not a factor (Jablonski & Chaplin, 2000; Overfield, 1995).

Skin color is probably the most significant biological variation in terms of nursing care. Nursing care delivery is based on accurate client assessment, and the darker the client's skin, the more difficult it becomes to assess changes in color. When caring for clients with highly pigmented skin, the nurse must first establish the baseline skin color, and daylight is the best light source for doing so. If possible, dark-skinned clients should always be given a bed by a window to provide access to sunlight. When daylight is not available to assess skin color, a lamp with at least a 60-watt bulb should be used. To establish the baseline skin color, the nurse must observe skin surfaces that have the least amount of pigmentation, which include the volar surfaces of the forearms, the palms of the hands, the soles of the feet, the abdomen, and the buttocks. When observing these areas, the nurse should look for an underlying red tone, which is typical of all skin, regardless of how dark its color. Absence of this red tone in a client may indicate pallor. Additional areas that are important to assess in dark-skinned clients include the mouth, the conjunctivae, and the nail beds. Generally speaking, the darkness of the oral mucosa correlates with the client's skin color. The darker the skin, the darker the mucosa; nevertheless, the mucosa is lighter than the skin.

The nurse must be aware that oral hyperpigmentation can occur on the tongue and the mucosa and can alter the value of the oral mucosa as a site for observation. The occurrence of oral hyperpigmentation is directly related to the darkness of a person's skin. Oral hyperpigmentation appears in 50% to 90% of African-Americans, compared with 10% to 50% of Whites. Another important consideration for the nurse is the appearance of a hard palate because it takes on a yellow discoloration, particularly in the presence of jaundice. The hard palate is frequently affected by hyperpigmentation in a manner similar to that of the oral mucosa and the tongue. The nurse should also assess the lips because they may be helpful in assessing skin-color changes (such as jaundice or cyanosis). It is important for the nurse to remember, however, that the lips of some Black people have a natural bluish hue (Rouch, 1977; Sommers, 2011). Thus, it is important for the nurse to have established the baseline color of the lips if they are to be of value in detecting cyanosis (Branch & Paxton, 1976; Sommers, 2011).

It is also important for the nurse to establish the normal color of the conjunctivae when working with persons from transcultural populations. The conjunctivae will reflect the color changes of cyanosis or pallor and are a good site for observing petechiae. Another excellent source for determining the presence of jaundice is the sclera. The nurse should first establish a baseline color for the sclerae because the sclerae of dark-skinned persons often have a yellow coloration caused by subconjunctival fatty deposits. A common finding in persons with highly pigmented skin is the presence of melanin deposits or "freckles" on the sclerae.

The final area of assessment should be the nail beds, which are useful for detecting cyanosis or pallor. In dark-skinned persons, it is difficult to assess the nail beds because they may be highly pigmented, thick, or lined or contain melanin deposits. Regardless of color, for baseline assessment, it is important for the nurse to notice how quickly the color returns to the nail bed after pressure has been released from the free edge of the nail. A slower return of color to the nail bed may indicate cyanosis or pallor. It is also difficult to detect rashes, inflammations, and ecchymoses in dark-skinned persons. It may be necessary to palpate rashes in dark-skinned persons because rashes may not be readily visible to the eye. When palpating the skin for rashes, the nurse should notice induration and warmth of the area.

Other Visible Physical Characteristics

In addition to looking for pallor and cyanosis, the nurse should note other aberrations in the skin. For example, mongolian spots may be present on the skin of African-American, Asian American, American Indian, or Mexican American newborns. Mongolian spots are bluish discolorations that vary tremendously in size and color and are often mistaken for bruises. Another aberration that is more common in African-Americans than in other racial groups is keloids. These ropelike scars represent an exaggeration of the wound-healing process and may result from any type of trauma, such as surgical incisions, ear piercing, or insertion of an intravenous catheter.

Enzymatic and Genetic Variations

The basic genetic makeup of an individual is determined from the moment of conception. Then, among other things, the upper limits of achievement are set; the "map," so to speak, is drawn. In other words, a person can be only what he or she is genetically determined to be. More specifically, growth and development cannot go beyond what the genes make possible. An individual will not grow 1 inch taller than the genetic structure allows, regardless of the amount of exercise or vitamins consumed. By the same token, an individual will be no more intelligent than genetic structure allows, despite the amount of tutoring or special schooling the individual receives (Burt, 1966; Lorton & Lorton, 1984).

In medical terms, a person's race represents his or her genetic makeup. Although race may be irrelevant in some situations, knowing the racial predisposition to a certain disease is often helpful in evaluating clients and diagnosing their illness, as well as in assessing risks (Divan, 1989). The genetic and enzymatic predisposition to certain diseases is discussed in this chapter in the Susceptibility to Disease section; lactose intolerance and glucose-6-phosphate dehydrogenase (G-6-PD) deficiency are discussed under Nutritional Deficiencies.

Genes are the working subunits of chemical information that carry a complete set of instructions for making the needed protein for a cell (Lewis, 2010). It is essential to remember that genes contain a particular set of instructions by way of coding for a particular protein (Jorde, Carey, & Bamshad, 2010). These coded instructions are known as *deoxyribonucleic acid* (DNA). DNA is composed of two long, paired strands that are spiraled into what is known as a *double helix* (Collins, 1997). Although there are only four chemical bases in DNA—adenine, thymine, cytosine, and guanine—the order in which these bases occur determines specifically what information is available in a manner similar to the way in which the specific letters in the alphabet combine to form particular words and connect to form sentences (Jorde et al., 2010). DNA itself resides in a core, or what is known as the *nucleus*, of each of the cells in the body. In fact, every human cell, with the one notable exception of mature red blood cells, which have no nucleus, has the same DNA. All somatic cells have 46 molecules of double-stranded DNA. Likewise, each molecule consists of 50 to 250 million bases, which are housed in a chromosome (Jorde et al., 2010).

There are several levels of genetic investigation, including molecular genetics and cytogenetics. *Molecular genetics* is the study of genes at a biochemical or cellular level (Lewis, 2010). A gene and its effects are often separable, and, as such, geneticists are able to distinguish the gene responsible for a trait or illness from the actual expression of a particular trait or illness (Lewis, 2010). For example, the genes themselves compose what is termed the *genotypes*, whereas the actual expression of these genes is called the *phenotype*. In contrast to molecular genetics, *cytogenetics* is the study of genes that involves matching phenotypes to chromosomal variants. As the twentieth century progressed, cytogenetics rapidly matured as geneticists built upon the mapping of all four chromosomes of the fruit fly. By 1950, the arduous task of mapping genes on the 22 pairs of autosomes was begun (Lewis, 2010). Today this process of sequencing a genetic map is known as the *Human Genome Project* (Jorde et al., 2010). Work relative to the

15-year international Human Genome Project was officially inaugurated in the United States on October 1, 1990, and the purpose of the Human Genome Project was to identify the 3 billion code letters of a representative human genome by the year 2005 (Gannett, 2008). At the same time, geneticists were to identify the exact location of all genes on the sequencing map. On April 14, 2003, work relative to the sequencing of the Human Genome Project was finally completed a full 2 years ahead of schedule (Gannett, 2008).

Another area of genetic study is termed *population genetics*. Population genetics is the study of allele frequencies in populations (Lewis, 2010). Population genetics is extremely important because human beings tend to marry or mate with people primarily like themselves—that is, the same racial, ethnic, and cultural groups. Because of this, there is a tendency for a frequency of certain alleles in that given population. For example, although 1 of 800 women in the general U.S. population is affected by the *BRCA1* breast cancer gene, this figure climbs dramatically to 1 of every 100 women among Ashkenazi Jews (Lewis, 2010).

Today the relative role that genetics plays in understanding the etiology of disease is becoming evident. It is important to remember that all diseases, except for trauma, have a genetic linkage. The earliest introduction to the concept of genetic inheritance comes from the nineteenth-century work of Gregor Mendel. Mendel's work involved the identification and breeding of a variety of pea plants (Lewis, 2010; Overfield, 1995). From his work, Mendel noted that these pea plants had two different expressions of an inherited trait. For example, Mendel noted that when short plants were bred with short plants they were "true breeding"—that is, giving rise to the production of only short plants. However, when tall plants were bred with short plants or another tall plant, the next generation resulted in only tall offspring. This phenomenon indicates that a gene can and does exist in alternative forms. In genetics, these alternative forms are called *alleles* (Lewis, 2010).

Ordinarily a gene is a stable entity, but over the course of time a gene can suffer a change in sequence (Lewis, 2010). This change is termed a *mutation*. The new form of the gene is inherited in a stable manner, as in the case of the previous form (Lewis, 2010). When a mutation occurs, the organism carrying the altered gene is called a *mutant*, whereas the organism that carries the normal, or unaltered, gene is called the *wild type*. The term *wild type* is used to describe either the genotype or the phenotype.

To understand how copies of a gene are transmitted, it is necessary to understand that the life cycle of an organism passes through a diploid phase and essentially has two copies of each gene. At conception, one of two copies is passed from the parent to a gamete (a germ cell, egg, or sperm). At this point, the gamete contains one copy of each gene of the organism, and this is called the *haploid set*. Consequently, the alternative types of gametes produced by the parents unite to form what is called the *zygote* (the fertilized egg) (Lewis, 2010).

With a mutation, new alleles arise. Generally, when a mutation occurs, the particular frequency is represented by only one copy among all the copies of that particular gene in the population (Nussbaum, McInnes, & Willard, 2007). The probability that a new mutation will survive from one generation to the next is largely dependent on both chance and natural selection. From one generation to the next, depending on chance, allele frequencies fluctuate (Nussbaum et al., 2007). This entire phenomenon is termed *genetic drift*.

When an individual has two identical alleles for a gene, this individual is said to be *homozygous* for that gene. Similarly, an individual with two different alleles is *heterozygous*. In other words, a person inherits essentially one allele from each parent. These alleles can be the same or different. Therefore, at any locus on a chromosome pair, there is a gene composed of two alleles. For example, the blood types A, B, and O are the alleles for the ABO blood type locus (Overfield, 1995). If there is only one allele at a particular locus, then the gene is said to be *monomorphic*. In contrast, when there are multiple alleles at a particular gene locus, the gene is said to be *polymorphic* (Overfield, 1995). An excellent example of this concept is found in the enzyme deficiency disorder G-6-PD deficiency, which is said to be caused by the most polymorphic genes known, with more than 400 alleles (Luzzatto & Poggi, 2008).

In Mendel's classic work, he noted that each of the genes identified had two alleles, which is suggestive of two obvious expressions. A gene may have many alleles (variants) as a result of changes in any of the hundreds or thousands of DNA base pairs that make up a gene. However, because the concept of DNA and DNA sequencing had not yet been identified, Mendel was able to detect a gene variant only if the phenotype was altered. For example, if a green pea produced a yellow pea, this phenomenon would be a phenotypic alteration (Lewis, 2010). As Mendel continued his work, he noted that in some instances one gene could mask the expression of another. In this case, the gene that masks the expression of the other is considered to be completely *dominant*, whereas the mask allele is considered to be *recessive*. An excellent example of this concept was noted when Mendel crossed a "true-breeding" tall plant with a short plant. In this case, the tall plant (or the tall allele) was completely dominant to the short plant (short allele), and thus all the plants in the next generation were tall (Lewis, 2010; Overfield, 1995). An inherited trait is said therefore

to be either dominant or recessive. Whether this trait is dominant or recessive depends on the particular nature of the phenotype. Often the heterozygote, on a biochemical level, is actually intermediate, or a mixture of the homozygous dominant and homozygous recessive, although the heterozygote and the homozygous-dominant genotypes are indistinguishable (Lewis, 2010; Overfield, 1995). For example, in the case of Tay-Sachs, a genetically inherited disease commonly found among Jews, the heterozygote (with one dominant and one recessive allele) actually produces half the normal amount of the enzyme that the gene encodes, yet this amount appears to be sufficient for normal function, and so that person remains as healthy as a person with two dominant alleles. A phenotypic (disease itself) expression of the gene would occur only if a person inherited two recessive alleles.

How a person inherits a particular gene depends on two basic characteristics: (1) the dominant or recessive nature of the allele and (2) the type of chromosome that the gene in question is part of (Lewis, 2010). If a person has dominant alleles—that is, has only one copy of the gene—this dominant allele can affect the phenotype. In contrast, a person who has a recessive allele must have two copies of the gene if the phenotype is to be expressed. For example, the cancer-predisposing alleles *BRCA1* and *BRCA2* are dominant. Therefore, an individual would need to inherit one copy of the gene from one parent to have a 1 in 2 chance of developing the disease. The second mode of inheritance depends on the chromosome location that the particular gene is a part of. For example, human beings have 46 chromosomes, including two that determine sex—X and Y (sex chromosomes). The presence or absence of a single gene on the Y chromosome is responsible for determining sex. The remaining chromosomes are termed *nonsex chromosomes*, or *autosomes*. Specifically, a female has 44 autosomes and two X chromosomes. In contrast, a male has 44 autosomes and one X and one Y chromosome. In other words, there are actually 23 pairs of chromosomes consisting of 22 pairs of autosomes, and one pair of X and Y chromosomes (Jorde et al., 2010; Lewis, 2010). Because there is a difference in sex chromosome constitution, it is believed that genes on the sex chromosomes follow different, sex-linked patterns of inheritances in the two sexes. In the case of X-linked dominant inheritance, it is essential to remember that male-to-male transmission never occurs because men cannot pass their X chromosomes to their sons. In addition, all daughters of an affected male with an X-linked gene will actually receive the gene either in a recessive or a dominant form (Harper, 1993; Jorde et al., 2010). For example, if the father passes an X-linked recessive gene to his daughter, the daughter will be a carrier. However, if the father passes an X-linked dominant gene to his daughter, the daughter will be affected (Harper, 1993; Jorde et al., 2010). Thus, modes of inheritance of a particular trait can depend on the recessive and dominant characteristics of the allele or on whether the gene is located on the sex chromosome or on an autosomal chromosome (Saito, Okui, Tokino, Oshimura, & Nakamura, 1992).

To understand the significance of genetics, it is essential to develop an awareness of the relative role of single mendelian traits in humans. Single mendelian traits in humans are associated with disorders or traits linked to a single gene. For example, the most prevalent mendelian disorders are believed to be cystic fibrosis, Tay-Sachs disease, and Duchenne muscular dystrophy (Lewis, 2010). Yet, although these mendelian traits are considered prevalent, they are extremely rare, affecting 1 in 10,000 or fewer births (Lewis, 2010). Today, about 2500 mendelian disorders are known, and some 2500 other identifiable conditions are suspected to be mendelian related because of their recurrence patterns in large families (Lewis, 2010).

Some disease cannot be explained by the single-gene mendelian-trait theory. Although every individual has two alleles for any autosomal gene (one allele for each chromosome), a gene can exist in a given population in more than two allelic forms (Lewis, 2010). This different allele combination often leads to variations in phenotype (Harper, 1993; Lewis, 2010). In addition, there is a difference in the dominance relationship of an allele. For example, as previously indicated, in the case of complete dominance, one allele is expressed, and the other is not. However, in some instances, some genes demonstrate what is termed *incomplete dominance,* which occurs when the heterozygous phenotype is intermediate between that of either homozygote (Harper, 1993; Lewis, 2010). For example, in the case of familial hypercholesterolemia, an individual with two disease-causing alleles actually lacks the liver receptors that take up cholesterol from the bloodstream (Lewis, 2010). In this case, the phenotype will actually parallel the number of receptors. Individuals with one mutant allele die in young adulthood, and those with two of the wild type (the most common expression of a particular gene in a given population) do not develop this inherited form of heart disease (Lewis, 2010).

Understanding genetics and its transcultural and racial implications is of paramount importance. Understanding race and the genetic implications is also important. There are scientists who recognize only Black, White, and Asians/American Indians as racial groups (Brues, 1977; Overfield, 1995; Polednak, 1986). Asians and American Indians are often placed by these scientists in one major group because of some genetic similarities (Brues, 1977; Overfield, 1995). *Race* is an important term because races of people are not static. What is implied by this is that all races have evolved over time as a direct response to environmental stimuli. Thus the characteristics that define a race will not necessarily define any specific individual from that particular race of people (Overfield, 1995). For example, the Yupik Eskimos are said to have a 75% gene frequency of M in the MN blood system and 61% in the O, 25% in the A, and 16% in the B within the ABO blood groups (Overfield, 1995). These same individuals are believed to have no prevalence for Rh-negative blood (Overfield, 1995). A health care professional working with this group of people might assume incorrectly therefore that the most common array of traits for the Yupiks would be blood types M and O and that these individuals would be invariably Rh positive. Although some Yupiks might actually display this array of traits, it must be remembered that because of genetic heterogeneity, some individual Yupiks might differ (Overfield, 1995).

It has been reported that the incidence of dizygotic twinning is highest in African-Americans, occurring in 4% of births. Dizygotic twinning occurs in approximately 2% of births in Whites and in 0.5% of births in Asians (Benirschke, Kaufmann, & Baergen, 2006; Giger, Davidhizar, & Wieczorek, 1993).

Some research interpretations (Jensen, 1969, 1974, 1977) have indicated that the small but persistent differences between the average intelligence quotients (IQs) of African-American children and those of White children reflect a genetic difference. In his classic work, Jensen (1969) claimed to have controlled for variables, including income and education. He reported that he found a difference in IQ that he believed to indicate a genetic difference. Others have refuted Jensen's claim (Sesardic, 2000). In 1977, Jensen conducted a study of children between 5 and 16 years of age in the rural South, which indicated that the IQs of African-American children, but not those of White children, drop substantially as they grow older. Jensen believed that this contrast between African-Americans and Whites possibly meant that the decrement in IQ was genetically determined. This has not been supported by others' research.

Drug Interactions and Metabolism

Reactions to drugs vary with race. Some evidence indicates that drugs are metabolized by different races in different ways and at different rates (Davidhizar & Giger, 2008; Weber, 1999). For example, Zhou, Adedoyin, and Woods (1992) demonstrated that Chinese subjects are more sensitive to the cardiovascular effects of propranolol than White subjects are. In the body there are three classes of reactions to foreign chemicals or drugs: hydrolysis, conjugation, and oxidation (Henderson 2010; Kalow, 1982, 1986, 1989; Weber, 1999).

A term that is essential to understanding how drugs work in the body is *pharmacokinetics,* which actually is intended to mean or to determine when a steady state of concentration of drugs and their metabolites is achieved in the body (Henderson, 2010). There are two levels of thought regarding pharmacokinetics. The first is that the pharmacokinetics of medication deals with metabolism, blood levels, absorption, distribution, and excretion. The second level of thought suggests that pharmacokinetics also involves other variables including conjugation, plasma protein binding, and oxidation by the cytochrome P (CYP) enzyme isoforms (Henderson, 2010). Most medications are generally metabolized in two phases. In Phase I, medications are subjected to oxidation and are mediated through the P-450 isozymes. The CYP-450 enzymes actually represent what are termed a *superfamily* of over 50 heme-containing microsomal drug-metabolizing isozymes (Henderson, 2010; Matthews & Johnson, 2006). CYP-450 is named from the characteristic maximum spectral absorbance at 450 mm in its reduced state (Henderson, 2010; Matthews & Johnson, 2006). The name was changed from *450 mm* to *CYP.* Every portion of the newly named CYP-450 is intended to indicate or specify the nomenclature further. For instance, *CYP* actually designates the human chromosome P-450, which is then followed by an Arabic number with an asterisk (*), which is intended to indicate allelic variation(s) and thus the new nomenclature (Matthews & Johnson, 2006). For example, CYP2D6*3 actually belongs to the family 2, as well as the subfamily D. In concert with these factors is that the gene that is actually encoding for the isozyme is 6, whereas the allelic variant is 3 and is preceded with an asterisk (*), further distinguishing it (Matthews & Johnson, 2006).

Phase II enzymes are transferases and are thought to be necessary to allow endogenous substances to conjugate with drugs and their metabolites. It is important to remember that the CYP-450 enzyme 2D6 (debrisoquine hydroxylase), while an important step to the metabolic pathway for a great number of medications, are also responsible for drug-to-drug interactions (Henderson, 2010). According to Henderson (2010), it is essential to understand the CYP-450 system because this knowledge will allow accurate predictions of potential drug interactions and known side effects based on a number of demographic variables for racially/ethnically diverse individuals.

A critical isoform is CYP2D6 because it is essential to metabolism (e.g., with antipsychotics). It is essential to remember that CYP2D6 isoenzyme is responsible for the metabolizing of 25% to 30% of all clinically used medications, which include antidepressants, β-blockers, antipsychotics, morphine derivatives, and a host of other drugs (Matthews & Johnson, 2006). It is also interesting to note

that the CYP2D6 isoenzyme was actually discovered in relationship to the polymorphic relation of debrisoquine, an antihypertensive agent. In fact, the discovery showed that there were two distinct phenotypes exhibited with a urinary ratio of debrisoquine in relationship to its main 4-hydroxy metabolites (Matthews & Johnson, 2006). In general, individuals are classified as poor metabolizers; intermediate, slow metabolizers; extensive metabolizers; or ultra-rapid metabolizers (Henderson, 2010). It is also interesting to note that the ability to metabolize, or the rate of metabolism of, CYP2D6 varies by race. For example, in the world, poor metabolization occurs in 0.5% to 2.4% of Asians, 3% to 7.3% of Whites, 3.3% of Mexican Americans, and 3.6% of Nicaraguans (Henderson, 2010). There are also a number of isoforms accounting for metabolism of specific classes of drugs such as CYP2C9, CYP2C10, and CYP3A4. The concept of understanding how race and drugs synergistically interact is termed *ethnopharmacology.* The following are examples of reactions to specific drugs.

Isoniazid is a drug commonly used to treat tuberculosis. People metabolize this drug in one of two ways: they inactivate it very slowly or very rapidly. Those who inactivate this drug very slowly are at risk for developing peripheral neuropathy during therapy (Onyebujoh et al., 2005). Rapid inactivation of this drug occurs in 40% of Whites, 60% of African-Americans, 60% to 90% of American Indians and Eskimos, and 85% to 90% of Asians (Iman et al., 2010; Weber, 1999). *Pyridoxine* is given with isoniazid, and the doses are spaced at larger intervals for slower reaction during treatment for tuberculosis. Primaquine is metabolized by oxidation and is used to treat malaria. When this drug is given to individuals who lack the enzymes necessary for glucose metabolism of the red blood cells, hemolysis of the red blood cells occurs. Approximately 100 million people in the world are affected by this particular enzyme deficiency and thus are unable to ingest primaquine. Approximately 35% of African-Americans have this particular enzyme deficiency.

Succinylcholine is a muscle relaxant used during surgery. It is inactivated by hydrolysis by the enzyme pseudocholinesterase. In most individuals it is rapidly inactivated, but some individuals have the atypical form of the enzyme and suffer prolonged muscle paralysis and an inability to breathe after administration of the drug. African-Americans, Asians, and American Indians are at risk for having pseudocholinesterase deficiency; Whites have a slightly higher risk than these groups. Some Jews and Alaskan Eskimos have a considerably greater risk: 1 of 135 Alaskan Eskimos cannot metabolize the drug succinylcholine normally (Lockridge, 1990; Weber, 1999).

Alcohol is metabolized differently, depending on race. Two enzymes are involved in the metabolism of alcohol: alcohol dehydrogenase (ADH) and acetaldehyde dehydrogenase (ALDH). Alcohol metabolism is a two-step process: ADH converts alcohol to acetaldehyde, and acetaldehyde ALDH converts acetaldehyde (a toxic substance) to acetic acid (a nontoxic substance). Both of these enzymes have more than one variant. ADH has a high-activity type, which converts alcohol to acetaldehyde rapidly, and a low-activity variant, which converts it slowly (Edenberg, 2007; Weber, 1999). ALDH has four variants (ALDH-1 through ALDH-4). ALDH-1 is considered "normal"; other types are less efficient in their ability to metabolize acetaldehyde (Israel, Quintanilla, Sapag, & Tampier, 2006).

In Whites with "normal" levels of both ADH and ALDH-1, alcohol is metabolized fairly efficiently. In contrast, American Indians and Asians have an excessive level of high-activity ADH and a low level of ALDH-1. Consequently, persons in these groups metabolize alcohol to acetaldehyde rapidly. However, the metabolism to acetic acid is delayed. Because acetaldehyde is toxic and acetic acid is not, the net result is unpleasant effects, such as facial flushing and palpitations (Kudzma, 1992; Ma & Allan, 2011). Data from some studies indicate that American Indians and Asians experience noticeable facial flushing and other vasomotor symptoms after ingesting alcohol; in contrast, Whites and African-Americans experience less severe reactions. Facial flushing after ingestion of alcohol occurs in 45% to 85% of Asians versus 3% to 29% of Whites (Chan, 1986; Collins & McNair, 2003).

In regard to alcohol use, recent data suggest that Hispanic Americans and Black Americans are also at an increased risk for death from liver cirrhosis. Although the reasons for this remain largely unknown, one study compared racial and ethnic aspartate aminotransferase and gamma-glutamyltransferase level elevations among these individuals who drank (Stewart, 2002). Findings from this study suggest that among current drinkers, Black and Mexican Americans were more likely to have a twofold elevation of aspartate aminotransferase level than their White counterparts. These elevated levels were even more pronounced among those who drank more frequently (Mexican American: odds ratio, 9.1 [95% confidence interval, 3.9–21]; Black Americans: odds ratio, 3.1 [95% confidence interval, 1.4–6.8]) than among those who drank less frequently or were abstainers (Stewart, 2002).

Caffeine, a component of many drugs as well as coffee, tea, and colas, appears to be metabolized and excreted faster by Whites than by Asians (Davidhizar & Giger, 2008; Kudzma, 1992). It is thought that the differences noted in caffeine metabolism are directly correlated with liver enzyme differences (Kudzma, 1992).

Antihypertensives are another category of drugs that are metabolized differently depending on race. Several studies suggest that there are notable differences between African-Americans and their White counterparts in the metabolism of antihypertensive drugs (Davidhizar & Giger, 2008; Freis, 1986; Moser & Lunn, 1982; Zhou et al., 1992). Freis (1986) noted that African-Americans tend to need higher doses of beta-adrenergic receptor–blocking agents such as propranolol (Inderal). In contrast, angiotensin-converting enzyme inhibitors (such as captopril) tend to be less effective as a single therapy for African-Americans than for Whites with the same treatment regimen (Beevers, Lee, & Lip, 2003; Davidhizar & Giger, 2008; Moser & Black, 1998). Given the plethora of information on African-Americans and their inability to efficiently metabolize some antihypertensive drugs adequately, there is a school of thought that suggests that these individuals must be treated aggressively with a combination of antihypertensive drugs (possibly three as a mean number). Batson, Belletti, and Wogen (2010) noted that even when African-Americans were prescribed an aggressive medication regimen, this did not necessarily correspond with satisfactory blood pressure control. It is also interesting to note that even when body surface area and body weight are considered, Chinese men tend to need only about half as much propranolol as White American men (Cohen et al., 2010; Kim, Johnson, & Derendorf, 2004; Palaniappian et al., 2010).

*Thiazide diuretics** are the drugs of choice for initial therapy in hypertension, but genes play a major role in sodium reabsorption and can affect a patient's response to diuretic therapy. African-Americans' response to antihypertensive therapy is associated with chromosome 12q15[30,31] where the FRS2 gene is located. This is involved in growth factor signaling. FRS2 plays a significant role in vascular smooth muscle cell regulation (Piatkov, 2013). Patients with a single nucleotide polymorphism of the T594M gene (epithelial sodium channel) variant are thought to respond more favorably to amiloride therapy for blood pressure control than to thiazide-based diuretic drugs. In case of severe hypokalemia, potassium-sparing diuretics such as amiloride or triamterene should be used according to serum sodium and potassium levels (Hollier et al., 2006; Piatkov, Jones, & McLean, 2013; Swift & Macgregor, 2004).

Psychotropic drugs are also metabolized differently depending on race. For example, Burroughs, Maxey, Crawley, and Levy (2002) conducted a comparative study between Chinese and White participants, where findings suggested that Chinese participants required lower doses of benzodiazepines (diazepam [Valium], alprazolam

---

*This paragraph contributed by Henry Lewis, III, PharmD.

[Zanax], tricyclic antidepressants, atropine, and propranolol [Inderal]). When doses were comparable by race, the Chinese participants had an increase in side effects. These researchers also found that Chinese individuals tended to have a lower dose/optimal response threshold for haloperidol (Haldol) than did their White counterparts.

It is important for the nurse to remember that certain psychotropic drugs can cause higher blood levels in certain individuals by virtue of race (such as Asian Americans). It is essential to modify the dosage of these drugs based not only on body surface area and weight but also on racial considerations.

Lawson (1986) noted that clients from developing countries are routinely given smaller doses of antipsychotics (or neuroleptics) because some racial groups metabolize drugs more slowly and therefore experience a greater drug effect. For neuroleptic medications, these same variations by race are found in the United States.

In a prospective classic study of tardive dyskinesia, Glazer, Morgenstern, and Doucette (1993) found that among psychiatric outpatients treated with neuroleptic medications, race was a probable factor for this iatrogenic movement disorder. The data indicated that non-White clients, 97% of whom were African-American, were about twice as likely to develop tardive dyskinesia as their White counterparts. To ensure the accuracy of the results, the researchers controlled for other demographic and clinical risk factors.

In a follow-up study, Glazer, Morgenstern, and Doucette (1994) found that, compared with Whites, non-Whites were younger, less skilled, more likely to be unmarried, and more likely to have a diagnosis of schizophrenia. Non-Whites were also more likely to receive higher doses of neuroleptics, principally because they were frequently given more high-potency depot medications. Despite the control for known tardive dyskinesia factors, the estimated rate of tardive dyskinesia was nearly twice as high for non-Whites as for Whites. According to Glazer et al. (1994), none of the other demographic, clinical, psychosocial, or general health variables measured in the study appeared to explain the association between race and the propensity for tardive dyskinesia. The correlation between race as a biological marker and the development of tardive dyskinesia remains unclear (Glazer et al., 1994). Habits such as drinking and smoking are known to speed drug metabolism, and thus the fact that some Whites and African-Americans drink significantly more alcohol than some Asian Americans is an important consideration.

Some researchers (Feisthamel & Schwartz, 2006; Lefley, 1990) contend that African-American clients are significantly misdiagnosed as psychotic. Because they are viewed as more violent, they receive more medication and spend more time in seclusion than Whites, Hispanics, or Asians (Lefley, 1990). The higher dose of medication prescribed for African-Americans may result more from staff perception than from a decision based on serum levels and careful observation (Keltner & Folks, 1992).

Gender is another cultural consideration that may have a profound effect on the metabolism of drugs. Yonkers, Kando, Cole, and Blumenthal (1992) suggest that women have the potential for higher blood plasma levels of psychotropic drugs, especially when used with oral contraceptives. In addition, they note that women have greater efficacy of antipsychotic agents and a greater likelihood of adverse reactions, such as hypothyroidism and, in older women, tardive dyskinesia. Although plausible explanations for these differences have been offered, women have traditionally been excluded from clinical trials measuring the efficacy and metabolism of certain drugs.

Electrocardiographic Patterns

A common finding in African-Americans, particularly in African-American men, is the occurrence of inverted T waves in the precordial leads of the electrocardiogram. This aberration is a normal variant in the African-American population but would indicate a pathological condition if found in other racial groups, such as Whites.

Susceptibility to Disease

Another category of differences between racial groups is susceptibility to disease. The increased or decreased incidence of a particular disease may be genetically determined.

Tuberculosis. Historically, some American Indians have had a tuberculosis incidence that is 7 to 15 times that of non-Indians, whereas African-Americans have had a tuberculosis incidence 3 times higher than that of White Americans (Giger, 2011). Urban American Jews have been the most resistant to tuberculosis (Overfield, 1995). The increased susceptibility of African-Americans to tuberculosis may be a result of their tendency toward overgrowth of connective tissue components concerned with protection against infection because tuberculosis is a granulomatous infection (Polednak, 1986).

At the turn of the twentieth century, tuberculosis was the leading cause of death in the United States. It remained the leading cause of death until the introduction of antituberculosis drug therapy in the 1940s and early 1950s (Phipps, 1993). The case rates for tuberculosis steadily declined from 83,304 reported cases in 1953 to 22,225 reported cases in 1984 (Centers for Disease Control and Prevention [CDC], 1991). Since 1986, there has been a decline in the total number of tuberculosis cases reported across all age groups, with only 11,545 cases reported in 2009 in the United States (CDC, Tuberculosis Surveillance Report, 2013). Further declines occurred in 2013, with only 9582 cases reported (CDC, Tuberculosis Surveillance Report, 2013). Between 1985 and 2013, the highest reported case rates occurred in Miami, Atlanta, San Francisco, Tampa, Newark, and New York City (CDC, Tuberculosis Surveillance Report, 2013). It is postulated that these cities and their states have higher case rates than other cities have because their states also report the highest number of human immunodeficiency virus (HIV)-positive persons, particularly among intravenous drug abusers. In addition, these states have a larger influx of immigrants from countries in which tuberculosis is endemic (CDC, HIV/AIDS Surveillance Report, 2013).

Many persons with HIV infection have organisms that are resistant to most of the chemotherapeutic agents used to treat this type of tuberculosis. When an individual has drug-resistant tuberculosis, he or she may pass the resistant organisms to others. In such cases, effective treatment of this type of tuberculosis becomes nearly impossible (Phipps, 1993).

The number of reported cases of tuberculosis among certain racial groups has changed dramatically over the past several years. For example, in 2007, the incidence of tuberculosis was seven times higher among African-Americans than among non-Hispanic Whites, nine times higher among Asians and Pacific Islanders, and four times higher among American Indians (CDC, Tuberculosis Surveillance Report, 2013). Ethnic minorities now account for more than two thirds of all the reported cases of tuberculosis in the United States, partly as a result of the increased incidence of tuberculosis among ethnic minorities infected with HIV (CDC, Tuberculosis Surveillance Report, 2013). For example, in 2013, the states reporting the most cases of tuberculosis included (1) California (2470 cases, of which 213 were in Whites, 219 were in Blacks, 916 were in Hispanics, 4 were in American Indians, and 1118 were in Asians or Pacific Islanders), (2) Florida (821 cases, of which 189 were in Whites, 342 were in Blacks, 211 were in Hispanics, 1 was in an American Indian, and 79 were in Asians or Pacific Islanders), (3) New York (1006 cases, of which 121 were in Whites, 231 were in Blacks, 306 were in Hispanics, 1 was in an American Indian, and 306 were in Asians or Pacific Islanders), and (4) Texas (1501 cases, of which 179 were in Whites, 309 were in Blacks, 773 were in Hispanics, 0 was in American Indians, and 239 were in Asians or Pacific Islanders) (CDC, Tuberculosis Surveillance Report, 2013). It is also interesting to note that of the cases of tuberculosis reported for children, ethnic minorities account for nearly 83% (CDC, Tuberculosis Surveillance Report, 2013).

It is important to remember that susceptibility to disease may also be environmental or a combination of both genetic and environmental factors. The evidence indicates that tuberculosis can occur in response to both socioenvironmental and psychological stress factors. In a classic study of clients in Seattle, Holmes, Hawkins, Bowerman, Clarke, and Joffe (1957) found that environmental factors appeared to be relevant in relation to the onset of tuberculosis. In this classic study, data in the life experiences of each client were plotted for a 12-year period preceding hospitalization. Analysis of the data revealed that in the majority of clients, there was a gradual increase in experiences that were perceived by the individual as significant and stressful. The combination of stressful life experiences and personal perception resulted in a psychological crisis situation that was evidenced in the 2-year period preceding hospitalization. Further analysis of the data indicated that clients who are poorly equipped to deal with social relationships, especially when a lot of tension is present, may be at risk for tuberculosis.

Blood Groups, Rh Factor, and Disease. Blood groups also differentiate people in certain racial groups. A prevalence for type O blood has been found among American Indians, with some incidence of type A blood and virtually no incidence of type B blood. Almost equal incidences of types A, B, and O blood are found in Japanese and Chinese people, with the AB blood type found in only about 10% of the Japanese and Chinese populations. African-Americans and Whites have been found to have equal incidences of A, B, and O blood types. The predominant blood types of African-Americans and Whites are A and O, with fewer incidences of AB and B types (Jick et al., 1969; Overfield, 1995).

Statistically, persons with type O blood are at a greater risk for duodenal ulcers, whereas persons with type A blood are more likely to develop cancer of the stomach. In addition, there is some evidence that women with type O blood have a diminished chance of getting thromboembolic disease, particularly when taking birth control pills, in comparison with women with other ABO blood types (Jick et al., 1969; Overfield, 1995).

The Rh-negative factor in blood is most common in Whites, much rarer in other racial groups, and apparently absent in Eskimos (Lewis, 1942). Because there are at least 27 different antigens in the Rh system, this system is complex and difficult to understand. Of clinical significance is the D antigen because it is more immunogenic than any other Rh antigen and is usually the antigen involved in hemolytic disease of the newborn. When antigen D is present, the term *Rh positive* is used. Approximately 85% of persons in the world have Rh-positive blood. The term *Rh negative* is used when antigen D is absent. Persons with the Rh-negative factor who are exposed to Rh-positive blood form Rh antibodies. After continued exposure to Rh-positive blood, the Rh antibody will bind to corresponding antigens on the surface of red blood cells, which contain the Rh antigen. Ordinarily, Rh antibodies do not fix complement. As a result, there is no immediate hemolysis, such as that occurring with ABO incompatibility. Rather, Rh-antigen red blood cells are broken down rapidly by macrophages in the spleen, resulting in a conversion of hemoglobin (Hb) to bilirubin, which causes jaundice. Thus the multigravida woman with Rh-negative factor who has a Rh-positive mate and has either delivered or aborted a Rh-positive infant will be more likely to have babies who are susceptible to jaundice. This condition can be prevented in subsequent pregnancies if the Rh-negative woman is given RhoGAM immediately after aborting or delivering an Rh-positive infant.

Diabetes. Other conditions that appear to have biocultural or racial prevalence include diabetes mellitus, hypertension, sickle cell disease (SCD), and systemic lupus erythematosus (SLE). Reportedly, there is a high incidence of diabetes mellitus in certain American Indian tribes, including the Seminole, Pima, and Papago. However, diabetes was once believed to be quite rare among Alaskan Eskimos (Westfall, 1971), and there are data available to suggest that this is no longer the case (Alaskan Native Tribal Health Consortium, 2013). Diabetes mellitus is a major health problem in the United States, with an incidence of more than 20.9 million diagnosed cases and more than 7 million undiagnosed cases, which accounts for more than 6.2% of the total population in the United States (American Diabetic Association, 2015; CDC, Diabetes Surveillance Report, 2015; National Center for Health Statistics, 2014). Each year more than 800,000 new cases of diabetes are reported in the United States (American Diabetic Association, 2015; CDC, Diabetes Surveillance Report, 2015). In fact, the incidence of diabetes mellitus is so widespread that it is postulated that for every person with diagnosed diabetes, there is another person who remains undiagnosed. Diabetes is so prevalent in the U.S. population that it was the seventh leading cause of death in the United States (American Diabetic Association, 2015; CDC, Diabetes Surveillance Report, 2015; Centers for Disease Control 2014; U.S. Department of Health and Human Services, Health United States, 2014). Diabetes was reported as the underlying cause for more than 40,000 deaths and a contributory factor in approximately 160,000 other deaths (U.S. Department of Health and Human Services, Health United States, 2014). Diabetes is so prevalent in U.S. society that it is estimated that some 10.2% (15.7 million) of all

non-Hispanic Whites 20 years of age or older have diabetes, as well as 18.7% (4.9 million) of Blacks and 11.8% (4.2 million) of Hispanics (U.S. Department of Health and Human Services, Health United States, 2014; National Diabetic Statistics, 2014).

By proportion of the population, American Indians have a disproportionately high incidence of diabetes at 15.1% of their population (105,000), and Alaska Natives have the lowest percentage with diabetes (5.3%). By geographical region, American Indians residing in the southeastern United States have the greatest incidence of diabetes at 25.7% (American Diabetic Association, 2015). By race, diabetes is ranked as the seventh leading cause of death in the United States among Whites, Blacks, Chinese, and Filipinos. Women in the general U.S. population have a higher mortality associated with diabetes than do their male counterparts. In 2007, the age-adjusted death rate for diabetes by race was as follows: Whites, 22.8; Blacks, 50.1; American Indians or Alaska Natives, 50.3; Asians or Pacific Islanders, 18.4; and Hispanics, 33.6 (U.S. Department of Health and Human Services, Health United States, 2014).

It is important to note that the prevalence of diabetes varies according to race and gender. It increases with age and at all ages is highest among African-American women. In 1999, the prevalence of diabetes for African-American women (50.9 per 1000) was twice as high as the rate for their White counterparts (23.4 per 1000) (Mirsa, 2002).

While the Institute of Medicine's report *Unequal Treatment* (Smedley et al., 2003) suggests that ethnic minorities sometimes receive unequal treatment with regard to health care, the report is further illuminating with regard to care for diabetes. Although Blacks, Hispanics, and American Indians have a 50% to 100% higher burden of illness and mortality because of diabetes than their White counterparts, the disease appears to be more profoundly undermanaged among these vulnerable populations. Chin, Zhang, and Merrell (1998) noted that even after adjustment for gender, education, and age, African-Americans were still less likely to undergo measurements of glycosylated Hb, lipid testing, ophthalmologic visits, and influenza vaccinations than their White counterparts. It is even more interesting to note that Blacks with type 2 diabetes are more likely to be treated with insulin as opposed to an oral antihyperglycemic agent than their White or Mexican counterparts (Cowie & Harris, 1997).

There are three types of diabetes: type 1 (formerly referred to as insulin-dependent) diabetes mellitus, type 2 (formerly referred to as non–insulin-dependent diabetes), and gestational diabetes mellitus. Type 1 diabetes has a peak incidence between 10 and 14 years of age, apparently affects boys somewhat more frequently than girls, has a higher incidence in Whites, and accounts for 10% to 20%

of cases (Krolewski & Warram, 2005). The incidence of type 2 diabetes dramatically increases with age, is more frequent in women, has a higher incidence in non-White persons (particularly Hispanics and American Indians), and accounts for 80% to 90% of cases (Carter Center, 1985). Gestational diabetes has been reported in 20% of all pregnant women, increases with maternal age, but is not affected by race or culture (Rifkin, 1984).

Hypertension. The incidence of hypertension has been reported to be significantly higher in African-Americans than in White Americans. The onset by age is earlier in African-Americans, and the hypertension is more severe and is associated with a higher mortality in African-Americans. Studies that demonstrated obvious differences in blood pressure between African-Americans and their White counterparts date back to 1932 (Adams, 1932). Since that time, other studies have also clearly indicated a remarkable difference in blood pressure between African-Americans and individuals of other races (Lerner & Kannel, 1986; Stokes, Kannel, Wolf, Cupples, & D'Agostino, 1987).

In 1972, the National High Blood Pressure Education Program, in concert with the National Heart, Lung, and Blood Institute (NHLBI) of the NIH, was implemented (Joint National Committee, 2003). Up to now, this program has succeeded in its original mission of increasing awareness, prevention, and treatment of hypertension. The trends in awareness, treatment, and control of hypertension have been positive among U.S. adults from 1976 to 1994 (Burt et al., 1995). Data from the Third National Health and Nutrition Examination Survey (NHANES III) (1991–1994) indicate a level of adult public awareness of hypertension that was 68.4% of the total population. Similarly, knowledge of the adult U.S. population regarding treatment of hypertension has increased from 31% (NHANES II, 1976–1980) to 53.6%. Likewise, knowledge of adults in the general U.S. population regarding control of hypertension in that population increased from 10% (NHANES II, 1976–1980) to 27.4% (NHANES III, 1991–1994) (Burt et al., 1995).

For many years, it was postulated that 35% of African-Americans older than 40 years of age are hypertensive (Tipton, 1974). In a study with a random sample of adults 18 to 79 years of age, 9% of non-Blacks and 22% of African-Americans were found to be hypertensive, according to standards set by the World Health Organization, wherein a diastolic blood pressure of 95 mm Hg or greater indicates hypertension (Boyle, 1970). In another study done by the Chicago Health Association, the analysis of the data confirmed previous findings of a higher prevalence of hypertension among African-Americans in all age groups than among White Americans. Further analysis of the data

indicated an equal prevalence of hypertension among both sexes in African-Americans and an increased incidence with advancing age (Merck, Sharp, & Dohme, 1974). However, contrasting opinions indicate that hypertension may occur slightly more often in men than in women (Joint National Committee, 2003).

Data from the 30-year follow-up study to the classic Framingham study indicate that hypertension may be an independent risk factor for coronary heart disease for both men and women between 35 and 64 years of age (Stokes et al., 1987). Other data indicate that the prevalence of hypertension may be highest among Black, non-Hispanic women (National Center for Health Statistics, 2014). In the Maryland Statewide Household Survey of 6425 adults 18 years of age and older, 28.2% of the African-American population showed a prevalence of mild to moderate hypertension (a systolic blood pressure greater than 160 mm Hg and a diastolic blood pressure greater than 95 mm Hg) compared with 20.1% of their White counterparts (Saunders, 1985; State of Maryland, 1984).

Because the traditional terms *mild hypertension* and *moderate hypertension* failed to convey the major influence of high blood pressure as a risk factor for cardiovascular disease (CVD), the Joint National Committee on Detection, Evaluation, and Treatment of High Blood Pressure (2003) attempted to clarify terminology. According to the committee's report, 50 million Americans have elevated blood pressure, which by current definition implies a systolic blood pressure of 140 mm Hg or greater, a diastolic blood pressure of 90 mm Hg or greater, or both (Joint National Committee, 2003). The Joint National Committee (2003) also added new guidelines for prehypertensive status that were absent in prior reports. In May 2003, the seventh report guidelines stated that an individual may be considered prehypertensive if the systolic blood pressure is 120 to 139 mm Hg or the diastolic blood pressure is 80 to 89 mm Hg. Treatment of prehypertension depends on compelling indications. If there are no compelling indications, the Joint National Committee (2003) suggests no antihypertensive drugs. However, in case of compelling indications, including heart failure, post–myocardial infarction, high risk for coronary heart disease, diabetes, chronic kidney disease, and recurrent stroke prevention, the Joint National Committee suggests that drugs to control these compelling indications should also be considered. The committee concluded that the prevalence of hypertension increases with age, is greater in African-Americans than in Whites, is greater in both races in less educated individuals than in more educated individuals, and is especially prevalent and devastating in lower socioeconomic groups (Joint National Committee, 2003). In addition, the data indicate that in young adulthood and early middle age, the prevalence of high blood pressure is greater in men than in women. However, after middle age the reverse is true (Joint National Committee, 2003; Roccella & Lenfant, 1989).

On December 18, 2003, the much anticipated results of the Antihypertensive and Lipid-Lowering Treatment to Prevent Heart Attack Trial (ALLHAT) were finally released. In this clinical trial, more than 40,000 subjects were enrolled. The primary objective of this study was to compare a diuretic (chlorthalidone), an angiotensin-converting enzyme inhibitor (lisinopril), a calcium-channel blocker (amlodipine), and a α-blocker (doxazosin). The findings from this study suggest that thiazide diuretics may now be the initial drug of choice for hypertension, primarily because of their benefits in preventing coronary heart disease and their associated low costs (ALLHAT Officers, 2002a, 2002b). In addition, for patients who are already receiving antihypertensives, findings from ALLHAT suggest that diuretics should be considered concomitantly. Moreover, most clients who have hypertension, particularly African-Americans, will require more than one drug to control blood pressure adequately.

The prevalence for hypertension is also greater by geographical region. For example, both African-Americans and Whites residing in the southeastern United States have a greater propensity for hypertension and a greater rate of stroke-related death as a direct result of the condition than

do African-Americans and Whites residing in other areas of the country (Roccella & Lenfant, 1989). The new classifications for hypertension as proposed by the Joint National Committee (2003) are shown in Box 7-1. As indicated previously, a diagnosis of hypertension is confirmed when systolic blood pressure is consistently 140 mm Hg or greater and diastolic blood pressure is consistently 90 mm Hg or greater (based on the average of two or more readings). Reportedly, as a result of this definition, hypertension is of concern for approximately 50 to 60 million Americans (Joint National Committee, 2003; Walsh, 1993). It is essential to remember that hypertension should never be diagnosed on the basis of a single measurement except when the systolic blood pressure is 210 mm Hg or greater and the diastolic blood pressure is 120 mm Hg, with average levels of diastolic blood pressure of 90 mm Hg or greater and systolic blood pressure levels of 140 mm Hg or greater (Joint National Committee, 2003).

Many individuals who are hypertensive remain symptom-free for a long time; thus, researchers at the NHLBI have estimated that more than 50% of persons with hypertension do not know that they are hypertensive. Hypertension continues to be the major cause of heart failure, kidney failure, aneurysm formation, and congestive heart failure. Primary hypertension is evidenced in 90% of reported cases, whereas only about 10% of reported cases are classified as secondary. The diagnosis for primary

BOX 7-1   Classifications of Hypertension*

Classification for Blood Pressure	SBP, mm Hg[†]	DBP, mm Hg[†]	Drug Therapy without Compelling Indications	Drug Therapy with Compelling Indications
Normal	<120	And <80	No antihypertensive drugs are indicated in this category.	Use drugs for compelling indications.
Prehypertension	120–139	Or 80–89	No antihypertensive drugs are indicated in this category.	Administer drugs for compelling indications.
Stage I hypertension	140–159	Or 90–99	Antihypertensive, including thiazide-type diuretics, for most cases. May also consider ACE inhibitors or drugs such as β-blockers and calcium-channel blockers.	Administer drugs for compelling indications; also consider other antihypertensives (e.g., diuretics, ACE inhibitors).
Stage 2 hypertension	≥160	Or ≥100	Two-drug combination (using both thiazide-type diuretics and ACE inhibitors or drugs such as β-blockers and calcium-channel blockers).	Use drugs for competing indications in addition to other antihypertensives.

ACE, Angiotensin-converting enzyme; DBP, diastolic blood pressure; SBP, systolic blood pressure.
*Excerpted from the Seventh Report of the National Committee on Detection, Evaluation, and Treatment of High Blood Pressure (2003). Bethesda, MD: National Institutes of Health—National Heart, Lung, and Blood Institute.
[†]Treatment determined by highest blood pressure category.

hypertension may be supported when the following risk factors are present:

1. Positive family history
2. Increased sensitivity to the renin-angiotensin system
3. Obesity
4. Hypercholesterolemia
5. Hyperglycemia
6. Smoking
7. Abnormal sodium and water retention

Secondary hypertension is diagnosed when the following causes are present (Walsh, 1993):

1. Coarctation of the aorta
2. Pheochromocytoma (a catecholamine-secreting tumor)
3. Cushing's disease
4. Chronic glomerulonephritis
5. Toxemia from pregnancy
6. Thyrotoxicosis
7. Effects of certain drugs such as contraceptives
8. Collagen disease

Primary hypertension affects more African-Americans than White Americans. The NHANES researchers indicated that in persons 24 to 34 years of age, 3.6% of non-Black men, and 12.5% of African-American men have primary hypertension, as well as 2.3% of non-Black women and 8.6% of African-American women. According to this study, these figures appear to rise steadily with age and at all ages are conspicuously higher in African-Americans. Thus, the overall ratio of incidence of primary hypertension among African-Americans compared with non-Blacks is estimated to be 2:1. In addition, primary hypertension is believed to be more severe for African-Americans regardless of age. The death rate for primary hypertension at all ages up to 85 years is higher in African-Americans than in non-Blacks. It was reported that among men between 24 and 44 years of age, mortality from primary hypertension was 14.8% for African-Americans and 1% for non-Blacks. In this same age group, female mortality from primary hypertension was reported to be 12.3% for African-Americans and 0.8% for non-Blacks (Merck et al., 1974). These data indicate that African-Americans succumb to primary hypertension almost 15 times more often than non-Blacks do. Furthermore, the death rate for hypertension is probably an underestimation. The nurse must be aware of the significant risk factors for hypertension to assist in early detection and continued maintenance and treatment, which can help reduce mortality.

Data indicate that African-Americans have a higher propensity for hypertension (CDC, 1992; Joint National Committee, 2003; Lerner & Kannel, 1986; National Center for Health Statistics, 2014; Stokes et al., 1987). In fact, the prevalence of hypertension among persons 20 years of age

and older was down from 48.1 per 1000 in 1960–1962 to 34.9 from 1988–1994, and back up to 41.4 from 2005–2008 in African-American males as compared with 39.3 in 1960–1962, 24.3 in 1988–1994, and up to 31.5 from 2005–2008 in their White counterparts (National Center for Health Statistics, 2014). African-American women do not fare any better than their male counterparts. The prevalence among African-American women 20 years of age from 1988–1994 was 30.6, down from 50.5 from 1960–1962, but increased to 44.4 from 2005–2008; among White women, the prevalence was 20.4 in 1988–1994, a decrease from 34.9 for 1960–1962, and was slightly up at 28.1 from 2005–2008 (National Center for Health Statistics, 2014). It remains controversial as to whether genetic markers, such as skin color, can be related to hypertension prevalence among African-Americans and other persons with dark skin color (Braithwaite & Taylor, 2001). However, a classic study of African-Americans residing in Charleston, South Carolina, showed a significant association between blood pressure and skin darkness among both men and women (Boyle, 1970). The effect for this study was independent of age but was minimized by consideration of socioeconomic status.

A later but totally different study was done with African-Americans in the population from the same geographical location. Contrary to the earlier study, the data indicated that skin color was not significantly associated with a 15-year incidence of hypertension noted in African-American women over 35 years of age in this geographical location (Keil, 1981). In this study, skin color was measured by a photoelectric reflectometer on the medial aspect of the upper arm. In addition, the effect for the study was independent of socioeconomic status. Both these studies differ remarkably from a study reported by Braithwaite and Taylor (2001) that was conducted in Detroit on African-American men. According to Braithwaite and Taylor (2001), the data from this study indicate that there is a significant relationship between high blood pressure and skin color as measured by subjective coding of skin color of the forehead, between the eyes.

Klag, Whelton, Coresh, Grim, and Kuller (1991) found an association between skin color and systolic and diastolic blood pressures, which were higher in darker skinned persons than that in lighter skinned persons. In the study, 457 African-Americans were surveyed in three U.S. cities by use of a reflectometer to note the intensity of skin color and the correlation with blood pressure. The findings from the study indicate that both systolic and diastolic blood pressures may be higher in darker persons than in lighter ones and increased by 2 mm Hg for every 1–standard deviation increase in skin darkness. However, the association was dependent on socioeconomic status, whether measured by education or on another index consisting of education, occupation, and ethnicity. Significant findings were present only in persons on the lower level of either index (Klag et al., 1991). Using multiple linear regression, the researchers found that both systolic and diastolic blood pressures remained significantly associated with darker skin in the lower socioeconomic status, independent of age and BMI and concentration of blood glucose. The researchers concluded that the findings may be attributed to one of two factors:

1. The inability of such groups to deal with psychosocial stress associated with darker skin *or*
2. An interaction between the environmental factors associated with low socioeconomic status and a susceptible gene that has a higher prevalence in persons with darker skin (Klag et al., 1991)

Regardless of the race of the client, to obtain blood pressure measurements that are representative of the client's usual levels, it is important that the individual be seated with the arm bared, supported, and at heart level. The client should not have smoked or ingested caffeine within 30 minutes before the measurement is taken (Joint National Committee, 2003). If the measurement must be repeated, it should not be taken for at least 5 minutes after the first reading. To ensure an accurate measurement, the appropriate cuff size must be used. In addition, the bladder of the cuff should nearly (at least 80%) or completely encircle the arm (Joint National Committee, 2003).

Sickle Cell Disease. The most common genetic disorder in the United States is SCD, which occurs predominantly in African-Americans. It has been projected that 72,000 African-Americans have SCD. In fact, it is thought that in the United States, approximately 1 in 500 African-Americans and 1 in 1200 Hispanic-Americans are born with SCD. It is also interesting to note that approximately 2 million Americans—including about 10% of the African-American population—carry one gene for SCD, the "sickle cell trait" (Genes and Disease, n.d.).

Sickle cell disease or the trait also occurs in people from Asia Minor, India, the Mediterranean, and the Caribbean area but to a lesser extent than what has been reported in African-Americans. Sickle cell disease is characterized by chronic hemolytic anemia and is a homozygous recessive disorder. In SCD the basic disorder lies within the globin of the Hb, where a single amino acid (valine) is substituted for another (glutamic acid) in the sixth position of the beta chain. It is believed that this single amino acid substitution profoundly alters the properties of the molecule; Hb S is formed instead of normal Hb A as a result of the intermolecular rearrangement. The normal oxygen-carrying capacity of the blood is found in Hb A. As a result of

deoxygenation, however, there is a change in the solubility of protein, which makes the Hb molecules lump together, thereby causing the cell membrane to contract. The result is a sickle cell shape.

The affected cells have a shortened life span of 7 to 20 days, which is profoundly different from the life span of normal cells, which is 105 to 120 days. Hb SA is the heterozygous state and is often an asymptomatic condition referred to as *sickle cell trait.*

Sickle cell disease is believed to have occurred for many years in Africa along the Nile valley as an adaptive disease. In Africa this disorder was believed to produce resistance to malaria transmission by the *Anopheles* mosquito (Williams, 1975). In Africa, SCD or the trait affects approximately 10% of the Black population, and the death rate before 21 years of age has been 100% in those affected with the disease. Before full recognition of the clinical significance of SCD in the United States, the death rate was almost of the same magnitude as that in Africa. Today in the United States, as a result of improved and comprehensive care, as well as early recognition of the crisis of the disease, persons with SCD may live through their third and fourth decades of life.

A differential diagnosis for SCD should be made for all African-American persons who have (1) chronic anemia of undetermined origin; (2) an increased susceptibility to infections; or (3) unexplained attacks of joint, bone, or abdominal pain. Sickle cell disease is diagnosed in the laboratory through a technique called *hemoglobin electrophoresis.* This method provides a definitive diagnosis. In addition, a complete history, including a physical examination and laboratory database, should be done. The laboratory database should include a complete blood cell count with a differential and reticulocyte count, electrolytes, blood urea nitrogen, glucose, direct bilirubin, and urinalysis (Satcher & Pope, 1974). In addition, radiographs of the chest, abdomen, and bones are indicated if there is evidence of pain or fever. However, a bone scan is preferable.

For persons with SCD, the indications for prompt admission to a hospital include the following (Benjamin, Swinson, & Nagel, 2000; Leffall, 1974):

1. Vaso-occlusive pain crisis that does not respond to analgesics within 4 hours of administration
2. Aplastic crisis
3. Splenic sequestration, a life-threatening condition that requires immediate admission to the intensive care unit for continuous observation and therapy
4. Hyperhemolytic crisis, which can occur if the Hb and hematocrit levels continue to drop
5. Infections indicated by a temperature greater than 101° F or a white blood cell count greater than 15,000

cells/L (although viral ear, nose, and throat infections may not indicate admission for pediatric clients)

6. Thromboembolic phenomena in the lungs, cerebrum, and long bones
7. Pregnancy, which indicates an increased risk

A common problem associated with SCD is drug use and abuse. In a classic intervention study, at the Martin Luther King Jr. Hospital, a team of health professionals working through the National Sickle Cell Center was involved in the care of clients with SCD. Their work revealed three kinds of problems (Satcher, 1973):

1. Clients with SCD were typically stereotyped as drug abusers by many health professionals.
2. The delay in seeking medical care during a sickle cell crisis was caused by the client's desire to tolerate pain and avoid drug dependence.
3. Drug abuse in clients with SCD was found in clients with severe and disabling conditions. These clients required drugs so frequently that they often became mentally and physically dependent.

The nurse must be able to identify early signs of sickle cell crisis and teach the client to recognize these symptoms when they occur. The nurse should impress on the client the significance of early recognition and treatment of crisis symptoms. Ongoing surveillance of signs and symptoms of sickle cell crisis can promote appropriate treatment and perhaps prevent early death (Platt et al., 1994).

Systemic Lupus Erythematosus. Systemic lupus erythematosus is a chronic disease of unknown cause that affects organs and systems individually or in a variety of combinations. The disease affects women 8 to 10 times more often than it does men. The age distribution for the disease spans 2 to 97 years. Systemic lupus erythematosus was named after the classic butterfly rash, which is erosive and thus "likened to the damage caused by a hungry wolf" (Hochberg, 1993). This disease was once believed to be relatively rare and always fatal. However, with the advent of better techniques for recognition, the disease is now considered fairly common, and its course can be controlled by corticosteroids. Even today, however, some clients do die as a result of lesions that affect major organs or as a result of secondary infections. Although the cause of the disease is still unknown, three major causative factors are being investigated: (1) an aberration of the immune system that causes immune complexes containing antibodies to be deposited in tissue, which in turn causes tissue damage; (2) a viral infection that is caused by or results from some immunological abnormality; and (3) the combination of the first two factors. In addition, some drugs are known to induce lupus-like syndromes, including procainamide

(Pronestyl), isonicotinic acid hydrazide (INH, isoniazid), and penicillin (Hochberg, 1993).

As previously indicated, SLE was believed to be a rare disease. However, because of sophisticated detection procedures, researchers now postulate that this is not so—its incidence has been estimated to be 2.6 per 100,000 population. Although it occurs more frequently in African-Americans than in non-Blacks, it is reported to be extremely rare among the Asian population.

The nurse who understands that signs and symptoms of arthritis may indicate SLE, especially when combined with weakness, fatigue, and weight loss, can assist in early detection. In addition, the nurse should look for symptoms of sensitivity to sunlight, including development of a rash or symptoms of fever or arthritis as a result of exposure to sunlight. The butterfly lesions of SLE generally appear over the cheeks and bridge of the nose. These lesions are often bright red and may extend beyond the hairline, thus causing alopecia (loss of hair), particularly above the ears. Lesions may also be noted on the neck and may spread slowly to the mucous membranes and other tissues of the body. These lesions generally do not ulcerate; however, they do cause degeneration and atrophy of tissues. Other clinical findings may also be present, depending on the organs involved, including glomerulonephritis, pleuritis, pericarditis, peritonitis, neuritis, and anemia. The most severe manifestations of SLE are renal and neurological in nature.

Laboratory tests used to diagnose SLE may need to be specific to the organs involved, such as proteinuria, abnormal cerebrospinal fluid, or radiographic evidence of pleural reactions. Before the advent of the lupus erythematosus (LE)-cell preparation, or what is commonly called the LE-cell test, the diagnosis was based on the presentation of the butterfly rash and systemic complications; the disease was generally fatal. However, as a result of the LE-cell test and other sensitive tests, including the antinuclear antibody or the antinuclear factor test, clients with more varied symptoms have been confirmed earlier. Thus, through early detection, appropriate treatment has been initiated. Client teaching by the nurse should include instructions on the need for appropriate exercise, appropriate balance of rest and activity, and the necessity of avoiding direct exposure to sunlight. As indicated earlier, SLE has a higher prevalence among some racial groups, and the nurse who recognizes the biocultural significance of the disease is more apt to give culturally appropriate nursing care.

AIDS. One fact that is emerging with clarity is the increasing incidence of acquired immunodeficiency syndrome (AIDS) among African-Americans and Hispanics. In the United States, 1 of every 8 Americans is African-American, but among Americans with AIDS, 1 of every 4

is African-American. These numbers reflect the fact that 24% of the total AIDS cases reported thus far involve African-American persons. In the United States, 1 of every 12 Americans is Hispanic, but 1 of every 7 Americans with AIDS is Hispanic (CDC, HIV/AIDS Surveillance Report, 2013).

From June 1981 through December 2013, there were 1,870,000 reported cases of AIDS in the United States (CDC, HIV/AIDS Surveillance Report 2013). Of this number, 757,740 cases have occurred in men, whereas 185,560 have been reported in women (CDC, HIV/AIDS Surveillance Report, 2013).

Of the number of reported cases of AIDS, 436,557 were Whites, 497,267 were Blacks, 215,685 were Hispanics, 10,567 were Asian/Pacific Islanders; and 3514 were American Indians/Alaska Natives. Similarly, of the number of reported AIDS cases among women in the United States through December 2013, 30,854 were in Whites, 84,681 were in Blacks, 28,554 were in Hispanics, 803 were in Asians/Pacific Islanders, and 480 were in American Indians/Alaska Natives (CDC, HIV/AIDS Surveillance Report, 2013).

While women represented just 17% of the total AIDS cases, this figure nearly doubles to 28% of all HIV cases. Proportionately, heterosexual women and in particular heterosexual African-American women continued to be the fastest growing segment of the population to be diagnosed with AIDS. In addition, proportionately by population size, African-Americans continue to be infected by HIV at a disproportionately high rate (CDC, HIV/AIDS Surveillance Report, 2013). In fact, over the past decade AIDS has moved ahead of CVD to become the leading cause of death among African-Americans 25 to 44 years of age (CDC, HIV/AIDS Surveillance Report 2013).

Of the number of pediatric cases reported in the United States through December 2013 that involve children under 13 years of age, 1579 were in Whites, 5337 were in Blacks, 1876 were in Hispanics, 54 were in Asians, 31 were in American Indians, and 16 were in persons of unknown races (CDC, HIV/AIDS Surveillance Report, 2013). Although these numbers are alarming, they do not accurately reflect the full scope of this widespread problem in the United States. It is estimated that the data available on reported cases of AIDS indicate that the prevalence of AIDS in the United States is so widespread that 1 of every 300 Americans has AIDS, representing 0.3% of the total population (CDC, HIV/AIDS Surveillance Report, 2013). Yet, by 2008, while all state where moving toward name-based reporting, only 28 states had initiated an integrated name-based reporting system for HIV and AIDS. These states include the following:

- Alabama
- Alaska
- Arizona
- Arkansas
- Colorado
- Connecticut
- Florida
- Georgia
- Idaho
- Indiana
- Louisiana
- Michigan
- Minnesota
- Mississippi
- Missouri
- Nebraska
- Nevada
- New Hampshire
- New Jersey
- North Dakota
- Ohio
- Oklahoma
- South Carolina
- South Dakota
- Tennessee
- Texas
- Utah
- Virginia

In 2013, the top five leading metropolitan areas reporting the highest number of AIDS cases are New York City (126,237), Los Angeles (43,488), Miami (25,357), San Francisco (28,438), and Washington, DC (24,844) (CDC, HIV/AIDS Surveillance, 2013).

From June 1981 through December 2007, 597,499 people succumbed to AIDS or AIDS-related conditions in the United States. This number includes 571,453 adults and adolescents and 4931 children less than 13 years of age (CDC, HIV/AIDS Surveillance, 2013). Of the total number of patients who died in 2007 alone (18,089), 4501 were White, 8041 were Black, 2882 were Hispanic, 100 were Asian/Pacific Islander, and 70 were American Indian/Alaska Native (CDC, HIV/AIDS Surveillance, 2013).

Glucose-6-Phosphate Dehydrogenase

Another enzyme-deficiency disorder that is more prevalent in certain racial or ethnic groups is G-6-PD deficiency. Although this disorder is more prevalent in certain groups, these groups may have different forms of the deficiency. Williams (1975) reported that the type A variety, which moves rapidly on starch-gel electrophoresis, is found in 35% of African-Americans who have the deficiency. The slow-moving type B variety is found in 65% of Blacks who have the deficiency and in nearly all non-Blacks who have the deficiency. However, all forms affect males more than females because the genetic inheritance is carried on the X chromosome. The Cantonese Chinese disorder of G-6-PD has been found among the Chinese and the people of Southeast Asia. The incidence of the Cantonese Chinese form ranges from 2% to 5% (Williams, 1975). Still another form of G-6-PD deficiency is the Mediterranean variety, which is the most clinically severe type. This form of G-6-PD deficiency affects up to 50% of male Greeks, Sardinians, and Sephardic Jews.

An enzyme constituent of the red blood cells, G-6-PD is involved in the hexose monophosphate pathway, which accounts for 10% of glucose metabolism of the red blood cells (Luzzatto & Poggi, 2008). Under normal circumstances the proportion of glucose metabolized through this pathway may increase greatly if the cells are subjected to oxidants causing metabolic stress. The result is the formation of increased methemoglobin and degradation of Hb. In addition, certain medications tend to overwhelm the protective mechanism, especially when older red blood cells are involved, because of a decline in G-6-PD activity with the aging of these cells. Red blood cells with a genetically determined deficiency of G-6-PD are unable to withstand lesser oxidative stresses, and as a result a hemolytic process ensues that precipitates a significant anemia.

In the presence of certain conditions, G-6-PD–deficient red blood cells hemolyze, resulting in hemolytic anemia. Conditions that precipitate hemolytic anemia in susceptible persons include the administration of certain drugs, such as quinine, aspirin, phenacetin, chloramphenicol, probenecid, sulfonamides, and thiazide diuretics. The presence of infection and the ingestion of fava beans (also called "broad beans" or "horse beans") are also linked to the precipitous onset of hemolytic anemia. The fava bean is a dietary staple in some of the Mediterranean countries, such as Greece, and those of northern Africa. Favism, a condition induced by ingestion of the fava bean, is one of the most severe forms of G-6-PD hemolysis (Schuurman, van Waardenburg, DaCosta, Niemarkt, & Leroy, 2009). In addition, G-6-PD deficiency has been related to an adaptive process that prevents malaria. The discerning nurse should assist the client in identifying substances that are likely to precipitate hemolytic episodes. In addition, the client should be taught to exercise caution to prevent serious infections. Until an exposure occurs, G-6-PD deficiency is a condition that remains asymptomatic. The nurse must understand that hemolytic episodes are the result of culturally related nutritional habits and geographical and environmental location.

Nutritional Preferences and Deficiencies

Another category of differences among cultural groups is nutritional preferences and deficiencies.

Nutritional Preferences. Nutritional preferences include habits and patterns. When it comes to food choices, people are creatures of habit. The term *habit* connotes inflexibility, although people do change their habits for many reasons. The term *food patterns* is more descriptive of food choices. Many factors are associated with the formation of food patterns and preferences. Food patterns are developed during childhood as a result of family lifestyle and ethnic or cultural, social, religious, geographical, economic, and psychological components. All of these variables influence an individual's attitudes, feelings, and beliefs about certain foods. However, the paramount factors that seem to determine food choices are cultural and ethnic in nature. Adults in a particular culture set the tone for cultural food patterns, which establish the foundation for a child's lifelong eating customs regarding the timing of meals, the number of meals per day, foods acceptable for specific meals, methods of preparation, dislikes and likes, and table manners. Over time, children develop a sense of stability and security in regard to certain food patterns and attitudes.

Schwerin, Stanton, and Smith (1982) indicated that people exhibit distinct patterns of consuming foods in different combinations or forms and that for the most part these patterns have remained constant. For example, many southern Americans would routinely choose grits as a food but would not routinely choose lentils. However, American diets have become more homogeneous because of many factors, including transportation, advertising, mobility, economic status, methods of production, and appreciation of other people's cultural heritage (Katz, Hediger, & Valleroy, 1974; Pangborn, 1975; Riggs, 1980; Saldana & Brown, 1984).

Some people, based on their culture, have not been traditionally known to make food choices solely on the basis of the nutritional and health values of food. For example, one of the most nutritious vegetables is broccoli; however, broccoli ranks twenty-first among vegetables consumed in the United States. On the other hand, the tomato, which is the most commonly eaten vegetable in the United States, ranks sixteenth as a source of vitamins and minerals (Farb & Armelagos, 1980).

When people relocate, they carry established food habits to the new location, but these habits are retained only if the foods are available in the new location and are affordable. Foods in various cultures have different prestige or status. For example, beef and certain seafoods, such as lobster, are regarded as high-status foods among people in the United States. Hindus from India consider cows to be sacred and therefore do not eat beef. In seafaring countries, seafoods have no status value because they are common. Foods obtain their status rating from various factors, including religious beliefs, availability, cost, cultural values, and traditions, or because a highly respected individual has endorsed them. Even today, in many cultures men and their opinions regarding food preferences are more highly regarded than women and their opinions. In fact, in certain cultures men are so highly regarded that they are served meals first, before women and children. As a result of this practice, women and children may receive insufficient quantities and fewer varieties of food.

Food also has symbolic meaning, in some cultures, that has nothing to do with nutritional value. In these cultures eating becomes associated with sentiments and assumptions about oneself and the world. Food becomes symbolic to people not only because of religious connotations but also because it can be used as a reward. For example, a mother who gives a child candy or ice cream as a reward for good behavior may be reinforcing that food as a good food. On the other hand, a mother who serves a particular food (such as broccoli or cabbage) and says she is doing so because of bad behavior may be reinforcing that food as a bad food or punishment.

Food patterns and nutrition among African-Americans. Food patterns among African-Americans are not significantly different from those of non–African-Americans living in the same geographical area. However, distinct differences do exist for African-Americans living and raised in the North as compared with those in the South. African-Americans, as a cultural group, are in the low socioeconomic groups, which may precipitate nutritional problems. As a result of nutritional deficiencies, African-Americans tend to have medical problems that are somewhat different from those of White Americans. As mentioned earlier, hypertension is a medical problem that is twice as great in African-Americans as in White Americans. Another medical problem, particularly in women, that has been

linked to food patterns and selections is obesity. Soul foods, which are generally cooked for long periods and well-seasoned, may also contribute to many of the medical problems that African-Americans encounter. Soul foods, which have their roots in southern African-Americans who saw their preparation as economical, are listed in Table 7-1.

A cultural pattern that has been established among African-American pregnant women is the consumption of nonfood items (pica), which supposedly originated because of nutritional needs. Another common practice among children under 3 years of age, pregnant women, and some men is the eating of earthy substances such as dirt or clay. This practice is known as geophagy and is practiced mainly in lower socioeconomic groups. For many years in African society, the biological need for calcium, iron, and other minerals, especially by pregnant and lactating women, was partially met by eating clays that were high in nutrients. An analysis of some clays has revealed significant amounts of calcium, magnesium, potassium, copper, zinc, and iron, which are the same substances that have been prescribed for pregnant and lactating women in modern societies (Davidhizar & Giger, 2008). Africans who were brought to the United States as slaves continued to eat clay, which is still bought in some areas of the South and shipped to relatives in the North. However, geophagy leads to iron deficiency, mainly because clay inhibits the absorption of iron, potassium, and zinc (Halsted, 1968). It is believed that geophagy is both a cause and a consequence of anemia. In areas where clay is not readily available, laundry starch is sometimes substituted, although it can irritate the stomach and is almost completely lacking in valuable minerals.

There are many clinical implications for the nurse in meeting the nutritional needs of African-Americans, who normally have lower Hb and hematocrit levels than non–African-Americans have (Orkins et al., 2009). Although

TABLE 7-1	Foods Enjoyed by African-Americans		
Name of Food	**Region**	**Type of Food**	**Description**
Poke salad	Southern U.S.	Young shoots of pokeweed	Prepared with spicy seasoning and fatback
Collard greens	Southern U.S.	Garden raised	Prepared with spicy seasoning and fatback
Fatback	Southern U.S.	Pork fat	Prepared from loin of pig
Chicken wings	Southern U.S.	Chicken	Prepared by frying with spicy seasoning
Chitterlings	Southern U.S.	Meat	Intestines of young pigs that are boiled or fried
Hog maws	Southern U.S.	Meat	Stomach of pig
Grits	Southern U.S.	Grain	Hulled and coarsely ground corn that is boiled and simmered
Hoppin' John	Southern U.S.	Combination	Black-eyed peas and rice
Dandelion	Southern U.S.	Wild greens	Prepared with a spicy seasoning and fatback
Ribs	Southern U.S.	Pork	Prepared with spicy seasoning and slow heat

these lower Hb and hematocrit levels are believed to be partially caused by genetics, some studies suggest that nutritional factors may also be responsible (Jackson, Sauberlich, Skala, Kretsch, & Nelson, 1983).

Another clinical implication for the nurse who cares for African-Americans is that of lactose intolerance. Many African-Americans are lactose-intolerant but can tolerate such milk products as buttermilk, yogurt, fermented cheese, and small quantities of milk. In addition, certain nutrients known to be low in the African-American diet include iron, calcium, and vitamin A.

Another clinical implication for African-Americans is the high incidence of hypertension, which may necessitate a low-sodium diet. Because African-Americans habitually use large amounts of salt and other spicy seasonings, special attention must be given to the importance of seasoning foods to make them acceptable and at the same time limiting the use of salt.

Food patterns and nutrition among Puerto Ricans. Many Puerto Ricans, like persons from other Latin American cultures, subscribe to the theory of "hot" and "cold." The major difference for Puerto Ricans is that they classify diseases as hot and cold and foods and medications as hot, cold, and cool. Both Indian and Spanish influences are reflected in Puerto Rican native dishes (Table 7-2).

The common fare of Puerto Ricans is rice, cooked grainy and dried, and red or white beans stewed with bacon or olive oil, garlic, and onions. Another common fare is *safrito*, which is a tasty mixture of tomatoes, green peppers, sweet chili peppers, onions, garlic, oregano, and fresh coriander cooked in lard or vegetable oil and used as a relish to season foods. Other foods eaten regularly in Puerto Rico include *viandas* (a starchy vegetable dish consisting of plantains, sweet potatoes, and green bananas), cassava, breadfruit, *acerola*, mango, avocado, corn, okra, chayotes, and tubers. The acerola, which is also called the "West Indian" or "Barbados cherry," is the highest known source of vitamin C. The acerola contains 1000 mg (1 g) of vitamin C per 100-g portion. Many of the food items that are common in the United States are very expensive because they have to be imported. Chicken, pork, and beef, which are normally fried, are usually limited in the diet because of their cost. Eggs are generally used as the main dish and may be served as omelets. Milk is a very popular food item in Puerto Rico but is seldom drunk as a beverage. The intake of milk is believed to be low in Puerto Rico because of its cost. A popular beverage is *cafe con leche*, which is a combination of coffee with 2 to 5 ounces of milk. This beverage constitutes the largest portion of milk that is consumed. For the most part, foods are cooked for very long periods, or they are fried. Lard and salt pork are commonly used to flavor many dishes. One food item that has an exaggerated reputation for being nutritious and is often given to children and lactating women is malt beer.

There are many clinical implications for the nurse in meeting the nutritional needs of Puerto Ricans. Pregnant Puerto Rican women have a high incidence of megaloblastic anemia and therefore should be instructed to increase their intake of foods high in folic acid (Parker & Bowering, 1976). For the client who needs to control carbohydrate intake, the nurse should instruct the client about the necessity of counting *viandas* as bread exchanges. The nurse must also be aware that the diet of Puerto Ricans who have moved to mainland cities may lack variety because of the inability of some Puerto Ricans to afford the native island foods that they were accustomed to getting previously. Therefore, the nurse and the client should look for acceptable food items that are comparable in health value.

Food patterns and nutrition among Cubans. A major portion of the Cuban diet includes cut-up vegetables, stews, and casseroles that have been flavored with sage, parsley, bay leaves, thyme, cinnamon, curry powder, capers, onions, cloves, garlic, and saffron. An integral part of Cuban food preparation is saffron, which is so heavily used in the Cuban diet that some dishes are considered anemic looking and unpalatable unless they have a deep golden saffron hue. Chicken, fish, or meat soup is served at least once a day, before each major meal. Salad is also served

TABLE 7-2 Foods Enjoyed by Puerto Ricans

Name of Food	Type of Food	Description
Acerola	Fruit	Barbados cherry (*Malpighia* and *Bunchosia* species)
Arroz blanco	Grain	Enriched white rice
Bacalao	Meat	Salted codfish
San cocho	Combination	Soup prepared with meat and viandas
Safrito	Seasoning	Specially treated tomato sauce
Viandas	Vegetable	Starchy tropical vegetable dish that includes plantains, green bananas, and sweet potatoes

every day, along with fried foods, especially fish, poultry, and eggs. Most Cuban people eat rice and beans of many different varieties. Although fruits and vegetables are plentiful, most Cuban refugees do not consume fruits and vegetables on a regular basis (Gorden, 1982). The typical breakfast of Cuban people consists of coffee and bread. Some Cuban adults drink a lot of strong coffee and rum. Foods enjoyed by Cubans include the following:

Name of Food	Type of Food	Description
Guava	Fruit	Small yellow or red sweet tropical fruit
Plantains	Fruit	Banana-like fruit that tastes like sweet potatoes and is boiled or fried

There are many clinical implications for the nurse in meeting the nutritional needs of Cuban people. The nurse should be aware that in most Cuban diets calcium intake is normally low; therefore, the nurse should instruct the client to incorporate some cheese and milk into the diet. In addition, the nurse should advise the client to replace frying foods with other methods of food preparation, such as boiling or broiling. In addition, the client should be advised that long cooking periods for some foods, such as pork, are beneficial.

Food patterns and nutrition among American Indians. A problem for American Indians living on reservations that is as prevalent today as it was in the past is food scarcity and a lack of food variety. For American Indians, fresh fruits, vegetables, and meats are very expensive, if they are available at all. Traditional foods may vary among tribes; however, the basic diet of American Indians consists of corn, beans, and squash. A status food for most tribes is corn. Chili pepper is widely used among tribes because it adds spice to the diet and is considered to be a good source of vitamin C. On some reservations and particularly among some tribes, diets are considered to be very poor, supplying less than two thirds of the recommended daily allowances for one or more nutrients (Miller, 1981). The diets tend to be inadequate in calories, calcium, iron, iodine, riboflavin, and vitamins A and C (Owens, Garry, Seymore, Harrison, & Acosta, 1981).

Poor nutrition has been directly related to several leading causes of death among American Indians, including heart disease and cirrhosis of the liver. Diabetes is three times more common among some American Indian tribes than in the general U.S. population (Miller, 1981). American Indians have the highest reported prevalence of type 2 diabetes mellitus. In the Pima tribe, hyperinsulinemia

reflects a resistance to insulin action (Nagulesparan, Savage, & Knowler, 1982). Among some American Indian tribes, low Hb values and mild thyroid deficiencies are prevalent (Interdepartmental Commission, 1964) (Table 7-3).

There are many clinical implications for the nurse in meeting the nutritional needs of American Indians. The nurse must recognize that the diets of most American Indian tribes tend to be inadequate in protein, calcium, and vitamins C and A, which may result from unavailability or economics. Another problem found among American Indian tribes is the prevalence of lactose deficiency. The nurse should advise the client to consume nonmilk foods that are high in calcium and riboflavin.

Food patterns and nutrition among the Japanese. Most Japanese dishes are ideally suited for American life because they are economical and nutritious. Japanese people take great pride in the visual effect of foods that they prepare. In the Japanese culture, the arrangement of food, color contrasts, and even shape are considered to be as important as the cooking and seasoning of a particular food. In addition, the rules for picking up chopsticks, holding bowls and teacups, and eating soups are traditions that are well established and regularly observed. These traditional rules of etiquette are as important to the Japanese people as the preparation of the food.

Most of the foods are cooked on a hibachi (a small earthen grill) by broiling, steaming, and stir-frying. It is thought by the Japanese that stir-frying preserves vitamins because the food is cooked only briefly. Meat, which is very expensive in Japan, is stretched with vegetables. Fish is used in some fascinating ways, such as being served raw. Soybean products, which are considered an important source of protein, and tofu are common fare of the Japanese people. In the Japanese culture, salads are rarely served with meals, and bread is often replaced by rice or noodles. The Japanese people have a tendency to use extraordinary flavors when cooking, such as wheat germ powder, which is called *aji-no-moto*. Another important seasoning in Japanese cooking is soy sauce. The common beverages included in the Japanese diet among adults are unsweetened green tea (which is the national beverage), beer, and *sake* (rice wine). Milk is often included in the children's diet in the Japanese culture but is rarely used by adults (Table 7-4).

There are many clinical implications for the nurse in meeting the nutritional needs of the Japanese people. A common clinical problem found among the Japanese people is lactose intolerance. In working with a Japanese client, the nurse should advise the client to consume sources of calcium other than milk, such as tofu. The nurse should also advise the client to use enriched rice and to avoid washing the grains before cooking to preserve the nutrient value. When working with a Japanese client who

TABLE 7-3   Foods Enjoyed by American Indians

Name of Food	Type of Food	Description
Acorns (from some oak trees)	Nut	Leached-out paste
Amaranth	Vegetable, cereal	Leaves, seeds
American lotus	Vegetable	Kernels, tuber
Arrowhead (*Sagittaria*)	Vegetable	Tuber
Arrowroot (*Maranta*)	Vegetable	Tuber
Basswood	Vegetable	Buds, flowers
Cattail shoots	Vegetable, salad	Spikes, pollen
Chicory	Cooked salad	Young leaves
Dandelion	Salad	Leaves
Ginseng (American ginseng)	Vegetable	Roots
Groundnut	Vegetable	Tuber
Jack-in-the-pulpit	Vegetable	Long-term roasted corn
Jerusalem artichoke	Vegetable	Tuber
Jícama	Vegetable	Tuber
Nettle (collected with gloves)	Vegetable	Cooked shoots
Pawpaw	Pie, pudding	Fruit
Pigweed	Vegetable	Tops of leaves
Pine nuts (piñons)	Nuts	Nuts in pinecones of neoza pine, stone pine, and piñon
Pokeweed	Vegetable	Boiled sprouts, boiled roots
Prickly pear (Spanish tuna)	Fruit	Red fruit of cactus
Rose salad	Jelly	Fruit high in vitamin C
Smartweed (knotweed)	Salad	Leaves
Sorrel	Salad	Leaves
Sumac (smooth sumac)	Beverage	Steeped berries
Violet	Vegetable	Leaves, entire plant
Watercress	Salad	Leaves
Wild ginger	Vegetable	Root
Yucca salad	Vegetable	Flowers, pods

TABLE 7-4   Foods Enjoyed by the Japanese

Name of Food	Type of Food	Description
Ajinomoto	Seasoning	Refined from wheat gluten
Sake	Beverage	Rice wine
Sashimi	Fish	Raw fish
Shoyu	Seasoning	Soy sauce
Tempura	Combination	Deep-fried seafoods and vegetables
Tofu (Chinese dòfu)	Vegetable	Soybean curds

is on a sodium-restricted diet, the nurse should teach the client to measure the amount of soy sauce used and to avoid eating the many types of pickles that are ordinarily eaten. Another important clinical implication the nurse should remember is the high incidence of stomach cancer among Japanese people, which has been associated with their high intake of raw fish (Qureshi, 1981). Eating raw fish is believed to carry the risk of infestation with fish tapeworms (Goldman, 1985) and has been associated with outbreaks of gastroenteritis (Morse, Guzewich, & Hanrahan, 1986).

Food patterns and nutrition among Koreans. Just as in other Asian cultures, the main staple of the Korean diet is rice, which is mixed with other grains. Korean people generally mix rice with barley, millet, and red beans because it is believed that a diet consisting of only white rice causes health problems. Most Korean people eat three meals daily, which are of equal proportions. Before cooking, foods are cut into small pieces to facilitate the use of chopsticks. Soups containing seaweed, meat, or fish are always served. One of the most popular condiments in Korea is ginseng; Korean people believe that ginseng has roots resembling the human fetus, is a panacea for curing illnesses regardless of age or sex, and is a supposed aphrodisiac.

Korea is surrounded on three sides by water; thus, fish products are plentiful and account for 85% of the nation's animal protein intake. Almost every conceivable kind of fish is served, whether raw, freshly steamed, or salted and dried. One of the most expensive food items in Korea is eggs because they are scarce. The preferred meat of Koreans is beef, which is prepared by marinating, with lots of sugar to provide a crispy coating.

Kimchi involves one of the most nutritious preservative processes available in Korea and does not require refrigeration. *Kimchi* is prepared with chopped vegetables that are highly seasoned, salted, and fermented underground or in a special earthenware container. *Kimchi* can also be prepared from naturally grown vegetables such as cabbage, turnips, cucumbers, and other seasonable vegetables that are soaked in salt water overnight and seasoned the next day with garlic, scallions, ginger, and hot pepper. *Kimchi* is fermented without disturbance for at least 1 month and is best after 2 or 3 months.

Many vegetables are grown in Korea; thus, Koreans serve both fresh vegetables and *kimchi* routinely. Vegetables are never overcooked and are seasoned with red and black pepper, garlic, sesame seed oil, and soy sauce. Because Korea is surrounded by water on three sides, seaweed is plentiful and is a food item highly prized for its nutritive value. In the Korean culture, seaweed is a must for the expectant mother. Another common fare in Korea is noodles made from rice flour. A Korean diet includes many products made from soybeans, such as soy sauce, soybean paste, bean sprouts, bean curds, and soybean milk. The dairy products of Korea include bean curd and soybean milk. Because Korea is a densely populated country, there is no room for a dairy industry; thus, milk is very expensive and scarce and is served only to children. Because milk is so scarce, babies are often weaned from the breast as late as 2 years of age.

Fresh fruits are readily available in Korea and include apples, peaches, strawberries, pears, watermelons, blackberries, pomegranates, currants, and cherries. Fruit is generally served with each meal. Pastries such as cakes and pies are usually not served with meals; however, they can be found in many small specialty shops.

The national beverage of Korea is made from ginseng; Korea has never been a tea-drinking nation. Another beverage that usually accompanies a Korean meal is barley water, which is served cold in the summer and warm in the winter. Barley water is prepared with grains that stick to the pan after the rice for the meal has been removed. A cup or two of water is added to this rice, and the liquid is allowed to simmer slowly while the meal is being eaten; it is then served after the meal. Foods enjoyed by Korean people include the following:

Name of Food	Type of Food	Description
Barley water	Beverage	Prepared from leftover rice grains
Ginseng	Condiment	Spice
Kimchi	Combination	Vegetables that are highly seasoned, salted, and fermented underground for 1 to 3 months

There are many clinical implications for the nurse in meeting the nutritional needs of Korean people. Up to now, the medicinal properties of ginseng have been poorly researched, and information is extremely dated (Barna, 1985). However, it is believed that the long-term abuse of ginseng may be a contributing factor to hypertension. Less frequent adverse reactions from the long-term abuse of ginseng include nervousness, sleeplessness, skin eruptions, morning diarrhea, edema (Siegel, 1979), and irregularities in blood glucose levels (Ginseng, 1980). The nurse who works with Korean-American clients must remember that in the United States rice is not commonly mixed with other grains, as is practiced in Korea. To increase the nutritional value of rice, the client should use whole-grain or enriched rice.

Because Korean people are accustomed to the taste of seaweed, which is expensive, the nurse should encourage the client to substitute stronger tasting greens such as turnip greens, kale, and mustard greens. Lactose intolerance is a common problem among adults in Korea. Thus, the nurse should encourage the client to substitute other dairy products for fresh milk, such as cottage cheese, yogurt, and aged cheese, as well as the nondairy product tofu. For a diabetic Korean client, a sugar substitute may be dissolved in hot water and poured over meat that is broiled until the crispy texture has been achieved (Maras & Adolphi, 1985). Although *kimchi* is a zesty accompaniment to plain, broiled foods, it is not readily available in the United States; therefore, a Mexican salsa may be used as a substitute (Maras & Adolphi, 1985).

Food patterns and nutrition among Middle Easterners. The Middle East is composed of nine separate countries around the eastern Mediterranean Sea: Greece, Turkey, Lebanon, Syria, Iraq, Iran, Israel, Jordan, and Egypt. These countries are bound together by foods and certain attitudes about foods. The common staples of Middle Eastern people are lamb and goat. Because of the climate and the lack of suitable pasture land, beef is uncommon in the Middle Eastern countries. In most Middle Eastern countries, *dolma*, a popular meat dish, is often served. *Dolma* is made of ground meat mixed with rice, herbs, and spices and then wrapped in leaves or stuffed in vegetables. Because many of these countries are contiguous to the eastern Mediterranean seaboard, all varieties of saltwater and freshwater fish, shellfish, and roe are served. In some of the Mediterranean countries bound by religious tradition, some foods are restricted. For example, many Muslims avoid eating pork and wild birds; the main dish of the Muslim people is vegetables and legumes.

For most Middle Eastern people, bread is the staple of life; for every mouthful of food, most Middle Easterners eat a mouthful of bread (Valassi, 1962). A meal without bread is unthinkable for most Middle Eastern people. Bread is generally homemade, fresh, and warm, and the more compact dark bread is preferred to refined white bread. *Pilaf* is a festive dish that is served throughout the Middle East. Other common fares of Middle Eastern countries include beans and lentils, which rank directly behind bread and rice.

In the Middle East, boiled beans are served cold with olive oil dressing and lemon juice. In addition, a variety of vegetables, both cooked and raw, are served. Seasonings commonly used by Middle Easterners in food preparation include onions, fresh tomato paste, olive oil, and parsley. There are more than 120 ways of preparing eggplant, which is a favorite of most Middle Easterners.

Baklava is one of the most popular sweets in the Middle East. However, sweets are generally served only on holidays or during social calls. Unlike Americans, Middle Easterners seldom serve sweets as dessert. Instead, a bowl of fresh fruit consisting of cucumbers, guavas, mangos, citrus fruits, dates, figs, pomegranates, or bananas is the usual dessert. Cooking fats used in Middle Eastern cooking include olive and sesame oils, butter, and ghee, which is a clarified butter made from goat's, sheep's, or camel's milk. Middle Easterners use animal fat to cook foods when the dish is to be eaten hot and oils when the dish is to be eaten cold. Meals are not considered tasteful and well prepared unless a large quantity of fat is used. Popular spices in the Middle East include mint, oregano, and cinnamon. The most popular herb is garlic. The exception to this is found in Iran, where garlic is considered vulgar. Olives in many shapes and colors are popular.

Milk is not commonly served to adults; however, it is given to children. Yogurt is considered a supreme health food that cures many ills, confers long life and good looks, prolongs youth, and fortifies the soul. Yogurt is served in many foods; for example, it is mixed with diced cucumbers and is used as a topping for rice, fried vegetables, and desserts. Thin yogurt that has been diluted with water is considered safer, less perishable, and more thirst-quenching than milk. A specialty cheese served by Greek people is feta, a white cheese made from sheep's or goat's milk.

Wine is a forbidden drink in the Muslim faith, Islam. Other than Christians and Jews, many Near Easterners do not drink alcoholic beverages of any kind. Every meal ends with coffee or tea; however, coffee takes precedence most of the time. The exception to this is found in Iran, where the favorite drink is tea served hot and sweet (Table 7-5).

There are many clinical implications for the nurse in working with people from the Middle East. Because fresh milk is not normally consumed by adults from most Middle Eastern countries, the protein and calcium content

TABLE 7-5 Foods Enjoyed by Middle Easterners

Name of Food	Culture	Type of Food	Description
Baklava	Greek	Dessert	Layered pastry made with honey
Bulgur	Middle Eastern	Grain	Granular wheat product with nutlike flavor
Dolmades (*dholmadhes*)	Greek	Combination	Grape leaves stuffed with beef
Feta	Greek	Dairy product	Soft, salty, white cheese made from sheep's or goat's milk
Kibbeh	Middle Eastern	Meat	Fresh, raw lamb, ground and seasoned, similar to meatloaf
Moussaka	Greek	Combination	Meat and eggplant casserole
Phyllo	Greek	Grain	Paper-thin pastry for meat, vegetable, cheese, and egg dishes and pastries

of the diet must be increased. The nurse should encourage the Middle Eastern client to substitute yogurt for fresh milk because yogurt is a favorite of most Middle Easterners. White cheese, cottage cheese, and aged sharp cheese can also be substituted for fresh milk. For the client on a carbohydrate-restricted diet, the nurse must remember that bread should be restricted or eliminated from the diet because it is high in carbohydrates. The elimination of bread from the diet of persons in cultures where bread is a main staple is difficult. However, the nurse must stress to the client the importance of reducing carbohydrate intake. Because fat is used in large quantities to add taste to meals, the amount of fat in the diet could pose problems for clients on low-calorie, diabetic, or low-fat diets. For clients using sodium-restricted diets, feta cheese and olives should be eliminated from the diet.

Nutritional Deficiencies. Racially related nutritional deficiencies include lactose intolerance. Lactose intolerance, or intolerance to milk, is a relatively common condition considered normal in many ethnic groups. It is found in more than 66% of Mexican Americans and is very common in African-Americans, some American Indian tribes, Asians, and Ashkenazi Jews (Bayless, 1975; Burns & Neubort, 1984; Kisch, 1953). In fact, it has been reported in approximately 90% of adult African Blacks and 79% of African-Americans, American Indians, and Asians. Although lactose intolerance is very common among these racial groups, it is reported to be much less common among Whites of northern European descent; only 5% to 15% of this population have the disorder. Yet the statistical significance reported among Whites of northern European descent indicates that this condition is more than a rare phenomenon.

The cause of lactose intolerance is an insufficient amount of lactase, the enzyme responsible for converting the nonabsorbable milk sugar, lactose, into the absorbable sugars glucose and galactose. With lactase deficiency, any undigested lactose will remain in the small intestine, where, because of its osmotic capacity, it draws water. When the lactose reaches the colon, it begins to combine acetic acid and hydrogen gas, which results in the symptoms of lactose intolerance: cramping, flatulence, abdominal bloating, and diarrhea. These symptoms are dose related—they occur only if the person ingests more food containing lactose than the person's supply of available lactase can metabolize. Foods containing large amounts of lactose include milk, yogurt, and milk chocolate. Of these food items, nonfat dry milk contains the most lactose. Foods containing moderate amounts of lactose include cream, cottage cheese, and most cheeses. Even unlikely foods such as dried soup, cookies made from prepared mixes, cold cuts, and bread and butter

contain small amounts of lactose (When Patients Can't Drink Milk, 1976).

The nurse must be cognizant of foods that can cause lactose intolerance symptoms, particularly when working with persons who are extremely lactose intolerant. For most clients, treatment of this condition is usually a matter of restricting lactose-containing foods rather than eliminating them altogether. An adult who is advised to restrict milk and milk products but otherwise eat a well-balanced diet should not need any nutritional supplements. However, for pregnant or lactating women, nutritional supplements (such as calcium tablets) may be necessary. Lactose intolerance does not generally develop until after childhood; children who are deficient in lactose should be encouraged to eat aged cheeses because the aging process changes lactase to lactic acid. In addition, some physicians may recommend a soybean-based milk substitute, as well as vitamins and calcium supplements. Even for the adult lactose-deficient client, the astute nurse can suggest alternatives to milk products, such as cheese aged over 60 days. The nurse should be aware that telling the client to drink milk may not necessarily be good advice for many adults in the world and should give special consideration to the pregnant or lactating woman because most racial groups, except Whites, cannot tolerate milk in adulthood (Bayless, 1975).

Psychological Characteristics

Gaitz and Scott (1974) have indicated that although cultural factors may influence mental health scores in research studies, such scores are not indicative of whether one cultural group has more or fewer incidences of mental illness than another. There are many different definitions of *mental health,* one of which postulates that a person is mentally healthy when there is a balance in the person's internal life and adaptation to reality. Thus it can be determined that normal behavior is relative to a specific culture and that different psychological characteristics are promoted by each culture. Other variables that influence mental health include family relationships, childbearing practices, language, attitudes toward illness, and social and economic status.

Some cultural groups have a low socioeconomic status, which consequently affects mental health. For example, some Mexican Americans have a low socioeconomic status in terms of substandard housing, education, physical health, political influence, communication, and social exclusion. The concept of social exclusion must be considered as a contributing factor in the failure of any particular cultural group to assimilate the culture of the wider society. Broad exposure to other lifestyles, cultures, environments, and ideas facilitates an understanding and flexibility on the part of an individual when dealing with other people or when solving problems. Feelings of insecurity may also be related to cultural background. For example, psychological adjustment may be difficult for an American Indian who has lived on a reservation and goes to a college where there are few other American Indians. The difficulty in adjustment may be attributable to the fact that this person has lived in an isolated environment that has not assimilated into the mainstream of society. Therefore, health care providers must consider both ethnicity and economic factors when assessing mental health status.

There has been no consistent attack on problems of mental illness around the world. Although no continent or island area has been immune from mental illness, the study of mental illness in relation to culture has been restricted and often localized. There may have been a hesitancy to study cultures and mental illness because of possible implications of racism (Griffith & Griffith, 1986; Hampton, Gullota, & Crowel, 2010). Some authorities cite that psychiatrists have also not seriously discussed the possibility that racism may be a manifestation of an individual psychological disorder (Hampton et al., 2010). In any case, research on mental illness from a broad world perspective has been seriously lacking.

Although research, for the most part, is lacking, some interesting cultural data and implications are available in the studies that have been reported. Not only do mental illnesses seem to vary among cultures, but treatment does also. In Japan, psychiatric institutions are small; in the United States, they are large. Societies also have differing demands on individuals emerging from the treatment milieu. Not only do hospitals and treatment milieus differ around the world, but the paths into illness also show a different pattern in each culture. Variations in class identity or in the pace of acculturation of class segments may produce differences in deviant types. Similarly, personalities seem to vary among persons from different geographical regions. There is some evidence that the cultural backgrounds and forms of illness vary apart from the question of how these illnesses are treated. Lawson (1986) reported findings suggesting that racial and ethnic differences exist in the clinical presentations of psychiatric disorders. Significant racial differences have been noted among proposed biological markers for various psychiatric disorders, such as serum creatinine phosphokinase, platelet serotonin, and HLA-A2 determinations. Racial and ethnic differences in response to psychotropic medication, such as higher blood levels of the drugs found among Asians, affect dosage requirements and potential side effects. All these developments underline the importance of considering ethnic and racial factors in caring for psychiatric clients.

In the United States, the incidence of mental illness has been found to vary among certain racial groups. For example, post-traumatic stress disorder (PTSD) has been studied among Vietnam veterans. Because of racism in the military and racial and social upheaval in the United States during the Vietnam War years, as well as limited opportunities for African-Americans in the postwar period, African-American veterans of the Vietnam War often have harbored conflicting feelings about their wartime experiences. African-American veterans have been found to suffer PTSD at a higher rate than White veterans have. Diagnosis and treatment of PTSD in African-Americans are complicated by a tendency to misdiagnose African-American clients; by the varied manifestations of PTSD; by clients' frequent alcohol and drug abuse; and by medical, legal, personality, and vocational problems (Allen, 1986).

Also, in the United States there is evidence that schizophrenia has been consistently overdiagnosed and affective disorders underdiagnosed, particularly in African-Americans and low-socioeconomic groups (Dixon et al., 2001). General causes of such misdiagnoses include over-reliance on the classic thought disorder symptoms pathognomonic of schizophrenia and, for affective disorders, lack of clearly defined boundaries between normal and abnormal mood, as well as failure to realize that clients with affective illness can manifest cognitive thought processes. In addition, according to Jones and Gray (1986), misdiagnoses among African-Americans result from such factors as cultural differences in language and mannerisms, difficulties in relating between African-American clients and White therapists and staff, and the myth that African-Americans rarely suffer from affective disorders. The effects of cultural and racial differences on baseline behaviors and symptoms have thus far received little consistent attention. Research is needed to investigate more closely how the general diagnostic problems in psychiatry affect certain racial groups. Research is also needed on how cultural and racial differences may affect diagnosis. Finally, baseline behaviors and symptoms for racial groups must be established.

Meinhardt and Vega (1987) have reported that most studies of use of mental health services by ethnic groups have used parity as a measure of whether members of ethnic groups are receiving a fair share of services. The level of service is assumed to be adequate if the percentage of ethnic group members in the treatment population is the same as the group's percentage in the general population. However, service planning based on achieving parity fails to consider that some groups may have higher levels of need than others. Equitable care among ethnic and racial groups based on need is another issue that mental health professionals are addressing (López, 1981).

A better understanding of the differences among various cultures in the area of mental health and treatment for mental illness will enable culturally appropriate mental health care. Griffith and Griffith (1986) have pointed out that mental health professionals should give more consideration to the fact that cultural issues such as racism can cause psychological injury. It is evident from the increasing quantities of literature on culture and mental health that there is a growing awareness among health professionals that care for clients with mental problems must be culturally appropriate and that cultural factors do affect mental health. Although rice and tea may not be the most potent tools of modern psychiatry, they may play an important role in making psychiatric care acceptable to the acutely disturbed Asian or Pacific Islander psychiatric client (Lu, 1987). It is important for the nurse to study what is available about the population groups being served and consider the important differences that may be required in the care provided. Not only must nurses appreciate that caring for clients from different cultural groups may require different care methods, but they must also assist other mental health workers in being sensitive to differing care needs.

Domestic Violence

In 2006, more than 232,960 women experienced some type of violent offense at the hand of an intimate (U.S. Department of Justice, Office of Justice Programs, 2006). This figure may be disproportionately low and actually as high as 1.8 million over the course of 1 year (U.S. Department of Justice, Office of Justice Programs, 2006). Other data suggest that the percentage of women who experience dating violence, including sexual assault, physical violence, or verbal or emotional abuse may be as high as 65% of all women (Heise, Ellsberg, & Gottemoeller, 1999). According to the U.S. Department of Justice, Bureau of Justice Statistics (Rennison & Welchans, 2000), *domestic violence* is defined as violent crimes by current or former spouses, boyfriends, and girlfriends. These violent crimes include lethal (homicide) and nonlethal (rape, sexual assault, robbery, aggravated assault, and simple assault) offenses (Rennison & Welchans, 2000). It is interesting to note that the Justice Department failed to mention other types of abuse, such as mental or emotional abuse, harassment, or stalking, all of which need to be factored into the equation to more fully understand the incidence of domestic violence (Rennison & Welchans, 2000). Pampel and Williams (2000) note that researchers who use the Justice Department database must recognize the need to address the problem of missing data. They conclude that missing data are typically the result of the failure to file, inconsistent filing of reports to the FBI by local police agencies, or incomplete records about the characteristics of specific incidents of homicide. They further noted that, in

particular, information about the perpetrators of the crimes may be missing even when reports of such crimes are filed, and this contributes significantly to skewed and vastly flawed data in many databases (Pampel & Williams, 2000).

By definition, the term *battering* implies that an individual is either physically or emotionally abused (Campbell, 1989; Flitcraft, 1991; Newman, 1993). Although there are reported cases of "male battering" perpetrated by women, the victims of abuse are women in more than 90% of all reported domestic violence cases (Flitcraft, 1991; Newman, 1993). Although battered women syndrome has been heavily documented in the literature (Campbell, 1989; Chez, 1988; Flitcraft, 1991; Newman, 1993; Pampel & Williams, 2000; Rennison & Welchans, 2000), it did not receive the adequate attention it needed as a social concern until 1994. Battered women syndrome moved to the forefront of social concerns with the murders of Nicole Brown Simpson (wife of famed running back O. J. Simpson) and her friend Ronald Goldman. Simpson, who pled "no contest" to "wife-beating" in 1989, was later acquitted of the murder of his ex-wife (Brown Simpson) and her friend (Goldman). However, in the civil trial brought by the estate of Nicole Brown Simpson and the father of Ronald Goldman, Simpson was found liable for the murders of Brown Simpson and Goldman. The plaintiffs were awarded an astounding $33 million. Because of Simpson's celebrity status, more attention was focused on battered women syndrome.

One in every three adult women experiences at least one physical assault by a partner during her adult lifetime (American Psychological Association, 2002). In fact, nearly 4 million American women will experience a serious physical assault by an intimate partner during a 12-month window (American Psychological Association, 2002). In addition, it is estimated that some 12 million women (25% of all women) will be abused in their lifetime (Pampel & Williams, 2000). Although it remains largely unknown how frequently domestic violence occurs, it has been suggested that it occurs 10 times more frequently than those statistics reported by the Bureau of Justice. Nonetheless, this report does help identify some interesting trends (Rennison & Welchans, 2000). In addition, the data suggest that there is a difference by race and ethnicity regarding the frequency of domestic violence. For example, Black women and their male counterparts have the highest rate of domestic violence. In fact, Black women experience domestic violence at a rate 35% higher than their White counterparts and 22 times higher than that of women of all other races (Rennison & Welchans, 2000). Domestic violence also appears to be prevalent among women 18 to 24 years of age (Rennison & Welchans, 2000). In addition, women of lower socioeconomic status are significantly more likely to experience domestic violence (Rennison & Welchans, 2000).

In the majority of cases involving "woman battering," the assailants were usually an intimate who was a family member, spouse, or boyfriend. The phenomenon of battered women syndrome has become so widespread that it is believed to be the leading cause of injury among women in the United States (Rennison & Welchans, 2000). Battering accounts for one in every five visits to the hospital emergency room by women in this country (Rennison & Welchans, 2000).

The incidence of battering may have a direct relationship to other violent crimes committed against women, such as rape and homicide. Homicide is the eleventh leading cause of death in the United States (National Center for Health Statistics, Health, United States, 2014). In fact, it is estimated that one of every six homicides in this country involves a family member (U.S. Department of Health and Human Services, 2002). Of the murders of women committed in the United States, about half are committed by a spouse. Although the number of people who were murdered by an intimate partner was down from the high in 1976 of 1600 women and 1357 men to 1219 women and 424 men in 1999, and continued to decline for women in 2008 to 1817 who were murdered in a single incident by an intimate partner, the number is still alarming (Violence Partner Center, 2008). In addition, about one third of all murdered females are likely to have been killed by intimates, as compared with 4% of male murder victims (Rennison & Welchans, 2000). Although most homicide statistics, by race, are only presented by White or Black racial categories, the data available suggest that homicides of women by intimates are declining. For White women, the number of homicides by an intimate declined from a high of 1600 women in 1976 to a low of 812 women in 1999. Similarly, the homicides of Black women declined from 714 murdered by an intimate in 1976 to a low of 338 women in 1999 (Rennison & Welchans, 2000).

In 2005, 191,670, or 1 in every 650, women were raped. Like the number of actual domestic violence cases, this number is greatly underestimated because 53% of women fail to report a rape (U.S. Department of Justice, Office of Justice Programs, 2006). In fact, according to the U.S. Bureau of Justice Statistics, 91% of U.S. rape victims are female and 9% are male, with 99% of the offenders often being male (U.S. Department of Justice, Office of Justice Programs, 2006c). The incidence of rape varies with race and ethnicity. Women who are raped are likely to be African-American women who have been raped by African-American men. Of the number of rapes, 65% occur at night (between the hours of 8 p.m. and 4 a.m.), 43% occur near the victim's home, and 15% occur at a friend's house. Although a greater number of women report "stranger rape," the incidence of acquaintance rape (date rape) and domestic violence rape is greatly underreported.

CASE STUDY

Sarah Jennings is a 21-year-old African-American married woman and the mother of a 12-month-old daughter. Mrs. Jennings was diagnosed at age 11 as having SCD. For the past 3 years, she has remained largely asymptomatic. She is admitted to the hospital in sickle cell crisis. Her admitting complaints include severe joint pains in both the upper and lower extremities, a temperature of 101.8° F, and shortness of breath. On physical examination, the nurse notes that Mrs. Jennings has coarse rales in the base of both lungs and that her lips are cyanotic and dry. Her nail beds are also cyanotic, and when they are blanched, capillary refill is slow. Initial laboratory examination reveals an Hb level of 8 g/dL. During the nursing history, it is revealed that Mrs. Jennings has also had problems drinking milk and eating certain dairy products for most of her adult life.

CLINICAL DECISION MAKING

1. List at least two contributing factors for Mrs. Jennings's SCD that relate to biological variations by race and ethnic heritage.
2. List at least one other racial group with a predisposition for sickle cell crisis.
3. List the basic causes of SCD.
4. List at least two other conditions that Mrs. Jennings could be at risk for developing because of her race and ethnic heritage.
5. Describe at least two differences noted when the nurse is assessing the skin color of dark-skinned individuals.

REVIEW QUESTIONS

1. Blood groups are said to differentiate people in different racial groups. You have a 29-year-old American Indian client admitted to your unit with diabetes. Based on what you know about American Indians, you might expect your patient's blood type to be which of the following?
   a. Type A
   b. Type B
   c. Type AB
   d. Type O

2. In making a correct nursing diagnosis regarding a rash on a patient, the nurse should complete which of the following tasks first?
   a. Become familiar with the patient's normal coloring to establish a baseline.
   b. Assess the skin in artificial lighting, not in sunlight.
   c. Assess darkly pigmented areas first, as it is less difficult to note color changes there.
   d. Assess lightly pigmented areas first, as it is less difficult to note color changes there.
3. Mongolian spots are a common finding in which of these groups? Mark all that apply.
   a. Black Americans
   b. White Americans
   c. Asian Americans
   d. American Indians

REFERENCES

Adams, J. M. (1932). Some racial differences in blood pressures and morbidity in groups of white and colored workmen. *American Journal of Medical Science, 184,* 342–350.

Alaskan Native Tribal Health Consortium. (2013). *Southeast Regional Health Profile.* Anchorage, Alaska: The Alaska Native Epidemiology Center.

Allen, I. (1986). Posttraumatic stress disorder among Black Vietnam veterans. *Hospital and Community Psychiatry, 37*(1), 55–60.

ALLHAT Officers and Coordinators for the ALLHAT Collaborative Research Group. (2002a). Major outcomes in high-risk hypertensive patients randomized to angiotensin-converting enzyme inhibitor or calcium channel blocker vs. diuretic. *Journal of the American Medical Association, 288,* 2981–2997.

ALLHAT Officers and Coordinators for the ALLHAT Collaborative Research Group. (2002b). Major outcomes in moderately hypercholesterolemic, hypertensive patients randomized to pravastatin vs. usual care. *Journal of the American Medical Association, 288,* 2998–3007.

Aloia, J. (2008). African Americans, 25-hydroxyvitamin D, and osteoporosis: a paradox. *American Journal of Clinical Nutrition, 88*(2), 545S–550S.

American Diabetic Association. (2015). *Vital statistics.* Alexandria, VA: American Diabetic Association.

American Psychological Association. (2002). *Facts about family.* Available at <www.apa.org>. Retrieved January 7, 2002.

Appel, S., Giger, J. N., & Davidhizar, R. (2005). Opportunity cost: the impact of contextual risk factors on the cardiovascular health on low income southern African American women. *Journal of Cardiovascular Nursing, 20*(50), 315–324.

Atrash, H., & Hunter, M. (2001). Health disparities in the United States: a continuing challenge. In D. Satcher & R. Pamies (Eds.), *Multicultural medicine and health disparities.* New York: McGraw-Hill.

Bandara, M. (2009). Exploring the link between culture and biodiversity in Sri Lanka. *Sansai: An Environmental Journal for the Global Community, 4,* 1–23.

Barker-Cummings, C., McClellan, W., Soucie, J. M., & Krisher, J. (1995). Ethnic differences in the use of peritoneal dialysis as initial treatment for end-stage renal disease. *Journal of the American Medical Association, 274,* 1858–1862.

Barna, P. (1985). Food or drug? The case of ginseng. *Lancet, 2,* 548.

Batson, B., Belletti, D., & Wogen, D. (2010, Autumn). Effect of African American race on hypertension management: a real-world observational study among 28 U.S. physician practices. *Ethnicity & Disease, 20,* 409–415.

Bayless, T. (1975). Lactose and milk intolerance: clinical implications. *New England Journal of Medicine, 292*(5), 1156–1159.

Beevers, D., Lee, K., & Lip, G. (2003). The antihypertensive and lipid-lowering treatment to prevent heart attack trial (ALLHAT): ALL predictable, and no big surprise out of a HAT? *Journal of Human Hypertension, 17,* 367–372.

Benirschke, K., Kaufmann, P., & Baergen, R. N. (2006). *Pathology of the human placenta* (5th ed.). New York: Springer.

Benjamin, L. J., Swinson, G. I., & Nagel, R. L. (2000). Sickle cell anemia in a day hospital: an approach for the management of uncomplicated painful crises. *Blood, 95*(4), 1130–1136.

Boyle, E. (1970). Biological patterns in hypertension by race, sex, body weight, and skin color. *Journal of the American Medical Association, 213,* 1637–1643.

Braithwaite, R., & Taylor, S. (2001). *Health issues in the Black community* (2nd ed.). San Francisco: Jossey-Bass.

Branch, M., & Paxton, P. (1976). *Providing safe nursing care for ethnic people of color.* New York: Appleton-Century-Crofts.

Brues, A. M. (1977). *People and race.* New York: Macmillan Publishing. (Reprinted 1990. Prospect Heights, IL: Waveland Press.).

Burns, E., & Neubort, S. (1984). Sodium content of koshered meat [letter]. *Journal of the American Medical Association, 252*(21), 2960.

Burroughs, V. J., Maxey, R. W., Crawley, L. M., & Levy, R. A. (2002). Racial and ethnic differences in response to medicines: towards individualized treatment. *Journal of the National Medical Association, 94*(10), 1–26.

Burt, C. (1966). The genetic determination of difference in intelligence: a study of monozygote twins reared together and apart. *British Journal of Psychology, 57,* 137–153.

Burt, V. L., et al. (1995). Trends in the prevalence, awareness, treatment, and control of hypertension in the adult U.S. population. *Radiology, 26*(1), 60–69.

Campbell, J. (1989). A test of two exploratory models of women's response to battering. *Nursing Research, 38*(1), 18–24.

Centers for Disease Control and Prevention (CDC). (1991). Nosocomial transmission of multi-drug resistant tuberculosis among HIV-infected persons—Florida and New York, 1988–1991. *Morbidity and Mortality Weekly Report, 40*(34), 585–591.

Centers for Disease Control and Prevention (CDC). (1992). Recommendations of the Advisory Council for the reduction of hypertension among minority populations. *Morbidity and Mortality Weekly Report, 40*, 1–7.

Centers for Disease Control (CDC). (2013). *Tuberculosis Surveillance Report*, Atlanta, GA.

Centers for Disease Control and Prevention (CDC). (2013). *HIV/AIDS surveillance report: U.S. HIV and AIDS cases reported through December 20*. Atlanta, GA: U.S. Department of Health and Human Services.

Centers for Disease Control. (2014). *National Diabetes Statistics Report 2014*, Centers for Disease Control, Atlanta, GA.

Centers for Disease Control (CDC). (2015). *Diabetes Surveillance Report* 2015, Atlanta, GA.

Chan, A. W. (1986). Racial differences in alcohol sensitivity. *Alcohol & Alcoholism, 21*(1), 93–104.

Chen, W., Bao, W., Begum, S., Elkasabany, A., Srinivasan, S. R., & Berenson, G. S. (2000). Age-related patterns of the clustering of cardiovascular risk variables of metabolic syndrome (syndrome X) from childhood to young adulthood in a population made up of black and white subjects. *Diabetes, 49*, 1042–1048.

Chez, R. (1988). Woman battering. *American Journal of Obstetrics and Gynecology, 156*, 1–4.

Chin, M., Zhang, J., & Merrell, K. (1998). Diabetes in the African-American Medicare population: morbidity, quality of care, and resource utilization. *Diabetes Care, 21*(7), 1090–1095.

Cohen, M., et al. (2010). Racial and ethnic differences in the treatment of acute myocardial infarction: findings from the Get With the Guidelines Coronary Artery Disease Program. *Circulation, 121*, 2294–2301.

Collins, F. (1997). Sequencing the human genome. *Hospital Practice, 32*(1), 35–55.

Collins, R., & McNair, L. (2003). *Minority women and alcohol use*. National Institute on Alcohol Abuse and Alcoholism. Available at: <http://pubs.niaaa.nih.gov/publications/arh26-4/251-256.htm>. Retrieved February 27, 2011.

Committee on the Review and Assessment of the NIH's Strategic Research Plan and Budget to Reduce and Ultimately Eliminate Health Disparities. (2006). *Examining the health disparities research plan of the National Institutes of Health: unfinished business*. <http://www.nap.edu/catalog/11602.html>.

Cowie, C., & Harris, M. (1997). Ambulatory medical care for non-Hispanic Whites, African-Americans and Mexican-Americans with NIDDM in the U.S. *Diabetes Care, 20*(2), 142–147.

Crawford, P., Story, M., Wang, M., Ritchie, L., & Sabry, Z. (2001). Ethnic issues in the epidemiology of childhood obesity. *Pediatric Clinics of North America, 48*(4), 855–878.

Davidhizar, R., & Giger, J. N. (2008). Understanding ethnopharmacology: implications for cultural relativism. *The Journal of the National Black Nurses Association, 19*(1), 63–68.

Davis, S., Northington, L., & Kolar, K. (2000). Cultural considerations for treatment of childhood obesity. *Journal of Cultural Diversity, 7*(4), 128–132.

Divan, D. (1989). Letter to the editor. *New England Journal of Medicine, 321*(4), 259.

Dixon, L., Green-Paden, L., Delahanty, J., Lucksted, A., Postrado, L., & Hall, J. (2001). Variables associated with disparities in treatment of patients with schizophrenia and comorbid mood and anxiety disorders. *Psychiatric Services, 52*, 1216–1222.

Edenberg, H. (2007). The genetics of alcohol metabolism: the role of alcohol dehydrogenase and aldehyde dehydrogenase variants. *Alcohol Research & Health, 30*(1), 1–13.

Farb, P., & Armelagos, G. (1980). *Consuming passions: the anthropology of eating*. Boston: Houghton Mifflin.

Feisthamel, K., & Schwartz, R. (2006). Racial bias in diagnosis: practical implications for psychotherapists. *Annals of the American Psychotherapy Association, 9*, 10–14.

Flitcraft, A. (1991). Domestic abuse: diagnosing, treating, and understanding its victims. *Clinical Nurse Practitioner, 9*(2), 3–5.

Freis, E. (1986). Antihypertensive agents. In W. Kalow, H. W. Goedde, & D. Agarwal (Eds.), *Ethnic differences in reactions to drugs and xenobiotics*. New York: Liss.

Gaitz, C., & Scott, J. (1974). Mental health of Mexican Americans: do ethnic factors make a difference? *Geriatrics, 1*(11), 110–113.

Gannett, L. (2008). *The human genome project. Stanford Encyclopedia of Philosophy*. Available at <http://plato.stanford.edu/entries/human-genome/>. Retrieved on February 27, 2011.

Genes and Disease. (n.d.). *Sickle cell anemia*. NCBI. Available at <http://www.ncbi.nlm.nih.gov/books/NBK22238>. Retrieved on July 24, 2011.

Giger, J. N. (2011). Defining health disparities from three viewpoints: reducing inequality in health care. In P. Cowen & S. Moorhead (Eds.), *Current issues in nursing* (8th ed.). St. Louis: Mosby.

Giger, J., Davidhizar, R., & Wieczorek, S. (1993). Culture and ethnicity. In I. Bobak & M. Jensen (Eds.), *Maternity and gynecologic care* (5th ed., pp. 43–67). St. Louis: Mosby.

Giger, J., Richardson, J., & Jones, D. (2002). African American children: a precious commodity at risk [editorial]. *Journal of National Black Nurses Association, 13*(1), vii–viii.

Ginseng. (1980). Medical letter drugs. *Therapy, 22*(17), 72.

Glazer, W. M., Morgenstern, H., & Doucette, J. T. (1993). Predicting the long-term risk of tardive dyskinesia in outpatients maintained on neuroleptic medications. *Journal of Clinical Psychiatry, 54*(4), 133–139.

Glazer, W. M., Morgenstern, H., & Doucette, J. T. (1994). Race and tardive dyskinesia among outpatients at a CMHC. *Hospital and Community Psychiatry, 45*(1), 38–45.

Goldman, D. R. (1985). Hold the sushi [letter]. *Journal of the American Medical Association, 253*(17), 2495.

Gorden, A. M. (1982). Nutritional status of Cuban refugees: a field study on the health and nutrition of refugees processed at Opa-Locka, Florida. *American Journal of Clinical Nutrition, 35*(3), 582.

Greaves, K., Puhl, J., Baranowski, T., Gruben, D., & Seale, D. (1989). Ethnic differences in anthropometrics characteristics and their parents. *Human Biology, 61*(3), 459.

Greenberg, J., Dintiman, G., & Oakes, B. (2004). *Physical fitness and wellness: changing the way you look, feel and perform* (3rd ed.). New York: Human Kinetics.

Griffith, E., & Griffith, E. (1986). Racism, psychological injury, and compensatory damages. *Hospital and Community Psychiatry, 37*(1), 71–75.

Halsted, J. A. (1968). Geophagia in man: its nature and nutritional effects. *American Journal of Clinical Nutrition, 21*(12), 1384.

Hampton, R. L., Gullotta, T. P., & Crowel, R. (2010). *Handbook of African American health.* New York: Guilford Press.

Harper, P. (1993). *Practical genetic counseling* (4th ed.). Oxford, England: Butterworth-Heinemann.

Heise, L., Ellsberg, M., & Gottemoeller, M. (1999). *Ending violence against women.* Baltimore: Johns Hopkins University School of Public Health. Population Information Program: Population reports, series L, no. 11.

Henderson, D. (2010). Pharmacology in African Americans. In R. L. Hampton, T. P. Gullotta, & R. Crowel (Eds.), *Handbook of African American health.* New York: Guilford Press.

Hochberg, M. C. (1993). The history of lupus erythematosus. In *The Lupus Foundation of America Newsletter* (pp. 93–102). Washington DC: LFA Patient Education Committee.

Hollier, J. M., et al. (2006). Epithelial sodium channel allele T594M is not associated with blood pressure or blood pressure response to amiloride. *Hypertension, 47*, 428–433.

Holmes, T. H., Hawkins, N. G., Bowerman, C. E., Clarke, E. R., & Joffe, J. R. (1957). Psychosocial and psychophysiological studies of tuberculosis. *Psychosomatic Medicine, 19*, 134–143.

Iman, F., Anwer, M. K., Iqbal, M., Alam, S., Khayyam, K. U., & Sarma, M. (2010). Tuberculosis: brief overview and its shifting paradigm for management in India. *International Journal of Pharmacology, 6*(6), 755–783.

Interdepartmental Commission on National Defense and Division of Indian Public Health (ICND & DIPH) (1964). *Fort Belknap Indian Reservation: nutrition survey.* Washington, DC: U.S. Public Health Service.

Israel, Y., Quintanilla, M., Sapag, A., & Tampier, L. (2006). *Combined effects of aldehyde dehydrogenase variants and maternal mitochondrial genes on alcohol consumption.* Department of Pathology and Cell Biology, faculty papers, 13. Available at <http://jdc.jefferson.edu/cgi/viewcontent.cgi?article=1013>. Retrieved July 24, 2011.

Jablonski, N., & Chaplin, G. (2000). The evolution of human skin coloration. *Journal of Human Evolution, 39*, 57–106.

Jackson, R. T., Sauberlich, H. S., Skala, J. H., Kretsch, J. J., & Nelson, R. A. (1983). Comparison of hemoglobin values in Black and White male U.S. military personnel. *Journal of Nutrition, 113*(1), 165.

Jensen, A. R. (1969). How much can we boost IQ and scholastic achievement? *Harvard Education Review, 29*, 1.

Jensen, A. R. (1974). Cumulative deficits: a testable hypothesis? *Developmental Psychology, 10*, 996.

Jensen, A. R. (1977). Cumulative deficit in IQ of Blacks in the rural South. *Developmental Psychology, 13*, 184.

Jick, H., et al. (1969). Venous thromboembolic disease and ABO blood type. *Lancet, 1*, 539–542.

Johe, R., Steinhart, T., Sado, N., Greenberg, B., & Jing, S. (2010). Intermaxillary tooth-size discrepancies in different sexes, malocclusion groups, and ethnicities. *American Journal of Orthodontics and Dentofacial Orthopedics, 13*(5), 600–607.

Joint National Committee. (2003). *The report of the Joint National Committee on Detection, Evaluation and Treatment of High Blood Pressure.* Washington, DC: National Institutes of Health, National Heart, Lung, and Blood Institute.

Jones, B., & Gray, B. (1986). Problems in diagnosing schizophrenia and affective disorders among Blacks. *Hospital and Community Psychiatry, 37*(1), 61–65.

Jorde, L., Carey, J., & Bamshad, M. (2010). *Medical genetics* (4th ed.). St. Louis: Mosby.

Kalow, W. (1982). The metabolism of xenobiotics in different populations. *Canadian Journal of Physiological Pharmacology, 60*, 1–19.

Kalow, W. (1986). Outlook of a pharmacologist. In W. Kalow, H. Goedde, & D. Agarwal (Eds.), *Ethnic differences in reactions to drugs and xenobiotics.* New York: Liss.

Kalow, W. (1989). Race and therapeutic drug response. *New England Journal of Medicine, 320*(9), 588–589.

Kasiske, B. (1998). Race and socio-economic factors influencing early placement on the kidney transplant waiting list. *Journal of the American Society of Nephrologists, 9*(11), 2142–2147.

Katz, S. H., Hediger, M. L., & Valleroy, L. A. (1974). Traditional maize processing techniques in the New World. *Science, 184*, 765.

Keil, J. (1981). Skin color and education effects on blood pressure. *American Journal of Public Health, 71*, 532–534.

Keltner, N., & Folks, G. (1992). Psychopharmacology update: culture as a variable in drug therapy. *Perspectives in Psychiatric Nursing, 28*(1), 33–35.

Khan, K. (2001). Physical activity in bone health. In K. Kakn, H. McKay, P. Kannus, & D. Bailey (Eds.), *Human Kinetics, British Journal of Sports Medicine 36* (pp. 76–77). Champaign, IL: Bennel.

Kim, K., Johnson, J., & Derendorf, H. (2004). Differences in drug pharmacokinetics between East Asians and Caucasians and the role of genetic polymorphisms. *Journal of Clinical Pharmacology, 44*, 1083–1104.

Kisch, B. (1953). Salt poor diet and Jewish dietary laws. *Journal of the American Medical Association, 153*(16), 1472.

Klag, M., Whelton, P., Coresh, J., Grim, C. E., & Kuller, L. H. (1991). The association of skin color with blood pressure in U.S. blacks with low socioeconomic status. *Journal of the American Medical Association, 265*(5), 599–602.

Krolewski, A., & Warram, G. (2005). Epidemiology of diabetes mellitus. In E. P. Joslin (Ed.), *Joslin's diabetes mellitus* (14th ed.). Philadelphia: Lippincott Williams & Wilkins.

Kudzma, E. (1992). Drug responses: all bodies are not created equal. *American Journal of Nursing, 92*, 48–50.

Lawson, W. (1986). Racial and ethnic factors in psychiatric research. *Hospital and Community Psychiatry, 37*(1), 50–54.

Leffall, L. D. (1974). Cancer mortality among Blacks. *CA: A Cancer Journal for Clinicians, 24,* 42–46.

Lefley, H. (1990). Culture and chronic mental illness. *Hospital and Community Psychiatry, 41,* 277.

Leininger, M. (2007). Theoretical questions and concerns: response from the theory of culture care diversity and universality perspective. *Nursing Science Quarterly, 20*(1), 9–13.

Lerner, D., & Kannel, W. (1986). Patterns of coronary heart disease morbidity and mortality in the sexes: a 26-year follow-up of the Framingham population. *American Heart Journal, 11,* 383–390.

Lewis, J. H. (1942). *The biology of the Negro* (Chicago University Monographs in Medicine). Chicago: University of Chicago Press.

Lewis, R. (2010). *Human genetics: concepts and applications* (9th ed.). Boston: McGraw-Hill Higher Education.

Lindquist, C., Reynolds, K., & Goran, M. (1999). Sociocultural determinants of physical activity among children. *Preventive Medicine, 29*(4), 305–312.

Lockridge, O. (1990). Genetic variants of human serum cholinesterase influence metabolism of the muscle relaxant succinylcholine. *Pharmacology and Therapeutics, 47*(1), 35–60.

López, S. (1981). Mexican Americans' usage of mental health facilities: underutilization reconsidered. In A. Baron (Ed.), *Explorations in Chicano psychology.* New York: Praeger.

Lorton, J., & Lorton, E. (1984). *Human development through the life span.* Belmont, CA: Brooks/Cole.

Lu, F. (1987). Culturally relevant inpatient care for minority and ethnic patients. *Hospital and Community Psychiatry, 38*(11), 1126–1127.

Luzzatto, L., & Poggi, V. (2008). Glucose-6-phosphate dehydrogenase deficiency. In S. Orkin, D. Fisher, T. Look, S. Lux, D. Ginsburg, & D. Nathan (Eds.), *Nathan and Oski's hematology of infancy and childhood.* Philadelphia: Saunders Elsevier.

Ma, I., & Allan, A. (2011). The role of human aldehyde dehydrogenase in normal and cancer stem cells. *Stem Cell Reviews, 7*(2), 292–306.

Maras, M., & Adolphi, C. L. (1985). Ethnic tailoring improves dietary compliance. *Diabetes Education, 11*(4), 47.

Matthews, D., Hosker, J. P., Rudenski, A., Naylor, B. A., Treacher, D. F., & Turner, R. C. (1985). Homeostasis model assessment: insulin resistance and beta-cell function from fasting plasma glucose and insulin concentrations in man. *Diabetologia, 28,* 412–429.

Matthews, H. W., & Johnson, J. L. (2006). Racial, ethnic, and sex differences in response to drugs. In R. Helms, D. J. Quan, E. T. Herfindal, & D. R. Gourley (Eds.), *Textbook of therapeutics: drugs and disease management* (8th ed.). Philadelphia: Lippincott Williams & Wilkins.

Meinhardt, K., & Vega, W. (1987). A method of estimating underutilization of mental health services by ethnic groups. *Hospital and Community Psychiatry, 38*(11), 1186–1190.

Melton, L., & Riggs, B. (2000). Epidemiology of age-related fractures. In L. Avioli (Ed.), *The osteoporotic syndrome: detection, prevention, and treatment* (4th ed.). San Diego, CA: Academic Press.

Merck, Sharp, & Dohme Inc. (1974). *Hypertension handbook for clinicians.* Westpoint, PA: Merck, Sharp, & Dohme Inc.

Miller, M. B. (1981). Supplementing and adding variety to the diets of Indians on a reservation in Minnesota. *Journal of the American Dietetic Association, 78*(6), 626.

Mirsa, D. (2002). *Women's health data book: a profile of women's health in the United States* (3rd ed., pp. 51–100). Washington, DC: Jacob's Institute of Women's Health and the Henry J. Kaiser Foundations.

Moser, M., & Black, H. (1998). The role of combination therapy in the treatment of hypertension. *American Journal of Hypertension, 11*(6 Suppl. 1), 73S–78S.

Morse, D. L., Guzewich, J. J., & Hanrahan, J. P. (1986). Widespread outbreaks of clam- and oyster-associated gastroenteritis. *New England Journal of Medicine, 314*(11), 678.

Moser, M., & Lunn, J. (1982). Responses to captopril and hydrochlorothiazide in black patients with hypertension. *Clinical Pharmacology Therapy, 32,* 307–312.

Nagulesparan, M., Savage, P. J., & Knowler, W. C. (1982). Increased in vivo insulin resistance in nondiabetic Pima Indians compared with Caucasians. *Diabetes, 31*(11), 952.

National Center for Health Statistics (2014). *Health, United States, 2014.* Hyattsville, MD: National Center for Health Statistics.

National Healthcare Disparities Report. (2014). Rockville, MD: Agency for Healthcare Research and Quality, U.S. Department of Health and Human Services.

National Institutes of Health. (2003). *National Institutes of Health strategic plan to reduce and ultimately eliminate health disparities 2002–2006.* Available at <http://ncmhd.nih.gov/our_programs/strategic/volumes.asp>. Accessed July 24, 2011.

Newman, K. (1993). Giving up: shelter experience of battered women. *Public Health Nursing, 10*(2), 108–113.

Nold, J., & Georgieff, M. (2004). Infants of diabetic mothers. *Pediatric Clinics of North America, 51,* 619–637.

Nussbaum, R., McInnes, R., & Willard, H. (2007). *Thompson and Thompson genetics in medicine* (7th ed.). Philadelphia: Saunders.

Ogden, O., Carroll, M. D., Curtin, L. R., McDowell, M. A., Tabak, C. J., & Flegel, K. M. (2006). Prevalence of overweight and obesity in the United States, 1999–2004. *Journal of the American Medical Association, 295*(13), 1549–1555.

Onyebujoh, P., et al. (2005). Treatment of tuberculosis: present status and future prospects. *Bulletin of the World Health Organization, 83*(11), 857–865. [Epub 2005 Nov 10].

Orkins, S., Nathan, D., Ginsberg, D., Look, T., Fisher, D., & Lux, S. (2009). *Nathan and Oski's hematology of infancy and childhood* (7th ed.). Philadelphia: Saunders.

Overfield, T. (1995). *Biologic variation in health and illness: race, age and sex differences* (2nd ed.). Boca Raton, FL: CRC Press.

Owens, G. M., Garry, P. J., Seymore, R. D., Harrison, G. G., & Acosta, P. B. (1981). Nutrition studies with White Mountain Apache preschool children in 1976 and 1969. *American Journal of Clinical Nutrition, 34*(2), 266.

Palaniappian, L., et al. (2010). Call to action: cardiovascular disease in Asian Americans: a science advisory from the American Heart Association. *Circulation, 122,* 1242–1252.

Pampel, F., & Williams, K. (2000). Intimacy and homicide: compensating for missing data in the SHR. *Criminology, 32*(2), 661–680.

Pangborn, R. M. (1975). Cross-cultural aspects of flavor preferences. *Food Technology, 29*(6), 34.

Parker, S. L., & Bowering, J. (1976). Folacin in diets of Puerto Ricans and Black women in relation to food practices. *Journal of Nutrition Education, 8*(2), 73.

Phipps, W. (1993). The patient with pulmonary problems. In B. C. Long, W. J. Phipps, & V. Cassmeyer (Eds.), *Medical surgical nursing: concepts and clinical practice* (4th ed.). St. Louis: Mosby.

Piatkov, I., Jones, T., & McLean, M. (2013). *Drug discovery,* ed. Hany A. El-Shemy, ISBN 978-53-51-0906-8.

Platt, O., et al. (1994). Mortality in sickle cell disease: life expectancy and risk factors for early death. *New England Journal of Medicine, 330*(23), 1639–1644.

Polednak, A. P. (1986). Connective tissue responses in Blacks in relation to disease: further observations. *American Journal of Physical Anthropology, 74,* 357–371.

Qureshi, B. A. (1981). Nutrition and multi-ethnic groups. *Royal Social Health Journal, 101*(5), 187.

Ravean, G. M. (2011). Insulin resistance: from bit player to centre stage. *Canadian Medical Association Journal, 183*(5), 536–537.

Rennison, M., & Welchans, W. (2000). *Intimate partner violence.* Washington, DC: U.S. Department of Justice, Office of Justice Programs, Bureau of Justice Statistics, NCJ178247, revised 1/14/00.

Rifkin, H. (Ed.), (1984). *The physician's guide to type II diabetes (NIDDM): diagnosis and treatment.* New York: American Diabetic Association.

Riggs, S. (1980). Tastes of America. *Regionality Institutions, 87*(12), 76.

Roccella, E. J., & Lenfant, C. (1989). Regional and racial differences among stroke victims in the United States. *Clinical Cardiology, 12*(4), 1213–1220.

Rouch, L. (1977). Color changes in dark skin. *Nursing, 7*(1), 48–51.

Saito, S., Okui, K., Tokino, T., Oshimura, M., & Nakamura, Y. (1992). Isolation and mapping of 68 RFLP markers on human chromosome 6. *American Journal of Human Genetics, 50*(1), 65–70.

Saldana, S., & Brown, H. E. (1984). Nutritional composition of corn and flour tortillas. *Journal of Food Science, 49*(4), 202.

Satcher, D. (Ed.). (1973). *Sickle cell counseling: a committee's study and recommendations.* New York: National Foundation—March of Dimes.

Satcher, D., & Pope, L. (1974). *Emergency evaluation and management of persons with sickle cell disease.* Bethesda, MD: National Institutes of Health.

Saunders, E. (1985). Special techniques for management of hypertension in Blacks. In W. D. Hall, E. Saunders, & N. B. Shulman (Eds.), *Hypertension in blacks: epidemiology, pathophysiology, and treatment* (pp. 209–236). St. Louis: Mosby.

Schuurman, M., van Waardenburg, D., Da Costa, J., Niemarkt, H., & Leroy, P. (2009). Severe hemolysis and methemoglobinemia following fava beans ingestion in glucose-6-phosphatase dehydrogenase deficiency: case report and literature review. *European Journal of Pediatrics, 168*(7), 779–782.

Schwerin, H. S., Stanton, J. L., & Smith, J. L. (1982). Food, eating habits, and health: a further examination of the relationships between food eating patterns and nutritional health. *American Journal of Clinical Nutrition, 35*(Suppl. 5), 1319–1335.

Selemenda, C., Peacock, M., Hui, S., Zhou, L., & Johnston, C. (1997). Reduced rates of skeletal remodeling are associated with increased bone mineral density during the development of peak skeletal mass. *Journal of Bone and Mineral Research, 12*(4), 676–681.

Sesardic, N. (2000). Philosophy of science that ignores science: race, IQ and heritability. *Philosophy of Science, 67,* 580–602.

Shaffer, J., et al. (2007). Genetic markers for ancestry are correlated with body composition traits in older African Americans. *Osteoporosis International, 18*(6), 733–734.

Siegel, R. K. (1979). Ginseng abuse syndrome: problems with the panacea. *Journal of the American Medical Association, 24*(15), 614.

Silventoinen, K. (2003). Determinants of variant in adult body weight. *Journal of Biosocial Science, 35,* 283–285.

Smedley, B., Stith, A., & Nelson, A. (2003). *Unequal treatment: confronting racial and ethnic disparities in health care.* Washington, DC: National Academy Press, Institute of Medicine.

Sommers, M. (2011). Color awareness: a must for patient assessment. *American Nurse Today, 6*(1).

Srinivasan, S., Myers, L., & Berenson, G. (2002). Predictability of childhood adiposity and insulin for developing insulin resistance syndrome (metabolic syndrome [syndrome X]) in young adulthood: the Bogalusa Heart Study. *Diabetes, 51,* 204–209.

State of Maryland demonstration of statewide coordination for the control of high blood pressure (1977-1983), October. (1984). NHLBI Contract No. 1-HV-2986.

Stewart, S. H. (2002). Racial and ethnic differences in alcohol-associated aspartate aminotransferase and gamma-glutamyltransferase elevation. *Archives of Internal Medicine, 162*(19), 2236–2239.

Stokes, J., Kannel, W., Wolf, P., Cupples, L. A., & D'Agostino, R. B. (1987). The relative importance of selected risk factors for various manifestations of cardiovascular disease among men and women from 35 to 64 years old: 30 years of follow-up in the Framingham study. *Circulation, 75*(6), 65–73.

Strauss, R., & Pollack, H. (2001). Epidemic increase in childhood overweight, 1986–1998. *Journal of the American Medical Association, 286*(22), 2845–2848.

Swift, P. A., & Macgregor, G. A. (2004). Genetic variations in the epithelial sodium channel: a risk factor for hypertension in people of African origin. *Advances in Renal Replacement Therapy, 4.*

The Carter Center. (1985). Closing the gap: the problem of diabetes mellitus in the United States. The Carter Center of Emory University. *Diabetes Care, 8*(4), 391–406.

Tipton, D. (1974). Physiological assessment of Black people. In *Care of black patients (X428.1).* A group of papers presented at a conference on care of the Black patient, sponsored by Continuing Education in Nursing. San Francisco: University of California.

Todd, K. H., Deaton, C., D'Adamo, A. P., & Goe, L. (2000). Ethnicity and analgesic practice. *Annals of Emergency Medicine, 35*(1), 11–16.

U.S. Department of Health and Human Services, *Healthy People 2000.* (2002). *National health promotion and disease prevention objectives.* Washington, DC: U.S. Government Printing Office, DHHS Publication No. PHS 91–50212.

U.S. Department of Health and Human Services. (2000). *Healthy People 2020: Understanding and improving health* (2nd ed.). Washington, DC: U.S. Government Printing Office.

U.S. Department of Health and Human Services. (2011). *CDC Health Disparities and Inequalities Report—United States, 2011.* Atlanta, GA: Centers for Disease Control.

U.S. Department of Health and Human Services, National Center for Health Statistics. (2014). *Health United States 2014.* Washington, DC: U.S. Government Printing Office.

U.S. Department of Health and Human Services. (2014). Youth Risk Behavior Surveillance—United States, 2009. *Morbidity and Mortality Report, 59*(ss–50), 1–148.

U.S. Department of Justice, Office of Justice Programs. (2006). *Criminal victimization in the United States, 2006, statistical tables.* Washington, DC: U.S. Government Printing Office.

Vaccarino, V., Gahbauer, E., Kasi, S., Charpentier, P., Acampora, D., & Krumholtz, H. (2002). *American Health Journal, 14396,* 1058–1067.

Valassi, K. H. (1962). Food habits of Greek Americans. *American Journal of Nursing, 11*(3), 240.

Violence Partner Center. (2008). *When men murder women: an analysis of the 2008 data.* Washington, DC: Violence Partner Center.

Wagner, D., & Heyward, V. (2000). Measures of body composition in blacks and whites: a comparative review. *American Journal of Clinical Nutrition, 71,* 1392–1402.

Walsh, E. (1993). The patient with peripheral vascular problems. In E. Long, B. C. Phipps, & W. J. Cassmeyer (Eds.), *Medical surgical nursing: concepts and clinical practice* (4th ed.). St. Louis: Mosby.

Weber, W. (1999). Population and genetic polymorphisms. *Molecular Diagnosis, 4*(4), 299–307.

Westfall, D. (1971). Diabetes mellitus among the Florida Seminoles. *HSMHA Health Reports, 86,* 1037–1041.

Wheeler, E. (2004). Racial disparities in hospitalized elderly patients with chronic heart failure. *Journal of Transcultural Nursing, 1594,* 291–297.

When patients can't drink milk. (1976). *Nursing Update,* 10–12.

White, S., & Pharoah, M. J. (2009). *Oral radiology: principles and interpretation* (6th ed.). St. Louis: Mosby.

Williams, R. A. (1975). *Textbook of Black-related disease.* New York: McGraw-Hill.

Winkleby, M., Robinson, T. N., Sundquist, J., & Kraemer, H. C. (1999). Ethnic variation in cardiovascular disease risk factors among children and young adults: findings from the third national health and nutrition examination survey, 1988–1994. *Journal of the American Medical Association, 281,* 1006–1013.

Witkop, C. J., Jr., & Barros, L. (1963). Oral and genetic studies of Chileans, 1960: 1. Oral anomalies. *American Journal of Physical Anthropology, 21,* 15–24.

Yonkers, K. A., Kando, J. C., Cole, J. O., & Blumenthal, S. (1992). Gender differences in pharmacokinetics and pharmacodynamics of psychotropic medication. *American Journal of Psychiatry, 149*(5), 587–595.

Zhou, H., Adedoyin, A., & Woods, A. (1992). Differing effect of atropine on heart rate in Chinese and White subjects. *Clinical Pharmacology Therapy, 52,* 120–124.

PART TWO

Application of Assessment and Intervention Techniques Specific to Cultural Groups

African-Americans

Brenda Cherry and Joyce Newman Giger

BEHAVIORAL OBJECTIVES

After reading this chapter, the nurse will be able to:

1. Identify ways in which the African-American culture influences African-American individuals and their health-seeking behaviors.
2. Recognize the need for an in-depth understanding of variables that are common within and across cultural groups to provide culturally appropriate nursing care when working with African-Americans.
3. Recognize physical and biological variances that exist within and across African-American groups to provide culturally appropriate nursing care.
4. Develop a sensitivity and an understanding for communication differences evidenced within and across African-American groups to avoid stereotyping and to provide culturally appropriate nursing care.
5. Develop a sensitivity and an understanding for psychological phenomena that influence the functioning of an African-American when providing nursing care.

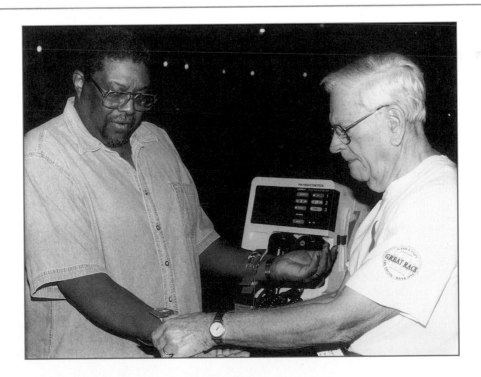

In a time when people are seeking to become more culturally aware, it is important to note distinctions in terminology regarding cultural groups. This is certainly true of African-Americans. Some African-American individuals and groups are encouraging the use of the term *Black Americans,* whereas others are encouraging the use of the term *African-Americans.* The term *African-Americans* is used to refer to a cultural heritage that is a combination of African and American. On the other hand, the term *Black Americans* is believed to place more focus on biological racial identity than on cultural heritage. The term *African-Americans* is used in this book except in instances where its descriptive characteristic is inappropriate, for example, Black skin, Black race, non-Black, Black English, and Black dialect. We have chosen these terms because they are now commonly used in the literature.

OVERVIEW OF AFRICAN-AMERICANS

According to the U.S. Census Bureau, there are approximately 45,562,000 African-Americans residing in the United States, representing approximately 14.4% of the American population (U.S. Department of Commerce, Bureau of the Census, U.S. Census Bureau, March 2015). Of the number of African-Americans residing in this country, 54.8% live in the South, 18.8% live in the Midwest, 17.6% live in the Northeast, and 8.8% live in the West (U.S. Department of Commerce, Bureau, American Community, 2015). Although African-Americans live throughout the United States, the states with the greatest number of African-Americans are New York (3,362,736), California (2,451,453), Texas (2,898,143), Florida (2,916,174), and Georgia (2,907,944) (U.S. Department of Commerce, Bureau of the Census, American Community Survey, 2015).

The cities with the most African-Americans are metropolitan New York City (3,362,616), Atlanta (1,707,913) Chicago (1,645,993), Detroit (980,451), Philadelphia (1,241,780, Houston (1,025,775), Memphis (414,928), and Dallas-Fort Worth (961,871) (U.S. Census Bureau, Bureau of the Census, American Community Survey, 2015). In 2014, African-Americans represented more than 50% of the total population in 10 U.S. cities: Gary, Indiana (84.0%), Detroit (82.8%), Birmingham, Alabama (73.5%), Jackson, Mississippi (70.6%), New Orleans (67.3%), Baltimore (64.3%), Atlanta (61.4%), Memphis (61.4%), Washington, DC (60.0%), and Richmond, Virginia (57.2%) (U.S. Department of Commerce, Bureau of the Census, American Community Survey, Brief on the Black Population, 2015).

In 2012, the median age of African-Americans residing in the United States was 32 years, compared with 35.3 years for the rest of the general population (U.S. Department of Commerce, Bureau of the Census, American Community Survey, 2015). This is up from 29.2 years of age in 1990 and 30.2 years of age in 2000. African-American men have a lower mean age than African-American women (29.62 versus 33.5 years). In 2009, only 8.4% of African-Americans were 65 years of age or older, compared with 14% of their White counterparts and 13% of the rest of the general population. The number of African-Americans 65 years of age or older was 2.5 million in 1990 (up from 2.1 million in 1980). It is interesting to note that in 2009 African-American women dominated the older age groups (62% versus 38% for their male counterparts). It is believed that the disproportionately low number of African-American males 65 years of age or older is a result of the higher mortality for African-American males (U.S. Department of Commerce, Bureau of the Census, American Community Survey, 2015; U.S. Department of Commerce, Bureau of the Census, The Older Population, 2000, 2001). Where age is concerned, an interesting phenomenon is thought to occur for African-Americans and is referred to as the *mortality crossover* ("crossover phenomenon"). This phenomenon is thought to occur in African-Americans at about 85 years of age. Many researchers postulate that the mortality for Blacks at this age is lower than that for Whites for the first time in the lifespan (LaVist, 2005).

In 2010, 84.1% of African-Americans 25 years of age or older held at least a high school diploma, compared with 91.6% of their White counterparts. In 2009, only 12.7% of African-Americans 25 years of age or older held a bachelor's degree or higher, which is down from 16.4% in 2000, compared with 21% for their White counterparts. Of the African-American males 25 years of age or older, 424,000 had less than a ninth-grade education; 1,178,000 had less than a high school degree with 9 to 12 years of education; 3,923,000 were high school graduates; 2,714,000 held an associate's degree or had some college; 1,169,000 held a bachelor's degree; and 610,000 held a graduate or professional degree. In contrast, of the African-American females 25 years of age or older, 544,000 had less than a ninth-grade education; 1,455,000 had less than a high school degree with 9 to 12 years of education; 4,086,000 were high school graduates; 3,906,000 held an associate's degree or had some college; 1,709,000 held a bachelor's degree; and 880,000 held graduate or equivalency or a professional degree (U.S. Department of Commerce, Bureau of the Census, American Community Survey, 2015).

Historical Account of African-Americans

From the sixteenth to the nineteenth centuries, more than 10 million Africans were brought to the United States and bonded into slavery (Leary, 2005). By historical accounts, nearly 600,000 slaves arrived in the United States in the sixteenth century, 2 million in the seventeenth century, 5 million in the eighteenth century, and 3 million in the nineteenth century (Ploski & Williams, 1989). Because of these historical accounts, the perception held by most Americans is that African-Americans may be the only cultural and ethnic group who reside in the United States today who did not immigrate to this country voluntarily. Although this perception has merit, in reality, the history of the arrival of Africans in the United States has become somewhat distorted throughout the years. In actuality, many Europeans (meaning those persons of English, German, and Scotch-Irish ancestry) voluntarily immigrated to the American colonies as laborers and became "indentured servants" (Public Broadcasting Service [PBS], n.d.). Many of these people were paupers or debtors who used indentured servitude to gain a better way of life. The first 20 African-Americans to land at Jamestown in 1619 (preceding the *Mayflower*) were accepted into the community as "indentured servants." Although it is true that these 20 African-Americans did not have freedom of choice in the decision to come to the colonies because they were systematically captured against their will, they nonetheless, over the same course of time as European indentured servants (7 years), enjoyed the same liberties and privileges of the "free working class," including the right to own property (PBS, n.d.).

Two of the most notable African-Americans who arrived in this country as "indentured servants" were Anthony Johnson, who became a "freeman" as early as 1622, and Richard Johnson. Anthony Johnson prospered so well that by 1651, he was able to acquire five "indentured servants." Likewise, Richard Johnson, having been given 100 acres of land of his own, acquired two indentured servants by 1654, two of whom were White (PBS, n.d.). However, it is appropriate to note that both of these men were the exception, not the rule. In fact, a fissure was cracking open, and African-American servitude and White servitude were beginning to be viewed differently. By 1640, African-Americans had ceased to be viewed as servants and were assigned the status of chattel (meaning one who remained a fixed item of personal property for the duration of life). More importantly, in some states, laws began to differentiate between races and the association of "servitude for natural life" with people of African descent (Leary, 2005; PBS, n.d.).

In 1661, the Virginia House of Burgesses formally recognized the institution of African-American slavery (PBS, n.d.; Virtual Jamestown Law, n.d.). Of the 13 original colonies, only Pennsylvania protested the system of slavery. By 1667, Virginia had written into its statutes that even purifying the African-American soul through baptism could not

alter the condition of the African-American regarding bondage or freedom. Thus, color became the real cutting edge that separated the African, now American, from the rest of the colonists (PBS, n.d.).

Even today, the cultural roots of African-Americans are entrenched in the African-American life experience. According to Bloch (1983), it is the African-American life experience that has established what has become known as the African-American view of the external world. The African-American life experience has shaped the internal attitudes and belief systems of African-Americans, and it continues to influence interactions of African-Americans with persons from other cultural groups.

Some of the health problems noted particularly in African-Americans are believed to be the result of varying genetic pools and hereditary immunity. However, many of these problems have been found to be more closely associated with economic status than with race. Three intervening and reinforcing variables are poverty, discrimination, and social and psychological barriers. These variables are regarded as being so profound in their effect on African-Americans that they tend to keep these individuals from using the health care services that are available. These variables may also explain why morbidity and mortality rates are higher among African-Americans than for the rest of the general population. Although underrepresented in the general population, African-Americans remain overrepresented among the health statistics for life-threatening illness.

The life expectancy for African-Americans, 75.1 years, continues to lag behind that for Whites, which is 78.9 years (National Center for Health Statistics, 2013). In 2013, the life expectancy for African-American men was 71.8 as compared with 76.5 for their White counterparts. Similarly, the life expectancy for African-American women was 78.1 compared with 81.2 for their White counterparts (National Center for Health Statistics, Health United States, 2014; *World Almanac*, 2015).

While overall the infant mortality rate in the United States declined slightly from 7.2 in 1990 to 5.96 in 2013, African-Americans continue to have a higher infant mortality rate (11.20 per 1000 live births in 2012) compared with White Americans (5.00 per 1000 live births in 2012) (National Center for Health Statistics, Health United States, 2014). Although the average life expectancy for African-Americans at birth edged upward to the middle 70s, and it improved ever so slightly for males, it is important to note that the life expectancy for African-American male babies born between 1986 and 2009 continues to shrink (National Center for Health Statistics, Health United States, 2014). A portion of the shrinkage is attributable to infant mortality, which is twice as high for African-American babies as for

White babies. Yet another portion of the shrinkage is attributable to disparities in health concerns, especially chronic illnesses, which contribute significantly to premature deaths (before 65 years of age) among African-American males. In fact, in 2012, the rate of deaths for African-American males was 55% higher for heart disease, 26% higher for cancer, 180% higher for stroke, and 100% higher for lung disease than for the rest of the general U.S. population (National Center for Health Statistics, Health United States 2014). Perhaps the greatest disparity was the rate of deaths or the potential for life lost for African-American males attributable to homicides, which was 630% higher, compared with White males (National Center for Health Statistics, Health United States, 2014). In health status disparities, African-American women do not fare much better than their male counterparts. When the life expectancy of White women is compared with the life expectancy of African-American women, African-American women have a shorter life expectancy (78 years versus 81.3 years) (National Center for Health Statistics, Health United States, 2014).

COMMUNICATION

Communication is the matrix for thought and relationship between all people regardless of cultural heritage (Murray & Huelskoetter, 1991). Verbal and nonverbal communication is learned in cultural settings. Difficulties arise if a person does not communicate in the way or manner prescribed by the culture because the individual cannot conform to social expectations. Communication, therefore, is basic to culturally appropriate nursing care.

Dialect

Dialect refers to the variations within a language. African-Americans speak English; however, there are widespread differences in the way English is spoken between African-Americans and other ethnic and cultural groups. Different linguistic norms evolve among groups of people who are socially or geographically separated. Social stratification alters the nature and frequency of intercommunication among groups. When social separation by factors such as ethnic origin or class is responsible for the origin and perpetuation of a particular dialect, the dialect is referred to as a *stratified dialect*. When differences in dialect emerge as a result of geographical separation of people, the dialect is called a *regional*, or *geographical*, dialect.

Origins of African-American Dialect in the United States.
Accurate and reliable data concerning the different dialects spoken by most African-Americans are unavailable to the public or to educators (Turner, 1948). The study of pidgin

and Creole language has facilitated an intelligent study of Black English and of the notable differences between Black English and Standard English (Deckart & Vickers, 2011). Research into the languages of Brazilians of African descent, as well as Haitians, Jamaicans, and the present-day African-American inhabitants off the seacoasts of South Carolina and Georgia, indicates a correlation of structural features of several of the languages spoken in parts of West Africa, as well as a similarity to the English spoken by Whites in the United States (Hymes, 1971; Kautzsch, 2012).

The first Africans brought to the United States as slaves were systematically separated during transportation, and this separation continued after arrival. African slaves may not have been forced to give up their African languages; however, they were thrown into situations in which learning a new language became a priority in establishing a way to communicate with slaves from other countries (Dillard, 2008; Hamlet, 2011). As a result, the various African languages combined with the languages of other cultural groups in the New World, such as the Dutch, the French, and the English. This combination of the different African languages with other languages fostered a need for a "common language" for all African-Americans, which ultimately led to the restructuring of grammar of all languages, including English. This process is referred to as "pidginization" and "creolization." Pidgin English is not a language but a dialect. Pidgin tends to be simple in grammar and limited in vocabulary. Typically, in communities where pidgin is spoken, its use is limited to trade purposes, task-oriented activities, and communication among cultural or ethnic groups (Deckert & Vickers, 2011). When a pidgin dialect undergoes internal expansion and extension of use, the results are creolization. It is from a pidgin dialect that a Creole language was born. In the United States, several Creole dialects still exist, particularly in the rural South and in such places as New Orleans, Louisiana; Hattiesburg and Vicksburg, Mississippi; and Mobile, Alabama. Furthermore, the migration of African-Americans from the South saw the development of pidginization and creolization in some northern cities such as New York, Chicago, and Detroit. Evidences of past migration and its effect on dialect and Black English remain obvious even today.

Language Usage. The dialect that is spoken by many African-Americans is sufficiently different from Standard English in pronunciation, grammar, and syntax to be classified as Black English. The use of Standard English versus Black English varies among African-Americans and in some instances may be related to educational level and socioeconomic status, although this is not always the case. The use of Standard English by African-Americans is important in terms of social and economic mobility. However, the use of Black English has served as a unifying factor for African-Americans in maintaining their cultural and ethnic identity. This may explain why many African-Americans continue to speak Black English despite the social, economic, and educational pressures that are often exerted by members of other cultures (Fisher & Lapp, 2013). Thus, it is not uncommon for some African-Americans to speak Standard English when serving in a professional capacity or when socializing with Whites and then revert to Black English when interacting in all–African-American settings. Some African-Americans who have not mastered Standard English may feel insecure in certain situations where they are required and expected to use Standard English. When confronted with such situations, they may become very quiet, with the result that they may be labeled hostile or submissive.

Pronunciation of Black English

There is a tendency for users of what is often referred to as "Black dialect" to pronounce certain syllables and consonants somewhat differently. For example, *th*, as in *the, these,* or *them,* may be pronounced as *d*, as in *de, dese,* and *dem* (Collins, 2008; Dillard, 1972; Kautzsch, 2012). In Black English there is also a tendency to drop the final *r* or *g* from words; thus *father* and *mother* become *fatha* and *motha*. The words *laughing, talking,* and *going* are pronounced *laughin, talkin,* and *goin*. Speakers of Black English may also place more emphasis on one syllable as opposed to another; for example, *brother* may be pronounced *brotha*. In addition, the final *th* of words is pronounced as *f* in Black English; thus *bath, birth, mouth,* and *with* are pronounced *baf, birf, mouf,* and *wif* (Collins, 2008; Kautzsch, 2012).

Copula deletion of the verb *to be* is a common omission in some environments; for example, the speaker of Black English might say, "He walking" or "She at work" in contrast to the Standard English "He is walking" or "She is at work." Black English speakers may also use the unconjugated form of the verb "to be" where Standard English speakers would use the conjugated form. An example of this would be "He be working" in contrast to the Standard English "He is working."

In Standard English every verb is in sequence and must be marked as either present or past tense. However, in Black English only past-tense verbs need to be marked. For example, in Black English the *s* marking the present tense may be omitted: thus "He go" or "She love." Attempts to correct this can result in phrases such as "goes" and "We loves." Speakers of Black English may also omit the possessive suffix. For example, in Black English one might say, "Richard dog bit me" or "Mary dress" in contrast to the Standard English "Richard's dog bit me" or "Mary's dress" (Collins, 2008; Kautzsch, 2012).

Speakers of Black English also have some words that are classified as slang. These words are different from slang words used in other dialects and may or may not convey the same meaning. For instance, African-Americans may use the word *chilly* or *chillin* to infer sophistication, whereas a White individual may use the word *cool* or (formerly) *groovy* to convey the same meaning. Some African-Americans may use the verb *to fix* to denote planned actions, for example, "I'm fixin to go home," whereas the user of Standard English would say, "I'm getting ready to go home."

The speech of some African-Americans is colorful and dynamic. For these persons, communication also involves body movement (kinesics). Some African-Americans tend to use a wide range of body movement, such as facial gestures, hand and arm movements, expressive stances, handshakes, and hand signals, along with verbal interaction. This repertoire of body movements can also be seen in sports and in dance, which is the highest communicative form of body language.

Some African-Americans use sounds that are not words to add expression to their conversation or to music, such as *oo-wee* or *uh huh,* which have analogies in some of the West African languages as expressed in the surviving Gullah dialect (Sea Islands, South Carolina) but not in English.

The term *signifying* describes an approach wherein one attempts to chide or correct someone indirectly. For example, one might correct someone who is not dressed properly by saying, "You sure are dressed up today."

Most African-Americans use Black English in a systematic way that can be predictably understood by others; thus Black English cannot and should not be regarded as substandard or ungrammatical. It is estimated that approximately 80% of African-Americans use Black English at least some of the time (Dillard, 1972).

Implications for Nursing Care

The nurse must develop a sensitivity to communication variances as a prerequisite for accurate nursing assessment and intervention in multicultural situations. In all nursing environments the potential for misunderstanding the client is accentuated when the nurse and the client are from different ethnic groups. Perhaps the most significant and obvious barrier occurs when two persons speak different languages. However, the nurse must be cognizant of the fact that barriers to communication exist even when individuals speak the same language. The nurse may have difficulty explaining things to a client in simple, jargon-free language to facilitate the client's understanding. The nurse must develop a familiarity with the language of the client because this is the best way to gain insight into the culture. Every language and dialect are special and have unique ways of looking at the world and at experiences (Kluckhohn, 2003). Every language also has a set of unconscious assumptions about the world and life. According to Kluckhohn (2003), people see and hear what the grammatical system of their language makes them sensitive to perceive.

The nurse who works with African-American clients may find that although the language is the same, the perception of what message is being sent and received by the nurse and the client may be different. The important variables that may pose a problem for the nurse is the client's interpretation of specific verbal and nonverbal messages, such as communication style, eye contact, and use of touch and space (Dayar-Berenson, 2014). Therefore, it is of the highest priority for the nurse who is working with African-Americans, particularly those who speak Black English, to understand as much of the context of the dialect as possible.

The nurse must bear in mind that Black English cannot be viewed as an unacceptable form of English. Thus it is important for the nurse to avoid labeling and stereotyping the client. The nurse should avoid chiding and correcting the speech of African-Americans because this behavior can result in the client's becoming quiet, passive, and, in some cases, aggressive or hostile. On the other hand, although the nurse should attempt to use words common to the client's vocabulary, mimicking the client's language can be interpreted as dehumanizing. For example, if a nurse were to say *dem* for *them* or *dese* for *these,* the client may perceive this as ridicule.

When working with persons who speak Black English, the nurse must keep in mind that the client may use slang to convey certain messages. However, slang terms often have different meanings among individuals and especially among cultural groups. For example, an African-American client's response to questioning about a diagnostic test, "It was a real bad experience," may actually mean that it was a unique and yet positive experience. The nurse working with this client will need to clarify the exact meaning of the word *bad.* In Black English the word *bad* is often used for the exact opposite, in other words, "good." In another example, an African-American client who states that the medication has been taken "behind the meal" may mean the medication has been taken "after eating." A nurse may interpret behind to mean "before" rather than "after" because the dictionary definition states that behind means "still to come." The nurse must be cautious about interpreting particular words each time an African-American uses certain terms.

It is essential that the nurse identify and clarify what is happening psychologically and physiologically to the African-American client. When possible, the nurse should substitute words commonly understood by the African-American client for more sophisticated medical terms. When this is done, the nurse will find that the African-American client is more receptive to instructions and more cooperative. Stokes (1977) offers a list of terms commonly used by nurses and equivalent words used by some African-Americans:

Conditions (Medical/Black English)	Functions (Medical/Black English)
Diabetes/sugar	Constipation/locked bowels
Pain/miseries	
Syphilis/bad blood, pox	Diarrhea/running off, grip
Anemia/low blood, tired blood	Menstruation/red flag, the curse
Vomiting/throwing up	Urinate, urine/pass water, tinkle, peepee

The nurse must remember that some African-Americans place a great deal of importance on nonverbal elements of communication and that the verbal pattern of some African-American clients may differ significantly from that of a non–African-American nurse. It is also important for the nurse to keep in mind that words used by some African-American clients may be the same as those used by the nurse but have different, idiosyncratic meanings. When working with African-American clients, the nurse must also remember that eye contact, nodding, and smiling are not necessarily essential or direct correlates that the African-American client is paying attention (Sue, 2003).

SPACE

According to Hall (1990), the degree to which people are sensorially involved with each other, along with how they use time, determines not only at what point they feel crowded or have a perception that their personal space is collapsing inwardly but the methods for alleviating crowding as well. For example, Puerto Ricans and African-Americans are reported to have a much higher involvement ratio than other cultural groups such as German Americans or Scandinavian Americans. It is believed that highly involved people, such as African-Americans, require a higher density than less involved people. However, highly involved people may at the same time require more protection or screening from outsiders than people with a lower level of involvement do.

To understand the variable of space, it is essential to understand time and the way it is handled because the variable of time influences the structuring of space. According to Hall (1990), there are two contrasting ways in which people handle time, monochronic and polychronic, and each affects the way in which an individual perceives space. People with low involvement are generally monochronic because such individuals tend to compartmentalize time; for example, they may schedule one thing at a time and tend to become disoriented if they have to deal with too many things at once. On the other hand, polychronic individuals tend to keep several operations going at once, almost like jugglers, and these individuals tend to be very involved with each other.

Implications for Nursing Care

The nurse who works with Latin Americans, Africans, African-Americans, or Indonesians may feel somewhat uncomfortable because these cultures generally dictate a much closer personal space when personal and social spaces are involved (Purnell, 2013). Because some African-Americans are perceived as polychronic individuals, it is important for the nurse to remember that polychronic individuals tend to collect activities.

When polychronic individuals interact with monochronic individuals, some difficulties may be experienced because of the different ways in which these individuals relate to space and to each other. An example of a difficulty encountered between monochronic and polychronic individuals is when monochronic individuals become upset or angry because of the constant interruptions of polychronic individuals.

Some monochronic individuals believe that there must be order to get things done. On the other hand, polychronic individuals, such as some African-Americans, do not believe that order is necessary to get things done. The nurse who works with African-Americans must keep in mind that to reduce polychronic effects, it is necessary to reduce multiple-activity involvements on the part of the client. The nurse can accomplish this by separating activities with as much screening and scrutiny as necessary (Hall, 1990). One goal of nursing intervention should be to help the client structure activities in a ranked order that will produce maximal benefits for the client.

SOCIAL ORGANIZATION

Social organization refers to how a cultural group organizes itself around particular units (such as family, racial or ethnic group, and community or social group). Most African-Americans have been socialized in predominantly African-American environments. Historically, because of legalized segregation, African-Americans were separated or isolated from the mainstream of society. Consequently, African-Americans are the only cultural group in the United States that has not been assimilated into the mainstream society. Even today, African-Americans maintain separate and in most cases unequal lifestyles compared with other Americans. Evidence of the failure to assimilate on the part of African-Americans is seen in the existence of predominantly African-American neighborhoods, churches, colleges and universities, and public elementary and high schools.

Historical Review of Slavery and Discrimination

Patterns of discrimination have existed in the United States since the inception of slavery. With the inception of slavery came the foundations of attitudes and beliefs that were and continue to be the pillars that support the institution of racism. Racism, discriminatory practices, and segregation combined have produced insularity or separatist feelings and attitudes on the part of some African-Americans. As a result, African-Americans are often accused of having more separate and more insular patterns of communication, which have restricted some African-Americans from participating in the wider White society. Thus some African-Americans prefer to maintain themselves within their own group. Accordingly, this insularity has promoted the retention of culturally seeded beliefs that differ from the beliefs held by the dominant culture. Lim (2015) noted that every cultural group has unique beliefs that influence their attitudes regarding health. These beliefs tend to determine the types of behavior and health care practices that a particular cultural group views as appropriate or inappropriate. In other words, the attitudes and beliefs regarding health and illness vary in the United States between African-Americans and Whites and even among African-Americans themselves.

Attitudes, beliefs, values, and morals are the basic structural units of any culture. Culture is an outward manifestation of a way of life; it is dynamic, fluid, and ever evolving. The family is the basic social unit of most cultures and is the means by which culture is passed down from one generation to the next. The inception of slavery in the United States precipitated the beginning of the destruction of the transplanted African culture. In Africa, Africans had been accustomed to a strictly regulated family life with rigidly enforced moral codes. The family unit was close knit, well organized, connected with kin and community, and highly functional for the economic, social, psychological, and spiritual well-being of the people (Jones, 1998). The family was the center of African civilization.

The destruction of the African family began with the capture of slaves for transplantation to the New World, which began in 1619. As slaves were captured, the young, healthy men, women, and children were forcibly removed from their families and tribes. This separation continued as these slaves journeyed to the New World because they were placed on ships without regard for family unity, tribe, or kinship. On the arrival of the slaves in the United States, this systematic separation of individuals from families persisted.

The cruelest form of emasculation of the Black Africans, now Americans, was the breeding of slaves for sale. Infants and children were taken from their mothers and sold as chattel. Marriage between slaves was not legally sanctioned and generally left to the discretion of the owners. Some slave owners assigned mates when slaves reached breeding age. Others would not permit their slaves to marry a slave from another plantation. Most slave owners sold husbands, wives, and children without consideration for family ties. The children who were produced of the slave union belonged to the slave owner, not to the parents. The African-American family in the United States during slavery lacked autonomy because the family members were someone else's property. The parents were unable to provide security or protection for their children. Husbands were unable to protect their wives. In a documentary of the lives of 75 African-American women, Angelou (1989) described the heartbreaking tenderness of African-American women and the majestic strength they needed to survive the subjugation and horror of the slavery experience.

In contrast to this view of the destruction of the African-American family during slavery, Gutman (1976) contends that the African-American family was not disaggregated because of slavery. In fact, Gutman (1976) presents compelling evidence to suggest not only that some African-American families remained intact during slavery but also that many slave marriages were officially documented, as were the names of their offspring. Gutman (1976) cautions, however, that no more misleading inference could be drawn from these data than to argue that the data alone show that slaves lived in stable families.

Changing Roles of the African-American Family

Under the system of slavery in the United States, the role of the African-American man as husband and father was obliterated. The African-American man was not the head of the household, nor was he the provider or the protector of his family. Instead, he was someone else's property. Under the system of slavery, the African-American man remained powerless to defend his wife and children from harm, particularly when they were beaten or sexually assaulted by the White overseer or owner or by any other White person. The African-American male slave was often referred to as "boy" until he reached a certain age, at which point he became "uncle." The only crucial function for the African-American man within the African-American family was siring children.

In the United States under the system of slavery, the African-American woman became the dominant force in the family. She was forced to work side-by-side with her male counterpart during the day and had the additional responsibility of caring for family members at night. The African-American woman was forced to bear children for sale and to care for other children, including those of the slave owner. Some African-American women during slavery were also forced to satisfy the sexual desires of any White man, and any children born out of this union were considered slaves. If the African-American woman had a husband, he was merely her sexual companion and was referred to as her "boy" by the slave owner and by White society in general. The inception of slavery, the division of the African family and subsequently the African-American family, and the subordinate role of the African-American man played a significant part in the establishment of the female-dominated African-American household that exists even today in the United States.

Even after slavery was abolished in the United States, the destructive forces against the African-American family persisted. Today, the residual effects of slavery are still evident in some parts of the country. After slavery was abolished and during the emancipation period and the years that followed, the African-American man was either denied jobs or given tasks that were demeaning and dehumanizing. From the time of the abolition of slavery until the mid-1960s, African-Americans in some parts of the country were attacked, lynched, and murdered. Sexual attacks on African-American women also continued. Such actions further served to drive some African-American men away from their families. Thus there was further weakening of the family and subsequently of the African-American male role (Leary, 2005). Despite the discriminatory practices and the continued hostile attacks against African-Americans, some African-American families nevertheless were able to establish themselves. As these African-American families were increasingly able to develop a secure economic status, they began to establish schools, churches, and other social organizations.

Characteristics of the African-American Family

In the United States, there are basically two types of family structures: the male-headed (patriarchal) family structure and the female-headed (matriarchal) family structure. In 2000, the number of African-American female-headed households was creeping slowly downward. In 2009, such families constituted 44% of African-American families. In addition, between 1950 and 2009, the number of African-American female-headed householders who had never been married quadrupled, from 9% in 1950 to 42.4% in 2012 (U.S. Department of Commerce, Bureau of the Census, American Community Survey, 2015). The fact that approximately half of the African-American families in the United States are female-headed is attributable in part to factors related to and carried over from slavery. For example, the African-American family has not been able to overcome deficits related to education and income. According to the U.S. Department of Commerce, Bureau of the Census (2015), the average income for African-American men, compared with men in other cultural groups with similar skills and educational levels, is significantly lower. African-American males, in particular, have not made significant strides in gaining entry into the workforce since the 1980 census (U.S. Department of Commerce, Bureau of the Census, American Community Survey, 2015). The annual labor participation rate for African-American males in 2009 dropped slightly from the 1990 and 2000 (65.3%) data to 63.2%, compared with 70.6% in 1980. In 2009, 65.5% of African-American men and 63.2% of African-American women participated in the workforce, compared with 74.3% of White men and 60.3% of White women (U.S. Department of Commerce, Bureau of the Census, American Community Survey, 2015). Overall, African-Americans are less likely to participate in the workforce than other racial and ethnic groups. Whereas the median household income (which takes into account all sources of income, including full- and part-time jobs and interest income, for a household) for the nation was $45,320, it was only $39,879 for African-Americans; in comparison, for their White counterparts the median income was $65,000. The median earnings figure for African-Americans for males (which takes into account only full-time work status) was only $36,171, as compared with $45,485 for the rest of the general population (U.S. Department of Commerce, Bureau of the Census, American Community Survey, 2015). In addition, the median earnings figure for African-American females ($31,546) was disproportionately lower than that of the rest of the general population ($35,299) (U.S. Department of Commerce, Bureau of the Census, American Community Survey, 2015).

Implications for Nursing Care

Even today, the African-American family is often oriented around women; in other words, it is matrifocal. This has implications for the nurse because within the African-American family structure, the wife or mother is often charged with the responsibility for protecting the health of the family members. The African-American woman is expected to assist each family member in maintaining good health and in determining treatment if a family member is ill. This responsibility has both positive and negative effects

because African-American clients often enter the health care delivery system at the advice of the matriarch of the family. The nurse must recognize the importance of the African-American woman in disseminating information and in assisting the client in making decisions. Although the African-American family may be matrifocal, it is nevertheless essential to include the African-American man in the decision-making process.

Some African-American families are composed of large networks and tend to be very supportive during times of crisis and illness. Large network groups can have both positive and negative effects on wellness, illness, and recovery behaviors (Dayar-Berenson, 2014; Lim, 2015). Jackson, Neighbors, and Gurin (1986) found that network size was positively related to distress: the more informal helpers there were, the higher the distress score on the instrument used in the survey. One conclusion of the study is that network size is not a good measure of perceived social support. According to the findings from the study, the more serious the problem, the more people within the network are consulted for help. But a greater number of people consulted does not necessarily reduce the severity of the problem; rather, an individual with an acute illness may spend so much time seeking assistance within the network that necessary and timely treatment is delayed. The nurse should include all the members of the network in planning and implementing health care because some members of the network may provide advice or care that could be detrimental to the client. For example, an African-American client who is admitted with an electrolyte imbalance and is brought laxatives from home by a relative may have additional electrolyte problems when the laxatives are taken without consulting members of the health care team. In this case the nurse must emphasize the importance of the nurse's role in providing health care. Once the family develops a feeling of trust, the nurse is more likely to be consulted should perceived health needs arise, for example, when the client needs a laxative.

TIME

Time is a concept that is universal and continuous. All emotional and perceptual experiences are interrelated with the concept of time. The perception of time is individual and determined by cultural experience (Hall, 1989). In the United States, time has become the most important organizing principle of the dominant culture (Hall, 1989). The majority of individuals of the dominant culture are time conscious and very future oriented; they make it a common practice to "plan ahead" and "save for a rainy day." Time has become very important and comparable to money in the American society. Doing things efficiently and faster has become the American way.

It is impossible to characterize African-Americans and their perceptions of time as one way or the other because African-Americans, just as individuals from other cultural groups, vary according to social and cultural factors. Some African-Americans who have become assimilated into the dominant culture are very time conscious and take pride in punctuality. These individuals are likely to be future oriented and believe that saving and planning are important. They are likely to be well educated and to hold professional positions, although this is not always the case, because some African-Americans who are not well educated and do not hold professional jobs still value time and have hopes for the future (and are likely to encourage their children to seek higher education and to save for the future) (Dayar-Berenson, 2014).

On the other hand, some African-Americans react to the present situation and are not future oriented; it is their belief that planning for the future is hopeless because of their previous experiences and encounters with racism and discrimination. They believe that their future will be the same as their present and their past (Dayar-Berenson, 2014). These individuals are likely to be jobless or have low-paying jobs. Educational levels may vary from junior high school to college degrees among persons who share this belief. Such individuals are unlikely to value time; thus they do not value the concept of punctuality and may not keep appointments or arrive much later than the scheduled time. It is the belief of some African-Americans that time is flexible and that events will begin when they arrive. This belief has been translated down through the years to imply an acceptable lateness among some African-Americans of 30 minutes to 1 hour. This perception of time can be traced back to West Africa, where the concept of time was elastic and encompassed events that had already taken place as well as those that would occur immediately (Mbiti, 1990).

Finally, some African-Americans have a future-oriented concept of time because of their strong religious beliefs. These individuals may be from all socioeconomic and educational levels. It is their belief that life on Earth, with all its pain and suffering, is bearable because there will be happiness and lack of pain after death. African-Americans who hold this belief plan their funerals and even purchase their grave plots long before their deaths (Smith, 1976).

Implications for Nursing Care

Because some African-Americans perceive time as flexible and elastic, it is essential for the nurse to include the client and family in the planning and implementation of nursing care. When planning nursing care with the client and family, the nurse should emphasize events that have

flexibility where time is concerned, such as morning care and bathing. On the other hand, the nurse must also emphasize events that have no flexibility where time is concerned and where delay in doing something, such as taking time-release medications or medications for certain conditions, would have serious implications for the client's well-being. For example, a client with high blood pressure must be made to understand that the medication must be taken as and when prescribed, not as and when desired. A medication missed today cannot be made up by taking double the amount tomorrow. As another example, a client with type 1 diabetes cannot delay the time between meals.

Some African-Americans are perceived as individuals with present-time orientations. Such persons may have a more flexible adherence to schedules and may believe that immediate concerns are more relevant than future concerns. Because appointment schedules may lack meaning, the nurse must emphasize the importance of adhering to the appointment schedule. If the nurse knows a particular client has a pattern of arriving late, the nurse may advise that client to arrive for scheduled appointments at least half an hour early. For the nurse who works with clients who are focused on the present, it is essential to avoid crisis-oriented nursing and promote preventive nursing (Sue, 2003).

ENVIRONMENTAL CONTROL

Health Care Benefits

In the United States the system of health care beliefs and practices is extremely complex and diverse among cultural groups. Variations in health care beliefs and practices cross ethnic and social boundaries. These variations are evidenced even within families. Culture influences individual expectations and perceptions regarding health, illness, disease, and symptoms related to disease. Accordingly, culture, cultural beliefs, and cultural values influence how one copes when confronted with illness, disease, or stress (Anderson & Bauwens, 1981).

In the United States, a distinction between "illness" and "disease" has been made by anthropologists and sociologists (Staples, 1976). *Illness* has been defined as an individual's perception of being sick, which is not necessarily related to the biomedical definition of disease. *Disease* has been defined as a condition that deviates from the norm. Thus illness may exist in the absence of disease and vice versa (Staples, 1976). Norms used to determine a disease condition, by Western standards, have for the most part been taken from studies conducted on White subjects. Thus, when these norms are applied to other cultural groups, such as African-Americans, the norm values may be meaningless and lead to erroneous conclusions. For example, to receive a 2 for color on the Apgar scoring system for newborns, the infant must be completely pink. Another example of a Western norm expectation is that an inverted T wave may be an ominous, pathological finding. However, in the case of African-Americans and particularly African-American men, such a finding should be the expectation, rather than being perceived as ominous and pathological. Also, growth as related to body size and physique is often normed by White Western standards. Thus African-Americans, who mature at an earlier age and typically have larger physiques than those of their White counterparts, may be perceived as being either overweight or oversized when White Western norms are applied.

Health Care Beliefs and the African-American Family

African-Americans in the United States are a highly heterogeneous group; thus, it is impossible to make a collective statement about their health care beliefs and practices. Many health care beliefs that are exhibited by African-Americans in the United States are derived from their African ancestry (Smith, 1976). For example, in West Africa, where most African-Americans originated, man was perceived as a monistic being, that is, a being from which the body and soul could not be separated (Smith, 1976). Man was also perceived as a holistic individual with many complex dimensions. Religion was interwoven into health care beliefs and practices. (West Africans continue even today to believe that illness is a natural occurrence resulting from disharmony and conflict in some area of the individual's life.) Because life was centered on the entire family, illness was perceived as a collective event and subsequently a disruption of the entire family system. The traditional West African healers always involved the individual's entire family in the healing process, even when the disorder was believed to be somatic. Thus, the traditional West African healer based treatment on the premise of wholeness, the necessity for reincorporation of the client into the family system, and involvement of the entire family system in the care and treatment of the individual (Treas & Wilkinson, 2014).

Perception of Illness. In the United States some African-Americans perceive illness as a natural occurrence resulting from disharmony and conflict in some aspect of an individual's life. This belief is a cultural value that has been passed down through the generations to African-Americans as a result of West African influences and tends to involve three general areas: (1) environmental hazards, (2) divine punishment, and (3) impaired social relationships (Snow, 1977). An example of an environmental hazard is injuries as the result of being struck by lightning or bitten by a snake. Divine punishment might include illnesses or diseases that the individual attributes to sin. Impaired social relationships may be caused by such factors as a spouse leaving or parents disowning a child (Snow, 1977).

Another belief held by some African-Americans is that everything has an opposite. For every birth, there must be a death; for every marriage, there must be a divorce; for every occurrence of illness, someone must be cured (Snow, 1978). Some African-Americans may not be able to distinguish between physical and mental illness and spiritual problems and as a result may present themselves for treatment with a variety or combination of somatic, psychological, and spiritual complaints (Smith, 1976). For example, a client may present real symptoms of an ulcer but relate the symptoms to past sins or grief over a financial loss. The client desires assistance not only for the somatic disorder but also for the psychological and spiritual complaints.

African-Americans who share mainstream attitudes about pain may respond to pain stoically out of a desire to be a perfect client. This means that they tend not to "bother" the nurse by calling for attention or for pain medication. For such clients the nurse must make it clear that the client has a right to relief from pain. On the other hand, some African-American clients exhibit a different form of stoicism. Hard experience has convinced them that trouble and pain are God's will. In this case the nurse needs to help the client understand that pain retards healing and is medically undesirable (Taylor, Lillis, & Lynn, 2015; Treas & Wilkinson, 2014).

Folk Medicine

Complementary alternative medicine, which includes folk medicine, is germane to many cultural and ethnic groups. Individuals from all aspects of society may use folk medicine either alone or with a scientifically based medical system. The importance of folk medicine and the level of practice vary among the different ethnic and cultural groups, depending on education and socioeconomic status. In contrast to the scientifically based health care system in the United States, folk medicine is characterized by a belief in supernatural forces. From this perspective, health and illness are characterized as natural and unnatural.

According to Snow (1983), it matters whether an African-American person comes from a rural background when it is necessary to select health care providers. Some African-Americans who were reared in the rural South may have grown up being treated by folk practitioners and may not have encountered a physician until they reached adulthood. Therefore, these people are more likely to turn to a neighborhood folk practitioner when they become ill.

According to Harley (2006), folk medicine is still used within the African-American community because of the humiliation encountered in the mainstream health care system, lack of money, and lack of trust in health care workers. Today, some African-Americans go to physicians in order to get prescribed medications, not because they believe the physician is superior in knowledge or training.

Witchcraft, voodoo, and magic are an integral aspect of folk medicine (McKenzie & Chrisman, 1977). Natural events are those that are in harmony with nature and provide individuals who believe in and practice folk medicine with a certain degree of predictability in the events of daily living. Unnatural events, on the other hand, represent disharmony with nature, and so the events of day-to-day living cannot be predicted (Harley, 2006). Another aspect of the folk medicine system is a belief in opposing forces—that everything has an opposite. For example, for every birth, there must be a death. Also incorporated into the system of folk medicine is the belief that health is a gift from God, whereas illness is a punishment from God or a retribution for sin and evil (Harley, 2006; Vaughn, Jacquez, & Baker, 2009). This concept is evidenced by the belief held by some African-Americans that if a child is born with a physical handicap, it is a punishment from God for the past wrongdoings of the parents. In this way, sins of the father and mother are passed on for retribution by the children (Snow, 1983). Such beliefs are not limited to African-Americans but are also found among other cultural groups in the United States; for example, some Mexican Americans believe that illness is a punishment for some sin or misdeed (Treas & Wilkinson, 2014).

Practice of African-American Folk Medicine. Some African-Americans in the rural South and in the urban northern ghettos still practice folk medicine based on spirituality, including witchcraft, voodoo, and magic (Harley, 2006). Some of these individuals may also use the orthodox medical system. Historically, such cities as New Orleans and Baton Rouge, Louisiana, were very much voodoo oriented, and such beliefs were held not only by African-Americans but also by members of other cultural groups. Even today, the African-American folk medicine system is practiced by the high-ranking voodoo queen in some Louisiana cities. The Louisiana Voodoo Society is a carryover from a combination of Haitian and French cultural influences (Dayar-Berenson, 2014; Lim, 2015). Voodoo and witchcraft are not restricted to Louisiana and are also practiced in such places as the Georgia sea islands, which are just off the coast of Savannah. Interestingly enough, some of the inhabitants of the Georgia sea islands remain pure-blooded descendants of West African ancestry. Even today,

some people there have refused to intermarry with members of other cultural groups, thus maintaining the tradition of "pure-blooded" lineage (Wolfram & Clark, 1971). Pure-blooded descendants of West Africans are also found off the coast of South Carolina. A few of these people still speak Gullah (English with an admixture of various African languages) and tend to isolate themselves when possible from the mainstream of society (Wolfram & Clark, 1971).

African-American Folk Medicine System Defined. In the system of African-American folk medicine, illness is perceived as either a natural or an unnatural occurrence. A natural illness may occur because of exposure to the elements of nature without protection (such as a cold, the flu, or pneumonia). Natural illnesses occur when dangerous elements in the environment enter the body through impurities in food, water, and air. However, the words *natural* and *unnatural* are connoted to mean more or less than the dictionary definitions of these words. For example, cancer, which is linked to such environmental hazards as smog, cigarette smoke, toxic waste, and other chemical irritants, is considered a natural illness in a professional medical system. However, those persons who share beliefs in African-American folk medicine might view cancer as an unnatural illness, perceiving it as a punishment from God or a spell cast by an evil person doing the work of the devil (Harley, 2006; Vaughn et al., 2009). Such persons may not readily acknowledge the fact that cancer, for example, may be caused by environmental factors such as cigarette smoking; thus they may continue smoking even after being diagnosed with cancer. Unnatural illnesses are perceived as either a punishment from God or the work of the devil. This perception is in contrast to the dictionary definition of illness as an unhealthy condition of the body or mind.

Types of Folk Practitioners. Jordan (1975) identified distinct types of folk practitioners. The first type is the "old lady" or "granny" who acts as a local consultant. This individual is knowledgeable about many different home remedies made from certain spices, herbs, and roots that can be used to treat common illnesses. Another duty of this individual is to give advice and make appropriate referrals to another type of practitioner when an illness or a particular medical condition extends beyond her practice (Jordan, 1975). The second type of practitioner is the "spiritualist," the most prevalent and diverse type of folk practitioner. This individual attempts to combine rituals, spiritual beliefs, and herbal medicines to effect a cure for certain illnesses or ailments. The third type of practitioner is the voodoo priest or priestess. In some West Indies islands, the voodoo practitioner can be a man, whereas in some rural southern areas of the United States, the voodoo practitioner must be a woman and may inherit this title only by birthright and a perceived special gift (Snow, 1974).

In contrast to the type of voodoo priest or priestess found in some West Indies islands and in some rural or urban southern U.S. areas is the type of voodoo priest or priestess found in some larger urban areas such as Chicago; Queens, especially the neighborhood of Jamaica, in New York City; or Los Angeles. In these cities the voodoo folk practitioner may be either male or female, does not have to inherit the right to practice by virtue of bloodline, and does not have to possess significantly powerful gifts (Snow, 1974). Historically, the voodoo priestess found in cities such as New Orleans must possess certain physical characteristics; that is, she must be African-American, and more specifically she must be of mixed ancestry, either an octoroon (a person of one eighth Black ancestry) or a quadroon (a person of one fourth Black ancestry) if her powers are to be superior (Snow, 1974).

Even today, some African-Americans still turn to one of these three types of practitioners when seeking medical advice. Educational level or socioeconomic status does not appear to alter or affect how some African-Americans perceive folk practitioners. Similar views are shared by some members of other cultural groups. In the summer of 1988, newspaper articles throughout the United States carried the story that the First Lady of the United States refused to make any moves or to allow her husband, the president of one of the most powerful countries in the world, to make decisions unless an astrologer was consulted.

Witchcraft: An Alternative Form of Folk Medicine. The practice of witchcraft is widespread and is not limited to the boundaries of the United States. Various degrees of witchcraft are practiced in countries throughout the world. In addition, the practice of witchcraft is not limited to any one particular cultural group. Persons who believe in witchcraft feel that it can be used not only to cure illness or disease but also to cause illness or disease. For example, strokes, dementia, and some gastrointestinal disorders may be perceived by some persons who believe in witchcraft to be the direct result or influence of witchcraft (Henderson & Primeaux, 1981).

The practice of witchcraft is based on the belief that there are some individuals who possess the ability to mobilize the forces of good and evil. These abilities are based on the principles of sympathetic magic, which underlie many of the beliefs of folk medicine practice. The basic premise of sympathetic magic is that everything in the universe is connected. There is a direct connection between the body and the forces of nature. Interpretation and direction of events are accomplished by understanding these connections. Sympathetic magic is categorized into *contagious* and *imitative magic*. The basic premise of contagious magic is the perception that physically connected objects can never be separated; therefore, any actions against the parts constitute an action against the whole (Henderson & Primeaux, 1981). Individuals who practice witchcraft may use a piece of clothing or nail clippings from someone to cast an "evil" spell or to protect the individual. The basic premise of imitative magic is that like follows like, or that one will imitate what one desires to achieve. For example, a knife placed under the bed will cut pain; an evil charm put on when the moon is waxing will increase the power of the charm.

A recurring theme in the practice of witchcraft is that of animals being in the body. Lizards, toads, snakes, and spiders are believed to be the most common types of intruders. These animals are dead and pulverized and are generally believed to enter the body by means of food or drink. It is not uncommon for persons who believe in witchcraft to refuse to eat or drink food prepared by someone they believe may have put a hex on them. Individuals who believe that such a spell has been cast on them may present themselves at health care facilities with symptoms described as "reptiles crawling over the body" or "snakes wiggling in their stomach." Some of these individuals may also share the belief that the physician is powerless to help them once they have been "hexed" (Jordan, 1979).

Perceptions Concerning Folk Medicine and Other Alternative Medical Solutions. The prevalence of the belief in and the use of folk medicine remedies and other alternative forms of health care is not fully understood (Jacques, 1976). It is impossible to generalize or postulate how widespread the use of folk medicine remedies is among African-Americans. However, evidence does exist that there are some African-Americans in all areas of the United States who believe in and practice folk medicine as well as other alternative forms of health care, such as witchcraft, voodoo, and spiritualism (Snow, 1983). There is also evidence to support the notion that different levels of folk medicine are practiced (Jacques, 1976). The boundaries of folk healers for some African-Americans may also vary. For example, the "granny" folk healer may possess the skills and knowledge to cure only simple illnesses or ailments. In contrast, a "witch doctor" is believed to possess supernatural powers that allow the "casting out of such things as animal demons" (Jordan, 1979). In addition, African-American folk medicine practitioners may have titles different from those of folk practitioners found in other cultural groups in the United States, such as "conjure doctor," "underworld man," "father divine," "root doctor," and "root worker" (Jacques, 1976).

Origins of African-American Folk Medicine. African-American folk medicine practices in the United States can be traced back to regions of West Africa (Harley, 2006). There are also influences on African-American folk medicine that originated in other countries, such as Haiti, Jamaica, and Trinidad (Smith, 1976). Because of slavery, there was a blending of various African tribes, particularly in slave cities and states such as New Orleans, Louisiana, and Savannah, Georgia, with other cultural groups such as the French, the Creoles, and the Indians. Various folk medicine practices found among some African-Americans in the North and the South have been handed down from generation to generation. Even today, the consistent use of some form of African-American folk medicine continues, and such continuity indicates that these practices have withstood the test of time and are presumed to be valid, although no empirical data exist that would indicate the validity or reliability of such practices.

Rationale for the Use of African-American Folk Medicine. Some African-Americans choose to use folk medicine because of tradition, whereas others have made this choice based on previous discriminatory practices and unfair treatments that have existed throughout some regions of the United States. In this regard, the deliveries of health care services were not exempt from Jim Crow laws, which were legally sanctioned until the mid-1960s throughout the South. However, the Northern regions of the United States also were not exempt from such discriminatory practices in regard to health care. This is evident in the passage of the Hill-Burton Act in 1946, which was not abolished until 1966 with the passage of the Federal Medicare Act (Bullough & Bullough, 1982).

The Hill-Burton Act, also known as the Hospital Construction Survey Act, provided federal grants for hospitals, both private and public, that admittedly did not serve African-Americans. Under this law, hospitals, whether private or public, were allowed to discriminatorily serve populations based on race. In addition, these same hospitals were allowed to continue these discriminatory practices in regard to hiring and staffing patterns. From such practices were born the all–African-American hospitals, which were found not only in the South but also in the North. Inclusions and exclusions for purposes of rendering health care services to those persons in need were left to the proprietors of the hospital. Thus patterns of admission and service to African-Americans varied throughout the country without regard to regional locale. In some northern and western states, admission to and service by some hospitals remained theoretically open to all races on equal terms, whereas in other states the courts upheld the rights of hospital proprietors to segregate as they saw fit.

This discriminatory practice was dramatically emphasized by the deaths of two famous African-Americans: Bessie Smith, in 1937, and Charles Drew, in 1950. Bessie Smith was a legendary blues singer who was critically injured in an automobile accident while traveling from Jackson, Mississippi, to Memphis, Tennessee. White attendants at the scene of the accident surmised correctly that Smith had a severed right arm and therefore needed immediate medical attention. The attendants took Smith to a hospital designated as "all White," and the administrators at the hospital refused to treat her despite the severity of her injuries. The ambulance attendants were forced to take Smith to Memphis, where she could be treated. On arrival, Smith was in profound shock, having lost a great quantity of blood. It has been said that despite Bessie Smith's obvious fame and the great admiration shown her by millions of fans, both African-American and White, the fact that she was African-American ultimately caused her death (Albertson, 2003).

Charles Drew, a surgeon, discovered blood plasma and developed the procedure for blood plasma transfusion. Even today, people throughout the world, regardless of race, benefit from his discovery. However, despite his profoundly important contribution to the medical field, the discovery of blood plasma was of no benefit to Drew when he, like Smith, was involved in an automobile accident and similarly was refused treatment in an "all-White" hospital. Although Drew was responsible for the technique of blood plasma transfusion, it was not used to save his life because he was taken to a hospital that legally had the right to refuse him treatment.

African-American folk medicine therefore took root not only as an offshoot of African cultural heritage but also as a necessity when African-Americans could not gain access to the traditional health care delivery system. Furthermore, some African-Americans turned to African-American folk medicine because they either could not afford the cost of medical assistance or were tired of the insensitive treatment by caregivers in the health care delivery system (Bullough & Bullough, 1982). Today African-Americans have access to the health care delivery system through legal channels. Some African-Americans still refuse to use the system, however, citing reasons such as past experiences, the escalating cost of health care, and the sometimes insensitive treatment on the part of non-Black caregivers in regard to the physiological and psychosocial differences evidenced among African-Americans.

Some African-Americans have a strong religious orientation, and most African-Americans belong to the Protestant faith. Although folk medicine and folk practices are widely documented in the literature as being common practices for the treatment of illnesses among

African-Americans, the most common and frequently cited method of treating illness remains prayer (Spector, 2008). According to Snow (1977), many of her informants found it impossible to separate religious beliefs from medical ones.

Death and Dying Rituals. It is important to note that there are variations in customs regarding death and dying rituals among African-Americans depending on country of origin, religious affiliation, geographic region, economic level, and educational background of each family member (Campinha-Bacote, 2013; Dowd, Poole, Davidhizar, & Giger, 1998). Many African-American families are composed of large networks, and often it is thought that such large networks tend to be very supportive during times of crises, such as during death and the dying process (Dowd et al., 1998). Some researchers have suggested that among many African-Americans there are varying ways that emotions are expressed about the death of a loved one (Campinha-Bacote, 2013). For example, while many people believe that African-Americans are quite expressive at the death of a loved one, this may not always be the case. For example, some African-Americans cry, whereas others remain silent and stoic (Campinha-Bacote, 2013). It is not unusual to see large gatherings at the time of death and during the burial process (Campinha-Bacote, 2013). Some African-Americans, and particularly those in the rural South, have maintained the tradition of keeping the body of the deceased in the home the evening before the funeral (Campinha-Bacote, 2013). This practice is probably what began the ritual of people coming to a home to help where they could. The church services for the deceased certainly depend on the religious affiliation. But regardless of the religious affiliation, it is not uncommon to see church "nurses" help family members view the body and deal with the stress of a funeral (Perry, 1993). African-Americans view death as a natural part of living, and their strong religious beliefs (which include seeing death as inevitable and a part of God's will, the sure and certain hope that the deceased is in God's hand, and the future hope that they will be reunited in heaven after death with the deceased) helped many of them deal effectively with death (Campinha-Bacote, 2013). Nonetheless, it is essential for the health care professional to remember that many bereaved African-Americans are more likely to seek help to adjust to the death from their clergy than from a health care professional (Neighbors, Musick, & Williams, 1998).

Implications for Nursing Care. Cultural health practices are often considered efficacious, neutral, or dysfunctional (Pillsbury, 1982). Practices that are considered efficacious are recognized by Western medicine as beneficial to health regardless of whether they are different from scientific practice. Practices the nurse regards as beneficial should be actively encouraged. The nurse should keep in mind that a treatment plan that is congruent with the client's own beliefs has a better chance of being successful. For example, some African-Americans believe that certain herbs and spices are essential in the treatment of certain disequilibriums in the body. In this case an herbal decoction could be used in place of water and might be just as beneficial for the treatment of specific conditions such as dehydration. Neutral practices (such as putting a knife under the bed to cut pain) are considered to be of no significance one way or the other to the health of an individual. However, psychological benefits may have a profound effect on the perception of pain. Dysfunctional health practices are viewed as harmful from a health point of view. For example, it is considered a dysfunctional health practice in Western medicine to use sugar and over-refined flour excessively. Dysfunctional health practices found among some African-Americans include such practices as using boiled goat's milk and cabbage juice for stomach infection.

Because some African-Americans tend to equate good health with luck or success, an illness may be viewed as undesirable and equated with bad luck, poverty, domestic turmoil, or even unemployment. As indicated previously, illnesses may be classified as natural or unnatural. Natural illnesses occur because a person is affected by natural forces without adequate protection. The nurse may be able to help the client more readily understand how these natural illnesses, such as colds and flu, can be avoided. Unnatural illnesses, which are believed to be the direct result of evil influences, are much more difficult for the nurse to combat. If the nurse has a client who believes that unnatural illness has resulted from witchcraft or voodoo or is a punishment from God, it may be very difficult to convince the client that a treatment can be implemented that will minimize or eliminate the problem. For example, a client may view breast cancer as a punishment from God. In this instance the client should be encouraged to seek medical treatment because unnecessary delay can have serious consequences. Although the nurse may not subscribe to cultural healing beliefs, it is essential that the nurse recognize their existence and their importance for some African-American clients. It is also important for the nurse to remember that effective nursing care cannot be implemented until the nurse acknowledges certain cultural health beliefs that have an effect on the client's behavior and recovery.

Among some African-Americans, it is believed that the maintenance of health is strongly associated with the ability to read the signs of nature. Subsumed in this belief is the idea that natural phenomena, such as the phases of the moon, the seasons of the year, and the planetary positions, all either singly or in combination affect the human body and human physiological functioning. Some African-Americans believe that the best days to wean babies, for example, or to have dental or surgical procedures can be found in the *Old Farmer's Almanac* (Snow, 1974). To the nurse, such beliefs may seem peculiar; however, the nurse must acknowledge the existence of such beliefs before culturally appropriate nursing care can be given. The nurse must also recognize that although some of these beliefs may be helpful, others may be neutral, and still others may be extremely dangerous for the client. The nurse must be able to sort beliefs into these three categories and assist the client in recognizing beliefs that may be dangerous.

Some African-Americans believe that cultural healing remedies help a person psychologically in dealing with discomfort. However, when these things fail, they believe a physician should be consulted. These same African-Americans may also believe that the nurse should recognize these cultural beliefs and use remedies based on these beliefs that prove to be helpful to the client (Bloch, 1976a). When an African-American client does arrive for professional health care, the nurse might assume that the client has tried all the cultural healing remedies known. While doing the initial assessment, the nurse needs to find out what the client has been using at home to minimize illness symptoms. This initial assessment will assist the nurse in determining whether these home remedies will interact or interfere with orthodox medical approaches. If the client has been using harmless home remedies, such remedies may continue to be used in the client's treatment. Other harmless remedies might be added to the client care plan at the client's suggestion (Bloch, 1976a).

Religion for some African-Americans has functioned primarily as an escape mechanism from the harsh realities of life. The African-American church functions to promote self-esteem among its membership as well as to act as a curator for maintaining the culture of many African-Americans. Therefore, the nurse cannot overlook the importance of the African-American minister and the African-American church in the recovery of the client. If there is no African-American minister within the hospital facility, the nurse should contact the client's own minister. It is essential for the nurse to remember that the African-American minister can essentially bridge the gap between the African-American client and other health care workers because the African-American minister understands the rituals, folkways, and difference in the mores of African-Americans (Smith, 1976).

BIOLOGICAL VARIATIONS

Until recently, the education of health care practitioners was based on the biopsychosocial characteristics of the dominant White culture. The lack of an in-depth understanding of biological and cultural differences resulted in less than optimum health care for persons who were not members of the dominant culture. When providing care to African-American clients, the nurse must realize that racial differences involve more than skin color and hair texture. African-American people have distinctive genotypes and phenotypes that characterize them as a racial group and as different from other racial groups. Moreover, the nurse must understand that African-Americans also have ethnic and cultural differences that distinguish them from other ethnic and cultural groups. It is essential for nurses and other health care providers to understand these biological variations in order to avoid racial and ethnic disparities in health care.

In 2002, a committee under the auspices of the Institute of Medicine released a seminal report titled *Unequal Treatment: Confronting Racial and Ethnic Disparities in Health Care*. The committee unequivocally noted that evidence of racial and ethnic disparities in health care is for the most part consistent regardless of the nature of the illness or the types of health care services rendered (Institute of Medicine, 2002). While it has been previously noted that socioeconomic status plays a major contributory factor in unequal treatment, particularly where African-Americans are concerned, Braithwaite and Taylor (2001) noted that even if income levels were standardized and if all impediments regarding access to care were eliminated, disparities in health outcomes might still exist. They contend that this argument gives credence to the need to eliminate cultural incompetence among health care providers. Seemingly, nurses would not be exempt from this argument, as they must serve as advocates for culturally competent care for all clients entrusted to their care.

Birth Weight

Data from previous epidemiological reports consistently reveal that there is a difference in the mean birth weight of approximately 200 g between African-American infants and White infants, with White infants weighing more. These differences persist even when socioeconomic status, maternal age, parity, and smoking are controlled for (Hulsey, Levkoff, & Alexander, 1991). Davis et al. (1993) used ultrasound examinations to compare biparietal diameter (BPD), head circumference (HC), abdominal circumference (AC), and femur length in 5405 African-American and White fetuses. They found no significant difference in the BPD, HC, and AC; however, femurs in

African-American fetuses were significantly longer. The birth weights of the infants were also compared, and these data again revealed differences in birth weight between African-American and White infants (3331 versus 3135 g; $P < 0.001$), with White infants being heavier.

It is postulated that birth weight contributes significantly to neonatal mortality among African-American neonates (Braithwaite & Taylor, 2001). It is clear that prematurity, which is defined as a birth weight under 2500 g, is twice as common for African-Americans as it is for Whites (Iyasu, Becerra, Rowley, & Hogue, 1992), and it has been suggested that the definition for prematurity be lowered from 2500 to 2200 g for African-Americans (Morton, 1977). The gestational period for African-Americans tends to be 9 days shorter than that for Whites, and a slowing down of gestational growth occurs in African-American infants after 35 weeks. Before 35 weeks of gestation, African-American infants are usually larger than White infants (Giger, Davidhizar, & Wieczorek, 1993; Pratt, Janus, & Sayal, 1977). The reasons for these differences in birth weights remain vague. Nonetheless, because the death rates for African-American infants are nearly three times the national average, some researchers have suggested that approximately three quarters of the disparity in infant mortality rates are primarily attributable to the larger proportion of babies with low birth weight and the very low birth weights (less than 1500 g) among these vulnerable neonates (Braithwaite & Taylor, 2001; Iyasu et al., 1992).

Growth and Development

African-American children tend to mature faster than White children. Today African-American children are more mature at birth in both the musculoskeletal and the neurological systems (Falkner & Tanner, 1978). Neurologically, African-American children tend to be more advanced until about 2 or 3 years of age, and in the musculoskeletal system they tend to be more advanced until puberty (Roche, Roberts, & Hamell, 1978). The differences in skeletal maturity are attributed to genetic and environmental factors.

Body size, height, weight, bone length, and body structure of African-Americans and Whites have been extensively studied in the United States. Studies done by Abraham, Clifford, and Najjar (1976) revealed that the average height and weight of African-American and White men 18 to 74 years of age are approximately the same; White men tend to be 0.5 cm taller than African-American men. The average height for African-American and White women is the same; however, African-American women are consistently heavier than White women at every age, and between 35 and 64 years of age they are typically an average of 20 lb heavier than their White counterparts.

Body Proportion

The body proportions of African-Americans differ from those of Whites, Asians, and American Indians. There are definitive differences in bone length that are obvious on study. African-Americans have shorter trunks than Whites and tend to have longer legs than Whites, Asians, and American Indians. African-American men tend to have wider shoulders and narrower hips than Asians, who tend to have narrow shoulders and wide hips. The long bones of African-Americans are significantly longer and narrower than those of Whites (Farrally & Moore, 1976). The bones of African-Americans are also denser. African-American men have the densest bones, followed by African-American women, White men, and finally, White women, who have the lowest bone density of the two races. The greater bone density explains why osteoporosis is rare in African-Americans and why White women have a greater incidence of osteoporosis. Bone curvature also varies among the different races. The femurs of African-Americans are quite straight; in comparison, the femurs of American Indians are anteriorly convex, and those of Whites have intermediate curvature. This characteristic appears to be genetically determined, but weight also seems to be a factor because obese African-Americans and Whites tend to demonstrate more curvature than other individuals do (Gilbert, 1977).

Body Fat

The amount and distribution of body fat are two other areas where there are pronounced differences by virtue of race and ethnic group. The racial differences are mostly related to socioeconomic status. Persons from the lower socioeconomic class tend to have more body fat than those from the middle class, and persons from the middle class tend to have more body fat than those from the upper class. There is some evidence indicating that fat distribution may vary according to race. African-American people tend to have smaller skinfold thickness in their arms than Whites have, but the distribution of fat on the trunk is similar for both Whites and African-Americans (Bagan, Robson, & Soderstrom, 1971). Whites have a larger chest volume than African-Americans; hence they have greater vital capacity and forced expiratory volume (Oscherwitz, 1972). African-Americans, on the other hand, have a larger chest volume than American Indians and Asians and thus greater vital capacity and forced expiratory volume than members of these racial groups (Oscherwitz, 1972).

Skin Color

Skin color, or pigmentation, is the most distinguishing physical difference among the various races and is determined by melanin. All people have some melanin, but some racial groups have more melanin than others. The greater the amount of melanin an individual has, the darker the skin pigmentation will be. The skin color of persons who are classified as African-Americans ranges from "white" to very dark brown or perhaps even black. Melanin provides protection from the effects of the sun; however, the risk of sunburn does exist. African-Americans do get sunburned but not as easily as Whites; repeated, prolonged sun exposure is a risk for cancer. Although African-Americans and other individuals with darker skin have a lower incidence of skin cancer, it is imperative that they receive education regarding risk reduction. Teaching should include the risk of prolonged sun exposure and when to use sunscreen (Campinha-Bacote, 2013).

The skin coloring should be uniform, but areas that are not exposed to the sun may be lighter, such as the buttocks, abdomen, and thorax. The exceptions to this rule for African-American people are the skinfolds in the groin, the genitalia, and the nipples, which tend to be darker than the rest of the body. (An old wives' tale suggests that to determine the true color of a newborn infant, one should look at the ears, which tend to be darker at birth than the rest of the body.) Except for the areas just mentioned, hypopigmentation and hyperpigmentation (unless it is a birthmark) are abnormal (Bloch, 1983). Pigmentation of the lips, nail beds, palmar surfaces, creases of the hands, and plantar surfaces and creases of the feet may vary, just as skin coloring does. The range of coloring for the lips of African-Americans may vary from pink to plum. The palmar and plantar surfaces may range from light pink to dark pink to a brown, and the creases may range from dark pink to dark brown, depending on the amount of pigmentation (Bloch, 1976b). The gums may have areas of hyperpigmentation, and the sclerae may have scattered areas of brown pigmentation that appear to be freckles.

Mongolian spots are a common variance found in African-American infants. They are migratory leftovers of melanocytes that have lingered in the lumbosacral region at a greater than normal depth, which accounts for their dark blue-green appearance. Mongolian spots occur in 90% of African-Americans, 80% of Asians and American Indians, and only 9% of Whites (Gupta & Thappa, 2013). Normally found on the buttocks, thighs, ankles, and arms, mongolian spots usually disappear in the first year of life and should not be mistaken for a bruise.

Birthmarks appear to be most common in African-American individuals, occurring in 20% of African-Americans, compared with 2% to 3% of Whites, Mexicans, and American Indians. These pigmented marks appear as sharply demarcated macules that vary from light tan to dark brown, depending on the skin color. They may be present anywhere on the body (Overfield, 1995).

Black skin is also more susceptible to an overgrowth of connective tissue in response to injury, or keloid formation. Keloids are raised areas of scar tissue that can result from minor injuries such as skin tears or punctures, from more major injuries such as burn injuries or traumatic lacerations, or from surgical incisions (Campinha-Bacote, 2013).

Normal, healthy skin should be warm, dry, and elastic. There should be a red glow present in Black skin. Color changes associated with abnormal conditions are rashes, which may be difficult or impossible to detect in the individual who is darkly pigmented. Darkly pigmented lips and nail beds with melanin deposits make nursing assessment even more difficult. When possible, the nurse should become familiar with the client's normal coloring to establish a baseline value. The skin assessment should be done in a well-lighted room. Sunlight is the best lighting; if artificial lighting is used, it should be nonglaring (Campinha-Bacote, 2013; Treas & Wilkinson, 2014). When assessing the darkly pigmented individual for specific color changes such as pallor, jaundice, or cyanosis, the nurse should inspect the conjunctivae and oral membranes of the buccal mucosa. Jaundice also appears as a yellowish discoloration of the sclerae if they are not pigmented. The mucous membranes of the buccal mucosa and the palmar and plantar surfaces may also be inspected for yellow discoloration.

The nurse may also rely on palpations and the client's history to detect the presence of bruises in the darkly pigmented client. The nurse should use the dorsal surface of the hand to assess for areas of increased warmth and tenderness. Questioning should include a history of recent trauma. The petechiae cannot be readily visualized on the dark-skinned individual. The nurse should inspect the sclerae for dark blue spots. The client history should include questioning about symptoms of conditions in which petechiae would be present. Palpation and the client history may also be used to detect the presence of a macular rash on the client who is dark skinned (Bloch, 1983).

Genetic Differences

Methylenetetrahydrofolate Reductase. Some researchers have noted that moderate hyperhomocysteinemia is a putative risk for the development of cardiovascular disease (CVD) (Cheng, 2013). Hyperhomocysteinemia is an independent risk factor for premature arteriosclerotic vascular disease and venous thrombosis (Cheng, 2013). Mutations in the gene, which code for methylenetetrahydrofolate reductase (MTHFR), account for reduced enzyme levels and elevated plasma homocysteine (Duca, 2013). The heterozygote state results in mild hyperhomocysteinemia, a risk factor for CVD. Homocysteine levels are also influenced by diet (Cheng, 2013). Dilley et al. (2002) attempted to determine whether the mutation $C \rightarrow T677$ in the

MTHFR gene or the TC833/844in68 and G→A919 mutations in the *CBS* gene were associated genetically with myocardial infarctions (MIs) among African-Americans. The analysis of the data suggested that 15% of the cases analyzed demonstrated that these individuals were heterozygous for C→T677 (*MTHFR*) mutation, whereas 1.8% of the subjects were homozygous. Further findings from this study showed that their controls were 15% heterozygous and 2.1% homozygous and suggested that there was no significant association with myocardial infarction among these African-Americans who participated in the study. Yet these researchers noted that, while no association was noted for T→C833 (*CBS*) among the experimental or controls and while there was no significant association between this mutation and MI, the prevalence of the heterozygous state among African-Americans (15%) was higher than that among their White counterparts (12%). These researchers concluded that the racial differences of these genes warranted further investigation.

Tumor Necrosis Factor Alpha. One candidate gene predisposing to type 2 diabetes within the major histocompatibility complex region is tumor necrosis factor alpha (TNFα), a cytokine. In rats, elevated levels of TNFα have been shown to produce "sustained increase in glucose production, utilization, and clearance," as well as an insulin resistance (IR) state (Bendtzen et al., 1988; Dilley et al., 2002; Fernandez-Real et al., 1997; Hotamisligil, Arner, Caro, Atkinson, & Spiegelman, 1995; Hotamisligil, Murray, Choy, Spiegelman, 1994; Hotamisligil, Shargill, & Spiegelman, 1993; Jongeneel et al., 1991). TNFα expression has also been observed in rodent models of obesity and diabetes. When TNFα was neutralized in obese fa/fa rats, a significant increase in peripheral uptake of glucose in response to insulin was observed. Treatment of adipocytes with TNFα resulted in downregulation of GLUT4 messenger ribonucleic acid. TNFα also interferes with the signaling of insulin and blocks its biological action (Hotamisligil et al., 1994; Hotamisligil et al., 1993). In humans, abnormal expression of TNFα appears to play a role in obesity-related IR (Rajkovic et al., 2014). A polymorphism in the TNFα promoter has been associated with increased levels of basal serum insulin and leptin (Hotamisligil et al., 1994; Hotamisligil et al., 1993; Kubaszek et al., 2003). The differences were greater in women than in men. TNFα has been linked to the development of IR among African-Americans and is considered to be one of the precursors to the development of metabolic syndrome (syndrome X).

Metabolic syndrome (syndrome X) is a clustering of abnormalities characterized by the primary defect of compensatory IR, glucose intolerance, dyslipidemia, and centrally distributed obesity (American Heart Association [AHA], Heart Disease and Stroke, 2015). Chen et al. (2000) conducted a study to examine the age-related patterns of cardiovascular risk factor clusters relative to the metabolic syndrome (syndrome X) among African-American and White children. The clusters in this study for the metabolic syndrome (syndrome X) included (1) insulin resistance index, (2) body mass index (BMI), (3) triglycerides/high-density lipoprotein (HDL) cholesterol ratio, and (4) mean arterial pressure. Regardless of age, four mediating factors contribute to the development of coronary heart disease (CHD): hyperinsulinemia (syndrome X), hypercholesterolemia, hypertension, and obesity. A sedentary lifestyle, the large percentage of fat consumed per day by African-American children, and the prevalence of obesity all may contribute to the development of metabolic syndrome (syndrome X) even among African-American children (DeBoer, 2011; Giger, Richardson, & Jones, 2001). In other words, African-American children are not exempt because of their tender years from developing syndrome X and starting the downward spiral toward diabetes and ultimately CHD.

Interestingly, findings from the study by Chen et al. (2000) suggest that overall, White children had a higher total of adverse clusters among the four indices measured (9.8; $P < 0.01$) than their African-American counterparts (7.4; $P < 0.01$). These follow-up findings to the Bogalusa Heart Study are interesting because prior and recent analyses of these data sets suggest that while predictability of childhood adiposity and insulin resistance syndrome is difficult to determine with certainty in children, the contributions of these adverse clusters can provide convincing evidence for the future development of syndrome X, thereby leading to the development of CHD in adulthood (Srinivasan, Myers, & Berenson, 2002). As African-Americans age, the adverse clusters outrank those of their White counterparts, and this ultimately leads to the development of syndrome X and CHD in adulthood. Srinivasan, Myers, and Berenson (2002) also examined the contributions of childhood adiposity and insulin as a weighed predictor to adulthood risk of developing metabolic syndrome (syndrome X) among African-American and White children with baseline ages of 8 to 17 years. Using a logistic regression model, these researchers noted that childhood BMI and insulin resistance served as significant predictors of adult clustering for metabolic syndrome (syndrome X). In this study, BMI was the strongest indicator, exhibiting a curvilinear relationship. Further findings from this study also suggest that childhood obesity often is a powerful predictor of the development of metabolic syndrome (syndrome X) later in life. These findings suggest that children, and particularly African-American children, can benefit tremendously from programs that underscore the importance of weight control and increased physical activity (Srinivasan et al., 2002). Tumor necrosis factor α has also been linked with human leiomyoma, of which African-American women tend to have a disproportionate prevalence (Ciavattini et al., 2013). In fact, Kurachi, Matsuo, Samoto, and Maruo (2001) were among the first researchers to demonstrate increased cellular levels of TNFα in leiomyoma cells.

Apolipoprotein E. Apolipoprotein E (ApoE) is a polymorphic protein involved in the catabolism of chylomicron remnants. Various ApoE phenotypes are related to the development of combined hyperlipidemia and familial combined hyperlipidemia, total and low-density lipoprotein (LDL) cholesterol, and insulin levels and are associated with CHD, stroke, and type 2 diabetes (Dallongeville et al., 1991; Ferrucci et al., 1995; Imaru, Koga, & Ibayashi, 1988; Margaglione et al., 1998; Valdez, Howard, Stern, & Haffner, 1995). The high frequency of the appearance of ApoE supports this gene as a candidate marker for CHD. It is thought that ApoE participates in the receptor-mediated clearance of blood lipids such as cholesterol, which is considered a major risk factor for CHD (Amemiya et al., 1996). In North America, it has been estimated that the variability of this gene (*ApoE* gene locus) accounts for up to 6% of the variation in CHD. The *ApoE* locus lies on chromosome 19 and has three common alleles ($_E$2, $_E$3, $_E$4), which are coded for the *E* isoforms *ApoE2, ApoE3,* and *ApoE4,* respectively (Amemiya et al., 1996). While the frequencies of these isoforms vary from race to race, it is thought that *ApoE3* shows the highest frequencies ($\geq$49%) and *ApoE2* the lowest ($\leq$15%). The frequency by population in North America is generally no higher than 6%. Among African-Americans there tends to be a direct correlation between the frequency of this candidate gene and the development of CHD (Dallongeville et al., 1991; Valdez et al., 1995).

C-Reactive Protein. C-reactive protein (CRP) is produced by the liver and released in response to inflammation. It is present in the serum within 24 to 48 hours after an inflammatory stimulus. C-reactive protein is a known predictor of increased risk for heart attacks, strokes, and peripheral vascular disease and is used to screen for atherosclerosis in middle-aged and elderly people. High-sensitivity CRP (hs-CRP) has been developed to detect low-grade inflammatory activity within the vascular system. An hs-CRP of <0.7 mg/dL denotes a low risk, 0.7 to 1.1 mg/dL indicates a mild risk, 1.2 to 1.9 mg/dL is a moderate risk, 2.0 to 3.8 mg/dL is high risk, and 3.9 to 15 mg/dL is very high risk. Data from several research studies have indicated that CRP values may vary according

to gender and race and in the presence of certain chronic disease states. In a multiethnic population-based study that examined CRP values in over 2500 White and Black subjects, which controlled for traditional cardiovascular risk factors such as BMI, estrogen, and statin use, findings suggested that CRP values above 3 mg were more common in White females (odds ratio [OR] 1.6; 95% confidence interval [CI], 1.1–2.5) and Black females (OR 1.7; 95% CI, 1.2–2.6). However, in male subjects, the CRP values were within the normal range. Nonetheless, conclusions from this study suggested that differences in race and gender existed (Khera et al., 2005).

Kraus et al. (2007) examined the relationship between hs-CRP and osteoarthritis in 662 subjects. The applicability of using CRP values in predicting risk for cardiovascular events was also evaluated in this study. The study suggested that hs-CRP values were higher in African-Americans, women who used pain medications, and individuals who had hypertension or chronic obstructive pulmonary disease. These researchers also found a correlation between the CRP values and BMI and waist circumference. But even given these findings, these researchers concluded that the pathogenic significance of hs-CRP elevations in women and African-Americans was unclear and that obesity, ethnicity, and gender confound the use of serum hs-CRP values in predicting CVD risk (Kraus et al., 2007). Similarly, Alley et al. (2006) studied the effects of socioeconomic status and CRP levels. Data for this study were obtained from the fourth wave of the National Health and Nutrition Examination Survey (NHANES) collected between 1999 and 2002. This survey included an oversampling of older persons, Blacks, and Hispanics who were predominantly Mexican. From the sample of 6946 individuals, demographic data suggested that persons with higher CRP levels were older, Black, or female or were living in poverty. These researchers concluded that the differences in extremely elevated CRP levels ($\geq$10 mg/dL) may be a reflection of high levels of poverty, which affect the ability to acquire adequate medical treatment. Nonetheless, chronic disease along with risky health behaviors that are associated with poverty were also cited as plausible causes for CRP elevations in this group.

Enzymatic Variations

Biochemical variations and their effects on health vary according to race. As with other racial variations, biochemical variations are attributed to genetic factors and environmental influences. Lactose intolerance is a well-known condition that is correlated with race: 90% of African Blacks and 75% of African-Americans have lactose intolerance (Center for Food Allergies, n.d.; Giger, Davidhizar, & Cherry, 1991; Lactose intolerance, n.d., National Institutes of Health [NIH], 2004). Individuals with lactose intolerance lack the enzyme to convert lactose to glucose and galactose, and as a result, gastrointestinal symptoms of bloating, cramping, and diarrhea occur. The condition is genetically transmitted, although the specific gene has not been identified (Johnson, Cole, & Abner, 1981). There appear to be two periods in life during which symptoms occur: infancy shortly after weaning and the teen years or early 20s. The condition is diagnosed on the basis of signs or symptoms that occur after the ingestion of milk or other products containing lactose. Treatment consists of avoidance of these products, with appropriate substitution of other products. In addition, there are products available on the market that can be taken to help alleviate symptoms associated with this condition. Some people report a degree of success with such products, whereas other people report little benefit from their use. The nursing implications for nurses caring for African-American clients include (1) knowledge of the condition and its prevalence among African-Americans and (2) education of clients with the condition to avoid products containing lactose. The education of these clients should include encouraging them to read labels and make appropriate food substitutions (National Institute of Diabetes and Digestive and Kidney Diseases, n.d.).

Susceptibility to Disease

Susceptibility, or the degree to which an individual is resistant to disease, is determined by genetics and environment. Technological advances in medicine have contributed to improvement in general health and increases in the lifespan of all Americans. Despite these advances, African-Americans, Hispanics, American Indians, and Asian Pacific Islanders continue to have alarming health disparities that ultimately lead to a shorter life expectancy. For African-Americans, death rates from heart disease, cancer, stroke, diabetes, and acquired immunodeficiency syndrome (AIDS) are much higher than those in the general population. Genetics and environmental factors play a major role in many of the 10 leading causes of death for African-Americans. For example, African-Americans experience higher morbidity and mortality rates from CVD, the number one cause of death for all Americans. Major risk factors for CVD are related to both hereditary predisposition and environmental factors such as diet and physical inactivity. African-Americans have a higher mortality for certain cancers, such as breast and colon cancer. In 2013, the Health United States Report, the age-adjusted death rates for cancer of the colon and rectum, prostate, and breast were higher for African-American males and females compared with individuals from other racial and ethnic groups. For White males and females, the mortality rate per

100,000 for all cancers was 208.2 and 150.6, respectively, compared with 264.8 for Black males and 167.1 for females. Similarly for Hispanics, the age-adjusted mortality rate for all ages was 149.4 for males and 99.4 for females (National Center for Health Statistics, Health United States, 2014). In females, the breast cancer mortality rate for Whites was 21.5 per 100,000 compared with 30.3 per 100,000 for Blacks and 14.4 per 100,000 for Hispanics (National Center for Health Statistics, Health United States, 2014). Hereditary predisposition and environmental factors such as diet, obesity, and physical inactivity have been identified as major risks for both types of cancers (National Center for Health Statistics, Health United States, 2014). Risk factors for type 2 diabetes, the fourth leading cause of death in African-Americans, have been linked to heredity and environment. Another major factor that has been associated with increased susceptibility to disease is disparities in health care. Numerous published reports relate disparities in health care and inequities in access and delivery of health care to higher mortality rates in African-Americans. The complex interaction between the environment, economics, and access to health care all interact to pose a tremendous physical and economic burden on society. In addition, the shortage of minority health care providers has been shown to have a significant impact on access to health care, the practice of specific health promotion behaviors, and the decisions to seek preventative care (Biello, Rawlings, Carrol-Scott, Browne, & Ickovics, 2010).

Cardiovascular Disease. Cardiovascular disease is a pandemic problem and continues to be the major cause of death worldwide. The primary cause for the increased prevalence of CVD in developing countries has been attributed to the westernization of native cultures (AHA, 2015). The World Health Organization (WHO) has identified CVD as the underlying cause of death in 17.3 individuals worldwide, or 30% of total global mortality. The WHO estimates that the number of deaths resulting from CVD will increase to 23.6 million people by the year 2030 (WHO 2015; AHA, Heart Disease and Stroke Statistics, 2015; Update World Health Organization [WHO], 2015).

Despite significant progress made in the treatment and prevention of CVD, MI, cerebrovascular accident (CVA) or stroke, and other forms of heart disease, CVD continues to be the leading cause of mortality and morbidity in the United States for adults in all demographic groups. Moreover, Americans suffer more than 1.5 million heart attacks and strokes annually (AHA, Fact Sheet, 2014). Cardiovascular disease claims more lives in the United States than the next five leading causes of death combined. Heart disease and stroke are the first and fourth leading causes of deaths, respectively, in the United States, accounting for one of every three deaths in the United States (AHA, Heart Disease and Stroke Statistics, 2015 Update). Data from the AHA Heart Disease and Stroke Statistics 2015 Update indicate that over 83.6 million adults in the United States are living with one or more types of CVD or the complications of a stroke. This statistic includes diseases of the heart, stroke, hypertension, heart failure, congenital cardiovascular defects, atherosclerosis, and other circulatory system diseases. Before 72 years of age, the average annual event rate for the first coronary event in men between 35 and 44 years of age is 3 per 1000. With advancing age, this figure rises dramatically to 74 per 1000 (AHA, Heart Disease and Stroke Statistics, 2015 Update). For women, age is the most important risk factor for developing coronary artery disease. According to the AHA, prior to menopause the death rates from CVD are lower than in men. Although overall death rates for women may actually be lower, rates may be perceived as somewhat comparable because of their sheer numbers; however, death tends to occur at a later age (AHA, 2015; Appel, Moore, & Giger, 2006; Giger et al., 2005, AHA; Heart Disease and Stroke Statistics, 2015 Update). Recent data from the American Heart Association Heart Disease and Stroke Statistics 2015; Update and NHANES III also indicate that over the past 3 decades more women have died of CVD than men.

Cardiovascular disease is the number one cause of deaths in African-Americans. In fact, coronary heart disease (CHD) and stroke together account for more than one third of all deaths in African-Americans (AHA, Heart Disease and Stroke Statistics, 2015 Update). It is interesting to note that nearly half of all African-American adults have some form of CVD, which includes heart disease and stroke. According the AHA 2014 Fact Sheet, among African-Americans, 44% of men and 49% of women affected have some form of CVD. The percentage of African-Americans with CHD is 10.7%, compared with 6% for non-Hispanic Whites. Further, African-Americans are more likely to die of a myocardial infarction than any other racial or ethnic group (AHA, Heart Disease and Stroke Statistics, 2015 Update). The disparity in death rates between African-Americans and Whites is partly due to hereditary predisposition for hypertension, type 2 diabetes, obesity, and lifestyle choices. Moreover, it has been well documented that African-Americans have more CVD risk factors such as hypertension, type 2 diabetes, and obesity, which places them at an increased risk for heart and cerebral vascular disease. Hypertension is a major independent risk factor for coronary artery disease, stroke, and peripheral arterial disease. The prevalence of hypertension in African-Americans is the highest in the world. In 2012, an estimated 70% of all CVD was attributed to hypertension; therefore, this condition is an extremely

important consideration for the African-American in the development of CVD (AHA, Heart Disease and Stroke Statistics, 2015 Update).

Since the 1900s, CVD has been the number one cause of death every year except 1918. Despite this well-known fact, the general public continues to have a misguided perception about the health risk of heart disease (AHA, Heart Disease and Stroke Statistics, 2015 Update; Mieszczanka & Velord, 2014). Most Americans still fear cancer more than heart disease. According to Blumenthal and Flack (2003), women rank breast cancer high on the list of personal health threats when in fact 1 death in 4.6 among women is due to breast cancer compared with 1 death in 3.2 due to CVD (AHA, Heart Disease and Stroke Statistics, 2015 Update). In African-American women, the greatest risk for CVD is the high prevalence of hypertension and type 2 diabetes. Despite advances in management of CVD, African-American women have a higher prevalence of hypertension compared with other ethnic and gender groups (Mieszczanka & Velord, 2014). The rate of hypertension in African-American women has reached epidemic proportions, with 46.1% of African-American women affected nationwide compared with 30.1% of White women (AHA, Heart Disease and Stroke Statistics, 2015 Update). African-American women have greater mortality and morbidity from hypertension compared with women from other racial and ethnic groups (AHA, Heart Disease and Stroke Statistics, 2015 Update). In 2010, the mortality rate from stroke was 49.2/100,000 in African-American women compared with 37.2/100,000 in White women (AHA, Heart Disease and Stroke Statistics, 2015 Update; National Center for Health Statistics, Health United States, 2014).

Coronary heart disease was once perceived as a disease that most commonly afflicted men. This perception probably developed because the condition strikes men more often in the middle years of life. This perception had been reinforced by the Framingham study, which was initiated in 1948. In this classic study, the data indicated that, on average, women develop the symptoms of heart disease a decade later than men. Work relative to this study is ongoing, and although earlier data show that the incidence of the disease was disproportionately higher among men than women, current data indicate that CHD is the number one killer of women and is more prevalent in African-American women than in African-American men (AHA, 2014; Mieszczanka & Velord, 2014).

An estimated 85.6 million American adults have one or more types of CVD. Of this number, 43.7 million are over the age of 60 (AHA, Heart Disease and Stroke Statistics, 2015 Update). It is estimated that over 2150 Americans die of CVD every day, an average of one death every 40 seconds. The majority of deaths from CVD are due to CHD. Further,

635,000 new myocardial infarctions and approximately 300,000 recurrent myocardial infarctions occur annually. An estimated additional 155,000 silent myocardial infarctions also occur each year (AHA, Heart Disease and Stroke Statistics, 2015 Update). From 2001 to 2011, the overall CVD death rate declined by approximately 30.8%, but African-American men and women continue to show higher rates of death from CVD compared with Whites. According to the AHA 2015 Update, the 2011 preliminary mortality rates from CVD were 229.1 per 100,000. Rates of death from CVD were 271.9 per 100,000 for White males compared with 352.4 per 100,000 for African-American males. In White and African-American females, the CVD mortality rates were 188.1 and 248.6 per 100,000, respectively. Data from this report also show that African-American women and Mexican American women have a higher prevalence of CVD risk factors than White women of comparable socioeconomic backgrounds. In 2011, the overall mortality rate from CHD was 109.2 per 100,000, with disproportionately higher rates for African-American males and females. Among African-American males, the CHD mortality rate was 161.5 per 100,000 compared with 146.5 per 100,000 for White males. Similarly African-American women did not fare much better than their male counterparts, with a disproportionately higher mortality rate (99. 7 per 100,000) compared with their White counterparts (80.1 per 100,000) (AHA, Heart Disease and Stroke Statistics, 2015 Update). According to Mieszczanka and Velord (2014), African-American women tend to develop CHD much earlier than White women do. Furthermore, the death rate for African-American women under 55 years of age is twice that of White women. Finally, until 75 years of age the mortality from CHD is higher in African-American women than in women of other racial backgrounds (National Center for Health Statistics, 2013).

There are nine easily measurable and potentially modifiable risk factors that account for over 90% of the risk of an initial acute myocardial infarction. The pathophysiological effects of the risk factors are seen in both men and women in different racial and ethnic groups. These nine risk factors are cigarette smoking, abnormal blood lipid levels, hypertension, diabetes, abdominal obesity, physical inactivity, poor daily dietary intake of fruits and vegetables, excessive alcohol consumption, and stress. Hypertension, obesity, and dyslipidemia continue to be the major independent risk factors for CHD and stroke (National Center for Health Statistics, Health United States, 2014). Hypertension is now identified as one of the components of metabolic syndrome, and it is recognized as a syndrome of vascular and metabolic disorders that occur along a continuum.

As indicated previously, the term *metabolic syndrome* or *dysmetabolic syndrome* refers to a cluster of risk factors leading to CVD and type 2 diabetes mellitus. This constellation of disorders have been identified as the underlying cause of end-stage vascular disease and metabolic derangements (AHA, Heart Disease and Stroke Statistics, 2015 Update). Clinical findings associated with a diagnosis of metabolic syndrome include a waist circumference greater than 88 cm in women and greater than 102 cm in men, dyslipidemia (triglycerides >150 mg/dL, HDL cholesterol <40 mg/dL in men and <50 mg/dL in women), blood pressure greater than 130/85 mm Hg, or receiving drug therapy for hypertension, and two elevated fasting glucose values greater than 100 mg/dL. The presence of three or more clinical findings are needed to confirm the diagnosis of metabolic syndrome (AHA, 2015).

Data from the NHANES collected between 2003 and 2006 indicated that ~34% of adults over the age of 20 met the new criteria for metabolic syndrome. More recent data from the AHA Heart Disease and Stroke Statistics 2015 Update show the age-adjusted prevalence was 21.8% of women and 23.69% of men. The age-adjusted prevalence of people with metabolic syndrome was higher in Mexican American men than non-Hispanic Black men (34.76% and 18.9%, respectively). For women, the prevalence was 31.5%, 38.8%, and 40.6%, respectively, for non-Hispanic white, non-Hispanic Black, and Mexican women. For non-Hispanic Black women, the age-adjusted prevalence was 53% higher than for non-Hispanic Black men and 22% higher for Mexican American women than Mexican American men. When compared with their counterparts, 50% of African-American adults had two or three risk factors, compared with less than one third of non-Hispanic Whites and Mexican Americans. Data from both the American Heart Association and the National Heart, Lung, and Blood Institute support the strong correlation between the identified risk factors and CVD morbidity and mortality (AHA, Heart Disease and Stroke Statistics, 2015 Update).

Hypertension. Hypertension is an independent risk factor for coronary artery disease. It is also associated with an increased risk for developing stroke, heart failure, renal insufficiency, and peripheral vascular disease (AHA, Heart Disease and Stroke Statistics, 2015 Update). Further, hypertension is a major independent risk factor for CVD morbidity and mortality. In the United States, hypertension remains poorly controlled despite major advances in pharmacological therapies, and as a result health care providers need heightened awareness of achieving tight blood pressure control to reduce morbidity and mortality from CVD (AHA, Heart Disease and Stroke Statistics, 2015 Update; NHANES, 2011–2012). Approximately 69% of individuals with a first myocardial infarction, 77% with a first stroke, and 74% with heart failure have blood pressure greater than 140/90 mm Hg (AHA, Heart Disease and Stroke Statistics, 2015 Update). The prevalence of hypertension among African-Americans and Whites in the southeastern United States is higher, and mortality due to myocardial infarction and stroke is greater than in any other region in the country (AHA, Heart Disease and Stroke Statistics, 2015 Update). According to the AHA (Heart Disease and Stroke Statistics 2015 Update), African-Americans have the poorest rate of hypertension control; as a result, the age-adjusted mortality rate from hypertension increased by 36.4%. In 2011, the death rates per 100,000 population from hypertension were 114.5 for White males, 212.8 for Black males, 92 for White females, and 157.9 for Black females (AHA, Heart Disease and Stroke Statistics, 2015 Update 2015; National Center for Health Statistics, 2013; AHA, Heart Disease and Stroke Statistics, 2015 Update). Of the four leading causes of death in African-Americans, hypertension can be associated with at least three of the four disease states: CHD is the leading cause of death in African-Americans, CVA is listed as third, and diabetes is listed as the fourth (AHA, Heart Disease and Stroke Statistics, 2015 Update). Ventricular hypertrophy, arteriosclerosis, and atherosclerosis occur as a direct result of pathological changes that are exacerbated as a result of sustained blood pressure elevation. Left ventricular hypertrophy causes myocardial ischemia, dysrhythmias, and heart failure (Leon & Bronas, 2009). Arteriosclerosis and atherosclerosis lead to CHD and CVAs. Individuals with diabetes have a higher risk of CHD and hypertension, and diabetes can accelerate pathophysiological vascular changes, thereby exacerbating both conditions (Lamendola & Mason, 2004).

Approximately 47.1% of all deaths in hypertensive Black males and 35.1% of all deaths in hypertensive Black females can be directly attributed to elevated blood pressure (AHA, Heart Disease and Stroke Statistics, 2015 Update). The earlier onset of hypertension, along with a greater percentage of individuals with stage 3 disease, is associated with an 80% higher mortality for stroke and a 50% increase in the prevalence of heart disease. Further, hypertensive African-Americans experience increased rates of end-stage renal failure. When compared with Whites, Black Americans have a 1.3 times higher incidence of non-fatal stroke, a 1.8 times higher incidence of fatal stroke, a 1.5 times higher incidence of fatal heart disease, and 4.2 times higher incidence of end-stage renal failure (AHA, Heart Disease and Stroke Statistics, 2015 Update). The prevalence of hypertension in Black women is more than three times that of White males and females. Compared with White females, Black females have an 81% higher rate of ambulatory medical visits for hypertension (AHA, Heart Disease and Stroke Statistics, 2015 Update).

Serum Cholesterol Levels. Elevated serum lipid levels, another major risk factor, is associated with increased risk for CVD. Elevated total cholesterol levels greater than 240 mg/dL have been shown to be an accurate predictor of CVD morbidity and mortality. The mean level of LDL cholesterol for American adults age 20 and older is 115.8 mg/dL. Levels of 130 mg/dL to 159 mg/dL are considered borderline high. Levels of 160 mg/dL to 189 mg/dL are classified as high, and levels above 190 mg/dL are very high (AHA, Heart Disease and Stroke Statistics, 2015 Update). Among non-Hispanic Whites, the mean cholesterol levels were 113.8 mg/dL for men and 116.8 mg/dL for women. In non-Hispanic Blacks, the mean cholesterol for males was 113.4 mg/dL and 115.5 mg/dL for women. According to data from the AHA's Heart Disease and Stroke Statistics 2015 Update, in individuals age 20 and older, total cholesterol was lower in Black American females and males compared with their White counterparts. For total serum cholesterol levels greater than 200 mg/dL, the prevalence was 38.6% for Black males and 40.7% for Black females as compared with 40.5% and 45.8%, respectively, for their White counterparts (AHA Fact Sheet, 2013). The prevalence of total cholesterol levels of 240 mg/dL or higher was 10.8% for Black males and 11.7% for Black females compared with 12.3% and 15.6% for White males and females, respectively (AHA, 2013). Although total serum cholesterol levels tend to be lower in Black adult males and females than in their White counterparts, some data indicate that Black Americans have higher rates of CVD because of a greater prevalence of comorbid conditions such as diabetes, obesity, and hypertension (AHA, Heart Disease and Stroke Statistics, 2015 Update). For example, in data available from 2000 to 2010, the age-adjusted values in individuals age 20 and older suggest that the prevalence of total serum cholesterol levels greater than 240 mg/dL is higher among White males and females (11.4% and 15.4%, respectively) than among their Black male and female counterparts (10.2% and 10.3%) (National Center for Health Statistics, Health United States, 2014).

It is interesting to note that high-density lipoprotein cholesterol (HDL) is considered cardioprotective. Higher HDL cholesterol levels are associated with greater protection against CVD. In adults, HDL cholesterol levels less than 40 mg/dL are a known risk factor for CVD. Men and women who have low HDL cholesterol and high total cholesterol levels have the highest risk for myocardial infarction. The mean level of HDL cholesterol in American adults age 20 and older is 52.9 mg/dL (AHA, Heart Disease and Stroke Statistics, 2015 Update). Data from the AHA's Heart Disease and Stroke Statistics 2015 Update indicated that mean HDL cholesterol levels for non-Hispanic whites was 47.7 mg/dL for males and

58.5 mg/dL for White females compared with 51.9 mg/dL for Black males, 57.4 mg/dL for Black females, 45.4 mg/dL for Hispanic American males, and 54.3 mg/dL for Mexican Hispanic females.

Although the proportion of women with cholesterol levels above 240 mg/dL has steadily declined, the number of women age 20 and older with elevated serum cholesterol levels remains alarmingly high. In fact, data from NHANES 2007–2010 estimate that 31.9 million adults have total serum cholesterol values greater than 240 mg/dL. Among the number of women with high serum cholesterol levels, 15.3% were White, 10.3% were Black, and 13.7% were Mexican American (AHA, Heart Disease and Stroke Statistics, 2015 Update). For African-American women, these numbers become more disconcerting because elevated LDL cholesterol, very low-density lipoprotein cholesterol, and triglyceride levels are positively associated with diabetes and obesity, and African-American women tend to have higher rates of diabetes and obesity. In Blacks, these conditions may negate estrogen's protective mechanism against CHD (AHA, Heart Disease and Stroke Statistics, 2015 Update; Mieszczanka & Velord, 2014).

Smoking. Tobacco use is the leading cause of preventable death and the underlying cause of approximately 5 million premature deaths per year worldwide and just under 500,000 deaths in the United States. Smoking is a powerful risk factor contributing to the development of CVD. Smoking has been linked to 35% of deaths from CVD (AHA, Heart Disease and Stroke Statistics, 2015 Update). Persons who smoke have a 25% higher risk of developing CHD than nonsmokers, and they have a higher incidence of sudden cardiac death. The risk for stroke and MI is two to four times higher in cigarette smokers than in nonsmokers. From 2005 to 2009, an estimated 443,100 Americans died each year of smoking-related illnesses; 35.3% of the deaths were due to CVD (AHA, Heart Disease and Stroke Statistics, 2015 Update). Data from the Heart Disease and Stroke Statistics 2015 Update illuminate the fact that even though the total number of individuals who smoke has dropped, smoking continues to be a prevalent problem among adolescents in high school. In 2013, 16.4% of male students and 15% of female students in grades 9 through 12 reported current tobacco use; 14.7% of males and 2.9% of females reported current smokeless tobacco use. Data from the AHA's Heart Disease and Stroke Statistics 2015 Update revealed that more White male and female students reported current cigarette smoking (19.1% and 18.1%, respectively) than Black male and female students (10.5% and 6.2%, respectively). Further, data in this report revealed that White youths 18 to 24 years of age from families with lower educational attainment had substantially higher rates

of smoking than African-American and Mexican American youths with similar educational attainment. Data from the AHA Heart Disease and Stroke Statistics 2015 Update indicated that in 2012, approximately 69.7 million Americans over the age of 12 were using some type of tobacco product. By race/ethnicity, the age-adjusted estimates for tobacco users 18 years and older was 31.2% for Whites, 27.7% for Blacks, 44.9% for American Indians and Alaska Natives, 28.5% for Native Hawaiians and other Pacific Islanders, 22.9% for Hispanics or Latinos, and 13.6% for Asians. American Indian/Native Alaskans have higher rates of smoking (37.7%) than Black males (24.8%), and American Indian/Native Alaskan females have higher rates of smoking (36%) than Black females (15.5%). For all cigarette smokers, there is a 1.5- to 3-fold increase in risk for myocardial infarction. However, in young women who smoke cigarettes, the risk may be increased as much as tenfold to 25% (AHA, Heart Disease and Stroke Statistics, 2015 Update). In the adult population, although other racial groups have higher smoking prevalence than do African-Americans, the potential effect of smoking appears to produce more devastating consequences among young premenopausal African-American women, including lowering HDL2-C, an associated risk for CVD and myocardial infarction (Forey et al., 2013).

Exposure to environmental smoke is also known to increase the risk for developing CVD and respiratory diseases. An estimated 33,951 nonsmokers die from CHD each year as a result of exposure to secondhand smoke. Data indicated that approximately 60% of children between 3 and 11 years of age are exposed to secondhand smoke (AHA, Heart Disease and Stroke Statistics, 2015 Update). Levels of cotinine, a biomarker indicating secondhand smoke exposure, declined from 52.5% in 1999 to 2000 to 40.1% in 2007 to 2008 for individuals in all age groups. From 2007 through 2008, levels in children ages 3 to 11 declined from 60.5% to 53.6% and from 55.4% to 46.5% in children and adolescents ages 12 to 19. In individuals ages 20 years and older levels dropped from 52.5% to 40.1%. During this same period, cotinine levels were higher in African-Americans (55.9%) compared with Whites (40.1%) and Mexican Americans (25.8%). Data continue to show that Blacks have higher levels of cotinine than non-Hispanic Whites, even though the percentage of exposure to environmental smoke is slightly higher. One plausible explanation for the differences is that Blacks may metabolize nicotine at a slower rate, leading to increased serum levels of cotinine. Another reason for higher levels in Black children is that they may actually experience greater exposure to environmental smoke (AHA, Heart Disease and Stroke Statistics, 2015 Update). The American Heart Association (2015) revealed that smoking rates were substantially higher in families with lower educational attainment. In the same report, data showed that smoking rates were highest among persons living below the poverty level. It is well documented that the percentage of African-Americans who live in poverty is higher than that for other racial and ethnic backgrounds. This may explain why poor African-American women have higher rates of smoking than their White counterparts.

Diabetes. Diabetes is defined as a heterogeneous group of chronic metabolic disorders caused by defects in insulin secretion or insulin action. The physical manifestations of diabetes are impaired glucose tolerance, hyperglycemia, and IR (Global Diabetes Plan, 2011; Pearson, 2015; Zettervall, 2005). In type 1 diabetes, which accounts for 1% to 5% of cases, there is an absolute deficiency of insulin secretion. In type 2 diabetes, which accounts for 90% to 95% of cases, the cause is a combination of resistance to insulin action and inadequate compensatory insulin secretory response (Global Diabetes Plan, 2011; Pearson, 2015). Hypertension is present in 20% to 60% of persons with diabetes. Hypertension often is an initial presenting symptom of IR and metabolic syndrome and may be a hallmark for the onset of type 2 diabetes. Diabetes is now a global epidemic with an estimated 366 million individuals affected by the disorder (Global Diabetes Plan, 2011). According to data from the Global Diabetes Plan, this number is expected to increase to 552 million within the next 20 years. In the United States, an estimated 29.1 million adults have a known diagnosis of diabetes, 8.1 million have undiagnosed diabetes, and 80.8 million have prediabetes (AHA, Heart Disease and Stroke Statistics, 2015 Update). From 2005 to 2012, the number of adults with diabetes increased from 20.6 million to 29.1 million (National Diabetes Statistics Report, 2014). In 2012, 1.7 million new cases were diagnosed, and the number of persons with diabetes is expected to continue to rise over the next decade (National Diabetes Statistics Report, 2014). The prevalence of diabetes varies according to race and gender, increases with age, and at all ages is highest among African-Americans (AHA, Heart Disease and Stroke Statistics, 2015 Update). In 2010, diabetes was recorded as the seventh leading cause of death in the United States. More recent data rank diabetes as the fourth leading cause of death (National Center for Health Statistics, 2013) for African-Americans (Office of Minority Health, n.d.). In 2011, diabetes was the cause of death for approximately 73,831 people, and it was identified as the contributing cause of death for another 239,189 individuals (AHA, Heart Disease and Stroke Statistics, 2015 Update; National Diabetes Statistics Report, 2014). The prevalence of type 2 diabetes is higher in African-Americans than in Whites, and the age-adjusted overall mortality is 2.2 times higher for African-Americans. African-American, American Indian, and Hispanic women experience the highest diabetes mortality rates (AHA, Heart Disease and Stroke Statistics, 2015 Update; Office of Minority Health, n.d.). In 2009, the overall age-adjusted rate of death from diabetes for African-American males and females was 44.9% and 35.8%, respectively, compared with 24.3% and 16.2%, respectively, for their White counterparts (AHA, Heart Disease and Stroke Statistics, 2015 Update). African-Americans with diabetes have a higher risk for coronary artery disease, stroke, and other major complications of diabetes (such as end-stage renal disease, limb amputations, and blindness) than their White counterparts (Office of Minority Health, n.d.).

Obesity and sedentary lifestyle. Obesity is another health condition that remains a pandemic problem. According to the WHO, worldwide obesity has increased by 27.5%. From 1980 to 2013, the number of people who are obese has increased from 857 million to 2.1 billion (Ng et al., 2014). According to Ng et al., the United States has seen the greatest increase in adult obesity, with one third of the population meeting the definition. In 2010, the WHO estimated that by 2015 the number of overweight people in the world would reach 2.3 billion and of this number, over 700 million would be obese. If current rates of obesity and overweight in individuals continue to grow, this number will surpass predictions. In the United States, slightly more than 300,000 deaths per year can be directly attributed to obesity, and the condition has been cited as second only to cigarette smoking as a major modifiable risk factor for all causes of death. It is a well-documented fact that obesity and inactivity are significant risk factors for CVD and diabetes (AHA, Heart Disease and Stroke Statistics, 2015 Update; Mieszczanka & Velord, 2014). Obesity leads to changes in systemic circulation resulting in increased platelet aggregation, increased activity of the sympathetic nervous system and the renin-angiotensin-aldosterone system, as well as endothelial dysfunction (Beaser et al., 2010; Samad & Ruf, 2013). Central adiposity, one of the components of metabolic syndrome, is associated with an increase in glucose abnormalities, hypertension, and atherosclerosis. Abdominal obesity is an independent risk factor for ischemic stroke in all racial and ethnic groups (AHA, Heart Disease and Stroke Statistics, 2015 Update). Overweight in children is defined as a value at or above the 95th percentile of the gender-specific BMI for age growth charts. Obesity among adults is defined as a BMI of 30 kg/m^2 or greater. Approximately 69% of Americans are overweight or obese, including 82% of African-American women over 40 years of age (Office of Minority Health, n.d.). Data from the NHANES III suggested that 23 million American children and adolescents 2 to 19 years of age are overweight and that 74.1 million American adults are obese. This change represents a significant increase in the prevalence of overweight children and adolescents and obesity among adults. Data from NHANES III revealed that obesity is more prevalent among certain racial and ethnic groups and that gender and age are contributing factors. This same study showed that rates of obesity were higher in African-American women (58%) compared with 33% for White women, 43% for Hispanic women, and 5.8% for Asian women. There is a direct link between obesity and the development of CVD, dyslipidemia, type 2 diabetes, sleep apnea, and numerous forms of cancers (AHA, Heart Disease and Stroke Statistics, 2015 Update; Ng et al., 2014).

Results from NHANES III revealed a positive correlation between obesity and hypertension in African-Americans. Persons who are overweight or obese have an increased risk of developing hypertension, type 2 diabetes, CHD, stroke, and sleep disorders (AHA, Heart Disease and Stroke Statistics, 2015 Update). There is a higher prevalence of obesity in women with lower incomes, and African-American women are more likely to be in a lower income bracket than White women (Centers for Disease Control and Prevention [CDC], 2014; National Center for Health Statistics, Health United States, 2014). This fact is also supported by recent data from the AHA Heart Disease and Stroke Statistics 2015 Update. This report showed that 82% of non-Hispanic Black females and 69% of non-Hispanic Black males are overweight, compared with 73% of White males and 61% of White females. Non-Hispanic Black females also have the highest rate of obesity (58%) compared with non-Hispanic Black males (38%), non-Hispanic White males (34%), and non-Hispanic White females (33%) (AHA, Heart Disease and Stroke Statistics, 2015 Update; CDC, 2014). Factors contributing to obesity include excessive dietary intake of calories and fatty foods and physical inactivity (AHA, Heart Disease and Stroke Statistics, 2015 Update; CDC, 2014; National Center for Health Statistics, 2014). Persons with lower incomes and less education typically have poorer dietary habits and are not as physically active as those who have high incomes and are better educated (AHA, Heart Disease and Stroke Statistics, 2015 Update; Levi et al., 2013; National Center for Health Statistics, 2013). African-Americans and Hispanics in general have lower incomes and are more likely to live in poverty than Whites (National Center for Health Statistics, 2014). In fact, 11,000,000 African-Americans live below the poverty index. If being overweight is a common problem in the general U.S. population, it is said to be at epidemic proportions in children in this country (Levi et al., 2013).

Childhood obesity continues to increase steadily and rapidly among African-American children (National Center for Health Statistics, Health United States, 2014; Ogden et al., 2010). Some researchers conclude that childhood obesity often serves as a primary marker for high-risk dietary and physical inactivity practices (Levi et al., 2013). Childhood obesity can also contribute to the development of metabolic syndrome, leading to early onset of CVD and type 2 diabetes.

Stroke. Strokes are the fourth leading cause of death in the United States. In African-Americans, it remains the third leading cause of death, and the rate of death from stroke is almost twice as high as for Whites because of a greater prevalence of comorbid conditions, along with an increased severity and a more rapid progression of disease processes. Cardiovascular disease, hypertension, and diabetes, the major risk factors for strokes, are seen in disproportionate numbers of African-Americans. Of the four leading causes of death in African-Americans, hypertension can be associated with at least three of the four disease states: CHD, the leading cause of death among African-Americans; CVAs, listed as third; and diabetes, listed as fourth. Coronary heart disease and CVAs can occur or are exacerbated as a result of hypertension. Individuals with diabetes have a higher risk of CHD and hypertension, and both conditions are exacerbated by diabetes (AHA, Heart Disease and Stroke Statistics, 2015 Update).

Sudden Cardiac Deaths. Significant differences have been noted in the incidence of sudden cardiac arrest among African-Americans. A 2015 report from the AHA indicated that the rate of sudden cardiac death was much higher for young African-Americans than for Whites. Not only are African-Americans more likely to experience sudden cardiac arrest, but they are also more likely to succumb to the arrest (AHA, Heart Disease and Stroke Statistics, 2015 Update). In fact, among African-Americans in all age groups, both men and women have higher rates of cardiac arrests than their White counterparts have. The survival rate for African-Americans, compared with Whites, was remarkably different (0.8% vs. 2.6%). The difference in survival rate can be attributed to the fact that the mortality rate for African-Americans with coronary artery disease, left ventricular hypertrophy, heart failure, and cardiomyopathy is higher than that for Whites (AHA, Heart Disease and Stroke Statistics, 2015 Update). Data from a New York City study of out-of-hospital cardiac arrests show that the age-adjusted incidence for cardiac arrest per 10,000 adults was higher in Blacks at 10.1 compared to 5.8 for Whites. In 2006, a Duke University study by Berger on age, sex, and racial disparities in heart hospital transfer patterns revealed that older, female, and minority patients rushed to community hospitals with acute MIs were less likely to be transferred to larger hospitals offering procedures to restore artery patency.

The authors also found that women were 16% less likely to be transferred than men; compared with White patients, African-Americans were 31% and Hispanics were 41% less likely to be transferred. In another Duke University study, researchers found that hypertrophic cardiomyopathy (HCM), a common cause of sudden cardiac death in young competitive athletes, was an important issue for African-Americans (Maron et al., 2003) also found a large discrepancy in clinical diagnosis of HCM in African-American compared with White athletes. Of 1986 patients clinically diagnosed with HCM, only 158 (8%) were African-American. Furthermore, among the 286 cardiovascular deaths, most were caused by HCM ($n = 102$). Results of this study showed that, of the 102 athletes who died from HCM, 42 were White (41%) and 56 were African-American (55%). These researchers concluded that HCM is under-diagnosed in African-American athletes and that the condition is a common cause of sudden death in this population.

More recent data continue to support the fact that African-American males experience higher mortality from sudden cardiac death than White males. In 2008, Mitchell et al. conducted the Sudden Cardiac Death in Heart Failure (SCD-HeFT) study to examine survival benefits from implantable cardiac defibrillator (ICD) therapy. In this study, 23% of the subjects were ethnic minorities and 17% were African-Americans. The investigators evaluated two major prespecified subgroups: heart failure cause (ischemic vs. nonischemic) and New York Heart Association class (II vs. III). The authors compared demographic, clinical variables, socioeconomic status, and long-term outcomes with the subject's race. The results of this study demonstrated that ICD therapy significantly improved survival compared with medical therapy alone in stable, moderately symptomatic heart failure patients with an ejection fraction of 35% or less. Data also supported the fact that African-Americans were younger and had more nonischemic heart failure, lower ejection fractions, worse New York Heart Association functional class, and higher prevalence of a history of nonsustained ventricular tachycardia when compared to Whites. Data also indicated that survival benefits from ICD therapy in SCD-HeFT were not dependent on race and that death rates were equally decreased in both racial groups receiving ICD therapy compared with placebo (hazard ratio, 0.65 in African-Americans and 0.73 in Whites). Although data support the fact that African-Americans are less likely to receive an ICD, in this clinical trial setting, there was no evidence that

they were less willing to accept ICD therapy than were Whites.

Other plausible explanations for the differences between the rates and lethality of sudden cardiac arrest for African-Americans and their White counterparts are as follows: (1) inexperience and lack of familiarity with basic cardiopulmonary resuscitation techniques of the persons at the site; (2) response time of the emergency ambulance to the site, particularly in "African-American neighborhoods"; (3) response time of the hospital emergency team to the African-American client in full cardiac arrest (AHA, Heart Disease and Stroke Statistics, 2015 Update; Braunwald, 2012; Sasson et al., 2012); and (4) inequities in quality of care for clients at risk for ventricular dysrhythmias (AHA, Heart Disease and Stroke Statistics, 2015 Update). The findings from this study, along with more recent data from the AHA, indicate that the incidence of cardiac arrest is significantly higher among African-Americans in every age group, and early intervention and prevention techniques to reduce the chronicity of CHD appear to be plausible mechanisms to prevent cardiac arrest in this population.

AIDS (HIV) Risk. While CVDs have been heralded as the single leading cause of death across all ethnic and racial groups, little attention has been paid to the growing incidence of deaths from AIDS among African-Americans under 35 years of age. Human immunodeficiency virus (HIV) and AIDS was once thought of as a disease that primarily affected gay single White males. According to data published by the CDC (2011; National Center for Health Statistics, 2013), the severity of the impact of HIV among homosexual and bisexual men of all races and ethnicities has been seriously underscored. Data from this report clearly show that within African-Americans, Hispanics, and Latinos, the disease has had the severest impact on homosexual or bisexual African-American and White males between ages 30 and 40. In 2010, an estimated 10,600 (72%) of new infections occurred among young homosexual and bisexual African-American males and other men who report having sex with other males occurred in African-American men. The greatest number of new infections, 4500 (45%), occurred in African-American gay and bisexual males ages 13 to 24 (CDC, 2014; Kaiser Family Foundation, 2014). This number was more than twice the rate among Whites, Hispanics, and Latinos; both groups had slightly less than 2000 new cases. African-American women continue to account for the largest number of new HIV infections (64%) when compared to infection rates for women of other races (Kaiser Family Foundation, 2014). In 2010, the incidence of infection for African-American women was 4 times the rate for Latin American women and 20 times the rate for White women. This same report indicated that the common mode of transmission for African-American women was through heterosexual contact compared with White women in whom the common mode of transmission was intravenous drug injection. Although there were fewer new HIV infections among African-American women compared to African-American men (6595 vs. 1776), the CDC Office of Minority Health's most recent analysis reveals that African-American women are far more affected than women of other races. The HIV incidence rate in African-American women (40 per 100,000) is nearly 20 times higher than that of White women (2 per 100,000) and five times higher than the rate of infection for Hispanic and Latino women (8 per 100,000). In 2011 alone, 23,168 African-Americans were diagnosed with HIV (CDC, 2011; Kaiser Family Foundation, 2014; National Center for Health Statistics, 2013; Office of Minority Health, n.d.).

In 2010, approximately 47,989 new cases of AIDS were reported in the United States—a much higher figure than the CDC's previous estimates (CDC, 2012c). According to the Statistics 2012 HIV Surveillance report, from 2008 to 2011, the number of deaths from AIDS remained stable among children under age 13 and in individuals in the age groups 13 to 14, 20 to 24, 55 to 59, and 60 to 64. The death rate decreased among children and adolescents ages 15 to 19, and in adults ages 25 to 29, 30 to 34, 35 to 39, 40 to 44, 45 to 49, and 50 to 54. The death rate increased in adults from ages 65 and older. Further, the estimated death rate for persons with a diagnosis of HIV infection was highest in persons aged 45 to 59. Although infections and deaths have decreased for all other races, African-Americans continue to have the highest rates of new infection and death compared with individuals of races and ethnic backgrounds. Among racial groups, African-Americans had the highest rates (58.3/100,000) compared with Whites (7/100,000) and Hispanic/Latinos (19.5/100,000) (CDC Statistics, 2013; Kaiser Family Foundation, 2014). With regard to race and ethnicity, the number of individuals living with HIV/AIDS is highest among African-Americans (44%), compared with Whites (33%) and Hispanics/Latinos (20%). Disparities are also seen in the number of persons diagnosed with HIV/AIDS; from 2008 through 2012, the rates of HIV/AIDS cases were 36.4 per 100,000 in African-Americans, 3.5 per 100,000 in Whites, 10.2 per 100,000 in Hispanics/Latinos, 4.9 per 100,000 in American Indians/Alaska Natives, 2.7 per 100,000 in Asians, and 6.2 per 100,000 in Native Hawaiians/other Pacific Islanders (CDC, 2012a). The impact of AIDS is disproportionately affecting minorities and women. In 2011, African-American females accounted for the greatest number of women diagnosed with AIDS (32.2/100,000 compared to White females

at 1.4/100,000). In 2012, approximately 50% of all reported new cases of AIDS (27,928) occurred in African-American women. In 2011, African-American women accounted for 25% of new cases of AIDS in women (Kaiser Family Foundation, 2014; Office of Minority Health, n.d.). Similarly, in 2011 nearly 80% of all new pediatric AIDS cases reported were among African-Americans (Child Trends Data Bank, 2012).

In 2011, although African-American males represented only 13% of U.S. males by proportion of the population, they disproportionately represented 44% of all reported cases of AIDS (Kaiser Family Foundation, 2014). In 2011 alone, 15,958 African-Americans had a confirmed diagnosis of stage 3 HIV/AIDS (Office of Minority Health, n.d.). Even more astounding is the number of African-American women who had AIDS (70,812) compared with their White counterparts (19,676). In addition, although by proportion of the population African-American women make up only 14% of U.S. females, these individuals disproportionately represent 36.4% of all reported cases of AIDS in women. In fact, overall, African-Americans now represent approximately 50% of all reported cases of AIDS in the United States to date (CDC, 2012c; Kaiser Family Foundation, 2014). Moreover, African-Americans between 13 and 19 years of age now account for 82% of newly reported AIDS cases in that age group as of 2011 (CDC, 2012c). Most recent data from the Kaiser Family Foundation (2014) indicate that 1 in 16 African-American men and 1 in 32 African-American women will be infected with HIV at some point in their lifetime. In addition, African-Americans between 13 and 24 years of age continue to account for a disproportionate rate of all HIV diagnoses (Kaiser Family Foundation, 2014; Health United States, 2012).

Men who have sex with men still represent the largest group of individuals with HIV/AIDS in the United States (CDC, 2012a; Kaiser Family Foundation, 2014). However, since the first reported case in 1981, HIV/AIDS has become a major cause of morbidity and mortality among African-Americans. Ward and Duchin reported in 1998 that for the first time the number of African-Americans with a diagnosis of AIDS was approximately equal to the number of reported cases in Whites. Since 1995, HIV infection has been cited as the leading cause of death in persons 24 to 44 years of age (Kaiser Family Foundation, 2014).

A disproportionate number of individuals with AIDS in this age range (22–44) are African-American (CDC, 2012c). According to the Statistics 2012 HIV Surveillance Report (CDC, 2012c), the rate of death from AIDS was greater for African-American males (16.5 per 100,000) than for White males (2.3 per 100,000). African-American females fare even worse (7.5 per 100,000), with a death rate significantly higher than that for White females (0.5 per 100,000) (CDC, 2012c). Statistical data from the CDC 2014 State HIV Prevention Report and Statistics 2012 HIV Surveillance Report (CDC, 2012c) support the fact that a greater percentage of African-Americans are infected with HIV and are dying of AIDS compared with other races. According to demographic data from the CDC Health Statistics 2012 HIV Surveillance Report, a total of 635,816 persons regardless of race/ethnicity have died of AIDS as of 2011. The cumulative estimated number of deaths of persons with an AIDS diagnosis in the United States and dependent areas, through 2011, was 659,068. In the 50 states and the District of Columbia, this included 643,254 adults and adolescents and 5175 children under age 13 years at death. Breaking those numbers out by race/ethnicity has become difficult since 2001. However, Table 8-1 depicts deaths from AIDS through 2011 by race/ethnicity and by gender.

Moore, Stanton, Gopalan, and Chaisson (1994), researchers at Johns Hopkins University School of Medicine, conducted a study on HIV-positive individuals to determine whether there were notable differences in the administration of antiretroviral drugs among Black and White clients. Findings from this study suggest that Black HIV-positive individuals are less likely than their White counterparts to be given antiretroviral drugs, including medication to prevent *Pneumocystis carinii* pneumonia (PCP). Of Blacks surveyed, only 58% of those medically eligible received drug therapy, compared with 82% of their White counterparts. Researchers found no significant differences in receipt of drug therapy with respect to such moderating variables as age, gender, mode of HIV

transmission, type of insurance, income, education, or place of residence. Similarly, Shapiro et al. (1999) noted that even after adjustment for insurance status, CD4 cell count, sex, age, methods of exposure to HIV, and region of the country, African-Americans, along with their Hispanic counterparts, were 24% less likely than their White counterparts to receive protease inhibitors or non-nucleoside reverse transcriptase inhibitors at the initial assessment by their health care providers.

Guidelines published by the U.S. Public Health Service (PHS) suggest that to effectively treat HIV-infected persons, antiretroviral therapy should begin when the client's CD4 cell count falls to 500 cells/mm³ or less. These PHS guidelines also suggest that prophylactic treatment for PCP should begin when the CD4 count reaches 200 cells/mm³ or less. Because CD4 cells are integral to the body's immune defense, reduction in CD4 cells is generally associated with a weakening in the immune system. This reduction, particularly among HIV-positive individuals, generally signals an onset of disease symptoms, including PCP (Sampson & Workman, 2013). Moore et al. (1994) also noted that among clients with a CD4 cell count of 500 cells/mm³ or less, only 48% of Blacks, compared with 68% of Whites, received antiretroviral therapy. Despite the PHS guidelines for administration of prophylactic therapy to all clients with a CD4 cell count of 200 cells/mm³ or less, researchers found an even greater disparity between Blacks and their White counterparts, with Blacks invariably receiving little intervention when CD4 cell counts dropped to 200 cells/mm³ or less.

Highly active antiretroviral therapy (HAART) has resulted in a significant decline in mortality from HIV disease in all racial and ethnic groups; however, data continue to show that racial, ethnic, and gender differences in HIV mortality persist. In 2013, Singh, Azuine, and Siahpush published results of a study examining inequities in access to health care provided to racial and ethnic minorities. They found that inequities in access persist and in fact may be widening. This document cited that disparities in HIV/AIDS mortality are reflective of higher incidence of infection rates and lack of access to antiretroviral therapy. This study along with a number of others continues to show that minorities are less likely to receive the most sophisticated treatment for HIV infection, which would slow the onset of AIDS. Current research evaluating population demographics for prescribed HAART suggests that Hispanics and African-Americans are less likely to have access to and to use HAART therapy compared with non-Hispanic White persons, and women are less likely to have access and use HAART therapy compared with men (National Center for Health Statistics, Health United States, 2013; Singh et al., 2013).

TABLE 8-1 Cumulative AIDS Mortalities Occurring through December 2012 in the United States

Demographic Variable	Male	Female	Pediatric
Non-Hispanic White	251,282	15,466	1002
Non-Hispanic Black	223,880	40,753	2912
Hispanic	84,709	14,236	1224
Asian Pacific Islander	3053	351	37
Native American	1630	216	21
Unknown origin	601	10	16

From the Centers for Disease Control and Prevention. (2013). *HIV surveillance report.* Atlanta: Centers for Disease Control and Prevention, 25(2). No further data on cumulative deaths are available at this time.

Asthma. The incidence of asthma in general, and in African-American children in particular, is a concern for all health care practitioners. Asthma has a high prevalence among African-American adults and children. For example, in 2011, 4,300,000 African-Americans reported suffering from asthma; in fact, African-American women were 30% more likely to have asthma than non-Hispanic White women (Akinbami et al., 2012; National Center for Health Statistics, Health United States, 2013; Office for Minority Health, n.d.). In 2011, data suggested that African-Americans were three times more likely to die from asthma-related causes than their White counterparts. African-American children appear especially vulnerable to asthma and its consequences and had a death rate seven times that of non-Hispanic White children from 2008 to 2010. In concert with this high death rate, African-Americans tend to experience asthma-related emergency room visits more often than their White counterparts and a higher death rate per 1000 persons. According to Elward and Pollart (2010), each year patients with asthma make approximately 1.8 million visits to the emergency room for treatment. For African-Americans, rate of emergency room visits is five times greater compared with visits by Whites. In fact, recent data continue to suggest that African-American children are twice as likely to have an emergency department (ED) visit for asthma, have a higher hospitalization rate, and have a death rate from asthma that is four times higher, compared with their White counterparts. Socioeconomic status tends to play a major role in the diagnosis and chronicity of asthma in African-American children. For example, African-American children in poor families are more likely to be diagnosed with asthma. Although all of the causes of asthma remain unclear, African-American children who are exposed to second-hand tobacco smoke appear to be at increased risk for acute lower respiratory tract infections and acute exacerbations of asthma. Of critical importance is the fact that children living below or near the poverty level are also more likely to have high blood cotinine levels, a breakdown product of nicotine, than children living in higher income families (CDC, 2012; National Center for Health Statistics, 2013; NIH, 2010; National Health Interview Survey, 2012; Federal Asthma Disparities Plan 2012).

Wright (2007, 2009) conducted studies to profile California's African-American children with asthma ranging from 1 to 11 years of age addressing their demographics, their health care access, their asthma severity, their disability resulting from asthma, and their health care utilization patterns. A sample of 137 African-American children ($n = 137$) with a medical doctor's diagnosis of asthma was used. A secondary analysis of parental reports of their children's asthma was performed using the California Health Interview Survey (2001). Findings from this study suggested that within the past 12 months, African-American children had increased ED use because of their asthma (33.9%) compared with visits to their regular care provider and took daily asthma control medication (64.5%). Most children had mild asthma severity (68.7%), and many were prevented from regular school attendance (16.1%) and from doing regular school work (16.2%), and sometimes their physical activity was limited (17.6%) because of asthma. A conclusion from this study suggests that California's African-American children with asthma have high utilization of health care services because of asthma. This finding is in concert with available data from the CDC and other reporting agencies (American Lung Association [ALA], 2012; National Center for Health Statistics, 2014).

Psychological Characteristics

Some studies depict the pattern of interaction in the African-American family as pathological and unstable. Findings from one study indicate that if there is stability in the African-American family, it is attributable to the presence of a controlling, domineering mother. The pathological family interaction that occurs in some African-American families is said to affect the son so profoundly that in later life he is unable to adjust to the role of husband and father. Consequently, in unstable African-American families, the African-American male is unable to form mature, lasting relationships with others (Culture of Poverty Revisited, n.d.). In studies done on African-American male alcoholics, these individuals were found to have the lowest scores on tests of personality integration, with a more passive and compliant coping style than any other ethnic group of male alcoholics (Carroll, Klein, & Santo, 1978). It is believed that this passive and compliant coping style was rooted in the slavery era. During slavery, African-American mothers were forced to teach their male children to be passive if they were to survive the authority of the slave master because to be "uppity" meant possible physical punishment or even death. Today it would seem essential that the African-American male display the same survival skills because the authority figure remains (police, educators, employers, and so forth).

A classic study done on African-American boys from father-absent homes found that dependency and a passive coping style were evident among these boys (Barclay & Cusumano, 1967). Other studies suggest that boys from father-absent homes tend to be more dependent on their peer groups, display fewer aggressive behaviors, have lower self-esteem, and are more likely to display overt masculine behavior. In some studies looking at psychological issues of father-absent homes, social class appeared to be an intervening variable. A more deleterious effect on sex-role orientation was found in boys who lived in father-absent homes before 5 years of age (Covell & Turnbull, 1982). Because there is a greater probability of an African-American male being reared in a female-headed household, it has become necessary for African-American mothers to encourage masculine traits in their sons. An earlier study found that mothers who encouraged masculine traits in their sons had more of an effect in father-absent homes than in father-present homes (Biller, 1969).

Some social scientists and health care providers contend that African-Americans are at risk for the development of mental health problems. Corrective steps have been taken to alleviate the development of mental health problems; however, the mental health system continues to struggle to meet the emotional needs of African-Americans (Snowden, 1982; Snowden & Todman, 1982). Bullough and Bullough (1982) reported that rates of admission to mental health hospitals are higher and the hospital stay is longer for African-Americans than for any other ethnic group in the United States. However, when socioeconomic status was carefully controlled for, psychosis rates among Whites and African-Americans appeared similar.

Alcohol Abuse. Alcoholism is one of the major health problems in the African-American community, contributing to reduced longevity. Among African-Americans, there are high incidence rates of acute and chronic alcohol-related diseases, such as alcoholic fatty liver; hepatitis; cirrhosis of the liver; heart disease; cancer of the mouth, larynx, tongue, esophagus, and lung; and unintentional injuries and homicide (American Association of Gastroenterology). In a classic study, Harper and Dawkins (1976) reported that of 16,000 articles on alcohol abuse published from 1944 to 1974, only 77 included references to African-Americans, and only 11 were specifically about African-Americans. King (1982) reported that most studies between 1977 and 1980 dealt only with patterns of alcohol use. Only one study at that time (Stalls, 1978) explored racial differences in patterns of alcohol metabolism. Chartier and Caetano (2010) reviewed recent advances in alcohol research focusing on consumption, disorders, consequences and treatment use among ethnic groups. The authors found that progress has been made in the preceding decade in researching alcohol consumption, its detrimental effects, and the use and treatment access for minorities. This study also showed that disparities in research and treatment options continue to exist for African-Americans. The authors concluded that measures to eliminate the disparities should be the focus of research along with the development of more effective targeted strategies for the prevention and treatment of alcohol disorders in African-Americans.

In a classic study, Stalls (1978) found an increasing incidence of alcohol abuse among African-American youth and women, with serious implications for fetal alcohol syndrome. Drinking appeared to peak between 16 and 23 years of age, and, among women, drinking was highest for divorced women younger than 45 years of age. In another classic study, Brisbane (1987) noted that women who drank were typically younger than 45 years of age, were employed, and considered themselves middle class. In yet another classic study, Williams (1986) noted a contradiction in the high incidence of alcohol-related diseases and drinking patterns reported in African-Americans: when age and socioeconomic levels were controlled, African-Americans actually abstained more, drank less frequently, and consumed less alcohol than their White counterparts. African-American women were the exception, with 11% of African-American women drinking heavily, compared with 4% of White women.

More recent data from the 2008 National Survey on Drug Use and Health (Substance Abuse and Mental Health Services, 2009) support the fact that alcohol consumption is lower in African-American men and women. According to the National Health Interview Survey conducted by the CDC (2011), the percentage of current and regular alcohol consumption by African-Americans is 39% compared with 57% for non-Hispanic Whites and 42% for Hispanic adults. This same study also revealed that racial and gender differences exist in lifetime abstinence from alcohol. Data from the CDC 2011 Health Interview Survey found that Hispanic and African-American females had the highest rates of lifetime abstinence at 40.4% and 35.4% compared to White females at 18.3%. African-American males also had higher rates of lifetime abstinence at 20.7% compared to Hispanic and White males at 19% and 11%, respectively. Several causes of alcohol abuse and misuse in African-Americans have been identified in the literature. A primary factor is economics. Many African-American men drink as a result of unemployment, which leads to depression and frustration because of their inability to meet financial commitments. Britt (2009) concluded that unemployment is correlated with a high risk for alcohol problems among African-Americans. Availability is also a factor (Britt, 2009). Brown and Tooley (2004) have reported that in Los Angeles there are approximately three liquor stores per city block. African-American peer pressure is also reported as a contributing factor; peers expect heavy drinking, and brand names and quantity are often status identifiers. Finally, heavy alcohol use may be related to a desire to escape unpleasant feelings. Sterne and Pittman (1972) have also pointed out themes that seem to be present in African-American alcohol use. They linked being paid on the weekend to Saturday relaxation and thus drinking. A second theme is the prevalence of taverns in the African-American community that serve as social centers. Finally, alcohol appears to be used as an escape from personal problems.

African-Americans are less likely to seek treatment for problem drinking than any other ethnic group in the United States (Chartier & Caetano, 2010). Research indicates that several areas must be addressed to increase the likelihood of successful treatment outcomes. The first step is to get the African-American alcoholic into a treatment program. Programs that are located within the community and are accessible to public transportation are more likely to be used, except by the upwardly mobile African-American person, who is more likely to seek private services outside the community. The African-American church can and in some instances does serve a dual role in this first step because it can provide a facility and at the same time act as a referral source (Britt, 2009; Giger, Appel, Davidhizar, & Davis, 2008). Most African-American churches are centrally located within the African-American community, and even as members relocate, they tend to maintain their roots in the African-American church. Also, prayer has been associated with the treatment modality and overall success rate for the recovering alcoholic. The church continues to be the mainstay of the African-American family, and rather than seeking outside help for alcoholism, the family often attempts to resolve problems by going to the minister. Some African-Americans have reported that they stopped drinking before seeking professional help because of their spirituality, which assisted with the transition (Brisbane, 1987; Britt, 2009; Giger et al., 2008; Hudson, 1986; Knox, 1986; Westermeyer, 1984).

When treating the recovering alcoholic, the nurse must remember that the family can often provide assistance in the form of shelter, food, money, or clothing. The extended family may also take on counseling roles that close relatives find too painful (Brisbane & Womble, 1986). The nurse must also have an awareness of the socioeconomic context and its effect on intrapsychic processes. The elimination of stereotypical bias by both the nurse and the client and the inclusion of social values and traditions are necessary to maximize intervention, give culturally appropriate nursing care, and affect recovery rates (Institute of Black Chemical Abuse, 1988).

Post-traumatic Stress Disorder. Many studies indicate that minority Vietnam veterans have experienced a greater degree of maladjustment after the Vietnam War than their White counterparts (National Alliance on Mental Health). Some of these studies have given a variety of reasons for this maladjustment, including the fact that minorities felt more conflict about participating in the war because they had less to gain than persons in the dominant culture. Another reason postulated by the researchers was that minorities were more likely to be identified with the enemy, who were also different in skin color from White Americans. Perhaps the most significant reason for post-traumatic stress disorder (PTSD) among minority Vietnam veterans was that minorities continued to experience discrimination after returning home from the war in Vietnam (Dohrenwend et al., 2008).

In a later study, Penk et al. (1989) also found that among Vietnam combat veterans, African-Americans appeared to be more maladjusted than their White counterparts. One conclusion of this study is that ethnicity emerges as a significant parameter in studies of PTSD, but the exact contributions of ethnicity have not been explained fully by current findings on the subject. Many researchers have postulated that significant increases in PTSD in African-American Vietnam veterans may be attributable in part to the fact that during the Vietnam War years (1964–1975), African-Americans suffered the major loss of a leader (through the assassination of Martin Luther King Jr. in 1968) and experienced the racial conflicts evidenced by rioting in Washington, DC, Watts (in Los Angeles), and other cities throughout the country (Karnow, 1997). Finally, a study mandated by Congress found that thousands of Vietnam veterans continue to suffer from PTSD 41 years after the war ended (Mooney, 2014).

Recent studies emphasize the importance of examining the prevalence PTSD in veterans of wars that have occurred since Vietnam as the disorder poses a significant public health problem among deployed and nondeployed veterans. In addition to PTSD among Vietnam veterans, there are thousands more who served in the Afghanistan and Iraq wars who have the disorder. The Afghanistan and Iraq wars are the longest United States combat operations since Vietnam, and veterans of both wars experienced multiple stressors that contribute to the risk for PTSDs. During combat, soldiers constantly face the risk of death or injury, witness death or injury of their comrades, and kill or wound numerous enemy soldiers. Further, prolonged lack of rest and sleep is another factor contributing to undue stress, as there are many instances when soldiers have to remain awake and alert for days on end (*Iraq War Clinician Guide*, n.d.).

A number of studies have examined the prevalence of PTSD in veterans of Operation Enduring Freedom (OEF) in Afghanistan and Operation Iraqi Freedom (OIF) in Iraq. Results of these studies evaluating OEF and OIF veterans for positive PTSD screens revealed a higher prevalence in male and female veterans from racial and ethnic minority groups. Two large studies, the National Health Study for a New Generation of U.S. Veterans (NewGen) (2015) and a second study conducted by investigators from the Veterans Affairs (VA) Office of Public Health (2014), sampled thousands of veterans in an effort to determine the prevalence of positive screens for PTSD in deployed and nondeployed veterans of OEF/OIF as well demographic subgroups of veterans using the VA health care system and those who received care outside of the system. The NewGen study included 30,000 veterans deployed to OEF or OIF who were sampled from a Defense Manpower Data Center personnel roster and 30,000 nondeployed veterans who served in the OEF/OIF era but were not deployed to either conflict. This 10-year study was initiated in 2009, and data collection for the first wave was completed in 2010.

Analysis of data from the first wave of the study found that 13.5% of OEF/OIF deployed and nondeployed veterans screened positive for PTSD. Results also showed that deployed males had a higher percentage of positive screens (16.2%) compared with nondeployed males (10.5%). Deployed females had slightly higher positive screens compared to their nondeployed counterparts (12.5% and 12.3%, respectively). In regard to race/ethnicity screening in deployed veterans, positive results were greater (23.5%) in deployed persons of unidentified race/ethnicity compared with African-American non-Hispanics (21.9%), Hispanics (19.7%), non-Hispanic other race (16.2%), and White non-Hispanics (14.1%). Positive screenings for nondeployed veterans were higher in African-American non-Hispanics (15.7%) compared with Hispanics (13.7%), White non-Hispanics (9.2%), non-Hispanics of another race (15.7%), and missing race/ethnicity (10.1%) (Dursa, Reinhard, Barth, & Schneiderman, 2014; VA Office of Public Health).

The VA Office of Public Health study was based on the National Health Study for New Generation of U.S. Veterans (NewGen). Results from this study revealed that the overall prevalence of probable PTSD was 13.5%, which was similar to findings in prior studies. The investigators also found that PTSD was higher among deployed (15.7%) compared with nondeployed (10.9%) veterans. Another finding was the increased risk of a positive screen for PTSD among VA health care users, African-Americans, those who served in the Army, and active duty OEF/OIF veterans. Finally, the investigators observed the same trend but to a lesser degree in veterans who had not been deployed (Mooney, 2014).

Maguen, Ren, and Bosch (2010) conducted a retrospective, cross-sectional study of veterans of OEF and OIF. This study examined gender differences in sociodemographic, military service, and mental health characteristics among the participants who were diagnosed with depression or PTSD. Findings of this study revealed that new users of the VA health care system were more likely to be Black women under 30 who had only one deployment to Iraq or Afghanistan. Results showed that females received depression diagnoses more frequently than their male counterparts. In contrast, males were more frequently diagnosed with PTSD and alcohol use disorder than their female counterparts. Other significant findings indicated that female veterans who sought care were more likely to be Black, single, and young. The investigators found that a larger number of older females were diagnosed with PTSD and depression compared with younger females. The opposite was true for males; a greater number of younger males tended to be diagnosed with depression and PTSD. Further, Black men and women were less likely than their White counterparts to receive a depression diagnosis. One plausible reason for this finding is that evidence suggests that ethnic minorities return home to more supportive communities and their welcome may differ as they re-enter their community. Finally the authors reported that a disproportionately large number of women in the military (30%) belong to an ethnic minority group. Fontana, Rosenheck, and Desai (2010) reported similar findings regarding the fact that a large percentage of females in the military are African-American and other ethnic minorities. These findings are supported by other studies showing under-representation of African-American women in research on females serving in the military.

Implications for Nursing

It is important for the nurse to be aware that African-American veterans may be at high risk for PTSD, depression, and other mental health disorders. The plan of care should begin with an assessment of the level of social support in relationships among families and community. Spirituality is also important as many African-Americans continue to heavily rely on religion (Greenawalt et al., 2011). Religious coping among African-American veterans should be assessed and incorporated into treatment plans.

The aftermath of Hurricanes Katrina and Rita in 2005 brought a heightened awareness of the social, economic, and health disparities in the United States. Hurricane Katrina has been cited as one of the worst natural disasters in U.S. history (Logan, 2010). Approximately 2000 people died as a result of the storm, and an untold number of people were forced to permanently relocate. African-Americans and the poor were most impacted by the devastation of Hurricane Katrina. Multiple stressors occurring during the storm and in its aftermath have resulted in immeasurable psychological and physiological suffering for the victims. During the storm, victims were forced to fight for survival, and many watched as their loved ones perished. In the days that followed the storm, while waiting to be evacuated, families suffered from inadequate amounts of food and water. Many individuals who were in shelters endured insufferable heat, poor ventilation, and unsafe and unsanitary conditions. During the evacuation period, adults and children were separated, tearing families apart for prolonged periods. The victims who found refuge at designated shelters were overwhelmingly African-Americans; in these shelters, some witnessed or experienced American Association of Gastroenterology violent physical assaults, including rape (MSNBC, 2010). More than 1000 people in Louisiana lost their lives, and of this number, the majority resided in New Orleans. According to the Louisiana Department of Health and Hospitals' 2006 report, 53% of the individuals who died were African-American, 39% were White, 2% were Hispanic, and the remaining 5% were Native Americans and unknown races. Data from the Center on Budget and Policy Priority (Shapiro & Sherman, 2005) indicated that African-Americans made up a disproportionate number of the victims who were most severely affected by the storm.

Hurricane Katrina destroyed the major psychiatric inpatient and crisis facilities that provided services to a large number of poor, uninsured, and African-American residents of New Orleans. Two years after the hurricane, 50% of the hospitals had not reopened, and 50% of physicians were no longer practicing in New Orleans (Health Disparities Mental Health Fact Sheet, 2010). Recovery from the hurricane has been an uphill battle for many of the storm victims. The loss of family members, close friends, personal belongings, employment, and community support, as well as forced relocation, have resulted in an exacerbation in mental health problems. Documented reports show that approximately 25% of New Orleans residents have experienced higher rates of mental health problems such as increased alcohol consumption, marital problems, higher rates of depression, PTSD, substance abuse, acute psychosis, and domestic violence (Health Disparities Mental Health Fact Sheet, 2010).

Other Psychological Characteristics. The psychiatric literature on the psychological characteristics of African-Americans and treatment of African-Americans by mental health professionals is controversial. The psychiatric literature has reported increased psychopathological disorders among African-Americans (Pasamanick, 1964). Anatomical, neurological, and endocrinological differences have been cited as signs of African-American inferiority (Thomas & Sillen, 1972; Tobias, 1970). Research has been done on African-Americans that would not have been considered for other ethnic groups. For example, in the Tuskegee project, African-American men with syphilis were intentionally denied treatment without being informed of their disease (Cave, 1975; Jones, 1993). Research on IQs has been used to support statements of genetic inferiority and justify

social policies such as selective immigration laws and school segregation (Hirsch, 1981). Such psychological research has added to racial stereotyping and bias among some mental health professionals.

According to Meyers and Weissman (1980–1981), some differences in phobias have been found between African-Americans and Whites. Robins, Helzer, Croughan, and Ratcliff (1981) noted that the lifetime prevalence of acrophobia was significantly higher for African-Americans than for Whites. Vernon and Roberts (1982) found that African-Americans, compared with Whites, had a significantly lower lifetime rate of both major and minor depression but had a rate of bipolar depression that was twice that of Whites. A possible explanation for the discrepancy in findings is the lack of national data on racial differences in diagnostic analogs. It is now widely accepted that on the Minnesota Multiphasic Personality Inventory, African-Americans tend to score higher on the paranoia and schizophrenia scales than Whites because the instrument was not standardized on an African-American population (Bell & Mehta, 1981; Gynther, 1981; Jones, Gray, & Parson, 1981). When standardized diagnostic systems are used today, African-Americans do not differ from Whites in the prevalence of most psychiatric disorders. Robins et al. (1981) and Meyers and Weissman (1980–1981) have reported finding no significant race differences for schizophrenia or affective disorders (Adebimpe, 1981; Lawson & Lawson, 2004; Mukherjee, Shukla, & Woodle, 1983; Spurlock, 1985).

Snow (1978) found that a belief in witchcraft was shared by a third of the African-American clients who were treated at a southern psychiatric center. African-Americans who believe they have a folk illness may use the services of a root worker, reader, spiritualist, or voodoo priest. It is important for the nurse to know that the client may have used the services of a folk practitioner before or with scientific mental health therapy. Wintrob (1973) has promoted the idea that individuals who believe in folk remedies such as root work or obeah (Black ritual) may regard scientific treatment only as palliative because curing the total condition requires neutralization by a specially skilled folk healer. Wintrob (1973), Kreisman (1975), Weclew (1975), and Sandoval (1977) have suggested that mental health professionals should attempt to complement the use of scientific medicine with folk practices for clients who believe mental disorders are attributed to folk causes.

Implications for Nursing Care. The best reason for including the concept of biological variations in nursing practice is that knowledge of scientific facts aids the nurse in giving culturally appropriate care. It is also essential for the nurse who cares for people from other cultures to know certain biological concepts not only to give culturally appropriate nursing care but also to give nonharmful nursing care.

Important biological variations that the nurse should be aware of are related to body size, birth weight, and body proportion. It is important for the nurse who works with African-American children to remember that at birth African-American children tend to weigh less and be shorter than their White counterparts and that these variations may be attributable in part to socioeconomic status. Therefore, the nurse, whether in a hospital or in a clinic setting, must carefully evaluate growth status in terms of height and weight for African-American children. Some nurses believe that because growth charts are White normed, data gleaned from these charts lack implications in regard to African-American children. It is important for the nurse to recognize that even for African-American children serious growth deviation can have implications for intervention for nutritional deficiencies. These variations between African-American and White children may continue as the child grows. For example, African-American preschoolers are neurologically more advanced than their White counterparts. In addition, African-American children tend to have less subcutaneous fat than White children but are taller and heavier by 2 years of age (Dayar-Berenson, 2014; Owen & Lubin, 1973) The fact that African-American preschoolers are taller and heavier may indicate a need for appropriate client teaching about the nutritional needs of the growing child.

Because the average weight for an African-American woman is consistently higher than that for her White counterpart at every age, the nurse must teach African-American clients the value of serving nutritionally sound meals. In addition, the nurse must emphasize the importance of exercise, not only to maintain ideal weight but also for cardiovascular purposes.

It is essential that the nurse develop a sensitivity for and familiarity with physical features that are common to African-Americans, as well as with African-American–related illnesses and diseases. If the nurse is unable to develop a familiarity with physical features common to African-Americans and with African-American illnesses or diseases, the nurse cannot possibly hope to recognize or diagnose conditions that may cause disequilibrium in the body. In addition, the nurse must be prepared to deal promptly, efficiently, and appropriately with clinical variables that are common to all African-American clients and yet have significant variability in some African-American clients, such as hypertension or sickle cell anemia. Some researchers assert that there is no clear correlation between hypertension and obesity in African-Americans as there is with other racial/ethnic groups such as Whites. On the other hand, there appears to be a direct correlation between the amount of skin pigmentation and the frequency of hypertension. Therefore, because it has been suggested that there is a direct relationship between skin pigmentation and hypertension, the nurse should emphasize the need for the African-American client to undergo hypertension screening (Boyle, 1970; Dayar-Berenson, 2014).

Because glucose-6-phosphate dehydrogenase (G-6-PD) deficiency is a hematological problem that is present in 35% of African-Americans, it is essential that the nurse stress the importance of the fluorescent spot test as a screening tool in diagnosing this deficiency. The nurse can serve as a client advocate and insist or mandate that this test be a routine part of laboratory testing for all African-American clients. Also, precautions should be taken to eliminate the transfusion of G-6-PD–deficient blood, particularly in transfusions for infants (Beutler, 1983).

In addition, the nurse should exercise caution when planning diets for African-American clients, particularly African-American infants, because they may be lactose intolerant. In these cases the nurse should plan diets that allow substituting more compatible products with the same nutritional value for milk and milk products (Bloch, 1981).

SUMMARY

Some researchers contend that the disproportionate morbidity and mortality rates in the African-American population are directly attributed to discriminatory practices in health care and to inequalities in social, economic, and educational opportunities rather than biological variations and genetics (Geronimus, Bound, Waidmann, Colen, & Steffick, 2001). It is a well-known fact that a greater percentage of African-Americans are more likely to live in poverty and have lower educational achievement than other racial and ethnic groups in the United States (U.S. Department of Commerce, Bureau of the Census, 2002). It is plausible to assume that inequalities in income and education underlie many health disparities in the United States. Population groups that experience the worst health problems are also those that have the highest poverty rates and the least education (U.S. Department of Health and Human Services, 2010). In addition, because disparities in income and educational levels are often associated with differences in rates of illness and death, including heart disease, diabetes, and obesity, it is conceivable that an overriding theme with health disparities may logically rest with socioeconomic status.

Educational achievement for African-Americans continues to lag behind that for Whites, Asians, and Pacific Islanders. Higher educational levels are associated with a greater likelihood of obtaining and comprehending the health-related information that is needed to develop health-promoting behaviors and beliefs in prevention. When educated, individuals are more likely to make informed choices regarding health promotion behaviors. Furthermore, educated individuals are more likely to have knowledge of disease symptoms and to comprehend the seriousness of the symptoms. Access to health care, delays in treatment, and inappropriate treatment contribute to increased morbidity and mortality for minorities, women, and the poor (Institute of Medicine, 2002; Richards, Funk, & Milner, 2000). These practices place a tremendous economic burden on society and contribute to the perpetuation of poverty, despair, and separation from mainstream society.

Braithwaite and Taylor (2001) conclude that even when holding socioeconomic status, access to care, and poverty rates constant, health disparities tend to remain constant along racial lines, particularly among African-Americans. Thus, it is plausible to assume that changing variables related to socioeconomic status and educational attainment, while admirable and laudable, by themselves with no attention to unequal treatment; cultural incompetence on the part of health care providers; and lack of knowledge about culture, cultural heritage, and biological variations will contribute only modestly to changing health outcomes and thereby eliminating health disparities.

In caring for the African-American client, the nurse must recognize and acknowledge the client's racial, cultural, and ethnic background because it is in these areas that the client's experiences occur. It is important not only for the nurse to consider necessary adjustments in client care when the client is from a different racial origin but also that the racial origin of the nurse be considered. In a classic and innovative study by Remington and DaCosta (1989), the effects of ethnocultural differences between supervisor and caregiver are dramatically illustrated. The nurse who denies or does not believe race is a factor denies a significant part of the client's being. It is important that nurses recognize the cultural, economic, and social barriers that inhibit the client's ability to articulate and comprehend the relevant symptoms. All aspects of care provided must be adapted to the client's cultural experiences and educational and socioeconomic background. As a client advocate, it is imperative that the nurse perform an accurate, culturally competent assessment; document findings; and clearly articulate data to other health care providers.

CASE STUDY

Initial Presentation

Mr. Ralph Hunt is a 48-year-old African-American male who was admitted to the hospital with exertional dyspnea, activity intolerance, and a persistent, nonproductive cough. Approximately 6 weeks prior to admission, Mr. Hunt was treated for a lower respiratory infection with antibiotics and over-the-counter antitussives. Mr. Hunt continued to experience dyspnea with activity, and on the day of admission he felt much worse. He went to the emergency department and was admitted to the hospital with a diagnosis of left-sided heart failure.

History

Mr. Hunt was diagnosed with primary hypertension 15 years ago and type 2 diabetes 5 years ago. He admits to smoking two packs of cigarettes per day for the past 30 years. His prescribed medications are as follows: hydrochlorothiazide 25 mg by mouth daily, diltiazem 240 mg by mouth daily, and metformin 1000 mg by mouth daily.

Six months ago Mr. Hunt was seen for an annual physical examination; his weight had increased from 175 lb to 225 lb and his blood pressure was 206/110. A hemoglobin A1c, coagulation panel, and lipid panel were drawn. Mr. Hunt was given a prescription for lisinopril 20 mg by mouth, two times a day, and he was instructed to continue taking his other prescribed medications. He was also given an appointment with the diabetes educator and instructed to return for follow-up in 2 weeks. Mr. Hunt told the office nurse that he really didn't want to take any more drugs. He stated that he felt okay and that he could control his blood pressure with daily garlic tablets and a glass of cider vinegar. After a lengthy explanation by the nurse regarding the serious complications of uncontrolled diabetes and hypertension, Mr. Hunt reluctantly agreed to have the prescription filled and said that he would see the diabetic educator. At the 2-week follow-up visit, Mr. Hunt was agitated about having to take time off from work because he didn't get paid leave time. He had not made an appointment with the diabetes educator but assured the office nurse that he would do

so. Mr. Hunt's blood pressure was 180/100, his hemoglobin A1c was 10%, and his fasting blood glucose was 280.

Prior history includes an inguinal hernia repair at age 20. Mr. Hunt has a positive family history of type 2 diabetes (both parents), CHD (father and brother), and hypertension (both parents). Mr. Hunt smokes two packs of cigarettes a day and admits to having an occasional beer with his friends. He eats fast food 5 days a week because of his hectic schedule, and he very rarely exercises because he does a lot of walking and heavy lifting on the job.

Physical Examination

- Vital signs: blood pressure, 150/100 mm Hg right arm, 160/102 mm Hg left arm; heart rate, 121 beats/min; temperature, 98.7°F; respirations, 28 breaths/min; height, 5'9"; weight, 225 lb; BMI, 32; waist circumference, 47 in.
- Pulmonary (PU): lungs, fine crackles throughout.
- Heart (COR): irregular rate; rhythm, S1S2S3S4 heart sounds, 0 murmurs; capillary refill <3 sec; right dorsalis +1; left dorsalis obtained by Doppler.
- Gastrointestinal (GI): abdomen soft, protuberant; active bowel sounds all four quadrants.
- Genitourinary (GU): normal male genitalia.
- Integument: warm, dry, hair loss on lower extremities; toenails thickened and overgrown.

Laboratory and Diagnostic Tests

- Electrocardiogram (ECG): atrial fibrillation at a rate of 123, left ventricular hypertrophy, and an old anterior MI. Chest x-ray: cardiomegaly and pulmonary vascular congestion.
- Blood glucose: 342 mg/dL.
- Urinalysis: negative for protein, red blood cells, white blood cells.
- Hemoglobin A1c, 10; creatinine, 1.9 mg/dL; sodium, 137 mEq/L; blood urea nitrogen (BUN), 30 mg/dL; low-density lipoprotein (LDL) cholesterol, 350 mg/dL; high-density lipoprotein (HDL) cholesterol, 30 mg/dL; triglycerides, 239 mg/dL.

◎ CARE PLAN

Nursing Diagnosis: Fluid volume excess related to left ventricular dysfunction and sodium and water retention

Client Outcome	Nursing Interventions
Client will demonstrate resolution of signs of fluid volume excess and an improvement in symptoms.	1. Measure intake and output every 4 hours and record. 2. Weigh daily at same time under same conditions; record and notify health care provider of weight gain of 2 lb or more in a 24-hour period. 3. Assess client knowledge of heart failure and therapeutic regimen. 4. Assess client's usual dietary intake. 5. Review specific foods that should be avoided with prescribed diet—2 g sodium, low cholesterol—with client. 6. Maintain prescribed fluid restriction of 2500 mL or less per 24-hour period.

Nursing Diagnosis: Activity intolerance related to imbalance between oxygen supply and demand

Client Outcome	Nursing Interventions
Client will report measurable increase in activity tolerance and demonstrate a decrease in physiological signs of activity intolerance (e.g., pulse, blood pressure will remain in client's normal range).	1. Assess client's perception of activity limitations and the severity of symptoms. 2. Assess client's cardiac and respiratory response to activity. 3. Cluster nursing intervention to allow adequate periods of rest between each care activity. 4. Gradually increase client's activity levels. 5. Teach client methods to conserve energy, such as sitting while bathing or brushing teeth. 6. Educate client and spouse about monitoring response to activity and recognition of symptoms that indicate a need to alter activity levels (e.g., dyspnea or chest discomfort). 7. Identify conflicts and differences between client and spouse expectations and prescribe the therapeutic regimen to establish individual goals.

Nursing Diagnosis: Nutrition, imbalanced: more than body requirements related to imbalance between caloric intake and metabolic needs

Client Outcomes	Nursing Interventions
1. Client will verbalize importance of complying with prescribed exercise program. 2. Client will verbalize importance of complying with prescribed diet.	1. Assess client's usual dietary intake. 2. Review prescribed diet with client. 3. Explore client's self-perception, including what being overweight means to client. 4. Discuss with client the motivation for weight loss. 5. Assess height, weight, and body build to obtain a comparative baseline. 6. Calculate caloric needs based on physical requirement and activity levels. 7. Work with client and spouse to develop realistic goals for weight loss. 8. Assess client barriers to exercise. 9. Explain the importance of regular exercise for weight loss and reduction of cardiovascular risks.

Continued

Nursing Diagnosis: Ineffective health maintenance related to inability to make thoughtful judgments about management of hypertension

Client Outcome	Nursing Interventions
Client and family will verbalize understanding of pathological condition, complications, and importance of lifelong management of hypertension.	1. Assess client knowledge level and readiness to learn. 2. Teach client and family symptoms that require immediate medical attention. 3. Teach client correct method of measuring blood pressure and importance of reporting values that are persistently above levels that have been predetermined by health care provider. 4. Discuss the complications of uncontrolled hypertension. 5. Explain pathophysiology of hypertension. 6. Explain the risk factors for developing hypertension. 7. Explain to client that there is no cure for hypertension. 8. Explain the actions and indications of antihypertensive medications.

Nursing Diagnosis: Risk for injury related to combined adverse effects of antihypertensive medications

Client Outcome	Nursing Interventions
Client will verbalize understanding the combined adverse effects of oral antihypertensive medications and the importance of notifying physician of symptoms rather than stopping medications.	1. Assess client knowledge of prescribed medications. 2. Provide client with information related to adverse effects of all prescribed antihypertensive medications, such as dizziness and fatigue. 3. Stress the importance of notifying the physician of adverse effects rather than stopping the medication abruptly.

Nursing Diagnosis: Anxiety related to change in health status (therapeutic regimen, lifestyle changes, lack of control of condition, and potential complications of hypertension)

Client Outcome	Nursing Interventions
Client will identify methods to promote physiological and emotional comfort and a sense of well-being.	1. Explore client's perception of hypertension and related lifestyle changes. 2. Ask client and family to discuss how hypertension has affected their lifestyle. 3. Assess stressors in client's life and effective coping mechanisms. 4. Assess family resources and support systems. 5. Involve client and family in goals to reduce anxiety and to develop effective coping methods.

Nursing Diagnosis: Knowledge deficit related to unfamiliarity with pathophysiological state and therapeutic regimen for hypertension

Client Outcome	Nursing Interventions
Client will be able to define hypertension; state the complications of hypertension; and explain the actions, indications, and side effects of medications as well as the necessity for lifelong compliance with therapy.	1. Assess client's knowledge of hypertension. 2. Assess client's knowledge of the therapeutic regimen for hypertension. 3. Provide oral and written instructions related to hypertension, including therapeutic management. 4. Discuss the possibility of complications such as heart failure and stroke if the prescribed medication, dietary restrictions, and exercise program are not adhered to. 5. Review the signs of complications of hypertension that require immediate medical intervention. 6. Elicit client and family input in measures to achieve compliance with lifelong therapy.

CLINICAL DECISION MAKING

1. Explain how obesity, physical inactivity, and poor dietary habits contribute to the development of CVD.
2. Explain how persistent elevation of blood pressure increases the risk for developing CHD.
3. List the complications of uncontrolled hypertension.
4. Explain why it is important for the nurse to get a detailed health history from Mr. Hunt.
5. Based on the information in the care plan, identify factors that place Mr. Hunt at high risk for developing CVD.
6. Identify measures for the nurse to use to help Mr. Hunt verbalize concerns related to noncompliance with medication, diet, weight reduction, and lifestyle changes.
7. List several strategies that may help health care providers develop and use culturally appropriate communication techniques for African-Americans.
8. Describe ways in which health care providers may show sensitivity and acceptance of African-American folk health care practices.
9. Compare and contrast the social organization of African-Americans from diverse social and economic backgrounds.
10. List several practices from ancient African ancestry that are a part of modern nursing philosophy.
11. Describe the importance of folk medicine practices and folk healers to African-Americans in the rural setting.
12. Describe the significance of the Institute of Medicine's report on unequal treatment to the development of culturally competent care.
13. List several strategies that assist in organization of time as a method of assisting in the adherence to treatment and medication regimens.

REVIEW QUESTIONS

1. When providing care for an African-American client, it is important for the nurse to remember that African-Americans are perceived as being which of the following?
   a. Polychronic
   b. Monochronic
   c. Polymorphic
   d. Monomorphic
2. To reduce polychronic effects while caring for an African-American client, the nurse should do which of the following?
   a. Permit the client to have frequent, constant interruptions.
   b. Allow the client to keep the perception of the need for order.

   c. Allow the client to structure activities in a ranked order that will produce maximal benefits.
   d. Assist the client to structure activities in a ranked order that will produce maximal benefits.
3. You are taking care of an African-American female who recently had a CVA, leaving her unable to talk. As you attempt to give her medications with her milk on her tray, she resists. After explaining the importance of taking her medications, and on time, your client reluctantly takes the medications with milk. Later she has a large diarrhea stool. What biological variation should have been considered with this client?
   a. Lactose intolerance is high among African-Americans.
   b. Hypertension is high among African-Americans.
   c. Tuberculosis is high among African-Americans.
   d. Dietary variations may cause diarrhea in African-Americans.

REFERENCES

Abraham, S. J., Clifford, L., & Najjar, M. F. (1976). Height and weight of adults 18–74 years of age in the United States. *Advance Data, 3*, 1–18.

Adebimpe, V. (1981). Overview: White norms and psychiatric diagnosis of Black patients. *American Journal of Psychiatry, 138*, 279–285.

Akinbami, L., et al. (2012). Centers for Disease Control and Prevention, National Center for Health Statistics. Trends in asthma prevalence, health care use, and mortality in the United States 2001–2010. Available at <www.cdc.gov/hchs/data/data.briefs> Accessed December 22, 2014.

Albertson, C. (2003). *Bessie*. New Haven, CT: Yale University Press.

Alley, D., Seeman, T., Kim, J., Karlamangla, A., Hu, P., & Crimmins, E. M. (2006). Socioeconomic status and C-reactive protein levels in the U.S. population: NHANES IV. *Science Direct Brain and Behavior Immunity, 20*, 498–504.

Amemiya, H., et al. (1996). Apolipoprotein(a) and pentanucleotide repeat polymorphisms are associated with the degree of atherosclerosis in coronary heart disease. *Atherosclerosis, 123*(1–2), 181–191.

American Heart Association (AHA) (2013). *Fact sheet*. <http://www.heart.org/idc/groups/heart-public/@wcm/@adv/documents/downloadable/ucm_461513.pdf> Accessed December 31, 2014.

American Heart Association (AHA) (2014). *Fact sheet*. <http://www.heart.org/idc/groups/heart-public/@wcm/@adv/documents/downloadable/ucm_461513.pdf> Accessed December 31, 2014.

American Heart Association (AHA) (2015). *Heart disease and stroke statistics 2015 update*. Dallas: American Heart Association.

American Lung Association (ALA) (2012). *Trends in asthma morbidity and mortality: American Lung Association epidemiology and statistics unit research and health education division.* Accessed December 2014.

Anderson, S. V., & Bauwens, E. E. (1981). *Chronic health problems: concepts and application.* St. Louis: Mosby.

Angelou, M. (1989). Maya Angelou (personal interview and portrait). In B. Lanker (Ed.), *I dream a world: portraits of Black women who changed America.* New York: Stewart, Tabori, & Chang.

Appel, S., Moore, T. M., & Giger, J. N. (2006). An overview and update on the metabolic syndrome: implications for identifying cardiometabolic risk among African-American women. *Journal of National Black Nurses Association, 17*(2), 47–62.

Bagan, M., Robson, J., & Soderstrom, R. (1971). Ethnic differences in skin fold thickness. *American Journal of Clinical Nutrition, 24,* 864–868.

Barclay, A., & Cusumano, D. R. (1967). Father absence, cross sex identity, and field-dependent behavior of male adolescents. *Child Development, 38,* 343–350.

Beaser, R., & Staff of the Joslin's Diabetes Center (2010). *Joslin's diabetes deskbook: a guide for primary care givers* (2nd ed., pp. 75–77). Boston: Joslin Diabetes Center.

Bell, C., & Mehta, H. (1981). The misdiagnosis of Black patients with manic depressive illness: second in a series. *Journal of the National Medical Association, 73,* 101–107.

Bendtzen, K., et al. (1988). Association between HLA-DR2 and production of tumor necrosis factor α and interleukin 1 by mononuclear cells activated by lipopolysaccharide. *Scandinavian Journal of Immunology, 28,* 599–606.

Berger, J. (2006). Age, sex, racial disparities in heart attack transfer patterns. *Duke Med News.* <http://news.bio-medicine.org/medicine-news-3/Age–sex–racial-disparities-in-heart-attack-hospital-transfer-patterns-5851-1/>.

Beutler, E. H. (1983). Glucose-6-phosphate dehydrogenase deficiency. In W. J. Williams (Ed.), *Hematology* (3rd ed.). New York: McGraw-Hill.

Biello, K., Rawlings, J., Carrol-Scott, A., Browne, R., & Ickovics, J. R. (2010). Racial disparities in age and preventable hospitalizations among U.S. adults. *American Journal of Preventative Medicine, 38*(1), 54–60.

Biller, H. B. (1969). Father absence, maternal encouragement, and sex role development in kindergarten boys. *Child Development, 40,* 539–546.

Bloch, B. (1976a). Health care from a minority viewpoint. San Francisco: University of California, School of Nursing. Unpublished study.

Bloch, B. (1976b). Nursing intervention in Black patient care. In D. Luckraft (Ed.), *Black awareness: implications for Black patient care* (pp. 27–35). New York: American Journal of Nursing Company.

Bloch, B. (1981). Black Americans and cross-cultural counseling experiences. In A. J. Marsella & P. B. Pedersen (Eds.), *Cross cultural counseling and psychotherapy.* New York: Pergamon Press.

Bloch, B. (1983). Bloch's assessment guide for ethnic/cultural variations. In M. S. Orque, B. Bloch, & L. S. A. Monrroy (Eds.), *Ethnic nursing care: a multicultural approach* (pp. 49–75). St. Louis: Mosby.

Blumenthal, B., & Flack, J. (2003). Establishing cardiovascular risk. In R. Blumenthal & J. Flack (Eds.), *Managing cardiovascular disease: a focus on hypertension and dyslipidemia* (pp. 1–16). Cleveland: Advanstar Medical Economics.

Boyle, B., Jr. (1970). Biological pattern in hypertension by race, sex, body weight, and skin color. *Journal of the American Medical Association, 213,* 1637–1643.

Braithwaite, R., & Taylor, S. (2001). *Health issues in the Black community* (2nd ed.). San Francisco: Jossey-Bass.

Braunwald, S. (2012). *Heart disease: a textbook of cardiovascular medicine* (9th ed., pp. 26–27, 448–449). Philadelphia: Elsevier–Sanders.

Brisbane, F. (1987). Divided feeling of Black alcoholic daughters. *Alcohol Health and Research World, 12,* 48–50.

Brisbane, F. L., & Womble, M. (1986). Afterthoughts and recommendations. *Alcoholism Treatment Quarterly, 2*(3–4), 249–270.

Britt, A. (2009). *African Americans, substance abuse and spirituality. Minority Nurse.* <http://minoritynurse.com/african-americans-substance-abuse-and-spirituality/> Accessed December 31, 2014.

Brown, F., & Tooley, J. (2004). Alcoholism in the Black community. In G. Lawson & A. Lawson (Eds.), *Alcohol and substance abuse in special populations.* Austin, TX: Pro-Ed.

Bullough, V. L., & Bullough, B. (1982). *Health care for the other Americans.* East Norwalk, CT: Appleton-Century-Crofts.

California Health Interview Survey (CHIS) (2001). *The UCLA Center for Health Policy.* Available at <www.chis.ucla.edu/publications.html> Retrieved September 10, 2011.

Campinha-Bacote, J. (2013). African Americans. In L. Purnell (Ed.), *Transcultural health care a culturally competent approach* (4th ed., pp. 91–114). Philadelphia: FA Davis.

Carroll, J. F., Klein, M. I., & Santo, Y. (1978). Comparison of the similarities and differences in the self-concepts of male alcoholics and addicts. *Journal of Consulting Clinical Psychology, 46,* 575–576.

Cave, V. (1975). Proper uses and abuses of the health care delivery system for minorities with special reference to the Tuskegee syphilis study. *Journal of the National Medical Association, 67,* 82–84.

Centers for Disease Control and Prevention (CDC) (2001). Sudden death in U.S. young adults: 1989–96 Centers for Disease Control AIDS hotline (1997). *National Center for Health Statistics monthly vital statistics report (1996), 45*(3), 10 (DHHS Publication No. PHS 3, 10). Hyattsville, MD: Public Health Services.

Centers for Disease Control and Prevention (CDC) (2003). Racial/ethnic and socioeconomic disparities in multiple risk factors for heart disease and stroke—United States. *MMRW Morbidity and Mortality Weekly Report, 54,* 113–117.

Centers for Disease Control and Prevention (CDC) (2006). *National Health and Nutrition Examination Survey.* Available at <http://www.cdc.gov/nchs/about/major/nhanes/datalink.htm> Accessed May 15, 2006.

Centers for Disease Control and Prevention (CDC) (2008). *HIV/AIDS, statistics and surveillance reports* (table 11a). Available at <www.cdc.gov/hiv/topics/surveillance/resources/reports/index> Accessed May 3, 2010.

Centers for Disease Control and Prevention (CDC) (2011). Summary of health statistics for U.S. adults: National Health Interview Survey. *U.S. Department of Health and Human Services Centers for Disease Control and Prevention Vital Statistics, 10*(256), 193–194.

Centers for Disease Control and Prevention (CDC) (2012a). *HIV/AIDS statistics and surveillance reports* (Tables 1–6). <http://www.cdc.gov/nchs/nhanes.htm> Accessed December 18, 2014.

Centers for Disease Control and Prevention (CDC) (2012b). *National Health and Nutrition Examination Survey.* Accessed December 31, 2014.

Centers for Disease Control and Prevention (CDC) (2012c). *Statistics 2012 HIV Surveillance Report, 24.* <http://www.cdc.gov/hiv/pdf/statistics_2012_HIV_Surveillance_Report_vol_24.pdf> Accessed December 20, 2014.

Centers for Disease Control and Prevention (CDC) (2012d). *Vital Health Statistics: National Surveillance of Asthma U.S. 2001–2010, 3*(35). <http://www.cdc.gov/mmwr/preview/mmwrhtml/mm6153a1.htm> Accessed January 2, 2015.

Centers for Disease Control and Prevention (2013). *HIV surveillance report.* Atlanta: Centers for Disease Control and Prevention. 25(2).

Centers for Disease Control and Prevention (CDC) (2014). *State HIV Progress Report.* <http://www.cdc.gov/hiv/pdf/statistics_2012_HIV_Surveillance_Report_vol_24.pdf> Accessed December 20, 2014.

Center for Food Allergies (n.d.). Available at www.CenterforFoodAllergies.com. Accessed January 2, 2015.

Chartier, K., & Caetano, R. (2010). Ethnicity and health disparities in alcohol research. *Alcohol Research and Health, 33*(1–2), 152–160.

Chen, W., Bao, W., Begum, S., Elkasabany, A., Srinivasan, S. R., & Berenson, G. S. (2000). Age-related patterns of the clustering of cardiovascular risk variables of syndrome X from childhood to young adulthood in a population made up of black and white subjects. *Diabetes, 49*, 1042–1048.

Cheng, X. (2013). Updating the relationship between hyperhomocysteinemia lowering therapy and cardiovascular events. *Cardiovascular Therapeutics, 31*, e19–e26.

Ciavattini, A., et al. (2013). Uterine fibroids: pathogenesis and interactions with endometrium and endomyometrial junction. *Obstetrics and Gynecology International.* Retrieved from <http://www.hindawi.com/journals/ogi/2013/173184/> Accessed January 3, 2013.

Child Trends Data Bank (2012). *Children and youth with AIDS.* Available at <www.childtrendsdatabank.org> Accessed January 3, 2015.

Collins, D. (2008). The issue of ebonics and the constructed national view of the Black American. *The Lamar University Electronic Journal of Student Research.* Available at <www.eric.ed.gov/contentdelivery/serv/et/ERICSERV/et> Accessed December 13, 2014.

Covell, K., & Turnbull, W. (1982). The long-term effects of father absence in childhood on male university students' sex-role identity and personal adjustment. *Journal of Genetic Psychology, 141*, 271–276.

Dallongeville, J., Roy, M., Lebouef, N., Xhignesse, M., Davignon, J., & Lussier-Cacan, S. (1991). Apolipoprotein E polymorphism association with lipoprotein profile in endogenous hypertriglyceridemia and familial hypercholesterolemia. *Arteriosclerosis and Thrombosis, 11*, 272–278.

Davis, R. O., Cutter, G. R., Goldenberg, R. L., Hoffman, H. J., Cliver, S. P., & Brumfield, C. G. (1993). Fetal biparietal diameter, head circumference, abdominal circumference and femur length: a comparison by race and sex. *Journal of Reproductive Medicine, 38*, 201–206.

Dayar-Berenson, L. (2014). *Cultural competencies for nurses: impact on health and illness* (2nd ed., pp. 133–159). Burlington, MA: Jones and Bartlett.

Deboer, M. (2011). Ethnicity, obesity and the metabolic syndrome: implications on assessing risk and targeting interventions. *Expert Review of Endocrinology Metabolism, 6*(2), 279–289.

Deckart, S., & Vickers, H. (2011). *An introduction to sociolinguistics: social identity* (pp. 46–57). New York: Continuum International.

Dillard, J. (2008, Winter). Sketch of history of black English. *Southern Quarterly, 45*(2), 53. Available at <www.docstoc.com/docs/39636183/A-Sketch-of-the-History-of-Black-English> Accessed April 30, 2010.

Dillard, J. L. (1972). *Black English: its history and usage in the United States.* New York: Random House.

Dilley, A., Hooper, W. C., El-Jamil, M., Renshaw, M., Wenger, N. K., & Evatt, B. L. (2002). Mutations in the genes regulating methylene tetrahydrofolate reductase (MTHFR C0T677) and cystathionine beta-synthase (CBS G0A919, CBS T0c833) are not associated with myocardial infarction in African Americans. *Thrombosis Research, 103*(2), 109–115.

Dohrenwend, B., Turner, J., Turse, N., Lewis-Fernandez, R., & Yager, T. J. (2008). War-related post-traumatic stress disorder in Black, Hispanic, and majority White Vietnam veterans: the roles of exposure and vulnerability. *Journal of Traumatic Stress, 21*(2), 133–141.

Dowd, S., Poole, V., Davidhizar, R., & Giger, J. N. (1998). Death, dying and grief in a transcultural context: application of the Giger and Davidhizar model. *The Hospice Journal, 13*(4), 33–56.

Duca, R. (2013). *Hyperhomocysteinemia as a result of the (MTHFR) C677T polymorphism causes an increased risk of cerebrovascular disease: a biochemical perspective.*

Dursa, E., Reinhard, M., Barth, S., & Schneiderman, A. (2014). Prevalence of a positive screen for PSTD among OEF/OIF and OEF/OIF–era veterans in a large population based cohort. *Journal of Traumatic Stress, 10*(27), 542–549.

Elward, K., & Pollart, S. (2010). Medical therapy for asthma: updates from the NAEPP guidelines. *American Family Physician, 82*(10), 1242–1251.

Falkner, F., & Tanner, J. (1978). *Human growth I: principles and prenatal growth.* New York: Plenum Press.

Farrally, M., & Moore, W. (1976). Anatomical differences in the femur and tibia between Negroids and Caucasians. *American Journal of Physiology and Anthropology, 43*(1), 63–69.

Fernandez-Real, J. M., et al. (1997). The TNA-α gene Nco 1 polymorphism influences the relationship among insulin resistance, percent body fat, and increased serum leptin levels. *Diabetes, 46*(9), 1469–1472.

Ferrucci, L., et al. (1995). Apolipoprotein E epsilon 2 allele and risk of stroke in the older population. *Stroke: A Journal of Cerebral Circulation, 28*(12), 2410–2416.

Fisher, D., & Lapp, D. (2013). Learning to talk like the test: guiding speakers of African American vernacular English. *Journal of Adolescent & Adult Literacy, 56*(8), 634–638.

Fontana, A., Rosenheck, R., & Desai, R. (2010). Female veterans of Iraq and Afghanistan seeking care from VA specialized PTSD programs: comparison with male veterans and female war zone veterans of previous eras. *Journal of Women's Health, 19*(4), 751–757.

Forey, B., Fry, J., Lee, P., Thornton, A. J., & Coombs, K. J. (2013). The effect of quitting smoking on HDL cholesterol—a review based on within-subject changes. *Biomarker Research, 1,* 26. Available at <www.biomarkersres.org/content> Accessed January 2, 2015.

Geronimus, A., Bound, J., Waidmann, T., Colen, C., & Steffick, D. (2001). Inequality in life expectancy, functional status, and active life expectancy across selected Black and White population in the United States. *Demography, 38*(2), 227–251.

Giger, J. N., Appel, S. J., Davidhizar, R., & Davis, C. (2008). Church and spirituality in the lives of the African American community. *Journal of Transcultural Nursing, 19*(4), 375–383. [Epub July 23, 2008].

Giger, J., Davidhizar, R., & Cherry, B. (1991). Biological variations in the Black patient. *Imprint, 38*(2), 97–98.

Giger, J., Davidhizar, R., & Wieczorek, S. (1993). Culture and ethnicity. In I. Bobak & M. Jensen (Eds.), *Maternity and gynecologic care* (5th ed., pp. 42–67). St. Louis: Mosby.

Giger, J. N., Strickland, O. L., Weaver, M., Taylor, H., & Acton, R. T. (2005). Genetic predictors of coronary heart disease risk factors in premenopausal African-American women. *Ethnicity and Disease, 15*(2), 221–232.

Giger, J., Richardson, J., & Jones, D. (2001). African-American children: a precious commodity at risk. *Journal of National Black Nurses Association, 13*(1), vii–viii.

Gilbert, B. M. (1977). Anterior femoral curvature: its probable basis and utility as a criterion for racial assessment. *American Journal of Physical Anthropology, 45*(3), 601–604.

Global Diabetes Plan 2011–2012 (2011). *International Federation of Diabetes.* Available at <www.idf/global-diabetes-plan-2011-2021> Accessed January 21, 2015.

Greenawalt, D., et al. (2011). Mental health treatment involvement and religious coping among African American, Hispanic and White veterans of the wars of Iraq and Afghanistan. *Depression Research and Treatment, 2011,* 192186. Accessed January 10, 2015.

Gupta, D., & Thappa, D. (2013). Mongolian spots: how important are they? *World Journal of Clinical Cases, 1*(8), 230–232. Accessed January 15, 2015.

Gutman, H. (1976). *The Black family in slavery and freedom: 1750–1925.* New York: Vintage Books.

Gynther, M. (1981). Is the MMPI an appropriate assessment device for Blacks? *Journal of Black Psychology, 7,* 67–75.

Hall, E. T. (1989). *Beyond culture.* New York: Anchor Books.

Hall, E. T. (1990). *The hidden dimension.* New York: Anchor Books.

Hamlet, J. (2011). Word! The African American oral tradition and its rhetorical impact on American popular culture. *Black History Bulletin, 74*(1), 27–29. Accessed December 20, 2015.

Harley, D. (2006). Indigenous healing practices among rural elderly African Americans. *International Journal of Disability, Development and Education, 53*(4), 433–452.

Harper, F., & Dawkins, M. (1976). Alcohol and Blacks: survey of periodical literature. *British Journal of Addiction, 71,* 327–334.

Health Disparities Mental Health Fact Sheet. (2010). Available at <www.ncmhd.nih.gov/hdFactSheet.asp> Accessed June 2, 2010.

Health United States (2012). *United States Department of Health and Human Services. Centers for Disease Control. National Center for Health Statistics.* Retrieved December 10, 2014.

Henderson, G., & Primeaux, M. (1981). *Transcultural health care.* Reading, MA: Addison-Wesley.

Hirsch, J. (1981). To "unfrock the charlatans." *Sage Race Relations Abstracts, 6,* 1–65.

Hotamisligil, G., Arner, P., Caro, J. F., Atkinson, R. L., & Spiegelman, B. M. (1995). Increased adipose tissue expression of tumor necrosis factor-α in human obesity and insulin resistance. *Journal of Clinical Investigation, 95,* 2409–2415.

Hotamisligil, G., Murray, D. L., Choy, L. N., & Spiegelman, B. M. (1994). Tumor necrosis factor inhibits signaling from the insulin receptor. *Proceedings of the National Academy of Sciences of the United States of America, 91*(11), 4854–4858.

Hotamisligil, G., Shargill, N., & Spiegelman, B. (1993). Adipose expression of tumor necrosis factor-α: direct role in obesity-linked insulin resistance. *Science, 259,* 87–91.

Hudson, H. L. (1986). How and why Alcoholics Anonymous works for Blacks. *Alcoholism Treatment Quarterly, 2*(314), 11–29.

Hulsey, T. C., Levkoff, A. H., & Alexander, G. R. (1991). Birth weight of infants of Black and White mothers without pregnancy complications. *American Journal of Obstetrics and Gynecology, 164,* 1299–1302.

Hymes, D. (1971). *Pidginization and creolization of languages.* London: Cambridge University Press.

Imaru, Y., Koga, S., & Ibayashi, H. (1988). Phenotypes of apolipoprotein E and abnormalities in lipid metabolism in patients with non-insulin dependent diabetes mellitus. *Metabolism: Clinical and Experimental, 37*(12), 1134–1138.

Institute of Black Chemical Abuse (1988). *Annual report.* Minneapolis, MN: Institute of Black Chemical Abuse.

Institute of Medicine (2002). *Unequal treatment: confronting racial and ethnic disparities in health care.* Washington, DC: National Academy Press.

Iraq war clinician guide (Appendix J-2: Warzone-related stress reactions: what veterans need to know) (n.d.). Washington, DC: U.S. Department of Veterans Affairs. Available at <http://www.ptsd.va.gov/professional/materials/manuals/iraq-war-clinician-guide.asp> Retrieved January 15, 2015.

Iyasu, S., Becerra, J. E., Rowley, D. H., & Houge, C. J. (1992). Impact of very low birth weight on the black-white infant mortality gap. *American Journal of Preventive Medicine, 8*(5), 271–277.

Jackson, J., Neighbors, H., & Gurin, G. (1986). *Findings from a national survey on Black mental health: implications for practice and training. National Institute of Mental Health: Mental health research and practice in minority communities.* Rockville, MD: U.S. Department of Health and Human Services.

Jacques, G. (1976). Cultural health traditions: a Black perspective. In M. F. Branch & P. P. Paxton (Eds.), *Providing safe nursing care for ethnic people of color.* East Norwalk, CT: Appleton-Century-Crofts.

Johnson, R., Cole, R., & Abner, F. (1981). Genetic interpretation of social/ethnic differences in lactose absorption and tolerance. *Human Biology, 53*(1), 1–3.

Jones, B., Gray, E., & Parson, E. (1981). Manic-depressive illness among poor urban Blacks. *Journal of the National Medical Association, 72,* 141–145.

Jones, L. (1993). *Bad blood: the Tuskegee syphilis experiment.* New York: Free Press.

Jones, L. (1998). *Home: social essays.* Hopewell, NJ: Ecco Press.

Jongeneel, V., Briant, L., Udalova, I. A., Sevin, A., Nedospasov, S. A., & Cambon-Thompson, A. (1991). Extensive genetic polymorphism in the human tumor necrosis factor α region and relation to extended HLA haplotypes immunology. *Proceedings of National Academy of Sciences of the United States of America, 88,* 9717–9721.

Jordan, W. C. (1975). Voodoo medicine. In R. A. Williams (Ed.), *Textbook of Black-related diseases* (pp. 115–138). New York: McGraw-Hill.

Jordan, W. C. (1979). The roots and practice of voodoo medicine in America. *Urban Health, 8,* 38–48.

Kaiser Family Foundation (2014). *The HIV/AIDS epidemic in the United States.* Available at <www.kff.org/hivaids/fact-sheet/the-hivaids-epidemic-in-the-united-states> Accessed November 29, 2014.

Karnow, S. (1997). *Vietnam: a history* (2nd ed.). New York: Penguin Books.

Kautzsch, A. (2012). Earlier African American vernacular English: socio-historical background. In K. Lunkenheimer & B. Kortmann (Eds.), *The Mouton world atlas of variation in English* (pp. 126–140). Berlin: DeGruyter.

Khera, A., et al. (2005). Clinical research: atherosclerosis race and gender differences in C-reactive protein levels. *Clinical Research: Journal of the American College of Cardiology, 46,* 464–469.

King, L. M. (1982). Alcoholism—studies regarding Black Americans: 1979–1980. *Alcohol and Health Monograph 4: Special Population Issues,* 385–407.

Kluckhohn, C. (2003). The gifts of tongues. In L. A. Samovar & R. E. Porter (Eds.), *Intercultural communication: a reader* (10th ed.). Belmont, CA: Wadsworth/Thompson Learning.

Knox, D. H. (1986). Spirituality: a tool in the assessment and treatment of Black alcoholics and their families. *Alcoholism Treatment Quarterly, 2*(3–4), 313–343.

Kraus, V. B., Stabler, T. V., Luta, G., Renner, J. B., Dragomir, A. D., & Jordan, J. M. (2007). Interpretation of C-reactive protein (CRP) levels for cardiovascular disease risk is complicated by race, pulmonary disease, body mass index, gender and osteoarthritis. *Cartilage, 15*(8), 966–971.

Kreisman, K. (1975). The curandero's apprentice: a therapeutic integration of folk and medical healing. *American Journal of Psychiatry, 132,* 81.

Kubaszek, A., Pihlajamäki, J., Punnonen, K., Karhapää, P., Vauhkonen, I., & Laakso, M. (2003). The C-174G promoter polymorphism of the IL-6 gene affects energy expenditure and insulin sensitivity. *Diabetes, 52*(2), 558–561.

Kurachi, O., Matsuo, H., Samoto, T., & Maruo, T. (2001). Tumor necrosis factor-alpha expression in human uterine leiomyoma and its down-regulation by progesterone. *Journal of Clinical Endocrinology & Metabolism, 86*(5), 2275–2280.

Lactose intolerance (n.d.). *Johns Hopkins Medicine Health Library.* Available at <www.johnshopkins.medicinehealth.library.html> Accessed January 15, 2014.

Lamendola, C., & Mason, C. (Eds.), (2004). *Reducing cardiovascular risk in the insulin resistant patient* (pp. 14–22). New York: Preventive Cardiovascular Nurses Association.

LaVist, T. (2005). *Minority populations in health: an introduction to health disparities in the United States.* San Francisco: Jossey Bass.

Lawson, G., & Lawson, A. (2004). *Alcoholism and substance abuse in special populations.* Austin, TX: Pro-Ed.

Leary, J. (2005). *Post traumatic slave syndrome: America's legacy of enduring injury and healing* (pp. 47–57). Milwaukee: Uptone Press.

Leon, A., & Bronas, U. (2009). Hypertension: life style modifications for its prevention and management. *American Journal of Lifestyle Medicine, 3*(6), 425–439.

Levi, J., et al. (2013). *Facts in fat how obesity threatens America.* Robert Wood Johnson Foundation. Available at <http://healthyamericans.org/report/108/> Retrieved January 2, 2015.

Lim, R. (2015). *Clinical manual of psychiatry* (2nd ed., pp. 77–119). Washington, DC: American Psychiatric Publishing.

Logan, J. (2010). *The impact of Katrina: race and class in storm damaged neighborhoods. Brown.*

Louisiana Department of Health and Hospitals (2006). *Hurricane Katrina: reports of missing and deceased.* Available at <www.dhh.state.la.us/news.asp> Accessed July 31, 2010.

Maguen, S., Ren, L., Bosch, J., Marmar, C. R., & Seal, K. H. (2010). Gender differences in mental health diagnoses among Iraq and Afghanistan veterans enrolled in Veterans

Affairs health care. *American Journal Public Health*, *100*(12), 2450–2456. Available at <www.medscape.com/viewarticle/777214> Accessed December 30 2014.

Margaglione, M., et al. (1998). Prevalence of apolipoprotein E alleles in healthy subjects and survivors of ischemic stroke: an Italian case-control study. *Stroke: A Journal of Cerebral Circulation*, *29*(2), 399–403.

Maron, B. J., et al. (2003). Relationship of race to sudden cardiac death in competitive athletes with hypertrophic cardiomyopathy. *Journal of the American College of Cardiology*, *41*(6), 974–980.

Mbiti, J. (1990). *African religions and philosophies* (2nd ed.). Portsmouth, NH: Heinemann.

McKenzie, J., & Chrisman, N. (1977). Healing herbs, gods, and magic. *Nursing Outlook*, *25*(5), 325–327.

Meyers, J., & Weissman, M. (1980–1981). The prevalence of psychiatric disorders (DSM-III in the community: 1980–1981) (Unpublished manuscript).

Mieszczanka, H., & Velord, G. (2014). *Management of cardiovascular disease in women* (pp. 3–12). London: Springer.

Mitchell, J., et al. (2008). Clinical investigation outcome in African Americans and other minorities in the Sudden Cardiac Death in Heart Failure Trial (SCD-HeFT). *American Heart Journal*, *155*(3), 501–506.

Mooney, B. (2014). *Study offers new statistics on how many OEF and OIF veterans have PTSD: condition not just related to deployment. US Medicine*. <http://www.usmedicine.com/current-issue/study-offers-new-statistics-on-how-many-oefoif-veterans-have-ptsd/> Retrieved December 30, 2014.

Moore, R., Stanton, D., Gopalan, R., & Chaisson, R. (1994). Racial differences in the use of drug therapy for HIV disease in the urban community. *New England Journal of Medicine*, *330*(11), 763–768.

Morton, N. E. (1977). Genetic aspects of prematurity. In D. M. Reed & F. J. Stanley (Eds.), *Epidemiology of prematurity*. Baltimore: Urban & Schwarzenberg.

MSNBC Nightly News (2010). *Hurricane Katrina five years later. MSNBC*. Available at <http//www.msnbc.com/id/38247215/ns/nightly_news> Accessed August 29, 2010.

Mukherjee, S., Shukla, S., & Woodle, J. (1983). Misdiagnosis of schizophrenia in bipolar patients: a multiethnic comparison. *American Journal of Psychiatry*, *140*, 1571–1574.

Murray, R. B., & Huelskoetter, M. W. (1991). In *Psychiatric/mental health nursing* (3rd ed.). East Norwalk, CT: Appleton & Lange.

National Center for Health Statistics (2010). *Health, United States, 2010, with urban and rural chartbook*. Hyattsville, MD: National Center for Health Statistics.

National Center for Health Statistics (2013). *Health United States, 2013, with special feature on prescription drugs*. U.S. Department of Health and Human Services Centers for Disease Control.

National Center for Health Statistics (2014). *Health United States 2014*. Hyattsville, MD: U.S. Government Printing Office.

National Diabetes Statistics Report. (2014). Available at <www.cdc.gov/diabetes/pubs/stats/report/4/national-diabetes/report> Accessed December 30, 2013.

National Health and Nutrition Examination Survey (NHANES) (1999–2002).

National Health and Nutrition Examination Survey (NHANES) (2005–2006, 2008). Documentation, codebook, and frequencies. Hyattsville, MD: U.S. Government Printing Office.

National Health and Nutrition Examination Survey (NHANES) (2011–2012). Accessed December 31, 2014.

National Health Study for a New Generation of U.S. Veterans (NewGen) (2015). U.S. Veterans Affairs. Public Health Service. Washington, DC.

National Heart Lung Blood Institute/American Heart Association (2014). <www.nhlbi.nih.gov/health/health-topics/cad> Accessed December 1, 2014.

National Institutes of Health (NIH), National Heart, Lung and Blood Institute (2004). *Morbidity and mortality chart book on cardiovascular, lung and blood diseases*. Bethesda, MD: National Heart, Lung, and Blood Institute.

National Institute of Diabetes and Digestive and Kidney Diseases. Available at <www.digestive.niddk.nih.gov> Retrieved December 31, 2014.

Neighbors, H. W., Musick, M. A., & Williams, D. R. (1998). The African American minister as a source of help for serious personal crises: bridge or barrier to mental health? *Health Education Behavior*, *25*(50), 759–767.

Ng, M., et al. (2014). Global, regional, and national prevalence of overweight and obesity in children and adults during 1980–2013: a systematic analysis for the Global Burden of Disease Study. *Lancet*, *384*, 766–781.

Office of Minority Health. *Minority population profiles*. Available at <www.minorityhealth.hhs.gov/omh/> Retrieved December 20, 2015.

Ogden, C., Lamb, M., Carroll, M., & Flegal, K. (2010). Obesity and socioeconomic status in adults: United States 2005–2008. *NCHS Data Brief* (50). Accessed December 20, 2014.

Oscherwitz, M. (1972). Differences in pulmonary function in various racial groups. *American Journal of Epidemiology*, *96*(5), 319–327.

Overfield, T. (1995). *Biologic variations in health and illness: race, age and sex differences* (2nd ed.). Reading, MA: Addison-Wesley.

Owen, G. M., & Lubin, A. (1973). Anthropometric differences between Black and White preschool children. *American Journal of Diseases in Children*, *126*, 168.

Pasamanick, B. (1964). Myths regarding prevalence of mental disease in the Negro. *Journal of the National Medical Association*, *58*, 6–17.

Pearson (2015). *Nursing: a concept based approach* (2nd ed., pp. 740–746). Boston: Pearson.

Penk, W. E., et al. (1989). Ethnicity: post-traumatic stress disorder (PTSD) differences among black, white, and Hispanic veterans who differ in degrees of exposure to combat in Vietnam. *Journal of Clinical Psychology*, *45*(5), 729–735.

Perry, H. L. (1993). Mourning and funeral customs of African Americans. In D. P. Irish, K. F. Lundquist, & V. J. Nelson (Eds.), *Ethnic variations in dying, death, and grief.* Washington, DC: Taylor & Francis.

Pillsbury, B. (1982). Doing the month: confinement and convalescence of Chinese women after childbirth. In M. Kay (Ed.), *Anthropology of human birth.* Philadelphia: F. A. Davis.

Ploski, H., & Williams, J. (1989). *The Negro almanac: a reference work on the African-American* (5th ed.). Detroit: Gale Research.

President's Task Force on Environmental Health Risks and Safety Risks to Children (2012). *Federal asthma disparities plan.* Available at <http://www.health.gov/environment/TaskForce/fin.pdf> Accessed December 31, 2014.

Pratt, M. W., Janus, Z. L., & Sayal, N. C. (1977). National variations in prematurity (1973 and 1974). In D. M. Reed & F. J. Stanley (Eds.), *The epidemiology of prematurity* (pp. 53–74). Baltimore: Urban & Schwarzenberg.

Public Broadcasting Service (PBS). *From indentured servitude to racial slavery. Part 1.* Available at <http://www.pbs.org/wgbh/aia/part1/1narr3.html>

Purnell, L. (2013). *Transcultural health: a culturally competent approach* (4th ed., pp. 91–114). Philadelphia: F. A. Davis.

Rajkovic, N., et al. (2014). Relationship between obesity, adipocytokines and inflammatory markers in type 2 diabetes: relevance for cardiovascular risk prevention. *International Journal of Environmental Research and Public Health*, 11, 4049–4065. Available at <www.mdpi.com/journal/ijerph> Accessed December 31, 2014.

Remington, G., & DaCosta, G. (1989). Ethnocultural factors in resident supervision: black and white supervisors. *American Journal of Psychotherapy*, 43(3), 343–355.

Richards, S., Funk, M., & Milner, K. (2000). Differences between blacks and whites with coronary heart disease in initial symptoms and delay in seeking care. *American Journal of Critical Care*, 9(4), 237–244.

Robins, L. N., Helzer, J. E., Croughan, J., & Ratcliff, K. S. (1981). National Institutes of Mental Health diagnostic interview schedule: its history, characteristics, and validity. *Archives of General Psychiatry*, 38, 381–389.

Roche, A. F., Roberts, J., & Hamell, P. V. (1978). Skeletal maturity of youths 12–17 years of age: racial, geographic and socioeconomic disproportions. *National Health*, 11(167), 1–98.

Samad, F., & Ruf, W. (2013). Inflammation, obesity and thrombosis. *Blood Journal*, 120(20). Available at <www.bloodjournal.org/content/early/2013/10/02/blood-2013-05-427708> Accessed January 10, 2015.

Sampson, J., & Workman, L. (2013). Care of patients with HIV disease and other immune deficiencies. In D. Ignatavicius & L. Workman (Eds.), *Medical surgical nursing patient-centered collaborative care* (7th ed., pp. 356–380). St. Louis: Elsevier.

Sandoval, M. (1977). Santería: Afro-Cuban concepts of disease and its treatment in Miami. *Journal of Operational Psychiatry*, 8(52), 48–53.

Sasson, C., et al. (2012). Association of neighborhood characteristics with bystander-initiated CPR. *New England Journal of Medicine*, 367(17), 1607–1615.

Shapiro, I., & Sherman, A. (2005). *Essential facts about the victims of Hurricane Katrina.* Center on Budget and Policy Priorities. Available at <http://www.cbpp.org/research/essential-facts-about-the-victims-of-hurricane-katrina> Accessed August 23, 2010.

Shapiro, M. F., et al. (1999). Variations in the care of HIV-infected adults in the United States: results from the HIV cost and services utilization study. *Journal of the American Medical Association*, 28(24), 2305–2315.

Singh, G., Azuine, R., & Siahpush, M. (2013). Widening socioeconomic, racial, and geographic disparities in HIV/AIDS mortality in the United States, 1987–2011. *Advances in Preventative Medicine*, 2013, 657961. Retrieved January 10, 2015.

Smith, J. A. (1976). The role of the Black clergy as allied health care professionals in working with the Black patients. In D. Luckcraft (Ed.), *Black awareness: implications for Black care* (pp. 12–15). New York: The American Journal of Nursing Company.

Snow, L. E. (1974). Folk medical beliefs and their implications for care of patients: a review based on studies among Black Americans. *Annals of Internal Medicine*, 81, 82–96.

Snow, L. E. (1977). Popular medicine in a Black neighborhood. In E. H. Spicer (Ed.), *Ethnic medicine in the Southwest.* Tucson: University of Arizona Press.

Snow, L. E. (1978). Sorcerers, saints, and charlatans: Black folk healers in urban America. *Culture, Medicine and Psychiatry*, 2, 69.

Snow, L. E. (1983). Traditional health beliefs and practice among lower class Black Americans. *Western Journal of Medicine*, 139(6), 820–828.

Snowden, L. (1982). *Reaching the underserved: mental health needs of neglected populations.* Newbury Park, CA: Sage.

Snowden, L., & Todman, P. A. (1982). The psychological assessment of Blacks: new and needed developments. In E. E. Johns & S. J. Korchin (Eds.), *Minority mental health* (pp. 193–226). New York: Praeger.

Spector, R. E. (2008). *Cultural diversity in health and illness* (7th ed.). Upper Saddle River, NJ: Pearson Prentice Hall.

Spurlock, J. (1985). Psychiatric states. In R. A. Williams (Ed.), *Textbook of Black-related diseases.* New York: McGraw-Hill.

Srinivasan, S., Myers, L., & Berenson, G. (2002). Predictability of childhood adiposity and insulin for developing insulin resistance syndrome (syndrome X) in young adulthood. *Diabetes*, 51, 204–209.

Stalls, F. A. (1978). Racial differences in alcohol metabolism. *Alcohol Clinical and Experimental Research*, 2(1), 10.

Staples, R. (1976). *Introduction to Black sociology.* New York: McGraw-Hill.

Sterne, M., & Pittman, D. J. (1972). *Drinking practices in the ghetto.* St. Louis: Washington University Social Science Institute.

Stokes, L. G. (1977). Delivering health services in a Black community. In A. M. Reinhardt & M. B. Quinn (Eds.), *Current practice in family-centered community nursing* (pp. 51–65). St. Louis: Mosby.

Strauss, R., & Pollack, H. (2001). Epidemic increase in childhood overweight, 1986–1998. *Journal of the American Medical Association, 286*(22), 2845–2848.

Substance Abuse and Mental Health Services Administration (2009). *Results from the 2008 National Survey on Drug Use and Health: National Findings.* (Office of Applied Studies, NSDUH Series H-36, HHS Publication No. SMA 09-4434). Rockville, MD.

Sue, D. (2003). *Counseling the culturally diverse: theory and practice* (4th ed.). New York: John Wiley.

Swank, A. M., & Fell, R. D. (1990). Effects of acute smoking and exercise on high-density lipoprotein-cholesterol and subfractions in Black female smokers. *Metabolism: Clinical and Experimental, 39*, 343–349.

Taylor, C., Lillis, C., & Lynn, P. (2015). *Fundamentals of nursing: the art and science of person centered nursing care* (pp. 1159–1161). Philadelphia: Wolters Kluwer.

Thomas, A., & Sillen, S. (1972). *Racism and psychiatry.* New York: Brunner/Mazel.

Time almanac. (2011). New York: Encyclopaedia Britannica.

Tobias, P. (1970). Brain-size, grey matter, and race: fact or fiction. *American Journal of Physical Anthropology, 32*, 3–26.

Treas, L., & Wilkinson, J. (2014). *Basic nursing concepts, skills and reasoning* (pp. 138, 322, 326–329). Philadelphia: F. A. Davis.

Turner, L. (1948). Problems confronting the investigation of Gullah. *American Dialect Society Publications, 9*, 78–84.

U.S. Department of Commerce, Bureau of the Census (2015). *American community survey.* Washington, DC: U.S. Government Printing Office.

U.S. Department of Commerce, Bureau of the Census (2011). *2010 Census briefs update.* Washington, DC: U.S. Government Printing Office.

U.S. Department of Commerce, Bureau of the Census (2002). *Population profiles by age, sex, race, and Hispanic origin.* Summary File 3. Washington, DC: U.S. Government Printing Office.

U.S. Department of Commerce, Bureau of the Census (2000). *The older population in the United States, 2000.* Washington, DC: U.S. Government Printing Office.

U.S. Department of Commerce, Bureau of the Census (2015). Washington, DC: U.S. Government Printing Office.

U.S. Department of Commerce, Bureau of the Census (2015). *Brief on the Black population.* Washington, DC: U.S. Government Printing Office.

U.S. Department of Commerce, Bureau of the Census (2001). *The 65 years and older population: 2000.* Washington, DC: U.S. Government Printing Office.

U.S. Department of Commerce, Bureau of the Census (2005). *We the people: Blacks in the United States: census brief.* Hyattsville, MD: U.S. Government Printing Office.

U.S. Department of Health and Human Services (2000). *Healthy People 2010: understanding and improving health* (2nd ed.). Washington, DC: U.S. Government Printing Office.

U.S. Census Bureau, Income and Poverty in the United States (2013). *Current population reports.* <http://www.cbpp.org/research/essential-facts-about-the-victims-of-hurricane-katrina> Accessed December 31, 2014.

U.S. Department of Health and Human Services (2007). *HIV in the United States.* Washington, DC: U.S. Government Printing Office, Centers for Disease Control.

U.S. Department of Health and Human Services (2010). *The Office of Minority Health.* Available at <http://www.dhss.mo.gov/MinorityHealth> Accessed March 10, 2010.

U.S. Department of Health and Human Services (2007). *A strategic framework for improving racial/ethnic minority health and eliminating racial/ethnic health disparities.* Available at <http://www.musc.edu/nursing/departments/researchoffice/documents/Graham%202008.pdf> Accessed July 8, 2014.

Valdez, R., Howard, B., Stern, M., & Haffner, S. (1995). Apolipoprotein E polymorphism and insulin levels in biethnic populations. *Diabetes Care, 18*(7), 992–1000.

Vaughn, L., Jacquez, F., & Baker, R. (2009). Cultural health attributions beliefs and practices: effects on healthcare and medical education. *The Open Medical Education Journal, 2*, 64–74. Retrieved December 10, 2014.

Vernon, S., & Roberts, R. (1982). *Use of the SAD-RDC in a triethnic community survey.* Springfield, MA: Merriam-Webster.

Veteran Affairs (2014). *Years of PTSD research, education and technology provides comprehensive mental health care for veterans.* Washington, DC: V terans Affairs Office.

Virtual Jamestown Law. Available at <http://www.virtualjamestown.org/Laws1> Accessed January 10, 2015.

Ward, J., & Duchin, J. (1998). U.S. epidemiology of HIV and AIDS. In P. A. Volberding & M. A. Jacobson (Eds.), *AIDS clinical review* (pp. 10–32). New York: Marcel Dekker Publications.

Warzone-related stress reactions: what veterans need to know. The Iraq War Clinician Guide. Available at <http://www.ptsd.va.gov/professional/materials/manuals/iraq-war-clinician-guide.asp> Retrieved January 15, 2015.

Weclew, R. (1975). The nature, prevalence, and level of awareness of curanderismo and some of its implications for community health. *Community Mental Health Journal, 11*, 145.

Westermeyer, J. (1984). The role of ethnicity in substance abuse. In B. Stimmel (Ed.), *Cultural and sociological aspects of alcoholism and substance abuse* (pp. 9–18). New York: Haworth Press.

Williams, M. (1986). Alcohol and ethnic minorities: Native Americans—an update. *Alcohol Health and Research Works, 11*(2), 5–6.

Wintrob, R. (1973). The influences of others: witchcraft and rootwork as explanations of behavior disturbances. *Journal of Nervous and Mental Disorders, 156*, 318.

Wolfram, W. A., & Clark, H. (Eds.), (1971). *Black–White speech relationships.* Washington, DC: Center for Applied Linguistics.

World Almanac (2015). *Infobase Learning*. New York.

World Health Organization (Updated January 2015). *Cardiovascular diseases (CVDs) Fact sheet No. 317*.

Wright, K. (2007). Examining racial and ethnic disparities and predictors of medication use among California's African American, Latino, and White children with asthma. *The Journal of the National Black Nurse's Association, 18*(2), 1–15.

Wright, K. (2009). Disparities and predictors of emergency department use among California's African American, Latino and White children with asthma, ages 1–11. *Ethnicity and Disease, 19*(1), 71–77.

Zettervall, D. (2005). A pragmatic approach to the management of diabetes and its complications. *CE Today for Nurse Practitioners, 4*(3), 17–27.

Mexican Americans

Linda McMurry, Huaxin Song, Donna C. Owen, Elizabeth W. Gonzalez, and Christina R. Esperat

BEHAVIORAL OBJECTIVES

After reading this chapter, the nurse will be able to:

1. Discuss the influence of Spanish-language usage by Mexican Americans in adapting to the mainstream U.S. culture.
2. Explain the distance and intimacy behaviors of Mexican Americans.
3. Describe the organization of the Mexican American family unit.
4. Explain the Mexican American orientation to time.
5. Describe the impact of locus of control on Mexican Americans' perceptions of the environment and their ability to control it.
6. Describe how the "hot–cold" beliefs of Mexican Americans influence their health and illness beliefs.
7. Identify the biological variations of Mexican Americans.

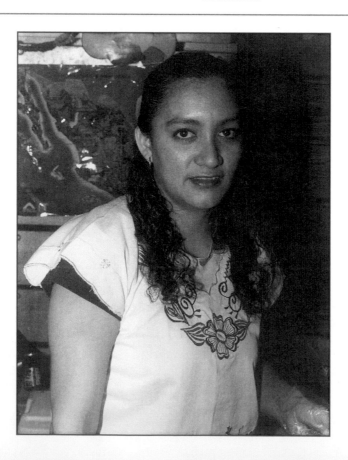

OVERVIEW OF MEXICO

Mexico, or what is officially referred to as the United Mexican States (*Estados Unidos Mexicanos*), is a country in the southern part of North America. Mexico consists of 31 states and a federal district (Central Intelligence Agency [CIA], 2014). The boundaries of Mexico extend southward from the United States to Guatemala and Belize in Central America. The western coast of Mexico borders on the Pacific Ocean, which includes the Gulf of California and the Gulf of Tehuantepec. The eastern coast of Mexico fronts on the Caribbean Sea and the Gulf of Mexico, which includes the Bay of Campeche. Mexico, which includes several outlying islands, has a total area of 758,449 square miles and is the third largest Latin American nation after Brazil and Argentina. Mexico is about one fifth the size of the United States (CIA, 2014).

Over 60% of Mexicans are mestizos, that is, of mixed Spanish and Amerindian descent (CIA, 2014). They trace their native heritage back to Indian groups that built great civilizations in Mexico long before the Spanish explorers arrived in the 1500s (Falicov, 2005). When the Spaniards came to Mexico in 1519, they found Indians who were skilled in writing, mathematics, astronomy, painting, sculpture, and architecture. Indian pottery, metalwork, and textiles were very highly developed for the period. Many Spaniards married women from the native Indian population. Spain's discovery and eventual conquest of Mexico marked the start of the destruction of many elements of existing civilizations (Villarruel & Leininger, 2004). Missionaries were sent to convert the Indians to Christianity. Many of the riches of the land were carried back to Spain. Catholicism is the dominant religion in Mexico, with about 82.7% of the population as of 2010 (CIA, 2014). In recent decades the number of Catholics has been declining, due to the growth of other Christian denominations, which constituted 9.7% of the population (CIA, 2014).

After centuries of Spanish rule, the people rose and a republic was declared in 1823. After numerous conflicts and the U.S.–Mexican War (1846–1848), Mexico lost the lands north of the Rio Grande to the United States. French invasions were also repulsed. However, internal conflict continued, with years of rebellion and factional fighting. A new constitution in 1917 finally brought social reform, as the Institutional Revolutionary Party assumed control and dominated politics from 1929 to the late 1990s. During 1983 and 1984, Mexico suffered its worst financial crisis in 50 years, leading to critically high unemployment and an inability to pay its foreign debt. The collapse of oil prices in 1986 cut into Mexico's export earnings and worsened the situation. Political and governmental conflict resulted in an unstable situation that contributed to many Mexicans seeking economic gain in the United States. Although the value of the peso fell drastically, an austerity plan and assistance from the United States saved Mexico's currency from complete collapse in 1995. Mexico's economic freedom score is 66.4, making its economy the fifty-ninth freest in the 2015 Index (CIA, 2014). The economic freedom in Mexico has declined by 1.4 points since 2011. Deteriorations in the fiscal and regulatory environments have occurred in an environment of slow economic growth despite a reform-minded leadership bent on increasing competition and opening the economy to trade and investment. Mexico's economic growth has been driven largely by integration with Canada and the United States in the North American Free Trade Agreement, but economic performance remains far below potential. Despite a more open economic environment, business regulations continue to undermine economic efficiency. Ensuring more dynamic growth will require broader based reforms to improve the investment climate and enhance the rule of law. Mexico is the major drug-producing and transit nation with the world's second largest opium poppy cultivator (CIA, 2014). The estimated annual wholesale earnings from illicit drug sales ranges from $13.6 billion to $39 billion (Cook, 2007; Fantz, 2012). At least 60,000 people were killed during the ongoing asymmetric war between the Mexican government and the drug cartels between 2006 and 2012; more than 18,000 additional people were reported missing (Booth, 2012; Miroff & Booth, 2012). The Merida Initiative, which provides $1.4 billion over 3 years for the United States to assist the Mexican government with training, equipment, and intelligence, has failed to make a difference (*Time Almanac*, 2011).

The estimated population of Mexico in 2014 was 120,286,655 (CIA, 2014). By a 2014 estimate, the average annual rate of natural increase was estimated at 1.21% (CIA, 2014). The birth rate in Mexico is 19.02 births per 1000 persons, whereas the infant mortality is estimated to be 12.58 deaths per 1000 live births (CIA, 2014). Over the past 4 decades, the life expectancy at birth has increased from 35 to 72.7 years for males and 78.3 years for females (CIA, 2014). Approximately 50% to 75% of the Mexican population suffer from malnutrition, making it one of the leading causes of death among children. On the other hand, the obesity rate was 32.1% in 2008, which ranked Mexico at the twenty-third highest obesity rate in the world; the United States was ranked eighteenth. The estimated child labor rate was 5%, or over 1.1 million child workers, in 2009. The gross domestic product (2013 estimate) is $1.33 trillion, with a per capita income of $15,600 (CIA, 2014). The unemployment rate was 4.9% (2013 estimate), and the population below the poverty line was 52.3% (2012 estimate) (CIA, 2014).

MEXICAN AMERICANS

The southwest region of the United States was settled by Spaniards in 1598 in what is today New Mexico. Later, citizens of the United States began settling in what was then Mexican territory. Mexicans helped establish many southwestern cities and taught the settlers skills in mining, farming, and ranching. After the U.S.–Mexican War, which separated Mexico, a treaty provided land and cultural rights to those of Mexican descent. Unfortunately, these rights were never fully honored, and Mexican Americans living in these areas have tended to become an economically segregated working-class group (Moore & Pachon, 1985).

Mexican Americans are Americans of full or partial Mexican descent. The estimated number of Mexican Americans in 2013 was over 34 million, which was 10.8% of the total population in the United States (U.S. Bureau of the Census, 2013). By 2015, the estimated number of Mexican Americans was roughly 54 million, accounting for 17.0 of the total U.S. population (U.S. Department of Commerce, Bureau of the Census, American Community Survey, 2015).

Over the years, numerous socioeconomic and political conditions in Mexico and the demand for cheap agricultural and industrial labor in the United States have contributed to the movement of Mexicans to the United States (Villarruel & Leininger, 2004). Because of the geographical closeness of Mexico and the United States and the permeability of the border, some Mexicans move back and forth between Mexico and the United States legally and some illegally. The movement back and forth across the border allows them to remain in contact with their families and native customs while seeking economic opportunities in the United States. The U.S. Department of Homeland Security (Hoefer, Rytina, & Campbell, 2009) reports that the heaviest concentration of illegal immigrants coming into the United States—69% of all undocumented individuals—come from Mexico; this represents a 57% change between 2000 and 2006. Lack of citizenship may present a significant barrier to psychosocial and physical health and to gaining education, skills, stable jobs, decent living conditions, and government benefits. Mexican Americans who are undocumented frequently experience tension regarding discovery and deportation back to Mexico. Preoccupation with possible discovery and deportation for illegal aliens serves to further augment the symptoms of post-traumatic stress disorder (PTSD) (Cervantes, Snyder, & Padilla, 1989). The plight of the illegal alien has worsened since enactment of the Immigration Reform and Control Act of 1986 (Gelfand & Bialik-Gilad, 1989). In an attempt to control illegal immigration to the United States, employers are now required to verify citizenship status within 24 hours after hiring an employee. Thus, undocumented aliens are often forced into low-paying day-labor jobs.

The Mexican immigrant populations have been concentrated mostly in the south and western portions of the United States, but more recently, the Midwest and East Coast have seen sizable increases in their populations. Thirteen states now have 100,000 or more residents who are Mexican immigrants, and California has the heaviest concentration (39%). Most Mexican Americans have rural agricultural backgrounds (U.S. Department of Commerce, Bureau of the Census, 2013). However, it is difficult to generalize about geographical location and the occupational background of people in this ethnic group. The diversity in Mexican Americans ranges from rural villagers in New Mexico and Colorado (Saunders, 1954; Weaver, 1970) to agricultural laborers in Texas (Rubel, 1966) to low-income residents in Arizona and to urban lower class individuals in California (Clark, 1970). Just as the people are diverse, studies often represent specific populations of Mexicans and offer differing definitions of Mexican Americans. Discussion of Mexican Americans is complicated by the diversity of this population (Bollenbacher, Heck, & Davidhizar, 2000; Davidhizar, 2001). Because of this, making general conclusions about Mexican Americans as a result of individual studies must be done with great caution. It bears noting, however, that of the estimated 54 million Latinos in the United States in 2013, 64% are of Mexican origin, followed by Puerto Ricans (9.5%), Central Americans (8.9%), South Americans (6.1%), Cubans (3.7%), Dominicans (3.2%), and other Hispanics and Latinos (4.6%) (U.S. Department of Commerce, Bureau of the Census, 2013).

The Hispanic American population is growing rapidly in the United States. In fact, in 2000 the number of Hispanics exceeded the number of African-Americans, escalating this group to the largest ethnic minority group in the United States. In 2010, 50 million Hispanic Americans were reported to live in the United States, and Hispanics now represent 16.8% of the total U.S. population (U.S. Department of Commerce, Bureau of the Census, 2013). As in the past, people of Hispanic origins, including Mexican Americans, Puerto Ricans, Cubans, and persons from Central or South America, could identify themselves as Hispanic (U.S. Department of Commerce, Bureau of the Census, 2013). However, in the 2000 census, the term *Latinos* was used for the first time on the census form (U.S. Department of Commerce, Bureau of the Census, 2000). The terms *Hispanic* or *Latino* may be used interchangeably. In fact, these terms now reflect new terminology set forth in standards issued by the Office of Management and Budget in 1997.

The Mexican American population has also been growing rapidly. According to the U.S. Department of

Commerce, Bureau of the Census, American Community Survey (2015), the Mexican American population nearly doubled between 1970 and 1980. Between 1980 and 2000, the number of Mexican Americans residing in the United States doubled again. The Mexican American population was increased from 20,640,178 in 2000 to 31,798,258 in 2010 (Ennis, Ríos-Vargas, & Albert, 2011). Today, there are some 54 million Mexican Americans residing in the United States, accounting for 17.0% of the total U.S. population (U.S. Department of Commerce, Bureau of the Census, American Community Survey, 2015).

The proximity of Mexico to the United States has resulted in a noteworthy amount of drug trafficking. The practice of smoking cannabis leaves came to the United States with Mexican immigrants who came north during the 1920s (Musto, 1991). Much of the cocaine that reaches the United States from Colombia comes by way of Mexico (Booth, 1996). Along with the drugs has come an increase in violence for border cities, creating problems for the judicial system by overcrowding jail cells, and for the health care system, which is often unprepared for the influx of health and socially related problems (Zong & Batalova, 2014).

Use of the health care system in America has been problematic for many Mexican Americans because of lack of insurance (Hahn, 1995). As estimated in the 2013 American Community Survey conducted by the U.S. Bureau of the Census, the uninsured rate for Hispanic or Latino individuals was 28.4%, which was much higher than the national average (14.5%), White non-Hispanic (10.2%), and Black (17.1%) (U.S. Department of Commerce, Bureau of the Census, 2013). Explanations for lack of insurance are partly related to communication difficulties and to lack of understanding that insurance is needed. Lack of health insurance is also related to culture, because most Hispanics who have recently immigrated do not understand the competitive health care market and the need for insurance, and many still place their trust in traditional herbal remedies (Ross, 1995; Villarruel & Leininger, 2004). Health care agencies are not eager to treat uninsured, indigent people since undocumented aliens do not qualify for Medicare or Medicaid funds. Angel, Angel, and Markides (2002) noted that most of the Mexican Americans who were uninsured are younger, female, poor, and foreign. These persons report that they make fewer health care visits, are less likely to have a usual source of care, and more often receive care in Mexico. Another complication regarding the use of the health care system is that many Mexican Americans live in crowded, substandard city housing, which has limited access to high-quality health care facilities (Ross, 1995). When comparing Mexican American, African-American, and White American low-income women, Keenan, Marshall, and Eve (2002)

noted that while psychosocial variables were significant predictors for health care use, for Mexican American women, psychosocial vulnerability was mediated by barriers that affected utilization in a more complex way. Borders, Xu, Rohrer, and Warner (2002) studied rural Mexican Americans living in Texas and noted that psychosocial variables including part-time employment, lack of continuous health insurance coverage, and poor health status could be related to levels of satisfaction with health care.

Immigration of Mexicans to the United States has created difficulties in schools, such as the special needs of teaching children who do not have English-speaking skills (Serrano, 1997). Yet another problem can be noted in California, where funds are not provided for educating children who are illegal aliens. The educational achievement of Mexican Americans is steadily rising. For example, the prevalence of the population with a high school diploma or higher educational attainment among Hispanics or Latinos has increased from 27% in the 1970s to over 64% in 2013 (U.S. Department of Commerce, Bureau of the Census, 2013). Illegal and legal immigrants from Mexico present other problems for the United States since many immigrants have relatives who are citizens and who participate in the debate about deportation and obstruction to the path to citizenship (Campo-Flores, 2006).

In general, it is estimated that Mexican Americans have less formal education than the national average. In fact, in 2013, approximately 64.7% of Hispanic or Latino individuals over 25 years of age have graduated from high school, and only 14% of Hispanics or Latinos have graduated from college. These figures are compared with national averages of 86.6% and 29.6%, respectively, for all racial groups in the United States (U.S. Department of Commerce, Bureau of the Census, 2013). Increased education has resulted in a decrease in problems related to poor housing, jobs, and discrimination. However, many customs in the United States, including needing a driver's license and insurance to avoid problems with the police, being quiet in the evening in a conservative neighborhood, and exhibiting polite behavior toward women are part of the socialization process that must be learned in order to adapt to most communities in the United States (Woodbury, 2000). While some Mexican Americans are positive about the socialization process, many Mexican Americans try to retain a cultural identity within the dominant population (Chávez, 1986).

"Cultural uniqueness" is not academic nomenclature for Mexican Americans. The phrase is used to describe physical, emotional, and behavioral distinctions unique to many Mexican Americans (Chávez, 1986). Unlike European immigrants, who often hasten to absorb the culture found in the United States, many Mexican Americans have not. In *Megatrends,* John Naisbitt (1984) states that "none of the new groups individually can begin to match the numbers and the potential influence of Spanish-speaking Americans." Concepts such as *machismo* (manliness), *confianza* (confidence), *respeto* (respect), *vergüenza* (shame), and *orgullo* (pride) predominate in the culture, and traditional gender and family roles continue to be part of the heritage that separates Mexican Americans from other cultural groups. Unfortunately, and perhaps because of the desire to retain cultural identity, many Mexican Americans have experienced discrimination in education, jobs, and housing. Skin color, language differences, and Spanish surnames have all contributed to discrimination (Zong & Batalova, 2014).

In 2013, 47.7% of Mexican American families were married couple families, 8.9% were single male household families, and 20.2% were female-headed households (U.S. Department of Commerce, Bureau of the Census, 2013). In addition, in 2010, Mexican American households had 3.52 people, compared with 2.38 people for the rest of the general population among non-Hispanic Whites. This increase in persons per household partly accounts for the rapid growth of both the Mexican Americans in particular and the Hispanic populations in the general population. Mexican Americans are a younger population; 32.8% of Mexican Americans are 18 years or younger compared with 21.4% of non-Hispanic Whites (U.S. Department of Commerce, Bureau of the Census, 2013). The median age for Hispanic and Latino individuals was 28 years, while the national average was 37.5 (U.S. Department of Commerce, Bureau of the Census, 2013).

In 2013, of the total number of Mexican American males (16 years and over) in the workforce, 15.9% held jobs in management, professional, or related occupations; 22.2% held jobs in service occupations; 14.7% held jobs in sales or office occupations; 3.1% held jobs in farming, fishing, or forestry occupations; 22.3% held jobs in construction, extraction, maintenance, and repair occupations; and 21.7% held jobs in production, transportation, or material moving occupations. Of the total number of Mexican American females (16 years and over) in the workforce, 24.6% held jobs in management, professional, or related occupations; 32.2% held jobs in service occupations; 12.5% held jobs in sales or office occupations; 1.4% held jobs in farming, fishing, or forestry occupations; and 9.5% held jobs in production, transportation, or material moving occupations (U.S. Department of Commerce, Bureau of the Census, 2013).

Despite the shift from jobs related to agriculture for the general population of Mexican Americans residing in the United States, in 2013 the median family income for Mexican Americans in general was only $42,897, as compared with $62,367 for all other races. The median per capita income for Mexican Americans was only $16,117 as compared with $45,320 for all other races (U.S. Department of Commerce, Bureau of the Census, 2013). Among all Mexican Americans at all ages, 24.7% live below the federally defined poverty level (U.S. Department of Commerce, Bureau of the Census, American Community Survey, 2015.

While Mexican Americans are merging into the general labor force, other than seasonal work, Kissam (1993) reported that except for southern Florida, 80% to 90% of all the migrant and seasonal labor force were foreign born and almost all were of Mexican origin (Mines, Gabbard, & Samardick, 1992). Kissam reported the following developments in the migrant Mexican labor force: (1) diffusion into other geographical areas of the United States, (2) greater ethnic and linguistic diversity than earlier workers, (3) increasing numbers of unaccompanied males supporting families who remain at home, (4) changing characteristics of reunited families settling in the United States after the father had migrated for 5 to 10 years (children of these families transfer to U.S. schools after years of school in Mexico, rather than having K–12 schooling in the United States, and these families experience a high level of stress in assimilating as a united family and as immigrants), (5) increasing numbers of very young and very old migrant workers, and (6) growing numbers of female-headed households. The changing demographics of Mexican migrant farm workers present many challenges to U.S. agencies in adequately meeting their needs.

COMMUNICATION

Spanish, the primary language for many Mexican Americans, is the fourth most commonly used language in the world, the second most commonly spoken language in the United States, and one of the six languages used by the United Nations (Lewis, Simons, & Fennig, 2014). Of the people in the United States who speak a second language, over 50% speak Spanish. Of U.S. Latinos, almost 90% speak Spanish (Lewis et al., 2014).

Dialect

The Spanish language is spoken in many dialects; Mexican Americans who have an Indian heritage may speak one of more than 50 Spanish dialects. Fortunately, the majority of words spoken have the same meaning (Zoucha & Purnell, 2003). Differences in dialect may be found in certain communities. Dialects may also be identified by their proximity to the Mexican border. In the nineteenth century, the dominant language in the barrios and rural settlements was that of Mexico, although some Tejanos also attained facility in English and thus became bilingual. Various linguistic codes characterize oral communications in present-day enclaves. However, because of continued emigration from Mexico, racial separation, and exposure to American mass culture, some Texas Mexicans speak formal Spanish only, just as there are those who communicate strictly in formal English. More common are those Spanish speakers using English loan words as they borrow from the lexicon of mainstream society. Another form of expression, referred to as *codeswitching,* involves the systematic mixing of the English and Spanish languages. Another mode of communication is *caló,* a hip code composed of innovative terminology and codeswitching used primarily by boys in their own groups (Rodolfo, 2007). This southwestern regional form of dialogue, now used across subculture groups of Mexican American teens, is also used to a lesser extent by older Mexican Americans (Cummings, 2003).

Touch

Adult Mexican Americans can be characterized as tactile in their relationships. Embracing or holding hands while walking is common among close friends of the same gender. Although female Mexican Americans may initiate more tactile behavior in communicating, there is a contradiction where modesty is concerned. Mexican American women have been taught to highly value female modesty and not to expose their bodies to men or even other women. Nakedness is avoided and will cause embarrassment, even among close family members. Consequently, being touched by health care providers is often a source of embarrassment (Katz, 2014; Lagana & Gonzalez-Ramirez, 2003). Women will generally prefer to receive care from a female health care provider, and adolescent girls may desire to have their mother or female relative present for pelvic examinations and other intimate aspects of a physical examination. Although religious beliefs may explain lack of birth control, discomfort with certain areas of the body may also explain why some Mexican American women avoid the use of a diaphragm. Men also have strong feelings about modesty and may feel threatened if expected to have a complete physical examination (Getrich et al., 2012). While this modesty may explain the reluctance of some Mexican American men to use condoms, this reluctance may also reflect the imbalance of power between men and women. Increasingly, women in committed relationships are being included in contraceptive decision making (Dehlendorf, Levy, Kelley, Grumbach, & Steinauer, 2013). Consideration of the Mexican American client's need for modesty suggests approaches for nurses doing physical assessments (Andrews, 2006). During the examination, care should be taken to uncover only the body part being examined and to allow only persons essential to the examination in the examination room.

Hispanic men who are asked to participate in prostate screening experience embarrassment, which poses a barrier to disease prevention behaviors (Getrich et al., 2012). Breast self-examinations are often perceived to be embarrassing but are done by Mexican American women who are more acculturated (Padilla & Villalobos, 2007). Education using breast models, videotapes, and community-based group discussion improves breast health knowledge and promotes screening behavior in Mexican American women (Calderón et al., 2010).

Context

When being interviewed, Mexican Americans may engage in small talk before approaching the business of the interview. It is important for the nurse to remember that small talk will often facilitate accomplishing nursing objectives for the interview and is therefore not a waste of time.

Traditionally, in communicating with others, Mexican Americans have used diplomacy and tactfulness. There is also pride in verbal expression, which is likely to be elaborate and indirect. Direct confrontation and arguments are considered rude and disrespectful. Self-disclosure is reserved for those whom the individual knows well. The Mexican American may appear agreeable on the surface regarding an issue because of the value of courtesy. However, the nurse may later be surprised and disappointed because agreements are not being carried out.

Kinesics

Eye behavior is important to Mexican Americans, especially when children are involved. *Mal ojo* (evil eye) is a folk illness described as a condition that affects infants and children and occurs because an individual who is believed to possess a special power voluntarily or involuntarily injures a child by looking at and admiring but not touching the child (Bayles & Katerndahl, 2009). With this condition the child cries, develops a fever, vomits, and loses his or her appetite. If one is admiring a child, this disorder may be prevented by also touching the child's head or arm. The spell is broken when the individual who has given the "evil eye" touches the child. Therefore, the nurse should touch the child when giving care because in the minds of Mexican Americans, this action can both prevent and treat the illness.

English as a Second Language

Most Mexican Americans can also speak some English and for those of Mexican descent born in the United States, 98% are fluent in English. The inability to speak English fluently has led to increased failure rates for school-aged Mexican Americans (Taylor, Lopez, Martinez, & Velasco, 2012). Lack of language fluency has a negative impact on psychological well-being and diminishes quality of life (Zhang, Hong, Takeuchi, & Mossakowski,

2012). The longer Mexican immigrants stay in the United States, the less likely they are to retain the mother language, which probably is most directly attributable to the fact that English is the language used in schools and at work. Increasing attention is being given to the need for bilingual education for Mexican American students, and as a result, more Mexican Americans are becoming bilingual. Telles and Ortiz (2009), in a unique study of acculturation of the same cohort of Mexican Americans followed across four generations, noted that by the fourth generation, almost all are English and Spanish speaking. Paradoxically the learning of English by Mexican immigrants who also attain greater economic well-being is associated with increased risk of cardiovascular disease (Salinas & Sheffield, 2011).

Some Mexican Americans still use English selectively. In an extensive study on language loyalty among various ethnic groups residing in the United States, it was found that Spanish remains the most persistent of all foreign languages. Although other ethnic groups may have lost the connection to their mother tongue over time, Mexican Americans have been more likely to retain their mother language in succeeding generations in the United States. Even today, some fluency in Spanish characterizes most Mexican Americans at all income levels. Another reason for the persistence of Spanish among Mexican Americans is that in the United States, the mass media for information and entertainment are permeated with Spanish. Spanish accounts for approximately 66% of the total foreign-language broadcasting in the United States. In 2009 there were over 1323 Spanish-language radio stations with Internet broadcasts (Guskin & Mitchell, 2011). This is significant for the provision of improved health care for those with limited English fluency.

It is not uncommon for people who speak different languages to use each language in different contexts or for different purposes. Perhaps the most frequent situation is that of Mexican Americans who use English in their work and Spanish at home or with their friends. In northern New Mexico it is common to find words retained from sixteenth- and seventeenth-century Spanish colonial times (Cobos, 2003) and some villages where the only English spoken is for official occasions, such as conferring with a government agency. Because of the remoteness of these communities, these Mexican Americans may retain Spanish as their principal language. Communication by Mexican Americans is also complicated because many Mexican Americans learn a language that blends English and Spanish. Mexican American adults use this blended form of language more often than children do. Consequently, a nurse who may know both English and Spanish may still have difficulty understanding this blended language.

Implications for Nursing Care

Because some Mexican Americans rely on Spanish to communicate with other people, it may be very frightening for them to participate in the American health care system, and it is frustrating for the nurses giving them care. Nurses caring for clients who do not speak English need to develop and use strategies that show respect for and comfort with cultural differences of these clients (Cioffi, 2003). In a metasynthesis of qualitative studies, having a translator present was not sufficient for nurses to connect with their Mexican American clients (Coffman, 2003). Friendly facial expressions, facing the client, and talking directly to the client even when using the services of an interpreter were found to be important (Coffman, 2003). The use of certified translators is designed to enhance the communication experience between clinician and clients. However, the translator and client sometimes engage in a separate conversation in an attempt to culturally advocate client concerns with the system or provider (Roat, 2006). Care should be taken to ensure that this experience does not undermine the client–provider relationship. Technology, through digital translators, has been designed to help the health care provider maintain direct interaction with Spanish-speaking clients. Digital translators enable translation, back translation, and the creation of a communication log. Schillinger et al. (2003) conducted a study of primary care physicians speaking with diabetics and reported that patients with low literacy in the primary language of the physician received less interactive communication about their disease process. Thus, while efforts should be increased to recruit Mexican Americans into the health professions and to encourage students and professionals to study Spanish in order to communicate with clients, attention to the social features of how people speak when languages differ is needed. The way people use language to motivate health behavior or persuade one another is affected by cultural differences (Pope, 2005). When professional staff cannot speak Spanish, interpretation services must be obtained in order to provide culturally competent care. Based on the recommendations of the Office of Minority Health National Standards for Culturally and Linguistically Appropriate Services in Health Care (CLAS Standards), family and friends should not be used as interpreters. Using children as translators should be avoided since children lack understanding of medical conditions, and as with other untrained interpreters, conflict of interest is likely to arise. Bilingual hospital staff members have as high as 50% inaccuracy when interpreting (Diamond, Wilson-Stronks, & Jacobs, 2010). Although the CLAS Standards recommend asking individuals to rate their primary language and capacity in English and to use qualified institutional interpreters, hospitals continue to find it challenging to comply.

It is important for the nurse to remember that language is a cultural factor that influences health care practices (Oliva, 2008). Mexican American clients view nurses who attempt to speak some Spanish as caring and respectful. It is uncommon for Mexican Americans to be aggressive or assertive when interacting with health care providers. Direct conflict or disagreement with a health care provider generally does not occur; rather, the Mexican American client will be silent or not adhere to the prescribed treatment plan. The nurse who works with bilingual Mexican Americans must remember that when under stress, these persons often may revert to their first language, Spanish. The nurse should explain that the nurse can be more helpful if the client communicates in the language that both the nurse and the client understand. When this is impossible because of high levels of stress on the part of the client, the nurse should find a translator. Understanding the profound effect of bilingualism on the client also requires appreciation of the dimension of language independence—the capacity to acquire, maintain, and use two separate language codes, each with its own lexical, syntactic, phonetic, semantic, and ideational components. Many Mexican Americans who are proficient in both Spanish and English operate parallel language codes, each with its own associations between message words and events in their ideational system (Javier & Marcos, 1989). A good example of language compartmentalization can be found in the saying of Emperor Charles V: "To God I speak in Spanish, to women in Italian, to men in French, and to my horse in German" (*Oxford Dictionary of Quotations*, 2009). In certain situations a client may speak to his or her family in Spanish, to the nurse in English, and, when extremely stressed, to both family and nurse in a combination of both English and Spanish (Sobralske & Katz, 2005).

It is also important for the nurse to keep in mind that Mexican Americans tend to describe emotional problems by using dramatic body language. In addition, research has shown that when Mexican Americans are interviewed in English, or across their language barrier, they are usually judged by experienced clinicians as showing more severe symptoms than when they are interviewed in their mother tongue (Favazza, 1983; Marcos, Alpert, Urcuyo, & Kesselman, 1973). The nurse should keep in mind that nonverbal communication differs among cultures; thus, it is important to work closely with the client and family in order to evaluate symptoms from a variety of perspectives.

The nurse must guard against the use of idioms and abstractions when dealing with clients who do not completely understand the language. The nurse should also avoid responding to the client in a joking manner. Jokes are easily misinterpreted, frequently based on nuances of communication or language, and for the most part are lost in translation. When working with a Mexican American client who lacks understanding of the language, statements using slang or colloquialisms should be avoided because they may be interpreted literally.

One of the most important roles of the nurse in caring for the Mexican American client is that of teacher. Teaching should begin with an assessment of the client's ability to communicate and understand, which will guide the nurse in deciding which other family members should be included in the teaching process. The home situation must be carefully evaluated to adapt care to the reality of the living situation. Instruction should include all aspects of the client's condition and treatment and should be communicated in simple, concrete terms with ample opportunity allowed to raise questions and validate understanding. There should be continuous evaluation of learning by questioning and return demonstrations, and problem solving should be encouraged. Throughout this process, the nurse must continue to build a trusting relationship with the client so that follow-up care will be maintained, helping to ensure that the client will seek medical care before future situations get out of control.

SPACE

Kluckhohn (1976) categorized people and the modalities of relationships as individualistic, collateral, or lineal. Some Mexican Americans are categorized as both collateral and lineal, implying that there may be a patron–peon system, such as a boss–worker relationship, or a family-versus-individual relationship.

In caring for Mexican Americans, *simpatia* and *personalismo* play a significant role. *Simpatia* is characterized by smooth or harmonious interpersonal relationships, described by courtesy, respect, and the absence of critical or confrontational behavior. Among Mexican Americans, a high degree of intimacy may lead to expectations of involving the nurse in the family system, with expectations of participation in familial activities and social functions (Andrews & Boyle, 2008). Mexican Americans as a group demonstrate a great need for group togetherness. Some Mexican Americans think of Anglos as distant because they require more personal space during conversation than Mexican Americans (Juckett, 2005). Ford and Graves (1977) found that when Mexican American second graders related to others, there was closer interpersonal distance and more touching among girls. Touching was of longer duration when spatial distances were closer. Boys tended to be less tactile when relating to others. It is believed that this pattern of socialization begins with the parent–child relationship and continues into adulthood. During the early years, the parents are permissive, warm, and caring with all their children. However, in later years, the girls remain much closer to home and are protected and guarded in their contacts. In contrast, the boys are allowed to be with other boys in informal social groups, where they develop their "machismo" (Murillo, 1978). (In delivering care to male clients, nurses must be aware of the concept of "machismo," a set of attitudes and identities associated with the Mexican concept of masculinity and manliness [Sobralske, 2006].) Gorek, Martin, White, Peters, and Hummel (2002) described issues encountered by Mexican American families trying to adapt to the placement of an older adult in long-term care settings and the concern for staff to create a living space for their parents that respected their cultural heritage and routines.

Implications for Nursing Care

The concepts of family obligation and spirituality are pervasive among Mexican American clients. *Personalismo* and *respeto* are expected from health providers; Mexican American patients expect a handshake in greeting and not offering this is considered rude (Andrews & Boyle, 2008).

The nurse who plans care delivery for Mexican American clients must keep in mind that Mexican Americans may resist care provided by those perceived as being different or from a different ethnic background (Monrroy, 1983). Some Mexican Americans may also have cultural biases that prohibit care being administered by persons of the opposite sex. For example, a male student nurse was assigned to a Mexican American client in labor. This assignment precipitated problems because the client, husband, and family were all very uncomfortable because "only her husband should see her like that." It was necessary to change the assignment in order to provide care. However, although same-sex health care providers are preferred, a health care provider of the opposite sex is usually acceptable by Mexican Americans as long as the care provider is sensitive to the modesty needs of the client (Lagana & Gonzalez-Ramirez, 2003).

SOCIAL ORGANIZATION

Within the Mexican culture, the family is the most valued institution and the main focus of social identification. Most Mexican Americans have nuclear families who live separately, although some extended family or other relatives often live in the same household (Glick, 1999). According to Chávez (1986), new immigrants (especially those who are undocumented) tend to live in a multiple-family arrangement, which offers the advantages of social and economic support. As the length of residency increases and the family becomes more financially independent, the nuclear family tends to find a singular arrangement for its household.

Traditional females display subdued qualities, while males have been the authority figure in the family, assuming responsibility for being head of the household and the decision maker (Sobralske, 2006). In a typical Mexican American family, male members usually display a strong sense of machismo that is irreconcilable with self-esteem or authority loss (Sobralske, 2006). The culture dictates that men need to be strong, reliable, virile, intelligent, and wise. They are expected to exhibit valor, dignity, self-confidence, and a high degree of individuality outside the family and be knowledgeable regarding sexual matters (Zoucha & Purnell, 2003). Men want to project the image of honesty, compassion, and integrity. The man of the family needs to be regarded as being proud, brave, courageous, devoted, loyal, honorable, and worthy of being the head of the household (Sobralske, 2006).

The male is considered the decision maker (Bonder, Martin, & Miracle, 2002). The mother of the family has the primary role of keeping the family cohesive. Although the mother may influence family decisions, she does not have a dominant role in the family. Increasing numbers of Mexican American women are finding work outside the home. Women who live in a rural setting often help with the family farming activities. Divorce is uncommon, but stable out-of-wedlock relationships are common in the lower socioeconomic levels. Meleis, Douglas, Eribes, Shih, and Messias (1996) reported on a group of employed, low-income Mexican women who worked in urban hospitals who experienced role overload and stress. There appeared to be difficulty reconciling the traditional cultural expectations of a woman's role in the changing society, which added the role of working outside the home.

Families are usually large, consisting of the parents and four or more children. Parent–child connectedness and respect for parental authority are valued over the husband–wife bond emphasized by the Western nuclear family. It is generally believed that Mexican Americans are familistic. *Familismo* or family interdependence is valued in the Mexican American culture. *Familismo* involves sharing by extended family members the responsibilities to nurture and discipline children, provide financial aid, provide companionship for lonely or isolated members, and engage in problem solving. There is low reliance on institutions and outsiders. Mexican families value behavior in children that denotes respect, responsibility, compliance, and being "well brought up" (Arcia & Johnson, 1998; Reese, Balzano, Gallimore, & Goldenberg, 1995; Sobralske, 2006). For some Mexican Americans, familism has been perceived as curtailing mobility by sustaining emotional attachment to people, places, and things. In the Mexican American culture, familism has been identified as the prime cause not only of low mobility but also of resistance to changes of all kinds. For Mexican Americans, familism, along with the specially assigned male role, is a source of collective pride. Nevertheless, Mexican Americans are believed to be deterred from collective and individual progress because of familism.

The major dominating theme of the traditional Mexican American family is the need for collective achievement of the family as a group. The collective needs of family supersede the needs of individual members. Also, any dishonor or shame that may occur for an individual member is considered a reflection on the entire family. The Mexican American family takes pride in family endeavors and generally does not seek help from outsiders to solve problems or meet needs. Mexican American families highly value having many relatives live nearby. The local extended family is tightly integrated, has frequent face-to-face encounters, and provides members with mutual aid (Glick, 1999). Mexican Americans have a mean network size of 5.78, which may include in-laws, grandparents, and a substantial number of other relatives, with some 69% of those studied reporting that most of their support was provided by immediate family members (Barnett, 2012; Lantican & Corona, 1989). The importance and obligation of Mexican Americans in meeting the needs of others indicate that there may be a higher priority placed on promoting and supporting the development of abilities to care for others than on abilities to care for self. Two other patterns, the "accepted obligation to perform roles within the family" and the "willingness to bear the burden so as not to cause pain for others" further indicate that caring for others is both expected and rewarded (Villarruel & Denyes, 1997; Villarruel & Leininger, 2004).

There is a high incidence of teenage pregnancy among Mexican Americans. The overall teen pregnancy rate in the United States has fallen 57% since 1991; however, in 2013, the birth rate for women between 15 and 19 years old for Hispanics (41.7 per 1000, total 92,960 births) was still the highest among all races and origins followed by non-Hispanic Blacks (39 per 1000, total 67,537 births) (Martin, Hamilton, Osterman, Curtin, & Matthews, 2015). In 2012, the birth rate for Mexican American teenagers (15–17 years old) was 24.8 per 1000 population, compared with 21.9 per 1000 for African-American teenagers and 8.4 per 1000 for White teenagers (Martin et al., 2015). Likewise, the teenage pregnancy rate in 2012 for Mexican Americans 18 to 19 years of age was 74.2, compared with 74.1 for African-Americans and 37.9 for Whites (Martin et al., 2015).

The entire family may contribute to the financial welfare of the family. Parental control in Mexican American families is strong. Older children contribute by caring for younger family members or animals or by helping with the production of food or other family enterprises. Children in migrant families often earn money by working along with other family members.

Children also assume other responsibilities in the family. For example, Valenzuela (1999) found that older children of immigrant families served multiple roles in assisting their parents to learn certain skills or activities that ranged from filing taxes to understanding difficult-to-read manuals and intervening or advocating on behalf of their parents or their household on complicated transactions. The elderly are respected and live with married children if they are not self-sufficient. The elderly also pass down cultural and folk medicine beliefs. Elder care among Mexican Americans is greatly influenced by the belief that the family is the most important and main source of assistance; thus, Mexican American elders turn to their children and other family members for assistance before seeking out any services in the community.

Váldez (1980) found that Mexican American families of a lower socioeconomic class tended to show more ethnic identification than those of a higher socioeconomic class. This phenomenon served to provide support for Mexican Americans of lower socioeconomic classes and a more positive adaptation to the mainstream U.S. culture. Smith (2002) investigated gender and academic success among Mexican Americans. The findings indicated that Mexican American females in New York City choose high schools that ensure academic success in spite of the expectation that they return home after school to care for their younger siblings and help with housework. Males, on the other hand, took little time in selecting a high school and after school had no responsibility, giving them unstructured time that often led to gang activity and eventually dropping out of high school. Smith noted that whereas this enabled Mexican women to be upwardly mobile, the opposite effect was noted in men.

An important institution in the Mexican heritage is the Catholic practice of *compadrazgo,* or co-parenthood (godparenthood), which was introduced to Mexico by the Spaniards. Godparents (*compadrazgos*) accept co-responsibilities for a child along with the parents. This kinship begins with the baptism of the child and continues throughout the child's life (Kemper, 1982); it is used for religious purposes and becomes an important resource for coping with the stresses of life (Gill-Hopple & Brage-Hudson, 2012). Frequently, a godparent is chosen from a higher socioeconomic level, which enables the child to have social resources that are more extensive than what the family could provide.

Another important tradition for many Mexican American families is the way in which holidays are celebrated with Mexican traditions. Others continue to celebrate Mexican holidays. During the celebration of the Mexican Christmas, called *Las Posadas*, the children are fond of breaking a piñata, a papier-mâché container filled with candy and gifts. Other important holidays are Cinco de Mayo (May 5) and Guadalupe Day (December 12), which is Mexico's most important religious holiday. Affluent Mexican Americans often spend significant amounts of money on special food and drink, decorations, and fireworks for a holiday festival. Holidays provide an opportunity for Mexican Americans to share with others.

Beliefs and Practices in Death and Dying

Death is a prevalent theme in Mexican culture, which may be influenced by the Aztec and Catholic beliefs that death is not the end but rather an entry into a new way of life (Paz, 1961). In a landmark study that examined the thoughts and behaviors about death, dying, and grief among Mexican American immigrants, Kalish and Reynolds (1981) found that religious symbols and rituals are important and that large, supportive Mexican American family networks provide comfort and practical aid while grieving. This is consistent with other findings that support the importance of *familismo* when coping with the death of a loved one. Many Mexican Americans believe that whatever the cause of death, it is the will of God, often referred to as *fatalism* (Beutter & Davidhizar, 1999). For example, Kalish and Reynolds (1981) found that 72% of Mexican Americans believed that accidental death was attributable to divine will, as compared with 56% of Anglo Americans. Additionally, they found that 27% of Mexican Americans thought of their own death daily, compared with 13% of Anglo Americans. Whereas none of the Anglo Americans believed that individuals should be allowed to die when they feel unproductive or unhappy, 3% of Mexican Americans reported they believed this should be allowed. Seventy-six percent of the Mexican Americans in this study reported that they are likely to touch the body of a deceased family member compared with 51% of Anglo Americans. In addition, 59% reported they would be likely to kiss the body of the deceased, compared with 33% of Anglo Americans. In addition, 59% of Mexican Americans believe that a person should visit the grave of his or her spouse at least six times during the first year, compared with 35% of Anglo Americans. Gelfand, Balcazar, Parzuchowski, and Lenox (2001) reported that Mexican Americans do not use hospice care because they are a close-knit community who prefer to take care of their own. On the other hand, Iwashyna and Chang (2002) examined differences in attitudes toward place of death among Whites, Mexican Americans, and Blacks that could not be explained by age, sex, income, education, and cause of death. After an inpatient hospital stay, 56% of Mexican Americans died, compared with 50% of Blacks and 43% of Whites. Twenty-two percent of Mexican Americans died in a nursing home compared with 18% of Blacks and 20% of Whites. Only 9% of Mexican Americans died in a private residence, compared with 18% of Blacks and 22% of Whites. Using an ethnographic approach Doran and Hansen (2006) interviewed Mexican American families about their bereavement experiences after the death of a child and found several themes reflecting the ways in which family members maintained an ongoing relationship with the deceased through dreams, storytelling, sense of presence ("I place a setting on the table for him on special occasions"), faith-based connections, proximity connections ("If I die I want to be buried here with him"), ongoing rituals ("I still prepare his favorite meal on his birthday"), and pictorial remembrances.

Because of strong family ties among Mexican Americans, the idea of truth telling and decision making during the end of life may have to be viewed differently from the traditional Western lens of individual autonomy and broadened to integrate the needs of the family. Religion and faith, and the role of the clergy, are important components of life in Mexican American families, and these components become intensified in the death and dying experience. Spiritual beliefs, the role of prayer, and the role of family in caregiving were predominant aspects in the end-of-life experience investigated in a sample of Mexican Americans (Gelfand, Balcazar, Parzuchowski, & Lenox, 2001). The study validated the need to focus on the role of religious institutions in Mexican American culture, where spirituality and religion are strong influences in the life experience. Pain and suffering are common aspects in the experience of death and dying. If the nurse and other health care providers do not understand Hispanic values about causes of pain, illness, and suffering, these experiences may go unrecognized or untreated (Valente, 2004). Differences in the expression of pain and suffering may exist even in the same culture. Hispanic males tend to be stoic and uncomplaining (Kemp, 2005), whereas among the women, moaning and crying are accepted means of expression of discomfort and pain.

Implications for Nursing Care

Of primary importance for the nurse caring for Mexican American clients is the concept that family values and roles are paramount in the client's treatment and recovery. Although the male head of the family should be consulted in health care decision making for other family members, clinicians need to focus more on engaging extended family and community supports. The inclusion of the entire family, both immediate and extended members, in the assessment, planning, and implementation of nursing care is critical if treatment is to be effective. Rather than viewing a large family who wishes to be with the client as an annoyance and frustration to staff, the nurse should discuss with the family how visits can be planned so that care can still be delivered and the client can obtain needed rest.

The family needs to be partners in the provision of care to clients. By integrating them into the provision of care, the family can provide assistance in feeding, bathing, or walking the client. Allowing the family to participate in the client's care builds trust and respect and encourages compliance and support for discharge planning and teaching. On the issue of medical information, Mexican American clients and families may not agree on who has the right to have this information. For example, in one study by researchers at the University of California, only two thirds (65%) of the Mexican Americans in the study believed that the patient should be told if there was a diagnosis of metastatic cancer. The other respondents believed that the giving of information and the decision-making responsibility and information should rest with the family (Ethics: Cultures Diverge, 1995). Thus, Mexican American clients and families may not agree on who has the right to have medical information.

When the nurse is experiencing difficulty in getting a client to follow a particular medical regimen, the nurse may suggest that the client solicit the opinions of other family members regarding proposed actions. This will demonstrate that the nurse understands the importance of the family in regard to health matters. Nurses can encourage Mexican American clients to use health-promoting behaviors, with the rationale that the family cares about their health and will support them in meeting their goals (Kerr & Richey, 1990). Furthermore, the nurse's actions should help to build a relationship of trust between the nurse and the client. Burk, Wieser, and Keegan (1995) note that to facilitate provision of culturally sensitive care to Mexican Americans at a birthing center on the Mexican border, prospective certified nurse-midwives are evaluated for their understanding of and desire to work with this particular population. New staff are required to read culture-specific information and are encouraged to attend Spanish classes to develop a familiarity with the language. Knowledge of the client's culture has been found to be a positive dimension in the client–provider process and important in providing culturally appropriate care.

TIME

Mexican Americans are usually characterized as having a present orientation of time and as being unable or reluctant to incorporate the future into their plans. An example of this orientation is that some Mexican Americans may spend several years' savings on an important religious festival. Also, the Mexican custom of the siesta in some ways represents the belief that rest (or the present) has a priority over continued work that could produce monies to safeguard the future. Individuals with this present orientation of time may appear to lack practical concern about the future or the need for deferring gratification to a future time. Many investigators believe that this orientation restrains Mexican Americans from upward social mobility. In addition, some regard the present orientation of time as a barrier to assimilation and integration into the mainstream of American culture. However, of particular significance in terms of time orientation is the fact that Mexican Americans place more value on the quality of interpersonal relationships than on the length of time in which they take place (Marín & Marín, 1991).

Khoury and Thurmond (1978) found few differences in the time perceptions of Mexican American and White American college students, despite the fact that the Mexican American students in the study were still maintaining cultural ties with the Mexican American culture. However, these findings cannot be generalized to Mexican Americans who are more immersed in their culture and less educated.

Implications for Nursing Care

Flexibility and creativity may be needed in order to work with differences in time orientation. It is important for the nurse to remember that personal ethnocentric attitudes toward time may negatively affect the planning of care for clients with a different time orientation. In the Western culture, health care settings tend to be future oriented, with weekly appointments, long-term treatment goals, and strict adherence to schedules. Scheduling can pose a barrier because patients and their families may not be able to leave work during the day to attend regular appointments. Because health care scheduling tends to be fixed and rigid, and traditional Hispanic culture time orientation tends to be more present oriented, Mexican American patients may encounter difficulties when trying to work within the schedules of the medical setting. A Mexican American client may be late for an appointment not because of reluctance or lack of respect but because the client may be more concerned with a current activity than with the activity of planning ahead to be on time. This concept, known as *elasticity,* implies that future-oriented activities can be recovered but present-oriented activities cannot.

Because Mexican Americans are likely to be present-time oriented, the nurse may experience difficulties in planning and implementing health care measures such as long-term planning. In addition, the nurse may experience difficulties in explaining why and when medications should be taken. When working with a client who has a condition such as hypertension, it is important for the nurse to emphasize the effects of this condition, as well as short-term problems that can occur if the medication is not taken on time. Emphasis on short-term problems is more likely to be beneficial because it is more likely to get results. Because Mexican Americans are present-time oriented, their perceptions and understanding of acute and chronic illness may be affected.

ENVIRONMENTAL CONTROL

Locus of Control

Many Mexican Americans have an external locus of control, believing that external forces operate in many social and individual circumstances. Some Mexican Americans perceive life as being under the constant influence of the divine will. There is also a fatalistic belief that one is at the mercy of the environment and has little control over what happens. Associated with this view is the belief that personal efforts are unlikely to influence the outcome of a situation; thus, some Mexican Americans do not believe that they are personally responsible for present or future successes or failures. This belief may precipitate feelings of hopelessness regarding the future and positive change. The effect of this fatalistic belief was noted in Sennott-Miller's (1994) study of Hispanic women who had difficulty maintaining cancer-prevention activities.

Effect on Personal Control. Data from transcultural studies have found that people with a belief in external control can be expected to have more distress as an outcome of this view (Hough, 1985). On the other hand, Mirowsky and Ross (1984) noted that distress was not observed in the Mexican culture as an outcome of a belief in an external locus of control. They also suggested that although distress can result from strong family ties, it is offset by the family's strong support and responsibility to the individual. A consequence of strong family ties is that the individual may have a greater feeling of personal control, which in turn deters anxiety. When Mexican Americans experience pain, they value stoicism and self-control. Calvillo and Flaskerud (1991) suggest that crying and moaning in these clients may serve the purpose of relieving pain rather than communicating that the pain is intolerable and intervention is desired.

Research has shown that health practices among Mexican Americans are influenced by psychosocial variables hypothesized in various models of health beliefs and behavior. Duffy, Rossow, and Hernandez (1996) reported that when the Health-Promoting Lifestyle Profile (HPLP)

was administered, Mexican American women had the highest total scores of all minority groups but lower scores than all predominantly White groups. HPLP self-actualization and interpersonal support scores were the highest subscale scores. Although Mexican American women in this study tended to practice more health-promoting lifestyle behaviors than other minority groups, it was also noted that a high number of the women worked in professional health care–related fields. However, their scores were lower than those reported for predominantly White groups, an indication that Mexican American women may lag substantially behind their White counterparts in the practice of "heart-healthy" lifestyles, even when the influence of socioeconomic status was removed. The exercise subscale was the lowest score for all groups, including minorities. Age, education, self-efficacy, health locus of control (internal and powerful others), and current health status made statistically significant contributions to the HPLP subscale scores. The Theory of Reasoned Action was tested by Poss (2000) in Mexican farm workers; this study revealed that certain constructs in the model predicted participation in health screenings for tuberculosis (TB), for which this group is at risk because of recent immigration history and exposure. Friedman-Koss, Crespo, Bellantoni, and Anderson (2002) noted that whereas 37% of all women over 60 use hormone replacement therapy, 24% of Mexican American women do so. On the other hand, Borrell, Lynch, Neighbors, Burt, and Gillespie (2002) conducted a study of prevalence and predictors of periodontitis. In a study of African-Americans, Mexican Americans, and non-Hispanic Whites, Mexican Americans had periodontal health profiles closer to those of non-Hispanic Whites than did African-Americans. These findings have significant implications for health professionals in terms of education related to health-promotion activities for Mexican Americans.

Skaff, Mullan, Fisher, and Chesla (2003) studied a sample of 74 Latino Americans and 115 European Americans with type 2 diabetes to determine if a sense of control was related to health. A model of control beliefs, disease-management behaviors, and health indicators was tested with two measures of control beliefs—one diabetes-specific (diabetes self-efficacy) and one global (mastery)—which were used to examine effects on management behaviors (diet and exercise) and on health (hemoglobin A_{1c} and general health). Results indicated that the relationship between control and management behaviors varied by measure of control and by group. For Latino participants, global mastery was related to management behaviors, whereas self-efficacy was related to such behaviors among European Americans. This study provides support for a diversified approach to control, behavior, and health, particularly in dealing with minority populations. A study on parental locus of control (PLOC) among parents of clinic-referred Mexican American preschoolers demonstrated that referred Mexican American parents exhibited a more external PLOC than non-referred Mexican American parents across a number of domains. Thus, similar to non-Hispanic Whites, preschoolers' behavioral problems are associated with an external PLOC among Mexican Americans (McCabe, Goehring, Yeh, & Lau, 2008).

Health Care Beliefs

Health care beliefs are determined by several factors inherent in an individual's history, environments, cultural norms and patterns, mores, and folkways. In turn, health behaviors are influenced by these health beliefs and determine how clients respond to interventions designed to improve health behaviors. Keller and Fleury (2006) reviewed literature on physical activity in Hispanic women and found that factors such as individual, social, and cultural influences can serve as promoting as well as hindering factors to physical activity among this group. For instance, self-efficacy and social support tend to be positively related to increased physical activity among Mexican American women; however, the likelihood of engaging in physical activity may be modulated by traditional values that consider this inappropriate for older women. This review supported the notion that ethnic groups cannot be considered heterogenous based upon a common language and that socioeconomic factors influence health behaviors significantly (Keller & Fleury, 2006).

The cultural belief in external locus of control influences the manner in which some Mexican Americans view health. Some Mexican Americans believe that health may be the result of good luck or a reward from God for good behavior. For some Mexican Americans, health represents a state of equilibrium in the universe wherein the forces of "hot," "cold," "wet," and "dry" must be balanced. This concept is believed to have originated with the early Hippocratic theory of health and the four humors. According to the Hippocratic theory, the body humors—blood, phlegm, black bile, and yellow bile—vary in both temperature and moisture (Harwood, 1971). Persons who subscribe to this theory believe that health exists only when these four humors are in balance. Thus, health can be maintained by diet and other practices that keep the four humors in balance. Illness, on the other hand, is believed to be misfortune or bad luck, a punishment from God for evil thoughts or actions, or a result of the imbalance of hot and cold or wet and dry. Cox (1986) found that a large number of elderly Hispanics attributed their health problems to old age and therefore did not seek any type of intervention.

Theory of Hot and Cold and Perception of Illness. One category of disease is hot and cold imbalance, in which illness is believed to be caused by prolonged exposure to hot or cold. To cure the illness, the opposite quality of the causative agent is applied to assimilate the hot or cold. Included in this category are illnesses that, rather than being caused by temperature itself, are associated with hot or cold aspects of substances found in medicines, elements, air, food, and bodily organs. Treatment is focused on such things as suggestions, practical advice, prayers, or indigenous herbs, with the goal of reestablishing balance (Juckett, 2013).

Although cold is believed to harm the body from without, excesses of heat developed from within the body itself and extending outward are believed to be related to such diseases as cancer, rheumatism, TB, and paralysis (Juckett, 2013) (Box 9-1). The focus of heat in the body is the stomach, whereas the head, arms, and legs are believed to be cool. Hot illnesses, such as skin ailments and fever, may be visible to the outside world. Many of the disorders caused by hot and cold imbalances are digestive in nature, which is related to the fact that an imbalance of hot and cold foods is believed to be damaging and suggests that to ensure good health, both hot and cold foods must be taken into the body. The quality of the food eaten determines whether diarrhea is a hot or cold condition. If the stool is green or yellow, the diarrhea is hot and the remedy is cold tea; if the stool is white, the diarrhea is cold and the remedy is hot tea.

Hot and cold are also associated with other aspects of life. Symbolically, cold is related to things that menace the individual, whereas hot is related to warmth and reassurance. In addition to air, water is seen as a source for cold. If an individual has participated in an activity that is considered hot, this person will not go near water because of its association with death. (At death, blood is believed to be turned into water.) The effort to balance hot and cold forces in the Mexican American belief system reflects the relationship between the individual and the environment. It is a symbolic attempt to attain a social order that is equitable (Juckett, 2013).

Theory of Hot and Cold and Effects on Growth and Development. Hot and cold Box 9-1 have symbolic significance for the nature and process of reproduction (Greene, 2007). During pregnancy, a woman may be advised not to eat hot foods. On the other hand, during menstruation or after childbirth, a woman might be told to avoid cold foods or avoid taking a bath. Infertility is associated with a "cold" womb, lack of intimacy, and rejection. A pregnant woman is believed to have an especially warm body, and to dissipate the warmth, she should bathe often and take short walks (Currier, 1966). The idea that warmth relates to intimacy follows in the relationship of

BOX 9-1 Hot–Cold Conditions, Foods, and Medicines and Herbs

Hot Conditions	Cold Conditions
Fever	Cancer
Infection	Pneumonia
Diarrhea	Malaria
Kidney problems	Joint pain
Rashes	Menstrual period
Skin ailments	Teething
Sore throat	Earache
Liver problems	Rheumatism
Ulcers	Tuberculosis
Constipation	Stomach cramps

Hot Foods	Cold Foods
Chocolate	Fresh vegetables
Cheese	Tropical fruits
Temperate-zone fruit	Dairy products
Eggs	Meats such as goats, fish, chicken
Peas	Honey
Onions	Cod
Aromatic beverages	Raisins
Hard liquor	Bottled milk
Oils	Barley water
Meats such as beef, waterfowl, mutton	
Goat's milk	
Cereal grains	
Chili peppers	

Hot Medicines and Herbs	Cold Medicines and Herbs
Penicillin	Orange flower water
Tobacco	Linden
Ginger root	Sage
Garlic	Milk of magnesia
Cinnamon	Bicarbonate of soda
Anise	
Vitamins	
Iron preparations	
Cod-liver oil	
Castor oil	
Aspirin	

Adapted from Wilson, H., Kneisl, C. (1996). *Psychiatric nursing* (ed. 5). Menlo Park, CA: Addison-Wesley.

mother and child. If a mother rejects her child, she is subject to an emotionally based disease called *bilis*, which can cause the infant to have chronic headaches and permanent injury. This belief indicates that the child may display chronic malnutrition, which Currier (1966) relates to a lack

of affection and support. Nursing of the child is also related to hot and cold characteristics (Galanti, 2008). A diminished milk flow is believed to result from coldness, whereas warmth is believed to increase the flow. An excess of warmth causes the child to become ill because the milk curdles and becomes indigestible.

Ensuring that there is a balance between hot and cold contributes to childrearing practices where worry over exposure to cold is mitigated by practices to promote warmth. During the first year of life, a child is kept physically close to the mother, either by being wrapped in her shawl or by sleeping in a bed next to her. This cultural practice has come under scrutiny because of concerns over the potential for infant death. An increase in infant bed sharing has been reported in Hispanic families, particularly those with lower household incomes and lower maternal education (Colson et al., 2013).

Folk Medicine

Use of folk medicine and folk practitioners is considered one of the most important variables leading to the underutilization of Western medicine by Mexican Americans (Ericksen, 2006; Lopez, 2005). The belief that health is a matter of chance and controlled by forces in nature is the basis of folk medicine. Folk medicine as practiced by Mexican Americans combines elements of the European Roman Catholic view and the view of the original Indians of Mexico. These beliefs have led to unique ways of accounting for physical and mental illnesses and their consequences and to unique methods of dealing with illnesses. This belief and practice system regarding health care is indigenous to the Mexican American community and is known as *curanderismo* (Andrews, Ybarra, & Matthews, 2013). Within this folk medicine system, illness is viewed from a religious and social context rather than the medical-scientific perspective of the dominant Western society (Lopez, 2005).

Types of Folk Practitioners. Operating within the curanderismo folklore system of beliefs and practices are several levels of healers. The first healer sought out is a member of the family; if the case is or becomes more complicated, healers within the community are sought out. Lopez (2005), in a study of 73 women with Latina surnames who were enrolled in a U.S. graduate social work program, found that between 20% and 40% had used some type of folk practitioner for their health care. Several levels of folk healers are described here, beginning with the lowest level, the family healer.

Family Folk Healer. The first person to be consulted at the time of illness is a key family member who is respected for her knowledge of folk medicine. This individual may be a wife, mother, grandmother, or other revered elderly relative. The healing practices are passed down in the family from mother to daughter. If the client does not improve, an intermediary person usually directs the client to the *curandero,* or Mexican folk healer.

Yerbero. The *yerbero* (or *herbero*) is a folk healer who specializes in using herbs and spices for preventive and curative purposes. This person grows and distributes herbs and spices and explains how to use them effectively (Volpato, Godínez, & Beyra, 2009).

Curandero and Curandera. The more serious physical and mental or emotional illnesses are brought to the *curandero* (or *curandera,* if a female). The *curandero* perceives life as being under the consistent influence of the divine will. People are believed to be born as sinners, with death being the result of their sins. The central focus of these healers' treatment is relieving clients of their sins. Suffering is seen as a component of illness, and death is seen as failure to be cured of sin (Andrews et al., 2013). The *curandero* believes that water, food, and air are important to the maintenance of health. Imbalance of these elements, imbalance between God and man, and imbalance between hot and cold are believed to contribute to illness.

Curanderos see clients with a wide range of both physical and psychological symptoms, such as gastrointestinal distress, back pain, headache, fever, depression, anxiety, irritability, fatigue, hostility, shame, guilt, sexual problems, alcoholism, and the common folk diseases (Titus, 2014). The diagnosis is made after a thorough assessment of all aspects of the client's life, including the family and even the supernatural. The treatment is provided in a room in the *curandero*'s home that is decorated with much religious paraphernalia. Treatments used include massage, diet, rest, suggestions, practical advice, indigenous herbs, prayers, magic, and supernatural rituals. Although *curanderos* generally use white magic, there are times when they may resort to black magic because the cure is difficult.

The *curandero,* who is believed to have the God-given gift of healing and is a full-time specialist, is often consulted before medical contact is made or may be consulted concomitantly with a medical contact. The effectiveness of curanderos seems to be in their ability to use their personality and healing regalia to encourage hope and trust on the part of the client. The beliefs and practices of this healer are supported by the family and the community, which tends to strengthen the client's sense of control over the situation. *Curanderos* are often preferred over the medical community because they are personal, are less dehumanizing, know the family, and are an integral part of the Mexican American community. *Curanderos* in most cases

are thought to have power over witches because they are believed to heal through the power of God (Titus, 2014).

Brujos and Brujas (Witches). The level of healers called *witches* may not be sought out until other forms of healing have been tried. The practitioners of witchcraft use several kinds of magic. Black magic is practiced by both male witches (*brujos*) and female witches (*brujas*), and red magic and green magic are believed to empower a witch to solve love problems by assuming an animal form. As mentioned previously, white magic is practiced by a *curandero,* is considered good magic, and is used in folk healing (Lopez, 2005). A motive for witchcraft may be hatred, jealousy, or envy. To cure, witches may use food or drink, imitative magic (such as dolls), evil air, or animal metamorphosis to bewitch (Wanderer & Rivera, 1986). There are many superstitions adhered to in this healing mode; for example, keeping black animals protects against witchcraft.

Among adult Mexican Americans, recourse to traditional healers is commonly encountered along with the use of Western medicine. The strongest predictors of use of traditional healers is limited English proficiency and dissatisfaction with medical practice (Andrews et al., 2013). Treatments involve traditional rituals, social reintegration, and penance (Lopez, 2005). The following are common folk illnesses observed among Mexican-Americans.

Folk-Related Illnesses. Concepts of disease among Mexican Americans relate to the negative effects of intensely emotional states and experiences, dislocation or malfunctions of organs or body parts, infant susceptibility, and magical thinking. Common childhood folk illnesses include *empacho, mal de ojo,* and *mollera caída* (Juckett, 2013). Folk illnesses have been linked to morbidity and mortality (Baer et al., 2003; Bledsoe, 2009).

Caída de la Mollera. *Caída de la mollera* refers to a fallen fontanel in infants caused by a fall, by rough bouncing of the child, or by removal of the nipple from the baby's mouth with too much force. This condition is viewed as an imbalance between the fontanel and the palate that blocks the passage of foods and liquids. Associated with *caída de la mollera* are the symptoms of inability to suck or grasp the nipple, vomiting, diarrhea, fever, restlessness, and crying spells (Juckett, 2013).

Before seeking out a physician, mothers often seek out older women in the community who seem to know how to treat this problem. Suggested remedies include pressing against the palate from inside the mouth, praying, applying eggs to the head and then pulling hairs, and holding the child with the head down. Lopez (2005) has noted that this condition is usually caused by severe dehydration and that correct medical treatment with intravenous fluids is essential.

Mal Ojo (Evil Eye). As mentioned earlier, *mal ojo* occurs when an individual who is believed to possess a special power admires or covets the child of another and looks at but does not touch the child. *Mal ojo* at times is associated with witchcraft and black magic. This condition is characterized by headaches, high fever, crying, diarrhea, restlessness, irritability, loss of weight and sleep, and sunken eyes (Lopez, 2005). The cure for the problem is to mix a hen's egg with water and place this under the head of the child's bed, which supposedly drives the bad influence out of the child's body. Another remedy is to have the person believed to be the source of the evil eye touch the afflicted individual. It is believed that the child will deteriorate, with severe coughing and vomiting, and possibly die if not treated. Families are known not to bring children with this problem to physicians because they fear the physician will misdiagnose the child and the child's condition will worsen.

Empacho (Obstacle). Children suffering from *empacho* are believed to have a chunk of food that they are unable to pass, causing a lot of abdominal pain. They are taken to an older woman who possesses the knowledge to treat this problem. To diagnose the illness, the client is held face down by the skin of the back. During this procedure, if a crack is heard, the diagnosis is *empacho.* Treatment then consists of body massages around the back and waist, which are given to restore the body's balance of hot and cold; this, in turn, allows the food chunk to pass through the intestine (Juckett, 2013).

Susto (Magical Fright). *Susto* is commonly observed among adults experiencing stress. It is caused by a frightening experience or event and leads to the temporary loss of one's spirit from the body. This condition may even affect an unborn child if the mother is frightened. *Susto* is associated with childhood epilepsy, is seen more often in females, and if left untreated is believed to develop into TB or even death. Symptoms of *susto* include crying, insomnia, anorexia, restlessness, nightmares, stomachache, diarrhea, high fever, and involuntary tics. Treatment for *susto* involves holding a ceremony known as *barrida,* in which a *curandero* sweeps the body with fresh herbs while the healer recites ritual prayers. A more severe form of *susto* is *espanto.* Studies have shown that individuals who suffer *espanto* long term have higher mortality and morbidity indices than those who suffer the less severe form (Permanente, 2001).

Nervios. *Nervios* refers to restlessness, insomnia, loss of appetite, headaches, and nonspecific aches and pains. This is linked to chronic experience of negative life circumstances, particularly revolving around interpersonal relationships (Juckett, 2013). *Nervios* is described as a culture-bound syndrome in the *Diagnostic and Statistical Manual of Mental Disorders,* fourth edition (DSM-IV) (American Psychiatric Association [APA], 1994). There is evidence that Mexican Americans would seek a medical provider for *nervios* but would seek folk healers or use home remedies for *susto* (Lopez, 2005).

Religious Views. Roman Catholicism is the predominant religion practiced by Mexican Americans. Common religious practices are baptism, confirmation, communion, weddings, and funerals. During times of crisis, Mexican Americans may rely on the priest and family for prayers. When a family member is ill, rituals that are practiced include making promises, lighting candles, visiting shrines, and offering prayers (Lopez, 2005).

Roman Catholic Mexican Americans may have beliefs that are influenced by ancient Indian practices of witchcraft and voodoo. As a result, some Mexican Americans may believe in demons. Incorporated in this system is a belief in witchcraft practices to manipulate evil forces. In the Mexican American community, witchcraft is called *brujería* and is seen as a magical or supernatural illness and occasionally as an emotional illness. *Brujería* has no scientific basis and is believed to be precipitated by opponents using the evil forces of hexes and spells. Symptoms of *brujería* include paranoia, delusions, hallucinations, feelings of being controlled by another person, mania, perverted and fitful behavior, depression, suspicion, and anxiety. Motives for witchcraft include envy, vengeance, hatred, and jealousy (Lopez, 2005).

Health Care Pluralism. Health care providers tend to consider folk beliefs and the Western biomedical viewpoint of health dualistically—"as mutually exclusive and in competition with one another," according to Kiesser, McFadden, and Belliard (2006), who also noted, "Patients, on the other hand, tend to make truly pluralistic health care decisions—moving freely between folk beliefs and biomedicine based on what they can access, what they can relate to, and what they believe works." Health care providers who understand, appreciate, and integrate into their practice how their patients make use of folk-based healing practices and beliefs with biomedical beliefs will maximize health care for their clients (Feldmann, Wiemann, Sever, & Hergenroeder, 2008).

Migrant Mexican American women have been reported to promote healthy behaviors, diagnose sick family members, and prescribe home remedies (Waldstein, 2010). These practices stem from a long tradition of self-care and family-care practices. There is also an increase in use of traditional healing practices among Mexican immigrants who have undocumented family members. The low cost of alternative health practices may be a primary factor in the choice to use traditional healers in lieu of Western health care providers (Andrews et al., 2013).

Implications for Nursing Care

It is important for the nurse to be aware that use of alternative therapies from Mexico is prevalent among Mexican Americans. Lopez (2005) reported that 44% of Mexican Americans in a study in the Texas Rio Grande Valley reported using alternative practitioners one or more times during the previous year. The most commonly sought therapies are herbal medicine, spiritual healing and prayer, massage, relaxation techniques, chiropractic, and visits to a curandero. The majority (66%) indicated that they never reported visits to alternative practitioners to their established primary health care provider. Lopez (2005) reported similar use of folk remedies in relatively acculturated Latina graduate students and the pluralistic belief in biomedical-based health care and folk medicine remedies.

The belief held by many Mexican Americans that external forces control the outcome of circumstances can influence adherence with medical or health care recommendations. This perspective may influence the practice of wellness programs in the U.S. health care system, such as smoking cessation, addiction programs, prenatal care, health-promotion activities, and chronic disease treatment by Mexican Americans. Because the traditional healing system of *curanderismo* incorporates religious beliefs, some Mexican Americans may also believe that they are more in touch with the divine will, and therefore the origin and healing of illness, when they enter the health care system. The nurse should understand that Mexican Americans will have more respect for the caregiver who accepts the spiritual and folk basis of their health beliefs.

The nurse should observe how the client is implementing health management; in particular, client self-management in chronic disease is key to the success of care. In cases of nonadherence to the management protocol, the nurse should discuss any issues with the client and family to determine if the basis for nonadherence is folk beliefs. For instance, beliefs regarding hot and cold characteristics will affect how the client accepts some of the treatment plan. The nurse might inquire if the condition is considered a hot or cold disease. The client may have some definite beliefs about this and about whether the medical treatment can restore the hot–cold balance within the body. If the treatment is incongruent with folk beliefs, the nurse should attempt to find compromises or solutions that will resolve the incongruence, and allow the client to maintain his or her belief system, while at the same time adhering to the prescribed medical or health care management. One can expect the older client or first-generation immigrant to be more attached to these beliefs; therefore, focusing health teaching on younger family members may be more useful in establishing adherence. Communication between the nurse and client enhances adherence (Miller & Davidhizar, 2001).

The healers in the folk medicine system are people with whom the Mexican Americans have established relationships and with whom they can easily communicate. These healers know and can treat the folk illnesses that the uninitiated health care worker may not recognize. It is helpful for the nurse to understand the respect this culture has for the *curandero,* who is often consulted simultaneously with the physician or nurse. The long-term goal of a nurse working in a Mexican American community should be to understand the folk medicine beliefs and to try to establish a relationship with the *curandero* in the hope of influencing acceptance and understanding of the rationale for modern health care practices and thereby gaining the community's confidence (Titus, 2014).

The nurse should recognize that the *curandero* is involved in relieving people of their sins so that they can experience healing and that a spiritual perspective is usually an integral part of the U.S. health care system. One might compare the healer's influence in this ethnic group to that of the clergy in the dominant U.S. society, wherein mutual cooperation is focused on meeting clients' spiritual and physical needs. Mexican American clients also need to be encouraged to practice their religious beliefs and to receive supportive visits from the clergy. Acknowledging the client's reliance on the folk health care system as well as on his or her religious beliefs and medical assistance will promote a more holistic focus for nursing care.

It is important to recognize the strong influence of hot and cold imbalance in folk beliefs. Some of these healing beliefs and practices are practical, such as massage, prayer, listening, or the application of cold for a fever. However, some practices can lead to missed clues for serious conditions that do not respond to these remedies, such as prolonged diarrhea, vomiting, dehydration, parasites, or malnutrition in children. For example, the nurse should suspect that malnutrition in a 1-year-old child may be caused by the practice of separating the child from the mother at the time of weaning. Teaching the mother about the child's physical and emotional needs may improve the malnutrition. When dealing with children, Leininger (2002) cautions the nurse to touch the children so that if the parents fear the evil eye, the cultural remedy of touch will cure the condition.

In dealing with folk-related diseases, the nurse needs to understand perceived causes for these conditions, for example, environmental influences, such as *caída de la mollera* or *empacho,* or evil influences, such as *mal ojo* or *susto.* Because these diseases are considered indigenous to the culture, they are usually seen and treated first by the *curandero.* Patients coming to the nurse's attention with these conditions probably have had these symptoms for a while and have already been treated unsuccessfully by the *curandero.* The nurse's physical assessment needs to be thorough. Cultural variables should be included in the assessment. In managing pain, important variables to assess are cultural, psychological, and social factors that affect attitudes and responses to pain and how pain is reported. Rather than showing disrespect for the folk healer, the nurse should develop the relationship with the client in such a way as to maintain the support of the folk healer. Respect should also be shown for amulets that the client might wear to protect against the evil eye or evil spirits. For example, the *mano milagroso* ("miraculous hand") is worn by many people of Mexican origin for luck and to ward off evil. Amulets worn by persons from Mexico may have red yarn attached (Spector, 2004). The nurse should allow the client to continue to wear the amulet rather than attempt to take it away. The nurse should appreciate that eating eggs and bread, drinking tea, and sleeping are methods that some persons from Mexico believe are effective to maintain health, and these beliefs should be respected (Spector, 2004). The nurse should take an integrative approach that allows the client to use and understand alternative health practices and biomedical practices. Client education should take into account the pluralistic views of clients and foster access to health care strategies from multiple belief systems. Respect, caring, understanding, and patience should be the hallmarks of care (Juckett, 2013). Mexican American adults vary in their willingness to be involved in their treatment decisions. Some younger, more assimilated clients are frequently willing to participate in decision making but are less likely to ask for or refuse specific treatments, while others prefer to let their provider make the decisions. Most important, creating a mutually respectful client–provider relationship will foster client-centered care that enables the client to feel heard and understood (Juckett, 2013).

Many older Mexican American adults are most familiar with a patriarchal model of care and may benefit from efforts to strengthen the client–provider relationship in a transition to a model of care that emphasizes client-centeredness. Although it is important to encourage client involvement in treatment decisions, it is essential to remember that because differences in clients' willingness to engage in client-directed care may exist, the use of shared decision making should be considered.

Skin Color

The skin color of Mexican Americans can vary from a natural tan to dark brown. Persons with lighter color have more Spanish ancestry, whereas darker-skinned persons have more Indian ancestry. It is more difficult to recognize vasodilatation or vasoconstriction in the darker-skinned client, in whom vasoconstriction and anemia are manifested as an ashen color rather than a bluish coloration. The mongolian spots (areas of darker skin found on the sacral area) found on infants usually disappear by 4 years of age. The hair of Mexican Americans is usually dark and may be curly and woolly, straight, or wavy (Monrroy, 1983).

Biological Variations and Susceptibility to Disease

Health disparities among subgroups within American society are influenced by many determinants, primarily socioeconomic and cultural. Significant health disparities among Mexican Americans have been observed; since this is one of the major ethnic groups in the United States, this phenomenon cannot be overlooked.

Diabetes. In 2007, about 2 million Mexican Americans had been diagnosed with diabetes, composing 10.2% of all Mexican Americans. On average, Mexican Americans are 1.9 times more likely to have diabetes than non-Hispanic Whites of similar age. Particularly common among middle-aged and older Mexican Americans, about 25% to 30% age 50 years or over have either diagnosed or undiagnosed diabetes (National Center for Health Statistics, 2010). Compared to non-Hispanic white adults, the risk of diagnosed diabetes was 18% higher among Asian Americans, 66% higher among Hispanics, and 77% higher among non-Hispanic blacks. Among Hispanics compared to non-Hispanic White adults, the risk of diagnosed diabetes was about the same for Cubans and for Central and South Americans, 87% higher for Mexican Americans, and 94% higher for Puerto Ricans (Centers for Disease Control and Prevention [CDC], 2014). Having risk factors for diabetes increases the chance that a Mexican American, as in all populations, will develop diabetes; risk factors seem to be more common among Hispanics than non-Hispanic Whites. These factors include a family history of diabetes, gestational diabetes, impaired glucose tolerance, hyperinsulinemia and insulin resistance, obesity, and physical inactivity. Higher rates of the diabetes complications nephropathy (kidney disease), retinopathy (eye disease), and peripheral vascular disease have been documented in studies of Mexican Americans, whereas lower rates of myocardial infarctions (heart attacks) have been found (CDC, 2014b).

Diabetes affects 8.5% of the adults in New Mexico (New Mexico Department of Health, 2010). Approximately 17% of people age 40 and over in New Mexico have diabetes (CARES Needs Assessment, 2003). Diabetes tends to be more severe in Hispanics than non-Hispanic Whites. Diabetes occurs at a younger age, more often requires insulin to be controlled, results in more limb amputations, contributes to eye disease, is responsible for a six times higher incidence of kidney failure, and results in a death rate two to four times the rate for non-Hispanic Whites (Otiniano, Black, Ray, Du, & Markides, 2002; Vásquez, 1997). The adverse impact of uncontrolled diabetes is compounded by lack of access to primary care and preventive services and by education of less than 12 years (Otiniano et al., 2002; Philis-Tsimikas et al., 2004). In a study of the impact of diabetes on employment and earnings outcomes of middle-aged and older Mexican Americans in the Southwest, Bastida and Pagan (2002) found men had a lower probability of employment but no effect on earnings, whereas women had lowered productivity and earnings but no significant change in their probability of employment. In a study by Luyas (1989), low-income Mexican American women with type 2 diabetes explained diabetes onset in terms of economic and family problems. Eid and Kraemer (1998) interviewed Mexican Americans with type 2 diabetes residing in California. Concerns about the cost were particularly expressed by the uninsured. Subjects tended to blend the treatment plan of conventional medicine with native customs. Mexican Americans with diabetes who had less than 12 years of education were more likely to report diabetic complications than those with more education. Both Philis-Tsimikas et al. (2004) and Davidson (2003) report the effectiveness of nurse-managed care for diabetic Hispanic patients in California.

Hypertension. The percentage of adults with prehypertension among Mexican Americans was increased from 23.7% in 2003 and 2004 to 31.4% in 2011 and 2012. However, the percentages of Stage I and Stage II hypertension among Mexican Americans were reduced from 40.6% and 25.1% in 2003 and 2004 to 39.7% and 15% in 2011 and 2012 due to increase of treatment, respectively (Yoon et al., 2015). A new statistics report in 2015 indicates Mexican Americans have lower risk of developing hypertension than non-Hispanic Whites and Blacks (CDC, 2015; Mozaffarian et al., 2015). Nelson, Norris, and Mangione (2002) found that even when Mexican Americans were diagnosed with high cholesterol requiring medication, they were less likely than their White

counterparts to take cholesterol-lowering agents. However, the percentage of people who received treatment among Mexican Americans has been increased from 55.6% between in 2006 to 71.5% in 2012 (Yoon et al., 2015). In a study using census figures from 1969 to 1971 and 1979 to 1981, Stern et al. (1987) reported less decline in the death rates of Mexican American men from total ischemic heart disease and myocardial infarction than in the death rates of other men.

Pernicious Anemia. Pernicious anemia, most often seen in the elderly, has been shown to occur in those of Latin American origin at a younger age than in White patients (Carmel, Johnson, & Weiner, 1987). Evidence shows that a low socioeconomic status has a strong effect on hemoglobin and hematocrit levels and that, given similar socioeconomic conditions, Mexican Americans tend to have higher hematocrit levels than their White counterparts have (Overfield, 1995).

Melanoma. Hispanics in the Southwest were found to have a poorer prognosis with melanoma because such melanoma arose from the palms, sublingual regions, mucous membranes, and soles; were more advanced in stage; occurred in older people; and metastasized (Black, Goldhahn, & Wiggins, 1987).

Communicable Diseases. Approximately 85% of the health problems common to Mexican Americans involve communicable diseases (National Center for Health Statistics, 2002) including respiratory tract infections, diarrhea, skin disorders, nutritional problems (particularly during the first year of life), macroscopic parasitosis, and amebiasis. One of the most severe medical problems facing nations throughout the world is TB, which is believed to occur in areas where there are crowded living conditions; low-income, substandard housing; and inadequate health care, such as that which existed for many in Mexico. In the United States, the population that is most at risk for the incidence and transmittal of TB is newly arrived immigrants, including Mexicans (Hood & Jackson, 1989; Phipps, 1993). Findings from a study of 7386 individuals revealed that higher prevalences of latent TB infections have been observed in foreign-born residents (18.7%), non-Hispanic Blacks/African-Americans (7.0%), Mexican Americans (9.4%), and individuals living in poverty (6.1%) (Bennett et al., 2008). Because there is a high prevalence of TB in Mexico, it is believed that Mexican Americans may have a predisposition to a higher prevalence of TB than other Americans (Phipps, 1993). McQuillan, Kruszon-Moran, Deforest, Chu, and Wharton (2002) noted that adult Mexican Americans were slightly less likely than other

Americans to have protective levels of antibody to diphtheria and tetanus.

Hepatitis C. Hepatitis C has also been found to occur at a higher rate among Mexican Americans. Although the rate among Whites in the United States is 1.5%, among Mexican Americans it is 2.1% (Cronin, 1997). Although an estimated 3.9 million persons in the United States have hepatitis C virus, this blood-borne virus, which can kill, was not identified until 1989. Since blood banks began screening for hepatitis C in 1990, the rate of new infections has declined. Although half of those who obtained the disease before 1990 are believed to have received it from blood, the other half probably did so by sharing needles or straws to inject drugs (Cronin, 1997). It is estimated that more people could die from the complications of hepatitis C than from acquired immunodeficiency syndrome (AIDS) (Cronin, 1997). Some 70% of the cases result in liver damage that leads to death. Once the disorder is diagnosed, lifestyle changes, such as avoiding alcohol, can prolong length and quality of life.

Childhood Obesity. In 2011 and 2012, the prevalence of overweight or obese (body mass index [BMI] for age ≥85th percentile of the CDC growth charts) for Hispanic children between 6 and 11 years old was 46.2%, which was higher than non-Hispanic Whites (29.4%) and non-Hispanic Blacks (38.1%) (Ogden, Carroll, Kit, & Flegal, 2014). In a classic study, Alexander and Blank (1988) suggested that the increasing incidence of obesity in Mexican American children may be a result of mothers believing that a fat baby is a healthy baby. The mothers in this study had a greater BMI than mothers in a control group did. These subjects also had "pushier" feeding practices with their children. To prevent the complications of adult obesity stemming from childhood obesity, nurses should identify mothers and their children who are at risk for obesity and encourage a weight-reduction program. The nurse should make an assessment of the potential need for nutritional education among Mexican American clients. Hispanic women may have cultural dietary variations prenatally. For example, antepartal cravings, including that for clay, are not denied. In the postpartum period, warm tea, broth, and corn gruel are acceptable foods, whereas citrus fruits, port (a wine), and tomatoes are avoided. It is believed harmful to eat and breastfeed simultaneously. The mother may believe stress and anger make bad milk, which makes a breastfeeding infant ill. Some Hispanics neutralize the bowel when weaning from breast to bottle by feeding only anise tea for 24 hours (White, Linhart, & Medley, 1996). Childhood obesity may lead to obesity in adulthood; 40.2% of Mexican American men 20 years and over are obese, compared to 45.2% of Mexican American women 20 years and older (CDC, 2014a).

HIV/AIDS. Nationwide, AIDS cases among Hispanics are occurring at triple the rate among non-Hispanics (National Center for Health Statistics, 2010). For Hispanic people, through 2008, the cumulative number of diagnosed AIDS cases was 180,061. Similarly, the total number of deaths reported from January 1999 through December 2008 was 81,793. The number of deaths has steadily risen in this vulnerable group. Among Hispanic men, the cumulative total of deaths through December 2001 was 67,557. For Hispanic males age 15 to 24, the number of deaths reported was 1373. For Hispanic women at all ages, the number of cumulative deaths reported through December 2001 was 14,236. The number of Hispanic women in the age range between 15 and 24 years—Mexican Americans are not listed separately—was 7, as compared with only 8 for Whites (National Center for Health Statistics, 2002). Because of the unsanitary working and housing conditions of migrant farmworkers and their limited opportunity to protect themselves, the opportunity for higher risk for human immunodeficiency virus (HIV) infection exists (Aplemis, 1996). According to the Centers for Disease Control and Prevention, Hispanics and Latinos make up 16% of the U.S. population but had 21% (9800) of all new HIV infections in 2010 (CIA, 2014). Marin (2003) reports an HIV prevention program in an American Hispanic community in which factors including marginalization, homophobia, poverty, and racism were addressed to increase feelings of empowerment.

Psychological Characteristics

Ethnic pride is an important cultural factor that needs to be considered in working with ethnic minority populations. Ethnic pride reflects positive feelings of connectedness and belongingness with regard to an individual's ethnic and cultural background, identity, and group. Although research on the relationship of ethnic pride to physical and mental health outcomes is limited, especially for Latino samples, a study involving ethnically diverse adolescents, including Mexican Americans, found that ethnic identity and cultural orientation mediate the relationship between perceived discrimination and depression. Specifically, when ethnic identity is strong, discrimination is not associated with depressive symptoms (Umaña-Taylor & Updegraff, 2007). The importance of family in the lives of Mexican Americans is well documented. Mexican Americans with depression often do not receive the help necessary to overcome depression (Interian, Martinez, Guarnaccia, Vega, & Escobar, 2007) and were likely to use psychotherapy or psychopharmacology (González et al.,

2010). Castro, Tein, and Kim (2009) found that family support mediated the relationship between ethnic pride and depression in Mexican American women. Keeler, Siegel, and Alvaro (2014) found that familistic values mediated the relationship between depressive symptoms and help-seeking behavior from family among Mexican Americans.

Various challenges confront Mexican Americans in this country. The process of immigration and acculturation can be stressful for Mexican Americans. Mexican immigrants to the United States experience significant stress related to being in a new and unfamiliar environment. The circumstances surrounding immigration can place Mexican immigrants at risk for psychological distress (Fortuna, Porche, & Alegria, 2008). Language barriers can lead to social isolation. Additionally, intergenerational tensions may occur as many Mexican Americans are confronted with traditional collectivist culture and the individualism valued by the majority culture in the United States, especially with the young generation (Donlan, 2011).

Discrimination in the United States has its psychological impact on families, especially for Mexican Americans. Several studies have documented the association between discrimination and mental health issues. Experiences of discrimination have been linked in Hispanics and Latinos to a range of negative mental health outcomes such as depression, anxiety, and psychological distress. For example, Crouter, Davis, Updegraff, Delgado, and Fortner (2006) found that high levels of discrimination are associated with poor mental health status among Mexican Americans. Specifically, depressive symptoms have been linked to discrimination among Mexican Americans. Racial discrimination has been identified as a risk factor in the development of PTSD and maladaptive alcohol use in persons of color (Cheng & Mallinckrodt, 2015). In another study, D'Anna-Hernandez, Aleman, and Flores (2015) found that perceived discrimination was positively associated with acculturative stress (cultural adaptation) and depression among Mexican American pregnant women. This is consistent with the findings of Beck (2006) indicating that Mexican American mothers have a higher rate of depression (17%) compared with the general population (10–15%). Little work has been done to address the role of acculturative stress on maternal mental health in this population.

There is a limited amount of research on mental health care for older Hispanic adults. Much of the current research focuses on adults aged 64 and younger. The research on older Hispanic mental health indicates their vulnerability as members of three minority groups: older adults, Hispanics, and the mentally ill. Mexican American elders are at risk for depression, and depression has been linked to chronic financial strain, gender (being a woman), and presence of health problems (Chiriboga, Jang, Banks, & Kim, 2007). According to Han, Gfroerer, Colpe, Barker, and Colliver (2011) Hispanic older adults were less likely to receive mental health services for serious psychological distress. The lifetime prevalence rates in older Hispanics for any depressive disorder is 16.4%, anxiety disorder 15.3%, and 26.8% for any psychiatric disorder (Jimenez, Alegría, Chen, Chan, & Laderman, 2010). With the growing aging population in this subgroup, additional research on mental health services in Hispanic older adults is warranted.

Alcohol and drug comorbidity poses a particular challenge for Mexican Americans. Because of their belief that alcohol consumption is a way of celebrating life, alcohol is consumed in all aspects of life and contributes to the increased incidence of accidents, violence, and unintentional injuries. Mexican Americans, together with Puerto Ricans, have the highest rate of binge drinking, driving under the influence of alcohol, alcohol abuse, and dependence (Caetano, Ramisetty-Mikler, & Rodriguez, 2008). Heavy drinking and drinking consequences (e.g., alcohol-related accidents) have been associated with racial discrimination and racial stigma among Hispanic community adults (Zemore, Karriker-Jaffe, Keithly, & Mulia, 2011). Vega, Scribney, and Achara-Abrahams (2003) examined co-occurrence of comorbid alcohol, drug, and non–substance use psychiatric disorders in a population sample of Mexican-origin adults for rural and urban areas of central California. They found that alcohol abuse or dependence with co-occurring psychiatric disorders is a primary disorder among Mexican-origin adult males, with a 7.5% lifetime prevalence. The co-occurring lifetime rates of alcohol and other drug disorders with non–substance use psychiatric disorders, or both, were 8.3% for men and 5.5% for women and were 12.3% for the U.S.-born and 3.5% for immigrants. Specifically, among male immigrants, dual diagnoses consist primarily of an alcohol disorder and a non–substance use disorder. Among U.S.-born males, dual diagnoses consist of alcohol abuse or dependence, an illicit drug abuse or dependence disorder, and an additional non–substance use disorder. Accelerating risk for alcohol and drug abuse or dependence disorders associated with either immigrant acculturation suggests that the prevalence of comorbidity involving alcohol and other drug disorders in the Mexican population will increase over time. In a study on the prevalence of psychiatric disorders, Alegría et al. (2007) found that lifetime psychiatric disorder was more prevalent among Latino American women. Dual diagnosis of substance abuse and other mental health disorders occurs at an earlier age for U.S.-born Latinos compared with Latino immigrants (Vega, Canino, Cao, & Alegria, 2009). The rate of drug use disorder among

U.S.-born Mexican Americans was 8.3 times greater than for foreign-born Mexican Americans, while for non-Hispanic Whites, the ratio was about 2.7:10. Other research has found, however, that when rates of substance abuse are considered among Mexican Americans, marijuana is the second most abused drug, with heroin and cocaine ranking third and fourth (Eden & Aguilar, 2004). Inhalants are also frequently abused among young Hispanics (Eden & Aguilar, 2004). Using a subset sample derived from an epidemiologic survey in the Mexican American Prevalence and Services Survey that examined the effects of immigration status on mental health status, Breslau et al. (2007) found that U.S.-born Mexican Americans had higher rates of any psychiatric disorder and PTSD than their foreign counterparts.

Estimates from the National Health and Nutrition Examination Survey indicate that 10% of Mexican Americans have had a major depressive episode (Jonas, Brody, Roper, & Narrow, 2003); another estimate suggests that depression is elevated in certain segments of the Mexican migrant farm workers to approximately 40% in the Upper Midwest (Magana & Hovey, 2003). Although immigrants tend to have lower rates of mental illness than their U.S. counterparts (Grant et al., 2004), evidence suggests that conditions such as anxiety disorder and substance abuse, in addition to depression, are common among immigrants from Mexico.

There is evidence that family structure and family functioning are important protective and risks factors for the Latinos. In Mexican American families, the family may serve as a buffering mechanism that encourages individual members to share, thereby reducing anxiety and stressful situations. For example, Bray, Adams, Getz, and Baer (2001) surveyed adolescent children in a 3-year longitudinal study to determine the influence of family cohesion, family conflict, and family separation on alcohol usage. They found that family cohesion was related to decrease in alcohol use whereas family separation and conflict increase alcohol use. Mexican Americans with psychiatric symptoms generally do not seek formal mental health services, unless the symptoms are seen as problematic (Bray, Adams, Getz & Baer, 2001). Mexican American women have been found to be more likely than men to access mental health (Kim, Jang, Chiriboga, Ma, & Schonfeld, 2010). Heilemann, Lee, and Kury (2002) found that women who spent all of their childhood years in Mexico before coming to the United States have a lower level of depressive symptoms and more satisfaction with life than women who were exposed to the United States in childhood. However, there is growing evidence that Mexican American adolescents may be at risk for depressive symptoms (Fornos et al., 2005). Social and cultural differences between the Mexican American and the dominant American society appear to be a recurring theme among Mexican Americans with symptoms of psychological disorders. Feelings of social isolation may serve to increase personal feelings of isolation. For some Mexican Americans, poverty, feelings of isolation, persecution, and discrimination can put them at risk for mental health problems. It is important for the nurse to be aware of factors that put Mexican Americans at risk for mental health problems. Knowledge of these factors will assist the nurse in making the diagnosis and planning preventive measures that will help lower the client's psychological risk.

Implications for Nursing Care

In providing health care education for the Mexican American, the nurse must remember to address cultural differences such as health values, ethnic care practices, family life patterns, dietary practices, the presence of insurance, and a usual source of care. It is also important to communicate the necessity of commitment by the whole family to making lifestyle changes if they are to be successful. Hispanic Americans in the San Antonio Heart Study were found to be less knowledgeable about preventing heart attacks and not engaging in risk-reducing behaviors as often as non-Hispanic Whites (Hazuda, Stern, Gaskill, Haffner, & Gardner, 1983). Derenowski (1990) noted that cardiovascular risk reduction and changes in lifestyle are necessary components of education for some Mexican Americans.

It is important for the nurse to recognize that the informal health care system in Mexico is generally composed of several elements, one of which is self-medication. In the early 1980s in Mexico, just as in the United States, prescriptions were required for all medications, such as antibiotics and steroids. However, during this time the sale of drugs in Mexico was uncontrolled, except for narcotics, barbiturates, and other addictive drugs. The pharmacist was, in effect, the chief physician's surrogate, and many Mexican American immigrants have been accustomed to receiving medication from a pharmacist without a prescription. In addition, some Mexican Americans consider medication to be always necessary and may not believe that their illness is being treated unless a particular medication is ordered.

The massive scale to which self-medication is practiced in Mexico is potentially dangerous (Anthony-Tkach, 1981; Cespedes & Larson, 2006; Gartin, Brewis, & Schwartz, 2010). To illustrate this point, in 1974 an outbreak of typhoid fever that was considered the worst in the century occurred in and around Mexico City. The causative agent was identified as chloramphenicol-resistant *Salmonella typhi*. Health officials in Mexico City believed that the indiscriminate use of antibiotics may have caused the organism to become resistant to the effects of chloramphenicol. It is important for the nurse to assess whether a

Mexican American client with a communicable disease is practicing self-medication for treatment. The assessment of the potential for self-medication as well as close follow-up study may be beneficial in reducing the drug-resistant causative organisms that can ensue from self-medication. The nurse who works with Mexican American clients with communicable diseases needs to emphasize that communicable diseases are preventable and that prompt care is essential to reducing exposure to, as well as morbidity from, communicable diseases.

Public health concerns are present in all ethnic minority groups, particularly those with recent immigration histories. This is particularly true among Mexican migrant farm workers in the United States, who, because of their highly mobile existence, may have difficulty accessing screening services for certain health conditions (Poss, 2000). In the U.S. population, 25% of all TB cases are Latino; however, they account for just 13% of the total population. The increased incidence of TB among Latinos has been attributed to the increasing number of Latino immigrants from the developing world, where TB is endemic (Ailinger, Armstrong, Nguyen, & Lasus, 2004). Because of the rise in TB, syphilis, and AIDS in Hispanic migrant workers, nurses should assess for these diseases and urge appropriate follow-up care. Nurses should be aware that the initial use of folk remedies can allow these diseases to spread and cause the delay of medical treatment.

Treatment of chemical dependency among Mexican Americans is a major challenge because of three central factors that inhibit treatment: integration of alcohol consumption within the Hispanic culture, the psychology of the Hispanic culture, and the family dynamics of the traditional Hispanic. Randolph, Stroup-Benham, Black, and Markides (1998) use the term *fiesta drinking* to refer to the consumption of large amounts of alcohol on special occasions. Drinking behavior is so ingrained in the Mexican culture that social functions ranging from baptisms to funerals generally include alcoholic beverages (Arrendondo, Weddige, Justice, & Fitz, 1987). Drinking occurs among Mexican Americans when the individual is coping with negative feelings as well as experiencing positive feelings. Although drinking and driving have substantially declined in the United States in the past two decades, this trend has not been seen among Hispanic drivers. Higher rates of driving while impaired, arrests, and alcohol-related crashes are particularly noted among Mexican Americans. The nurse must remember that the fatalistic element of Hispanic psychology helps to incorporate and at the same time augment drinking problems among Mexican Americans. When a drinking problem is described by a Mexican American in an intake interview, it may be followed by the client saying, "That's life" or "This is our cross to bear." For the most part, this external locus of control serves to block the identified alcoholic, and the family as well, from assuming a more active role in the recovery process.

Rather than seeking outside professional help for the treatment of alcohol abuse, Mexican Americans may collaborate with the *curandero* in treating the alcoholism or may try self-medication. The nurse must assess whether the client who is a substance abuser is using a *curandero* or is self-medicating with other drugs because these factors may further intensify the problem. The nurse must also assess carefully whether a client with a drug-abuse problem would be best suited for individual, group, or family therapy. This determination can be made only after a thorough intake interview. Because the Mexican American family is built on a system of family orientation, it is believed that perhaps the best mode of treatment for Mexican Americans is family therapy. The initial purpose of family therapy for Mexican American substance abusers should be to evaluate the family's influence on the client's chemical dependency problems. The nurse should incorporate both the nuclear and the extended family in the evaluation. Preventive interventions among youths, adults, and families may offer the best hope of preventing first use or progression of drug dependence and secondary substance disorders among individuals with signs of mood and anxiety disorders. In addition, more school- and community-based programs are needed in English and Spanish that can reach the Mexican American population with effective intervention strategies, limit alcohol access to adolescents, and reduce social marketing to this population. Treatment interventions that communicate knowledge and promote skills assist immigrant parents to counteract the health risk trends of acculturation on substance use.

To plan safe, effective, individualized nursing care for members of the Mexican American community that is appropriate and congruent with their lifestyles and cultural beliefs, nurses must know and understand the cultural patterns and belief systems of this ethnic group (Murillo-Rohde, 1977). Conway and Carmona (1990) caution nurses that Mexican American beliefs in traditional health and home remedies are often perceived by Mexican Americans as a wealth of options that decrease their need for using the modern health care system.

Mexican American farm workers are at risk for mental and physical health conditions because of social isolation, poverty, depression, and ongoing seasonal mobility. Mexican migrants (those who moved from Mexico to live or work in the United States for a limited or undefined period) reported more sexual partners and are at higher risk for HIV than Mexicans who do not migrate to the United States (Magis-Rodriquez et al., 2009). Mexican migrants living and working in the United States often enter into a society with cultural norms that differ from those in their own cities or hometowns. They are exposed to a social culture that is often more open and permissive with regard to sexual and drug-using behaviors, which may be unique to the local settings where they live. The exposure to different cultural norms combined with more opportunities to engage in high-risk behavior may influence some to adopt drug use behaviors and increase the number of sex partners. In another study, O'Brien (1983) relates that if Mexican American farm workers have worked as migrants since childhood, they frequently experience debilitating back pain and arthritis. In addition to other chronic health problems, short-term illnesses present problems (such as hemorrhaging after childbirth or abortion, dental problems), and nutritional illnesses occur because of inadequate food supplies. Nurses should be aware of local migrant programs that can assist in meeting their various health needs.

To date, the elevated risk behaviors among migrants do not seem to have translated into a detectable rise in HIV infection in this population. However, given the historical impact of migration on HIV transmission in other countries, it would be wise to carefully monitor future HIV incidence and prevalence among migrant farm workers. Magis-Rodriquez et al., (2009) suggest that new forms of service delivery system must be developed that offer services to the migrant population, regardless of their place of origin or current status and location.

Kerr and Richey (1990) suggest that Mexican American migrant farm workers have the following potential needs for improved health: improved access to health resources, improved knowledge of health-promoting behaviors, and fewer language barriers. Taking portable equipment (such as cholesterol screening equipment) to the migrant camps would improve accessibility. Health-promoting behaviors could be improved by assessment of the migrants for their current knowledge and healthful practices. Language barriers could be decreased if English classes were taught and if nutritional labeling in Spanish were instituted.

It is important for the nurse to remember that Mexican Americans differ from other cultural groups in their expression of symptoms and in how the ill person is perceived and treated by others. For example, in the Mexican American culture, epilepsy carries far less social stigma than in other ethnic and cultural groups.

SUMMARY

To provide appropriate health care for the Mexican American population, it is crucial for nurses to be aware of the stereotypes that commonly are held in viewing minority groups. This is especially true for Mexican Americans, who are often stereotyped as "Hispanic" despite the fact that there are many Hispanic subgroups with their own demographic characteristics and beliefs (Hahn, 1995). It is critical for the culturally sensitive nurse to evaluate each client as a unique individual despite the client's cultural group. It is also essential to consider that Mexican Americans are one of the major ethnic groups in the United States in whom health disparities exist and contribute to chronic health conditions and death (Esperat, Feng, Owen, & Green, 2005).

Mexican American immigrants present many special needs and potential problems in adjustment. Many males have left their families in Mexico and face the difficulty of separation. Some families are reunited after separation but experience difficulty in readjusting as a family and in negotiating the U.S. educational system, health care system, and other aspects of the new American culture. The Mexican American community in the United States is rich in cultural beliefs and values. This group has adhered to traditional beliefs and values more than other minority groups have. Because this group is growing rapidly in size and now is gradually moving to areas of the country other than the Southwest, more nurses will be coming into contact with Mexican Americans through community and health care systems and need to respond to the challenges this presents. Nurses who do not understand the culture of their clients are less likely to be positive in their views and consequently less effective. By understanding the cultural diversity unique to Mexican Americans and accepting beliefs that affect health care, nurses can plan effective, culturally appropriate care.

CASE STUDY*

George García, a 23-year-old migrant farm worker, and his wife, Anita, age 20, bring their 4-month-old daughter to the emergency room of a small community hospital. They speak only broken English. They have another small child with them, as well as two older women. They are very worried about the infant, who they say has been unable to retain feedings of diluted cow's milk. Now, because of poor sucking and increased sleeping, the infant has not had anything by mouth for the past 24 hours. When asked, the parents indicate that the infant has had only three wet diapers since yesterday. The nurse notices that the infant's eyes are sunken, she is listless, and her fontanels are depressed. When asked, the parents say the infant has been sick for 3 or 4 days. One of the older women makes a pushing-up motion with her hand as she points to the infant's mouth. Further assessment reveals a rectal temperature of 103° F. The family has not taken the temperature at all in the past 3 to 4 days. Skin turgor is good; mucous membranes are tacky. Diarrhea is not present. The infant's heart rate is 120 and regular but thready. Respirations are 12 per minute at rest. The infant does not cry during rectal temperature taking or when touched with a cold stethoscope.

*Stacie Hitt, RN, MSN, assisted in developing this case study and care plan.

◎ CARE PLAN*

Nursing Diagnosis: Fluid-volume deficit related to active fluid loss (vomiting and no intake for 24 hours)

Client Outcome	Nursing Interventions
Infant will exhibit signs of adequate hydration.	1. Offer appropriate fluids as tolerated. Maintain accurate record of intake. 2. Weigh daily. 3. Assess all parameters (such as vital signs, skin character) for hydration. 4. Apply urine collection device if indicated. 5. Measure urine volume and specific gravity.

Nursing Diagnosis: Imbalanced nutrition, less than body requirements related to inability to ingest nutrients

Client Outcome	Nursing Interventions
Infant will consume and retain appropriate number of calories per weight per day.	1. Gradually reintroduce foods as indicated—clear liquids, then formula (give samples) or breast milk. 2. Determine family's source of water and refrigeration for milk products. 3. Determine if mother had been breastfeeding prior to giving diluted cow's milk. 4. Encourage her to resume breastfeeding. 5. Observe infant while feeding. 6. If unable to suck, consult physician for intravenous order.

Nursing Diagnosis: Ineffective infant feeding pattern related to neurological impairment as evidenced by listlessness

Client Outcome	Nursing Interventions
Infant will progress to normal feeding pattern.	1. Assess infant's oral reflexes (root, gag, suck, swallow). 2. Record intervals of sleep and wakefulness; observe infant's level of activity when awake. 3. Provide pacifier to encourage sucking if infant must receive hyperalimentation. 4. Assess ease of arousal. 5. Encourage family to participate in holding, caring for, and talking with infant.

Continued

◎ CARE PLAN—cont'd

Nursing Diagnosis: Communication, impaired verbally, related to cultural differences (foreign-language barriers)

Client Outcome	Nursing Interventions
Family will be able to communicate basic needs and understanding of infant's condition and care.	1. Assess language spoken best by family. 2. Assess family's ability to comprehend English. 3. Talk more slowly than normal to family. 4. Use gestures or drawings for clarity. 5. Be careful to touch children after looking directly at them. 6. Make a conscious effort to address father when explaining care. 7. Show respect to older women. 8. Obtain a fluent, consistent, certified translator.

Nursing Diagnosis: Health maintenance, ineffective related to inability to make thoughtful judgments in regard to health of infant

Client Outcome	Nursing Interventions
Family will demonstrate understanding and ability to perform skills necessary for care of infant at home.	1. Determine what information the family needs. 2. Determine folklore beliefs related to health care. Initiate the teaching. 3. Determine influence older women have on family's health care beliefs. 4. Determine medication practices, including use of self-prescription of antibiotics. 5. Determine equipment needed for home care. 6. Seek social service referral. 7. Seek assistance from agencies.

*Stacie Hitt, RN, MSN, assisted in developing this case study and care plan.

CLINICAL DECISION MAKING

1. Which family member is likely to make the decision about whether to allow the infant to be hospitalized?
2. What might the nurse do to encourage the best communication with this family?
3. What kinds of data should be obtained in the history?
4. What folk disease does the family probably believe the infant has?
5. How should the nurse explain to the family why the infant needs to be hospitalized?
6. Why would it be advantageous for the nurse to touch both the infant and the other child while relating to them?
7. How could the nurse show acceptance of the folk remedies that may have already been tried with the infant?
8. The infant is admitted to the hospital. What could be expected in terms of family visitation?
9. What teaching goals should the nurse have for this family?

REVIEW QUESTIONS

1. Mexican Americans tend to subscribe to which of the following beliefs?
   a. Hot and cold and wet and dry
   b. Yin and yang and light and dark
   c. Smooth and dark
   d. Black and white
2. Mrs. M., a Mexican American who just gave birth, tells the nurse not to include certain foods on her meal tray because her mother told her to avoid those

foods while breastfeeding. The nurse tells her that she doesn't have to avoid any foods and should eat whatever she desires. This demonstrates which of the following?

a. Ethnocentrism
b. Cultural relativism
c. Assimilation
d. Subculture

3. To plan effective care, the nurse needs to understand that the family characteristic reflecting the worldview of a Mexican American family that will most affect how decisions are made about care is probably which of the following?

a. The father as the authority figure.
b. The mother as head of household.
c. Giving considerable freedom to women.
d. Using emotional communication styles.

REFERENCES

Ailinger, R., Armstrong, R., Nguyen, N., & Lasus, H. (2004). Latino immigrants' knowledge of tuberculosis. *Public Health Nursing*, 21(6), 519–523.

Alegría, M., Mulvaney-Day, N., Torres, M., Polo, A., Cao, Z., & Canino, G. (2007). Prevalence of psychiatric disorders across Latino subgroups in the United States. *American Journal of Public Health*, 97(1), 68–75.

Alexander, M., & Blank, J. (1988). Factors related to obesity in Mexican American preschool children. *Image: Journal of Nursing Scholarship*, 20(2), 79–82.

American Psychiatric Association (APA) (1994). *Diagnostic and statistical manual of mental disorders* (4th ed.). Washington, DC: American Psychiatric Association.

Andrews, C. S. (2006). Modesty and healthcare for women: understanding cultural sensitivities. *Community Oncology*, 3(7), 443–446.

Andrews, M. M., & Boyle, J. S. (2008). *Transcultural concepts in nursing care*. Philadelphia: Wolters Kluwer Health/Lippincott Williams & Wilkins.

Andrews, T. J., Ybarra, V., & Matthews, L. L. (2013). For the sake of our children: Hispanic immigrant and migrant families' use of folk healing and biomedicine. *Medical Anthropology Quarterly*, 27(3), 385–413.

Angel, R., Angel, J., & Markides, K. (2002). Stability and change in health insurance among older Mexican Americans. *American Journal of Public Health*, 92, 1264–1271.

Anthony-Tkach, C. (1981). Care of the Mexican American patient. *Nursing and Health Care*, 24, 424–427.

Aplemis, L. (1996). Migrant health care: creativity in primary care. *Advanced Practice Nursing Quarterly*, 2, 45–49.

Arcia, E., & Johnson, A. (1998). When respect means to obey: immigrant Mexican mothers' values for their children. *Journal of Child and Family Studies*, 7, 79–95.

Arrendondo, R., Weddige, R., Justice, C., & Fitz, J. (1987). Alcoholism in Mexican Americans: intervention and treatment. *Hospital and Community Psychiatry*, 38(2), 180–183.

Baer, R., et al. (2003). A cross-cultural approach to the study of folk illness nervios. *Culture, Medicine and Psychiatry*, 27, 315–337.

Barnett, M. A. (2012). *Extended family support networks of Mexican American mothers of toddlers*. Retrieved from <http://www.firelands.bgsu.edu/content/dam/BGSU/college-of-arts-and-sciences/NCFMR/documents/WP/WP-12-07.pdf>.

Bastida, E., & Pagan, J. (2002). The impact of diabetes on adult employment and earnings of Mexican Americans: findings from a community based study. *Health Economics*, 11(5), 403–413.

Bayles, B. P., & Katerndahl, D. A. (2009). Culture-bound syndromes in Hispanic primary care patients. *The International Journal of Psychiatry in Medicine*, 39(1), 15–31.

Beck, C. T. (2006). Acculturation: implications for perinatal research. *MCN. The American Journal of Maternal Child Nursing*, 31(2), 114–120.

Bennett, D. E., et al. (2008). Prevalence of tuberculosis infection in the United States population: the National Health and Nutrition Examination Survey, 1999–2000. *American Journal of Respiratory and Critical Care Medicine*, 177(3), 348–355.

Beutter, M., & Davidhizar, R. (1999). A home care provider's challenge: caring for the Hispanic client in the home. *Journal of Practical Nursing*, 49(3), 26–36.

Black, W., Goldhahn, R., & Wiggins, C. (1987). Melanoma within a southwestern Hispanic population. *Archives of Internal Medicine*, 123(10), 1331–1334.

Bledsoe, B. E. (2009). Faith in a cure: understanding the role folk medicine plays in prehospital care of many Mexican-Americans. *JEMS: A Journal of Emergency Medical Services*, 34(12), 62–65.

Bollenbacher, L., Heck, J., & Davidhizar, R. (2000). Maternity nurse's attitudes towards Mexican-American clients. *Journal of Practical Nursing*, 50(3), 14–16.

Bonder, B., Martin, L., & Miracle, A. (2002). *Culture in clinical care*. Thorofare, NJ: Slack.

Booth, C. (1996). Caribbean blizzard. *Time*, 46–48.

Booth, W. (2012). *Mexico's crime wave has left about 25,000 missing, government documents show*. Retrieved from <http://www.washingtonpost.com/world/the_americas/mexicos-crime-wave-has-left-up-to-25000-missing-government-documents-show/2012/11/29/7ca4ee44-3a6a-11e2-9258-ac7c78d5c680_story.html> Accessed March 28, 2015.

Borders, T., Xu, K., Rohrer, J., & Warner, R. (2002). Are rural residents and Hispanics less satisfied with medical care? Evidence from the Permian Basin. *Journal of Rural Health*, 18(1), 84–92.

Borrell, L., Lynch, J., Neighbors, H., Burt, B. A., & Gillespie, B. W. (2002). Is there homogeneity in periodontal health between African Americans and Mexican Americans? *Ethnicity and Disease*, 12(1), 97–110.

Bray, J., Adams, G., Getz, G., & Baer, P. (2001). Development, family, and ethnic influences on adolescent alcohol usage: a growth curve approach. *Journal of Family Psychology, 15*(2), 301–314.

Breslau, J., Aguilar-Gaxiola, S., Borges, G., Kendler, K. S., Su, M., & Kessler, R. C. (2007). Risk for psychiatric disorder among immigrants and their US-born descendants: evidence from the National Comorbidity Survey Replication. *Journal of Nervous and Mental Disease, 195*, 189–195.

Burk, M. E., Wieser, P. C., & Keegan, L. (1995). Cultural beliefs and health behaviors of pregnant Mexican-American women: implications for primary care. *Advances in Nursing Science, 17*(4), 37–52.

Caetano, R., Ramisetty-Mikler, S., & Rodriguez, L. A. (2008). The Hispanic Americans Baseline Alcohol Survey (HABLAS): rates and predictors of DUI across Hispanic national groups. *Accident Analysis & Prevention, 40*(2), 733–741.

Calderón, J. L., Bazargan, M., Sangasubana, N., Hays, R. D., Hardigan, P., & Baker, R. S. (2010). A comparison of two educational methods on immigrant Latinas breast cancer knowledge and screening behaviors. *Journal of Health Care for the Poor and Underserved, 21*(3), 76–90.

Calvillo, E., & Flaskerud, J. (1991). Review of literature on culture and pain of adults with focus on Mexican-Americans. *Journal of Transcultural Nursing, 2*(2), 16–23.

Campo-Flores, A. (2006). Immigration. *Newsweek*, 28–38.

CARES Needs Assessment (2003). *Community actions resource enhancement strategies community wide needs assessment in Taos County.* Taos, NM: Community Coalition.

Carmel, R., Johnson, C., & Weiner, J. (1987). Pernicious anemia in Latin Americans is not a disease of the elderly. *Ethnology, 147*(11), 1995–1996.

Castro, K. F., Tein, J., & Kim, S. (2009). Cultural predictors of physical and mental health status among Mexican American women: a mediation model. *American Journal of Community Psychology, 43*, 35–48.

Centers for Disease Control and Prevention [CDC] (2014a). *Childhood obesity facts.* Retrieved from <http://www.cdc.gov/obesity/data/childhood.html> Accessed March 28, 2015.

Centers for Disease Control and Prevention [CDC] (2014b). *National diabetes statistics report, 2014.* National Center for Chronic Disease Prevention and Health Promotion. Retrieved from <http://www.cdc.gov/diabetes/pubs/statsreport14/national-diabetes-report-web.pdf>.

Centers for Disease Control and Prevention [CDC] (2015). *High blood pressure facts.* Retrieved from <http://www.cdc.gov/bloodpressure/facts.htm> Accessed April 10, 2015.

Central Intelligence Agency (CIA) (2014). *The world factbook: Mexico.* Retrieved from <https://www.cia.gov/library/publications/the-world-factbook/geos/mx.html> Accessed March 28, 2015.

Cervantes, R., Snyder, S., & Padilla, A. (1989). Posttraumatic stress in immigrants from Central America and Mexico. *Hospital and Community Psychiatry, 40*(6), 615–619.

Cespedes, A., & Larson, E. (2006). Knowledge, attitudes, and practices regarding antibiotic use among Latinos in the United States: review and recommendations. *American Journal of Infection Control, 34*, 495–502.

Chávez, N. (1986). Mental health services delivery to minority populations: Hispanics—a perspective. In M. Miranda & H. Kitano (Eds.), *Mental health research and practice in minority communities.* Rockville, MD: National Institute of Mental Health.

Cheng, H. L., & Mallinckrodt, B. (2015). Racial/ethnic discrimination, posttraumatic stress symptoms, and alcohol problems in a longitudinal study of Hispanic/Latino college students. *Journal of Counseling Psychology, 62*(1), 38.

Chiriboga, D. A., Jang, Y., Banks, S., & Kim, G. (2007). Acculturation and its effect on depressive symptom structure in a sample of Mexican American elders. *Hispanic Journal of Behavioral Sciences, 29*(1), 83–100.

Cioffi, R. J. (2003). Communicating with culturally and linguistically diverse patients in an acute care setting: nurses' experiences. *International Journal of Nursing Studies, 40*(3), 299–306.

Clark, M. (1970). *Health in the Mexican American culture.* Berkeley: University of California Press.

Cobos, R. (2003). *A dictionary of New Mexico & Southern Colorado Spanish.* Albuquerque: Museum of New Mexico Press.

Coffman, M. J. (2003). Cultural caring in nursing practice: a meta-synthesis of qualitative research. *Journal of Cultural Diversity, 11*(3), 100–109.

Colson, E. R., et al. (2013). Trends and factors associated with infant bed sharing, 1993–2010: the National Infant Sleep Position Study. *Journal of the American Medical Association Pediatrics, 167*(11), 1032–1037.

Conway, R., & Carmona, P. (1990). Cultural complexity: the hidden stressors. *Journal of Advanced Medical-Surgical Nursing, 1*(4), 65–72.

Cook, C. W. (2007). *CRS report for Congress: Mexico's drug cartels.* Washington, DC: Analyst in Latin American Affairs/Foreign Affairs, Defense, and Trade Division.

Cox, C. (1986). Physician utilization by three groups of ethnic elderly. *Medical Care, 24*(8), 667–676.

Cronin, M. (1997). Billboard campaign spotlights growing hepatitis C epidemic. *The Seattle Times*, A1.

Crouter, A. C., Davis, K. D., Updegraff, K., Delgado, M., & Fortner, M. (2006). Mexican American fathers' occupational conditions: links to family members' psychological adjustment. *Journal of Marriage and Family, 68*(4), 843–858.

Cummings, L. L. (2003). Cloth-wrapped people, trouble, and power: pachuco culture in the greater Southwest. *Journal of the Southwest, 45*, 329–348.

Currier, R. L. (1966). The hot-cold syndrome and symbolic balance in Mexican and Spanish-American folk medicine. *Ethnology, 5*, 251–263.

D'Anna-Hernandez, K. L., Aleman, B., & Flores, A. M. (2015). Acculturative stress negatively impacts maternal depressive symptoms in Mexican-American women during pregnancy. *Journal of Affective Disorders, 176*, 35–42.

Davidhizar, R. (2001). So your patient is Latino. *Journal of Practical Nursing, 51*(1), 18–20.

Davidson, M. (2003). Effect of nurse-directed diabetes care in a minority population. *Diabetes Care, 26*(8), 2281–2287.

Dehlendorf, C., Levy, K., Kelley, A., Grumbach, K., & Steinauer, J. (2013). Women's preferences for contraceptive counseling and decision making. *Contraception*, 88(2), 250–256.

Derenowski, J. (1990). Coronary artery disease in Hispanics. *Cardiovascular Nursing*, 4(4), 13–21.

Diamond, L. C., Wilson-Stronks, A., & Jacobs, E. A. (2010). Do hospitals measure up to the national culturally and linguistically appropriate services standards? *Medical Care*, 48(12), 1080–1087.

Donlan, W. (2011). The meaning of community-based care for frail Mexican American elders. *International Social Work*, 54(3), 388–403.

Doran, C., & Hansen, N. (2006). Constructions of Mexican American family grief after the death of a child: an exploratory study. *Cultural Diversity and Ethnic Minority Psychology*, 12(2), 199–211.

Duffy, M., Rossow, R., & Hernandez, M. (1996). Correlates of health-promotion activities in employed Mexican American women. *Nursing Research*, 45(1), 18–24.

Eden, S., & Aguilar, R. (2004). The Hispanic chemically dependent client: considerations for diagnosis and treatment. In G. Lawson & A. Lawson (Eds.), *Alcoholism and substance abuse in special populations*. Austin, TX: Pro-Ed.

Eid, J., & Kraemer, H. (1998). Mexican-Americans experience with diabetes. *Image: Journal of Nursing Scholarship*, 30(4), 393.

Ennis, S. R., Ríos-Vargas, M., & Albert, N. G. (2011). The Hispanic population: 2010. *2010 Census Briefs*. Retrieved from <http://www.census.gov/prod/cen2010/briefs/c2010br-04.pdf>.

Ericksen, A. (2006). Hispanic healthcare. *Healthcare Traveler*, 15–21.

Esperat, M. C., Feng, D., Owen, D., & Green, A. (2005). Transformation for health: a framework for health disparities research. *Nursing Outlook*, 53, 113–120.

Ethics. (1995). Cultures diverge on patient autonomy. *AJN The American Journal of Nursing*, 95(11), 10–11.

Falicov, C. (2005). Mexican families. In M. McGoldrick, J. K. Pearce, & J. Giordano (Eds.), *Ethnicity and family therapy* (3rd ed.). New York: Guilford Press.

Fantz, A. (2012). *The Mexico drug war: bodies for billions*. Retrieved from <http://edition.cnn.com/2012/01/15/world/mexico-drug-war-essay/index.html> Accessed March 28, 2015.

Favazza, A. (1983). Cultural factors in diagnosis and treatment. *ACP Psychiatric Update*. New York: Medical Information Systems.

Feldmann, J. M., Wiemann, C. M., Sever, L., & Hergenroeder, A. C. (2008). Folk and traditional medicine use by a subset of Hispanic adolescents. *International Journal of Adolescent Medicine and Health*, 20(1), 41–51.

Ford, J., & Graves, J. (1977). Differences between Mexican American and White children in interpersonal distance and social touching. *Perceptual and Motor Skills*, 45(3), 779–785.

Fornos, L., Mika, V., Bayles, B., Serrano, A. C., Jimenez, R. L., & Villarreal, R. (2005). A qualitative study of Mexican American adolescents and depression. *Journal of School Health*, 75(5), 162–169.

Fortuna, L. R., Porche, M. V., & Alegria, M. (2008). Political violence, psychosocial trauma, and the context of mental health services use among immigrant Latinos in the United States. *Ethnicity & Health*, 13(5), 435–463.

Friedman-Koss, D., Crespo, C., Bellantoni, M., & Anderson, R. (2002). The relationship of race/ethnicity and social class to hormone replacement therapy. *Menopause: The Journal of the North American Menopause Society*, 9(4), 264–272.

Galanti, G. A. (2008). *Caring for patients from different cultures* (4th ed.). Philadelphia: University of Pennsylvania Press.

Gartin, A., Brewis, N., & Schwartz, N. (2010). Nonprescription antibiotic therapy: cultural models on both sides of the counter and both sides of the border. *Medical Anthropology Quarterly*, 24, 85–107.

Gelfand, D., Balcazar, H., Parzuchowski, J., & Lenox, S. (2001). Mexicans and care for the terminally ill: family, hospice and the church. *American Journal of Hospice and Palliative Care*, 18(6), 391–396.

Gelfand, D., & Bialik-Gilad, R. (1989). Immigration reform and social work. *Social Work*, 34(1), 23–27.

Getrich, C. M., et al. (2012). Expressions of machismo in colorectal cancer screening among New Mexico Hispanic subpopulations. *Qualitative Health Research*, 22(4), 546–559.

Gill-Hopple, K., & Brage-Hudson, D. (2012). Compadrazgo: a literature review. *Journal of Transcultural Nursing*, 23(2), 117–123.

Glick, J. (1999). Economic support from and to extended kin: a comparison of Mexican Americans and Mexican immigrants. *International Migration Review*, 33(3), 745–765.

González, H. M., Vega, W. A., Williams, D. R., Tarraf, W., West, B. T., & Neighbors, H. W. (2010). Depression care in the United States: too little for too few. *Archives of General Psychiatry*, 67(1), 37–46.

Gorek, B., Martin, J., White, N., Peters, D., & Hummel, F. (2002). Culturally competent care for Latino elders in long-term care settings. *Geriatric Nursing*, 23, 272–275.

Grant, B., Stinson, F., Hasin, D., Dawson, D. A., Chou, S. P., & Anderson, K. (2004). Immigration and lifetime prevalence of DSM-IV psychiatric disorders among Mexican Americans and non-Hispanic whites in the United States. *Archives of General Psychiatry*, 61, 1226–1233.

Greene, M. J. (2007). Strategies for incorporating cultural competence into childbirth education curriculum. *The Journal of Perinatal Education*, 16(2), 33–37.

Guskin, E., & Mitchell, A. (2011). Hispanic media: faring better than mainstream media. *The State of the News Media 2011. Pew Research Center's Project for Excellence in Journalism*. Retrieved from <http://www.stateofthemedia.org/2011/hispanic-media-fairing-better-than-the-mainstream-media/>.

Hahn, M. (1995). Providing health care in a culturally complex world. *Advances for Nurse Practitioners*, 3, 43–45.

Han, B., Gfroerer, J. C., Colpe, L. J., Barker, P. R., & Colliver, J. D. (2011). Serious psychological distress and mental health service use among community-dwelling older US adults. *Psychiatric Services, 62*(3), 291–298.

Harwood, A. (1971). The hot-cold theory of disease. *Journal of the American Medical Association, 216*(7), 1153–1158.

Hazuda, H. P., Stern, M. P., Gaskill, S., Haffner, S. M., & Gardner, L. I. (1983). Ethnic differences in health knowledge and behaviors related to the prevention and treatment of coronary heart disease. *American Journal of Epidemiology, 117,* 717–728.

Heilemann, M. V., Lee, K. A., & Kury, F. S. (2002). Strengths and vulnerabilities of women of Mexican descent in relation to depressive symptoms. *Nursing Research, 51*(3), 175–182.

Hoefer, M., Rytina, N., & Campbell, C. (2009). *Estimates of the unauthorized immigrant population residing in the United States: January 2006.* Washington, DC: U.S. Department of Homeland Security.

Hood, L., & Jackson, N. (1989). Caring for the patient with TB. *Advancing Clinical Care, 4*(4), 14–18.

Hough, R. (1985). Life events and stress in Mexican-American culture. In *Stress and Hispanic mental health: relating research to service delivery* (pp. 110–146). Rockville, MD: U.S. Government Printing Office.

Interian, A., Martinez, I. E., Guarnaccia, P. J., Vega, W. A., & Escobar, J. I. (2007). A qualitative analysis of the perception of stigma among Latinos receiving antidepressants. *Psychiatric Services, 58*(12), 1591–1594.

Iwashyna, T., & Chang, V. (2002). Racial and ethnic differences in place of death: United States, 1993. *Journal of the American Geriatrics Society, 50*(6), 1113–1117.

Javier, R. A., & Marcos, L. R. (1989). The role of stress on the language-independence and code-switching phenomena. *Journal of Psycholinguistic Research, 18*(5), 449–472.

Jimenez, D. E., Alegría, M., Chen, C. N., Chan, D., & Laderman, M. (2010). Prevalence of psychiatric illnesses in older ethnic minority adults. *Journal of the American Geriatrics Society, 58*(2), 256–264.

Jonas, B., Brody, D., Roper, M., & Narrow, W. (2003). Prevalence of mood disorders in a national sample of young American adults. *Social Psychiatry and Psychiatric Epidemiology, 38*(11), 618–624.

Juckett, G. (2005). Cross-cultural medicine. *American Family Physician, 72,* 2267–2274.

Juckett, G. (2013). Caring for Latino patients. *American Family Physician, 87*(1), 48–54.

Kalish, R., & Reynolds, D. (1981). *Death and ethnicity: a psychocultural study.* Los Angeles: USC.

Katz, V. (2014). Children as brokers of their immigrant families' health-care connections. *Social Problems, 61*(2), 194–215.

Keeler, A. R., Siegel, J. T., & Alvaro, E. M. (2014). Depression and help seeking among Mexican-Americans: the mediating role of familism. *Journal of Immigrant and Minority Health, 16*(6), 1225–1231.

Keenan, L., Marshall, L., & Eve, S. (2002). Extension of the behavioral model of healthcare utilization with ethnically diverse, low-income women. *Ethnicity and Disease, 12*(1), 111–123.

Keller, C., & Fleury, J. (2006). Factors related to physical activity in Hispanic women. *Journal of Cardiovascular Nursing, 21*(2), 142–145.

Kemp, C. (2005). Cultural issues in palliative care. *Seminars in Oncology Nursing, 21*(1), 44–52.

Kemper, R. (1982). The compadrazgo in urban Mexico. *Anthropological Quarterly, 55*(1), 17–30.

Kerr, M., & Richey, D. (1990). Health-promoting lifestyles of English-speaking and Spanish-speaking Mexican-American migrant farm workers. *Public Health Nursing, 7*(2), 80–87.

Khoury, R., & Thurmond, G. (1978). Ethnic differences in time perception: a comparison of Anglo and Mexican Americans. *Perceptual and Motor Skills, 47*(3), 1183–1188.

Kiesser, M., McFadden, J., & Belliard, J. (2006). An interdisciplinary view of medical pluralism among Mexican-Americans. *Journal of Interprofessional Care, 20,* 223–234.

Kim, G., Jang, Y., Chiriboga, D. A., Ma, G. X., & Schonfeld, L. (2010). Factors associated with mental health service use in Latino and Asian immigrant elders. *Aging & Mental Health, 14*(5), 535–542.

Kissam, R. (1993). *Everyday realities and effective public policy: the case of migrant and seasonal farmworkers.* Paper presented at the meeting of the National Conference on Migrant and Seasonal Farmworkers, Denver, CO.

Kluckhohn, F. (1976). Dominant and variant value orientations. In P. J. Brink (Ed.), *Transcultural nursing: a book of readings* (pp. 63–81). Englewood Cliffs, NJ: Prentice Hall.

Lagana, K., & Gonzalez-Ramirez, L. (2003). Mexican Americans. In P. F. St. Hill, J. G. Lipson, & A. I. Meleis (Eds.), *Caring for women cross-culturally* (pp. 218–235). Philadelphia: F. A. Davis.

Lantican, L., & Corona, D. (1989). *A comparison of the social support networks of Filipino and Mexican American primigravidas.* Paper presented at the Sigma Theta Tau International Conference, Indianapolis, IN.

Leininger, M. (2002). *Transcultural nursing: concept, theories, research and practice* (3rd ed.). New York: McGraw-Hill.

Lewis, M. P., Simons, G. F., & Fennig, C. D. (2014). *Ethnologue: languages of the world* (17th ed.). Dallas: SIL International.

Lopez, R. A. (2005). Use of alternative folk medicine by Mexican American women. *Journal of Immigrant Health, 7*(1), 23–31.

Luyas, G. (1989). *An explanatory model of diabetes by Mexican American women.* Paper presented at the Sigma Theta Tau International Conference, Indianapolis, IN.

Magana, C., & Hovey, J. (2003). Psychosocial stressors associated with Mexican migrant farmworkers in the Midwest United States. *Journal of Immigrant Health, 5*(2), 75–86.

Magis-Rodriquez, C., Lemp, G., Hernandez, M., Sanchez, M. A., Estrada, F., & Bravo-García, E. (2009). Going North: Mexican migrants and their vulnerability to HIV. *Journal of Acquired Immune Deficiency Syndrome, 51*(S1), S21–S24.

Marcos, L. R., Alpert, M., Urcuyo, L., & Kesselman, M. (1973). The effect of interview language on the evaluation of psychopathology in Spanish-American schizophrenic patients. *American Journal of Psychiatry, 130,* 549–553.

Marin, B. (2003). HIV prevention in the Hispanic community: sex, culture, and empowerment. *Journal of Transcultural Nursing, 14*(3), 186–192.

Marín, G., & Marín, B. V. (1991). *Research with Hispanic populations*. Newbury Park, CA: Sage.

Martin, J. A., Hamilton, B. E., Osterman, M., Curtin, S. C., & Matthews, T. (2015). Births: final data for 2013. *National Vital Statistics Reports: From the Centers for Disease Control and Prevention, National Center for Health Statistics, National Vital Statistics System, 64*(1), 1.

McCabe, K., Goehring, K., Yeh, M., & Lau, A. (2008). Parental locus of control and externalizing behavior among Mexican American Preschoolers. *Journal of Emotional and Behavioral Disorders, 16*(2), 118–126.

McQuillan, G., Kruszon-Moran, D., Deforest, A., Chu, S. Y., & Wharton, M. (2002). Serologic immunity to diphtheria and tetanus in the United States. *Annals of Internal Medicine, 136*(9), 660–666.

Meleis, A., Douglas, M., Eribes, C., Shih, F., & Messias, D. K. (1996). Employed Mexican women as mothers and partners: valued, empowered, and overloaded. *Journal of Advanced Nursing, 23*(1), 82–90.

Miller, S., & Davidhizar, R. (2001). Sociocultural aspects of adherence to medical regimens for Mexican Americans. *Care Management*, 44–48.

Mines, R., Gabbard, S., & Samardick, R. (1992). *Harvest worker analysis*. Los Angeles: Commission on Agricultural Workers.

Miroff, N., & Booth, W. (2012). *Mexico's drug war is at a stalemate as Calderon's presidency ends*. Retrieved from <http://www.washingtonpost.com/world/the_americas/calderon-finishes-his-six-year-drug-war-at-stalemate/2012/11/26/82c90a94-31eb-11e2-92f0-496af208bf23_story_1.html> Accessed March 28, 2015.

Mirowsky, J., & Ross, C. (1984). Mexican culture and its emotional contradictions. *Journal of Health and Social Behavior, 25*(1), 2–13.

Monrroy, L. S. A. (1983). Nursing care of Raza/Latina patients. In M. S. Orque, B. Block, & L. S. A. Monrroy (Eds.), *Ethnic nursing care: a multicultural approach* (pp. 115–148). St. Louis: Mosby.

Moore, J., & Pachon, H. (1985). *Hispanics in the United States*. Englewood Cliffs, NJ: Prentice-Hall.

Mozaffarian, D., et al. (2015). Executive summary: heart disease and stroke statistics—2015 update a report from the American Heart Association. *Circulation, 131*(4), 434–441.

Murillo, N. (1978). The Mexican American family. In C. A. Hernández, M. J. Haug, & N. N. Wagner (Eds.), *Chicanos: social and psychological perspectives* (2nd ed., pp. 15–25). St. Louis: Mosby.

Murillo-Rohde, I. (1977). Care for all colors. *Imprint, 24*(4), 29–32, 50.

Musto, D. (1991). Opium, cocaine and marijuana in American history. *Scientific American, 265*, 40–47.

Naisbitt, J. (1984). *Megatrends*. New York: Warner Books.

National Center for Health Statistics (2002). *Health United States, 2002 with urban and rural chartbook*. Hyattsville, MD: National Center for Health Statistics.

National Center for Health Statistics (2010). *Health United States, 2010 with urban and rural chartbook*. Hyattsville, MD: National Center for Health Statistics.

Nelson, K., Norris, K., & Mangione, C. (2002). Disparities in the diagnosis and pharmacologic treatment of high serum cholesterol by race and ethnicity data from the Third National Health and Nutrition Examination Survey. *Archives of Internal Medicine, 162*(8), 929–935.

New Mexico Department of Health (2010). *Statistics on New Mexico health issues*. Albuquerque.

O'Brien, E. (1983). Reaching the migrant worker. *American Journal of Nursing, 83a*(6), 895–897.

Ogden, C. L., Carroll, M. D., Kit, B. K., & Flegal, K. M. (2014). Prevalence of childhood and adult obesity in the United States, 2011–2012. *Journal of the American Medical Association, 311*(8), 806–814.

Oliva, N. L. (2008). When language intervenes. *AJN The American Journal of Nursing, 108*(3), 73–75.

Otiniano, M., Black, S., Ray, L., Du, X., & Markides, K. S. (2002). Correlates of diabetic complications in Mexican-American elders. *Ethnicity and Disease, 12*(2), 252–258.

Overfield, T. (1995). *Biologic variations in health and illness: race, age, and sex differences* (2nd ed.). New York: CRC Press.

Oxford Dictionary of Quotations. (2009). New York: Oxford University Press.

Padilla, Y., & Villalobos, G. (2007). Cultural responses to health among Mexican American women and their families. *Family and Community Health, 30*(18), s24–s33.

Paz, O. (1961). *The labyrinth of solitude*. New York: Grove Press.

Permanente, K. (2001). *A provider's handbook on culturally competent care: Latino population* (2nd ed.). Santa Clara, CA: National Diversity Dept.

Philis-Tsimikas, A., et al. (2004). Improvement in diabetes care of underinsured patients enrolled in Project Dulce. *Diabetes Care, 27*(1), 110–115.

Phipps, W. (1993). The patient with pulmonary problems. In B. C. Long, W. J. Phipps, & V. Cassmeyer (Eds.), *Medical surgical nursing: concepts and clinical practice* (3rd ed.). St. Louis: Mosby.

Pope, C. (2005). Addressing limited English proficiency and disparities for Hispanic postpartum women. *Journal of Obstetric, Gynecologic, and Neonatal Nursing, 34*, 512–520.

Poss, J. (2000). Factors associated with participation by Mexican migrant farmworkers in a tuberculosis screening program. *Nursing Research, 49*(1), 20–28.

Randolph, W., Stroup-Benham, C., Black, S., & Markides, K. (1998). Alcohol use among Cuban-Americans, Mexican-Americans, and Puerto Ricans. *Alcohol Health and Research World, 22*, 265–269.

Reese, L., Balzano, S., Gallimore, R., & Goldenberg, C. (1995). The concept of education: Latino family values and American schooling. *International Journal of Educational Research, 23*(1), 57–81.

Roat, C. E. (2006). *Certification of health care interpreters in the United States: a primer, a status report, and considerations for national certification*. Retrieved from

<http://www.calendow.org/uploadedFiles/certification_of_
health_care_interpretors.pdf>.

Rodolfo, A. (2007). *Occupied American: a history of Chicanos* (6th ed.). New York: Pearson Longman.

Ross, J. (1995). Who are they, where are they and how do we talk to them? Hispanic Americans. *Hospitals and Health Networks, 69*(19), 65.

Rubel, A. (1966). *Across the tracks: Mexican Americans in a Texas city.* Austin, TX: University of Texas Press.

Salinas, J. J., & Sheffield, K. M. (2011). English language use, health and mortality in older Mexican Americans. *Journal of Immigrant and Minority Health, 13*(2), 232–238.

Saunders, L. (1954). *Cultural difference and medical care.* New York: Russell Sage Foundation.

Schillinger, D., et al. (2003). Closing the loop: physician communication with diabetic patients who have low health literacy. *Archives of Internal Medicine, 163*, 83–90.

Sennott-Miller, L. (1994). Using theory to plan appropriate interventions: cancer prevention for older Hispanic and non-Hispanic White women. *Journal of Advanced Nursing, 20*(5), 809–814.

Serrano, B. (1997). A lesson in inequality: districts in wealthy areas, where school levies are common, often have better schools. *The Seattle Times*, A-1.

Skaff, M., Mullan, J., Fisher, L., & Chesla, C. (2003). A contextual model of control beliefs, behavior and health: Latinos and European Americans with Type 2 diabetes. *Psychology & Health, 18*(3), 295–312.

Smith, R. (2002). Barnard study links gender, academic success among Mexican-Americans. *Black Issues in Higher Education, 19*(8), 16.

Sobralske, M. (2006). Machismo sustains health beliefs of Mexican American men. *Journal of the American Academy of Nurse Practitioners, 18*, 348–350.

Sobralske, M., & Katz, J. (2005). Culturally competent care of patients with acute chest pain. *Journal of the American Academy of Nurse Practitioners, 173*, 342–349.

Spector, R. (2004). *Cultural diversity in health and illness* (6th ed.). Englewood Cliffs, NJ: Prentice Hall Health.

Stern, M. P., Bradshaw, B., Eifler, C. W., Fong, D. S., Hazuda, H. P., & Rosenthal, M. (1987). Secular decline in death rates due to ischemic heart disease in Mexican Americans and non-Hispanic Whites in Texas, 1970–1980. *Circulation, 76*(6), 1245–1250.

Taylor, P., Lopez, M. H., Martinez, J., & Velasco, G. (2012). *Language use among Latinos. Pew Research Center: Hispanic Trends.* Retrieved from <http://www.pewhispanic.org/2012/04/04/iv-language-use-among-latinos> Accessed March 30, 2012.

Telles, E. E., & Ortiz, V. (2009). *Generations of exclusion: Mexican Americans, assimilation and race.* New York: Russell Sage Publications.

Time Almanac (2011). *Time Almanac powered by Encyclopedia Britannica 2011.* Chicago, IL: Encyclopedia Britannica.

Titus, S. K. F. (2014). Seeking and utilizing a curandero in the United States: a literature review. *Journal of Holistic Nursing, 32*(3), 189–201.

Umaña-Taylor, A. J., & Updegraff, K. A. (2007). Latino adolescents' mental health: exploring the interrelations among discrimination, ethnic identity, cultural orientation, self-esteem, and depressive symptoms. *Journal of Adolescence, 30*(4), 549–567.

U.S. Department of Commerce, Bureau of the Census (2000). *Population Census, Race and Hispanic Origins.* Hyattsville, MD: U.S. Government Printing Office.

U.S. Department of Commerce, Bureau of the Census (2013). *2013 American Community Survey 1-year estimate.* Retrieved from U.S. Bureau of the Census <http://factfinder.census.gov/faces/nav/jsf/pages/index.xhtml> Accessed March 28, 2015.

U.S. Department of Commerce, Bureau of the Census (2015). *American Community Survey,* Washington, DC: U.S. Government Printing Office.

Váldez, A. (1980). *Ethnic maintenance among Mexicans and Puerto Ricans.* Waco, TX: Report to Southwestern Sociological Association.

Valente, S. (2004). End of life and ethnicity. *Journal for Nurses in Staff Development, 20*(6), 285–293.

Valenzuela, A. (1999). Gender roles and settlement activities among children and their immigrant families. *The American Behavioral Scientist, 42*(4), 720–742.

Vásquez, S. (1997). Diabetes alert: high-fat, genetics make Hispanics prone to the disease. *Rocky Mountain News*, 3d.

Vega, W., Scribney, W., & Achara-Abrahams, L. (2003). Cooccurring alcohol, drug, and other psychiatric disorders among Mexican-origin people in the United States. *American Journal of Public Health, 93*(7), 1057–1064.

Vega, W. A., Canino, G., Cao, Z., & Alegria, M. (2009). Prevalence and correlates of dual diagnoses in US Latinos. *Drug and Alcohol Dependence, 100*(1), 32–38.

Villarruel, A., & Denyes, M. (1997). Testing Orem's theory with Mexican Americans. *Image: Journal of Nursing Scholarship, 29*(3), 283–288.

Villarruel, A., & Leininger, M. (2004). Culture care of Mexican Americans. In M. Leininger (Ed.), *Transcultural nursing* (3rd ed.). New York: McGraw-Hill.

Volpato, G., Godínez, D., & Beyra, A. (2009). Migration and ethnobotanical practices: the case of *Tifey* among Haitian immigrants in Cuba. *Human Ecology, 37*(1), 43–53.

Waldstein, A. (2010). Popular medicine and self-care in a Mexican migrant community: toward an explanation of an epidemiological paradox. *Medical Anthropology, 29*, 71–107.

Wanderer, J., & Rivera, G. (1986). Black magic beliefs and white magic practice: the common structures of intimacy, tradition and power. *The Social Science Journal, 23*(4), 419–430.

Weaver, T. (1970). Use of hypothetical situations in a study of Spanish-American illness referral systems. *Human Organisms, 29*, 140.

White, J., Linhart, J., & Medley, L. (1996). Culture, diet and maternity. *Advances for Nurse Practitioners, 4*, 26–28.

Wilson, H., & Kneisl, C. (1996). *Psychiatric nursing* (5th ed.). Menlo Park, CA: Addison-Wesley.

Woodbury, R. (2000). A class for strangers in a strange land. *Time*, 8.

Yoon, S. S., Gu, Q., Nwankwo, T., Wright, J. D., Hong, Y., & Burt, V. (2015). Trends in blood pressure among adults with hypertension: United States, 2003 to 2012. *Hypertension*, 65(1), 54–61.

Zemore, S. E., Karriker-Jaffe, K. J., Keithly, S., & Mulia, N. (2011). Racial prejudice and unfair treatment: interactive effects with poverty and foreign nativity on problem drinking. *Journal of Studies on Alcohol and Drugs*, 72(3), 361.

Zhang, W., Hong, S., Takeuchi, D. T., & Mossakowski, K. N. (2012). Limited English proficiency and psychological distress among Latinos and Asian Americans. *Social Science & Medicine*, 75(6), 1006–1014.

Zong, J., & Batalova, J. (2014). *Mexican immigrants in the United States*. Retrieved from <http://www.migrationpolicy.org/article/mexican-immigrants-united-states> Accessed March 28, 2015.

Zoucha, R., & Purnell, L. D. (2003). People of Mexican heritage. In L. D. Purnell & B. J. Paulanka (Eds.), *Transcultural health care* (pp. 264–278). Philadelphia: F. A. Davis.

10

Navajos

Catherine E. Hanley

BEHAVIORAL OBJECTIVES

After reading this chapter, the nurse will be able to:

1. Identify ways in which the Navajo culture influences Navajo individuals and health-seeking behaviors.
2. Recognize physical and biological variances that exist in and across Navajo groups to provide culturally appropriate care.
3. Develop a sensitivity and understanding for communication differences as evidenced within and across Navajo groups to avoid stereotyping and to provide culturally appropriate nursing care.
4. Develop a sensitivity and understanding for psychological phenomena that influence the functioning of a Navajo when nursing care is being provided.
5. Describe the influence of traditional Navajo folk medicine and the relationship to health-seeking behaviors.

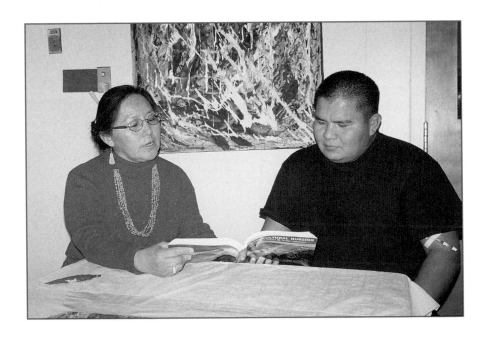

OVERVIEW OF THE NAVAJOS

Archeological evidence places Navajos in the Gobernador Canyon area of northwestern New Mexico by the late 1400s or early 1500s. By the early 1600s, some Navajos had migrated as far as the Black Mesa country of northern Arizona (Iverson, 2002). The first written historical observations of the Navajos have been attributed to Arate Salmerón (1626) and Father Benavides (1630).

According to (Schwartz, 2004; Iverson 2002), the various Pueblo peoples exerted a tremendous influence on the evolution of the Navajo culture in the new region. There is historical evidence indicating that the Navajos and Pueblos were at times foes. However, Brugge (1968) suggested a number of instances when Navajo and Pueblo villages allied themselves against the Spanish and other outside groups. Schwartz (2004) and Young (1961) concluded that the Navajos and the Pueblos existed together in a relationship that was more peaceful than hostile. Regardless of whether the Pueblos and the Navajos lived peacefully, the Pueblos probably did influence change in the Navajo lifestyle in some critical ways. For example, the Navajos have a matrilineal clan system that still exists today and dictates that a Navajo inherits the clan and thus the lineage from the mother (Iverson, 2002; Schwartz, 2004). The implication is that people from the same clan are considered relatives with varying responsibilities to one another.

For the western Pueblos, the clan traditions were strong, and it is probable that they influenced the Navajos in the direction of clan formation (Iverson, 2002). In addition, the Pueblo people were sedentary and had agricultural ways that undoubtedly also had some effect on the Navajos. As a consequence of these influences, the Navajos gradually adopted a way of life that was significantly less nomadic, with less emphasis on hunting than that of other Apachean groups. Seemingly, the Navajos learned trades such as weaving, pottery making, silversmithing, and agriculture from the Pueblo people en route to the Southwest. According to Iverson (2002), the Navajos credit "Spiderwoman" with their instruction in weaving. Differences existed in that Pueblo men traditionally were weavers, whereas Navajo men rarely became weavers.

During the sixteenth, seventeenth, and eighteenth centuries, the Navajo people underwent tremendous expansion, cultural acquisition, and social change. According to Weirto (2010), the Navajos have always had a great capacity to absorb and elaborate on cultural traits adopted from other people. For example, the Pueblo weaving tradition is responsible for producing the Navajo blanket, which is unmistakably the product of the *Diné* (the Navajo word for *people*). The language, although distinctively Navajo (from the entirely different Athapaskan family of languages), was learned by other Indians; however, few Navajos attempted to master a foreign tongue (Weirto, 2010). The Navajo people lived freely on the land of their forefathers, located between the four sacred mountains: Mount Blanca (Colorado) to the east, Mount Taylor (New Mexico) to the south, San Francisco Peak (Arizona) to the west, and Mount Hesperus (Colorado) to the north. Four directional colors were associated with the four sacred mountains: white with Mount Blanca, blue with Mount Taylor, yellow with San Francisco Peak, and black with Mount Hesperus. To understand the history of the Navajo people, it is important to understand the significance of the four sacred mountains, which historically were considered the cardinal boundary peaks surrounding the Navajo country. Even today, Navajo people believe that the four sacred mountains were gifts from the "Holy People" (*diyín dine`é*, or *haashch`ééh dine`é*); therefore, traditions, prayers, songs, and sacred trust are embodied in these mountains (Navajo Health Systems Agency, 1985; Schwartz, 2004; Weirto, 2010).

Perhaps one of the most significant periods of Navajo history occurred during 1864, when more than 9000 Navajo people were captured in what is now Arizona and forced to journey to Fort Sumner on the Bosque Redondo Reservation in what is now New Mexico. During this long journey (known in Navajo history as the "long walk") and internment at Fort Sumner, more than 2000 Navajo men, women, and children died of respiratory tract diseases, gastrointestinal disorders, and exhaustion.

During May 1868, the fourth year of their forced internment, the Navajos' elected leader, Chief Barboncito, told a Washington delegation appointed by President Andrew Johnson, "I hope to God you will not ask me to go to any other country except my own." In speaking these words, Chief Barboncito expressed the feelings, beliefs, traditions, and desires of the Navajo people. On May 28, 1868, the United States of America and the Navajo tribe entered into a treaty that was ratified on August 12, 1868, by President Andrew Johnson (Iverson, 2002; Schwartz, 2004; Treaty, 1973).

After the signing of the 1868 treaty, the Navajos moved progressively in the direction of the Four Sacred Mountains. Gradual as it might have seemed, the call from the Four Sacred Mountains for the return to Navajo ways reflected the futuristic response of self-determination, self-governance, and self-actualization (Hanley, 1987; Iverson, 2002). Although the treaty signed at Fort Sumner was not the first treaty but the eighth treaty made between the Navajo people and the United States in 22 years, it was historically significant because it led to their release from Fort Sumner and to the establishment of their first reservation at Fort Defiance, Arizona. (At that time Arizona was a separate territory; it became the forty-eighth state in 1912.) After the Navajo people were released from their internment at Fort Sumner, they began to develop a diversified economy. For the Navajo, raising livestock was an important element of the economy but not the only element. From early and later historical accounts, it appears that the Navajos have always been perceived as great farmers. A reemerging question about the Navajo people concerns why they traditionally needed such a diverse economy; another reemerging question concerns why livestock took on a more essential role within the Navajo economy. The answers to these questions seemingly overlap and are mutually reinforcing: for the Navajo people, a diversified economy made more thorough and efficient use of the different opportunities provided by various soils, altitudes, and vegetations.

Three different climatic zones exist in the area in which the Navajo people live. The humid, or mountain, zones account for roughly 8% of the total Navajo area; the mesas and high plains, with their intermediate steppe climate, account for roughly 37% of the Navajo area; and the comparatively warm desert regions account for roughly 55% of the Navajo area. Winter temperatures in these regions range from an average minimum of 4° to 15° F in the humid zone, to 10° to 25° F in the steppe zone, to 11° to 30° F in the desert zone. Summer temperatures in these regions range from an average maximum of 70° to 80° F in the humid zone, to 80° to 88° F in the steppe zone, to 100° F or higher in the desert. The average rainfall in all three areas is concentrated in the late summer period, which extends from July to September, with great variation in amount within each zone. The desert and humid zones each receive an additional 41% of precipitation in the form of winter snow.

The soils in the Navajo region may be classified as excellent, good, or fair in terms of runoff, grass-producing ability, and erosion. Only about one third of the area is considered excellent or good in terms of soil productivity, and about 15% of the soil is unproductive, with little vegetation cover. The vegetation includes grassland, meadows, sagebrush, browse (shrub), and woodland (which is inaccessible and barren in some places). More Navajo land is covered with coniferous timber than with sagebrush (Iverson, 2002).

It was believed that the conflicts between the Navajos and their neighbors were contributing factors to their economic diversification. For example, historical accounts suggest that as raiding by and against the Navajo people grew in intensity, it consequently complicated agricultural pursuits and led to an increased need for mobility. In addition, the steady growth of the Navajo population figured greatly in the economic diversification: as the Navajo tribe grew in number, so did the quantity of livestock. Two principal periods of growth occurred in the Navajo tribe. The first period came in the last years of the eighteenth century and in the early years of the nineteenth century, before the White American campaign against the Navajos. The second principal period of growth followed the Navajo return from Bosque Redondo. It was during the first period of expansion that livestock was established as an economically important commodity (Brugge, 1964; Iverson, 2002).

Life Today among the Navajos

The spectacular growth of the Navajo population began during the post–Fort Sumner era. In 1870 the Navajo population numbered 15,000 (Boyce, 1942; Iverson, 2002). By 1900 the Navajo population had grown to 21,000, and by 1935 the population had grown to 35,500. The population has grown steadily ever since. In 1981 there were approximately 151,000 Navajo Indians, who resided primarily in rural areas on or near the 27,000-square-mile reservation that is located in Arizona, New Mexico, Colorado, and Utah (U.S. Department of Commerce, Bureau of the Census, 2002). By 1986, the Navajo population had grown to 171,097, making the Navajo tribe the largest Indian tribe in the continental United States. Today, the Navajo continues to be the largest tribe in the United States, with a population of 362,4888. The Cherokees are the second largest at 273,192 (U.S. Department of Commerce, Bureau of the Census, American Community Survey, 2015). These new figures represent an increase of 546,891 or 27.1% between 1990 and 2009 for the American Indian population alone (not in conjunction with Alaska Natives) (U.S. Department of Commerce, Bureau of the Census, American Community Survey, 2015). If the American Indian population was used in conjunction with other races—for example, Alaska Natives—the 2000 Census data suggest that there was an increase in that population by as many as 2.2 million people or 110% (U.S. Department of Commerce, Bureau of the Census, American Community Survey, 2015).

The 2010 census found that approximately 500 Indian tribes (2,540,309 people) reside in 26 states, with most American Indians residing in the western part of the United States as a consequence of the forced western migration of the tribes (U.S. Department of Commerce, Bureau of the Census, American Community Survey, 2015). In fact, according to the Bureau of the Census, in 2010, 43% of American Indians reported living in the West, 31% lived in the South, 17% lived in the Midwest, and 9% lived in the Northeast (U.S. Department of Commerce, Bureau of the Census, American Community Survey, 2015).

According to the 2010 census, the Navajo nation is dominated by those who are under 18 years of age. In fact, the Navajos have a median age of 28.0 years of age as compared with the rest of the general U.S. population at 36.7 years (U.S. Department of Commerce, Bureau of the Census, American Community Survey, 2015). Women outnumber the men in the Navajo population (51.4% vs. 48.6%). Married-couple families represent only 37.5% of all Navajo families compared with 49.3% of families in the rest of the general population. Similarly, 27.5% of families are female-headed with no father present compared with only 12.5% of the rest of the general population. Of the number of Navajos, 27.9% had less than a high school diploma; 32% had a least a high school diploma; 31.6% had some college education or an associate degree; 6% had a bachelor's degree, and only 2.6% had a graduate or a professional degree (U.S. Department of Commerce, Bureau of the Census, American Community Survey, 2015).

It should be noted that there is a clear distinction between American Indians and the Alaska Natives. The term *Native American* is intended to imply tribes residing in the continental United States (in contrast to Native Canadians). Today, although many American Indians remain on reservations and in rural areas, an equal number reside in cities, especially in Oklahoma, California, New Mexico, and Alaska (U.S. Department of Commerce, Bureau of the Census, American Community Survey, 2015).

In 2013, the median family income for the American Indians was $27,389, as compared with $62,367 for the U.S. White population (U.S. Department of Commerce, Bureau of the Census, American Community Survey, 2015). American Indian women fared worse than the rest of the general population, with a median per capita income of $27,570 compared with $35,299, respectively. American Indian men barely made more than White women and made considerably less than the rest of the general population, with a median income of $32,723, compared with $45,320, respectively (U.S. Department of Commerce, Bureau of the Census, American Community Survey, 2015). The Navajo tribe derives revenue from oil, coal, uranium, and federal grants and contracts. Nevertheless, high unemployment rates continue to be a major problem among the Navajos (Iverson, 2002).

COMMUNICATION

Dialect and Style

The Navajo language is classified as Athapaskan because historically it has been shown to be derived from the languages used by the people of Lake Athabasca in northwestern Canada. The Navajo language is also similar to the languages spoken by some peoples living in Alaska, some on the northern coast of the Pacific Ocean, and some in northern California (such as the Hupas). In addition, Navajo and the 12 groups of Apache dialects form a dialect continuum of one single language. These separate groups speaking a language similar to the Navajo language are referred to as *Athapaskans.* Among the Navajo, 39.2% speak English only at home; 60.7% speak a language other than English at home; and 15% speak English less than very well (U.S. Department of Commerce, Bureau of the Census, American Community Survey, 2015).

The language of the Navajo people involves tonal speech in which pitch is of great importance. All vowels and consonants are fully sounded, regardless of how many times they are doubled or tripled in the same word. Vowels are often interchanged, creating several variations and meanings of the same word.

The Navajo language is believed to reflect a concept of the universe that is constantly in motion. In the Navajo language, position is defined as a withdrawal from motion. For example, a person speaking English says "on," whereas a Navajo person says something directly opposite in meaning for the word "on": the Navajo speaker says "at rest." Whereas an English speaker says, "I dressed" or "One dresses," the Navajo speaker says, "I moved into my clothes" or "One moves into clothes." The language directly parallels mythological thought in that not only is the language in motion but so too are cultural and spiritual heroes (Iverson, 2002; Sobralske, 1985).

When Navajo people speak, most of the sentences contain the concept *good.* For some Navajo people, the concept *good* may be defined as a favorable or desirable quality that promotes prosperity and happiness. Therefore, the word *good* is synonymous with other words, such as *agreeable, attractive,* or *beautiful* (*nizhóní*). The concept of goodness is directly related to the ideology of health and is even found in the Blessingway healing ceremony. This ceremony is viewed by the Navajos as a "good" event because it promotes everlasting harmony or perfection.

Even today the majority of Navajo people still speak the native language. Although many Navajo Indians are fluent in both the Navajo language and the English language, there are also many who do not speak English and therefore require the assistance of a Navajo interpreter when seeking or receiving health care. The Navajo language does not always have an equivalent single word for an English word; instead, the language uses a description of all occurrences affecting what is being said.

Until recently the Navajo language was unwritten. In World War II, a special branch of the U.S. Marine Corps was developed for Navajos who served as Navajo code talkers. It has been estimated that this highly esteemed group saved millions of lives because the enemy was unable to understand the Navajo language or infiltrate its code.

Touch

Instead of shaking hands on meeting another person, as it is practiced in the dominant U.S. culture, Navajos extend a hand and lightly touch the hand of the person they are greeting. Other examples of the use of touch in the Navajo culture include the tradition of massaging a newborn baby as a bonding experience between mother and baby and the tradition of giving a small gift and preparing a small feast for the family when the baby laughs for the first time because this token of esteem touches the heart of all the people around the baby. Another example is the taboo against touching a dead person or an animal killed by lightning, which is extended to touching articles associated with the deceased individual or animal. This taboo is not extended to animals whose death resulted from other natural causes.

Use of Silence and the Importance of Names

On initially meeting strangers, Navajo people may appear silent and reserved. Once the Navajo individual becomes familiar with the other person, warm behavior is usually demonstrated. In addition, when introducing themselves by name, Navajos give honor to ancestors by stating the clan and the location of their home.

Kinesics

Kinesics practiced within the Navajo culture includes the avoidance of eye contact. In dominant cultures in the United States, eye contact is considered important and if not present may cause suspicion. However, the opposite is true in the Navajo culture, where eye contact is considered a sign of disrespect.

In earlier days, Navajo people frowned on pointing anything at another person because pointing was considered insulting. Some Navajos believed that an object being passed to another person should be held upright so that an end would not point at the other person.

Language Lateralization

In a classic study of language lateralization in Navajo reservation children, one group of Navajo children was tested by a researcher who spoke only Navajo (McKeever, Hunt, Wells, & Yazzie, 1989). Another group of Navajo and White children was tested by a researcher who spoke only English. Findings from the study indicate that there appeared to be a strong right-ear advantage for the White children tested by the English-speaking researcher. A similar right-ear advantage was found in the Navajo children when they were tested by the Navajo-speaking researcher, whereas the Navajo children tested by the English-speaking researcher revealed minimal, nonsignificant right-ear advantage. Most of the previous research has suggested that Navajos and other Native Americans have an absence of right-ear advantage. The results of this study were found to be inconsistent with the view that Navajos and other Native Americans are right-brain-hemisphere dominant and thus have a left-ear advantage as a function of the appositional mode of language and thought (McKeever, Hunt, Wells, & Yazzie, 1989).

Implications for Nursing Care. Because the Navajo language does not always have one single word that is similar to one English word in meaning, to do a nursing assessment and develop a nursing diagnosis, goals, and interventions, the nurse must remember that what is being said must be interpreted by approximation. Because some Navajo people do not speak English, it may be necessary to provide a person who is fluent in the Navajo language. When a Navajo interpreter is used, this person must be knowledgeable about medical terminology as well as the cultural aspects of the Navajo lifestyle.

It is also important to remember that the first encounter is not always made to deal with official matters. It is meant to provide an opportunity for the nurse to become acquainted with the family and vice versa. Future rapport with the family is based on this consideration.

Navajo individuals who enter the profession of nursing may experience a cultural shock when care must be provided for a dying patient because of the taboo against touching a dead or dying person and items associated with death. Because of the taboos associated with death, some Navajo nurses may have a healing ceremony performed after contact with a dead person.

Space

Time and space are bound to each other; therefore, it must be remembered that the elimination of time alters spatial concepts (Hall, 1990). For some Navajo people there is no such thing as imaginary space. Space is so real a concept that it may not be located in any dimension other than real space. For example, space may not be located in the realm of thought; there is no abstract space. For the Navajo Indian, a space such as that found in a room or a house is the same as a small universe (Hall, 1990).

For the Navajo people, personal living space, or that of the traditional Navajo dwelling (*hooghan, hogan*), is surrounded with many traditions and superstitions or taboos. The hogan is a round, open room with distinct functional areas. Many Navajo people believe that shared space provides a spiritual security and a sense of trust. Sheepskins, with the head facing the fire, are used for sleeping. A wood-burning stove, situated center front with the vent pipe extending through the ceiling, provides a means of cooking food. Taboos associated with death in a *hogan* include the need to seal the entry, warning other Navajos to stay away, and frequently the need to abandon or burn the *hogan* when a death has occurred. Another event that renders a *hogan* unusable is lightning striking in proximity; even wood from such a *hogan* is never used for any purpose by a Navajo, except for a Navajo medicine man in relation to ceremonies. Before a new *hogan* is occupied, it is usually blessed by a hired Navajo medicine man, who either strews pollen along the cardinal points or performs a formal ceremony. The *hogan* is so important to the Navajo culture that all Navajo ceremonies are performed in it. Although the *hogan* is often crowded with members of both nuclear and extended families, the Navajo need for extension of space is demonstrated by the fact that miles often separate one *hogan* from another or one camp from another.

Implications for Nursing Care. Because personal space is so important and has no imaginary boundaries, it is important for the nurse to remember that some Navajo clients may have difficulty adapting to situations that place them in spaces that are not familiar. It is important for the nurse to familiarize the client with the space provided during hospitalization and when personal space is limited during health care administration. The nurse should be sensitive to the fact that a hospital might be unfamiliar to some Navajo people, with new things and experiences, such as different types of foods, different buildings and equipment, different varieties of uniforms, different types of health professionals and support staff, and different types of communication. This situation is particularly true when Navajo clients are hospitalized off the reservation, where Navajo interpreters are unavailable, or when great distances from their home prevent visitation from their extended family.

The nurse may encounter other health concerns and problems related to life in the cramped environment of a *hogan,* such as infectious diseases from the lack of indoor plumbing and water supply and burns related to the indoor stoves. Lack of food and food storage may contribute to nutritional deficiencies. In addition, the distance between *hogans* has a public health implication because isolation from the mainstream creates barriers in the delivery of health care. One main barrier is the lack of public transportation. Non–Navajo-speaking public health nurses cope with this barrier with the assistance of Navajo interpreters traveling as a team in a four-wheel-drive vehicle over treacherous terrain and unpaved roads.

SOCIAL ORGANIZATION

Family

The Navajo culture is extremely family oriented, but the term *family* has a much broader meaning than just referring to the nuclear family of father, mother, and children. The biological family is the center of social organization and includes all members of the extended family. The Navajo people are traditionally a matriarchal society, which means that when a couple marries, the husband makes his home with his wife's relatives, and his family becomes one of several units that live in a group of adjacent *hogans* or other types of dwellings.

There is no set numbers or types of relatives limiting the extended family, and their focus is to help one another grow, to collaborate on resources that will provide an adequate livelihood, and to participate in daily life occurrences. Assistance with ceremonies, particularly those associated with birth, death, marriage, or sickness, is shared and has great importance. Usually a male family member who is looked on as having the greatest amount of prestige will rise as leader for the extended family and provide necessary direction. However, in settling issues, all sides are listened to and the entire group determines the outcome.

The family is considered so important in the Navajo culture that to be without relatives is to be really poor; children learn from infancy that the family and the tribe are of paramount importance. In the Navajo culture, being available for a family member is extremely important, and it is common practice for many members of the extended family to come to the hospital and stay with the client or in proximity to the client until discharge. This situation is particularly true of mothers who have a child in the pediatric unit. All efforts should be made to provide overnight accommodations for the mother in the same room with the child if this is not medically contraindicated.

Family Roles and Structure

In the traditional nuclear family, the mother is responsible for the domestic duties associated with the home. The father, on the other hand, is responsible for any outside work necessary to maintain the family and the home. Children are responsible for assisting both parents (Iverson, 2002; Roessel, 1981). Within Navajo families, children are viewed as assets, not liabilities. Navajo Indian children are rarely told they cannot do something but instead are frequently told of the consequences of doing a particular thing (Iverson, 2002; Primeaux, 1977). Children are encouraged by their parents and members of the extended family to live and learn by their decisions. Because the Navajo traditions are passed down by the elderly, Navajo children are taught to respect tradition and to honor wisdom (Iverson, 2002; Primeaux, 1977).

Despite the role assumed in the family, family support is critical to the Navajos. Epple, Wright, Joish, and Bauer (2003) examined active family nutritional support to determine if there was an association with improved metabolic outcomes for the Diné (Navajo) individuals who had Type 2 diabetes. Findings from this study suggested that active family nutritional support is significantly associated with specific indices for maintenance of diabetes such as control of triglyceride, cholesterol, and hemoglobin A_{1c} levels. Further findings of this study suggested that the Navajo family in its aggregate is a more useful unit of intervention compared with the individual alone, especially when designing diabetes care interventions.

Marriage

Some Navajo marriages are still arranged. In any case, marriage and the family are considered the foundation of Navajo life. In Navajo society, women are expected not to excel or achieve more success than their husbands (Iverson, 2002; Roessel, 1981). This is even the case among some female Navajo nurses, who may be cautious about excelling in the profession at the risk of their marriages. In earlier times, divorce among traditional Navajos occurred when the wife placed her husband's belongings outside the *hogan* (Iverson, 2002; Roessel, 1981). Skogrand et al. (2008) conducted a qualitative study among two Navajo Nation chapters to determine factors that made these Navajo marriages strong. The sample consisted of 21 couples who believed they had strong marriages. Factors for strong marriages were identified and included (1) the ability to maintain open lines of communication, (2) taking the opportunity to learn about the importance of marriage, (3) providing time to nurture the relationship, and finally (4) providing the opportunity to build a solid and strong foundation.

Traditional Navajo Dress

The dress of traditional Navajo women has been adapted from the dress of the Spaniards encountered during the internment of the Navajo people at Fort Sumner. The dress usually consists of long, gathered calico skirts and brightly colored velveteen blouses. Because of the harsh terrain and great amount of walking done by Navajo women to get from one place to the other, sneakers and socks are the primary type of footwear.

Traditional Navajo men have adapted the western type of garb, which includes jeans, cotton western shirts, boots, and wide-brimmed hats. Both men and women commonly carry woolen blankets and wear large amounts of turquoise, coral, and silver jewelry as well as ornate buttons and belts. Also, both men and women traditionally wear their long hair tied in a knot behind their head; the knot is covered with rows of white woolen yarn.

Religion

Historically the Navajo people have been guided by sacred myths and legends that describe the tribe's evolution from inception to the present. Supernatural beings portrayed in these stories symbolize the Navajo culture, in which religion and healing practices are blended. Values and beliefs intrinsic to their culture and religion form the Navajo day-to-day living experiences.

Implications for Nursing Care

It is important for the nurse to remember that both the nuclear family and the extended family are of paramount importance to the Navajo client. Because Navajo people believe that family members are responsible for each other, it is not uncommon for many relatives to come to the hospital to care for the Navajo client. Restrictive hospital rules that allow only two visitors at a time or only immediate relatives have no meaning for some Navajo people. The nurse and other members of the health care team should be sensitive to the reality that *hogans* and camps are at times located a great distance from one another and that visiting a sick relative in the hospital may necessitate travel for many miles, with other family sacrifices needed to obtain funding for this journey. Referral to appropriate available resources will have a positive influence on family-centered care. The presence of family members also provides an ideal opportunity for their inclusion in discharge-planning sessions. Flexibility in scheduling follow-up clinic appointments should also be considered.

Because the Indian kinship or clan system is unfamiliar to most nurses in the United States, it is important for the nurse to develop a sensitivity to and an understanding of the significance of Indian clanships. For example, not only does one inherit lineage from one's mother, but it is also common for a Navajo child to have several sets of grandparents, uncles, cousins, brothers, and sisters. Among the Navajo people, first cousins may be treated as brothers and sisters, and great aunts and uncles as grandparents. The whole system of clanship may prove to be thoroughly confusing to the nurse because several sets of grandparents, brothers, sisters, uncles, and aunts may show up at the hospital, all claiming close relationship to the client.

TIME

The cultural interpretation of time has a temporal focus that views human life as existing in a three-point range that includes past, present, and future (Kluckhohn & Strodtbeck, 1973). Navajo Indians are viewed as being primarily present-time oriented. However, it should be noted that some Navajo Indians are perceived as being both past- and present-time oriented. The common orientation regarding the man–nature theme is a mixed perception that espouses that man is subjugated to nature and at the same time is suggestive that man should learn to live in harmony with nature. In a classic study by Kluckhohn and Strodtbeck (1973), it was noted that the present-time orientation was the preferred mode of time orientation for the population of Rimrock Navajos sampled. The findings of the study also suggested that past-time orientation was somewhat more preferable than future-time orientation but that the difference in preference was not statistically significant. In the study it was also noted that although some of the respondents preferred to be perceived as being subjugated to nature, the one significant preference was a perception of being in harmony with nature.

Implications for Nursing Care

Most people in the dominant culture in the United States are regulated by clocks and are therefore very time conscious. Future-oriented individuals may have a great deal of difficulty with some Navajo people because of their present-time orientation. It is important for the nurse to remember that because Navajo Indians are perceived as being present-time oriented, time is viewed as being on a continuum, with no beginning and no end (Primeaux, 1977). In some Navajo homes there are no clocks because Navajo time is casual, present-time oriented, and relative to present needs that must be accomplished in a present-time frame. Because certain tasks are associated with present needs, it may be difficult for the nurse to counsel and advise a Navajo client about crucial future events, such as taking medications. The present-time orientation of a Navajo client may cause this person to eat two meals today, four meals tomorrow, no meals the next day, and three meals the day after. This becomes an important nursing implication if a client is told to take the medicine with meals, particularly if the medication is to be taken three times a day. Another indication of the Navajo present-time orientation is related to the failure to keep clinical appointments.

ENVIRONMENTAL CONTROL

Some Navajo Indians are perceived as having an external locus of control; although they believe that man is not subjugated to the effects of nature, they also believe that it is essential for man to live in harmony with nature and its elements. As mentioned earlier, Kluckhohn and Strodtbeck (1973) noted that the Rimrock Navajos sampled preferred the orientation theme of "man in harmony with nature." One conclusion from the study was that some Navajo Indians had a mixed locus of control that was suggestive of both a "being"-oriented and a "doing"-oriented culture.

In the past, self-esteem and a health-oriented locus of control have been postulated as predictors of attitudes and behaviors directly related to children's health. A classic study by Lamarine (1987) was done to measure the relationship between self-esteem, a health-oriented locus of control, and health attitudes of Navajo children in the fourth to sixth grades. The analysis of the data indicates that there is a statistically significant relationship between self-esteem and positive attitudes toward health. In addition, the study found that self-esteem was a modest predictor of health attitudes and health behavior intentions among Navajo and Pueblo children.

A craniofacial team at the University of New Mexico Medical Center at Albuquerque were successful in the treatment of a large population of Navajos because of team awareness of the Navajo concept of health (Smoot, Kucan, Cope, & Asse, 1988). This understanding of the Navajo concept of health, in which man is viewed as being in balance with the environment (and therefore an understanding of the Navajo concerns with ghosts, "skinwalkers," and rules for orderly living), allowed team members to integrate the family, as well as the Navajo medicine man, into the care and treatment of children with craniofacial diseases. In addition, to provide culturally appropriate care, the craniofacial team had to develop an understanding of traditional Navajo healing ceremonies and the need for special handling of disposed body parts during surgery.

Illness and Wellness Behaviors

Traditional Navajo concepts espouse the need for the Navajo people to be in harmony with the surrounding environment and with the family. Some Navajo Indians have a perception of health that is not limited to the physical body but encompasses congruency with the family, environment, livestock, supernatural forces, and community. To maintain spiritual health, some Navajo people believe that it is essential to be in harmony with supernatural forces. Iverson (2002) concluded that health and religion cannot be separated in the Navajo world; rather, the link between traditional religion and healing ceremonies found among Navajo Indians is obvious.

Traditional Navajo concepts of health and disease have a fundamental place in the Navajo concept of man and his place in the universe. Native healing ceremonies encompass traditional Navajo medicine and general native healing practices and form the foundation of Navajo culture. These ceremonies are central to the attitudes, beliefs, values, and perceptions of the Navajo people.

Blessingway is the main philosophy from which more than 35 major and minor ceremonial variations are derived. This Navajo practice attempts to remove ill health by means of stories, songs, rituals, prayers, symbols, and sand paintings (Iverson, 2002; Sobralske, 1985). In the Blessingway ceremony, the importance of family and clan members is emphasized in the healing process. The mother is considered particularly important because she can relate prenatal incidents of ill nature that affect health.

Native Healers

Navajo medicine men and medicine women spend many years learning their skills and serving as apprentices. There are several types of medicine men and women:

1. *Diagnosticians* are those who diagnose illness or the cause of disharmony. Their title may be "crystal gazer" or "hand trembler," depending on the method used in diagnosing the patient.
2. *Singers* (*hataaii,* an undifferentiated singular-plural noun) are those who perform and direct the elaborate and complex healing ceremonies.
3. *Herbalists* are those specialized practitioners who use herbs to treat patients and who may also diagnose illness and causes of ailments.

Medicine men and medicine women have *jish,* or medicine bundles, containing symbolic and sacred items, including corn pollen, feathers, stones, arrowheads, and other instruments used for healing and blessing. Many of these sacred objects and plants are found on the sacred mountains that border the Navajo reservation and are gathered only by medicine people (Iverson, 2002; Navajo Health Systems Agency, 1985).

There is great effort on the part of the Indian Health Service and the traditional Navajo healers to work together in a collaborative and cooperative way. It is not uncommon to observe a medicine man or medicine woman in the hospital speaking with a physician regarding the care of a client. When medically indicated, clients may also receive passes to participate in a healing ceremony held outside the hospital. There has been a continued and sustained mutual respect on the part of these two groups for the expertise of the other (Navajo Health Systems Agency, 1985).

In 1984, in a classic study, the Navajo Health Systems Agency conducted a research study to investigate the types of traditional healing services being provided and the types of cultural orientations to traditional healing practices being provided for newly hired Indian Health Service care providers. The conclusions of the survey reiterated the need for continued and improved collaboration and cooperation between traditional medicine people and Western physicians. For example, serious cases of injury and illness are often referred to the hospital by medicine people, and physicians have sent clients to medicine people when deemed appropriate, particularly in cases of psychological or behavioral disorders (Navajo Health Systems Agency, 1985).

Death and Dying Rituals

The Navajos are considered a traditional people. They have often been characterized as being very respectful of death and the dead (Iverson, 2002; Kluckhohn & Leighton, 1974; Lewis & Bourne, 1989). Yet it is essential to remember that the beliefs held by the Navajos depend on personal experience; the level of acculturation into traditional U.S. society; and beliefs in traditional religion, Christianity, and/or in the Native American Church. Traditional Navajos are so respectful of the dead that they do not touch the body (Braun, Pietsch, & Blanchette, 2005). In fact, when a Navajos dies, it is suggested by tradition that other Navajos not touch the body (Braun et al., 2005). It is thought that if a Navajos touches the body of the dead, the spirit of the deceased might contaminate that person and thus the individual would require what is known as a "cleansing ceremony" (Braun et al., 2005). Some Navajos believe that the ghost of the dead might possibly return to his or her home, so traditional Navajos may build a temporary home or *hogan* away from the main home and move the dying person to this new structure (Braun et al., 2005). It is essential to remember that even traditional Navajos may send terminally ill Navajos to the hospital. The dead are usually quickly buried by the Navajos (Braun et al., 2005). The Navajos tend to avoid discussion of death and dying as it is a revered experience, and the name of the dead is not spoken out loud (Braun et al., 2005). The afterlife for most Navajos is not necessarily equated with reward, good behavior, or a quality of one's life (Braun et al., 2005). Some researchers contend that while the Navajos believe in the afterlife, it is perceived as only a very "shadowy and uninviting phenomenon" (Braun et al., 2005; Kluckhohn & Leighton, 1974). For Navajos who commit suicide, such an individual is believed to be destined to carry the object used to commit the suicide in the afterlife (Braun et al., 2005). The Navajos have been slow to embrace the concepts of advance directives or truth in disclosure of terminal illness. For example, Carrese and Rhodes (1995) found that because the Navajos believe that thought and language shape reality, discussions of negative information such as the disclosure of risk in informed consent, truth in telling about terminal illness, and advance directives for future illness may all possibly be a violation of traditional Navajo values.

Implications for Nursing Care

To a Navajo Indian, *being* is a fundamental concept; as mentioned earlier, Navajos are considered more "being" oriented than achievement oriented. Individuals are perceived as being more important than possessions, wealth, or other material things. If something is perceived as good, it is only as good as its value to other people. It is important, therefore, for the nurse to remember that some Navajo

Indians believe that goodness is found only when one is in complete harmony with the surrounding environment. The nurse should also keep in mind that if a Navajo is to have the perception of being in harmony with the environment, the environment must be structured in such a way that harmony is promoted. If a nurse were to deny or not allow the client the opportunity to achieve harmony with other people, animals, plants, nature, weather, and supernatural forces, the client would not be able to obtain a sense of assuredness in relation to physical, social, psychological, and spiritual health.

It is important for the nurse to determine which cultural health practices are beneficial, neutral, or harmful to the client to provide culturally appropriate care. If a cultural practice is considered either beneficial or neutral, the practice should be incorporated into the plan of care. However, if a cultural practice is considered harmful, the nurse should devise a teaching strategy that will assist the client in developing an understanding of the implications of the practice on continued health maintenance. For example, after delivery the umbilical cord is taken from the newborn, dried, and buried near an object or place that symbolizes what the parents want for the child's future. Burial close to the home of the infant signifies the continued tie or relationship with the child's home and Mother Earth. Because this neutral practice does not negatively affect health care, it should be acknowledged, accepted, and incorporated into the plan of care. Also, to provide culturally appropriate nursing care, it is essential that the nurse respect the need for Navajo people to maintain traditional rituals even when hospitalized. For example, it would not be uncommon for a Navajo individual to sprinkle certain foods, such as corn and cornmeal, around the bedside during a curative ritualistic ceremony. The nurse who comes in the room and finds cornmeal around the bedside may initially be disturbed and insist that it be removed. However, the nurse should keep in mind that this cornmeal (as well as other rituals) is extremely important in the ritual and that, because it does not have any negative health-related implications, it should be left at the bedside until the client and the family desire its removal (Primeaux, 1977).

The U.S. government has passed numerous acts and implemented numerous programs specifically to address health-related issues among the Navajo people and their involvement in the determination of their health care. The 1975 Indian Self-Determination Act provides that any federal program serving the health needs of Navajo people may be either self-determined or contracted for by the Navajo tribe or its designee. Services contracted for must be comparable to or exceed existing services under the direction of federally operated programs, such as the Indian Health Service. Through collaborative efforts, the commitment to improve the health status of the Navajo population and to increase tribal involvement in health care management has been enhanced, reconfirmed, and extended to other components of health care (Hanley, 1987).

The basic authority for health care for American Indians and Alaskans is provided by the Snyder Act of 1921. The Bureau of Indian Affairs assumed responsibility as a federal branch for providing health care services for the Navajo people until 1954. At that time, the responsibility was transferred to the Indian Health Service as a result of the U.S. Transfer Act of 1954. In 1967 the Navajo area of the Indian Health Service was established to address the health care needs of Navajos. Today, the Navajo area is one of 12 areas within the Indian Health Service and has its administrative location in Window Rock, Arizona.

BIOLOGICAL VARIATIONS

Many American Indians are faced with a number of health-related problems. Some of the contributing factors include the fact that many of the old ways of diagnosing and treating illness have not outlasted the migration and changing ways of most American Indians. It has been estimated that at least one third of all American Indians live in a state of absolute poverty. As a direct result of this poverty, the compounded problems of lost skills and economic endeavors, and the increased complexity of disease entities, many American Indians are in a health-related crisis. In addition, many illnesses and diseases are related to such factors as poor living conditions and malnutrition. American Indians are believed to be at risk for tuberculosis, maternal and infant deaths, diabetes, and malnutrition.

In the past, American Indians continuously had the highest infant mortality in the United States. While it is true that the infant mortality rate for American Indians declined from an average of 13.9 per 1000 live births from 1983 to 1985, to an average of 12.6 per 1000 live births between 1989 and 1991, to 8.3 per 1000 live births in 2010, these rates are all disproportionately high compared with the national average of 6.15 in 2010 (National Center for Health Statistics, 2010). The infant, child, and youth death rates also remain disproportionately high for American Indians, led only by African-Americans. In 2010, the overall infant mortality rate for children younger than 1 year of age was 690.7 per 100,000, as compared with 564.2 for their White counterparts. Similarly, the death rate for American Indian children 1 to 4 years of age was 54.5 per 100,000, as compared with 25 for their White counterparts. In addition, the death rate for American Indian children 5 to 14 years of age was 16.9 per 100,000, as compared with 14 for their White counterparts. The rate for deaths for American Indians adolescents 15 to 19 years of age was also disproportionately high at 95.54 per 100,000 population, as compared with 59.1 per 100,000 for their White counterparts (Child Trends, 2014).

In 2010, the age-adjusted death rate for all causes of death for the American Indian population was 641.9 per 100,000 population (National Center for Health Statistics, Health United States, 2014. The life expectancy at birth overall for American Indians is 74.5 years compared with 76.9 years for the rest of the general population (National Center for Health Statistics, Health United States, 2014). For American Indian males, the life expectancy is again disproportionately low at 69.1 years (77.5 years for females) (National Center for Health Statistics, Health United States, 2014).

However, although American Indians have had an increase in life expectancy, the rate still lags behind that for all other races in the United States (National Center for Health Statistics, Health United States, 2014). In 2010, the leading causes of death in the American Indian population included (1) heart disease, (2) cancer, (3) unintentional injuries, (4) diabetes, (5) stroke, (6) chronic liver disease and cirrhosis, (7) chronic lower respiratory disease, (8) suicide, (9) influenza and pneumonia, and (10) homicide (National Center for Health Statistics 2014). The leading causes of death and the figures change dramatically when American Indian data are reviewed by age. For example, in 2010-2011, the leading causes of death (adjusted rate) for American Indians 25 to 44 years of age were (1) unintentional injuries at 117.6 per 100,000 population (compared with 2.5 per 100,000 for Whites), (2) chronic liver disease and cirrhosis at 31.6 per 100,000 population (compared with 7.5 per 100,000 population for Whites), (3) suicide at 31.5 per 100,000 population (compared with 2 per 100,000 for Whites), and (4) diseases of the heart at 30 per 100,000 population (compared with 1.7 per 100,000 population for Whites) (National Center for Health Statistics, Health United States, 2014).

Body Size and Structure

Navajo children tend to have low length-for-age and high weight-for-length measures. These reference indicators suggest a suboptimal nutritional status among Navajo Indians. Navajo children with birth weights of less than 2500 g tend to be shorter, lighter, and thinner than children with birth weights of over 2500 g. In a classic study by Peck, Marks, Dibley, Lee, and Trowbridge (1988), the analysis of the data indicates that much of the nutritional risk, as indicated by growth abnormality among Navajo infants, is most directly attributable to the persistent effects of intrauterine growth retardation and low birth weights.

There is documented evidence of a high prevalence of obesity in American Indian children. For example, Lohman et al. (1999) found a high prevalence of obesity among American Indian children representing six different Indian nations. Similarly, White et al. (1997) noted that weight, body mass index (BMI), skinfolds, and waist circumference were greatest among participants 40 to 59 years of age and lowest in participants 60 years of age and older. Among American Indian men who participated in the study, the prevalence of overweight was 37% among those 20 to 39 years of age. Similarly, it was 50% among male American Indians 30 to 59 years of age but was only 15% for male American Indians over 60 years of age (White et al., 1997).

Skin Color

Skin color is perhaps the most recognizable way in which people are categorized. Although other surface characteristics subtly add to this categorization, skin color is perhaps one of the most obvious ways in which people vary across ethnic and cultural barriers. Skin-color variability is caused by a pigment that is produced by the melanocytes located in the epidermal layer of the skin. According to classic work of Wasserman (1974), the melanocytes originate in the neural crest, which is near the embryonic central nervous system, and seemingly migrate into the fetal epidermis. This origin explains the significance of pigmentation. Mongolian spots are therefore leftovers that somehow linger in the lumbosacral region at a somewhat greater than ordinary depth and cause the bluish effect seen on the skin surface. Mongolian spots are obvious in 90% of Blacks, 80% of Asians and American Indians, and 9% of Whites (Jacobs & Walton, 1976). Mongolian spots are commonly found on the buttocks and back and occasionally on the abdomen, thighs, and arms. Mongolian spots appear so ominous on inspection that a nurse who is unfamiliar with this type of discoloration may easily mistake them for child abuse. The neural origin of melanocytes explains the shape. Mongolian spots resemble neurons with dendritic appendages that insert themselves well up into the epidermal cells. These appendages inject melanosome granules containing melanin pigments into the epidermal cells (Szabó, 1975).

Dark-skinned individuals are seemingly protected from the effects of sunlight to a greater degree than light-skinned individuals are. One reason for this may be the dispersal of the melanosomes from the basal cells directly to the stratum granulosum. Therefore, when inspecting the skin of Whites, Asians, and American Indians, the nurse will find that melanosomes are incorporated singly (Szabó, Gerald, Pathak, & Fitzpatrick, 1969).

Other Visible Physical Characteristics

One visible physical difference that appears to be a startling finding for the nurse is the cleft uvula, wherein the uvula may be separated at the tip, thereby giving it a fishtail appearance. Although this is the most common variation, the separation can also occur as a complete division into two uvulas (Meskin, Gorlin, & Isaacson, 1964). Although this condition is rare in Blacks and Whites, it occurs in about 10% of Asians and as many as 18% of American Indians (Schaumann, Peagler, & Gorlin, 1970).

Another visible physical difference is associated with age-related increases in earlobe creasing. A study of Eskimos, Navajos, and Whites by Overfield and Call (1983) found no differences among the groups in the frequency of age-related earlobe creasing. However, findings from the study did indicate a difference in relation to age and onset of earlobe creasing across ethnic and cultural barriers. Whites were found to have earlobe creases at least a decade earlier than Navajos were.

Enzymatic Variations

Lactose intolerance occurs among the majority of the populations of the world. In fact, it affects 94% of Asians, 90% of African Blacks, 79% of American Indians, 75% of American Blacks, 50% of Mexican Americans, and 17% of White Americans (Bose & Welsh, 1973; Leichter & Lee, 1971; McCracken, 1971; Sowers & Winterfeldt, 1975).

Susceptibility to Disease

Tuberculosis. The role of socioeconomic factors in the incidence of tuberculosis, which includes conditions such as overcrowding and poor nutrition, cannot be disregarded. However, ethnicity also appears to be an important factor in the incidence of tuberculosis. Numerous studies suggest a high incidence of tuberculosis among American Indians (Delien, 1951; Heath, 1980). The incidence of tuberculosis varies among tribes, from a low of 2% for Apaches to 4.6% for Navajos (Reifel, 1949). In the 1980s, the previously high incidence of tuberculosis among American Indians was greatly decreased, but the incidence is still considered high compared with the general population.

Type 2 Diabetes. Type 2 diabetes mellitus is a major health problem for American Indians, occurring as early as the teens or early 20s. The earlier onset has led to an earlier onset of complications, as well as excessive mortality in the early and middle adult years. Age-specific death rates for diabetes appear to be 2.6 times higher for American Indians between 25 and 54 years of age compared with the rest of the general U.S. population (National Center for Health Statistics, Health United States, 2014). The age-adjusted death rate for diabetes as the single underlying cause

among American Indians was 34.8, as compared with 19.5 for White Americans, 26.9 for Hispanics, and 13.1 for Asian Americans (U.S. Department of Health and Human Services, National Diabetes Statistics Report, 2014). In addition, the complications from diabetes among American Indians are appearing with distressing frequency. The National Diabetes Advisory Board noted in 2002 that complications such as amputations have a rate of occurrence 2 to 3 times that of the general U.S. population and a renal failure rate 20 times that of the general U.S. population.

According to the U.S. Department of Health and Human Services, National Center for Health Statistics (2014), 45% of outpatient visits in some facilities for Indian health services are for diabetes-related problems. In addition, in some Indian tribes the rate of newly diagnosed diabetes is as high as 25%. (It is interesting to note, however, that before the 1940s, the occurrence of diabetes among Indians was rare [Tom-Orme, 1984].) The highest prevalence rates of diabetes among American Indians are found among the Pimas of Arizona, the Senecas of Oklahoma, and the Cherokees of North Carolina; the lowest rates are found in the Navajos, Hopis, and Apaches (Tom-Orme, 1984).

It is uncertain as to why diabetes mellitus is so prevalent among American Indians. One hypothesis suggests that some American Indians have a genetic predisposition for diabetes that is seemingly triggered by changes in dietary practices and increasing obesity (Neel, 1962). Another hypothesis, called the "thrifty-gene" hypothesis, suggests that during the centuries when American Indians lived a migratory life characterized by periods of feast and famine, a "thrifty gene" developed as a result of natural selection. It has been proposed that this gene might have affected carbohydrate metabolism and storage so that during times when food was readily available, carbohydrates could be more readily stored in the body to be used during periods of scarcity. This theory proposes that, even today, some American Indians continue to store carbohydrates in excess, but because periods of food scarcities or famine no longer occur as they once did, American Indians tend to become obese, which ultimately leads to the development of diabetes (Andrews & Boyle, 2003).

Numerous studies support the idea that American Indians have a predisposition for diabetes mellitus. In a classic study by Sugarman (1989), 177 cases of gestational diabetes and 13 cases of preexisting diabetes were identified in a retrospective analysis of 4094 deliveries among Navajo women. The findings of the study therefore suggest a prevalence of 4.6% for gestational diabetes. The study also noted that when women with preexisting diabetes or previously documented gestational diabetes were excluded, the prevalence of gestational diabetes was 3.4%. Although each data source independently failed to identify 20% to 40% of diabetic pregnancies, more than 97% of cases were identified when the data sources were used collectively (Sugarman, 1989).

In a similar classic study, 181 pregnant Navajo women were screened for gestational diabetes (Massion et al., 1987). The findings of this study indicated that the 50-g oral glucose screening test was greater than 7.2 mmol/L or 130 mg/dL in 44 of the subjects, or approximately 24.3% of the women. In addition, the test was greater than 8.3 mmol/L or 150 mg/dL in 23 of the subjects, or approximately 12.7%. With the use of standard oral glucose tolerance testing, the incidence of gestational diabetes in the study population was 6.1%. Therefore, the study concluded that universal screening of gestational diabetes is recommended among Navajo women because they are perceived as a high-risk population (Massion et al., 1987).

Sugarman and Percy (1989) noted an age- and sex-adjusted prevalence of type 2 diabetes of 10.2% among the approximately 76% of Navajo adults living on reservations. This figure was approximately 60% greater than the estimated prevalence of 6.4% for the general U.S. population. In addition, findings from the study suggest that Navajo people are more overweight than the general U.S. population (Sugarman & Percy, 1989).

O'Connor, Fragneto, Coulehan, and Crabtree (1987) conducted a classic cross-sectional study to assess the association of various demographics and medical care variables with metabolic outcomes in Navajos with type 2 diabetes. In the study, the dependent variable was identified as metabolic control and was measured as the mean of all random plasma glucose values obtained at scheduled clinic visits for diabetes over a 2-year period. Using multivariate analysis, the researchers noted that better metabolic control was most strongly associated with compliance with appointments. In addition, the study noted an association between the mode of treatment and metabolic control.

More recently, researchers have begun to examine the relationship between the use of select oral contraceptives and the development of diabetes among American Indian women. For example, Kim, Seidel, Begier, and Kwok (2001) found that American Indian women who use depot medroxyprogesterone are more likely to develop diabetes than patients who had used combination estrogen-progestin oral contraceptives (odds ratio, 3.8; confidence interval, 1.8–1.9). Further findings suggest that even after adjustment for BMI, the excess risk for the development of diabetes by these women persisted (Kim et al., 2001).

It is postulated that Navajos with diabetes mellitus are at great risk to develop other life-threatening illnesses. For example, Donahue and Orchard (1992) noted that, as with all other racial populations, Navajos with diabetes mellitus are at a high risk to develop atherosclerotic macrovascular complications. Hoy, Light, and McGill (1995) noted that about one fourth of all the Navajos enrolled in their study over 20 years of age who attended an Indian Health Service clinic had cardiac disease. Further findings from this study suggest that this figure represented more than five times the prevalence for heart disease in their age-matched counterparts without diabetes.

O'Connor, Crabtree, and Nakamura (1997) found that there is a greater incidence in mortality experiences of Navajos with type 1 diabetes mellitus. Findings from this study suggest that among the Navajos enrolled in the study, there were 30 deaths among the 154 study subjects (39%) from the diabetic groups, as compared with 13 (17%) from their age-matched controls (O'Connor et al., 1997).

Hypertension. Hypertension is rapidly becoming an increasingly important health problem among American Indians and in particular the Navajos. Percy et al. (1997) conducted a community-based study in 1991 and 1992 that included three standardized measurements of blood pressure on the Navajo reservation. Findings from this study indicated that the overall age-standardized prevalence of hypertension among the 780 adults examined (systolic >140 mm Hg; diastolic >90 mm Hg) was 19%, with a 24% prevalence noted among men and a 15% prevalence noted among women. Further findings from this study suggest that among the subjects surveyed, the prevalence of hypertension increased with age and relative weight, was more prevalent among men, and was associated with diabetes mellitus (Percy et al., 1997).

Shigella.   The resistance to trimethoprim-sulfamethoxazole (TMP-SMX) emerged among *Shigella* isolates from the Navajo reservation in the southwestern United States in 1985 and consequently was of paramount importance to health care workers (Griffin et al., 1989). In 1983 TMP-SMX resistance was noted at a rate of 3%; however, by 1985 this rate had increased significantly to 21%. The findings of the study indicated that all the respondents who were studied and examined were resistant to ampicillin and streptomycin and had minimal inhibitory concentrations resistant to sulfamethoxazole. The findings also indicated that polyclonal, highly TMP-SMX–resistant *Shigella* emerged through transfer of trimethoprim-resistant genes from aerobic bowel flora to endemic *Shigella* strains. Therefore, the findings indicated that the use of antimicrobials can lead to symptomatic shigellosis.

Myocardial Infarction. Klain, Coulehan, Arena, and Janett (1988) noted that the myocardial infarction rate for Navajo men had more than doubled in comparison with an earlier study by the researchers. In addition, they noted that there was a gradual increase in myocardial infarctions among Navajo women. The study concluded that the majority of the Navajos who sustained acute myocardial infarctions were hypertensive (51%), diabetic (50%), or both (31%). However, it was noted that very few of the respondents in the study admitted that they smoked cigarettes.

Arthritis. There appears to be a high prevalence of arthritis, including rheumatoid arthritis, among selected American Indian tribes as compared with non-Indian populations (Ng, Chatman, & Young, 2011). Rheumatoid arthritis was found at a rate of 6.8% in Chippewa Indians, and Willkens et al. (1982) noted in a study on Yakima Indians in Washington State that Chippewa women had an arthritis incidence of 3.4%. Although it has been suggested that Navajo Indians have a unique form of arthritis, the findings of one study suggest that Navajos have the same type of arthritis as that of the rest of the U.S. population (Rate, Morse, Bonnell, & Kuberski, 1980). Nurses should also be aware that there have been notable findings of arthritis in the presence of negative blood studies in the Navajo population. Although it has been suggested that geographical location is one major contributing factor to the problem of arthritis, tribes that reside in one location and then move to another do not exhibit any changes in prevalence rates (Overfield, 1995).

HIV and AIDS. American Indians and Alaska Natives in a 13-state area had twice the reported gonorrhea and syphilis morbidity than the rest of the general population. In addition, in some states, they also had the highest incidence of hepatitis B. Among these populations, there was also an increase in epidemic intravenous methamphetamine use in one rural American Indian–Alaska Native community. The number of persons who are seropositive for human immunodeficiency virus (HIV) is reported to be low in these groups. However, this low number is believed to be somewhat distorted because of the racial misclassification of these individuals (CDC Surveillance Report, 2009; Kaiser Foundation, 2009). Although only 3700 American Indians have been diagnosed with acquired immunodeficiency syndrome (AIDS), it is interesting to note that more than 1790 have died (Fauci, 2011). Of this number, 1480 were male and 310 were female. By proportion of the population, the number of American Indians and Alaska Natives who survive after an AIDS diagnosis is statistically smaller than that of any other U.S. racial or ethnic group in the United States (CDC, 2009). In 2006, when compared by proportion of the population, and especially with Whites, American Indians and Alaska Natives have a disproportionately higher rate of HIV infection—14.6 cases versus 11.5 cases per 100,000 (CDC, 2009). It is important to remember, however, that although there has been a relatively lower number of cumulative AIDS cases among American Indians and Alaska Natives, the incidence of AIDS is steadily increasing among this population (CDC, 2009).

Colorectal Cancer. Among all cancers, colorectal cancer is one of the deadliest and is now the third leading cause of death for American Indians and Alaska Natives (Espey et al., 2007). Like some other ethnic minority groups, American Indians and Alaska Natives are less likely to be diagnosed at early stages of this disease (59.6%) as compared with their White counterparts (66.5%) (Espey et al., 2007; Purdue et al., 2008). Wiggins et al. (2008) noted that the age-adjusted incidence rate of colon and rectal cancer of 46 per 100,000, reported for the counties and states in Indian Health Service Contract Health Service Delivery Area, was often misclassified as being much lower than it actually was for the American Indian and Alaska Native. In fact, when this rate was compared with that of Whites, it was noticeably lower (46 per 100,000 vs. 50.8 per 100,000, respectively). The percentage of these individuals 50 years of age or older who undergo diagnostic tests for colorectal cancer is also extremely low. For example, only about 12% of American Indians and Alaska Natives residing in the Southwest have undergone tests for fecal occult blood within the past year; only about 21% reported having an endoscopy in the past 5 years (CDC, Surveillance Report, 2013).

Nutritional Preferences

Because there are more than 500 different American Indian tribes, American Indian dietary practices vary widely. However, it should be noted that contemporary American Indian diets combine foods indigenous to the areas with modern processed foods. Food practices are also influenced by tribal beliefs and practices, geographical area, and local availability of selected foods. In certain tribal areas where game and fish are plentiful, these foods are important dietary sources. Although fruits, berries, roots, and wild greens are perceived to have important nutritional value, they are scarce in many federally defined Indian geographical regions. They are also scarce in urban centers such as large cities, except when found in season in supermarkets (Andrews & Boyle, 2003; U.S. Department of Agriculture, Food and Nutrition Service, 1984).

Foods preferred by many Navajos include meat and blue cornmeal. Milk, on the other hand, is usually not listed by Navajo people as a preferred food, and this lack of preference for milk has contributed to protein malnutrition among Navajos. One study reporting protein malnutrition among elderly Navajo clients indicates that protein malnutrition is present and is more common in males, hospitalized clients, and the elderly (Williams & Boyce, 1989). The importance of cultural dietary preferences among Navajos in relation to client teaching has been identified by Koehler, Harris, and Davis (1989). According to these researchers, dietitians and nutritionists should be aware of the rich ethnic diversity among American Indians and use this knowledge accordingly in nutritional counseling.

After 6 months of ethnographic research, Wolfe and Sanjur (1988) conducted a study on 107 Navajo women who for the most part were in the food assistance program. With its primary purpose being to describe and evaluate the contemporary Navajo diet, the study was done on the basis of a 1-day dietary recall. Using data from this 1-day dietary recall, mean nutrient intakes were found to be below the recommended daily allowances for calcium, phosphorus, iron, and vitamin A. Analysis of the data also suggested that 63% of the women in the sample were overweight or obese. Although overall percentages of energy from fat, carbohydrates, and protein were closer to those recommended in the dietary allowances than the percentages found in the general U.S. population, the fat intake appeared to be primarily saturated, and fiber intake was lower than the average for the rest of the general U.S. population. In addition, among the Navajo women sampled in the study, traditional foods were infrequently consumed. Another significant finding indicated that women with higher incomes tended to have better diets. The study also noted that commodity foods supplied by the U.S. Department of Agriculture's food distribution program provided approximately 43% of caloric intake and 37% to 57% of the intake of all nutrients except for fat and vitamin C for 72% of the population sampled. Thus a significant finding of the study was the important contribution that the food distribution program makes to the contemporary Navajo diet.

Alcohol Metabolism

For many years behavioral scientists have been searching for the biological reason why certain racial or ethnic groups such as Asians and American Indians react to alcohol differently from the way other racial or ethnic groups do, and they have noted that alcohol metabolism varies as a result of ethnic heritage. For example, some Asians and American Indians have reported physical symptoms, such as profound facial flushing and other vasomotor symptoms, after drinking alcohol. Wolff (1973) noted that most Whites do not experience similar symptoms. It has also been suggested that a high incidence of alcoholism is found in some ethnic groups, such as American Indians, Blacks, and Whites (Klatsky, Friedman, Siegelaub, & Gérard, 1977).

As indicated in Chapter 7, there are two different enzymes involved in alcohol metabolism, both of which are variations of alcohol dehydrogenase (ADH): a high-activity type of ADH, which converts alcohol to acetaldehyde rapidly, and a low-activity variant, which converts it slowly (Kalow, 1982, 1986, 1989; Stamatoyannopoulos, Chen, & Fukui, 1975). The enzyme involved in metabolism of acetaldehyde to acetic acid also has several varieties, including acetaldehyde dehydrogenase 1 through 4. Acetaldehyde dehydrogenase 1 (ALDH-1) is considered "normal"; other types are considered "deficient" in their ability to metabolize acetaldehyde (Goedde, 1983, 1986; Keltner, personal communication, 1994).

In Whites, alcohol is metabolized "fairly efficiently" by the liver enzyme ADH, whereas in American Indians and Asians it is metabolized by ALDH, which works faster, often causing circulatory and unpleasant effects such as facial flushing and palpitations (Kudzma, 1992). Studies have indicated that American Indians and Asians experience noticeable facial flushing and other vasomotor symptoms after ingesting alcohol as compared with their White and African-American counterparts, who experience less severe reactions.

Although attempts have been made to explain biological variations of metabolic absorption of alcohol in different racial or ethnic groups, it is not meant in this context to explain the causes of alcoholism. Alcoholism exists among American Indians in very high percentages.

Psychological Characteristics

There appears to be one interesting racial difference in brain development in regard to cerebral speech-lateralization differences noted among Asians, American Indians, and other races. It has been suggested that Hopi, Navajo, and Japanese individuals either process linguistic information in both hemispheres or have right-hemisphere dominance (Overfield, 1995; Scott, 1979). Among Navajos, this finding is demonstrable, particularly when one is given a dichotic listening task. Navajos appear to have a left-ear advantage, which is suggestive of right-cerebral-hemisphere dominance, as opposed to their White counterparts, who have the usual right-ear advantage suggestive of left-cerebral-hemisphere dominance. For the nurse who is working with an aphasic client, possible racial differences in cerebral dominance cannot be overlooked (Overfield, 1995).

Implications for Nursing Care

It is important for the nurse to remember that although many researchers have implicated socioeconomic factors as a causative agent in tuberculosis, other researchers have related ethnicity to the high incidence of tuberculosis. Regardless of the causation, nurses need to assist Navajo people in learning about the significance of tuberculosis. Teaching should be clear and attempt to clarify any misunderstandings about tuberculosis. The nurse should use straightforward and easy-to-understand language. For example, the nurse might teach the client and the family how tuberculosis is spread and demonstrate how the organism can actually be seen through a microscope. The nurse should also make every effort to explain the symptoms of tuberculosis in simple terms so that the client and the family develop an understanding of the condition. For example, the nurse might begin by telling the client and the family that the symptoms begin with the client losing weight, then developing a cough, and then starting to spit up blood. In addition, the nurse might lessen the anxiety created by the need for radiographs by saying that the taking of radiographs is just like the taking of photographs (Wauneka, 1962).

Harris, Davis, Ford, and Tso (1988) designed and tested a cardiovascular health education curriculum using 215 fifth-grade students from rural New Mexico, including Navajo, Pueblo, and Hispanic children. The teaching effort of the program was augmented by materials, examples, and exercises relevant to these particular cultures. The findings of the study suggested a significant increase in knowledge among these students about the cardiovascular system, obesity, tobacco use, and the need for exercise, nutrition, and habit change. The study concluded that a culturally oriented program can be valuable in promoting a healthful lifestyle in minority children.

SUMMARY

Today, the Navajo nation is a culture in transition. As changes occur in educational levels, employment, and environment, the Navajo people find themselves assimilating more with the dominant culture of the United States. The need to be able to blend their traditional culture with the dominant culture of the United States is creating conflict for some Navajo people. When providing health care to Navajo clients, nurses are being challenged to seek ways to bridge the gap between traditional cultural practices and Western medical practices to provide culturally appropriate nursing care.

CASE STUDY

Mary Littlejohn, a 20-year-old Navajo Indian, is admitted to the hospital for a high-risk pregnancy related to gestational diabetes. This is Mrs. Littlejohn's second pregnancy. She is married and has a 2-year-old daughter at home. She lives in a *hogan* with her daughter, husband, mother, father, and two aunts. There is no running water, electricity, or plumbing in the home. When Mrs. Littlejohn arrives at the hospital for admission, 12 of her family members are with her. Once she has been admitted to her room and is in bed, her grandmother sprinkles cornmeal around her bed. When the nurse takes the client's history, Mrs. Littlejohn relates that she had the same problem last time she was pregnant. Mrs. Littlejohn also relates to the nurse that she has felt tired and very weak, has had some spots before her eyes, and headaches. In addition, she has to urinate frequently at night and does not appear to be able to get enough water or food. The nurse notes on examination that the client's blood pressure is 140/88, her temperature is 99.8° F, her pulse is 102, and her tongue appears coated. The laboratory test done at Mrs. Littlejohn's last clinic visit 1 week ago revealed that her serum glucose level was 160 mg/dL.

CARE PLAN

Nursing Diagnosis: Health maintenance, ineffective, related to inability to make thoughtful judgments regarding a high-risk pregnancy

Client Outcomes	Nursing Interventions
1. Client and family will verbalize a desire to learn more about high-risk pregnancies, diabetes, gestational diabetes, and appropriate techniques to reduce symptoms.	1. Identify with client and family sociocultural factors that influence health-seeking behaviors.
2. Client and family will verbalize a willingness to comply with a medical therapeutic regimen to control gestational diabetes.	2. Determine client's and family's knowledge level about diabetes, gestational diabetes, and implications for high-risk pregnancies.
3. Client and family will verbalize an understanding of the need to comply with routine, scheduled follow-up care to prevent an at-risk delivery.	

Continued

◎ CARE PLAN—cont'd

Nursing Diagnosis: Communication, impaired verbal, related to cultural difference

Client Outcomes	Nursing Interventions
1. Family will be able to communicate personal and family-related needs to health care personnel. 2. Family will be able to communicate feelings about diabetes, gestational diabetes, and treatment regimen. 3. Each family member will be able to send precise, understandable messages to one another through appropriate verbal and nonverbal communication.	1. Assist family in developing adequate communication techniques to communicate feelings and anxieties to one another and to health care personnel. 2. Assist family in developing the ability to determine discrepancies in communicated verbal and nonverbal behavior. 3. Assist family in developing appropriate language skills and nonverbal perception to decrease the possibility of faulty perception.

Nursing Diagnosis: Family processes interrupted, related to shift in health status of family member because of gestational diabetes and high-risk pregnancy

Client Outcome	Nursing Interventions
1. Family will participate in care and maintenance of client. 2. Family will assist nurse in helping client return to a high level of wellness. 3. Family will verbalize difficulties encountered in seeking appropriate external resources.	1. Determine family's understanding of client's condition. 2. Determine support systems available to family from external resources. 3. Determine with family supportive networks of friends and extended family members. Involve family in care and management of client. 4. Encourage family to verbalize fears and anxieties.

Nursing Diagnoses—Definitions and Classifications 2012–2014. Copyright © 2012, 1994–2012 by NANDA International. Used by arrangement with Wiley-Blackwell Publishing, a company of John Wiley and Sons, Inc. In order to make safe and effective judgments using NANDA-I nursing diagnoses it is essential that nurses refer to the definitions and defining characteristics of the diagnoses listed in the work.

CLINICAL DECISION MAKING

1. List several factors that may contribute to diabetes among Navajos.
2. Identify at least one reason why Mrs. Littlejohn's grandmother sprinkled cornmeal around the client's bed.
3. Describe at least two communication barriers encountered by nurses in the dominant society when providing care to Navajo clients.
4. Describe at least one health practice that Mrs. Littlejohn may adhere to that may be perceived as negative.
5. Describe the structure of the traditional Navajo family and the relationship to health-seeking behaviors.
6. Identify the possible negative effects of the environment and spatial relationships in a *hogan* on health and health-seeking behaviors.

REVIEW QUESTIONS

1. John Ahiga, a Navajo, often arrives late when medications are being dispensed on a psychiatric unit. As his nurse, you understand that this patient is doing which of the following?
   a. Receiving hallucinogenic drugs.
   b. Demonstrating present-time orientation.
   c. Demonstrating past-time orientation.
   d. Demonstrating future-time orientation.
2. The style of communication that would be most effective for a culturally competent nurse to adopt during an assessment interview with a 30-year-old Navajo client would be:
   a. The frequent use of nonverbal behaviors such as gesturing, smiling, and making wry faces.

b. A loud voice, unbroken eye contact, minimal gesturing, and straight-to-the-point questions.

c. To be open and friendly, ask direct questions, and touch the client's arm or hand occasionally for reassurance.

d. A soft voice, avoiding eye contact, with general leads and reflective techniques.

3. When providing nursing care for someone of the Navajo Indian culture, the nurse should remember which of the following?

a. To make frequent eye contact.

b. To avoid eye contact.

c. To shake hands firmly.

d. To use pointing to assist with communication.

REFERENCES

Andrews, M. M., & Boyle, J. S. (2003). *Transcultural concepts in nursing care* (4th ed.). Philadelphia: Lippincott Williams & Wilkins.

Bose, D. P., & Welsh, J. D. (1973). Lactose malabsorption in Oklahoma Indians. *American Journal of Clinical Nutrition, 26,* 1320–1322.

Boyce, G. (1942). *A primer of Navajo economic problems.* Mimeographed material. Window Rock, AZ: Navajo Service, Bureau of Indian Affairs.

Braun, K. L., Pietsch, J. H., & Blanchette, P. L. (2005). *Cultural issues in end-of-life decision making.* Thousand Oaks, CA: Sage.

Brugge, D. (1964). Navajo land usage: a study in progressive diversification. In C. S. Knowlton (Ed.), *Indian and Spanish adjustments to arid and semiarid environments.* Lubbock, TX: Texas Technological College Committee on Desert and Arid Zone Research, Contribution No. 7.

Brugge, D. (1968). Pueblo factionalism and external relations. *Ethnohistory (Columbus, Ohio), 191*–200.

Carrese, J. A., & Rhodes, L. A. (1995). Western bioethics on the Navajo reservation. *Journal of the American Medical Association, 274,* 826–829.

Centers for Disease Control and Prevention (CDC) (2009). *HIV/AIDS Surveillance Report, 2007, 19,* Table 4.

Child Trends Databank (2015). *Infant, child, and teen mortality.* Available at: <http://www.childtrends.org/?indicators=infant-child-and-teen-mortality>-See more at: <http://www.childtrends.org/?indicators=infant-child-and-teen-mortality#sthash.WErqQLlR.dpuf>.

Delien, H. (1951). Continuity of program—a necessity of tuberculosis control among American Indians. *Lancet, 71*(4), 136–137.

Donahue, R., & Orchard, T. (1992). Diabetes mellitus and macrovascular complications. *Diabetes Care, 15,* 1141–1155.

Epple, C., Wright, A. L., Joish, V. N., & Bauer, M. (2003). The role of active family nutritional support in Navajos' type 2 diabetes metabolic control. *Diabetes Care, 26*(10), 2829–2834.

Espey, D. K., et al. (2007). Annual report to the nation on the status of cancer, 1975–2004, featuring cancer in American Indians and Alaska Natives. *Cancer, 110*(10), 2119–2152.

Fauci, A. S. (2011). AIDS: let science inform policy. *Science, 333*(6038), 13.

Goedde, H. (1983). Population genetic studies on aldehyde dehydrogenase isozyme deficiency and alcohol sensitivity. *American Journal of Human Genetics, 35,* 769–772.

Goedde, H. (1986). Ethnic differences in reactions to drugs and other xenobiotics: outlook of a geneticist. In W. Kalow, H. W. Goedde, & D. P. Agarwal (Eds.), *Ethnic differences in reactions to drug and xenobiotics* (pp. 9–20). New York: Alan R. Liss.

Griffin, P. M., Tauxe, R. V., Redd, S. C., Puhr, N. D., Hargrett-Bean, N., & Blake, P. A. (1989). Emergence of highly trimethoprim-sulfamethoxazole-resistant *Shigella* in a Native American population: an epidemiologic study. *American Journal of Epidemiology, 129*(5), 1042–1051.

Hall, E. (1990). *The hidden dimension.* New York: Anchor Books.

Hanley, C. E. (1987). Changing patterns of health care on the Western Navajo reservation (Unpublished thesis). American College of Healthcare, Chicago.

Harris, M. B., Davis, S. M., Ford, V. L., & Tso, H. (1988). The checkerboard cardiovascular curriculum: a culturally oriented program. *Journal of School Health, 58*(3), 104–107.

Heath, C. (1980). A descriptive and evaluative study of the tuberculosis occurring in American Indians residing in Shannon and Washabaugh Counties, South Dakota, 1970 through 1978 (Master's thesis). University of Texas, Houston.

Hoy, W., Light, A., & McGill, D. (1995). Cardiovascular disease in Navajo Indians with type II diabetes. *Public Health Reports, 110*(1), 87–94.

Iverson, P. (2002). *The Diné: a history of the Navajo.* Albuquerque, NM: University of New Mexico Press.

Jacobs, A. H., & Walton, R. G. (1976). Incidence of birthmarks in the neonate. *Pediatrics, 58,* 218–222.

Kaiser Foundation (2009). *A profile of American Indians and Alaska Natives and their health coverage. Race, ethnicity, & health care: issue brief.* Menlo Park, CA: The Kaiser Foundation. Available at <http://www.kff.org/minorityhealth/upload/7977.pdf>.

Kalow, W. (1982). The metabolism of xenobiotics in different populations. *Canadian Journal of Physiological Pharmacology, 60,* 1–19.

Kalow, W. (1986). Outlook of a pharmacologist. In W. Kalow, H. W. Goedde, & D. P. Agarwal (Eds.), *Ethnic differences in reactions to drugs and xenobiotics.* New York: Liss.

Kalow, W. (1989). Race and therapeutic drug response. *New England Journal of Medicine, 320*(9), 588–589.

Kim, C., Seidel, K., Begier, E., & Kwok, Y. (2001). Diabetes and depot medroxyprogesterone contraception in Navajo women. *Archives of Internal Medicine, 161*(14), 1766–1771.

Klain, M., Coulehan, J. L., Arena, V. C., & Janett, R. (1988). More frequent diagnosis of acute myocardial infarction among Navajo Indians. *American Journal of Public Health, 78*(10), 1351–1352.

Klatsky, A. L., Friedman, G. D., Siegelaub, A. B., & Gérard, M. J. (1977). Alcohol consumption among White, Black, or

Oriental men and women: Kaiser-Permanente multiphasic health examination data. *American Journal of Epidemiology*, *105*(4), 311–323.

Kluckhohn, C., & Leighton, D. (1974). *The Navajo*. Cambridge, MA: Harvard University Press.

Kluckhohn, F., & Strodtbeck, F. (1973). *Variations in value orientations*. Westport, CT: Greenwood.

Koehler, K. M., Harris, M. B., & Davis, S. M. (1989). Core, secondary, and peripheral foods in the diets of Hispanic, Navajo, and Jemez Indian children. *Journal of American Dietary Association*, *89*(4), 638–640.

Kudzma, E. (1992). Drug responses: all bodies are not created equal. *American Journal of Nursing*, *92*, 48–50.

Lamarine, R. J. (1987). Self-esteem, health locus of control, and health attitudes among Native American children. *Journal of School Nursing*, *57*(9), 371–374.

Leichter, J., & Lee, M. (1971). Lactose intolerance in Canadian West Coast Indians. *Journal of Digestive Diseases*, *16*(9), 809–813.

Lewis, E., & Bourne, S. (1989). Perinatal death. *Bailliére's Clinical Obstetrics and Gynaecology*, *13*(4), 935–953.

Lohman, T., et al. (1999). Body composition assessment in American Indian children. *The American Journal of Clinical Nutrition*, *69*(4), 764S–766S.

Massion, C., O'Connor, P., Gorab, R., Crabtree, B. F., Nakamura, R. M., & Coulehan, J. L. (1987). Screening for gestational diabetes in a high-risk population. *Journal of Family Practice*, *25*(6), 569–575.

McCracken, R. (1971). Lactase deficiency: an example of dietary evolution. *Curriculum Anthropology*, *12*(4–5), 479–517.

McKeever, W. F., Hunt, L. J., Wells, S., & Yazzie, C. (1989). Language laterality in Navajo reservation children: dichotic test results depend on the language context of the testing. *Brain and Language*, *36*(1), 148–158.

Meskin, L. H., Gorlin, R. J., & Isaacson, R. J. (1964). Abnormal morphology of the soft palate: the prevalence of cleft uvula. *The Cleft Palate Journal*, *1*, 342–346.

National Center for Health Statistics (2010). *Health United States, 2010 with rural chartbooks*. Hyattsville, MD: U.S. Government Printing Office.

National Center for Health Statistics (2014). *Health United States, 2014 with rural chartbooks*. Hyattsville, MD: U.S. Government Printing Office.

Navajo Health Systems Agency (1985). *Report on traditional medicine survey*. Window Rock, AZ: Navajo Health Systems Agency.

Neel, J. V. (1962). Diabetes mellitus: a "thrifty" genotype rendered detrimental by progress. *American Journal of Human Genetics*, *14*, 353–362.

Ng, C., Chatwood, S., & Young, T. K. (2011). Arthritis in the Canadian Aboriginal population: north-south differences in prevalence and correlates. *Preventing Chronic Disease*, *8*(1), A04. [Epub 2010 Jun 15].

O'Connor, P., Crabtree, B., & Nakamura, R. (1997). Mortality experiences of Navajo with type 2 diabetes mellitus. *Ethnicity and Health*, *2*(3), 155–162.

O'Connor, P. J., Fragneto, R., Coulehan, J., & Crabtree, B. F. (1987). Metabolic control in non–insulin-dependent diabetes mellitus: factors associated with patient outcomes. *Diabetes Care*, *10*(6), 697–701.

Overfield, T. (1995). *Biologic variation in health and illness* (2nd ed.). Reading, MA: Addison-Wesley.

Overfield, T., & Call, E. B. (1983). Earlobe type, race, and age: effects on earlobe creasing. *Journal of American Geriatric Society*, *31*(8), 479–481.

Peck, R., Marks, J., Dibley, M., Lee, S., & Trowbridge, F. L. (1988). Birth weight and subsequent growth among Navajo children. *Public Health Reports*, *33*, 88.

Percy, C., Freedman, D. S., Gilbert, T. J., White, L., Ballew, C., & Mokdad, A. (1997). Prevalence of hypertension among Navajo Indians. *Journal of Nutrition*, *127*(Suppl. 10), 2114S–2119S.

Primeaux, M. (1977). Caring for the American Indian patient. *American Journal of Nursing*, *77*(1), 91–94.

Purdue, D. G., et al. (2008). Regional differences in colorectal cancer incidence, stage, and subsite among American Indians and Alaska Natives, 1999–2004. *Cancer*, *113*(Suppl. 5), 1179–1190.

Rate, R. G., Morse, H. G., Bonnell, M. D., & Kuberski, T. T. (1980). Navajo arthritis reconsidered: relationship to HLA-B27. *Arthritis and Rheumatism*, *23*(11), 1299–1302.

Reifel, A. (1949). Tuberculosis among Indians of the United States. *Diseases of the Chest*, *16*, 234–249.

Roessel, R. (1981). *Women in Navajo society*. Rough Rock, Navajo Nation, AZ: Navajo Resources Center.

Schaumann, B. F., Peagler, F. D., & Gorlin, R. J. (1970). Minor orofacial anomalies among a Negro population. *Oral Surgery, Oral Medicine, and Oral Pathology*, *29*(4), 566–575.

Scott, S. (1979). Cerebral speech lateralization in the Native American Navajo. *Neuropsychologia*, *17*(1), 89–92.

Skogrand, L., et al. (2008). Strong Navajo marriages. *American Indian and Alaska Native Mental Health Research: The Journal of the National Center American Indian and Alaskan Native Programs*, The University of Utah, 25–41.

Smoot, E. C., Kucan, J. O., Cope, J. S., & Asse, J. M. (1988). The craniofacial team and the Navajo patient. *The Cleft Palate Journal*, *25*(4), 395–402.

Sobralske, M. (1985). Perceptions of health: Navajo Indians. *Topics in Clinical Nursing*, *7*(3), 32–39.

Sowers, M., & Winterfeldt, E. (1975). Lactose intolerance among Mexican Americans. *American Journal of Clinical Nutrition*, *28*, 704–705.

Stamatoyannopoulos, G., Chen, S., & Fukui, M. (1975). Liver alcohol dehydrogenase in Japanese: high population frequency of atypical form and its possible role in alcohol sensitivity. *American Journal of Human Genetics*, *27*, 789–796.

Sugarman, J. R. (1989). Incidence of gestational diabetes in a Navajo Indian community. *Western Journal of Medicine*, *150*(5), 648–651.

Sugarman, J. R., & Percy, C. (1989). Prevalence of diabetes in a Navajo Indian community. *American Journal of Public Health*, *79*(4), 511–513.

Szabó, G. (1975). The human skin as an adaptive organ. In A. Damon (Ed.), *Physiological anthropology*. New York: Oxford University Press.

Szabó, G., Gerald, A. B., Pathak, M. A., & Fitzpatrick, T. B. (1969). Racial differences in the fate of melanosomes in human epidermis. *Nature, 222*, 1081–1082.

Tom-Orme, L. (1984). Diabetes intervention on the Uintah-Ouray reservation. In M. Carter (Ed.), *Proceedings of the ninth annual Transcultural Nursing Conference*. Salt Lake City, UT: Transcultural Nursing Society.

(1973). *Treaty between the United States of America and the Navajo tribe of Indians*. Las Vegas: KC Publications.

U.S. Department of Agriculture, Food and Nutrition Service (1984). *American Indians: a guide for nutrition educators*. Washington, DC: U.S. Government Printing Office.

U.S. Department of Commerce, Bureau of the Census (2000). *The American Indians and Alaska Native population, 2000 census brief*. Washington, DC: U.S. Government Printing Office.

U.S. Department of Commerce, Bureau of the Census (2002). *Population profiles by age, sex, race and Hispanic origin, Summary File 3*. Hyattsville, MD: U.S. Government Printing Office.

U.S. Department of Commerce, Bureau of the Census (2009). *American Community Survey, Population Profiles, The Navajo*. Washington, DC: U.S. Government Printing Office.

U.S. Department of Commerce, Bureau of the Census (2011). *The 2010 Census Brief*. Washington, DC: U.S. Government Printing Office.

U.S. Department of Commerce, Bureau of the Census (2015). American Community Survey. Washington, DC: U.S. Government Printing Office.

U.S. Department of Health and Human Services (2014). *National Diabetes Statistics Report*, 2014.

U.S. Department of Health and Human Services (2014). *Health, United States, 2014: Urban and rural health chartbook*. Hyattsville, MD: National Center for Health Statistics.

U.S. Department of Health and Human Services, Centers for Disease Control and Prevention (2013). *Diabetes surveillance report*. Atlanta: Centers for Disease Control and Prevention, U.S. Department of Health and Human Services.

Wasserman, H. P. (1974). *Ethnic pigmentation: historical, physiological and chemical aspects*. New York: Elsevier.

Wauneka, A. (1962). Helping a people to understand. *American Journal of Nursing, 62*(2), 88–96.

Weirto, V. (2010). *The racialization of the Diné youth in education*. Albuquerque, NM: University of New Mexico.

White, L. M., Ballew, C., Gilber, T., Mendlein, J. M., Mokdad, A. H., & Strauss, K. F. (1997). Weight, body image, and weight control practices of Navajo Indians: findings from the Navajo Health and Nutrition Survey. *Journal of Nutrition, 127*(10), 2094s–2098s.

Wiggins, C. L., et al. (2008). Cancer among American Indians and Alaska Natives in the United States, 1999–2004. *Cancer, 113*(Suppl. 5), 1142–1152.

Williams, R., & Boyce, W. T. (1989). Protein malnutrition in elderly Navajo patients. *Journal of American Geriatrics and Sociology, 37*(5), 397–406.

Willkens, R. F., Hansen, J. A., Malmgren, J. A., Nisperos, B., Mickelson, E. M., & Watson, M. A. (1982). HLA antigens in Yakima Indians with rheumatoid arthritis. *Arthritis and Rheumatism, 25*(12), 1435–1439.

Wolfe, W. S., & Sanjur, D. (1988). Contemporary diet and body weight of Navajo women receiving food assistance: an ethnographic and nutritional investigation. *Journal of American Dietary Association, 88*(7), 822–827.

Wolff, P. (1973). Dietary habits and cancer epidemiology. *Cancer, 43*, 1955–1961.

Young, R. (1961). The origin and development of Navajo tribal government. In R. W. Young (Ed.), *The Navajo yearbook* (Vol. 8, pp. 371–411). Window Rock, AZ: Bureau of Indian Albuquerque Affairs.

11

Appalachians

Cynthia C. Small

BEHAVIORAL OBJECTIVES

After reading this chapter, the nurse will be able to:

1. Describe the history of the Appalachian region.
2. Describe Appalachian communication patterns.
3. Describe the Appalachian orientation to time and space.
4. Explain values related to family that may be held by persons with Appalachian heritage.
5. Describe the Appalachian traditional health care system, including folk beliefs, herbal remedies, and lay practitioners.
6. Describe factors affecting Appalachian use of biomedical health services.
7. Discuss illnesses that tend to have higher mortality among Appalachians.

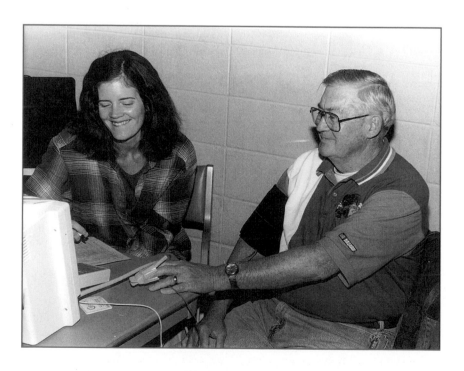

OVERVIEW OF APPALACHIA

In 1963 the President's Appalachian Regional Commission (PARC) report concluded that "Appalachia is a region apart—geographically and statistically" (PARC, 1963, p. xvii). The basis for this distinction in socioeconomic terms was Appalachia's poverty, deficits in living standards and education, and lack of urbanization. Since this report, dramatic changes have occurred in economic development, resulting in associated social and cultural transitions. Yet Appalachians, especially in the central region, are characterized by unique features.

Approximately 27 million people live in the federally defined Appalachian region, which is nearly 200,000 square miles across 410 counties in 13 states, including all of West Virginia and selected counties in Alabama, Georgia, Kentucky, Maryland, Mississippi, New York, North Carolina, Ohio, Pennsylvania, South Carolina, Tennessee, and Virginia (Appalachian Regional Commission, 2013; Obermiller & Maloney, 2007; U.S. Department of Commerce, Bureau of the Census, American Community Survey, 2015). Originally, the Appalachian region was defined as 360 counties in 11 states in a bill enacted by the U.S. Congress in 1965, titled the *Appalachian Regional Act,* and subsequently revised. Today, data on the Appalachian region are collected with federal authority by the Appalachian Regional Commission (U.S. Department of Commerce, Bureau of the Census, American Community Survey, 2015).

The Appalachian area has three subregions: Northern, Central, and Southern Appalachia. Northern Appalachia is the largest region and consists of portions of New York, Pennsylvania, Ohio, and Maryland and most of West Virginia. It is the most urbanized, populated, and relatively economically advantaged of the three subregions. Southern Appalachia includes counties in southern Virginia, eastern Alabama, Georgia, Tennessee, Mississippi, and North and South Carolina. Of the 13 states, West Virginia is the most rural and the only state residing entirely within the Appalachian region.

Central Appalachia includes parts of Kentucky, Tennessee, Virginia, and the southern area of West Virginia. It is the smallest and poorest of the three areas, is predominantly rural, and has a coal mining economic base. Central Appalachia, particularly the rural areas, stands out most distinctly as a severely distressed economic area, along with particular areas of Northern Appalachia (the rest of West Virginia and portions of Ohio) and Southern Appalachia (clusters of counties in northern Mississippi and Alabama) (Cushing & Rogers, 1996; Obermiller & Maloney, 2007). In 2000 the Appalachian Regional Commission identified nine Appalachian states as having distressed counties—that is, counties with immediate concerns because of the high infant mortality rate, poverty, unemployment, and low income.

Originally home to American Indian tribes such as the Cherokee, the Appalachian area is now populated overwhelmingly by non-Hispanic Whites, with only 1% of the population American Indian and 8% African-American. Most African-American Appalachians reside in the urban areas or in the rural counties in Southern Appalachia. However, the population is experiencing rapid demographic change, with an increase of nearly 50% in the minority population in the last decadal census, with increases of 239.3% for the Hispanic population and 18.7% for the African-American population. Minority population growth surpassed that of Whites for all Appalachian states and was particularly high for children with persons of younger working ages (18–43 years) (Obermiller & Maloney, 2007; Pollard, 2004).

For the most part, the Appalachian region is classified as a rural, nonfarming area, although some large cities are encompassed in the area, including Pittsburgh, Pennsylvania; Charleston, West Virginia; Knoxville and Chattanooga, Tennessee; and Birmingham and Montgomery, Alabama. Many Appalachians live in and around the rocky, mountainous terrain, and the roads to their small homes are long, rough, steep, narrow, and often difficult to navigate. Because of the terrain, many communities have only recently been able to support public utilities, such as municipal heating, water, and sewage systems. Only until the 1980s were paved primary highways, telephones, electricity, and running water widely accessible.

Because of the isolation, lack of distinguishing physical characteristics, and low visibility of the people, Appalachians have been relatively overlooked as an American ethnic minority. Although the Appalachian region is federally designated, the Appalachian people are not awarded the status of a federally defined ethnic/minority group. Further, Appalachians do not generally identify themselves as being "Appalachian" or "mountaineers" or any other ethnic designation. Yet this designation may be useful to providers because of the shared history, core values, beliefs, and behavioral patterns that have been identified for this group. Although persons who are considered Appalachian generally reside in the Appalachian region, some have migrated to other parts of the United States. On the other hand, some Americans from other areas have migrated to Appalachia; however, migration to the region does not in itself result in classification as an Appalachian.

History

In 1749, Thomas Walker was the first known European American to penetrate the Appalachian maze of hogback ridges and deep valleys. Some 20 years later Daniel Boone blazed the Wilderness Trail through the Cumberland Gap, soon to be followed by more than 100,000 settlers (MacAvoy & Lippman, 2001; Obermiller & Maloney, 2007). The forefathers of the new settlers came from Northern European countries such as England, Wales, Scotland, Germany, and France, often seeking religious or personal freedom and available land (Obermiller & Maloney, 2007; Tripp-Reimer, 1982). Life in the rural wilderness areas and the continuing isolation of Appalachians, particularly the central and southern mountaineers, has distinguished Appalachians from the mainstream of American society (Obermiller & Maloney, 2007; Simon, 1987).

Historically, like many ethnic groups, Appalachians have borne the brunt of discriminatory characterizations. As with much labeling of minority groups, this stereotyping has emphasized negative behaviors and serves as a barrier to our understanding the health needs, core values, beliefs, and behaviors that the Anglo-Celtic rural mountain-dwelling people may share. This holds true not only for those who live in Appalachia but also for the approximately 4 million Appalachian people who migrated to major urban areas of the North Central United States beginning in the late 1950s and peaking in the 1980s (Obermiller & Malony, 2007). Early migrants from the Appalachian region to urban areas such as Cincinnati, Columbus, Detroit, and Cleveland often remained at the poverty level and often congregated with other persons from Appalachia (Obermiller & Maloney, 2007; Tripp-Reimer, 1982); more recently, they continue to be absorbed into working- and middle-class neighborhoods because of their increased access to employment and education.

Economy

Historically, Appalachia was a rural, agricultural area. Then, beginning in the late 1800s, the economic base and the landscape were changed by the dominant industries of mining, lumber, and textiles. The local communities were often not advantaged by these industries. Generally, the wealth that was generated was not reinvested in the region but exported to the urban areas, largely in the East. This resulted in a low tax base and high rates of poverty (Barnett, Halverson, Elmes, & Braham, 2000; Obermiller & Maloney, 2007). Often there was corporate ownership of the resource-rich land; in some counties in West Virginia, coal companies and railroads own up to 90% of the surface land. As a result, much of the usable land was unavailable to the local Appalachians. In addition, health services, schools, and other public services were underfunded because of the lack of a solid tax base (resulting from incentives given to the corporations) (Burkhardt, 1991).

In general, rural populations across the United States tend to be poorer, older, less educated, and more likely to be uninsured. Rural residents generally have poorer overall health status, less access to care, and difficulty with paying for services (even if they have insurance), and they participate in fewer health promotion activities (Appalachian Regional Commission, 2013; Friedell et al., 2001; Huttlinger, Schaller-Ayers, Kenny, & Ayers, 2004; Huttlinger, Schaller-Ayers, & Lawson, 2004; Obermiller & Maloney, 2007). In contrast, metropolitan areas have more public utilities and better health infrastructure, the population is generally better educated, and more are employed at higher paying jobs (Barnett et al., 2000).

In 2013, the per capita income of those persons residing in the federally defined Appalachian regions was approximately $4000 less than the per capita income for the rest of the general United States (Appalachian Regional Commission, 2013). Yet taken at face value, these figures are somewhat misleading. Appalachia is characterized by extremes of wealth and poverty. Because the per capita income is slightly lower than the national average, the poverty rate is at least twice the national average at 15.4%. In 2013, the unemployment figure for persons identified as rural Appalachian was 8.1% compared with 6.7% for the rest of the general U.S. population (Appalachian Regional Commission, 2013; Barnett et al., 2000; Muratova, Islam, Demerath, Minor, & Neal, 2001; U.S. Department of Labor, 2002). With increasing environmental concerns and international competition, there has been a loss of mining and textile jobs.

Education

In 1970, the proportion of the adult population that completed high school in the Appalachian region was 27% in the rural areas and 52% in the metropolitan areas; by 2000, this proportion had risen to 53% and 79%, respectively (Appalachian Regional Commission, 2013). Currently, in all of Appalachia, 11.4% of persons 25 years of age or older have less than an eighth-grade education; 35.4% have some high school education but no diploma; 84.6% hold a high school diploma or general equivalency diploma (GED); and 21.7% hold a 4-year college degree or higher (Appalachian Regional Commission, 2015). Although more Appalachian children now graduate from high school, the 17% dropout rate is still higher than that for children of other ethnic groups (Appalachian Regional Commission, 2013; Obermiller & Maloney, 1990; Penn, Borman, & Hoeweler, 1994). Although education is increasingly seen as important, school attendance may also tax a family's meager resources. Denham (1999a) noted that the need for new clothing, transportation, homework, and peer conflicts placed additional burdens on many families.

Public Services

In the 1960s, 39% of persons in all of Appalachia (and 63% in rural areas) lived in houses without complete indoor plumbing, yet by 1990, this figure had transitioned to only 2%. Even in the rural areas of Central Appalachia, only 5% of homes today are without complete indoor plumbing (Isserman, 1997). Yet according to the Bureau of the Census (American Community Survey, 2015; U.S. Department of Commerce, Bureau of the Census, 2015; Appalachian Regional Commission, 2013), nearly 630,000 occupied households in Appalachia lack complete plumbing facilities, which means that they are without one or more of the following: a toilet, a tub or shower, or running water. Similarly, the proportion of households with telephones has now risen, so that only 10% to 15% of occupied housing units currently lack phones (Cushing & Rogers, 1996). In Central Appalachia, 14% of occupied homes do not have a vehicle or any available means of public transportation (Cushing & Rogers, 1996).

Core Cultural Patterns

Four interacting core cultural patterns provide the underlying structure of much that will be discussed throughout this chapter, but first, two caveats: the intention here is not to provide a rigid stereotype of Appalachians but to identify patterns that may serve as guides to understanding. Furthermore, cultural value patterns are identified for aggregates and, as such, are not directly transferable to individuals (Dreher & MacNaughton, 2002; Tripp-Reimer & Fox, 2001). Rather, these patterns provide a contextual understanding by which health care providers may assess an individual's unique health care abilities and needs.

In the classic work of Tripp-Reimer (1980), four interacting Appalachian cultural patterns were identified: independence, the ethic of neutrality, familism, and personalism. Independence developed out of a history of escaping religious persecution and as a survival mechanism. There is a pride in self-sufficiency (Blakeney, 1987). At a time when most people hire others to fix their cars or build their homes, Appalachians take pride in doing things for themselves. This helps explain the difficulty encountered by many Appalachians when it is necessary to ask for financial help or welfare. However, this pattern is context specific and may not apply in unfamiliar clinical settings, particularly in a crisis. For example, while Appalachian nurses wanted to promote more decisional control for hospitalized patients, Appalachian patients reported a desire for much less control (Rosswurm, Dent, Armstrong-Persily, Woodburn, & Davis, 1996). Hunsucker, Frank, and Flannery (1999) found that interdependence, not independence, characterized rural Southern Appalachian family

members who had a member in the intensive care unit. Other rural Appalachian family member needs that were different from urban families included a preference for informal support systems (family, friends, and religion) over formal systems, close personal relationships and a desire for frequent communication with professionals, flexible visiting hours, permission for emotions, and provision for time alone.

In his early ethnographic work, Hicks (1976) reported that Appalachians demonstrate what he termed an *ethic of neutrality*. This is evidenced in four behavioral imperatives: (1) avoiding aggression or assertiveness, (2) not interfering in another person's business unless requested to do so, (3) avoiding domination over other people, and (4) avoiding arguments and seeking agreement. Consequently, there may be low tolerance for paternalistic or prescriptive behavior patterns. Rather than messages attacking an organization or individual, politeness is valued (Denham, Meyer, Toborg, & Mande, 2004). For example, according to Blakeney (1987), an occupational therapist and native of Appalachia, "It is more important to get along with others than to make conflicting true feelings known" (p. 62).

Familism emphasizes the importance of relationships with consanguineous nuclear and extended family members rather than self-actualization through individual accomplishments (Tripp-Reimer, 1980). The high reliance on family may influence choice of employment, religious affiliation, marriage partners, and health care practices. A sense of family is central to the Appalachian sense of self, which in turn is intricately linked with the land, homestead, and trusted neighbors (Blakeney, 1987; Rowles, 1991). Appalachians who have migrated elsewhere often strongly continue to value their connection to the "hills" and homeland and go to great lengths to maintain those connections (Blakeney, 1987).

While trust is extended cautiously, it may be built through a personal orientation in contrast to a bureaucratic or service-oriented relationship (Tripp-Reimer, 1980). In health interactions, a person-focused rather than disease-focused approach is preferred. This preference for a personal orientation may explain why nursing care has been noted to be preferred to medical-based cure modalities (Blakeney, 1987).

COMMUNICATION

Appalachians are English-speaking people; however, they have several idiomatic differences in the meanings of specific words. Throughout the Appalachian region, there are various dialects with high concentrations of words of Scottish or Elizabethan English heritage (Dial, 1975). Thus

TABLE 11-1   Comparison of How High- and Low-Context Cultures Differ in Negotiations

	Low-Context Cultures	High-Context Cultures
Mode	Direct	Indirect
Style	Control/confrontation	Accommodation/avoidance
Strategy	Competition	Collaboration
Explanation	Linear, analysis	Nonlinear, synthesis
Problem exposure	Direct/confrontational	Indirect/nonconfrontational
Orientation	Action and solution focused	Relationship oriented and process focused

phrases used by some Appalachians may be interpreted entirely differently by non-Appalachians. For example, an Appalachian person may say "running off," which may be interpreted by a non-Appalachian as leaving home or running away but may actually mean diarrhea. These examples of stylistic differences represent generally rare opportunities for miscommunication. On the other hand, the Appalachians' use of folk categories of illness may be the basis for greater misunderstanding. As will be described in greater detail in the folk belief section, "Appalachian Folk Health System," several illnesses sound like, but are conceptually distinct from, the biomedical terms. For example, *high blood pressure* and *hypertension* are two folk illness categories in the Appalachian region that are distinct from the biomedical category of hypertension.

Variations in metacommunication patterns are generally more important than the idiomatic differences just described. Metacommunication patterns include mode, style, strategy, explanation, problem exposure, and orientation. Hall (1989, 2006) typified cultures on the basis of high- or low-context communication. For high-context cultures (HCCs), most of the meaning of a communication comes from the context; it is unspoken. For low-context cultures (LCCs), most of the meaning comes from the actual words used. Gudykunst and Ting-Toomey (1988) provide a framework for comparing how high- and low-context cultures differ in their approach to negotiation (Table 11-1). Because the dominant communication mode for Appalachians is high context and that for health providers is low context, opportunities for misunderstandings are maximized.

Nonverbal communication patterns may also vary. Although common among many groups, direct eye contact is often viewed by Appalachians as impolite or lacking good manners (Hicks, 1976; Mullen & Phillips, 1998) or even as aggressive or hostile behavior (Helton, 1995; Murray & Huelskoetter, 1991). Many Appalachians use a verbal pattern that is much more concrete than the patterns displayed by middle-class Americans, who tend to be more abstract. For example, in health education materials,

politeness, succinct facts presented without "sugar coating it" or "getting preachy," and "Talk … just like one-on-one" was preferred (Denham, Meyer, Toborg, & Mande, 2004, p. 299).

Implications for Nursing Care

As the textile, mining, and lumber industries began to grow in the Appalachian regions, many Appalachian persons were stripped of their land and other natural resources. Company towns controlled the stores, educational systems, and financial capital, exploiting the people and the land. This historical context fostered mistrust of outsiders. Positive interactions between an Appalachian person and an outsider often require that a trusting relationship first be established. Strategies to improve communication include making the time to listen and talk about matters that are important to the individual and the family. It may be helpful to use a direct approach, giving the facts, discussing within the context of prior family experiences, and soliciting the opinion and advice of family members before making recommendations.

Again, the nurse should be aware that some Appalachians, because of the ethic of neutrality, might wish to avoid confrontation and tell nurses what they believe the nurse wants to hear. The nurse can diminish this possibility by adopting a high-context communication style: speaking indirectly, emphasizing collaboration, avoiding confrontation, and developing the relationship (Lewis, Messner, & McDowell, 1985; Tripp-Reimer, 1980). Finally, because many Appalachian folk illnesses sound like biomedical disease categories, nurses need to take special care to understand what clients truly mean in their use of illness categories.

SPACE

Personal space is very important to Appalachians, which is evident in their maintaining a personal distance when interacting (Purnell & Counts, 2003). As addressed earlier, familism and the sense of self are intimately linked to the land and homestead (Blakeney, 1987; Rosswurm et al., 1996; Rowles, 1991). Appalachians love the land, and some prefer to live apart from the rest of society, nestled in the privacy of the hollows and hills. Appalachians are considered present-oriented (Blakeney, 1987) and focused on "being" rather than "doing" (Lewis et al., 1985; Purnell & Counts, 2003; Rowles, 1991, 2000; Tripp-Reimer, 1982). They have been described as believing that because tomorrow is not promised, they must live for today. While this has been interpreted as fatalism, it may also be interpreted as a realistic understanding of life circumstances. Poverty, harsh living conditions, rudimentary municipal supports, and isolation may make "unhurried" adaptive patterns of behavior necessary to conserve energy and accomplish the everyday work necessary to meet basic needs for survival.

Implications for Nursing Care

In contrast to the typical behavioral characteristics of Appalachians, which is to be family oriented and concerned with the well-being of others, when an Appalachian is ill, personal space collapses inwardly (Simpkins, 1979), meaning that the Appalachian person expects to be waited on and cared for by others. Thus the focus of both the individual and the members of the family is on the ill person. In a hospital setting, this may create obstacles to planning and executing nursing care because it is not unusual for a large number of family members to arrive with the client and to expect to maintain proximity with the client throughout the duration of the hospitalization. This desire for proximity is also evidenced when a client is scheduled for a clinic appointment, even if the condition is perceived by the health care professionals as minor.

SOCIAL ORGANIZATION

Family

The major unit of Appalachian social organization and group identity is generally the family rather than the community or Appalachian region (Blakeney, 1987; Obermiller & Maloney, 2007). The nuclear and extended families are both very important. Some Appalachians are so intensely loyal that they feel a personal responsibility for in-laws, nieces, and nephews, as well as other distant family members. Appalachians tend to place a greater importance on the extended family than do most middle-class Americans; the extended family is considered important regardless of the social, educational, or economic level of the individual. Thus relatives are sought for advice, validation, and support on many matters, particularly those pertaining to health and illness (Culture of Poverty Revisited,

1977; LaFargue, 1980). Kinship groups are the major social organizing force in the region (Tripp-Reimer & Friedl, 1977) on which to build community-level involvement. The dedication to family is of such paramount importance to most Appalachians that Purnell and Counts (2003) note most Appalachians rarely move more than 30 miles from their families.

The extensive ties to the nuclear and extended family are evident when a family member becomes ill or dies, in that members of the entire family may take leave from their jobs to be with the ill or dying relative for the duration of the crisis. This tendency to miss work for a family illness may have negative job consequences. If a family member is chronically ill, continued employment may be sacrificed for the "good" of the family (Jones, 1983). This intense loyalty for being with ill family members may remain long after an Appalachian person migrates from the region (Helton, 1995). This loyalty is also carried over into housing in northern areas; a landlord may find a property deserted, with all personal belongings intact, because the tenant had returned to the Appalachian region to be with a sick relative.

The Appalachian family is basically patriarchal (Murdock, 1982; Tripp-Reimer, 1982), but mothers and grandmothers make most health decisions (Denham et al., 2004). Denham (1999a, 2002) conducted three ethnographic studies over a 5-year period in two southeastern Ohio counties. She found that most families focused on present rather than future health. The concept of "family health routines" involves multiple interacting individuals that constitute a family perspective. She notes that for the Appalachian families studied, mothers assume primary roles in establishing the behaviors viewed as important for children's health needs. Mothers are the main health care teachers and decision makers and are pragmatic in caring for family health. For example, mothers are more likely to encourage family members to incorporate health information into family routines when it is viewed as meaningful, aligned with family values, and applicable to members' needs and when adequate resources or supports are available (Denham, 2002). Determination of need for medical care was made after a "wait and see" time period, upon the counsel of close friends and family, and based on the mother's judgment (Denham, 1999b).

Children are viewed as security for the future (Tripp-Reimer, 1982). While marriage before childbirth is preferred, in the case of an early pregnancy, the family tends to become more cohesive, providing love and security to the expectant mother. The grandparents often care for grandchildren, particularly if both parents work. The children appear to have a sense of who they are and a greater sense of belonging. The desired family size has decreased dramatically; the norm is now two to three children (Murray & Huelskoetter, 1991; Obermiller & Maloney, 2007).

Elderly family members are generally respected and often reside with their children or nearby. The attitude among Appalachians toward elders is reported to be one of honor, attributable to the elders' role in cultural transmission to later generations. Rowles (1983) found that spatial separation of elders from their adult children when they relocated generated critical dilemmas for the Appalachian elders. It was difficult to reconcile their fear of leaving the familiar environment (with its physical, social, and emotional support) with their desire to be close to the family. The study was based on a 4-year observation of elderly persons in a rural northern Appalachian community and was intended primarily to explore the tensions between factors that reinforced locational stability and factors that encouraged relocating to the homes of children residing outside the Appalachian region.

Religion

Initially on arrival in the United States, many Appalachian persons were Presbyterians, Episcopalians, or members of some other formally organized denomination. However, these churches required educated clergy and a centralized organization, both of which proved to be impractical in the wilderness (Burkhardt, 1991). As a result, in rural areas locally autonomous nondenominational churches emerged throughout the Appalachian region. For the most part, these individualistic churches stress the centrality of grace, authority of the Bible, religious experience, a call to preach, and local church governance (Simpson & King, 1999). Whereas some social reformers have viewed the local churches as a hindrance to social progress, others recognize their adaptive features, making life worth living in grim situations (Jones, 1983). Mainstream denominations, particularly Southern Baptist and United Methodist, are more prevalent in the urban areas of Appalachia and generally attended by more economically advantaged congregations.

Simpson and King (1999) explored health-related and religious activities in the local autonomous churches to include prayer requests, anointing, and testimony. They proposed that religious health partnerships could provide a channel for health promotion effects in rural Appalachia. On the other hand, churches differ in their willingness to engage in progress that is "of the world" and not inspired by God.

Implications for Nursing Care

Rather than an individualist experience, health and illness are a family affair, negotiated and understood within a family context and often under the purview of women, especially mothers. In health care, family members' involvement may include consultation regarding etiology, severity, and treatment options. Integration of concrete examples of risk behavior, health problems, and treatments within the experiences of the nuclear and extended family system may be an effective health care strategy for providers (Denham et al., 2004).

In contrast to the well Appalachians' emphasis on independence, ill Appalachian interdependence is emphasized. The family surrounds the person and often provides needed care (Hunsucker et al., 1999; Rosswurm et al., 1996). In a hospital or clinic setting, it is not unusual for a large number of family members to arrive with the client and expect to maintain proximity with the client throughout the duration of the hospitalization. Consequently, mechanisms for family involvement need to be incorporated into the plan of care and hospital policies.

Familism, the ethic of neutrality, and poverty may influence health behaviors. Because Appalachians tend to be family oriented, it may be important to elicit family opinions in regard to health care. If the family's ideas and opinions are not incorporated into the plan of care, the family and client may not accept the health care recommendations or services. It may be helpful to blend the informal and formal systems (Ramey, 1993) or recruit family members or other trusted care providers as care brokers.

It may be helpful to develop mechanisms for supporting and encouraging family involvement in care (Maas et al., 2004; Specht et al., 2000). Minimally, the nurse must recognize that changes in health behaviors affect the entire family system, and consequently the nurse should incorporate family members in health education. For example, if a person is admitted to the hospital for diabetes, not only should the client be given instructions on diabetes care, but the family members should also be given the same level of instruction. Instruction must take into account the resources the family has in the home, including the informal care network and assets such as running water, finances to purchase supplies, and refrigeration.

In addition, since the family context, health beliefs, practices, and religion are often intertwined, it is important that an assessment of these be done on admission to the health care system. For example, a study done with Appalachian women found that premature birth is associated with a woman's negative feelings about pregnancy, low self-esteem, and depression (Jesse, Seaver, & Wallace, 2003). On the other hand, Appalachian pregnant women who had a greater sense of spirituality and lower levels of personal stress were found to participate in fewer risky health behaviors (e.g., smoking) (Jesse & Reed, 2004). As such, integrating stress reduction and spirituality in prenatal health care promotion visits may be helpful. This may be particularly important for Medicaid-supported pregnant women who were found to have an increased incidence of smoking, depressive symptoms, and physical abuse compared with private-pay pregnant women (Jesse, 2003). Confusion regarding professional stereotyping of fatalism for clients' lack of personal resources of time, money, or access to health care beliefs must be recognized and avoided. Finally, church–health partnerships may be useful in the delivery of health promotion information.

TIME

Tripp-Reimer (1982) found a strong difference in interpretations of time perceptions between Appalachians and non-Appalachian health care providers. Non-Appalachian health care professionals interpreted missed appointments negatively and were judgmental in their characterization of Appalachians as not having skills for long-term planning. On the other hand, the Appalachian professionals understood that Appalachians focus on the present to meet overwhelming needs and the uncertainty of what tomorrow will bring. Furthermore, Appalachian professionals understood that Appalachian persons may miss appointments or be late because they are working to meet everyday needs, may lack transportation, or are concerned about being fired if they take off from work.

The way in which rural Appalachians structure time differs from the urban population. Blakeney (1987) explains that the Appalachians view modern humans as having lost the technique of enjoying time for oneself, the art of "sitting for a spell" to visit with another person or to cherish a moment in solitude. An isolated, self-sufficient lifestyle still requires hard work and offers few modern conveniences. However, those people in Appalachia who continue this lifestyle achieve a self-directed balance in their lives and establish their own individualized patterns of work, leisure, self-care, and rest.

Implications for Nursing Care

Because of Appalachians' perspectives on time, they may live at a pace that facilitates an awareness of body rhythms as opposed to clock time. Because some Appalachians are present-time oriented, it is best and often necessary for the nurse to assess kinesthetic needs and gently access personal and emotional space by visiting with the client before an examination or treatment is performed. Another consideration is that it is common for some Appalachian clients to arrive for an appointment at a time that is different from when the appointment is scheduled. If they are turned away, they may not access those services again. There are a number of alternative methods for delivery of health

services that are being explored and tested. Modes of health care delivery to facilitate community-level and client access to health care include family involvement in care planning, teleconferencing and telehealth, assistance with transportation, flexible scheduling and extended clinic hours, open walk-in clinics, outreach clinics close to clients' homes, home visits, parish nursing, and clinics done in association with churches and other sites of congregation (Calico, 1996; Edwards, Lenz, & East-Odom, 1993; Friedell et al., 2001; Hunsucker et al., 1999; Hurley, Turner, & Floyd, 2000; Simpson & King, 1999; Wallace, Tuck, Boland, & Witucki, 2002).

ENVIRONMENTAL CONTROL

Environmental Health Threats

Factors contributing to the Appalachians' having health status lower than the U.S. average include low-paying jobs, lack of employment, lack of health insurance, environmental toxins, noise, and numerous occupational health hazards. Workers in the textile mills were often exposed to high levels of cotton, flax, or hemp dust, leading to the highest rates of "brown lung disease" in the country. Brown lung disease, or byssinosis, is irreversible and characterized by shortness of breath, coughing, and wheezing (Levenstein, Delaurier, & Dunn, 2002). Analogously, between 1950 and 1970, the mines were locations where "black choking death was accepted as normal and inevitable" (Caudill, 1976, p. 145). The high-impact machines created inches of dust on the tunnel floors that covered the miners' bodies. Lung disease incapacitated the miners. Black lung disease (pneumoconiosis) is a progressive incurable condition that is characterized by extreme shortness of breath. In addition, approximately 90% of coal miners over the age of 54 report hearing problems (Murray-Johnson et al., 2004). Although coal miners identified that hearing loss is a serious concern and voiced the importance of protective devices, they also reported a greater need for unencumbered hearing while in the mine. It was perceived to be important to remain aware of "roof talk," or noises that warn of the mine ceiling caving in (Murray-Johnson et al., 2004, p. 748). In addition to decreasing noise from the machinery, miners recommended that information be given to miners about decibel noise exposure throughout the mine, ongoing hearing screening services, and public campaigns to increase awareness about the problems and need for prevention to decrease hearing loss.

Death, Dying, and Death Rituals

While there is increasing and considerable diversity, Appalachian death rituals have been well characterized by Crissman (1994) and Sherrod (2005). When death is imminent, a vigil sometimes called a "death watch" is held by family and friends either in the home or, more commonly today, in the hospital. Participants in the vigil often observe for signs of impending death, such as premonitions, visions, and the death rattle. Usually the evening before the funeral, a wake or visitation period is often held at a funeral home or church; this is a time for paying respects to the dead and his or her family and to view the deceased. Funeral services are generally held in funeral homes or churches; these often include prayer, music, scriptural reading, and a sermon or eulogy. Following the funeral service, close mourners may proceed to the site of interment—sometimes on foot, but more often by car. Today, graves are typically dug by service workers rather than friends. Before the casket is lowered, ministers may preside over a committal service. Graves are often marked with headstones with chiseled writing (name, birth and death dates, and sometimes an epitaph) and sometimes a picture (Crissman, 1994; Sherrod, 2005).

Barriers to Care

Lack of available services; ethnocentric providers; difficult terrain; geographic isolation; cost; and lack of transportation, insurance, and telephones are common barriers to utilization of health care services by Appalachians (Beck, Jijon, & Edwards, 1996; Elnicki, Douglas, Morris, & Shockcor, 1995; Hall, Uhler, Coughlin, & Miller, 2002; Hansen & Resick, 1990).

In rural areas of Appalachia, 67% of the counties are federally designated shortage areas; the proportion of primary care physicians per population is less than half that in the rest of the United States (Barnett et al., 2000; Friedell et al., 2001). Rural clinic offices are often staffed by single providers with no laboratory support (Hesselgrave, 2001). In one study, most family members indicated they were unable to access primary care physicians because few providers accepted medical cards (Medicaid/Medicare) as payment; further, 80% had no or unreliable transportation (Denham, 1999b). In addition, the ethnocentrism of many providers and the higher proportion of foreign-trained physicians in underserved areas may deter Appalachians from returning for services (Tripp-Reimer, 1982).

Locus of Control

Appalachians' locus of control has been characterized as fatalistic, with strong roots in fundamentalist religion. Many Appalachians believe that God has control over their lives and that however things turn out, it is the "Lord's will." While most middle-class Americans believe that science can most often control events and health, many Appalachians do not believe that they have control over their future or their health. However, this idea of fatalism

is more complex than usually described and may not be related to lack of health efforts. Several studies report that while Appalachians may believe they cannot prevent an illness, they have strong self-determination about coping with and managing an illness (Ford, 1967; Hansen & Resick, 1990; Hunsucker, Flannery, & Frank, 2000; Rosswurm et al., 1996). This has been termed by Rosswurm et al. (1996) as "adaptive acceptance" (p. 456). This interpretation fits well with other research indicating a strong sense of self-reliance and inner strength among Appalachians (Burkhardt, 1993).

While Appalachians may not believe they are capable of maintaining their health without God's help, many believe they may be to blame for many chronic illnesses (such as diabetes). Smith and Tessaro (2005) documented that diabetes is often perceived by Appalachians as a self-induced illness, indicating a moral weakness and brought on by "laziness and lack of self discipline" (p. 295). Sometimes, if they believe that nothing can be done about a serious health condition, Appalachians may prefer not to be told the diagnosis (Sortet & Banks, 1997). Finally, when hospitalized, Appalachian patients may desire less decisional control than what nurses view as ideal (notably, in this study, physicians and patients preferred about the same level of patient decisional control) (Rosswurm et al., 1996).

In addition, we see variations in reports related to the coping styles of the Appalachians when confronted with critical illnesses of family members. In a study of the critical care coping styles of 30 family members of critically ill patients in two rural Appalachian hospitals, dominant coping styles were supportive, optimistic, confrontational, and self-reliant, with fatalism and evasive styles being ranked much lower (Hunsucker et al., 2000). Supportive strategies emphasizing the importance of close personal contacts were key. Action-focused coping centered on seeking information about the problem, handling things one step at a time, and keeping busy.

In contrast to middle-class America's "doing" activity orientation, Appalachians are considered "being" oriented, which means they focus more on interpersonal relationships than on personal accomplishments. In contrast with middle-class individualistic emphasis, Appalachian culture emphasizes the lineal-collateral orientation, indicating that an individual's most significant relationships are with family-related groups, kinship groups, or close neighbors. Many middle-class Americans seek self-actualization through individual accomplishments and autonomously set goals, whereas Appalachians tend to seek fulfillment through kin and neighbor interactions.

The "being" and lineal-collateral orientations, coupled with the present-time orientation, may influence health care practices, promoting a reactive rather than proactive stance. A nurse's initial encounter with an Appalachian client may be an emergency situation, such as a birth.

Appalachian Folk Health System

The Appalachian folk health system encompasses traditional beliefs about how to maintain health; the definition, nature, cause, and treatment of illnesses; traditional remedies; and lay health specialists. Again, many of these elements are in transition.

Beliefs. Illnesses are thought to result from the "will of God," a natural imbalance, or the body's response to personal habits, specific situations, or external exposures, particularly cold weather or "the cold" in general. Lack of "personal care" is an additional cause of illness. It includes (1) keeping the body strong, (2) eating right, and (3) taking fluids (Hansen & Resick, 1990). There are several Appalachian folk illnesses; three are discussed in more detail next.

High blood. One of the major health concerns of the Appalachian region is the state of the blood. The characteristics of the blood at issue may include whether it is thick or thin, good or bad, and high or low. Among Appalachians, the characteristic of *high* or *low blood* is a measure of blood viscosity and/or increased blood volume rushing to the head. High blood can be caused by diet, particularly pork and rich meats, fatty foods, and salt. These foods increase the viscosity of the blood by thickening it (pork and rich foods) or drying it up (salt). Many believe that emotions (anger, nervousness, stress) contribute to the etiology. Leading symptoms include dizziness, followed by headaches, visual disturbances, red or hot face, nausea, and nervousness.

Treatment focuses on restoring the proper balance so the blood is the right consistency. Keeping calm is thought to prevent a future attack. Some report an astringent (pickle brine, vinegar, Epson salts, garlic) may be an effective treatment; others do not find that (Nations, Camino, & Walker, 1985; Snow, 1976). High blood is distinguished from hypertension, which is a high "tension" or stress state (Nations et al., 1985).

Nerves. A lay idiom of distress, *nerves* is most often characterized by stressful social situations or events. Symptoms may include disturbed sleep patterns (falling and staying asleep), nervousness, tiredness, abdominal pain, shortness of breath, and anxiety attacks (Nations et al., 1985).

Sugar or sweet blood. The disorder of *sugar* or *sweet blood* results from the accumulation of sugar particles in the blood through one's life from eating sweet foods. Symptoms include dizziness, visual disturbances, and aching feet. The hazy vision is believed to be caused by the accumulation of sugar particles in the blood, which eventually settle in the eyes. Lay diagnostic signs include bruises that do not heal and having ants attracted to one's urine. Bitter herbs and foods (vinegar, gentian, Cerasee, or aloe teas) may be used to temporarily restore balance (Nations et al., 1985).

Knowledge of Biomedical Diseases

The level of biomedical health information and knowledge, particularly in rural Central Appalachia, is often very low (Hansen & Resick, 1990). There may be little knowledge of the biomedical explanations for how persons become ill, the complication of pregnancy, or how to prevent cardiovascular illness or diabetes. This unfamiliarity with the biomedical system may explain what has been termed "lack of interest" in the specifics of a biomedical diagnosis or interpreted as "denial" (Hansen & Resick, 1990; Lewis et al., 1985; Messner, Lewis, & Webb, 1984).

Medicinal Plants. Herbal remedies used in Appalachia are an integration of remedies derived from three primary sources: (1) American Indians, (2) nineteenth-century standard medical practice, and (3) ancestral practices rooted in northern Europe. The text *Medicinal Plants and Home Remedies of Appalachia* is an extensive resource. In this book, Boylard (1981) details the medicinal use of 90 plants in Central Appalachia and compares uses of each plant there with uses by American Indians, nineteenth-century medical practitioners, and Appalachians in the southern region. For example, *Lycoperdaceae* (puffball, devil's puff) spores are used as a hemostat to stop bleeding in all groups. *Phytolaccaceae* (pokeweed) is used to treat rheumatism by all groups and as a spring tonic in Central and Southern Appalachia. Other common remedies include white pine as an antiseptic, black pine as a cough medicine, ginseng for infant colic and general health, windroot for pleurisy, may apple root for rheumatism, elderberry as a disinfectant, and boneset (fever wort) tea for rheumatism or the flu, all of which have been shown to have some medicinal value (Boylard, 1981). However, the strength of the drugs that are used in home remedies is more variable than that of the drugs used in pharmaceutical preparations (Lewis et al., 1985). Herbs and over-the-counter medications may also be used in combination or sequentially.

In this domain, as in most other ethnic communities across the country, there is a shift from home remedies and use of wild medicinal herbs to over-the-counter remedies. This pattern was reported in the research of Denham (1999b), Mullen and Phillips (1998), and Rosswurm et al. (1996). Importantly, in the study of ethnomedical beliefs and clinic visits for folk illnesses, over-the-counter therapies were the most commonly used treatments (40%) prior to coming to the clinic. Further, the patients with ethno-medical conditions did not use home remedies or self-treat more than the others who presented only with biomedicine conditions (Nations et al., 1985).

Chronic illness management often integrates financial exigencies; norms of self-reliance; and a preference for "natural" foods, herbs, and vitamins over processed substances such as prescription medications (Smith & Tessaro, 2005). Noted are chromium, garlic, and vitamins to control blood glucose levels.

Lay Practitioners. The Appalachian folk medicine system had a tradition of folk healers commonly referred to as "granny women" and "herb doctors." These folk healers were commonly used because they were accessible, familiar with the culture, and well known to the family; lived in close proximity; used personalized interactions; and provided accepted remedies. However, lay practitioners are used much less frequently today. In a group of clinic patients in which nearly half reported ethnomedical complaints, only 4% reported consulting a faith healer or other alternative practitioner prior to their clinic visit (Nations et al., 1985).

Illness and Wellness Behaviors

Risk Behaviors. Several lifestyle factors place Appalachians at risk for health problems. These include a diet that is high in fats and carbohydrates, higher use of tobacco, lack of a regular exercise program, low use of seat belts, coal mining–associated hearing loss, and the poorest oral health in the United States, with the highest rate of toothlessness among elders (Murray-Johnson et al., 2004; Reed, Wineman, & Bechtel, 1995). For example, smoking is initiated earlier and more widely than in the general U.S. population. Although aware of the antismoking lung cancer health campaigns, some Appalachians ignore this information because of personal experiences. They know neighbors who have "smoked all their lives" and do not have lung cancer, and others who never smoked but died of lung cancer or other lung ailments. The proportion of Appalachian smokers in the "precontemplation" stage of the trans-theoretical model (TTM) of behavior change is higher than in the United States as a whole (Macnee & McCabe, 2004). Denham, Meyer, and Toborg (2004) investigated patterns of smoking among Appalachian adolescents in Ohio, Tennessee, and Virginia. They found that (1) the social community in tobacco-growing communities is a significant influence in tobacco use; (2) the family is important among young people in tobacco-growing communities and influences cessation positively and negatively; (3) parental smoking was an influence to smoking; (4) whereas some parents condone and even facilitate tobacco use by their children, others actively discourage use; and (5) concern for the health of younger brothers and sisters elicits a strongly protective reaction from youth in discussions of health risks related to secondhand smoke. Further, smoking is often used to relieve stress and is viewed as positive for weight control and alleviating boredom (Ahijevych et al., 2003). Thus, the benefits of smoking may be perceived to outweigh future health risks (Denham, 1999b).

Health Screening. Appalachian providers and consumers participate less often in preventive health screening programs. In a focus group study of rural Appalachian primary care providers, the perceived barriers to performing cancer screening were as follows: (1) provider-perceived patient barriers, including patients' fatalistic view of cancer; religious beliefs; low educational attainment; lack of cancer knowledge; a present, day-to-day orientation; and patients' not considering screening and health prevention a priority, and (2) provider-driven barriers, including a lack of time, lack of screening as part of the regular routine, a lack of provider continuity, and conflicting guidelines. Conversely, consumers' reasons for low participation in accessing preventive and routine health care include a lack of primary and/or specialty care providers, geographic or financial accessibility, long waiting periods for appointments, and level of health knowledge (Denham, 1999b; Elnicki et al., 1995; Huttlinger et al., 2004). In addition, a recent study reported considerable knowledge deficits for breast cancer screening and personal risk factors among even well-educated Appalachian women (Leslie et al., 2003).

Another perspective on cancer screening comes from studies reporting high rates of participation by low-income Appalachian women in preventive screening programs (cervical, breast, and rectal screens) when resources (clinics) were geographically and financially available (Reed et al., 1995). Further, the lack of mammography screening (less than half of the other screens) was largely attributed to lack of availability of those services at the same facilities. Innovative practice settings have demonstrated that Appalachians will use preventive services if they are available, accessible, and affordable (Edwards et al., 1993). Recent structures, such as community coalitions (Garland et al., 2004) and the Appalachian Cancer Network (Lengerich et al., 2004), show particular promise.

Illness Behaviors. When ill, Appalachians expect and receive aid from family members (Hansen & Resick, 1990). In a study of 257 randomly selected rural and urban Appalachian patients in eight hospitals in West Virginia, a significantly larger proportion of rural Appalachians reported that family help would be available at home for recovery.

In follow-up interviews, there was generally at least one adult child who was available to assist a parent (Rosswurm et al., 1996).

Nations et al. (1985) conducted a study to determine if ethnomedical beliefs and practices play an important role in primary care. In their study, 33 of 73 clients from a rural Appalachian area who presented themselves at a university primary care internal medicine program had 54 ethnomedical complaints. Of the ethnomedical complaints presented, 24.1% were of high blood pressure, 22.2% were of feeling weak and dizzy, 16.7% were of "nerves," 5.6% were of "sugar," and 3.7% were of "falling out." These 33 clients also reported biomedical complaints; the remaining 40 clients had biomedical complaints only, without evidence of ethnomedical complaints. No clients presented ethnomedical complaints alone. In the study, approximately two thirds of the clients consulted laypersons, primarily family members and friends, for their complaints, and at least 70% engaged in self-treatment before any clinical consultation. About 4% consulted a lay specialist. Approximately 130 biomedical complaints were presented and recorded by the clients' physicians; however, none of the 54 ethnomedical complaints was formally recorded. The high incidence of ethnomedical complaints among Appalachians and the failure of physicians to recognize these complaints indicate the need for providers to improve their history-taking skills, particularly regarding ethnomedical illnesses.

Mullen and Phillips (1998) used Giger and Davidhizar's Transcultural Assessment Model to identify six cultural phenomena of interest among Appalachians in southern Ohio. Results indicated that these participants had some characteristics commonly identified as *Appalachian,* such as having strong character, being stoic, being nonassertive, and having a strong belief in a Supreme Being. However, they also were found to communicate more openly, have a greater internal locus of control, be more future oriented, use no significant home remedies, be more time-conscientious about appointments, and be more likely to follow medical protocols than the stereotypic view of Appalachians. These findings may reflect the rapid transition occurring in the Appalachian region and provide a caution to practitioners not to forget about the dynamic nature of culture.

Implications for Nursing Care

The traditional Appalachian folk health system is in transition. While some traditional practices remain, others are diminishing. The health beliefs and any herbal therapies should be explored in depth in relation to the current clinical situation. Appalachians have a high need for health information and actively seek information resources.

Aiding the client to find an appropriate level of health information is a central function of the nursing role. Folk therapies that are neutral or beneficial should be encouraged. In the case where folk therapies or over-the-counter combinations may prove harmful, the nurse should provide health information in a clear, nonjudgmental manner.

BIOLOGICAL VARIATIONS

Health Disparities

Appalachia is one of the areas in the United States with excess mortality, morbidity, and disability (Geronimus, Bound, Waidmann, Colen, & Steffick, 2001); it has the highest concentration of regional Social Security Administration Disability claims and Supplemental Security Income (SSI) for persons age 18 to 64 (Litcher & Campbell, 2005; McCoy, Davis, & Hudson, 1994). The disability rates are high largely because of dangerous or toxic occupations, such as mining and textiles; poverty; and insufficient insurance coverage to screen and treat depression, as well as dental, vision, and hearing problems (Huttlinger, Schaller-Ayers, & Lawson, 2004).

Traumatic Injuries. In rural Appalachian Kentucky, males across all age groups have a higher risk for death from traumatic injury (Kerney, 2000). For children in rural Appalachian Kentucky, burns and child abuse were the most frequent cause for traumatic death for children under the age of 1, whereas motor vehicle accidents accounted for most of the injuries over the age of 1 (Svenson, Spurlock, & Nypaver, 1996). The higher rural death rate was attributed to factors such as decreased access to prehospital care, delayed acute care because of geographic isolation, and the need for provider training in pediatric advanced life support.

Respiratory Tract Diseases. Mortality from tuberculosis among Appalachians remains about 50% higher than the national average (National Center for Health Statistics, Health United States, 2014). High-risk occupations, such as those in the mining, timber, and textile industries, increase the number of respiratory and other disabling physical health problems. These diseases, such as black lung, are incurable, progressive, and debilitating (Carroll, 1999), contributing to disabilities that are far greater than the national average (McCoy et al., 1994). In addition, tobacco, a local industry, is widely used and contributes to lung disease (Ramey, 1993).

Coronary Artery and Coronary Heart Disease. The incidence of coronary artery disease, coronary heart disease, and mortality from heart disease and stroke among

Appalachians exceeds the national average (Browne & Richardson, 2006), especially in the central and southern regions of Appalachia (Dzik, 1997; Huttlinger et al., 2004; Neal et al., 2001). Ramsey and Glenn (1998) investigated medical records in one poor, underserved, rural Appalachian county in Tennessee. This county of approximately 7000 residents was found to have the highest poverty level in the state, with an unadjusted mortality rate for heart disease of 531.9 per 100,000, compared with the state mean of 318.1 per 100,000. The findings indicated that excessive smoking, lack of exercise, a high-fat diet, and abnormal serum lipid levels were key risk factors associated with heart disease. This supported an earlier study of middle-aged Appalachian women in an isolated county in northeast Tennessee, which identified that past or present smoking, history of lung disease, physical inactivity, obesity, and hypercholesterolemia were health risk factors leading to mortality (Edwards, Shuman, & Glenn, 1996). A relationship was found between the risk factors and low formal education levels, poverty, and limited access to health care. Thus, a better understanding of risk factors through education, more access to health care, and increased resources for adequate diet must all be addressed if heart disease is to be decreased among Appalachians. Neal et al. (2001) discuss the Coronary Artery Risk Detection in Appalachian Communities (CARDIAC) and the West Virginia Rural Health Education Partnerships (WVRHEP) as community-level screening and school-based health promotion programs to influence both children and parental health behavior.

Cancer. Although breast cancer rates are lower than the national average, cervical cancer remains higher for both Black and White Appalachian women (Hall, Rogers, Weir, Miller, & Uhler, 2000; Hopenhayn, Bush, Christian, & Shelton, 2005). White women in Appalachia have twice the incidence of cervical cancer than the national average, approaching the national rate for Black women (Erikson, 2001). African-American Appalachians (Newell-Withrow, 2000) were found to be actively engaged in health promotion and prevention. In particular, Fisher and Page (1987) found that women participated in Pap smear health screening if it was convenient, required, or requested. Huttlinger et al. (2004) found that a major barrier is the cost that insurance plans will not cover for health screening.

Infant Mortality

The high infant mortality rate, which is 9.3% (National Center for Health Statistics, Health United States, 2014), corresponds closely to the level of poverty. Spurlock, Moser, and Flynn (1989) conducted a study to examine differences in postnatal mortalities between the Appalachian portions of Kentucky and the remainder of the state. A key factor related to increased infant mortality in the Appalachian region was maternal education. Three types of postnatal deaths were disproportionately high among infants in the Appalachian region: sudden infant death syndrome, congenital malformations, and infections.

Nutrition

Food patterns in the Appalachian region have been described as "unpretentious, solid, and filling" (Flasher, 2002). Consequently, obesity is a considerable problem among all ages (Demerath et al., 2003). The Appalachian diet tends to be high in fats, carbohydrates, and salt. A wide variety of domestic and wild meats are eaten, and bread is generally served at each meal. Cornbread, biscuits and gravy, fried potatoes, and beans are staple food items (Flasher, 2002; Tribe & Oliveri, 2000).

While little work has been conducted on the provision of nutritional advice to children who are overweight/obese, Demerath et al. (2003) describe the promise and potential of school-based obesity screening and nutritional counseling program, the CARDIAC program.

SUMMARY

Although access to health care remains problematic, community intervention programs and practice models are being developed to help address this problem (Baker, McKenzie, & Harrison, 2005; Glisson & Schoenwald, 2005; Huttlinger et al., 2004). One example of a successful community-based project to increase awareness of remote rural Appalachian health needs and provide access to health care services is the collaborative Remote Area Medical (RAM) project (Huttlinger et al., 2004). This collaborative project provided primary, dental, and vision health care services to 3310 persons during July and October 2002 in the Wise, Virginia, and Mountain City, Tennessee, areas. Participants reported high satisfaction with each of the events, after driving 1.5 to 250 miles (Wise attendees) and 0.5 to 240 miles (Mountain City attendees) to attend. Although most of the participants had health insurance, this did not ensure affordability of health care. The events did demonstrate the desire and drive to acquire and provide culturally appropriate, consumer-based health care services.

The Appalachian people have a rich heritage that has been in dramatic transition over the past half-century. For generations, these beliefs and values were passed down and have persevered. In recent years, some Appalachians, especially the young, have moved to urban areas, and health providers are now more likely to come into contact with

Appalachian people through the conventional medical system. When working with persons from the Appalachian region, the nurse can build on some of the positive aspects inherent in the people, such as strength, independence, interdependence, sensitivity, and faith, to foster a therapeutic nurse–client relationship. In addition, knowledge of the traditional health care beliefs and the importance of the family can aid the nurse in giving culturally sensitive, individualized nursing care.

CASE STUDY

Sarah James, an 89-year-old widow who lives alone next door to one of her sons in Sweetwater, Tennessee, is seen at the clinic by the family clinical nurse specialist because she "feels bad." She arrives at the clinic with her three sons and their families, who are concerned because Sarah has been "running off" several times a day and will not eat. The clinical nurse specialist visits "for a spell" and then begins to take a health history. When the clinical nurse specialist asks what has brought Mrs. James to the clinic, the eldest son reveals that Sarah has "run off" six or seven times since yesterday and cannot drink her tea. Also, according to the eldest son, Mrs. James has not recently traveled out of Sweetwater, does not have proper refrigeration, and has recently eaten some "tater" salad that had sat out all day in the hot weather. It is determined that the diarrhea is watery, brown, and nonodorous. Mrs. James also had dry heaves but has not vomited and does not verbalize symptoms of pain.

Further assessment by the clinical nurse specialist reveals that Mrs. James has generalized weakness, poor skin turgor, dark circles around the eyes, sticky mucous membranes, pale skin, rectal temperature of 101° F, generalized abdominal tenderness, hyperactive bowel sounds, thready but regular heart rate of 100, blood pressure of 110/60 mm Hg, respirations of 24, and weight of 110 lbs.

After a complete physical examination, the clinical nurse specialist orders a stool culture, electrolytes, and a complete blood cell count. After collaboration with the clinic physician, the eldest son approves Mrs. James's admission to the hospital with her entire family in attendance. Mrs. James is crying as she enters the hospital. A diagnosis of dehydration and *Salmonella* poisoning is made. Arrangements are made for follow-up examination after discharge from the hospital

CLINICAL DECISION MAKING

1. List some strategies that may help the nurse communicate with an Appalachian family.
2. Describe the significance of the extended family and the roles within the Appalachian family structure.
3. Compare and contrast the differences in illness beliefs between middle-class Americans and Appalachians.
4. Describe the possible importance of home remedies to persons from Appalachian regions.
5. Identify three major barriers to health screening by rural Appalachians.
6. Describe how nurses can aid Appalachian patients in obtaining health information.
7. Indicate resources that health care providers can use to facilitate wellness.
8. List at least three major conditions for which Appalachians are at greater risk than the general U.S. population.

REVIEW QUESTIONS

1. While taking a history on an Appalachian patient, Mrs. Brown tells the nurse that she has had "high blood." The competent nurse interprets this to mean the patient has a history of which of the following?
   a. Increased low-density lipoproteins
   b. Hypercholesterolemia
   c. Hypertension
   d. Hemodilution
2. When an Appalachian client is ill, personal space collapses inwardly. For the nurse providing nursing care, this means:
   a. The person will try to be independent and self-sufficient.
   b. The person expects to be waited on and cared for by others.
   c. The person wants to be cared for by the family only.
   d. The person expects that health care decisions will be made by the family.
3. In planning health care screening for rural Appalachians, which of the following would be of least concern for the nurse?
   a. Tuberculosis
   b. Coronary heart disease
   c. Cervical cancer
   d. Breast cancer

◎ CARE PLAN

Nursing Diagnosis: Diarrhea related to infectious processes (*Salmonella*) as a result of inadequate refrigeration of food, as evidenced by six to seven watery, brown stools per day

Client Outcomes	Nursing Interventions
1. Client will exhibit signs of adequate hydration within 24 hours. 2. Client will resume normal elimination and peristaltic action within the next 24 to 48 hours.	1. Measure daily weight. 2. Record amount, character, and volume of stools. 3. Record intake and output. 4. Obtain stool culture. 5. Assess pain status. 6. Explain specific reason for problem (that is, lack of refrigeration of potato salad and other foods that need refrigeration). 7. Note results of complete blood count and electrolytes.

Nursing Diagnosis: Communication, impaired verbal, related to cultural differences

Client Outcome	Nursing Interventions
Communication will be established between client, nurse, and family to understand health condition and needs.	1. Determine meaning of verbal and nonverbal cues. 2. Establish rapport with client and family. 3. Be aware of cultural factors, such as avoiding eye contact. 4. Communicate with client in an unhurried manner. 5. Communicate in specific terms. 6. Ask client and family for their advice. 7. Avoid criticism and spend extra time with client. 8. Communicate on a first-name basis.

Nursing Diagnosis: Anxiety related to perceived threat of death

Client Outcome	Nursing Interventions
Client will show signs of decreased anxiety.	1. Involve family in nursing care. 2. Provide arrangement for one family member to stay during the night. 3. Exhibit a calm and unhurried manner. 4. Reassure client. 5. Be flexible in visiting regulations. 6. Be accepting of client's cultural differences. 7. Explain procedures to client in specific terms. 8. Arrange for a social service worker to visit for planning financial issues.

Nursing Diagnosis: Nutrition, altered: Less than body requirements, related to inability to absorb nutrients (diarrhea), as evidenced by absence of food intake for the past 48 hours

Client Outcome	Nursing Interventions
Client will consume a balanced diet for body size and maintain present weight before discharge.	1. Monitor weight. 2. Provide nutritionally balanced diet at times client feels like eating. 3. Document food intake. 4. Explain necessity for proper diet in specific terms. 5. Determine what foods she prefers to eat. 6. Encourage rest.

Nursing Diagnoses—Definitions and Classifications 2012–2014. Copyright © 2012, 1994–2012 by NANDA International. Used by arrangement with Wiley-Blackwell Publishing, a company of John Wiley and Sons, Inc. In order to make safe and effective judgments using NANDA-I nursing diagnoses it is essential that nurses refer to the definitions and defining characteristics of the diagnoses listed in the work.

REFERENCES

Ahijevych, I., Kuun, P., Christman, S., Wood, T., Browning, K., & Wewers, M. E. (2003). Beliefs about tobacco among Appalachian current and former users. *Applied Nursing Research, 16*(2), 93–102.

Appalachian Regional Commission. (2013). The new Appalachian subregions and their development strategies. *Appalachian: A Journal of the Appalachian Regional Commission, 8*(1), 11–27.

Appalachian Regional Commission (2015). *The Appalachian Region: A data overview from 2009-2013.* American Community Survey Chartbook.

Baker, G., McKenzie, A., & Harrison, P. (2005). Local physicians caring for their communities: an innovative model to meeting the needs of the uninsured. *North Carolina Medical Journal, 66*(2), 130–133.

Barnett, E., Halverson, J. A., Elmes, G. A., & Braham, V. E. (2000). Metropolitan and non-metropolitan trends in coronary heart disease mortality within Appalachia, 1980–1997. *Annual Epidemiology, 10*, 370–379.

Beck, R. W., Jijon, C. R., & Edwards, J. B. (1996). The relationships among gender, perceived financial barriers to care, and health status in a rural population. *The Journal of Rural Health, 12*(3), 188–196.

Blakeney, A. B. (1987). Appalachian values: implications for occupational therapists. *Occupational Therapy in Health Care, 4*(1), 57–72.

Boylard, J. L. (1981). *Medicinal plants and home remedies of Appalachia.* Springfield, IL: Charles C Thomas.

Browne, C., & Richardson, V. (2006). Older adults in minority groups. In B. Beckman & S. Ambrusco (Eds.), *Handbook of social work in health and aging* (pp. 304–309). New York: Oxford University Press.

Burkhardt, M. (1991). Exploring understandings of spirituality among women in Appalachia (Dissertation). Ann Arbor, MI: University Microfilms International.

Burkhardt, M. (1993). Characteristics of spirituality in the lives of women in a rural Appalachian community. *Journal of Transcultural Nursing, 4*(2), 12–18.

Calico, F. (1996). Home health moving toward "high touch, high tech": Appalachian regional healthcare pioneers homecare technology. *Health Management Technology, 17*(11), 22–25, 27.

Carroll, M. (1999). Viewpoint: Appalachian coal miners mutual help and advocacy. *Public Health Reports, 114*, 326–327.

Caudill, H. M. (1976). *The watches of the night.* Boston: Little, Brown.

Crissman, J. K. (1994). *Death and dying in central Appalachia: changing attitudes and practices.* Chicago: University of Illinois Press.

Culture of poverty revisited: a critique by the Mental Health Committee against Racism. (1977). New York: Mental Health Committee against Racism.

Cushing, B. J., & Rogers, C. (1996). *Income and poverty in Appalachia: a report to the Appalachian Regional Commission (research paper 9511).* Morgantown, WV: West Virginia University, Regional Research Institute.

Demerath, E., Muratova, V., Spangler, E., Li, J., Minor, V. E., & Neal, W. A. (2003). School-based obesity screening in rural Appalachia. *Preventive Medicine, 37*, 553–560.

Denham, S. (1999a). Epilogue: summary of three studies on family health with Appalachian families. *Journal of Family Nursing, 5*(2), 214.

Denham, S. (1999b). Part III: family health in an economically disadvantaged population. *Journal of Family Nursing, 5*(2), 184–213.

Denham, S. (2002). Family routines: a structural perspective for viewing family health. *Advances of Nursing Science, 24*(4), 60–74.

Denham, S. A., Meyer, M. G., & Toborg, M. A. (2004). Tobacco cessation in adolescent females in Appalachian communities. *Family & Community Health, 27*(2), 170–181.

Denham, S. A., Meyer, M. G., Toborg, M. A., & Mande, M. J. (2004). Providing health education to Appalachia populations. *Holistic Nursing Practice, 18*(6), 293–301.

Dial, W. (1975). The dialect of the Appalachian people. In B. Maurer (Ed.), *Mountain heritage.* Ripley, WV: Mountain State Art and Craft Fair.

Dreher, M., & MacNaughton, N. (2002). Cultural competence in nursing: foundation or fallacy? *Nursing Outlook, 50*(5), 181–186.

Dzik, A. J. (1997). Looking for dangerous places: some aspects of medical geography and disease mapping. *West Virginia Medical Journal, 93*(5), 250–253.

Edwards, J. B., Lenz, C. L., & East-Odom, J. (1993). Nurse-managed primary care: serving a rural Appalachian population. *Family Community Health, 16*(2), 50–56.

Edwards, J. B., Shuman, P., & Glenn, L. L. (1996). Relationships among health risk factors and objective physical findings in well rural Appalachian women. *Family Community Health, 18*(4), 67–80.

Elnicki, D., Douglas, K., Morris, M., & Shockcor, W. (1995). Patient-perceived barriers to preventive health care among indigent, rural Appalachian patients. *Archives of Internal Medicine, 155*(4), 421–424.

Erikson, J. (2001). Cervical cancer in Appalachia focus of study by new NCI Center. *Oncology Times, 23*(5), 46–51.

Fisher, S., & Page, A. I. (1987). Women and preventive health care: an exploratory study of the use of Pap smears in a potentially high-risk Appalachian population. *Women's Health, 11*(3/4), 83–99.

Flasher, W. C. (2002). *Cultural diversity: eating in America.* Columbus, OH: Ohio State University Extension Office.

Ford, T. (1967). The passing of provincialism. In T. Ford (Ed.), *The southern Appalachian region.* Lexington, KY: University of Kentucky Press.

Friedell, G. H., et al. (2001). Community cancer control in a rural, underserved population: the Appalachian leadership initiative on cancer project. *Journal of Health Care for the Poor and Underserved, 12*(1), 5–19.

Garland, B., Crane, M., Marino, C., Stone-Wiggins, B., Ward, A., & Friedell, G. (2004). Effect of community coalition structure and preparation on the subsequent implementation of cancer control activities. *American Journal of Health Promotion, 18*(6), 424–434.

Geronimus, A. T., Bound, J., Waidmann, T. A., Colen, C. G., & Steffick, D. (2001). Inequality in life expectancy, functional status, and active life expectancy across selected black and white populations in the United States. *Demography, 38*(2), 227–251.

Glisson, C., & Schoenwald, S. (2005). The ARC organizational and community intervention strategy for implementing evidence-based children's mental health treatments. *Mental Health Services Research, 7*(4), 243–259.

Gudykunst, W., & Ting-Toomey, S. (1988). *Culture and interpersonal communication.* Newbury Park, CA: Sage.

Hall, E. T. (1989). *Beyond culture.* New York: Anchor Books.

Hall, E. T. (2006). Context and meaning. In L. Samovar, K. Porter, & E. McDaniel (Eds.), *Intercultural communication: a reader* (7th ed., pp. 60–70). Belmont, CA: Thomson/Wadsworth.

Hall, H. I., Rogers, J. D., Weir, H. K., Miller, D. S., & Uhler, R. J. (2000). Breast and cervical carcinoma mortality among women in the Appalachian region of the U.S., 1976–1996. *Cancer, 89*(7), 1593–1602.

Hall, H. I., Uhler, R. J., Coughlin, S. S., & Miller, D. S. (2002). Breast and cervical cancer screening among Appalachian women. *Cancer Epidemiology, Biomarkers and Prevention, 11*, 137–142.

Hansen, M. M., & Resick, L. K. (1990). Health beliefs, health care, and rural Appalachian subcultures from an ethnographic perspective. *Family Community Health, 13*(1), 1–10.

Helton, L. (1995). Intervention with Appalachians: strategies for a culturally specific practice. *Journal of Cultural Diversity, 2*(1), 20–26.

Hesselgrave, B. (2001). Polypharmacy. *Managed Care Quarterly, 9*(4), 9–15.

Hicks, G. (1976). *Appalachian valley.* New York: Holt, Rinehart, & Winston.

Hopenhayn, C., Bush, H., Christian, A., & Shelton, B. (2005). Comparative analysis of invasive cervical cancer incidence rates in three Appalachian states. *Preventive Medicine, 41*, 859–864.

Hunsucker, S., Flannery, J., & Frank, D. (2000). Coping strategies of rural families of critically ill patients. *Journal of the American Academy of Nurse Practitioners, 12*(4), 123–127.

Hunsucker, S., Frank, D., & Flannery, J. (1999). Meeting the needs of rural families during critical illness: the APN's role. *Dimensions of Critical Care Nursing, 18*(3), 24–32.

Hurley, J., Turner, S., & Floyd, D. (2000). Development of a health service at a rural community college in Appalachia. *Journal of American College Health, 48*, 181–185.

Huttlinger, K., Schaller-Ayers, J., Kenny, B., & Ayers, J. (2004). Research and collaboration in rural community health. *Online Journal of Rural Nursing and Health Care, 4*(1), Retrieved on June 15, 2007 [Online]. Available at <http://www.rno.org/journal/issues/Vol-4/issue-1/Huttlinger_article.htm>.

Huttlinger, K., Schaller-Ayers, J., & Lawson, T. (2004). Health care in Appalachia: a population-based approach. *Public Health Nursing, 21*(2), 103–110.

Isserman, A. M. (1997). Appalachia then and now: an update of "the realities of deprivation" reported to the President in 1964. *Journal of Appalachian Studies, 3*(4), 43–73.

Jesse, D. E. (2003). Prenatal psychosocial needs: differences between a TennCare group and a privately insured group in Appalachia. *Journal of Health Care for the Poor and Underserved, 14*(4), 535–549.

Jesse, D. E., & Reed, P. G. (2004). Effects of spirituality and psychosocial well-being on health risk behaviors in Appalachian pregnant women. *Journal of Obstetric, Gynecologic, & Neonatal Nursing, 33*(6), 739–747.

Jesse, D. E., Seaver, W., & Wallace, D. (2003). Maternal psychosocial risks predict preterm birth in a group of women from Appalachia. *Midwifery, 19*, 191–202.

Jones, L. (1983). Appalachian values. In D. Whisnant (Ed.), *All that is native and fine: the politics of culture in an American region.* Chapel Hill, NC: University of North Carolina Press.

Kerney, K. B. (2000). Appalachia: the place, the people, and home care. *Home Health Care Management and Practice, 12*(6), 56–61.

LaFargue, J. P. (1980). A survival strategy: kinship networks. *American Journal of Nursing, 80*(9), 1636–1640.

Lengerich, E. J., et al. (2004). The Appalachia Cancer Network: cancer control research among a rural, medically underserved population. *The Journal of Rural Health, 20*(2), 181–187.

Leslie, N. S., Deiriggi, P., Gross, S., DuRant, E., Smith, C., & Veshnesky, J. G. (2003). Knowledge, attitudes, and practices surrounding breast cancer screening in educated Appalachian women. *Oncology Nursing Forum, 30*(4), 659–667.

Levenstein, C., DeLaurier, G. F., & Dunn, M. L. (2002). *The cotton dust papers: science, politics, and power in the "discovery" of byssinosis in the U.S.* Amityville, NY: Baywood.

Lewis, S., Messner, R., & McDowell, W. (1985). An unchanging culture. *Journal of Gerontological Nursing, 11*(8), 20–26.

Litcher, D., & Campbell, L. (2005). *Changing patterns of poverty and spatial inequality in Appalachia.* Washington, DC: The Appalachian Regional Commission.

Maas, L. M., et al. (2004). Outcomes of family involvement in care for caregivers of individuals with dementia. *Nursing Research, 53*(2), 76–86.

MacAvoy, S., & Lippman, D. (2001). Teaching culturally competent care: nursing students experience rural Appalachia. *Journal of Transcultural Nursing, 12*(3), 221–227.

Macnee, C. L., & McCabe, S. (2004). The transtheoretical model of behavior change and smokers in Southern Appalachia. *Nursing Research, 53*(4), 243–250.

McCoy, J. L., Davis, M., & Hudson, R. E. (1994). Geographic patterns of disability in the United States. *Social Security Bulletin, 57*(1), 25–26.

Messner, R., Lewis, S., & Webb, D. D. (1984). Unique problems and approaches in Appalachian patients with Crohn's disease. *The Society of Gastrointestinal Assistants Journal, 7,* 38–46.

Mullen, S., & Phillips, C. (1998). *Cultural beliefs of southeastern Ohio Appalachians. Proceedings of the Fourth Interdisciplinary Health Research Symposium.* Morgantown, WV: Health Care and Culture.

Muratova, V. N., Islam, S. S., Demerath, E. W., Minor, V. E., & Neal, W. A. (2001). Cholesterol screening among children and their parents. *Preventive Medicine, 33,* 1–6.

Murdock, G. (1982). *Outline of cultural materials* (5th ed.). New Haven, CN: Human Relations Area Files.

Murray, R. B., & Huelskoetter, M. W. (1991). *Psychiatric/mental health nursing* (3rd ed.). East Norwalk, CN: Appleton & Lange.

Murray-Johnson, L., et al. (2004). Using the extended parallel process model to prevent noise-induced hearing loss among coal miners in Appalachia. *Health Education & Behavior, 31*(6), 741–755.

National Center for Health Statistics (2014). *Health United States 2014.* Washington, DC: U.S. Government Printing Office.

Nations, M. K., Camino, L. A., & Walker, F. B. (1985). "Hidden" popular illnesses in primary care: resident's recognition and clinical implications. *Culture, Medicine and Psychiatry, 9*(3), 223–240.

Neal, W. A., et al. (2001). Coronary Artery Risk Detection in Appalachian Communities (CARDIAC): preliminary findings. *The West Virginia Medical Journal, 97,* 102–105.

Newell-Withrow, C. (2000). Health protecting and health promoting behaviors of African Americans living in Appalachia. *Public Health Nursing, 17*(5), 392–397.

Obermiller, P. J., & Maloney, M. (1990). The current status and future prospects of urban Appalachians. *Urban Advocate, 7.*

Obermiller, P., & Maloney, M. (2007). Living city, feeling country: the current status and future prospects of urban Appalachians. In K. M. Borman & P. J. Obermiller (Eds.), *From mountain to metropolis: Appalachian migrants in American cities* (pp. 3–12). Westport, CT: Greenwood.

Penn, E. M., Borman, K. M., & Hoeweler, F. (1994). Echoes from the hill: urban Appalachian youths and educational reform. In K. M. Borman & P. J. Obermiller (Eds.), *From mountain to metropolis: Appalachian migrants in American cities* (pp. 83–92). Westport, CT: Bergin & Garvey.

Pollard, K. M. (2004). The 1990s: an era of increasing diversity within Appalachia. In K. M. Pollard (Ed.), *A "new diversity": race and ethnicity in the Appalachian region* (pp. 5–15). Washington, DC: Population Reference Bureau.

President's Appalachian Regional Commission (PARC) (1963). *Appalachia: a report by the President's Appalachian Regional Commission.* Washington, DC: U.S. Government Printing Office.

Purnell, L., & Counts, M. (2003). Appalachians. In L. Purnell & B. Paulanka (Eds.), *Transcultural health care: a culturally competent approach* (2nd ed.). Philadelphia: F. A. Davis.

Ramey, R. (1993). COPD in rural Appalachia: a model for pulmonary rehabilitation. *Tar Heel Nurse,* 32–35.

Ramsey, P. W., & Glenn, L. L. (1998). Risk factors for heart disease in rural Appalachia. *Family Community Health, 20*(4), 71–82.

Reed, B. W., Wineman, J., & Bechtel, G. A. (1995). Using a health risk appraisal to determine an Appalachian community's health care needs. *Journal of Cultural Diversity, 2*(4), 131–135.

Rosswurm, M., Dent, D., Armstrong-Persily, C., Woodburn, P., & Davis, B. (1996). Illness experiences and health recovery behaviors of patients in Southern Appalachia. *Western Journal of Nursing Research, 18*(4), 441–459.

Rowles, G. D. (1983). Between worlds: a relocation dilemma for the Appalachian elderly. *International Journal of Aging Human Development, 17*(4), 301–314.

Rowles, G. D. (1991). Beyond performance: being in place as a component of occupational therapy. *American Journal of Occupational Therapy, 45*(3), 265–271.

Rowles, G. D. (2000). Habituation and being in place. *Occupational Therapy Journal of Research, 20,* 52S–67S.

Sherrod, M. (2005). Remembering the dead, comforting the living: adapting Christian ministry to Appalachian death practices. In S. E. Keefe (Ed.), *Appalachian cultural competency: a guide for medical, mental health, and social service professionals* (pp. 89–113). Knoxville, TN: University of Tennessee Press.

Simon, J. M. (1987). Health care of the elderly in Appalachia. *Journal of Gerontological Nursing, 13*(7), 32–35.

Simpkins, O. (1979). Appalachian culture. In B. Maurer (Ed.), *Rural and Appalachian health.* Springfield, IL: Charles C Thomas.

Simpson, M. R., & King, M. G. (1999). "God brought all these churches together": issues in developing religion-health partnerships in an Appalachian community. *Public Health Nursing, 16*(1), 41–49.

Smith, S. L., & Tessaro, I. A. (2005). Cultural perspectives on diabetes in an Appalachian population. *American Journal of Health Behavior, 29*(4), 291–301.

Snow, L. (1976). "High blood" is not high blood pressure. *Urban Health, 5,* 54–55.

Sortet, J. P., & Banks, S. R. (1997). Health beliefs of rural Appalachian women and the practice of breast self-examination. *Cancer Nursing, 20*(4), 231–235.

Specht, J. P., Kelley, L. S., Manion, P., Maas, M. L., Reed, D., & Rantz, M. J. (2000). Who's the boss? Family/staff partnership in care of persons with dementia. *Nursing Administration Quarterly, 24*(3), 64–77.

Spurlock, C. W., Moser, M., & Flynn, L. J. (1989). Regional differences in death rates among postneonatal infants in Kentucky, 1982–1985. *Journal of the Kentucky Medical Association, 87*(3), 119.

Svenson, J. E., Spurlock, C., & Nypaver, M. (1996). Factors associated with the higher traumatic death rate among rural children. *Annals of Emergency Medicine, 27*(5), 625–632.

Tribe, D. I., & Oliveri, C. S. (2000). *Changing Appalachian foodways: perceived changes and rationale for food habits of Appalachian Ohioans.* Columbus, OH: Ohio State University Extension Office.

Tripp-Reimer, T. (1980). Appalachian health care: from research to practice. *Transcultural Nursing Care, 5,* 48–59.

Tripp-Reimer, T. (1982). Barriers to health care: variations in interpretation of Appalachian client behavior by Appalachian and non-Appalachian health professionals. *Western Journal of Nursing Research, 4*(2), 179–191.

Tripp-Reimer, T., & Fox, S. S. (2001). Beyond the concept of culture: or, how knowing the cultural formula does not predict clinical success. In J. McCloskey & H. Grace (Eds.), *Current issues in nursing* (6th ed.). St. Louis: Mosby.

Tripp-Reimer, T., & Friedl, M. C. (1977). Appalachians: a neglected minority. *Nursing Clinics of North America, 12*(1), 41–54.

U.S. Department of Commerce, Bureau of the Census (2009). *American Community Survey.* Washington, DC: U.S. Government Printing Office.

U.S. Department of Commerce, Bureau of the Census (2015). *American Community Survey.* Washington, DC: U.S. Government Printing Office.

U.S. Department of Labor (2002). *Labor profiles of the United States: 2001.* Washington, DC: U.S. Government Printing Office.

Wallace, D. C., Tuck, I., Boland, C. S., & Witucki, J. M. (2002). Client perceptions of parish nursing. *Public Health Nursing, 19*(2), 128–135.

American Eskimos: The Yup'ik and Inupiat*

Tina D. DeLapp

BEHAVIORAL OBJECTIVES

After reading this chapter, the nurse will be able to:

1. Outline verbal and nonverbal communication barriers that may affect health care for the Yup'ik and Inupiat.
2. Describe values related to space that may be found among the Yup'ik and Inupiat.
3. Discuss the value and role of elders for the Yup'ik and Inupiat.
4. Explain how traditional time orientation may affect compliance with a health regimen of individuals of Yup'ik and Inupiat descent.
5. Discuss attitudes and beliefs of the Yup'ik and Inupiat that relate to health and illness.
6. Identify the impact of the adoption of a Western diet and lifestyle on health and illness patterns apparent in persons of Eskimo descent.

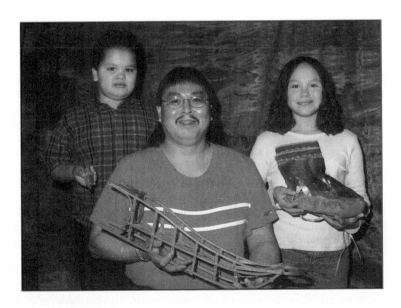

*Special appreciation is extended to Dr. Nancy Sanders for her contributions to this chapter.

Settlements of Eskimos are found in diverse locations, including the northern territories of Canada, Alaska, Russia, and Greenland. Although Eskimos may be found throughout the world, this chapter focuses on Alaskan Yup'ik and Inupiat Eskimos who have remained in their native land and those who have migrated to the mainland United States. To provide culturally appropriate nursing care, it is necessary for the nurse to understand the culture and heritage of the Eskimo people.

OVERVIEW OF ALASKA

The Land

Alaska is often described in superlatives. One fifth the size of the continental United States, Alaska has more coastline than the other 49 states combined and is by far the largest state in the continental United States. With a land area of 570,641 square miles, it is more than twice the size of Texas. Everything in Alaska appears to be on a grand scale. It is the home of the largest mountain in North America, Mount McKinley (also known as *Denali,* an Athabascan word meaning "The High One"), which rises to a height of 20,320 feet (*World Almanac and Book of Facts,* 2015) and is joined by six other peaks that are over 14,500 feet high. Alaska is also the home of the Bering Glacier, which, together with the Bagley Oil Field, covers 2000 square miles, an area larger than the state of Delaware (National Snow and Ice Data Center, 2014). There are more than 100,000 other glaciers in Alaska, only a few of which are named. Across Alaska, large mammals, including bear, moose, and caribou, roam largely undisturbed, providing for the subsistence needs of the Alaska Native population.

The chief influences on the climate in Alaska are its northern latitude, its large landmass, and its coastal waters. In the southern part of Alaska, the warm marine currents cause the climate to be temperate and damp, resulting in spruce rain forests on Kodiak Island and in the southern panhandle of the state. On the Aleutian Islands, where the climate is also temperate, grasses and shrubs predominate.

The interior of Alaska is bordered on the north by the Brooks Range, on the south by the Alaska Range, and on the west by the Arctic environment of the coast. The boreal forests of the interior consist of "relatively small specimens of white and black spruce, alder, birch and aspen [which] cover most of the rolling hills" (Langdon, 2014, pp. 6–7). The river drainages are marshy and flat and attract many species of waterfowl important to the Athabaskan Indians who live in this area. The temperature in interior Alaska varies dramatically from lows of −50° F in the winter to more than 90° F in the summer.

A 200-mile-wide band extending along the western coast of Alaska from Bristol Bay to the border of Alaska and Canada is the Arctic region (Langdon, 2014). This area is drained by the Yukon and Kuskokwim rivers and their tributaries. It is in this area that Eskimos live. The Inupiat Eskimos live in the northern section from the Seward Peninsula north to the Canadian border. Yup'ik Eskimos live south of the Seward Peninsula to Bristol Bay in southwestern Alaska, both along the coast and inland along the Yukon and Kuskokwim Rivers. Winters in this area are long, and summers are short and cool.

An unusual feature of Alaska's terrain is permafrost, or permanently frozen ground. In the Arctic region, continuous permafrost underlies surface dirt in depths of about 2000 feet. Some buildings and highways have been erected on permafrost; when the permafrost thaws, those structures sink. More recently, climate change has accelerated permafrost thawing, impacting the stability of infrastructure and ecosystems. Loss of sea ice has negatively impacted several animal species on which Inupiat peoples depend for subsistence, and coastal erosion has forced some villages to relocate for safety reasons (Environmental Protection Agency, 2013).

Over most of the arctic, annual snowfall is quite light, as little as 4 to 6 inches. While actual snowstorms are rare, ground blizzards, which whip up dry snow already on the ground, may persist for days (Lopez, 2001). At cold temperatures, wind speeds the rate of heat loss from the skin, thus increasing the risk of freezing injury (Varnado, 2008).

Alaska has 33,000 miles of coastline (Langdon, 2014; *World Almanac,* 2015). Migratory marine mammals (walrus, seals, and whales), fish (particularly salmon), and birds return to birthing grounds in Alaska during the summer. The Bering Sea, the Yukon and Kuskokwim Rivers and their tributaries, and the migratory bird nesting areas make the hunting and fishing resources an important source of subsistence food for the Alaskan Native population, including the Yup'ik and the Inupiat Eskimos (Langdon, 2014). Limited income-generating opportunities in rural villages make subsistence activities crucial for survival.

For many years the Eskimos claimed that certain lands belonged to them without effect. However, when oil was discovered in the state, the U.S. government recognized the right of Eskimos to their traditional lifestyle. The 1971 Alaska Native Claims Settlement Act (ANCSA) created 12 regional Native corporations and provided for the allocation of lab and monies to those corporations and to 200 Native villages. While any Alaska Native who lived in the geographic region of the corporation could become a shareholder, the shareholders of four of the corporations are primarily of Yup'ik or Inupiat ethnic origin; a fifth describes its shareholders as being of Yup'ik, Alutiiq, Aleut, or Athabascan origin.

Eskimos, individually and through their regional corporations, have varied in their responses to resource development proposals. In 2002, when the Bush Administration proposed drilling in the Arctic National Wildlife Refuge (ANWR), where the Inupiat Eskimos hold title to 92,000 acres, the Natives sided with the state and labor unions in favor of drilling. Environmentalists have argued that, while other Alaskan oil projects had not harmed the region's polar bears and caribou, ANWR drilling could threaten those species (Freddoso, 2002). To date, drilling in ANWR has not occurred. However, the polar bear population in the Beaufort Sea has dropped by nearly 40%, presumably due to reductions in polar sea ice (Rosen, 2014).

In contrast to their response to ANWR drilling proposals, Native groups have been largely united in their opposition to the proposed Pebble Mine, which they have argued would negatively impact important salmon streams in the Bristol Bay region (Langlois, 2014). There continues to be tension as various groups struggle to achieve a balance between income-generating resource development and culturally relevant subsistence activities (Chythlook-Sifsof, 2013).

In the former Soviet Union, Eskimo communities near the Bering Strait were moved inland to limit contact with the communities in Alaska. As relationships improved between the United States and the Soviet Union, visits by friends and relatives across the Bering Sea were resumed between 1988 and 1999. However, after a father and son drowned while returning home from Alaska, Russia restricted such trips until 2014, when a group of 12 men traveled in two aluminum skiffs from Provideniya, Russia, to Gambel, Alaska, to visit U.S. relatives for several days (Hopkins, 2014). Still, visits between relatives living in Russia and Alaska are infrequent.

OVERVIEW OF THE PEOPLE

Archeologists believe that the ancestors of the Eskimos came across the Bering Strait from Asia about 30,000 years ago (Haggett, 2002). The results of a genetic study of five populations of Eskimos suggested that at least four separate migrant groups crossed the Bering Strait at various times (Schanfield, Crawford, Dossetor, & Gershowitz, 1990). For centuries, the native people of Alaska lived in isolated regions and were undisturbed by outside cultures. Archeologists have estimated that 48,000 Eskimos lived along the Arctic region of North America from 1750 to 1800 A.D., with the majority (26,000) living in the area now known as Alaska. Approximately two fifths of these early Alaskans spoke Yup'ik and lived in southwestern Alaska, with the Yukon River as the natural dividing line between

this group and the Inupiat, who occupied the more northern coastal areas (Milan, 1980; *World Almanac*, 2015).

Significant population change occurred with the U.S. purchase of Alaska from Russia in 1867. Beginning in 1883, missionaries began to convert the Alaska Native population to Christianity and introduced limited health services (Nord, 1995). In the early 1900s, "outsiders" discovered the wealth of Alaska's natural resources, and the long-undisturbed culture of the natives residing in rural areas came face to face with elements of the Western culture brought by Alaska's new occupants. Outsiders also brought infectious diseases, including smallpox, influenza, hepatitis, and measles, to which the native people had no immunity (Fortuine, 1989; Morris, 1985). Epidemics killed thousands of the native people.

The gold rushes in the early 1900s brought miners and their families. In the 1940s and 1950s, military personnel came to Alaska because of its strategic geographical location. Between 1941 and 1945 over $1 billion was pumped into Alaska by the federal government to develop transportation systems including railroads, highways, airfields, docks, and breakwaters. The most recent influx of westerners arrived after 1968, when a large oil and gas reservoir, estimated to be twice as large as any other oil field in North America, was found on Alaska's north slope. The 800-mile Trans-Alaskan pipeline was completed in 1977 at a cost of $7.7 billion (Vassilou, 2009; *World Almanac*, 2015).

Today, Alaska has a diverse population. In 2013, Alaska's population was estimated to be 735,132 (U.S. Department of Commerce, Bureau of the Census, 2011, Census Briefs, 2015). Of those, 67.3% were White, 3.9% were Black, 14.7% were Alaska Native or American Indian, 5.8% were Asian or Pacific Islander, and 6.6% were Hispanic (U.S. Department of Commerce, Bureau of the Census, 2013).

Members of the indigenous population are often referred to collectively as *Alaska Natives*, and when such things as employment rates, educational levels, and disease incidence rates are discussed, the numbers and percentages generally refer to all Native groups (i.e., Indians and Eskimos); thus the poverty rate is known for Alaska Natives in general but not for the Yup'ik and Inupiat subgroups. In fact, the Native population is divided culturally and linguistically into five major groupings: Interior Indians (Athabaskans), Aleuts, Southeast Coastal Indians (Tlingit, Haida, and Tsimshian peoples, which have disparate languages), Northern Eskimos (Inupiat), and Southern Eskimos (Yup'ik) (Langdon, 2014). In 2010, Eskimos composed 56.8% of the Alaska Native population, with those of Yup'ik descent predominating slightly (30,868 compared to 25,687 of Inupiat descent). The median age for all Alaska Natives in 2010 was just 26.7 years, compared to 33.8 years for the state's entire population. This may be partly attributable to a fertility rate of 3 among Alaska Natives compared to a rate of less than 2.5 for non-Natives in Alaska (Hunsinger & Sandberg, 2013). Although Alaska Natives are a young population, in 2010 their life expectancy at birth was only 70.7 years, compared with 78.1 years for all Alaskans and 78.7 years for all U.S. people (Alaska Department of Labor & Workforce Development, 2013).

The seasonally adjusted unemployment rate in Alaska in September 2014 was 6.8% and ranked forty-first in the nation (U.S. Department of Labor, 2014a), while the national rate for the same month was 5.9% (U.S. Department of Labor, 2014b). Unemployment among Alaska Natives during the first half of 2013 was 11.7%, compared with a rate of 5.5% among white Alaskans (Austin, 2013). From 2007 through 2013, when the U.S. poverty rate was 14.3%, the rate among Alaska Natives living in Alaska was 21% (Macartney, Bishaw, & Fontenot, 2013).

CULTURE AND HERITAGE OF THE ESKIMOS

The word *Eskimo* is from the French *esquimau(x)*. The term refers to peoples living in arctic and subarctic regions from Greenland, through Canada and Alaska, to extreme northeast Siberia. The term is sometimes considered derogatory because it was erroneously thought to mean "eaters of raw meat" (*Random House Webster's College Dictionary*, 2000). As controversies about the naming of various sports teams have emerged in recent years and possibly because some Eskimos believe that the "eaters of raw flesh" attribution puts them in a poor light with modern audiences (DeMarban, 2014), exhibits at the Alaska Native Heritage Center (www.alaskanative.net) and the Smithsonian Arctic Studies Center at the Anchorage Museum (www.anchoragemuseum.org/exhibits-events/permanent-exhibits/alaska-native-culture/) are simply identified as being of either Yup'ik/Cup'ik or Inupiat origin. In Canada, the term *Inuit* has largely replaced the use of the word *Eskimo* (*Random House Webster's College Dictionary*, 2000).

Although some customs, traditions, and heritages are shared among Alaska Native groups, the groups have traditionally been enemies. Disputes over territorial rights to land or game resulted in the development of an animosity that has been carried on through the generations. These animosities are kept alive through the retelling of tales, and when things were missing from an Eskimo village, "the Indians" were blamed (Damas, 1984; Hall, 1975; Morris, 1985).

The Eskimo people have managed to preserve artifacts and many unique and interesting customs. Artifacts of Eskimo and other Alaska Native groups can be found at the Smithsonian Arctic Studies Center, which opened at the

Anchorage Museum in Spring 2010. Yup'ik and Inupiat elders have provided commentary on many of the artifacts included in the Center exhibits. Additionally, a full list of Alaska museums, many of which contain artifacts of Alaska Native peoples, can be found at www.museumsalaska.org. However, the traditional way of life is changing for the Eskimo as they have assimilated into the dominant culture, taken on mechanical trades and professional roles, and moved away from reliance on the land. Many young Eskimos are leaving rural villages to go away to school and are returning with new knowledge of the outside world. Some do not return (Hinsley, 2001).

The Eskimo people have lived in the harsh and frigid regions of northern and southwestern Alaska. Until recently, parkas and footgear (*mukluks*) made of animal skins were worn to survive the temperature, wind, and blizzards (Langdon, 2014). To survive in this frozen, non–crop-producing region, the Eskimos have hunted, fished, trapped, and gathered food on the tundra. Thus the dietary mainstay of the people traditionally consisted mainly of wild meat, such as caribou, and seafood, including seal, fish, and whale. A century ago the government brought reindeer to Alaska from Russia and Scandinavia in an effort to improve the meat supply. Under the terms of the Reindeer Act of 1937, which is still in effect today, only Alaska Natives were permitted to own reindeer (Bucki, 2004). However, commercial ranching has remained small; herders participate in the Kawerak Reindeer Herders Association (www.kawerak.org/reindeer.html), which provides administrative, logistical, advocacy, and field support toward the development of a self-sustaining reindeer industry.

Traditionally, dog teams were used for traveling, but this is no longer common. When dog teams were used, they had to be chained for the safety of villagers and to reduce the risk of dogs catching rabies from Arctic foxes. One tradition that remains from dogsled days is the annual Iditarod Trail sled dog race across Alaska from Seward to Nome. However, dogsled racing has been almost entirely taken over by non-Natives who can afford to pay the high cost of competition, estimated to be at least $30,000. Although animal rights activists annually oppose the race, it is a special event for many Alaskans and is promoted around the world as a tourist attraction (Rosen, 1997). Instead, many rurally residing Eskimos use snow machines and all-terrain vehicles (ATVs) for transportation. The reliance on mechanized transportation carries risks. Between 2000 and 2007, Alaska had an ATV mortality rate of 2.67/100,000, more than twice that of the next nearest state (Helmkamp, Aitken, Graham, & Campbell, 2012). The impact on Alaska Natives is disproportionately high (Snyder, Muensterer, Sacco, & Safford, 2014).

Traditionally, kayaking served as water transportation, and whaling was an important component of the economy for Eskimos who lived near the ocean (Lubbock, 1937; Stefansson, 1969); walrus and bearded seals were also important in the Inupiat diet. Today, tightly regulated whaling still occurs along the northern coastlines. When a whale is landed, the entire village participates in butchering the animal and the meat is shared. Salmon, other fish, seal, and migratory birds and their eggs were and are important components of the traditional diet of Eskimos who lived away from the ocean (Langdon, 2014). Reliance on foods obtained from water sources (i.e., oceans and rivers) is, however, a two-edged sword. Between 1996 and 1998, Alaska's drowning rate was three times higher than the national average. Within the state, the drowning rate for Alaska Natives was almost three times that of non-Native Alaskans (43 vs. 15/100,000 population). From 2000 through 2006, when Alaska Natives made up only 17% of the state's population, they accounted for 44% of drowning deaths in the state. Examination of individual drowning deaths indicated that the use of personal flotation devices (i.e., life vests) was substantially lower among Alaska Natives compared with non-Native Alaskans (Strayer, Lucas, Hill-Jilly, & Lincoln, 2010). Further, because Alaskan waters are so cold, the primary benefit of a life vest is largely that it aids efforts to find the body later.

Eskimos, as well as members of other Alaska Native groups, have traditionally shared a common set of values and beliefs that guide their behavior and that sometimes conflict with Western beliefs and values. These have included honesty, prioritizing communal and family needs over individual considerations, valuing sharing over accumulating, and respecting spirituality and interconnectedness with the natural world (Barnhardt, 2001; Hippler, 1974). In the northwest United States, the *potlatch*, a festive gathering of friends and neighbors among coastal Indians, would involve sharing not only food but also blankets and other useful items (Jilek-Aall, 1981).

It is a misconception that Eskimos live in dome-shaped ice-block shelters called *igloos*. In fact, such shelters were used primarily as emergency bivouacs by the Canadian Eskimos. The early Alaskan Eskimos lived in dwellings that were partially underground and covered with sod. Both the ice igloo and the sod huts had long, dipped tunnels as entrances so that the cold air, which is heavier, was caught in a natural trap, thus permitting the interior of the hut to be heated more easily. However, with the passage of the ANCSA in 1971, rapid and continuing change has occurred in many Alaskan Native villages (Wind, Van Sickle, & Wright, 2004). Today, wood frame houses, heated with wood or fuel oil, predominate in small villages that are scattered widely along the coast and major river systems.

Originally, "honey buckets" were used for sewage disposal. Later, honey buckets became black polyethylene bags that, when full, were tied and placed outside the door to be collected and transported to a dump outside the village (Fienup-Riordan, 2001). Also houses may have water storage tanks that allow running water as well as sewage storage tanks; both require regular servicing, with water tanks being filled and sewage tanks being emptied at regular intervals.

Today, because of government projects, many of the larger villages have a sewage treatment plant that includes a piping system where central water tanks supply water to houses via insulated plastic pipe, and raw sewage is piped out to sewage holding and treatment areas. However, winter temperatures play havoc with such systems, causing frozen lines and a need to temporarily revert to the old honey bucket system.

Permanent villages range in population from 20 to 1000 persons, with an average of 400 persons. Most of these villages share community water supplies, electricity, churches, stores, and irregular mail service by airplane.

Rapid changes have impacted Eskimos in recent years and caused social disorganization and cultural conflict. Those issues, in combination with the subsistence lifestyles, severe climate, and harsh terrain characteristic of remote areas, contributed to increased health risks for all ages of Eskimos (Taylor, 1988). From 1999 through 2009, the four leading causes of death among Alaska Natives (all groups) were malignancies, unintentional injuries, heart disease, and suicide; for all of those causes, the death rate was considerably higher when Alaska Natives were compared with White Alaskans (Espey et al., 2014). Using a slightly narrower time frame, from 2004 through 2007, the Alaska Native Epidemiology Center reported cancer to be the leading cause of Alaska Native deaths, accounting for 20.7% of deaths. Heart disease was reported as the second leading (14.2%) cause of death, followed by unintentional injury (13.1%, third) and suicide (6.8%, fourth). Among U.S. Whites, unintentional injuries ranked fifth and tenth, respectively, as the cause of death. Neither chronic liver disease nor homicide was among the top ten causes of death among U.S. Whites; among Alaska Natives, they ranked seventh and tenth (Alaska Native Epidemiology Center, 2009). Indeed, death rates for a wide range of causes differ significantly for Alaska Natives compared with White Alaskans, as examination of Table 12-1 makes clear.

Jackson (2000) noted that American Indians and Alaska Natives have the highest rate of reported disability of any racial or ethnic group in the United States. In the mid-1990s, 63% of American Indians and Alaska Natives over age 64 acknowledged having a disability; 52% reported their disability as severe. In the general population only

TABLE 12-1   Comparative Death Rates of Alaska Native American Indian versus Non-Native Alaskans, 1999–2009

Mortality Cause	Alaska Native Rate	Non-native Rate	Difference/Significance
Unintentional Injury (1990–2009)[a]	122.59	44.84	2.73*
Motor Vehicle Accidents	17.42	19.11	1.72*
Poisoning	33.76	12.11	2.79*
Falls	6.60	5.54	1.19
Suffocation	5.77	2.46	2.34*
Drowning	12.60	2.05	6.14*
Fire/burns	4.85	1.56	3.11*
Infectious Disease (1999–2009)			
0–19 years	9.40	2.00	4.67*
20–49 years	21.0	5.30	3.98*
≥50 years	255.20	104.10	2.45*
Cancer (1999–2009)[c]			
Males	298.70	207.20	1.44*
Females	232.60	155.50	1.50*
Stroke (1999–2009)[d]			
All	144.30	95.60	1.51*
Males	150.30	95.60	1.57*
Females	138.00	94.60	1.46*
Heart Disease (1990–2009)[e]			
All	413.50	325.0	1.27*
Males	519.50	406.20	1.28*
Females	329.50	249.10	1.32*
Chronic Liver Disease (1999–2009)[f]			
All	39.10	16.90	2.30*
Males	32.30	21.70	1.50*
Females	45.60	11.80	3.90*

*Significant at $P < 0.05$; all rates are per 100,000 population. [a]Murphy et al., 2014; [b]Cheek, Holman, Redd, Haberliine, & Hennessy, 2014; [c]White et al., 2014; [d]Schieb, Ayala, Valderrama, & Veazie, 2014; [e]Veazie et al., 2014; [f]Suryaprasad et al., 2014.

52.5% and 33.4% reported having any or severe disability, respectively (Jackson, 2000). Jackson concluded that Alaska Native elders constitute a major risk group for poor health, chronic disease, high medical expenditures, and institutionalization.

Death by violence is a significant concern among Alaska Natives, whose rate of suicide from 2004 through 2007 was 43.1 per 100,000, more than twice the rate for all Alaskan Whites (17.3 per 100,000) and considerably higher than that for U.S. Whites (12 per 100,000). During the same period, the homicide rate for Alaska Natives was 10.9, compared with 4.3 for Alaskan Whites and 3.8 for U.S. Whites; however, the homicide death rate among Alaska Natives has decreased by 70% since 1980 (Alaska Native Epidemiology Center, 2009).

Great strides have been made in reducing both infant and postneonatal mortality among the Alaska Native pop-

ulation. From 2004 to 2007, the adjusted infant mortality rate among Alaska Natives was 9 per 1000 live births; between 1980 and 1983, the rate was 17.2/1000. Despite substantial improvement over the past 25 years, the Alaska Native infant mortality rate compared unfavorably to the rates for Alaska Whites (4/1000) and for U.S. Whites (5.8/1000) (Alaska Native Epidemiology Center, 2009). Among the leading causes of infant mortality for both U.S. Whites and Alaska Natives from 1999 through 2009 were congenital anomalies (first leading cause, 243.6/100,000 population) and sudden infant death syndrome (SIDS) (second for Alaska Natives and third for U.S. Whites). However, the rate of congenital malformations among Alaska Native children was more than twice that of U.S. Whites (213.7 vs. 134.9/100,000), and the Alaska Native rate of SIDS was nearly four times the rate among U.S. Whites (240 vs. 54.3/100,000). Among Alaska Native children, unintentional injuries were the fourth leading cause of death (192.3/100,000); among U.S. Whites, the rate was only 23.4/100,000 (Wong et al., 2014a; Wong et al., 2014b).

Over the years, the Indian Health Service (IHS) has targeted specific health problems, such as the high rate of maternal and child health problems, with specific programs. For example, in 1984, Alaska was one of 10 states to receive a Child and Adolescent Service System Program to improve state services for troubled youth (VanDenBerg & Minton, 1987).

Until recently, medical care was provided to Yup'iks and Inupiats by the U.S. IHS as a treaty right. Doctors assigned to the IHS hospitals in Bethel, Nome, Kotzebue, and Barrow, and to the Alaska Native Medical Center (ANMC) in Anchorage provided inpatient and outpatient care. The physicians also traveled at least one time per year to the villages, where most Yup'ik and Inupiat people live, to provide medical care. In addition, the State of Alaska provides preventive health services using public health nurses who travel to each village at least once a year and as needed.

Over time, a system of health care, using indigenous residents located in each village, was instituted by the IHS. These "health aides" work in conjunction with the IHS and regional corporation doctors through the regional hospitals by using standing orders and consulting with the doctors via telephone. The level of care provided by the village health aides has increased substantially in recent years, partly as a result of the successful use of telemedicine technology in the areas occupied by Yup'iks and Inupiats. All of these approaches in providing health care fall within the Western biomedical paradigm, although some facilities also rely on indigenous providers, or "tribal doctors," to collaborate in caregiving.

After the ANCSA passed in 1971, a number of regional for-profit Native corporations established nonprofit health corporations programs to work on many health concerns (Dixon, 1998; Dixon & Roubideaux, 2001). In 1999, the health care of Alaska Natives came under the control of the regional native health corporations as a result of the adoption of the Alaska Tribal Health Compact, a self-governance agreement with the IHS. In the rural areas, the regional hospitals and clinics came under the management of the regional health corporations. In Anchorage, the Alaska Native Tribal Health Consortium (ANTHC), a body of tribal organization representatives, manages the ANMC, which opened a new state-of-the-art comprehensive medical facility in the late 1990s. In this way, decisions about how to allocate funds are made by the Alaska Native recipients of care, which allows direct input into the prioritization of health concerns to be addressed. In 2014, seven tribally managed hospitals, 44 tribal health centers, and 160 tribal community health aide clinics provided services to meet the health care needs of Alaska Natives, some of whom also take advantage of other health care options available in the state (Indian Health Service, 2014).

COMMUNICATION

Language

Although some authorities have related the language of persons native to the Arctic to the Athabaskan or Algonquian language groups (Szathmary, 1984), others have asserted that they are related only to the Aleut language. There are two branches of the Eskimo language: Inupiaq and Yup'ik. While Inupiaq is a single language with different dialects, there are actually three distinct Yup'ik languages in Alaska, including Central Yup'ik, Alutiiq, and Siberian Yupic. Until recently, children were discouraged from speaking any Eskimo language (Kaplan, 1984). In recent years, several schools serving Yup'ik or Inupiat Eskimo students have initiated various form of bilingual and/or Eskimo language immersion study options. Also, students enrolled at campuses of the University of Alaska Fairbanks (UAF) are able to complete a bachelor of arts degree in either Inupiat or Yup'ik.

Originally the Eskimo language did not exist in written form; thus the recounting of events in story form and in dance provided the only record of Eskimo life. Indeed, both the Inupiat and Yup'ik peoples had a rich tradition of storytelling with myths, stories, histories and songs being passed across generations (Jacobson, 1984; Kaplan, 1984). Today a phonetically written form of the Eskimo language, initially developed by missionaries, exists and is under continued study at the Alaska Native Language Center on the UAF campus.

In the oral language spoken by Eskimos, pronouns have no gender distinctions; the same word is used to convey that he, she, or it is eating. Further, intonation rather than words are used to convey questions. Thus English phrasing of an individual whose primary language is Eskimo may sound somewhat unusual. The word "let" may be used to express causation, permission, or obligation; for example, *my mother let me bring in wood* rather than *my mother made me bring in some wood*. Articles may be missing from spoken phrases: *He went to party* instead of *He went to a party* (Jacobson, 1984; Kaplan, 1984). Verb phrasing may differ from that typical of primary English speakers; for example, it is not uncommon to hear an Eskimo saying *I will eat my pills* rather than *I will take my pills*. Unlike children learning English, who generally begin to effectively use the passive structure of the language around the age of 4 years, children learning *Inuktitut* (one dialect of the Eskimo language) learn a simple and complex form of passive vocabulary as early as the age of 2 years (Allen & Crago, 1996).

In the past, each person in the Eskimo culture had a defined role in the group; therefore, the anticipation of each person's action required little verbal communication. Also, individuals who learned English as a second language seldom understood common English idioms (Jacobson, 1984; Kaplan, 1984; Vaudrin, n.d.). However, with English as a primary language of the young people and with the exposure to the world via satellite television, the Internet, and schools, idioms and abstract ideas have begun to have meaning. Still, the nurse who cares for Eskimo clients from the "bush" (i.e., remote areas) should avoid the extensive use of idioms, such as "a bull in a china shop," "out in left field," or "robbing Peter to pay Paul," which may lack meaning, especially for elders.

The language of the Eskimo people reflects their dominant concerns and interests. Certain words take on a more significant meaning than do other words. Because Alaska is seasonally a land of snow and ice, those words take on a more significant meaning. For example, there are three different Eskimo words for *snow* for which there are no single-word equivalents in the English language; different words are used for falling snow, soft snow on the ground, and drifting snow. Another important word for the Eskimo is *ice*. Different words describe freshwater ice, saltwater ice, and icebergs because ice also serves different and important purposes in those cultures (Armstrong, Roberts, & Swithinbank, 1973).

For the older generation, English is the second language. When one is speaking to an older person, comprehension can be facilitated by speaking slowly and in literal terms. Children who know only English may have trouble communicating with their grandparents who know only Eskimo (Taylor, 1988). Translators may be helpful, but it is important to remember that the Eskimo language has no translation for the future or for abstract ideas. When providing care to an Eskimo client, the nurse should provide an explanation about specific therapeutic interventions in English and, if a translator is available, in Eskimo. The need for a trained medical translator fluent in the appropriate dialect of the Eskimo language cannot be overemphasized, especially when working with elders; translation services are an integral part of services provided by most of the regional Native hospitals.

Use of Silence

Eskimos tolerate periods of silence more easily than do people in Western society (Kleinfeld, 1971). In fact, it is considered rude to fill silences with chatter because it prevents one from having the space to express viewpoints. The perceived Western intolerance of silence serves to increase

the Eskimo's feelings of being dominated and inferior (Kleinfeld, 1971; Vaudrin, n.d.). Traditionally in Eskimo culture, each adult is given the opportunity to express a viewpoint without a time limit. For example, an Eskimo may go to see a White person for some reason and just sit in silence for many minutes before saying why he or she has come. However, individuals in Western society may be insensitive to this mode of communication and interpret silence as nonparticipation or passive acceptance (Vaudrin, n.d.). Generally, Eskimos are a polite people who are unlikely to criticize other people's opinions and actions unless such actions cause a threat to the social group. There appears to be a proscription against verbal expression of negative effect (Kost-Grant, 1983; Lantis, 1960). In dealing with people in Western society, the younger generation of Eskimos has, for the most part, adopted Western ways, which includes becoming more verbal.

Touch

There is a wide range of acceptable open demonstration of affection displayed in public among various subgroups in the Eskimo culture. However, the handshake is considered universally acceptable and a mandatory politeness. Hugging is an acceptable greeting between family members and between women friends. Eskimo men are more reserved in their expressions of affection, using a handshake with only one movement, not up and down, as a common way to greet friends and family.

Elders asked about traditional healing practices reported that massage was commonly employed as a technique to treat both pain and constipation (DeLapp & Ward, 1981). The late Eskimo healer Della Keats (1985) healed many people through the use of massage, manipulation, herbal medicines, and love (Book, Dixon, & Kirchner, 1983; DeLapp, personal communication, 1979; Juul, 1979). According to Keats, she inherited the skill of her hands and learned the use of herbs for healing from her mother and other Eskimo elders. Through love, touch, and a combination of old and new medicines, Keats reportedly healed her people (DeLapp, personal communication, 1979).

Traditional Eskimos are very modest about exposing the body, and it is often difficult to persuade older Eskimo people to undergo complete physical examinations, particularly for diagnostic purposes. The nurse who cares for Eskimo clients needs to establish a trust relationship before diagnostic examinations are initiated. In the presence of pain and illness, however, there is less resistance to physical examination (Schaefer, 1973).

Kinesics

Eskimos use nonverbal communication extensively through body posture and facial expression (Alaska Department of

Health & Social Services, 2006). Years of watching animal behavior for survival needs have made the Eskimo people experts in the interpretation of nonverbal language. The nurse who understands the Eskimo culture will look for nonverbal clues, such as watching the face for raised eyebrows or blinking (indicating "yes") or a wrinkled nose (indicating "no"). Older Eskimos seldom disagree publicly with others. Although smiles and head nods in the Western culture may indicate agreement, for Eskimos, they may simply acknowledge the other person's words. Among Eskimos, actual agreement is determined by action. Insincerity and deceptiveness are quickly perceived through body talk and lead to distrust and eventually to social ostracism. Thus, others are evaluated by body language, and this evaluation is nonverbally communicated back by inclusion or exclusion of the person in future activities. The nurse who lives and works among the Eskimo people will eventually understand the nonverbal language of Eskimos and its significance.

Implications for Nursing Care

For effective communication to occur, the nurse must develop a trust relationship with the client that in time will give rise to acceptance of the nurse. When the nurse works in an Alaskan village, the villagers may appraise the nurse not on skills but on the nurse's endorsement of the community. Some villagers may perceive acceptance in terms of the nurse's willingness to visit in homes, to take time to have a cup of coffee, and to participate in village activities. It is important for the nurse to recognize that some Eskimos have a need to know they are accepted as individuals and as a community. Thus, insincerity may be inferred by a discrepancy between nonverbal and verbal language and will cause mistrust and block communication. When dealing with Eskimo clients, whether in villages or in an integrated mainland U.S. society, the nurse should be assertive but not aggressive and use a suggestive rather than a directive approach (Davidhizar & Giger, 2000). Time should be provided for a slower pace of communication with Eskimo clients. The nurse should be aware that Eskimos are sensitive to comments that indicate lack of respect and that Eskimos report feelings of racism and lack of respect by health care workers (Whalen, 1999).

Some Eskimos respect the right of personal choice and self-determination as long as these actions do not affect the welfare of the family or community. The culturally sensitive nurse will avoid issuing direct orders, which may be viewed as being "bossy." When working with Eskimo clients, it is may be most effective to approach nonemergency situations in a roundabout way. For example, a public health nurse making a home visit may notice a baby's bottle rolling around on a dirty floor. Later the nurse may see the toddler pick the bottle up, take a few sips, and throw it back on the floor. If the nurse corrects the mother about failure to protect the child from the dangers of unrefrigerated milk and bottle-mouth syndrome, that mother may not come to the clinic or allow the nurse in the house again. However, the advice may be more readily accepted if the nurse waits until the mother brings the child in for health care, where teaching can be implemented and emphasis placed on the importance of refrigerated milk and dental hygiene to prevent bottle-mouth syndrome.

Eskimos are very sensitive to the power of the dominant culture (Vaudrin, n.d.) and may withdraw when they sense judgment by health care providers. Thus, it is of little value to lecture about alcohol use, chewing tobacco, or dipping or pinching snuff, which some Yup'ik women may "chew" several times daily. The development of trust and acceptance is the best form of demonstrating support for the community. This approach will allow the village community to educate itself and seek to change unhealthy lifestyles of community members. Health care providers should not fall into the trap of thinking that they alone can effect change; rather, change results from collaborative interaction, support, and nonjudgment between providers and the community.

When providing health teaching for a client who lacks English-language skills, the nurse should use educational material that can be understood. Many educational materials available for children in English do not address the specific kinds of injuries encountered in Alaska. The Emergency Medical Services program at the Yukon-Kuskokwim Health Corporation has developed four educational curricula with a specific focus on safety and first-aid issues appropriate for the Alaskan Eskimos. Two sets of books were created, one written in English and the other in Yup'ik, to ensure that culturally and linguistically appropriate materials were available (Taylor, 1988).

It is also important for the nurse to be aware that some Eskimos have been found to have chronic otitis media, which has impaired their ability to hear self-care instructions delivered verbally. Audiological services, including access to hearing aides, are available through the regional health corporations.

SPACE

In the Eskimo culture, individual space is often shared with family members (Lange, 1988; Roberts & Ross, 1979). What is perceived as crowded living conditions by individuals in Western society may be viewed by the Eskimo as living in the warmth and security of the family group. The Western cultural need to be territorial by owning private space was not a traditional value of the Eskimo people. Instead, the

Eskimo people valued sharing and perceived it as a preferable norm (Barnhardt, 2001). Acculturation has weakened this particular value system, but family rights still take precedence over individual rights. For example, if a family member desires the privacy of a room for a few hours, this request may be accepted as a personal need. However, if this same individual demands such privacy continuously in a two-room house with five members, ridicule and accusations of selfishness may result. As the need for individual space arises, individual family members may go on hunting, fishing, or camping trips to meet privacy needs as well as to return to nature.

A handshake distance between two people is considered the acceptable space for socialization on a daily basis. Closer approaches without permission are perceived as threatening, while greater distances are perceived as rude. An outsider who desires input from the Eskimos in a public meeting must recognize the decision-making process of the people and the effect that spatial requirements have on the decision-making process. The public zone for communication incorporates an intimate physical space where people sit in a circle, without a leader dominating the group. Some Eskimos view Westerners as masters of the savior attitude, which can serve to block communication with an impenetrable wall (Damas, 1984).

Implications for Nursing Care

The nurse who cares for Eskimo clients should remember that certain requirements for spatial distances must be observed. Requirements for space must take into account that the client may have unique beliefs about space and may be disturbed when a nurse ventures into personal space to do such routine procedures as give a bed bath or provide oral care, especially if a trust relationship has not been established. The nurse must determine how much self-care can be implemented by the client and how much must be implemented by the nurse. When self-care is threatened, clients who are protective of space may become withdrawn, overly aggressive, or overly passive. The nurse must be careful to allow the client to make decisions about care, and thorough explanations should be given when the nurse must venture into the intimate or personal zone without blocking communication.

SOCIAL ORGANIZATION

Family

The family unit, with its kinship ties, was paramount to survival in the harsh Arctic environment. The survival of the group traditionally was considered more important than the survival of the individual members. Several family units would band together in a migrating social group.

These social groups were not permanent because families could disband and join other groups during a lifetime. However, the roles for individuals and for families within a social group were clearly delineated, so that the groups were not weakened by the shifting of members (Nida, 1954). In fact, this shifting may have strengthened the culture by extending kinships. Extended families consisted of parents, their children (from a current or previous marriage or from adoption), grandparents, and single blood relatives. The husband was the head of the family, but the responsibility of bonding the family into a strong unit belonged to the mother. Thus, if the family was unsuccessful, the blame was placed on the woman. The woman's role for family bonding has continued into the modern cultural adaptation. However, in recent years, some male members of the Eskimo society find themselves at a loss with the diminution of the role of hunter and subsistence gatherer. Inactivity and lack of jobs for men have led to alcoholism and family dysfunction.

The role of Eskimo elders in the family had been one of respect, honor, and inclusion in the family unit. Branch and Heyano (2002) noted that when Eskimo elders are relocated to nursing or assisted living homes, considerable stress on both the family and the elder occurs. They described a Marrulet Eniit (Yup'ik for "Grandmother's house"), which opened in Dillingham, Alaska, in February 2000; the facility has provided a model for other Native-serving assisted living facilities in Alaska.

Kinships were vital social relationships when Eskimos lived in isolated areas. Kinship boundaries extended beyond blood relations through such practices as wife sharing, hunting partnerships, and the adoption of children. The code of behavior between kin was as binding as that between blood relatives (Langdon, 2014). These extensive kinship relationships were partially responsible for the cultural similarities in Eskimos that spread across the vast Arctic regions. History has recorded incidents of lost Eskimo hunters who crossed paths with another Eskimo band and were killed if the lost person could not prove kinship to a member of the new group (Williamson, 1974).

In Eskimo culture today, the extended family plays a very important role (Gallinek, 2006). Survival no longer depends on kinships, but these relationships are far from dead. There still is a linking of families, which is evidenced by the sharing of Native foods or the formation of business partnerships. Eskimo villages have multigenerational families living in the same household or in a household in close approximation. Conflict has begun to occur because of the impact of members of the younger generation adopting dominant culture views toward elders instead of maintaining the strong influence of the views of elders in guiding family functioning.

The extended family involves the informal adoption of babies between families. If someone finds it impossible to care for a baby, adoption is an accepted practice. In the past, adoptions were frequently carried out with little or no litigation. Over the past decades, the informal process has been replaced with a more formal process. In addition, the Indian Child Welfare Act strictly limits adoption of Alaska Native babies by non-Natives (Legal Information Institute, n.d.). An adopted child is fully incorporated into the extended family. Because of close family ties, the child is often related to the adoptive parents.

The rapid entry of the Eskimo into the American cash economy and value system has led to the restructuring of the Eskimo social and economic system. The nurse who interacts with persons from these cultures should recognize that partially accepted Western values may be superimposed over Eskimo values that are still practiced. The new elite class in Eskimo society is based on the ability to earn money without regard for old, established kinships and extended families, and a disregard for and severance of family and kinship ties underlie conflicts that may be found in villages today (Klausner & Foulks, 1982).

Individual Freedom Exists within the Family or Group. Eskimo cultures maintain respect for individual thought and personal freedom for behavior and decisions. At times, this individual freedom appears extreme because others in the society take on a noninterference attitude. For example, a husband may beat his wife without anyone lifting a finger to stop the beating, or a person may drink to oblivion day after day, and no one will take the bottle away (Roberts & Ross, 1979). The value of individual choice of behavior is honored as long as the integrity of the group is not in jeopardy. However, the Eskimos have decided as a group that alcoholism is destroying the fabric of their culture. A sobriety movement that urges Natives to become and stay sober has emerged within the group and become widespread across the region. The importance of the community as part of the pathway to sobriety has been operationalized by implementation of a local community option regarding the legality of possessing and purchasing alcoholic beverages by the State of Alaska. Of the 475 communities listed in the State of Alaska Community database, 20.6% ($n = 98$) have opted to impose limiting conditions on the sale and/or importation of alcohol. Of those 98 communities, 78 (80%) are described by the state as being traditional Yup'ik or Inupiat communities. Of the 78 Eskimo communities, 75 (96%) have chosen one of three limitations, including banning (1) sale ($n = 9$; 12%), (2) sale and importation ($n = 39$; 52%), and (3) sale and importation and possession ($n = 27$; 36%) of alcohol (Alaska

Community Database, n.d.). Further, efforts to understand pathways to sobriety among Alaska Natives have led to the recognition that prevention and treatment efforts should include attention to the importance of family and community in promoting sobriety (Hazel & Mohatt, 2001; Mohatt et al., 2004b; Seale, Shellenberger, & Spence, 2006).

Social Status within the Family Structure. Formerly, social status was attained by successful hunters who could provide food and skins not only for their own families but also for others. Successful hunters soon were recognized as leaders in the social group by the members. The opinions of successful hunters were given precedence over the opinions of others. A woman's status was secondary to her husband's and was gained through her own skills in keeping her family well fed and clothed. Each family member had an expected role to play. Grandparents were the primary educators of the children and imparted knowledge and skills required for survival. Children learned skills through play activities that also contributed to family needs, such as finding birds' nests for the eggs or challenging a playmate in picking the most berries.

Some Eskimo parents do not punish or even correct their small children because tradition says that the spirits of a deceased relative guide each youngster. In the Eskimo cultures the spirit of the deceased relative was considered so paramount to the survival of the young child that while a woman was in labor an old woman was brought to the bedside to recite the names of the child's dead relatives. The name that was uttered at the time the child became visible was regarded as the appropriate name, and thereafter that deceased ancestor was believed to become the guardian spirit of the child (Nida, 1954; Polk, 1987). Many Eskimos still believe that the essence of a dead relative is found in children born around the time of the death of a relative. For this reason many new babies may have the same name of a recently deceased family member.

For the Eskimo child, praise from parents and grandparents provides a positive learning experience and a strong self-concept (Polk, 1987). In Eskimo culture undesirable behavior traditionally was ignored, and if the behavior continued, the child was shamed through teasing and ridicule. Social controls within the community followed a similar pattern. There were no rigid rules. If a social standard was broken, it was assumed that the individual had a valid reason for the breach of conduct. Behavior was kept in control through teasing, gossip, and ridicule. If the behavior threatened group survival, the person was ostracized. To be isolated from the group meant certain death because an individual could not survive alone for long in the Arctic. The traditional Eskimo society is an example of a society that bases status on sharing and contributing to the well-being of the group that employs a positive feedback system to control its members (Gove, 1982; Williamson, 1974).

Traditional Eskimos did not have any formal recognition of puberty (Polk, 1987). This was in contrast to other primitive societies where formal rituals frequently marked the coming of age. Boys are recognized by a feast at the first kill, which is shared with the family. In traditional Yup'ik Eskimo culture, girls were recognized when they danced with the older women for the first time.

For the nurse to give culturally appropriate nursing care to the client whose cultural makeup encompasses traditional values regarding social status, it is necessary for the nurse to appreciate traditional family roles. In most cases, it is also necessary to involve both nuclear and extended family members in the planning, implementation, and evaluation of nursing care.

Political Structure

The political development of Eskimos has evolved into the development of councils, native corporations, and health care corporations. The Alaska Native Land Claims Act of 1971 spurred a political development pattern loosely similar to the political system in other states. Where once each community had an informal social structure that revolved around family and kin, now most villages have a decision-making council headed by an elected spokesperson.

Implications for Nursing Care

Extended family ties can be used to encourage noncompliant clients into following recommended therapy. These ties can also be used to find reasons for noncompliance because the client may not feel free to contradict the nurse. In Eskimo culture it is considered impolite to openly disagree with others. Cooperation, patience, and nonaggression are important values. Attempts to persuade or counsel another person, even to keep that person from doing something dangerous or foolish, are considered rude and are not tolerated. Attempts by health care staff to "help" through advising and counseling may be seen as meddling, which may be resisted by the client (Lange, 1988). The nurse may need to resolve a difficult situation by asking other family members for guidance. With the increased educational levels of the younger people and with the help of the nurse as an advocate, some Eskimos are beginning to assume autonomy in questioning medical therapy and social programs. It is essential that the nurse encourage the Eskimo client to take personal responsibility for health or illness in consultation with the appropriate family members. As appropriate, the nurse should directly involve the client in planning health care and in activities that pursue solutions to health needs.

Childrearing Practices

Eskimo parents have been observed to be highly sensitive to their children's behavior cues and appropriately responsive to those cues. At the same time, development was more likely to be promoted through child-initiated rather than parent-structured learning activities and positive reinforcement was the norm (MacDonald-Clark & Boffman, 1995). Children are considered individuals as soon as they learn to express themselves. What this means for the nurse is that a child is given the right to refuse or accept health-related care. Some parents will not force a child to do something that the child refuses to do. For example, a parent may make a statement such as, "I tell Sam to brush his teeth, but he won't do it" or "JoJo won't let me put drops in her ear." The parent may tease, shame, or ridicule the child in an attempt to persuade the child, but the parent will seldom demand the appropriate behavior. This is consistent with the findings of a study that used predominantly Eskimo focus groups in the Yukon-Kuskokwim delta to ascertain attitudes to ward tobacco use. The authors concluded that, for Eskimos, it was culturally inappropriate to tell others, including their own children, what to do (Renner et al., 2004).

Implications for Nursing Care

Nurses working with Eskimo families should recognize the "unusual strength of their sensitivity to the child and the gentle nature of discipline" (MacDonald-Clark & Boffman, 1995, p. 455) and to reinforce those strengths as an abuse prevention. At the same time, the nurse needs to emphasize that certain health care behaviors, such as brushing teeth or appropriately using medications, are important in preventing more serious problems, such as dental caries and otitis media. However, the implementation of these health-related practices may be difficult in view of culturally based childrearing practices.

In fact, dental caries is a significant problem among rural-residing Alaska Native children, where incidence rates as high as 87% among 4- and 5-year-old children and 91% among 12- to 15-year-old adolescents have been reported, with incidence being higher in villages without fluoridated community water systems (Centers for Disease Control, 2011). The high prevalence of dental caries imposes high intervention costs (Bruerd, 1997). In response, the ANTHC initiated a Dental Health Aide Therapist Program in 2004; graduates, who practice only in rural communities, provide both preventive and treatment services, including education, and sealing, fluoridating, cleaning, filling, and extracting teeth as needed (Native Health News Alliance, 2014).

TIME

The Arctic Circle marks the point at which there is no sunrise on December 21, the winter solstice (or the shortest day of the year), and no sunset on June 21, the summer solstice (or the longest day of the year). This factor gives rise to a unique phenomenon that occurs in the northernmost part of North America. When the sun rises on May 10 in Barrow, Alaska, North America's northernmost city, it does not set again until August 2, resulting in 84 days of continuous sunlight. When the sun sets on November 18 in Barrow, it does not rise again until January 24. Thus Barrow residents have 67 days of continuous semidarkness during which there are 3 to 5 hours of winter daylight, when the sun does not rise over the horizon.

The extended periods of daylight and darkness give rise to seasonal, geographically related behavior. During the summer months, it is not uncommon to see small children playing outside quite late in the evening and adults take advantage of the extended hours of daylight for fishing. Likewise, because of the extended periods of darkness in the winter, rural northerners tend to sleep late. Although most northerners have rearranged their lives in recent times to synchronize themselves with the Western day–night rhythm, some Eskimos remain on "Eskimo time," which is a result of both the unusual daylight pattern and a present-time orientation. Rather than being structured by the clock, time is cyclical, based on naturally recurring phenomena: sunrise, sunset, days, nights, moons (months), and seasons (Lewis & Ho, 1975). This time perspective as well as the reliance on subsistence activities to ensure the family's food supply may prompt Eskimo families to keep their children out of school to be in fish camp for a time after school officially opens. Fish camp, a present-time oriented activity, may be viewed as a time to be enjoyed, whereas school, a future-time oriented activity, prepares children for future, nontraditional goals. Similarly, committing to year-round jobs is difficult for some Eskimo adults because of the strong tradition of spending summer and fall in fish camps.

The present-time orientation of culture is sometimes reflected in the ways in which money is spent. There is an emphasis on consumable things that give immediate benefit. Budgeting and investing for the future may not be motivating concepts. Some Eskimos who have been away from the village and have earned a large sum of money during a season may come home and blow it in one spending spree for the family. This action exemplifies both the value of sharing with others and the common present-time orientation.

Implications for Nursing Care

It is important for the nurse to remember that Eskimo village residents may have a different time orientation from that of health care providers from the majority culture (Lange, 1988). During the summer, when it is daylight most of the time, villagers may sleep only when they become tired, and children may stay up very late. This may present real challenges for the nurse, in either clinic or hospital settings, because the lack of a definitive schedule interferes with clients keeping appointments and taking medications correctly. The nurse learns to take medical histories by village events and seasons. In any setting, it is important to know about the client's daily routine if nursing care is to be effectively implemented. Because schedules are flexible and time is relative, the nurse needs to inquire about daily schedules before requiring medication to be taken at a certain time. Many families do not eat meals together and may eat only twice a day. Therefore, telling a client to take a medication, intended for dosing three times a day, at mealtimes may result in only two doses being consumed.

"Eskimo time" requires readjustment by the nurse for such things as scheduling appointments for health care. A nurse who works effectively in a remote area of Alaska would avoid scheduling clinic appointments before 9 or 10 a.m., instead extending the work day into the evening hours. A visiting nurse on a tight schedule who insists that the villagers accept a Western time frame may hear comments such as, "You are always rushed" or "You must not like our village because you are always in a hurry to leave."

ENVIRONMENTAL CONTROL

The early Eskimos believed that the individual had three parts: body, soul, and name. All of these were considered of equal importance and combined to make the whole person. Early Eskimos also believed that everything, such as earth, wind, flowers, animals, and birds, had a spirit. In Yup'ik culture, a set of rules for living guided individual action (Sanders, 2000). Each family inherited a specific taboo system, and each person had a guiding spirit to help him or her during his or her lifetime. When a girl married, she had to abide by the taboos of both families (Gove, 1982). The spiritual leader, called a *shaman,* had the vital role of keeping the group healthy by persuading the spiritual world to continue smiling on the people. When famine struck or illness occurred, the shaman communicated with the spiritual world during trances to learn what taboo had been broken and who needed to appease the spirits.

Appeasement often meant that the guilty person confessed to breaking the taboo and suffered humiliation. It is interesting to understand that the shaman was not blamed if the shaman failed to find the cause for negative events. The people accepted their situation as a matter of fate (Blodgett, 1978; Lantis, 1960). Famine, bad luck, and failure in hunting meant the spirits were displeased with the Eskimo people, whereas successful hunting and times of plenty meant the spirits were pleased. Consequently, each Eskimo perceived his or her relationship with nature as being in or out of harmony with the spiritual world. Since shamanism has been largely replaced by Christianity (Blodgett, 1978), it is common for Eskimos to be Christian, depending on the denomination of the missionaries in a particular part of Alaska. Examples include the Catholic, Moravian, Russian Orthodox, and Presbyterian religions. Death is accepted as a part of life, which makes an enormous difference in attitudes about suffering, stress, and even acculturation. In the past, Eskimos were buried in wooden boxes above the ground because of the difficulty in digging graves; people are now buried in graves dug with jackhammers. Whereas wood was once at a premium and one cross contained many names, imported wood is now readily available (Morris, 1985).

Illness and Wellness Behaviors

Early Eskimos believed that each person had a spiritual healer who could be offended by the person's breaking a taboo. A broken taboo was manifested by the person's becoming ill. Possession by harmful spirits was recognized as a cause of illness. For example, it was considered taboo to eat polar bear liver, and any Eskimo who offended the bear spirit in this manner became ill or died. Studies in the 1940s indicated that vitamin A toxicity, rather than the ill effects of the broken taboo, was the cause of illnesses associated with eating polar bear liver (Rodahl, 1964). Regardless, the taboo protected the people by discouraging the consumption of polar bear liver.

Written information on shamanism is limited because of the prohibition of this religion by early missionaries. Folklore indicates that the shaman had predicted the coming of the strangers who would cause the death of the Eskimo; the prophecy was fulfilled when nearly one half of the Eskimos died of diseases brought by the early traders, whalers, and missionaries, to which the Eskimos were not immune (Fortuine, 1989). With the influx of Westerners, the lifestyles of the Eskimos also changed, as they moved into permanent settlements to take advantage of schools, churches, and medical care. The spread of communicable disease became rampant among the people, who now lived in permanent houses occupied by many people in close proximity. Before the influx of Westerners, the constant

moving of living sites prevented the hygiene problems that were now incurred by permanent villages.

Shamanism lost influence as Eskimos turned to the magic of medicine brought by the Westerners to cure the devastating infectious diseases. Many of the medical people were missionaries who implied that illness was related to the people's sinfulness and that the cure depended partly on their confession and acceptance of Western religion. The early Eskimos did not oppose the switch to the new religion because it seemed similar to shamanism. Medical treatment by Westerners was often restricted to the Eskimos whose names appeared on the church roster.

Eskimos often viewed illness stoically and not always as something for which treatment was needed. In a study of traditional Inupiat health practices, analysis of interviews with elders indicated that many clinical conditions were not viewed as "illness" but rather as an expected consequence of aging or merely as a temporary variation of normal bodily functions. The term *illness* seemed to be reserved largely for infectious conditions (DeLapp & Ward, 1981).

In the Eskimo cultures, there is a generation gap in health and illness concepts. An older person may have a more holistic view of health and believe that a happy person is less likely to develop physical ills, whereas a younger person may assign illness to direct physical causes. For example, in the case of suicidal behavior, a young person may blame alcohol, stating that if the person did not drink he or she would not commit suicide. Therefore, the treatment for the prevention of suicide is to take the alcohol away. On the other hand, older Eskimos may see suicidal behavior as an illness of the spirit that creates disharmony, leading to the choice of drinking. When the spirit is healed, the need for alcohol will disappear.

Implications for Nursing Care

When giving culturally appropriate nursing care to Eskimo clients, whether in remote areas of Alaska or in the mainland United States, the nurse must realize that an individual's feelings of environmental control are an important factor in the nursing assessment of client status. Illness and wellness behaviors among some Eskimo clients may be attributable to past belief systems and a belief in supernatural powers. The nurse may need to combat some superstitious beliefs to avoid delays in seeking medical treatment. It is also important for the nurse to appreciate that lifestyle changes, social change, and changes in society and the environment are all major determinants of health among the Inuit (Bjerregaard, Young, Dewailly, & Ebbesson, 2004).

Because some Eskimos tend to view nature as an entity that can be in equilibrium or disequilibrium, the nurse can build on this concept and teach the client that certain illness conditions in the body can also result from disequilibrium. Coupling the theory of equilibrium or disequilibrium with supernatural beliefs, the nurse may be able to adequately explain an illness in terms that are acceptable to the patient.

BIOLOGICAL VARIATIONS

Body Size and Structure

Ancestors of the Indians and Eskimos originated from the Asian race (Zegura, 1984). Anthropologists believe that there was a land bridge between Asia and Alaska that was crossed by the early Native people. Genetic studies have related the origin of Eskimos to a population of Asiatic Beringia (Szathmary, 1984). The Mongolian racial traits seen in the Eskimos include a short muscular body, large oblong skull with a definite occipital protuberance, well-developed lower jaw and maxillary bone, epicanthal folds, little or no body hair, dark-pigmented skin, and lumbar mongolian spots (Mann et al., 1962).

Early medical research noted the short stature and heavier weight per height of Eskimos, which was greatly different from that of Europeans and other circumpolar people (Milan, 1980). Three theories were proposed to explain this difference: (1) a genetic inheritance, (2) a combination of genetic inheritance and environmental adaptation, and (3) a condition of long-term nutritional deficiency. Part of the weight difference was attributed to the Eskimo's thicker bony skeleton and muscular chest and arms. Researchers demonstrated by the use of triceps and body skin-fold measurements that the extra weight was not caused by an extra layer of fat, negating the adaptation theory that Eskimos carried extra fat to protect the body from the cold. Muscular development resulting from an active lifestyle and genetic inheritance contributed to the early Eskimo's body structure (Milan, 1980).

The birth weights and heights of today's Eskimos are statistically similar to those of their White counterparts (Johnston, Laughlin, Harper, & Ensroth, 1982). However, Schaefer (1970) noted that some groups of Canadian Eskimos had demonstrated a pattern of height increase of greater than 1 cm per decade. Noting the emergence of nutritional anemia as a problem during the same period, Schaefer attributed the growth pattern increase to increased consumption of refined carbohydrates rather than improved nutrition. In 1970, in a classic work, Schaefer presented convincing data directly linking the growth rate to sugar consumption. Presumably because the traditional diet was nutrient dense, composed of low levels of simple carbohydrates and high proportions of protein and omega-3–containing fats, diabetes and cardiovascular disease were

uncommon. This has changed as the diet has changed; health problems, including cardiovascular disease, diabetes, and obesity now occur more commonly (McGrath-Hanna, Green, Tavernier & Bult-Ito, 2003).

However, in a classic work, Petersen & Bryant (1984) examined the nutritional status of Eskimo children living in Wainwright, Alaska. They found that, between 1968 and 1977, the stature of young children increased while the incidence of anemia decreased; the authors attributed these changes to improvements in health care and preventive health activities, including nutrition education.

In addition to encouraging clients to follow a traditional diet pattern, the nurse should also keep in mind that the growth charts commonly used in conducting health assessments of Eskimo children were based on White averages. Rather than relying on single measures, health and nutritional assessments of Eskimo children should rely on sequential growth patterns over time.

Skin Color

Eskimos have a "tanned" complexion that becomes deep brown to black with continuous exposure to the sun. This pigmentation is part of their mongoloid heritage. However, evolutionary selection may also explain this feature. Skin cancer research indicates that deeply pigmented skin has some natural protection from the ultraviolet rays of the sun. Therefore, the evolutionary conclusion is that Eskimos are more protected from skin cancer because of their deep skin pigmentation (Young, 1986). Wiggins et al. (2008) confirmed that Alaska Natives overall have a significantly lower risk of dying of melanoma compared with non-Hispanic Whites.

Other Visible Physical Characteristics

Mongoloid heritage among Alaskan Eskimos is reflected in the lumbar pigmented spots (Cordova, 1981) and the epicanthal eye folds. However, neither of these characteristics gives rise to significant health problems. The nurse who cares for Eskimo children needs to be able to distinguish between mongolian spots and those bruises that might be associated with child abuse. Child abuse may be reported to health care providers by well-meaning Westerners who notice "bruises" on an infant's arms and buttocks when these are only mongolian spots. However, during physical assessment it is important for the nurse to remember to document unusual placement of mongolian spots on areas such as the wrist, legs, and chest.

Enzymatic Variations

Enzyme deficiencies in lactase and sucrase have been documented in Eskimos. When given a lactose load equivalent to 3 to 4 cups of milk, 80% of Eskimo adults and 70% of

Eskimo children demonstrated intolerance symptoms of flatulence and diarrhea (Bell, Draper, & Bergan, 1973; Duncan & Scott, 1972). However, most could tolerate a daily glass of milk without symptoms. In the past, Eskimos had no dietary source of milk after being weaned from the breast, and nutritional analysis of traditional foods indicates that the diet of adult Eskimos remains quite low in calcium. Research is needed to determine if there is a genetic protective factor for calcium metabolism or if this population is at risk for osteoporosis from calcium-deficient diets. The nurse who works with Eskimo clients should encourage the use of alternative forms of milk, such as cheese (the preferred alternative), yogurt, and powdered milk. In addition, the nurse should be aware that another source of readily available calcium are the fish bones that are canned with the flesh.

Some Alaskan (approximately 5%) and Greenland Eskimos (approximately 10%) are intolerant of sucrose. Some classic research studies indicate that a can of soda or a piece of cake can cause debilitating diarrhea in some Eskimos (Bell et al., 1973); in children the intolerance becomes apparent when an exclusively breastfed child begins ingesting other food items, including in some cases, infant formula that contains corn syrup (Marcadier et al., 2014). The intolerance resulted from reduced or absent activity of the enzyme sucrase. Traditionally, diagnosis confirmation required small bowel tissue biopsy. Chronic sucrose intolerance has long been hypothesized to be genetic in origin, following an autosomal recessive transmission pattern (Meier, Draper, & Milan, 1991). Recently the specific genetic mutation responsible for sucrase deficiency has been identified, and a blood test for the disorder has become available (Marcadier et al., 2014).

Recently another genetic mutation that results in a glycogen storage disease (type 3a) in the Inuit has been identified. The disorder, which follows an autosomal recessive transmission pattern, is the result of a frameshift deletion that results in reduced activity of glycogen-debranching enzyme. The disorder ultimately causes hypoglycemia, hepatomegaly, and skeletal and cardiac muscle enlargement (Rousseau-Nepton et al., 2015).

Susceptibility to Disease

The isolation of Eskimos caused them to be susceptible to the devastating effects of infections brought to Alaska by outsiders. Eskimos who lacked exposure to certain diseases had no antibodies to these diseases. Since it has been documented that Eskimos develop antibodies to antigens as well as their Western counterparts do, the rapid spread of communicable disease among Eskimos is believed to have occurred because of the short incubation time of the organisms (Fortuine, 1989) and because of a lack of

knowledge about hygiene techniques necessary to stop the spread of communicable disease (Young, 1986).

Communicable Disease. Today, a higher incidence of communicable diseases is still being reported among some populations of Eskimos. For example, in an epidemiological study of streptococcal disease that affected 706 Alaskan Eskimo children, throat cultures were obtained during a long-term surveillance program. The factors significantly associated with streptococcal colonization among the Eskimo children included age, past colonization, competence of the local health aide in providing care, and the region in which the care was provided. However, gender and the number of children in overcrowded homes were excluded as factors important to the incidence of streptococcal colonization (Brant, Bender, & Marnell, 1982). Holman et al. (2004) reported that while respiratory syncytial virus (RSV) infection is one of the leading causes of hospitalization among all infants in the United States (27.4 per 1000 infants), the rate was higher among Alaska Native and American Indian infants across the United States (34.4 per 1000 infants). Singleton (2006) reported even higher rates for infants residing in the Yukon-Kuskokwim Delta, an area where Eskimos constitute a large proportion of the population. Incidence rates were as high as 384 infants per 1000 population between 1999 and 2000. Palivizumab prophylaxis resulted in a reduction in RSV hospitalizations for both premature infants (123 per 1000 population) and term infants (101 per 1000 infants) (Singleton, 2006).

In some remote villages in Alaska, hygiene techniques remain a nursing priority. When working with Eskimos, the nurse must implement teaching programs emphasizing hygienic practices and medical asepsis. Because some villages are extremely crowded and lack running water and proper sanitation systems, susceptibility to disease is augmented; thus, the nurse should also emphasize hygienic practices with residents. Indeed, the importance of in-home water and sanitation capacity in reducing the risk of respiratory, skin, and gastrointestinal tract infection among rural Alaska Natives has been confirmed (Hennessy et al., 2008). Lum et al. (1986) reported the significant effect that improved immunization programs, prenatal care, and improved health care have had on infant mortality. Deaths from infectious diseases, measles, and pertussis were dramatically reduced as health care was improved among southwestern Alaskan Eskimos between 1960 and 1980. Still another problem for Eskimo infants is exposure to *Haemophilus influenzae* type B (Hib) disease (Hall et al., 1987). Alaskan Eskimos have the greatest known endemic risk for this disease, which seems to have genetic factors that contribute to susceptibility (Petersen et al., 1987; Ward, Lum, Hall, & Silimperi, 1986). Petersen, Silimperi,

Chiu, and Ward (1991) noted that living in extended families at the time of disease onset was significantly associated with Hib disease.

In 1991, effective Hib vaccines were first used in Alaska. Prior to that time, Alaska Native children experienced Hib disease at disproportionately high rates compared to similarly aged children across the United States (400–700 vs. 60–100/100,000). While the number of cases has declined dramatically since Hib vaccination was introduced, Alaska Native children continue to experience higher rates of infection compared with non-Native Alaska children (6 vs. 0.4/100,000). The majority of cases that occurred between 1992 and 2009 occurred in the Yukon-Kuskokwim Delta, which is primarily peopled by Eskimos (Singleton, Bruce, Zulz, & Klejka, 2009).

Tuberculosis. Tuberculosis has a long history in Alaska. Fortuine (1989), a physician and historian, classified tuberculosis as an "introduced" disease. Some of the earliest written references to symptoms of tuberculosis are from the late 1700s and early 1800s, after the Russian explorers and fur traders had contact with the Alaska Native population.

It is difficult to quantify the extent of tuberculosis in the Yup'ik and Inupiat populations because the data are reported for Alaska Natives overall rather than specifically for Yup'iks and Inupiats. There is, however, historical evidence that the incidence of tuberculosis was greatest in the southwestern and northern regions of the state, where Yup'iks and Inupiats predominate. In 1952 there were 1853 cases of tuberculosis per 100,000 Alaska Natives, resulting in a huge impact on the Alaska Native population. By 2004, the rate of new cases was 39.2 per 100,000 population, almost eight times the overall U.S. rate (Indian Health Service, 2008). The rate remains disproportionately high among the native population of Alaska. Between 1999 and 2008, 64% of diagnosed cases occurred in Alaska Natives, despite the fact that they represented only about 16% of the state's population (Funk, 2009). The incidence of tuberculosis is related to environmental and socioeconomic issues, such as cramped overcrowded houses, poor availability of clean water (Stevenson, 1984), alcohol abuse, and poor nutrition, with high rates of type 2 diabetes mellitus, and deterioration of the public health infrastructure also contributing to the high rates in the state (Butler et al., 2001). Effective intervention includes both prevention and curtailment of possible spread once a case is present. Health education is essential and must include not only direct information on tuberculosis but also information on predisposing factors. Butler et al. (2001) stated that tuberculosis is an example of a disease that has reemerged and is now in decline but that continues to

disproportionately affect Alaska Natives. The annual incidence for Native Americans (including Alaska Natives) is twice as high as for the U.S. population overall (Indian Health Service, 2008).

Sexually Transmitted Diseases. Alaska Natives have higher rates of gonorrhea, chlamydia, and syphilis than individuals of all other ethnicities (Cecere & Jones, 2013, 2014a, 2014b). In contrast, with regard to human immunodeficiency virus (HIV), in 2013 Alaska Natives accounted for only 11.8% ($n = 7$) of the 59 new cases in the state. However, between 1982 and 2013, Alaska Natives accounted for 20.3% of all reported cases of HIV (Bovette & Harvill, 2014), despite comprising only about 15% of the population. There is some concern about the potential for an increase in HIV and acquired immunodeficiency syndrome cases among Alaska Natives because of alcohol and drug use, the effects of long-term unemployment and poverty, and lack of prevention activities. Because the *Chlamydia* bacteria allow for a possible entrance for HIV, the high chlamydia rate is cause for concern in relation to additional cases of HIV, especially among Alaska Native women in whom the *Chlamydia* rate is highest among the state's ethnic groups.

Glaucoma and Other Visual Disorders. While open-angle glaucoma is rare (Arkell et al., 1987), Eskimos are susceptible to primary narrow-angle glaucoma. In persons with primary narrow-angle glaucoma, the eyes have a shallow chamber angle and a thicker lens. Increasing age, especially in women, is believed to be an associated factor. Both genetic and environmental components appear to play a major role in the development of primary narrow-angle glaucoma (Van Rens, Arkell, Charlton, & Doesburg, 1988). In a recent audio computer-assisted survey of 3793 individuals receiving services at a regional health facility, 61.7% of whom self-identified as being Eskimo, 2.5% self-reported as having glaucoma; other eye disorders self-reported included cataracts (5.9%), diabetes-related eye disease (1.3%), and visual impairment (8.7%) (Haymes, Leston, Ferucci, Etzel, & Lanier, 2009).

Diabetes Mellitus. In Alaska, the prevalence of diabetes is increasing rapidly. In 2001, Hall, Sberna, and Utermole commented that the prevalence of diabetes among Alaska Natives had increased by 80% over the previous two decades. Alaska Native diabetes mortality from 1994 to 1998 was 250% greater than diabetes mortality from 1979 to 1983, raising the prevalence rate to be approximately equal to the U.S. rate for Whites; however, from 1981 to 1996, the diabetes mortality among U.S. Whites increased only 35% (Day & Lanier, 2003).

In a review of literature, Naylor et al. (2003) noted that the increasing prevalence had occurred concurrently with the increased intake of a higher proportion of dietary carbohydrate intake and decreased physical exercise related to a decline in subsistence activities. Although some research studies suggest that a normal glucose response is found among Eskimos (Bell, Draper, & Bergan, 1973), it is essential for the nurse to keep the increasing diabetes prevalence in mind and to implement preventive educational interventions that emphasize the importance of exercise and eating right. The effectiveness of prevention was evident in a diabetes prevention project that combined an educational intervention with personal diabetes risk counseling annually for 3 consecutive years in two Eskimo villages. Counseling emphasized the consumption of traditional foods high in omega-3 fatty acids and avoidance of certain store-bought foods high in palmitic acid, which is associated with glucose intolerance. Compared with two "control" villages, participants in the intervention had significant reductions (all $P < 0.01$) in total plasma cholesterol, low-density lipoprotein cholesterol, fasting glucose, and diastolic blood pressures as well as improved glucose tolerance (Ebbesson, Ebbesson, Swenson, Kennish, & Robbins, 2005).

Cardiovascular Disease. Fifty years ago, non-Natives died from cardiovascular disease at a rate three times higher than that of Alaska Natives. At that time, the major cause of death for Alaska Natives was infectious diseases. Between 2004 and 2007, the rate of death from heart disease for Alaska Natives was 178.9 per 100,000, approaching the overall rate of 209.5 per 100,000 for U.S. Whites. In contrast, during the same period, the death rate from cerebrovascular disease among Alaska Natives (all groups) was 60.1 per 100,000, slightly below the rate for the IHS (63.7) overall and clearly exceeding the rate for U.S. Whites (46.1) (Alaska Native Epidemiology Center, 2009; Indian Health Service, 2008).

Hypertension has long been known as a risk factor for cardiovascular disease. Worldwide, the Inuit populations are thought generally to have comparably lower blood pressures than those of most European populations. And when the blood pressures of four different Inuit groups residing in Canada, Alaska, and Greenland were studied, the Alaskan Eskimos were found to have lower pressures than the other three groups. Interestingly, the Alaskan Eskimos were also the most likely to be receiving antihypertensive treatment (Bjerregaard et al., 2003), a fact that may help to explain the relatively low rate of chronic kidney disease in Alaska Natives overall (Bassett & O'Malley, 2014).

Tobacco use has been identified as a risk factor for both heart disease and stroke. Smoking is prevalent among Alaska Natives in general and in Eskimos in particular. The results of the 2009 Alaska Behavioral Risk Factor Survey indicated that 39% of Alaska Native adults currently used cigarettes, with prevalence rates being higher among rural dwellers as well as lower income and less educated respondents (Alaska Behavioral Risk Factor Survey, 2011). In addition, 11% of Alaska Native adults admitted to current use of smokeless tobacco, including *Igmik* (a smokeless tobacco variant), with more men (8%) than women (1%) chewing.

Tobacco use is also high among Alaska Native youth; data from the 2003 Alaska Risk Behavior Survey indicated current cigarette smoking by 44% of Alaska Native high school students, with 24% using smokeless tobacco (Alaska Department of Health and Social Services, 2007). Still, use of tobacco declined significantly among both Alaska Native and non-Native youth in the state between 1995 and 2003. However, nearly twice as many Native high school students reported having ever smoked compared to non-Native high schoolers (Alaska Department of Health & Social Services, 2007). A number of tobacco prevention and cessation programs have been implemented in Alaska; nurses should encourage Eskimo clients to adopt a healthy lifestyle that excludes use of tobacco in any form.

The diet of Alaska Natives has been suggested as a protective factor for both cardiovascular and cerebrovascular disorders. Traditionally, the Eskimo people subsisted on a diet that was 44% protein (sea and land animals, fish, and birds), 47% fat (polyunsaturated), and 8% carbohydrates (berries, beach greens, and roots). Analysis of the dietary intake of Eskimos indicated protein intake of 26%, fat intake of 37%, and carbohydrate intake of 37% (Mann et al., 1962). Protein and fat intake decreased significantly while carbohydrate intake increased significantly. For some Eskimos the significant increase in carbohydrates is attributable to high intake of sugar.

Traditionally, in certain seasons early Eskimos ate foods that were high in cholesterol. In other seasons their diet was devoid of cholesterol. Today, fewer Eskimos continue to follow a seasonal pattern of dietary habits, and their dietary changes have had a negative impact on both cardiovascular and cerebrovascular health. Thus, the nurse is well advised to caution against excessive cholesterol intake.

In a study involving a Bering Strait Eskimo population, similar heart rates and heart-rate rhythmicity and almost identical acrophases were found in the Eskimo, the Aymara Indian, and the French populations. The study also found that Alaskan Eskimos had heart-rate means that varied by approximately 15 beats per minute (Rode & Shephard, 1984). This variation can have serious implications for the nurse who is monitoring heart rhythms. Thus, when monitoring the pulse rate of an Eskimo client, the nurse should, when possible, take an apical pulse and count the heart rate for 1 full minute.

Anemia. Iron deficiency anemia has been a prevalent problem among Alaska Native schoolchildren; common wisdom suggested that this was due to nutritional deficiency resulting from iron-poor food choices. However, a survey of 19 Native villages in western Alaska confirmed both the prevalence of iron deficiency anemia and reduced iron storage in males and females of all ages. Petersen, Parkinson, Nobmann, Bulkow, Yip, and Mokdad (1996) also found that participants had iron intake in amounts greater than those necessary to replace daily iron losses. An alternative explanation for the occurrence of anemia was found when higher concentrations of heme were found in the stools of 23 adults from two villages in the study. The authors concluded that the anemia might be the result of fecal loss rather than inadequate intake (Petersen et al., 1996). Later, Parkinson et al. (2000) noted a high prevalence of *Helicobacter pylori* in Alaska Natives, with prevalence increasing with age as well as a significant association between *H. pylori* seropositivity and low serum ferritin levels.

The high prevalence of anemia in Eskimo infants and children suggests that nutrition education should be provided to Eskimo mothers. Nurses working in infant programs should ensure that mothers of infants receive vitamin and iron supplements along with information on how to use them. Women who elect to not breastfeed should also be directed to the use of iron-fortified infant formulas, which can now be found even in remote areas in Alaska.

Cancer. Cancer statistics typically group all indigenous Alaska Native groups together, making it difficult to describe the incidence among Eskimos; the incidences described in this chapter are for all Alaska Native groups in Alaska. In Alaska, cancer is the second leading cause of death among Alaska Natives; the age-adjusted cancer death rate for Alaska Natives between 2004 and 2007 was 236.8 per 100,000, higher than rates for all IHS regions (184.1) and for U.S. Whites (183.4) (Alaska Native Epidemiology Center, 2009; Indian Health Service, 2008). Wiggins et al. (2008) reported specific rates of cancer incidence sites between 1999 and 2004; during those years, the most common cancer sites among Alaska Native men were prostate, lung, and colorectal. Furthermore, compared with non-Hispanic White males, Alaska Native males had higher rates of lung, colorectal, renal, stomach, liver, pancreatic, and biliary tract cancers. Among women, the incidence of cancer was slightly but significantly higher compared with non-Hispanic Whites, with breast, lung,

and colorectal cancers being the most common (Wiggins et al., 2008). Among Eskimo children under 20 years of age, overall cancer rates are not significantly different when compared with White children in the United States. However, Alaskan Eskimo children have significantly higher rates of hepatocellular cancer (Lanier, Holck, Day, & Key, 2003). Apart from risk factors such as smoking and diet, there is considerable interest in the role that infectious agents play as carcinogens. For example, hepatitis B virus (HBV) has been identified as a risk factor for the development of hepatocellular carcinoma (McCance & Huether, 2014). One longitudinal study followed 335 children who had received a three-dose series of hepatitis B vaccine beginning at birth for a median time of 10 years and concluded that immunization was effective in preventing development of clinical signs of hepatitis B and of chronic HBV infection (Dentinger et al., 2005); presumably the risk for those children to develop hepatocellular cancer was also reduced. The Epstein-Barr virus (EBV) has been implicated in the development of nasopharyngeal cancers, which occur at high rates in Alaska Natives (Lanier et al., 1980). The virus been found in more than 90% of cases of Burkitt's lymphoma in endemic regions, although only 15% of cases in nonendemic regions show evidence of infection (Gaffey & Weiss, 1990). It is suspected that the transmission of viral agents may require a susceptible genotype or other promotional events (Lynch, Schuelke, & O'Hara, 1984). It has been reported that Greenland Eskimos have the highest documented EBV titers in the world (Lanier & Alberts, 1996; Young, 1986). In Alaskan Eskimos a distinct variant of EBV type 2 was found in nasopharyngeal carcinoma and carcinoma of the parotid gland (Abdel-Hamid et al., 1992). Other risk factors associated with this type of cancer include the widespread lifestyle habits of smoking, alcohol, and chewing tobacco. Young (1986) reported a significant rise in nasopharyngeal cancer among teenagers and young adults seen at Alaska Native hospitals; epidemiologists attributed the increase in nasopharyngeal cancer to tobacco habits (snuff and cigarettes) that begin in preschool-aged groups rather than to the EBV. Between 1999 and 2004, cancers of the mouth and pharynx ranked eighth among Alaska Natives overall, with a risk ratio of 1.33 compared with non-Hispanic Whites (Wiggins et al., 2008).

Dietary habits such as the consumption of heavily smoked fish and fermented, salted foods may also add some carcinogenic risks. Insufficient data currently exist to determine whether genetic factors contribute to the cancer patterns of the Eskimo people. Wilson, Rausch, McMahon, and Schantz (1992) noted that chemotherapy effectively treated alveolar hydatid disease in Alaskan Eskimos.

Arthritis. According to a study reported in the *Morbidity and Mortality Weekly* (Centers for Disease Control, 1996), the American Indian and Alaska Native elders have the highest estimated age- and sex-adjusted annual prevalence of arthritis of all ethnic groups, including Asians, Pacific Islanders, Hispanics, and Blacks. American Indian and Alaska Native elders also reported the highest activity limitation caused by arthritis of any group (4.2%).

Asthma. Wind, Van Sickle, and Wright (2004) examined the perceptions of Yup'ik parents of asthmatic children using data from semistructured ethnographic interviews conducted in five villages and one town of the Yukon-Kuskokwim delta of southwest Alaska. Two interpretations of the increase in asthma among Yup'ik children were presented: (1) that there is a weakening of the collective physical body due to cold air, physical exertion, and dust and (2) that the Yup'ik consider asthma an embodiment of the degradation of the environment in which they live. "The fact that childhood asthma is seen as having a multiplicity of causes rather than being linked to a single source of environmental pollution suggests that community consensus about the relationship between locale and chronic disease for the Yup'ik may remain elusive" (p. 83).

Blood Variations. Rh-negative blood is rare in American Indians, particularly as they approach full blood quantum (Overfield, 1977); the same may be true of Alaskan Eskimos. However, because intermarriage has promoted genetic admixture, Rh-negative blood may occur in some Eskimos of mixed race. A survey of blood types and Rh factor in Canadian Eskimos residing in several sites in the Eastern Arctic, Jordan (1946) identified only three individuals who presented with Rh-negative blood, and all were of what he described as "mixed blood" (p. 433). More recently, a certified nurse midwife who works with an Alaska Native clientele related that she fairly regularly cared for Rh-negative mothers (Sarcone, personal communication, 2015). Thus, the nurse who counsels a woman during pregnancy or following a spontaneous abortion must be alert to her Rh factor. It is probable that, as genetic admixture increases in frequency, so too will the risk of Rh sensitization.

Nutritional and Lifestyle Preferences

After the control of infectious diseases among Alaskan Eskimos, the health–illness pattern shifted to reflect an increase in chronic disease. This increase in chronic disease may be attributable to the fact that the Eskimo diet and lifestyle changed as people assimilated many of the Western culture's bad habits, such as a sedentary lifestyle and a diet high in sugar, salt, and fat. Many Eskimos now use some form of locomotion, such as four-wheelers or snow machines, to get around villages that are less than a mile long or wide, minimizing needed exercise.

Clean water is sometimes a difficult commodity to obtain in Alaska. In some villages on the ocean, drinking water must be brought in as ice from several miles up the river. In the process of being brought to the village, the chunks of ice are often handled by many people and must then be melted, boiled, and cooled. Yet another concern for Inuits is that departure from the traditional Inuit diet lowers iodine intake. Urinary iodine excretion may be a useful biomarker of traditional Inuit food frequency (Andersen, Hvingel, Kleinschmidt, Jorgensen, & Laurberg, 2005).

Psychological Characteristics

"The suicide epidemic in Bush Alaska continues" is a frequent headline seen in Alaskan newspapers. The mental health status of Eskimos is complicated by the pressures created by traditional cultural demands, attempts at assimilation of Western values, and the harsh geographic region. Alcohol and drug abuse are the major causes of injury, accidents, and death among Alaskan Eskimos. Suicide is associated with alcohol abuse, which in turn is a symptom of a people attempting to assimilate in a rapidly changing society (Kettl & Bixler, 1993; VanDenberg & Minton, 1987). The IHS (2008) reported that the suicide death rate between 1999 and 2001 among Alaska Natives was 38.5, nearly four times the U.S. rate of 10.6 per 100,000. More recently, the Juneau *Empire* reported that the 2008 rate of 24.6 per 100,000 represented a 25% increase since 2005, with the state's Suicide Prevention Coordinator attributing the increase to stresses fueled by the high price of fuel and food in rural Alaska (2009 Alaska suicide rate, 2009). From May 23 to July 10, 2010, nine residents of rural, traditional Yup'ik villages ranging in age from 15 to 22 years committed suicide, with the youngest being the only female (Hopkins, 2010).

The suicidal behavior in Eskimo populations is believed to have changed in pattern and quantity. The rate of attempted suicide among Eskimos has more than quadrupled, and the incidence of completed suicides among young people has increased. To understand the psychological makeup and characteristics of the Eskimo people, the nurse needs to have an awareness of their history, its relationship to self-destructive behavior as evidenced among some Eskimos, and their present stress of acculturation.

For many Eskimos the rapid breakdown of traditional values, religion, lifestyle, and social relationships has led to an inability to find a meaningful role in the modern world. For example, a young Eskimo villager who is a student in a modern school, works on computers, and studies world events may become disillusioned at home, where the old roles and lack of employment may still exist. In this situation the parents may feel inadequate because they are unable to relate to the child as a result of the knowledge that the child has acquired at school. On the other hand, the child may see little importance in subsistence skills, such as fishing or hunting, in which the parents excel. After high school, the student may leave the village to attend college or trade school but may be underprepared in those larger settings. The student may be unable to tolerate living away from the village or family and return to the village after several months or years. When the adolescent returns to the village, reacceptance of village life may be difficult, giving rise to disillusionment, depression, and self-destructive behavior. Because they find that their own views and values have changed as a result of the outside experience, village life becomes stifling for many. Also, the trade or occupation learned while at school (such as computer science or even nursing) often has little relevance to life in the village. The result of all of this is that the village now has a frustrated, angry individual with incomplete readaptation to village life. These factors may lead to depression and to alcohol and drug use (Seltzer, 1980).

Males are at higher risk of suicide. During the 1980s, 86% of the suicide victims were male. The rate of suicide in men between the ages of 20 and 24 was in excess of 30 times the national rate for all age groups combined (Institute for Social and Economic Research, 1998). Many Eskimo women, on the other hand, attach meaning and purpose to life through the possibility of motherhood. Thus, Eskimo women are less likely than their male counterparts to become severely depressed. However, for Eskimo men, life may be perceived as purposeless because of their detachment from the family.

In a study that compared 567 Alaska Native criminal offenders referred to mental health professionals with 939 White offenders, it was found that alcohol abuse, the dominant social problem for some Alaska Natives, was not clearly associated with the degree of sociocultural change. Living in larger communities and higher educational achievement were associated with greater psychosocial maladjustment than the incidence of alcohol abuse. The region of residence had a stronger influence on the rate and type of maladjustment than did the ethnic group (i.e., Eskimo, Indian, or Aleut) or the ethnic density of the community of residence (i.e., the proportion of Alaska Natives in the population) (Phillips & Inui, 1986).

For some Eskimos, alcohol use has become an acceptable way to escape. Binge drinking has been related to the stress of acculturation (Kettl & Bixler, 1993; VanDenberg & Minton, 1987) and is at least partly related to the

fact that alcohol consumption was not a part of the traditional lifestyle. Because binge drinking is directly related to morbidity and mortality in Alaska, programs have been set up to deal with this problem. However, programs such as Alcoholics Anonymous have been relatively unsuccessful in Eskimo treatment, as have other forms of treatment designed for and by White people (Lange, 1988). Rather, culturally relevant programs have proved to be more effective (Mohatt, et al., 2004a; Mohatt, et al., 2004b).

Some reports have identified a biological predisposition of some Canadian Eskimos to be more susceptible to the deleterious effects of alcohol (Akins, Lanfear, Cline, & Mosher, 2013). Canadian Eskimos are rapid acetylators, as tested with isoniazid (Overfield, 1995; Schaefer, 1986). Phenytoin metabolism by Eskimos also differs from metabolism by Whites (Schaefer, 1986). Although the work with biological predisposition and alcohol metabolism has been done with Canadian Eskimos, the results are likely to be appropriately generalizable to the Alaskan Eskimos.

Implications for Nursing Care

Seltzer (1983) has reported three interesting cases of Eskimos who claimed to be possessed by spirits. The spirits appeared to represent culture-bound defense mechanisms and attempts at problem solving in Eskimos who had unresolved cultural conflicts. Although reports of spiritual possession are uncommon among mental health professionals in Alaska, Seltzer's report does emphasize the importance of knowledge of myths and customs, as well as culturally significant methods of healing, on the part of health care providers. Napoleon (1991) suggested that the large numbers of deaths and displacements resulting from epidemics of influenza, tuberculosis, and other communicable diseases in the early twentieth century and resulting rapid cultural change have led to a form of post-traumatic stress disorder among Yup'ik Eskimos.

Eschiti (2004) asserted that holistic nursing presents an ideal framework to foster promotion and maintenance of health for Alaskan Natives. Understanding cultural differences will allow the nurse to relate in a positive way to persons from varied cultural backgrounds. If nursing interventions are to be successful, they must not oppose a particular cultural practice. On the other hand, if the cultural practice is detrimental to the health status of the people, the nurse must devise a teaching plan and alternative strategies to combat the negative practice. If the nurse is to use time and energy efficiently, nursing care measures must be planned and implemented cooperatively with the client and family so that it is perceived as being culturally relevant. Community efforts are also important. For example, the Alaska Native Community Suicide

Prevention Center is an example of a community-based program that has shown promising results in reducing suicides among young adults (DeBruyn, Wilkins, Stetter-Burns, & Nelson, 1997).

The nurse who works with Eskimo clients must know certain biological concepts that are germane to the Eskimo people in order to give not only adequate care but also to avoid harmful care. As Western culture has influenced Eskimo people, behaviors have changed. For example, Eskimos now consume large quantities of carbohydrates, bottle-feed instead of breastfeed their infants, consume large quantities of alcohol, use tobacco extensively, and have assumed a more sedentary lifestyle. As the behaviors and health care needs of these individuals change, the nurse must modify approaches to client care accordingly.

SUMMARY

Despite the apparent Westernization of Eskimos, they have retained many of their traditional perceptions and responses to life situations. Whether in an Alaskan village or in a clinic or hospital in the mainland United States, the nurse who encounters an Eskimo client must incorporate a theoretical framework that encompasses knowledge of communication, spatial requirements, social organization, time, environmental control, and biological variations to enhance quality nursing care.

CASE STUDY

Rachel, a 6-year-old Eskimo girl, has chronic otitis media, anemia, poor dietary habits, noncompliance with prescribed medication, and low self-esteem, resulting in failure to adjust to school. The mother brings the child to the village clinic for treatment. When taking the history from the mother, the nurse notes that the child has six siblings and comes from a home where the father is frequently absent and, when present, is often drunk. The nurse observes that the mother provides inconsistent direction and resorts to threats and ridicule when attempting to correct or change the child's behavior. For example, when the child does not sit still, the mother states, "You be good, or the nurse will give you a shot." The nurse notes that both the child's ears have a gluelike discharge, which the mother states is being treated with eardrops given at the clinic 2 weeks earlier. However, the mother also states that the child refuses to allow the eardrops to be instilled because they "hurt" her ears. The nurse notes that only a small amount of the bottle has been used.

This is the second clinic visit. At the first visit, when asked about what the child ate, the mother responded that most food items came from hunting or fishing or the village store and that they usually had fish soup, pilot bread with shortening, and black, sugared tea. With a hemoglobinometer, the nurse now determines that the child's hemoglobin remains at the same low level as at the previous visit. The iron-supplement tablets given at the last visit have not been taken. When questioned about whether she eats the school lunch provided by the public lunch program, the child replies that no one likes her and that the other children take her food, and so she does not get much.

On examination of the child, the nurse finds a pale mucous membrane and poor muscle tone with decreased muscle activity. The child's temperature is 102° F, her pulse is 75, her blood pressure is 100/66 mm Hg, and her respirations are 22. The nurse notes that the child complains of a sharp, constant pain in both ears and frequently pulls or tugs at both ears, seemingly in an attempt to gain relief. On examination of the ears, the nurse notes that the external canal is free of wax and that the mastoid process behind the ear is not tender to touch. However, the tympanic membrane appears inflamed.

⊚ CARE PLAN

Nursing Diagnosis: Nutrition altered, less than body requirements

Client Outcomes	Nursing Interventions
1. Client will have increased iron level. 2. Client will have an adequate oral dietary intake. 3. Mother and client will describe causative factors related to inadequate nutrition. 4. Mother will verbalize safety measures related to oral iron medication.	1. Obtain height and weight measurements, and plot on a standard chart that has been normed for Eskimo children. 2. Do a 24-hour dietary recall. 3. Educate mother and client about iron-rich foods, including eggs, dates, and raisins. 4. Involve mother in designing a diet plan that emphasizes intake of adequate amounts of protein- and iron-rich foods. 5. Use an easy-to-understand nutrition brochure to illustrate how to make healthy food choices. 6. Encourage mother to seek additional assistance for dietary requirements, such as the WIC program. 7. Encourage mother to talk with teachers about lunchtime intake. 8. Reinforce with mother and client the need for taking appropriate dose of iron supplements. 9. Instruct mother to be certain to put iron supplements in a safe place so that other children cannot take the medication indiscriminately, thus avoiding iron toxicity.

Nursing Diagnosis: Management of therapeutic regimen related to decisional conflicts, as evidenced by mother stating that child refuses to use eardrops because they hurt her ears

Client Outcomes	Nursing Interventions
1. Parental knowledge about condition will be increased. 2. Mother and client will learn value of washing hands and not placing foreign bodies into the ear. 3. Mother and client will learn value of taking prescribed antibiotic for the full amount of time. 4. Measures will be taken to prevent the possibility of a tympanic membrane rupture. 5. Client will have increased comfort. 6. Measures will be taken to prevent recurrence.	1. Assess for hearing impairment or loss. 2. Examine external auditory canal and tympanic membrane. 3. Teach mother and child to wash hands to prevent illness. 4. Teach mother and client not to put hard or sharp things into the ear. 5. Teach mother and client to seek early medical care for pharyngitis to prevent spread of infection through eustachian tube to middle ear. 6. Teach mother and client that antibiotic must be taken as prescribed. 7. Teach mother and client signs and symptoms of tympanic membrane rupture, which include sudden relief of pain, and to call the clinic. 8. Teach mother and client the value of soft and liquid foods when chewing is extremely painful because of movement of the eustachian tube.

Continued

◎ **CARE PLAN—cont'd**

Nursing Diagnosis: Coping, ineffective individual (mother and child)
1. Related to complex self-care regimens
2. As evidenced by nonassertive response patterns, allows child to refuse medications and allows child to be taken advantage of

Client Outcomes	Nursing Interventions
1. Client will describe experiences that cause her to alter prescribed behavior. 2. Mother will develop an appropriate alternative for previous plan for medication administration.	1. Assess causative or contributing factors for noncompliance with prescribed therapy. 2. Assess client's rationale for noncompliance with medication. 3. Teach mother and client how to administer eardrops (room temperature). 4. Watch as mother administers eardrops. 5. Observe mother–child interactions. 6. Explain if modifications are needed. 7. Praise mother and child when medications are administered correctly.

Nursing Diagnosis: Self-esteem disturbance

Client Outcomes	Nursing Interventions
1. Client will verbalize positive feelings about self. 2. Client will take part in activities with other children in a confident manner. 3. Client will achieve grade-level objectives of school age.	1. Encourage client to express both positive and negative feelings. 2. Encourage mother to set limits on problematic behavior, such as poor hygiene, noncompliance with medication, and other negative behaviors. 3. Accept silence of client, but let her know that the nurse is there for support.

Nursing Diagnosis: Family process, altered; alcoholism coping, ineffective family: disabling related to impaired ability to constructively manage stressors secondary to alcoholism of father, as evidenced by actions that are detrimental to family well-being, child allowed to be taken advantage of at school, child not treated with ear medications

Client Outcome	Nursing Interventions
Mother relates expectations for what she will do in regard to child not being allowed to eat lunch at school, going to Al-Anon meetings.	1. Explore with the mother and the 6-year-old how their behavior has negatively affected the physical well-being of the 6-year-old girl (refusing ear treatment, allowing others to take away lunch). 2. Explore characteristics of families affected by alcoholism. 3. Provide information on community resources, such as Al-Anon, Alcoholics Anonymous, and family therapy.

CLINICAL DECISION MAKING

1. Explain the importance of silence in communication with Eskimo clients.
2. Identify why otitis media may be a common illness among Eskimo children.
3. Identify cultural factors that affect the treatment of otitis media in Eskimo children.
4. List factors that predispose Eskimos to risk as a result of consumption of large quantities of sugar.
5. List several contributing factors related to alcoholism among Alaskan Eskimos.
6. Formerly, tuberculosis was a disease condition to which Eskimos were believed to have inherited susceptibility. Today, however, this is considered untrue. List two factors cited that do have contributing significance.
7. Relate the sobriety movement to the worldview and values of Eskimos, and cite a problem in which this movement has been especially useful.

REVIEW QUESTIONS

1. The nurse is caring for a family in which five family members have tuberculosis. The family describes its health belief to the nurse, which included shamanic healing. The nurse knows the patient will be more compliant if she includes use of antituberculin medication as well as which of the following?
   a. Services of a folk healer
   b. Behavior therapy
   c. Acupuncture
   d. Yoga
2. A nurse caring for an Eskimo child observes dark spots in the lumbar area as well as other dark areas on the body. The nurse should do which of the following?
   a. Have the parents investigated for child abuse.
   b. Assess the areas to determine if they are mongolian spots.
   c. Recognize these areas as being related to coining.
   d. Ignore the difference in color.
3. As you explain your patient's condition to her husband, you notice that he is leaning toward you and raising his eyebrows. Knowing that he is an Eskimo, your most appropriate response to this behavior is to do what?
   a. Tell him that you understand his need to be alone.
   b. Ask whether he has any questions.
   c. Ask whether he would prefer to speak to the physician.
   d. Understand he is agreeing.

REFERENCES

2009 Alaska suicide rate increases yet again: experts say economic downturn may be a factor in high rates. (2009). *Juneau Empire*. Available at <http://juneauempire.com/stories/052909/sta_445021341.shtml> Retrieved September 28, 2014.

Abdel-Hamid, M., Chen, J., Constantine, N., Massoud, M., & Raab-Traub, N. (1992). EBV strain variation: geographical distribution and relation to disease state. *Virology*, *190*(1), 168–175.

Akin, S., Lanfear, C., Cline, S., & Mosher, C. (2013). Patterns and correlates of adult American Indian substance abuse. *Journal of Drug Issues*, *43*(4), 497–516.

Alaska Behavioral Risk Behavior Survey (2011). *Health risks in Alaska among adults: 2009 annual report*. Juneau, AK: Alaska Department of Health and Social Services. Available at <http://dhss.alaska.gov/dph/Chronic/Documents/brfss/pubs/BRFSS09_FullReport.pdf> Retrieved January 15, 2015.

Alaska Community Database (n.d.). *Community profiles*. Available at <https://www.commerce.alaska.gov/web/dcra/> Retrieved December 11, 2014.

Alaska Department of Health & Social Services (2006). Diversity and cultural issues in Alaska. In *Alaska Air Medical Escort training manual* (ch. 12, 4th ed.). Juneau, AK: Department of Health & Soial Services, Division of Public Health, Section of Injury Prevention and EMS.

Alaska Department of Health & Social Services (2007, March). *What state surveys tell us about tobacco smoking among Alaska natives: implications for program planning*. Available at <http://dhss.alaska.gov/dph/Chronic/Documents/Tobacco/PDF/AKNativeTobaccoReport.pdf> Retrieved January 16, 2015.

Alaska Department of Labor and Workforce Development (2013). *Alaska population overview: 2012 estimates*. Available at <http://labor.alaska.gov/research/pop/estimates/pub/popover.pdf> Retrieved November 19, 2014.

Alaska Native Epidemiology Center (2009). *Alaska Native health status report*. Anchorage, AK: Alaska Native Tribal Health Consortium. Alaska Native Tribal Health Consortium. Available at <http://www.anthc.org/chs/epicenter/upload/ANHSR.pdf> Retrieved on November 25, 2014.

Allen, E., & Crago, M. (1996). Early passive acquisition in Inuktitut. *Journal of Child Language*, *23*(1), 129–155.

Andersen, S., Hvingel, B., Kleinschmidt, K., Jorgensen, T., & Laurberg, P. (2005). Changes in iodine excretion in 50–69 year old denizens of an Arctic society in transition and iodine excretion as a biomarker of the frequency of consumption of traditional Inuit foods. *American Journal of Clinical Nutrition*, *81*(3), 656–663.

Arkell, S. M., Lightman, D. A., Sommer, A., Taylor, H. R., Korshin, O. M., & Tielsch, M. (1987). The prevalence of glaucoma among Eskimos of northwest Alaska. *Archives of Ophthalmology*, *105*(4), 482–485.

Armstrong, T., Roberts, B., & Swithinbank, C. (Eds.), (1973). *Illustrated glossary of snow and ice*. Cambridge, England: Scott Polar Research Institute.

Austin, A. (2013). *High unemployment means Native Americans are still waiting for an economic recovery*, Economic Policy Institute. Available at <http://www.epi.org/publication/high-unemployment-means-native-americans/> Retrieved November 20, 2014.

Barnhardt, C. (2001). A history of schooling for Alaska Native people. *Journal of American Indian Education, 40*(1), 1–30.

Bassett, R., & O'Malley, M. (2014). Chronic kidney disease in an Alaska Native/American Indian statewide healthcare network. *Nephrology Nursing Journal, 41*(4), 409–414.

Bell, R., Draper, H., & Bergan, J. (1973). Sucrose, lactose, and glucose tolerance in northern Alaskan Eskimos. *American Journal of Clinical Nutrition, 26*, 1185–1190.

Bjerregaard, P., et al. (2003). Blood pressure among the Inuit (Eskimo) populations in the Arctic. *Scandinavian Journal of Public Health, 31*(2), 92–99.

Bjerregaard, P., Young, T., Dewailly, E., & Ebbesson, S. (2004). Indigenous health in the Arctic, an overview of the circumpolar Inuit population. *Scandinavian Journal of Public Health, 32*(5), 390–395.

Blodgett, J. (1978). *The coming and going of shaman: Eskimo shamanism and art*. Winnipeg, Manitoba: Winnipeg Art Gallery.

Book, P. A., Dixon, M., & Kirchner, S. (1983). Native health in Alaska: report from Serpentine Hot Springs. In Cross-cultural medicine. *Western Journal of Medicine, 139*, 923–927.

Bovette, M. H., & Harvill, J. (2014). *Summary of HIV infection: Alaska 1982–2013*. Anchorage, AK: Alaska Section of Epidemiology. Available at <http://www.epi.hss.state.ak.us/bulletins/docs/b2014_05.pdf> Retrieved January 15, 2015.

Branch, K., & Heyano, R. (2002). Rural affordable assisted living in Dillingham, Alaska. *The IHS Primary Care Provider, 27*(5), 1–3.

Brant, L. J., Bender, T. R., & Marnell, R. W. (1982). Factors affecting streptococcal colonization among children in selected areas of Alaska. *Public Health Reports, 97*(5), 460–464.

Bruerd, B. (1997). Preventing baby bottle tooth decay and early childhood caries among AI/AN infants and children. *The IHS Primary Care Provider, 22*(3), 37–39.

Bucki, C. (2004). *Reindeer roundup! A K–12 educator's guide to reindeer in Alaska*. Fairbanks, AK: Reindeer Research Program, University of Alaska Fairbanks. Available at <http://www.uaf.edu/files/snre/MP_04_07.pdf> Retrieved November 20, 2014.

Butler, J. C., et al. (2001). Emerging infectious diseases among indigenous peoples. *Emerging Infectious Diseases, 7*(3), Suppl. Available at <http://wwwnc.cdc.gov/eid/article/7/7/pdfs/01-7732.pdf> Retrieved January 15, 2015.

Cecere, D., & Jones, S. A. (2013). *Syphilis outbreak update—Alaska, 2011–2013*. Anchorage, AK: Alaska Section of Epidemiology. Available at <http://www.epi.hss.state.ak.us/bulletins/docs/b2013_25.pdf> Retrieved January 15, 2015.

Cecere, D., & Jones, S. A. (2014a). *Chlamydial infection—Alaska, 2013*. Anchorage, AK: Alaska Section of Epidemiology. Available at <http://www.epi.hss.state.ak.us/bulletins/docs/b2014_10.pdf> Retrieved January 15, 2015.

Cecere, D., & Jones, S. A. (2014b). *Gonococcal infection—Alaska, 2013*. Anchorage, AK: Alaska Section of Epidemiology. Available at <http://www.epi.hss.state.ak.us/bulletins/docs/b2014_11.pdf> Retrieved January 15, 2015.

Centers for Disease Control (1996). Prevalence and impact of arthritis by race and ethnicity—United States, 1989–1991. *Morbidity and Mortality Weekly Report, 45*(18), 373–378.

Centers for Disease Control (2011). Dental caries in rural Alaska Native children—Alaska, 2008. *Morbidity and Mortality Weekly Report, 60*(37), 1275–1278.

Cheek, J. E., Holman, R. C., Redd, J. T., Haberline, D., & Hennessy, T. W. (2014). Infectious disease mortality among American Indians and Alaska Natives, 1999–2009. *American Journal of Public Health, Suppl 3, 104*(53), S446–S452.

Chythlook-Sifsof, C. J. (2013). Native Alaska, under threat: Commentary. *New York Times*, A-27.

Cordova, A. (1981). The mongolian spot: a study of ethnic differences and a literature review. *Clinical Pediatrics, 20*(11), 714–719.

Damas, D. (1984). *Arctic: handbook of North American Indians* (Vol. 5). Washington, DC: Smithsonian Institute.

Davidhizar, R., & Giger, J. (2000). Culture and care: profiling Alaskan Eskimos. *Health Traveler, 4*(12), 43–47.

Day, G. E., & Lanier, A. P. (2003). Alaska Native mortality, 1979–1998. *Public Health Reports, 118*(November–December), 518–530.

DeBruyn, L., Wilkins, B., Stetter-Burns, M., & Nelson, S. (1997). Violence and violence prevention. *The IHS Primary Care Provider, 22*(4), 58–60.

DeLapp, T., & Ward, E. (1981). *Traditional Inupiat health practices*. Proceedings of the Fifth International Symposium on Circumpolar Health, August 9–13, 1981, Copenhagen, Denmark, 69–70.

DeMarban, A. (2014). *As Washington Redskins controversy ramps up, complicated term "Eskimo" is reconsidered*, Alaska Dispatch News. Available at <http://www.adn.com/article/20140626/washington-redskins-controversy-ramps-complicated-term-eskimo-reconsidered> Retrieved August 2, 2014.

Dentinger, C. M., et al. (2005). Persistence of antibody to hepatitis B and protection from disease among Alaska Natives immunized at birth. *The Pediatric Infectious Disease Journal, 24*(9), 786–792.

Dixon, M. (1998). *Managed care in American Indian and Alaska Native communities*. Washington, DC: American Public Health Association.

Dixon, M., & Roubideaux, Y. (Eds.), (2001). *Promises to keep: public health policy for American Indians and Alaska Natives in the 21st century*. Washington, DC: American Public Health Association.

Duncan, I., & Scott, E. (1972). Lactose intolerance in Alaska Indian and Eskimo. *American Journal of Clinical Nutrition, 25*, 867–868.

Ebbesson, S. O. E., Ebbesson, L. O. E., Swenson, M., Kennish, J. M., & Robbins, D. C. (2005). A successful diabetes prevention study in Eskimos: the Alaska Siberia project. *International Journal of Circumpolar Health, 64*(4), 409–424.

Environmental Protection Agency (2013). *Climate change: Alaska*. Available at <http://www.epa.gov/climatechange/impacts-adaptation/alaska.html> Retrieved September 30, 2014.

Eschiti, V. (2004). Holistic approach to resolving American Indian/Alaska Native health care disparities. *Journal of Holistic Nursing, 22*(3), 201–208.

Espey, D. K., et al. (2014). Leading causes of death and all-cause mortality in American Indians and Alaska Natives. *American Journal of Public Health Suppl 3, 104*(53), S303–S311.

Fienup-Riordan, A. (2001). A guest on the table: ecology from the Yup'ik Eskimo point of view. In J. Grim (Ed.), *Indigenous traditions and ecology: the interbeing of cosmology and community* (pp. 541–558). Cambridge: Harvard University Press for the Center for the Study of World Religions, Harvard Divinity School.

Fortuine, R. (1989). *Chills and fever: health and disease in the early history of Alaska*. Fairbanks: University of Alaska Press.

Freddoso, D. (2002). Unions support Bush on Alaska drilling. *Human Events, 58*(9), 5.

Funk, B. (2009). *Tuberculosis in Alaska, 1999–2008. State of Alaska Epidemiology Bulletin # 31*. Anchorage, AK: Alaska Section of Epidemiology. Available at <http://www.epi.hss.state.ak.us/bulletins/docs/b2009_31.pdf> Retrieved January 15, 2015.

Gaffey, M. J., & Weiss, L. M. (1990). Viral oncogenesis: Epstein-Barr virus. *American Journal of Otolaryngology, 11*(6), 375–381.

Gallinek, P. (2006). Communities of compassion. *Healthcare Traveler, 7*(1), 33–37.

Gove, C. (1982). *The conflict between cultural persistence and acculturation as it affects individual behavior of northwestern Alaskan Eskimo*. San Diego, CA: Dissertation presented to graduate faculty of the School of Human Behavior, U.S. International University.

Haggett, P. (2002). *Encyclopedia of world geography, United States I* (2nd ed.). New York: Marshall Cavendish.

Hall, D. B., Lum, M. K., Knutson, L. R., Knutson, L. R., Heyward, W. L., & Ward, J. I. (1987). Pharyngeal carriage and acquisition of anticapsular antibody to *Haemophilus influenzae* type B in a high risk population in southwestern Alaska. *American Journal of Epidemiology, 126*(6), 1190–1197.

Hall, E. (1975). *The Eskimo storyteller: folktales from Noatak, Alaska*. Knoxville, TN: University of Tennessee Press.

Hall, L. D., Sberna, J., & Utermohle, C. (2001). *Diabetes in Alaska: 1991–2000*. Anchorage, AK: Alaska Section of Epidemiology. *State of Alaska Epidemiology Bulletin, 5*(4). Available at <http://www.epi.hss.state.ak.us/bulletins/docs/rr2001_4.pdf> Retrieved January 16, 2015.

Haymes, S. A., Leston, J. D., Ferucci, E. D., Etzel, R. A., & Lanier, A. P. (2009). Visual impairment and eye care among Alaska Native people. *Ophthalmic Epidemiology, 16*, 163–174.

Hazel, K. L., & Mohatt, G. V. (2001). Cultural and spiritual coping in sobriety: informing substance abuse prevention for Alaska Native communities. *Journal of Community Psychology, 29*(5), 541–562.

Helmkamp, J. C., Aitken, M. E., Graham, J., & Campbell, C. R. (2012). State-specific ATV-related fatality rates: an update in the new millennium. *Public Health Reports, 127*(4), 364–374.

Hennessey, T. W., et al. (2008). The relationship between in-home water service and the risk of respiratory tract, skin and gastrointestinal tract infections among rural Alaska Natives. *American Journal of Public Health, 98*(11), 2072–2078.

Hinsley, K. (2001). *Give me my father's body: the life of Minik, the New York Eskimo*. New York: Pocket Books.

Hippler, A. E. (1974). The North Alaska Eskimos: a culture and personality perspective. *American Ethnologist, 1*(3), 440–469.

Holman, R. C., et al. (2004). Respiratory syncytial virus hospitalizations among American Indian and Alaska Native infants and the general United States infant population. *Pediatrics, 114*(4), e437–e444.

Hopkins, K. (2010). Suicides, attempts spike again in Western Alaska villages, *Anchorage Daily News*. Available at <http://www.adn.com/20100714/suicides-attempts-spike-again-western-alaska-villages> Retrieved January 19, 2015.

Hopkins, K. (2014). *After 14 years, Russians boat across Bering Strait to visit Alaska relatives*. Alaska Dispatch News. Available at <http://www.adn.com/article/20140726/after-14-years-russians-boat-across-bering-strait-visit-alaska-relatives> Retrieved September 30, 2014.

Hunsinger, E., & Sandberg, E. (2013). The Alaska Native population: steady growth for original Alaskans through years of change. *Alaska Economic Trends, 33*(4), 4–9, 13. Available at <http://laborstats.alska.gov/trends/apr13art1.pdf> Retrieved November 19, 2014.

Indian Health Service (2008). *Regional differences in Indian Health 2002–2003*. Available at <http://www.ihs.gov/dps/files/RD_entirebook.pdf> Retrieved December 7, 2014.

Indian Health Service (2014). *Alaska area*. Available at <http://www.ihs.gov/alaska/> Retrieved December 8, 2014.

Institute for Social and Economic Research, University of Alaska, Anchorage (1998). *Physical and behavioral health statistics from the Alaska Natives Commission*. Available at <http://www.alaskool.org/resources/anc2/ANC2_sec1.html> Retrieved January 19, 2015.

Jackson, M. (2000). Healthy People 2010: reaching American Indian/Alaska Native elders. *The IHS Primary Care Provider, 25*(5), 1–2. Available at <http://www.ihs.gov/provider/documents/2000_2009/PROV0500.pdf> Retrieved December 7, 2014.

Jacobson, S. A. (1984). *Central Yup'ik and the schools: a handbook for teachers*. Juneau, AK: Alaska Department of Education, Bilingual/Bicultural Education Programs. Available at <http://sesa.org/search/node/Jacobson> Retrieved December 10, 2014.

Jilek-Aall, L. (1981). Acculturation, alcoholism, and Indian-style Alcoholics Anonymous. *Journal of Studies on Alcohol, 43*(Suppl. 9), 143–158.

Johnston, F. E., Laughlin, W. S., Harper, A. B., & Ensroth, A. E. (1982). Physical growth of St. Lawrence Island Eskimos: body size, proportion, and composition. *American Journal of Physical Anthropology, 58*(4), 397–401.

Jordan, D. (1946). Survey of blood grouping and Rh factor in the Eskimos of the Eastern Arctic, 1945. *The Canadian Medical Association Journal (CMAJ)*, 54(5), 429–434.

Juul, S. (1979). Portrait of an Eskimo tribal health doctor. *Alaska Medicine*, 21(6), 66–71.

Kaplan, L. D. (1984). *Inupiaq and the schools: a handbook for teachers*. Juneau, AK: Alaska Department of Education, Bilingual/Bicultural Education Programs. Available at <http://sesa.org/search/node/Kaplan> Retrieved December 10, 2014.

Keats, D. (1985). *Della Keats: Eskimo healer* (video). Kotzebue, AK: Manillnaq.

Kettl, P., & Bixler, E. O. (1993). Alcohol and suicide in Alaska Natives. *American Indian and Alaska Native Mental Health Research*, 5(2), 35–45. Available at <http://dx.doi.org/10.5820/aian.0502.1993.34> Retrieved January 21, 2015.

Klausner, A., & Foulks, E. F. (1982). *Eskimo capitalists: oil, politics, and alcohol*. Englewood Cliffs, NJ: Prentice Hall.

Kleinfeld, J. S. (1971). *Some instructional strategies for the cross-cultural classroom*. Juneau: Alaska Department of Education.

Kost-Grant, B. L. (1983). Self-inflicted gunshot wounds among Alaska Natives. *Public Health Reports*, 98(1), 72–78.

Langdon, S. J. (2014). *The Native people of Alaska*. Anchorage, AK: Greatland Graphics.

Lange, B. (1988). Ethnographic interview: an occupational therapy needs assessment tool for American Indian and Alaska Native alcoholics. *Occupational Therapy in Mental Health*, 8(2), 61–80.

Langlois, K. (2014). Pebble Mine: Alaska sides with mining corporation, tribes back EPA. *High Country News*. Available at <http://www.hcn.org/blogs/goat/the-fight-for-bristol-bay-alaska-sides-with-mining-corporation-tribes-back-epa> Retrieved November 27, 2014.

Lanier, A., & Alberts, S. (1996). Cancers of the buccal cavity and pharynx in circumpolar Inuit. *Acta Oncologica*, 35(5), 545–552.

Lanier, A., et al. (1980). Nasopharyngeal carcinoma in Alaskan Eskimos, Indians, and Aleuts: a review of cases and study of Epstein-Barr virus, HLA, and environmental risk factors. *Cancer*, 46(9), 2100–2106.

Lanier, A. P., Holck, P., Day, G. E., & Key, C. (2003). Childhood cancers among Alaska Natives. *Pediatrics*, 112(5), e396–e403.

Lantis, M. (1960). *Eskimo childhood and interpersonal relationships*. New York: AMS Press.

Legal Information Institute (n.d.). *U.S. code collection*, title 25, chapter 21, section 1915. Available at <http://www.law.cornell.edu/uscode/text/25/1915> Retrieved December 11, 2014.

Lewis, D., & Ho, M. (1975). Social work with Native Americans. *Social Work*, 20, 379–382.

Lopez, B. H. (2001). *Arctic dreams*. New York: Scribner.

Lubbock, B. (1937). *The Arctic whalers*. Glasgow, Scotland: Brown, Son & Ferguson.

Lum, M. K., Knutson, L. R., Hall, D. B., Margolis, H. S., & Bender, T. R. (1986). Decline in infant mortality of Alaskan Yup'ik Eskimos from 1960 to 1980. *Public Health Reports*, 101(3), 309–314.

Lynch, H., Schuelke, G., & O'Hara, M. (1984). Is cancer communicable? *Medical Hypotheses*, 14(2), 181–198.

Macartney, S., Bishaw, A., & Fontenot, K. (2013). *Poverty rates for selected detailed race and Hispanic groups by state and place: 2007–2011*. American Community Survey Briefs. U.S. Bureau of the Census. Available at <http://www.census.gov/prod/2013pubs/acsbr11-17.pdf> Retrieved November 20, 2014.

MacDonald-Clark, N., & Boffman, J. (1995). Mother-child interaction among the Alaskan Eskimos. *Journal of Obstetric, Gynecologic, and Neonatal Nursing*, 24(5), 450–457.

Mann, G. V., Scott, E., Hursh, L. M., Heller, C. A., Youmans, J. B., & Colsolazsio, F. (1962). The health and nutritional status of Alaskan Eskimos. *American Journal of Clinical Nutrition*, 11(1), 31–76.

Marcadier, J. L., et al. (2014). Congenital sucrose-isomaltase deficiency: identification of a common Inuit founder mutation. *Canadian Medical Association Journal (CMAJ)*, 187(2), 102–107. Available at <www.cmaj.ca/content/187/2/102.full>.

McCance, K. L., & Huether, S. E. (Eds.), (2014). *Pathophysiology: the biologic basis of disease in adults and children* (7th ed.). St. Louis: Mosby Elsevier.

McGrath-Hanna, N. K., Greene, D. D., Tavenier, R. J., & Bult-Ito, A. (2003). Diet and mental health in the Arctic: is diet an important risk factor for mental health in circumpolar peoples? A review. *International Journal of Circumpolar Health*, 62(3), 228–241.

Meier, R. J., Draper, H., & Milan, F. (1991). Pedigree analysis of sucrose intolerance among Native Alaskans. *Arctic Medical Research*, 50, 8–12.

Milan, F. A. (Ed.) (1980). *The human biology of circumpolar populations*. Cambridge: Cambridge University Press.

Mohatt, G. V., Hazel, K. L., Allen, J., Stachelrodt, M., Hensel, C., & Fath, R. (2004a). Unheard Alaska: Anchorage participatory action research on sobriety with Alaska Natives. *American Journal of Community Psychology*, 33(3–4), 263–273.

Mohatt, G. V., Rasmus, S. M., Thomas, L., Allen, J., Hazel, K., & Hensel, C. (2004b). "Tied together like a woven hat": protective pathways to Alaska native sobriety. *Harm Reduction Journal*, 1, doi:10.1186/1477-7517-1-10. Available at <http://www.harmreductionjournal.com/content/1/1/10> Retrieved January 15, 2015.

Morris, J. (1985). Caribou and ketchup—health implications. *Nursing Practice*, 1(2), 98–101.

Murphy, T., Pokhrel, P., Worthington, A., Billie, H., Sewell, M., & Bill, N. (2014). Unintentional injury mortality among American Indians and Alaska Natives in the United States, 1990–2009. *American Journal of Public Health Suppl 3*, 104(53), S470–S480.

Napoleon, H. (1991). *Yuuyaraq: the way of the human being*. Fairbanks, AK: University of Alaska, Fairbanks.

National Snow and Ice Data Center (2014). *Facts about glaciers*. Boulder, CO: National Snow and Ice Data Center. Available at <http://nsidc.org/cryosphere/glaciers/quickfacts.html> Retrieved December 9, 2014.

Native Health News Alliance (2014). Alaska dental health aide therapists mark 10 years in practice: provided expanded access to 40,000 Alaska Native people (Online only). Available at <http://www.nativehealthnews.com/alaska-dental-health-aide-therapists-mark-10-years-in-practice-provided-expanded-access-to-40000-alaska-native-people/> Retrieved January 5, 2015.

Naylor, J. L., Schraer, C. D., Mayer, A. M., Lanier, A. P., Treat, C. A., & Murphy, N. J. (2003). Diabetes among Alaska Natives: a review. *International Journal of Circumpolar Health*, 62(4), 363–387.

Nida, E. (1954). *Customs and cultures*. New York: Harper & Brothers.

Nord, E. (1995). Evolution of a public health nursing program, Yukon Kuskokwim Delta, Alaska, 1893–1993. *Public Health Nursing*, 12(4), 249–255.

Overfield, T. (1977). Biological variations: concepts from physical anthropology. *Nursing Clinics of North America*, 12(1), 19–27.

Overfield, T. (1995). *Biologic variation in health and illness* (2nd ed.). Reading, MA: Addison-Wesley.

Parkinson, A. J., et al. (2000). High prevalence of *Helicobacter pylori* in the Alaska Native population and association with low serum ferritin levels in young adults. *Clinical and Diagnostic Laboratory Immunology*, 7(6), 885–888.

Petersen, K., & Bryant, L. J. (1984). Growth and hematological changes in the Eskimo children of Wainwright, Alaska: 1968 to 1977. *American Journal of Clinical Nutrition*, 39(3), 460–465.

Petersen, K. M., Parkinson, A. J., Nobmann, E. D., Bulkow, L., Yip, R., & Mokdad, A. (1996). Iron deficiency anemia among Alaska Natives may be due to fecal loss rather than inadequate intake. *Journal of Nutrition*, 126(11), 2774–2783.

Petersen, G. M., Silimperi, D. R., Chiu, C. Y., & Ward, J. I. (1991). Effects of age, breast feeding, and household structure on *Haemophilus influenzae* type B disease risk and antibody acquisition in Alaskan Eskimos. *American Journal of Epidemiology*, 134(10), 1212–1221.

Petersen, G. M., et al. (1987). Genetic factors in *Haemophilus influenzae* type B disease susceptibility and antibody acquisition. *Journal of Pediatrics*, 110(2), 228–233.

Phillips, M. R., & Inui, T. S. (1986). The interaction of mental illness, criminal behavior and culture: Native Alaskan mentally ill criminal offenders. *Culture, Medicine and Psychiatry*, 10(2), 123–149.

Polk, S. (1987). Helping our children. *Children Today*, 16(5), 19–20.

Random House Webster's college dictionary. (2000). New York: Random House.

Renner, C. C., et al. (2004). Focus groups of Y-K delta Alaska Natives: attitudes toward tobacco use and tobacco dependence programs. *Preventive Medicine*, 38(4), 421–431.

Roberts, L., & Ross, C. (1979). Nursing north of sixty. *Canadian Nurse*, 75(5), 26–29.

Rodahl, K. (1964). *Between two worlds*. London: Heinemann.

Rode, A., & Shephard, R. J. (1984). Ten years of "civilization": fitness of Canadian Inuit. *Journal of Physiology*, 56(6), 1472–1477.

Rosen, Y. (1997). Iditarod trail leads to more pros, fewer native racers. *Christian Science Monitor*, 1.

Rosen, Y. (2014). Beaufort Sea polar bear population took big hit in early 2000, study says. *Alaska Dispatch News*, A-1.

Rousseau-Nepton, I., et al. (2015). A founder AGL mutation causing glycogen storage disease type IIIa in Inuit identified through whole-exome sequencing: a case series. *Canadian Medical Association Journal (CMAJ)*, 187(2), E68–E72. Available at <http://www.cmaj.ca/content/187/2/E68.full>.

Sanders, N. (2000). The relationship of spirituality and health among the Yup'ik of southwestern Alaska: an exploratory study. (Unpublished doctoral dissertation). Wayne State University, Detroit, MI.

Schaefer, O. (1970). Pre- and postnatal growth acceleration and increased sugar consumption in Canadian Eskimos. *Canadian Medical Association Journal*, 103(10), 1059–1068.

Schaefer, O. (1973). The changing health picture in the Canadian north. *Canadian Journal of Ophthalmology*, 8, 196–204.

Schaefer, O. (1986). Adverse reactions to drugs and metabolic problems perceived in northern Canadian Indians and Eskimos. *Progress in Clinical and Biological Research*, 214, 77–83.

Schanfield, M., Crawford, M., Dossetor, J., & Gershowitz, H. (1990). Immunoglobulin allotypes in several North American Eskimo populations. *Human Biology: An International Record of Research*, 62(6), 773–789.

Schieb, L. J., Ayala, C., Valderrama, A. L., & Veazie, M. A. (2014). Trends and disparities in stroke mortality by region for American Indians and Alaska Natives. *American Journal of Public Health Suppl 3*, 104(53), S368–S376.

Seale, J. P., Shellenberger, S., & Spence, J. (2006). Alcohol problems in Alaska Natives: lessons from the Inuit. *American Indian and Alaska Native Mental Health Research. (Online)*, 13(1). Available at <http://proquest.umi.com.proxy.consortiumlibrary.org/pqdlink?did=1075791431&Fmt=3&clientId=23364&RQT=309&VName=PQD> Accessed July 22, 2010.

Seltzer, A. (1980). Acculturation and mental disorders in the Inuit. *Canadian Journal of Psychiatry*, 25(2), 173–181.

Seltzer, A. (1983). Psychodynamics of spirit possession among the Inuit. *Canadian Journal of Psychiatry*, 28(1), 52–56.

Singleton, R. J. (2006). Decline in respiratory synctial virus hospitalization in a region with high hospitalization rates and prolonged season. *Pediatric Infectious Disease Journal*, 25(12), 1116–1122.

Singleton, R., Bruce, M., Zulz, T., & Klejka, J. (2009). *Four cases of* Haemophilus influenzae *type B—southwestern Alaska, 2009*. Anchorage, AK: Alaska Section of Epidemiology. Available at <http://www.epi.hss.state.ak.us/bulletins/docs/b2009_19.pdf> Retrieved January 21, 2015.

Snyder, C. W., Muensterer, O. J., Sacco, F., & Safford, S. D. (2014). Helmet use among Alaskan children involved in off-road motorized vehicle crashes. *International Journal of Circumpolar Health, 73*, 1–6. doi:10.3402/ijch.v73.25191.

Stefansson, V. (1969). *The friendly Arctic.* New York: Greenwood.

Stevenson, M. (1984). Tuberculosis in the North: a lifestyle issue. *Canadian Nurse, 80*(1), 41–43.

Strayer, H. D., Lucas, D. L., Hill-Jilly, D. C., & Lincoln, J. M. (2010). Drowning in Alaska: Progress and persistent problems. *International Journal of Circumpolar Health, 69*(3), 253–264.

Suryaprasad, A., Byrd, K. K., Redd, J. T., Perdue, D. G., Manos, M. M., & McMahon, B. J. (2014). Mortality caused by chronic liver disease among American Indians and Alaska Natives in the United States, 1999–2009. *American Journal of Public Health Suppl 3, 104*(53), S350–S357.

Szathmary, E. J. E. (1984). Peopling of northern North America: clues from genetic studies. *Acta Anthropogenetica, 8*(1 & 2), 79–109.

Taylor, C. (1988). Trauma prevention in rural Alaska. *Journal of Emergency Nursing, 14*(5), 36A–39A.

U.S. Department of Commerce, Bureau of the Census (2013). *State & County Quick Facts: Alaska.* Available at <http://quickfacts.census.gov/qfd/states/02000.html> Retrieved November 18, 2014.

U.S. Department of Labor (2014a). *Local area unemployment statistics.* Available at <http://www.bls.gov/laus/laumstrh.htm> Retrieved November 20, 2014.

U.S. Department of Labor (2014b). Unemployment in September 2014, *TED: The Economics Daily.* Available at <http://www.bls.gov/opub/ted/2014/ted_20141007.htm> Retrieved November 20, 2014.

VanDenBerg, J., & Minton, B. (1987). Alaska native youth. *Children Today, 16*(5), 15–18.

Van Rens, G. H., Arkell, S. M., Charlton, W., & Doesburg, W. (1988). Primary angle-closure glaucoma among Alaskan Eskimos. *Documenta Ophthalmologica, 70*(2–3), 265–276.

Varnado, M. (2008). Frostbite. *Journal of Wound, Ostomy, and Continence Nursing, 35*(3), 341–346.

Vassilou, M. S. (2009). *Historical dictionary of the petroleum industry.* Lanham, MD: Scarecrow.

Vaudrin, B. (n.d.). *Native/non-Native communication: creating a two-way flow.* Accessed through the Alaska Special Service Agency Education Library at <http://sesa.org/search/node/Vaudrin> Retrieved December 10, 2014.

Veazie, M., Ayala, C., Schieb, L., Dai, S., Henderson, J. A., & Cho, P. (2014). Trends and disparities in heart disease mortality among American Indians and Alaska Natives, 1990–2009. *American Journal of Public Health Suppl 3, 104*(53), S359–S367.

Ward, J. I., Lum, M. K., Hall, D. B., Silimperi, D. R., & Bender, T. R. (1986). Invasive *Haemophilus influenzae* type B disease in Alaska: background epidemiology for a vaccine efficacy trial. *Journal of Infectious Diseases, 153*(1), 17–26.

Whalen, D. (1999). Cultural sensitivity: a matter of respect. *Canadian Nurse,* 43–44.

Wiggins, C. L., et al. (2008). Cancer among American Indians and Alaska Natives in the United States, 1999–2004. *Cancer, 113*(S5), 1142–1152.

Williamson, R. (1974). *Eskimo underground social-cultural change in the Canadian central Arctic. Occasional papers* (Vol. 2). Uppsala, Sweden: Institutet för Allmän och Jämförande, Etnografi, Uppsala University.

Wilson, J., Rausch, R., McMahon, B., & Schantz, P. (1992). Parasiticidal effect of chemotherapy in alveolar hydatic disease: review of experience with mebendazole and albendazole in Alaskan Eskimos. *Clinical Infectious Diseases, 15*(2), 234–249.

Wind, S., Van Sickle, D., & Wright, A. (2004). Health, place and childhood asthma in southwest Alaska. *Social Science & Medicine, 58*(1), 75–88.

Wong, C. A., et al. (2014a). American Indian and Alaska Native infant and pediatric mortality, United States, 1999–2009. *American Journal of Public Health, Suppl 3, 104*(53), S320–S328.

Wong, C. A., et al. (2014b). Supplemental materials to American Indian and Alaska Native infant and pediatric mortality, United States, 1999–2009. *American Journal of Public Health, Suppl 3, 104*(53), S320–S328. Available at <http://ajph.aphapublications.org/doi/suppl/10.2105/AJPH.2013.301598> Retrieved December 8, 2014.

World Almanac and Book of Facts. (2015). New York: Infobase.

Young, T. K. (1986). Epidemiology and control of chronic disease in circumpolar Eskimos/Inuit populations. *Arctic Medical Research, 42*, 25–47.

Zegura, S. L. (1984). The initial peopling of the Americas: an overview from the perspective of physical anthropology. *Acta Anthropogenetica, 8*(1–2), 1–21.

Japanese Americans

Dawn Liam Doutrich and Yoshiko Yamashita Colclough

BEHAVIORAL OBJECTIVES

After reading this chapter, the nurse will be able to do the following:

1. Describe the influence of acculturation on Japanese Americans.
2. Develop sensitivity and understanding of the communication styles within and across the Japanese American culture to avoid stereotyping and to provide culturally appropriate care.
3. Describe the time orientation of some Japanese American people and its influence on wellness and illness behavior.
4. Discuss the spatial needs and implications for culturally appropriate care for the Japanese American client.
5. Discuss the influence of family and social organization on behavior.
6. Explain the health care beliefs, folk beliefs, and folk practices of Japanese Americans and their influence on health-seeking behaviors.
7. Recognize physical, biological, and psychological variances that exist within and across the Japanese American culture to provide culturally appropriate care.

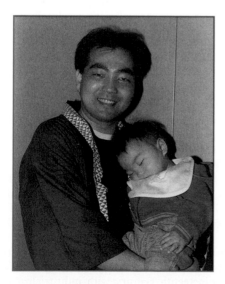

OVERVIEW OF JAPAN

Japan is a chain of islands that stretches in an arc more than 145,914 square miles (377,914 square km) long from the twenty-fourth parallel, off Taiwan, north to the forty-fifth parallel, just below Sakhalin Island (*World Almanac*, 2015). Japan lies just east of the Asian mainland. The Ryukyu chain, which lies southwest, was once United States–occupied territory. Similarly, the Kuriles, which are northwest, are Russian occupied. The Tsushima Strait separates Japan from Korea.

Japan is composed of four large, closely grouped islands—Hokkaido, Honshu, Shikoku, and Kyushu—and 4000 smaller islands. In landmass, Japan is 145,898 square miles. The four main islands constitute approximately 98% of the total landmass of the country. By comparison, Japan is just slightly smaller than California (*World Almanac*, 2015). The habitable and uninhabitable terrain of Japan roughly composes 0.3% of the world's total landmass, yet the population of this country accounts for 3% of the world's population. In 2014, Japan had the tenth largest population in the world, with 127,103,388 people (*World Almanac,* 2015). Because the Japanese landscape is mountainous with angled slopes, only 15% of the total land area is habitable (*World Almanac,* 2015), which accounts for the density of the population in certain regions of the country. In fact, the population of Japan is so dense that there are 873 people per square mile (320 square km). If the uninhabitable areas of Japan were excluded from this equation, a more realistic figure of 3885 people for every 1500 square yards (1760 yards equals a mile) would emerge (*World Almanac,* 2015).

The population explosion of Japan is attributed to industrialization; the population reached 65 million by 1930. After World War II, the Japanese government initiated a population policy to lower the rate of increase. Since the mid-1950s, the population growth rate has corresponded to those in Western European countries (*World Almanac,* 2015). In 2014, the birth rate for Japan was reported to be 6.07 per 1000, with the infant mortality at 2.13 per 1000 live births (Central Intelligence Agency [CIA], 2015). The average life expectancy at birth was 79.5 years for males and 86.3 years for females in 2010 (Ministry of Health, Labour, and Welfare, 2014). A declining rate of population growth, coupled with an increased average life expectancy, has resulted in the Japanese population becoming the most rapidly aging population in the world (*World Almanac,* 2015). This has prompted the Japanese government to develop long-term care insurance, to explore incentives for child-bearing, and to look carefully at current exclusionary immigration policies, a contentious political issue (McNeill, 2006; Onishi, 2005).

The capital of Japan is Tokyo, and with a population of 8.946 million (Statistics Bureau, 2014) and 3.533 million in the urban surrounding areas, Tokyo is among the largest cities by population in the world (United Nations, 2014; World Population Review, 2014). Although Tokyo–Yokohama (often considered together) is a densely populated city, it sprawls over only 800 square miles (2000 square kilometers) (*Time Almanac,* 2013; *World Almanac,* 2015). Tokyo is largely industrial and is the home of the Tokyo Stock Exchange (the Nikkei counterpart to the New York Stock Exchange), which is a barometer for the economic climate throughout the world.

Hokkaido is the least populated island in Japan. It is an industrial site where agriculture, leisure activities, and brew-making dominate the economy. Honshu is the island on which approximately 80% of the Japanese people reside, with the majority concentrated in the plains of Kanto (Tokyo) and Kansai (Kyoto-Osaka). Honshu is known for its distinctive business culture, major ports, and multiple airports (*World Almanac,* 2015). Shikoku is devoted primarily to agriculture. It is a subtropical island, and the

people are reputedly the most outgoing of all Japanese. Kyushu, the third largest island of Japan, is located in the southwest and close to Korea and China. There are bullet train services to anywhere in Honshu and Kagoshima in Kyushu.

The Ryukyu chain of islands was occupied by the United States from World War II until 1972 and is perhaps the poorest of all the regions in Japan. Several of the islands in the Ryukyus are uninhabited. Okinawa is one of the major islands in the Ryukyus and a major staging base for the U.S. Air Force and Army, another political issue for many Japanese (*World Almanac,* 2015).

In Japan, there are approximately 60 active volcanoes. In addition, Japan sustains approximately 1000 earthquakes a year, although most result only in minor damage (*World Almanac,* 2015). Three significant exceptions are the Great Kanto Earthquake of 1923, which killed over 100,000 people in the Tokyo and Yokohama area; the Great Hanshin Earthquake of 1995, which killed 6000 and injured 415,000 people in the Kobe area (CIA, 2015; *World Almanac,* 2015); and the third, the Tōhoku earthquake (also called the Great East Japan Earthquake), which registered a 9.0-magnitude and hit Japan on March 11, 2011. It triggered a large tsunami. According to the Japanese National Police Agency (2014), 15,889 people lost their lives due to the combined earthquake and 30-foot tsunami. The Tōhoku earthquake was the most powerful earthquake ever recorded to hit Japan, and the tsunami it triggered resulted in nuclear reactor core damage and meltdowns in the Fukushima prefecture, disasters taken together that shocked the world. Other than earthquakes and occasional typhoons, climatic conditions in the Japan archipelago are usually mild, with sufficient warmth and humidity in the summer for cultivation. Winters are cool and dry, unlike the subtropical and tropical winters of much of the rest of Asia. Significant seasonal changes vary with the direction of the prevailing wind, like much of monsoon Asia (*World Almanac,* 2015).

Although more than 67% of the total land area of Japan is forested, not all forests have commercial value because soil erosion is a problem. The sea provides the major portion of protein in the Japanese diet. Both the Sea of Japan and the Pacific Ocean are rich fishing grounds. Japan's fishing catch has been the world's largest since 1972. Japan has few mineral resources and depends on imports of raw materials and fuel (*World Almanac,* 2015).

Historically, Japan has primarily had an agriculture-based economy. The economy has changed rapidly since the late nineteenth century with industrialization, especially after World War II. Today, Japan is considered the most urbanized country in Asia.

The *Ainu,* whose name means "human," are known to be the original inhabitants of Japan. Nakamura (2005) contends that although official estimates place Ainu populations around 2% (23,000) of the Japanese, these are likely underestimates and there are more contemporary Ainu who chose not to self-identify because of fears of racism and discrimination. The ancestors of the Japanese are believed to have come from mainland Asia, crossing over from Korea. These early settlers moved eastward from Kyushu and settled in the Kansai Plain (Kyoto–Osaka regions). Eventually, they established an ordered society under chieftains who were dedicated to the cult of the sun. Buddhism was later introduced in the sixth century. The ethics of Confucianism were added to the practice of sun worship and animism (*Shinto*) (Storry, 1993). The Ainu once maintained a culture and language that are different from the rest of the Japanese; however, the Ainu language is now almost extinct.

Except for the Ainu, the Japanese population tends to perceive itself as ethnically and linguistically homogeneous (Yamamura, 2008). Yet there are significant numbers of long-term resident foreigners now living in Japan—over 2 million as of 2012 (Immigration Bureau of Japan, 2014). Included are Chinese (674,879), Koreans (545,879), Japanese-Brazilians (210,032), Filipinos (209,376), and 52,843 Peruvians in 2011 (Immigration Bureau of Japan, 2014). The foreign-born labor force in Japan is estimated at 686,000 in 2011 (Ministry of Health, Labour, and Welfare, 2014). Although this is not a large percentage of the population, it does suggest the homogenous label may be misleading.

IMMIGRATION

Today the ability of Japanese Americans to identify with Japanese culture depends largely on when they arrived, their historical trajectory, whether they were born in the United States, where they live, and how much acculturation and assimilation have occurred. The term *Nikkei* refers to all individuals of Japanese ancestry and includes Japanese Americans who have been in the United States for many generations and those who came recently (Machizawa & Lau, 2010). Among the various ethnic groups in the United States, a clear generational distinction among Japanese American groups is not only unique but also meaningful (Fugita & O'Brian, 1991; Machizawa & Lau, 2010). This distinction highlights different characteristics of Japanese Americans, including values and beliefs the immigrants from Japan brought with them, what they retained and passed on to their offspring, and the impact of historical events and laws on their experience and acculturation.

Before the 1890s a few Japanese scholars and businessmen came to the United States and settled along the East Coast. Because of their small numbers and desire to be acculturated and assimilated into the mainstream society in the United States, they were more readily accepted than later immigrants. The large influx of Japanese immigrants between 1890 and 1924 settled primarily along the West Coast and in Hawaii. Because of the prejudice they experienced, their lack of knowledge about the new country, and the language barrier, they tended to keep to themselves and formed relatively self-sufficient communities where they were able to retain familiar cultural values. *Nisei,* second-generation Japanese Americans, were largely influenced by the values and norms of their parents. However, third- and fourth-generation Japanese Americans may be less familiar with the Japanese language and customs.

To recap, the Japanese American people are the only immigrant group to identify themselves by the generation in which they were born, and these generation groups are distinguishable by the individual's age, experience, language, and values. The generation groups are the *issei,* the first generation to live in the United States; the *nisei,* the second generation; the *sansei,* the third generation; the *yonsei,* the fourth generation; the *gosei,* the fifth generation; and the *rokusei,* the sixth generation (Hashizume & Takano, 1983). These generational categories provide a framework for understanding family-related cultural values. For the *issei,* the family provided the anchor for the values and traditions of Japan. Today the family remains one of the most important factors in the lives of the Japanese people. The *issei* withstood extreme hardships and made personal sacrifices for the benefit of their children. Before the 1890s, the majority of Japanese persons who immigrated to the United States were men. Generally speaking, it often took many years before a Japanese man was able to afford a wife or family. These men might have been 30 or 40 years of age before they looked back to Japan to find their brides through the exchange of photographs and letters. Thus these Japanese women were often 10 to 20 years younger than their husbands. For the *issei* descendants, there was a strong, stable family support system. The exclusion law of 1924 prevented some of the early Japanese male immigrants from finding a spouse, which resulted in a group of single elderly men; however, most of these are no longer living.

The *nisei* were born in the United States during the pre–World War II period. Although this generation tended to have a higher educational level and was more fluent in English than their parents, they still faced intense racial discrimination in housing and employment (Sato & Takano, 1983). Hostile feelings on the part of many U.S. citizens intensified in 1942 with the declaration of the war with Japan. This sentiment climaxed with the evacuation and internment of Japanese Americans when President Roosevelt signed executive orders 9066 and 9102. Although restrictions applied to Japanese, German, and Italian aliens on the West Coast, only the Japanese, both alien and U.S.-born, were removed from their homes in California, Washington, Oregon, Arizona, and Hawaii and forcibly placed in internment camps (Daniels, Taylor, & Kitano, 1991; Strazar & Fisher, 1996). More than 120,000 persons were imprisoned. The experiences of those who survived are well documented (Houston & Houston, 2002; Yates, Kuwada, Potter, Cameron, & Hoshino, 2007; Yoo, 2000). Missing, however, are the accounts by those who did not survive or whose lives were broken and warped by this experience. During the internment, 6485 Japanese Americans were born in the camps, and 1990 Japanese Americans died in the camps (Daniels et al., 1991).

The evacuation and internment of the Japanese in U.S. camps have been described as the most dehumanizing experience for Japanese Americans. It not only disrupted their families and way of life but also had enormous financial implications that were largely created from the loss of their homes and businesses. To prove their loyalty as Americans and combat the racism that confronted them, an overwhelming number of *nisei* volunteered for the all-*nisei* 100th Infantry Battalion and its larger unit of Japanese Americans, the 442nd Regimental Combat Team (Kakesako, 1993; Yoshishige, 1993). These volunteers, who came from Hawaii and mainland internment camps, emerged as the most decorated unit for its size and duration of service (Chang, 1993).

After the war, the employment and cultural expectations of Japanese Americans from the *nisei* became more aligned with their American background. As this new generation became more acculturated, they began to rely less on the economic sanction of their *issei* fathers. These individuals sought a better way of life and upward mobility. The GI Bill offered many veterans a chance at a first-class education. Japanese Americans have been extremely successful in the assimilation process, particularly in certain states. In Hawaii, successful inroads have been made, particularly in the political arena (Burris, 1993; Okamura, 2014). Succeeding generations of Japanese Americans have benefited tremendously from the efforts of these earlier immigrants. Recognition of Japanese American rights and political power occurred, after a decade-long campaign, when the U.S. Congress passed the Civil Liberties Act of 1988 to make redress payments of $20,000 to each survivor who had been incarcerated during World War II (Daniels, 1991). Formal apologies occurred around this time. And, in 1993, then President Bill Clinton signed a presidential letter of apology that stated the "nation's actions were

rooted deeply in racial prejudice, wartime hysteria, and a lack of political leadership" (Dickerson, 2010, p. 230). In 2001, Congress appropriated funding to preserve ten of the detention sites, including Manzanar and Tule Lake. Besides lasting long-term psychological consequences like post-traumatic stress syndrome, health consequences of internment included increased cardiovascular disease and mortality. It is important to remember that the history of forced internment is a primary difference between early Japanese Americans and their descendants and recent Japanese immigrants

In 1965, with the lifting of the immigration restrictions based on race, creed, and nationality, Japanese immigrants were able to reestablish the continuity of family life (Kobata, 1979). Japanese Americans who immigrated after World War II may be called *shin-issei*, which means "new first generation." Many *shin-issei* came for business reasons or as brides of servicemen after World War II, the Korean Conflict, or the Vietnam War. Others immigrated more recently and some married U.S. citizens. Since these individuals grew up in Japan, their lives, values, and beliefs tend to differ somewhat from those of the descendants of the original *issei* (Fugita & O'Brien, 1991; Machizawa & Lau, 2010).

Life in the United States

In 2010, 763,325 Japanese Americans (designated as *Asian alone* on the census) resided in the United States (U.S. Department of Commerce, Bureau of the Census, Asian Population, 2012). This number represents a 0.3% increase in the population of Japanese Americans since the 1990 census, currently the slowest growth among Asians in the United States. When Japanese and one other Asian group are reported, however, 1,304,286 people designated themselves in the 2010 census survey as Japanese. This number includes multiracial individuals. Japanese Americans are reported as having the highest proportion (41%) of interracial identity among all Asian Americans (Pew Research Center, 2012). Overall, multiracial Japanese Americans represent 13.9% of the total Asian American population. Of the number of Japanese Americans residing in the United States, for the first time, geographic distribution has changed: 71% live in the West, 22.1% live in the South, 8% live in the Midwest, and 8.5% live in the Northeast. By state, the largest populations of Japanese Americans are found in California (33%), Hawaii (24%), New York (4%), and Washington (5.2%). They tend to live in the larger West Coast cities (U.S. Department of Commerce, Bureau of the Census, 2012; U.S. Department of Commerce, Bureau of the Census, 2012).

Whereas the median age of Asian Americans is 36.8 years, it is approximately 38.2 years for Japanese Americans in 2008 (Yamamura, 2008). In the United States, Japanese Americans are the oldest group of Asians by median age, and with one of the longest life expectancies of any American racial/ethnic group, "Japanese Americans constitute the country's oldest racial/ethnic group with almost 22% age 65 and older compared to about 13% in the overall U.S. population" (Lau, Machizawa, & Doi, 2012, p. 150). Of the number of Japanese Americans residing in the United States between 1980 and 2009, 20% were foreign born, compared with 12.4% of Japanese Americans living in the United States before 1975. These data suggest that immigration has played a major role in the increase in numbers of Japanese Americans in the United States (U.S. Department of Commerce, Bureau of the Census, Asian Population, 2012).

Japanese Americans, on the average, have 2.4 persons per family, compared with the national average of 2.6 persons per family. This number is in stark contrast to some other Asian groups whose family size may be considerably larger (Pew Research Center, 2012).

In 2010, the median family income for Japanese Americans was $65,050 as compared with $49,800 (Pew Research Center, 2012) for all other races/ethnicities. Likewise, Japanese Americans tend to be better educated than the U.S. population, with 46% of Japanese American adults 25 or older having earned a bachelor's degree or higher, while only 28% of the U.S. population has obtained this (Pew Research Center, 2012).

Asian Americans enjoy the longest life expectancy compared with other racial and ethnic groups residing in the United States. The life expectancy of Asian Americans regardless of gender is 83 years. By subpopulations, the life expectancy is 86 years for Chinese Americans, 85 years for Filipino Americans, and 85 years for Japanese Americans (National Center for Health Statistics, Health, United States, 2014).

COMMUNICATION

Communication and Culture

The official language in Japan, which is spoken by some 190 million inhabitants, is Japanese. Three systems (glyphs) are used concurrently to communicate in writing in Japanese. In the Japanese language, one system includes the *kanji*, or *honji*, ideographic or pictographic characters borrowed from the Chinese and used to express chief meanings of words, such as substantive and root meanings of verbs and adjectives (Iwasaki, 2006). *Kanji* characters may have concepts embedded. For example, the *kanji* for human, *hito*, implies "an individual who is supported by another" (Minami, 1985, p. 316). The kanji is composed of two sticks leaning inward against each other; without one,

the other falls, pictographically signifying the interconnectedness of the Japanese self. In addition to *kanji*, there are two syllabic scripts, *hiragana* and *katakana* (Iwasaki, 2006). *Hirigana* is the phonetic "alphabet" used to represent Japanese words, whereas *katakana* is used as the phonetic representation of foreign words (Unger, 2006). The *katakana* are also used in official documents and advertisements. Today, *Romaji*, from the Latin alphabet, is often used in modern Japanese, particularly for such things as company names and advertising, and especially for inputting Japanese into the computer. Western-style Arabic numbers are more commonly used for numbers when used in a left-to-right writing style, whereas traditional Chinese and Japanese numberings are more commonplace in the verbal communication of 1 to 10 and an up-and-down writing style in Japanese language.

Of the number of Japanese Americans residing in the United States, 0.7% speak an Asian or a Pacific Islander language at home, 84.9% speak English "very well" or "well," and 15.1% are linguistically isolated (Ryan, 2013).

Style. Japanese characteristics in language and behavior reflect characteristics of some of the values inherent in this ethnic group. A side note about the citations included in the sections of this chapter concerning culture and values is included here. Many of the citations come from classic anthropological or intercultural communication studies. These are dated, yet culture and values tend to remain stable and constant with change occurring incrementally over generations. In particular, cultural consistency has tended to be valued by the Japanese. For these reasons, the classic findings should still be considered relevant. The Japanese culture is known as the "culture of anticipatory perception" or "culture of consideration" because of the importance of empathizing with the speaker (Lebra, 1976). A concept central to the issue of communication is "empathic identification." The speaker identifies with and views the listener from the listener's point of view. The expectation is that the listener will also empathize with the speaker. Thus, verbal communication can be held to a minimum. For some Japanese Americans, constant verbal communication is seen as unnecessary. Many Japanese Americans value communication that is implicit, nonverbal, and intuitive over explicit, verbal, and rational (Hsu, Tseng, Ashton, McDermott, & Char, 1985). Therefore, communication may be seen by outsiders as less direct, somewhat vague, and somewhat concealing. A talkative person may be considered a "show-off" or insincere (Rogers & Izutsu, 1980). There is an underlying assumption that when true connected caring communication is happening, there is little need for words (Doutrich, 2000).

Behavior and communication are defined by role expectancy and status and by an attempt to preassess the listener's feelings or wishes. According to Schon and Ja (2005), the content of communication depends on the characteristics of the persons involved. Factors such as age, sex, education, social status, family background, and marital status often influence specific behaviors. Behaviors that may be seen as negative or resistive in Western culture may, in fact, be reflective of proper upbringing for some Japanese Americans. Openness may be construed as a sign of immaturity or lack of self-control, which may bring shame to the family.

Context. In a high-context culture such as Japanese, implicit nonverbal messages are of central importance; in multiethnic low-context cultures, explicit verbal messages are emphasized (Hall, 1976). Behaviors of individuals in a high-context culture tend to reflect the value of thinking before speaking, of modesty in acts and speech. In this sense, context is also viewed as intuitive. This concept is related to the context of empathy, with its value on sensitivity and responsiveness. It is essential for the speaker to avoid superficiality and poor subtleties of speech if intuitive understanding is to occur (Lebra, 1976). In addition, in a high-context culture, esthetic refinement and sophistication are evident in nonverbal, indirect, implicit, subtle messages. Thus, it is not surprising that some Japanese Americans may be threatened by or avoid ambiguous situations (Matsumoto, 1989).

Linguistics. The grammatical structure of a language frequently reflects the major theme of a culture (Johnson, Marsella, & Johnson, 1974). Four themes relating to verbal behaviors in Japanese Americans govern interactions: (1) a strong sense of gender differences, (2) a concern for hierarchy and status that manifests itself as deference toward authority, (3) an emphasis on self-effacement, and (4) a focus on nonverbal communication. These themes can be seen in the primacy of hierarchical status in the Japanese culture, where themes of the Meiji era (post-1868) of Japan and Confucian doctrines still dominate social behavior among many Japanese Americans.

Oral Language. The Japanese culture stresses nonverbal communication, and for some Japanese Americans there may be a general mistrust of spoken words (Leong, 1986). Lebra (1976) attributes this characteristic to a belief held by some Japanese Americans that indicates that the *ma-gokoro* ("true-heart," thus the innermost self) is incapable of being adequately or sincerely expressed through an outer part of the body such as the mouth, which is inclined toward deception. Directly related to the *ma-gokoro* is the importance of personal self as the monitor of self-identity.

Again, words are perceived as a poor substitute for the adequate expression of sincere feelings.

Self-abasement, modesty, and apology used by Japanese Americans when communicating are viewed by some health care professionals as self-effacing behaviors. Many health care professionals believe that this type of behavior is open to misunderstanding. Yet the complex meanings behind these attitudes and behaviors can be understood by the concept of *enryo,* which directs Japanese Americans to be modest, to defer to others, to play down personal accomplishments and achievements, and to direct attention away from oneself (Adler, 1998; Akimoto & Sanbonmatsu, 1999). *Enryo* by near translation means "restraint," "holding back," or "hesitancy" (Doi, 1973; Machizawa & Lau, 2010). It also may be thought of as "ritualized verbal self-deprecation used to maintain group harmony" (Gudykunst & Nishida, 1994, p. 29). For some Japanese Americans, self-praise or the acceptance of praise is considered poor manners, resulting in denying, ignoring, or negating another trait or behavior. To many Westerners, this behavior may be interpreted as lack of self-esteem or belittling (Chang, 1981).

The concepts of hierarchy and status also dictate communication patterns. For some Japanese Americans, it is considered impolite to disagree publicly with a person of higher status for fear of making this individual lose face. In traditional Japanese society, gender differences are reflected by males tending to be more economical in speech, particularly in public situations, and more direct in their delivery of opinions or ideas than their female counterparts (Johnson, Marsella, & Johnson, 1974). Oral expression is focused on increasing harmony and avoiding conflict (Chang, 1981; Fisher, 1996). Therefore, answering "yes" to questions may be a way of avoiding embarrassment or shame and does not necessarily imply that communication is agreed with, clear, or understood (Fisher, 1996). Leong (1986) concluded that Asian Americans are more likely to avoid having to express themselves verbally.

In studying communication apprehension among individuals in Japan, Korea, and the United States, Klopf, Cambra, and Ishii (1981) found that the Japanese frequently expressed feelings of nervousness and anxiousness. In some instances, these feelings made some of these individuals generally awkward and unsociable when communicating with strangers, particularly persons from different cultures. Furthermore, when some Japanese Americans become distressed, their communication may default to metaphors and idioms (Marsella, 1993).

Voice Quality. Vocal qualifiers include intensity, volume, pitch, and rate or speed (Ishii, 1987). In general, Japanese speak in a high-pitched voice, which may relate to the love of traditional folk songs (*minyo*) and sentimental nostalgic songs (*enka*), which call for high-pitched voices. Gender differences are also manifested in the manner in which women are expected to speak.

Nonverbal Communication

The Japanese culture is a relatively non–eye contact culture, and this is quite noticeable in public speaking and in the communication process (Ishii, 1987). Most Asian Americans consider it disrespectful to look someone directly in the eyes, especially if that person is in a superior position (Galanti, 1997). In nonverbal communication, integral quality and explicitness of feelings are involved in the process itself and are communicated paraverbally rather than directly. High awareness of nonverbal gestures and facial mimetic nuances exist among Japanese Americans (Johnson, Marsella, & Johnson, 1974). For some Japanese Americans, emotional expression of anger is unusual, and a stoic reaction is often manifested as a response to pain. *Gaman* is a Japanese concept that stems from the verb *gamansuru*, which translates as "to bear, to endure, to tolerate" and which has to do with self-control and endurance (Katada, 1991; Kinoshita & Gallagher-Thompson, 2004). Machizawa and Lau's study (2010) of Japanese American elders found that *gaman* had importance in help-seeking behaviors among *nisei* who tended to value enduring pain and discomfort with perseverance and dignity. *Gaman* is also considered a valuable social skill to be learned in childhood and used later in life when facing hardships, such as when in pain.

Related to the development of *gaman*, Katada (1991) noted that nonverbal communication is an emphasized Japanese socialization pattern. Bearing up with quiet self-control is valued and expected to be learned at a young age. In a study of preschool Japanese children, Katada found that some Japanese as young as 4 years old could verbalize the need for *gaman*. In this study, one child was able to suggest strategies (e.g., adequate information about what to expect with surgery) that would have aided him in his struggle to achieve *gaman*. Thus, there is cultural value placed on "bearing up," or doing *gaman*, which can be described as stoicism in the face of hardships such as pain and uncertainty. Japanese behavior patterns require that an individual be trained to recognize subtle cues of nonverbal communications and finely nuanced choices of words. Although cultural values for *gaman* and expectations for highly acute nonverbal perception are based upon traditional Japanese values, these values have meaning for many Japanese Americans.

Kinesics. Mehrabian (1968) estimates that, for Japanese Americans, communication of feelings and attitudes is 5% verbal, 38% vocal, and 55% facial expression. Thus, facial expression plays a crucial role in communicating emotions

and attitudes. It is essential to remember that the traditional behavior of some Japanese Americans is to control emotions, especially in formal and public situations. This value is believed to have originated in *heijo-shin* ("ordinary state of mind") in Zen Buddhism, which advocates controlling emotions and maintaining a neutral presence. An inappropriate smile may sometimes be seen as an unconscious and reflective attempt to avoid troubling others by showing one's true feelings.

Touch. Japanese culture is viewed as a nontouch culture. A hug is rarely offered and hugging is not common practice. There is close contact with infants but less touch or physical contact among adults (Ishii, 1987). Barnlund (1989) found that Japanese Americans touch family members less frequently than people in other cultures do. Physical contact may be perceived negatively and introduce tension into relationships (Marsella, 1993).

Silence. The ideal and ultimate pattern of communication in Japanese society is silent communication. Some Japanese Americans do not appreciate aggressive or spoken forms of communication and instead place a premium on intuitive understanding of what is being communicated (Doutrich, 2000; Marsella, 1993). Findings from several studies suggest that Japanese adults spend only half as much time in conversation per weekday as their U.S. counterparts (Ishii, 1987; Klopf & Ishii, 1976). The data further suggested that Japanese couples, especially those who had been married for some time and were happy in the relationship, usually remained silent with each other because they had developed *sasshi* ("guesswork" or "intuitive sensitivity"). In other words, they understand each other without speaking. *Sasshi* is also highly appreciated in other situations.

Implications for Nursing Care

Because it is impolite to think of personal needs, some Japanese Americans, when asked if they want something to eat or drink, may respond negatively. In such instances, if the nurse does not try to persuade the client to eat or drink, the nurse may be perceived as insensitive. The nurse should offer at least two to three times, even after receiving a negative reply the first time.

The nurse can learn to anticipate needs and accurately assess discomforts by relying on astute interpretation of the meaning of nonverbal expressions and behaviors. It is essential to remember that subtle facial expressions and gestures are expected to be understood. Japanese American clients may wait silently rather than ask questions because they believe health care providers know best and will meet their needs without being asked (Sato & Takano, 1983). This relates to a high regard for "anticipatory care" and the concept of *omakase* (Wenger, 2007). *Omakase* refers to a coping style that allows the patient to place his or her trust in the physician or nurse; therefore, the health care provider carries the burden for the patient. For the Japanese, health professionals are authority figures and are to be trusted (Suzuki, Kirschling, & Inoue, 1993), although there is recent evidence that this attitude has changed (Tarn et al., 2005). While Suzuki, Kirschling, and Inoue (1993) identified concepts specific to Japan, there are values embedded in the concepts that have migrated with the Japanese Americans. These include a value for hierarchy and trusting authority, an expectation that one will be cared for, and an expectation that one will not have to ask verbally for what one needs but that it will be anticipated by a caring other (Doutrich, 2000, 2001).

Because direct expression of negative feelings is an unusual behavior for some Japanese Americans, indirect messages should not be mistaken for agreement. For example, rather than verbalize to the staff discontent with the health care, the client may have the family request a unit change. Nurses who expect clients to express their feelings through direct action may be surprised when they encounter a Japanese American client who is withdrawn and silent. For the nurse who is unfamiliar with the cultural behaviors of the Japanese American, behaviors in ambiguous, embarrassing, or anxiety-producing situations may be difficult to understand, and the client may be labeled as passive or nonresponsive. For some Japanese Americans, it is extremely important to control expressions of anger or pain. The nurse should be aware of situations that may cause discomfort, such as the exclusion of the family from the plan of care. The nurse must also remember that some Japanese Americans consider it insulting to be addressed by their first names, especially the first generation, who tend to follow strict hierarchical rules of deference and respect.

SPACE

Although there are variations in spatial requirements among individuals, Japanese Americans tend to have a higher tolerance for crowding in public spaces than other Americans (Watson, 1980). Even in relative proximity, a personal space can be created. Time and attention are given to the organization of their living space and perception by the senses (Hall, 1976). Privacy is generally maintained by family members by limiting self-disclosure to persons in binding or trusting relationships (Baker, 1993). For some Japanese Americans, well-manicured gardens can provide a degree of tranquility and peace that tends to expand personal spatial boundaries.

Japanese Americans, like other Asian Americans, tend to use less physical contact when interacting. They may also appear reserved and formal in new situations as they maintain their social zones. However, a contemporary study found that while Asian Americans compared with White Americans differ in the way they perceive crowding, all suffer similar negative psychological distress at high-density housing, independent of household income (Evans, Lepore, & Allen, 2000).

Implications for Nursing Care

Nurses should not misinterpret the reserved and formal behavior manifested by some Japanese Americans as a dysfunctional sign. The nurse should remember that these clients need to establish a caring, trusting relationship before they engage in self-disclosure. Japanese Americans may feel uncomfortable with the overuse of physical contact or the invasion of personal space when interacting. When some Japanese Americans are hospitalized, the nurse can help the client by identifying territorial boundaries within the room. Identification of these territorial boundaries may reduce conflicts created from the invasion of privacy of others, particularly when more than one client shares a room.

SOCIAL ORGANIZATION

Effect of Immigration on Social Organization

Most early Japanese immigrants who remained in the United States, the *issei*, eventually brought their future families to the United States. As their numbers increased, many Japanese immigrants experienced increased racial prejudice. Their fairly self-sufficient subcommunities often served as a buffer and provided for their needs and social support. The traditional Japanese value system places emphasis on the family, group orientation, harmony, and mutual aid (Cheung, Leung, & Tsui, 2013; Fugita & O'Brien, 1991; Yoo, 2000). This value system has allowed the families and communities to survive, particularly during and after World War II. Japanese behaviors and values, such as not imposing on others or standing out, preserving harmony, controlling emotions, persevering, and respecting authority, have allowed them to acculturate rapidly (Adler, 1998). For many Japanese Americans, interdependence and dependence on each other are perceived as very important (Doi, 1973).

As increasing numbers of the *nisei* generation entered adulthood, they sought ways to overcome the personal, economic, and legal barriers that their parents endured. For example, at one point in American history, Japanese Americans were prevented from buying homes in desirable parts of town, using public swimming pools, and entering many professions (Kitano & Daniels, 2001). The early *nisei*, some of them recent college graduates but most still teenagers, wanted to prove their loyalty as Americans and thus combat anti-Japanese sentiment. Citizen organizations sprang up in various West Coast cities in the early 1920s. In 1930, the Japanese-American Citizens League became a national organization (Hosokawa, 2002). Some of the political clout of these organizations can be seen in the successful enactment of an amendment to the Cable Act to permit *nisei* girls who married alien Japanese to regain their citizenship. In addition, a bill was passed to allow foreign-born Asian men who served in the U.S. armed forces in World War I to be granted citizenship. The passage of this bill enabled 700 *issei* to become naturalized citizens (Hosokawa, 2002). And, as mentioned previously, the U.S. Congress has passed laws that specifically address reparations of Japanese Americans interned during World War II.

Ethnic community organizations, such as long-term care services established and expanded by the *nisei* and maintained by the *sansei*, are examples of ways that traditional Japanese values and culture are expressed (Young, McCormick, & Vitaliano, 2002). Japanese American descendants of the *issei* continue to emphasize the importance of caring for their elderly parents. Interestingly, it is important to note that the *issei* generation rarely experienced caring for their own parents because in most cases their parents were in Japan. Increased intermarriage among Japanese Americans and dispersed residency suggest that it might be difficult to pass on aspects of Japanese tradition and ethnicity to future generations. Yet in a recent comparative study of social service environments for elders, 230 Japanese American baby boomers preferred a mixed service environment that included both Japanese-specific and nonethnic-specific activities, preferences that suggest a value related to maintaining elements of Japanese culture (Miyawaki, 2013).

Family Systems

Intergenerational relations are close among most Japanese Americans. There continues to be a flow of goods, money, and services among the generations. The general pattern of the Japanese family is the vertical family structure, with the father and other male members in the topmost position. "Vertical" social structure means that relationships are clearly defined to those above or below, a clearly determined line of social status (Padilla, Wagatsuma, & Lindholm, 1985). In contrast, social structures in the United States have been described as more "horizontal," implying less differentiation among social classes. The phrase *kodomo no tame ni* ("for the sake of the children") reflects the sacrifices and hardships families would endure to ensure the success of the next generation. Many of the activities in the

Japanese family occur in both the nuclear family and the extended family. Problems are handled within this structure, and the achievement or accomplishment of the individual member is a reflection on the entire family (Akiyama, 2008; Jeong & You, 2008; Kitano, 1976).

The younger generation continues to be willing to assist and give more than what is requested and expected by the older generation (Machizawa & Lau, 2010; Osaka, 1979). Yet despite a long-standing tradition of family connection and caregiving, Japanese American families face challenges similar to those of other populations—aging parents, fewer available caregivers, more women in the workforce, and geographic mobility (Lau, Machizawa, & Doi, 2012; McCormick, Imai, & Rubenstein, 1995; Young et al., 2002).

Machizawa and Lau (2010) studied the psychological needs of Japanese American elders. Among other things, they found that there was heterogeneity among this group and that the elders tended to want contact and connection with family but did not want to be burdensome. Many hesitated to directly verbalize need and valued family and social networks. A newer study of community-dwelling Japanese American elders living alone in "Chicagoland" was conducted by Lau, Machizawa, and Doi (2012). This in-depth qualitative study added a more detailed explanation about aspects of support for this population. The authors found the elders relied on family for homemaking and health management but hesitated to lean on family for other types of support. This was primarily due to concerns of being burdensome, worries that there could not be reciprocation of support, and a sense of self-reliance on the part of the elder. Other perceived barriers included family-related interpersonal circumstances like poor communication, distance, and intergenerational differences. The elders relied on partners for emotional and emergency support, on friends for transportation assistance and emotional support, and on neighbors for emergency support. But they also described issues with friend and neighbor interpersonal situations, including difficulty in making "real" friends, relocation, health declines, and the death of friends and neighbors. The authors stated the formal support system (e.g., adult day care and cultural programs) was used by the elders for socializing and learning, and the in-home care formal support was used by the elders "for personal/homemaking assistance and companionship" (p. 149).

For some Japanese Americans, the self is viewed as part of a set of interpersonal relationships, of which the family system is the central core (Fugita, Ito, Abe, & Takeuchi, 1991). In this sense, the self is subordinate to the family social unit, and consequently most Japanese Americans find it difficult to stand out publicly as individuals. This difficulty is evidenced by the reluctance of some Japanese

Americans to give speeches, talk about themselves in casual conversations, or engage in self-serving behaviors.

Fostering of *amae,* or "interdependency," is also seen as a method of enhancing group solidarity and social relationships. This concept is also based on preservation of harmony and the suppression of conflict (Fugita et al., 1991; Kinoshita & Gallagher-Thompson, 2004). *Amae* ("passive love"), as defined by Doi (1962), means "to depend and presume upon the benevolence of others" and is often associated with the Japanese word for "sweet" (*amai*). This relationship may also exist between two people. Some data indicate that this concept is significant for Japanese American families living in the United States (Adler, 1998; Ching et al., 1995; Kinoshita & Gallagher-Thompson, 2004; Kobayashi-Winata & Powers, 1989). In traditional U.S. society, assertiveness is seen by Americans as a characteristic of well-behaved children. For some Japanese-American parents, assertiveness is interpreted instead as a characteristic of the poorly behaved child (Kobayashi-Winata & Powers, 1989). *On* (a sense of obligation within the Japanese hierarchy) forms the basis of reciprocal relationships among peers and within social networks (Fugita et al., 1991).

While intervention and assistance are taken for granted within the family, the in-depth qualitative study of Japanese American elders mentioned previously revealed that a sense of reciprocity is an important component for elder Japanese Americans related to their willingness to receive family support (Lau et al., 2012). Casual help from outsiders is usually avoided because of the concern of becoming entwined in reciprocal relationships with them. The reluctance to accept help from social service agencies may reflect this concern as well as values of stoicism, privacy, and frugality (Lau et al., 2012). According to Kitano (1969), Japanese families traditionally value authoritarian styles of leadership, where the father makes unilateral family decisions. Sue (2004) described the family lifestyle of Chinese and Japanese Americans as patriarchal, with authority and communication exercised from the top down. Sue (2004) also noted that within these families there is a need for interdependent roles, strict adherence to traditional norms, and minimization of conflict by suppression of overt emotion. In a study comparing Japanese and White American couples, Japanese American couples tended to make more unilateral decisions and showed more restraint and less self-disclosure (Hsu et al., 1985). The concepts or values related to guilt and shame may be used to control family members.

Japanese American individuals tend to exhibit close contact among the generations. For some Japanese American families, family obligations take precedence over individual desires. Problems are generally handled within the family, and negative behaviors, such as delinquency, school failure, unemployment, or mental illness, are considered family failures that disrupt the desired harmony of family life and reflect badly on the family. The care of the elderly is generally the responsibility of the oldest son or an unmarried child. Yet there is a rapidly changing context for elderly care in Japan based on the changing demographics and the economic requirement that women work outside the home. Similarly, in the United States, according to a study by Young et al. (2002), changes are taking place in the context and to some degree in the underlying core values related to caretaking among generations of Japanese Americans.

Active discouragement of verbal communication, avoidance of discussion of personal problems, and limited expression of emotion have also been noted as common patterns in the traditional Japanese family (Hsu et al., 1985; McDermott, Tseng, & Maretzki, 1980). However, a number of other studies (Kobayashi-Winata & Powers, 1989; Morris, 1990) have found that a process of cultural change in family norms has become more prevalent across generations of Japanese Americans. There is a tendency to adopt more White American family norms and behaviors. This may be especially due to the higher rate of inter-racial marriages.

This tendency may not be true among elderly Japanese Americans, however. An elders study (Asian American Federation of New York, 2003) in New York City with a sample size of 25 and a mean age of 70 found that study participants endorsed traditional values such as respect and obedience (76%). Decision-making authority continues to primarily rest with the eldest son (96%), the concept of *on* is still important, and approval of their children's mate (96%) and avoidance of divorce for family reasons (92%) are also important. They also viewed generational differences in traditional values as minimal (86.4%).

Among Japanese Americans, there is evidence that participation in U.S. culture may shift personality dimensions toward those endorsed by monocultural U.S. Euro-Americans. A recent study (Güngör, Bornstein, De Leersnyder, Cote, & Mesquita, 2012) indicates that first-generation Japanese American immigrants tend to score in between U.S. Euro-Americans and Japanese nationals on several personality dimensions, including openness to experience, extraversion, conscientiousness, agreeableness, and neuroticism. The Japanese American participants report becoming more "American" and less "Japanese" in their personalities as they participate more with the U.S. culture (Güngör, Bornstein, De Leersnyder, Cote, & Mesquita, 2012). While the Güngör et al. (2012) study explores personality dimensions and the first-generation Japanese

American immigrant experience, Tsuda's (2014) paper, "'I'm not Japanese, I'm American!': The Struggle for Racial Citizenship among Later-Generation Japanese Americans," analyzes the experience of third- and fourth-generation Japanese Americans. Tsuda states that the third and fourth generation are still seen by "mainstream Americans" as "perpetual foreigners" (p. 406). Their Asian phenotype causes them to be challenged and marginalized and threatens their identity as they struggle for national inclusion. Clearly, stereotyping, generalizations, and discrimination by the majority culture continue to be a concern to some Japanese Americans.

Parent–Child Interaction. Methods of child care are inextricably linked not only to the tradition and customs of a culture but also to its systems of values. These methods appear to persist from generation to generation despite the acculturation process. For both the *issei* and the *nisei*, parent–child relationships tended to be intense, with few open expressions of emotion displayed. For these generational groups, there was much tolerance and permissiveness for the child until 5 or 6 years of age, at which time parents began to place emphasis on having the child learn emotional reserve and control.

In a classic study, Caudill and Frost (1974) compared the maternal and child care habits of Japanese Americans with those of Japanese nationals and White Americans to determine the effect on infant behavior. Findings from the study suggest that Japanese American mothers have a closer behavioral style to other Americans than to their Japanese national counterparts. The data also indicate that certain patterns of behavior from their Japanese cultural heritage were retained by these Japanese American mothers and babies. Nonetheless, in contrast to their Japanese counterparts, Japanese American mothers tended to play with their babies for longer times, held their babies more often, and sang to their babies more often (Caudill & Frost, 1974). Further findings from this study also suggested that Japanese American babies did less finger sucking than White American babies and spent less time playing alone (Caudill & Frost, 1974).

In another classic study, in interviews conducted with Japanese Americans in California, Connor (1974) found that the *sansei* were more likely to have a sense of closer family ties; a greater sense of duty, obligation, and deference; less need to dominate; a greater tendency to affiliate; less aggressiveness; a greater need for succor and order; and a greater fear of failure in social role performance than other Americans. These individuals also valued the importance of family and the preservation of the *ie,* which, translated, literally, means "household." However, it can also imply a continuum from past to future members (including the present generation, the dead, and the unborn, as well as a hierarchical structure with the father as head). Notable differences were found in child-rearing practices between Japanese and American parents (Kobayashi-Winata & Powers, 1989). The respondents in this study were Japanese businessmen who lived in Houston. Findings from the study suggested that Japanese parents were less likely than their American counterparts to report the use of external types of punishments, such as time-out or physically and socially punishing the child. A plausible explanation for these differences is the assimilation of American cultural values that place emphasis on independence and individuality. It is believed that insistence on individuality makes it necessary to use powerful, external techniques to ensure compliance in some situations (Kobayashi-Winata & Powers, 1989). In a summary of the literature on the grandparent caregiving role in ethnically diverse families, Kataoka-Yahiro, Ceria, and Caulfield (2004) reviewed grandparents as caregivers in three broad ethnic categories: African-American, Hispanic, and Asian American. They summarized results from 22 articles and three chapters published from 1980 to 2003 and stated that approximately 6 million grandparents are living with their grandchildren. While clearly this role is on the rise in many populations, information on Asian grandparents giving care was limited. In a comparative study of Asian grandparenting, Phua and Kaufman (2008) found younger, U.S.-born, householding grandparents were more likely than to be responsible for their grandchildren, and Asian Indians are less likely than Japanese grandparents to take on this responsibility. Research specifically on Japanese American grandparent caregivers was notable for its absence.

Strazar and Fisher (1996) note that, among Japanese Americans, abortion is not generally condoned but may not be uncommon for numerous reasons. First, some Japanese believe that an unwed mother brings great shame to the family. Second, adoption has become more common in recent times, and often some Japanese Americans will adopt a boy to carry on the family name (Strazar & Fisher, 1996).

Family Role in Education Attainment

The model-minority thesis surfaced in the mid-1960s because of publicity regarding high educational attainment levels, high median family incomes, low crime rates, and absence of juvenile delinquency and mental health problems among Asian Americans (Petersen, 1966). Asian Americans have been portrayed as extraordinary achievers. Mordkowitz and Ginsberg (1987) found that Japanese Americans often reported that their families emphasized educational accomplishment, and this is borne out by the fact that 46% of Japanese Americans 25 or older have at least a bachelor's degree (Pew Research Center, 2012). Many Asian immigrants are willing to sacrifice their own socioeconomic standing in exchange for giving the next generation a better chance to be successful in the world (Chan, 1991). As a result, these students held high expectations of themselves. More importantly, they were able to control their behavior because of the direct relationship between appropriate behavior and personal achievement.

Dornbusch, Ritter, Leiderman, Roberts, and Fraleigh (1987) found that Asian American responses were not significantly different from those of other groups regarding the value of working hard, parental pressures for academic achievement, need for students to make their parents proud, and, most important, avoiding embarrassment to the family. Significant group differences were noted in only one area. Asian Americans were more likely to believe that success in life depends on what is studied in school, which was directly related to the grades they received in high school. According to Sue and Okazaki (1990), a plausible explanation for this behavior is the belief held by some Asian Americans that educational attainment provides opportunities for upward mobility. To the extent that upward mobility is limited in noneducational avenues, education becomes increasingly important as a means for advancement. In addition, education is perceived by some Japanese Americans as a feasible means for mobility in view of limitations for success in other areas. Sue and Okazaki (1990) concluded that the effects of culture have been confused with the consequences of society.

Religion

Some of the ingrained cultural values evident in Japanese Americans are derived from Zen Buddhism, Confucianism, and Shintoism. Today, these values are seemingly manifested in Japanese Americans whether they practice Catholicism, Buddhism, Protestantism, or another religion. From the earliest immigrants, who came from mostly Buddhist backgrounds, the Japanese tended to adopt the religion of the area in which they lived, which resulted in divergent religious beliefs and practices among Japanese Americans in different locales. Religion and the church have both played an important role in acculturating the Japanese within their communities (Adler, 1998; Sato & Takano, 1983).

Shintoism and Buddhism are subscribed to by more than 80% of the Japanese culture in Japan. Christianity is also well established in Japan. In the United States, a great number of Japanese Americans are Christians. Nonetheless, funerals for some Japanese Americans, despite this Christian orientation, are likely to be Buddhist, particularly for the *issei* and the *nisei. Obon,* an important Buddhist observance honoring the ancestors, is celebrated by many Japanese American communities and has spiritual, cultural, and community significance (Nakao, 2005). In addition, for some Japanese Americans, births and marriages are colored by Shinto rituals but to a lesser extent for *yonsei* and *gosei* (Strazar & Fisher, 1996).

Implications for Nursing Care

Because many Japanese Americans place a high value on the family system, the nurse should be aware of the significant role the family plays in providing support, interdependence, and the fulfillment of duties. Respect is also greatly valued, and the linear relationship apparent in families and in casual relationships should be maintained and supported when providing care for the Japanese-American client and family support system. Although these values are the strength of the Japanese-American family, they can create stress and disharmony not only for the client but also for the family unit, especially with inter-racially married offspring. For example, the son- or daughter-in-law may not understand Japanese family values and beliefs well (Lau et al., 2012). It is essential for the nurse to remember that some Japanese American families may want to provide support to the hospitalized family member by keeping a bedside vigil, especially if the individual is elderly and doing poorly. Married men, especially *issei* and *nisei* Japanese Americans, may expect their wives to serve in the traditional caretaker role. Therefore, the wife (or daughter) may be expected to be available at the bedside so that the client does not have to bother the nurses, especially with intimate care or requests for assistance. The nurse must be alert to the overextension and lack of self-care of family members in providing for the client. The nurse should make every effort to assist the family to identify resources, both financial and human, to reduce the stress created when a family member is ill. In addition, the family should be assured that they are not alone. The nurse should not be discouraged if the family initially refuses outside help but rather realize that timing is important. In a study of attitudes toward community-based services among Japanese American families, Young et al. (2002) found that timing and pacing of the resource information were facilitating factors for Japanese Americans in considering services. Moreover, they found that health care providers could play a more active role in assisting families with service identification, information, and evaluation. Because family name and honor are important for this group, the nurse should be especially cognizant of the issue of confidentiality and respect. Information should not be shared with outsiders, even with extended family members who may appear close to the client. Information concerning illness is often kept within the immediate family.

TIME

In a classic 1962 study, Caudill and Scarr examined Kluckhohn's value orientations in Tokyo-area high schools and concluded that time orientations differed by context, with a future focus in technology and a present focus in social relations. The greatest number of generational changes in these values occurred in political considerations, whereas the smallest number occurred in the religious area. In contrast, Chang (1981) believed that this future orientation originated from a religious, philosophical view of life. Buddhism teaches that death in all living things is inevitable. People are instructed not to make plans in this world without reckoning with death. According to Sato and Takano (1983), time is considered valuable and must be used wisely. Hard work in the present is seen as important for future successes (Adler, 1998). For Japanese Americans, the time-person perspective with regard to past, present, and future is perceived in terms of generational distance from Japan. This is reflected in the geo-generational grouping of *issei, nisei,* and so forth (Lyman, 1994). Gudykunst and Nishida (1994) noted that in the United States, monochronic time predominates, which places emphasis on meeting deadlines, making plans, and being prompt. Polychronic time is associated with doing many things at once and is concerned with relationship rather than task completion. They suggest that the Japanese tend to use monochronic time when dealing with outsiders but polychronic time in their interpersonal relations.

Decisions are not necessarily made in relation to individual needs or benefits. Sato and Takano (1983) state that the *issei* perception of time was related to death, in which death is seen as continuous and suprapersonal. This view is in stark contrast to the Western view of death as personal and discontinuous. Depending on the degree of acculturation, the *nisei* also accept death more readily than the *sansei* and the *yonsei,* who are more like Americans in their attitudes toward death and time.

Implications for Nursing Care

Because Japanese Americans are both present and future oriented, the nurse must consider the context of the current situation. The Japanese American client is usually prompt and adheres to fixed schedules. However, Japanese American clients tend to be more prompt with persons they hold in high regard such as physicians than with persons not held in high regard. They generally follow directions concerning medications and treatments. Because of future orientation regarding their children, care must be taken with the children's diet and health. Japanese Americans will work hard with little regard for their health in the hope that future generations will have a better life.

ENVIRONMENTAL CONTROL

Locus of Control

Locus of control refers to the extent to which persons ascribe their successes or failures to internal or external causes. Japanese Americans tend to place more importance on relationships and familial commitments. As such, they tend to also be more externally influenced than persons from Western cultures (Yeh & Huang, 1996). Takemura (2007) noted that the concept of the individual is culturally bound and needs to be understood from an emic or cultural insider's perspective. In the classic work of Hofstede (1984), cultural interpretations using distinct dichotomies such as "individualism-collectivism" and perhaps the internal/external dichotomies of locus of control may assume a Western concept of individualism (consisting of autonomous individuals) as the starting point for the self. Takemura (2007) observed that the Japanese are often portrayed in the greater society as "soldier ants" or "worker bees" who will willingly sacrifice their interests as individuals to contribute to the group. Takemura (2007) cautions against interpreting culture based on false dichotomies, and quotes Hamaguchi (1977) who notes that the concept of the "individual" is not universal. The Japanese self is defined in relation to nature and other persons. In this sense, the Japanese culture is contextual, situational, and relational, rather than collectivistic (Takemura, 2007). In Japanese, the word for "individualism" (*kojin-shugi*) is an ambivalent word, one "suggesting selfishness rather than personal responsibility" (Reischauer, 1977). Noting these fundamental differences in the concept of the self is important when exploring locus of control. Gotay et al. (2004) compared Japanese, Japanese Americans, and European Americans in health attitudes and behaviors. They found that both American groups (Japanese Americans and European Americans) were similar but the Japanese respondents placed less priority on health, had less belief in the efficacy of health screening tests, had lower levels of internal health locus of control (HLOC), and had higher levels of "chance" and "powerful-other" HLOC. The difference in the sense of self to a more individualistic one may in part explain the differences in HLOC.

Illness and Wellness Behaviors and Folk Medicine

Major beliefs that have contributed to medicine in Japan influence the Japanese-American person's view of health and illness. In the Shinto religion, people are seen as inherently good. Evil is caused by outside spirits that cause humans to succumb to temptation and harm, which can be alleviated through purification rites. Disease is believed to be caused by contact with polluting agents, such as blood, corpses, and skin diseases, which accounts for the emphasis on cleanliness (Sato & Takano, 1983; Strazar & Fisher, 1996).

Another important belief held by some Japanese Americans is based on the traditional Chinese concept of harmony and balance among oneself, society, and the universe. Some Japanese Americans believe disharmony (with society or family) or imbalance (as from lack of sleep or exercise or because of poor diet) can cause disease. Therefore, restoration of balance should be the major focus of treatment. In addition, some Japanese Americans believe that illness may cause energy to slow or stop along the meridians of the body. Thus acupuncture, acupressure, massage, or moxibustion may be used to restore the flow of energy (Sato & Takano, 1983).

The *kampo* ("Chinese medicine") medical system was developed around the belief that forces of the universe affect an individual's body processes and activities. Health depends on maintaining a harmonious relationship with the universe. *Kampo* practitioners believe that dietary precautions and preventive measures help resist illness (Ishihara, 1962; Strazar & Fisher, 1996).

Certain foods have special symbolic meaning for Japanese Americans. Special foods, such as soft boiled rice and miso soup (a soup made with fermented soybean paste), may be eaten during illness as well as to promote good health. Traditionally, on their most important holiday, New Year's Day, most Japanese Americans eat special foods that have symbolic meaning for good health, prosperity, and happiness. Such foods include *kazu-no-ko* (dried herring roe) for fertility, *mochi* (steamed rice cake) for longevity and prosperity, *soba* (buckwheat noodles) served in clear broth for longevity and prosperity, and *kuromame* (black beans) for good health (Corum, 2000; Engle, 1993). Other symbolic foods include *ozoni* (a soup with *mochi,* vegetables, and/or meats) for prosperity, *gobo* (burdock root) symbolic of deep family roots, and *tai* (sea bream, a large red fish served whole) for happy occasions.

Although Asian medical traditions recently have regained popularity with the holistic and preventive health movement, most Japanese Americans tend to rely on Western medicine. Some use both Asian and Western medicine, depending on the illness and the efficacy of Western medicine. Yet for those who still subscribe to the Old World traditional health care practices brought with them from Japan, the basis for health practices may include a mixture of traditional medical practices (*kampo*) brought to Japan from China, Shinto beliefs, and Western medical practices (Strazar & Fisher, 1996). Albright et al. (2012) explored sociodemographic and ethnic differences in Hawaii and California for taking dietary supplements. The authors reported the main reasons Japanese Americans take dietary supplements were (1) to maintain a healthy life, (2) because of recommendations by a health professional, and (3) to prevent a disease or medical problem. Japanese Americans participating in the study also believed dietary supplements were as important as prescription medications.

When considering wellness, it is also useful to consider health risk behaviors. Maxwell, Crespi, Alano, Sudan, and Bastani (2012) analyzed health risk behaviors among five Asian American groups (age over 18) in California. Using data from the California Health Interview Survey, they estimated about 80% of Japanese American men had body mass indices (BMIs) of "increased/high risk" by Asian-specific BMI categories, and Japanese American women had one of the highest smoking and binge drinking prevalences among the five Asian American groups. These are concerning findings and can be helpful to inform priority setting for health promotion.

Death, Dying, Death Rituals, and Customs Observed

Meaning of Death and the Afterlife. Many Asian Americans believe death is a natural part of the life cycle; thus, death cannot be overcome through human intervention (Bowman & Singer, 2001; Braun & Nichols, 1997). This is a fundamental Buddhist belief. According to Tsuchida (2007), traditionally the Japanese have an animistic reverence; nature, *shizen,* means "a force that transcends human control and follows its own course of changes or processes." In this sense, for many Japanese, mechanical interventions to prolong life may be difficult to accept. Likewise the acceptance, or recognition, of brain death without an arrested heart may be problematic. In Japan, unlike in the United States, cardiopulmonary resuscitation is not commonly performed out of the hospital or by laypersons. Some Japanese make pilgrimages to Buddhist temples, which are associated with the belief that prayers made at the specific temples will assist the pilgrim in procuring a sudden death. The Japanese preference for a quick death is desired not only because there is less suffering involved but also because a prolonged illness may be a burden to the family (*meiwaku*), whether financially, physically, or psychologically (Bito et al., 2007).

The concepts of *karma* and reincarnation are based on the premise that one's conduct in a previous life affects the condition of the present life. This is also a part of the belief system of some Asian Americans (Braun & Nichols, 1997). For Japanese Americans, an individual's identity and the interpretation of the meaning of life are closely tied to their belief in their ancestors' spirit (Tsuchida, 2007). Therefore, because death is viewed as a natural phenomenon, some Japanese Americans may be better able to accept it when it comes. The Samurai ethos expects one to maintain an attitude of indifference to the minutiae of daily life. Thus, bravery and silent endurance are typical Japanese virtues (Ohara, 2000). Coupled with this is the notion that the bereaved should understand the dying person's last true wishes without there being verbal expression. Because of a strong feeling of connection to offspring consistent with an interdependent self, implicit rather than explicit expression has more weight and value. A strong interrelated society makes it possible to let the dying go without explicitly knowing his or her wishes. Moreover, the Japanese American family may accept the challenge of understanding the wishes of a dying person without explicit discussion since it is viewed as evidence of the closeness of their relationship. *Ishin denshin* (mind-to-mind communication or thought transference) is then put into practice.

Dying Process. Traditionally, the Japanese are willing to discuss death and dying while they are healthy. However, once someone becomes seriously ill, such discussion is difficult. In addition, anything relating to the number four (which has the same pronunciation, *shi,* as the Japanese word for death) and the number nine (pronounced *ku,* which also means suffering) should be avoided. Although fresh flowers are acceptable to give to the dying or the bereaved, a plant gift is considered taboo and is associated with long-term illness. This may be so because for the Japanese, the word for rooting, *ne-zuku,* is similar to the word that means "bedridden." Visiting of the sick by a religious leader is accepted in the United States but may indicate bad luck for some Buddhist Japanese because Buddhist monks are associated with death or funeral rituals. Whether Japanese Americans know their illness and prognosis depends greatly on their own and their family's acculturation level (Bito et al., 2007; Colclough, 2005).

Colclough (2005) and Colclough and Young (2007), in a qualitative study of 16 Japanese Americans, found that although most Japanese Americans preferred family decision making, the older family members tended to share implicit understanding with the ill patient about his or her end-of-life wishes. In contrast, the younger members tended to discuss end-of-life wishes explicitly. Further findings from this study suggest that there are times when the Japanese American patients kept their diagnosis or poor prognosis from their family to protect the family members from psychological burden. Hattori and Ishida (2012), in their qualitative study of elderly Japanese American beliefs about death, found that their participants ($n = 18$), Japanese Americans in Hawaii, highly valued not being a burden to family. Although they expected certain support from family and friends, the participants tried to prepare

their living arrangements and finances to avoid being a burden at the time of death. This avoidance of burdening others was a large component of what they considered "a good death."

Japanese Americans on the West Coast now have options for culturally sensitive long-term care and assisted living facilities (with Japanese language and culturally sensitive providers), and there has been an increased use of these types of care among the Japanese American population. Today, more hospice care is being used among this population (McCormick et al., 1996; Young et al., 2002) although they had a shorter length of stay than other groups of patients (21 days, compared with 32 days for Filipino Americans and 26 days for Whites (Ngo-Metzger, Phillips, & McCarthy, 2008). These researchers indicated that reasons for this were likely related to culture and included a lack of, or delayed, informed consent and a family willingness or sense of obligation to provide care. A possible issue for Japanese and Japanese American families is the practice of *diagnostic disclosure,* the discussion of a terminal diagnosis or poor prognosis with the patient. In the United States, diagnostic truth-telling is based on a concept wherein the patient is considered an autonomous individual, which is a key aspect of informed consent. Diagnostic disclosure is not the norm in all cultures and until recently was not common in Japan where typically the family would be informed first of a terminal diagnosis and they would decide how, when, and whether to inform the patient (Wros, Doutrich, & Izumi, 2004). In a Hawaiian study, Matsui and Braun (2009) surveyed 112 Japanese Americans (mean age 74.7 years, 71% women) and found that the preferred place to receive end-of-life care by their participants was hospice (40%) and home (39%), and more than half (53%) had discussed end-of-life issues with their physician and/or family. Clearly, these patients were aware of their diagnoses and diagnostic disclosure was not an issue.

Death Rituals. For traditional Japanese in the prefuneral period just after death, the body is bathed, dressed, and laid out with the deceased's head pointed toward the North without a pillow. A monk recites *sutras* (Buddhist prayers) at the bedside and gives the deceased a posthumous Buddhist name. This name is later inscribed on the tombstone and on the family's memorial tablet, which is kept in the home in a Buddhist altar. An overnight vigil is held at the home or a funeral site. During the vigil, it is important to keep incense burning, and visitors reminisce about the deceased. Acquaintances visit the site with "incense money" and offer incense during the vigil and/or funeral. Usually, a funeral lasts 2 hours. Cremation occurs right after the funeral, and a reception is held during the cremation. Then immediate family members go back to the crematorium to collect pieces of bones, which are placed into a small jar (urn) and are put under the tombstone or kept on an altar. Weekly ceremonies occur up to the seventh week, and an annual ceremony takes place up to the fiftieth year (not every year). The celebrations occur on the death date, equinox days, and the summer *Obon* festival. The extent to which Japanese Americans follow the traditional rituals depends on their level of religious practice and connections with traditional Japanese culture.

Implications for Nursing Care

Because some Japanese Americans hold traditional value orientations regarding fatalism, they often are perceived as having an external locus of control. The nurse must also remember that some Japanese Americans value self-control, particularly in areas they believe may reflect weakness or inadequacy. The loss of "face" and dignity should be especially considered in procedures and treatment. The desire to *gaman* may affect the Japanese American's willingness to request pain medications. Nurses can offer their time and practice attentive listening skills. Nurses also can make sure the patients and their families understand that it is expected that they express concerns and feelings. One approach from the nurse (particularly to offer pain medications) may not be enough for the patients and their families. Instead it is important to be particularly sensitive with these patients and multiple approaches to offer medications and care are recommended.

The nurse should inquire about treatments the client is using at home and what measures are most helpful. Special foods, tea, or herbal decoctions may be important for the client to have if there are no contraindications. It is very common for family or friends to bring fruit or special Japanese food when visiting. The client and family are likely to show hospitality by offering food to the nurse and visitors. Although it is unusual for the family and the client to hold special religious ceremonies at the bedside, privacy will be needed if such ceremonies are held.

Nagata and Cheng (2003) found that there was difficulty in bringing up a sensitive topic such as the internment experience between *nisei* and *sansei*. The results suggested that it could be difficult to talk about end-of-life issues. Health care providers may need to initiate such a discussion with a gentle suggestion.

BIOLOGICAL VARIATIONS

Body Size

Body size and body composition between Japanese Americans and Japanese nationals were compared in the 1980s. The body fat of males and females in both groups was similar; however, Japanese Americans had significantly greater body weight, fat-free mass, and BMI than Japanese nationals (Tahara, Moji, Muraki, Honda, & Aoyagi, 2003). Japanese Americans tend to be of smaller stature than their Euro-American counterparts. However, rapid Westernization has brought major changes in diet and lifestyle in Japan. As a result, the height of the average Japanese male has increased 4 inches over the past 35 years, with an average height of 5 feet, 7 inches (Ministry of Health, Labour, and Welfare, 2014). Likewise, the height of the average Japanese female has increased 2.7 inches over the past 30 years. In body proportions, Japanese, like other Asian Americans, tend to have longer trunks and shorter limbs than White Americans. They also tend to have wide hips and narrow shoulders (Overfield, 1995). According to the results of a U.S. national health survey, Asian Americans, compared with other ethnic/racial groups in the United States, have the lowest rates of obesity (10.8% vs. 32.6–47.8% [Ogden, Carroll, Kit, & Flegal, 2014]). These data are aggregated Asian American data and do not separate the Japanese American population. Although the percentage of Asian Americans with obesity is low, it appears that the more years a foreign-born Asian American spends in the United States, the higher the risk for being overweight or obese. Among U.S.-born Asian Americans, Japanese Americans are significantly more likely to be obese or overweight than foreign-born Asian Americans (Lauderdale & Rathouz, 2000). These higher incidences may be a result of a combination of diet and lifestyle. Concerns are raised that health risks begin at a lower BMI among Asian Americans compared with others, and a World Health Organization (WHO) expert committee has recommended lower cutoffs for Asians as points for "public health action" (Jih et al., 2014; WHO, 2004).

Skin Color

Skin color varies among Japanese Americans. Some Japanese Americans have more yellow tone than others. One can assess jaundice by looking at the sclerae of the eyes. The amount of sun exposure can make a noticeable difference in the skin color of the same individual.

Other Visible Physical Characteristics

Mongolian spots (bluish pigment from fetal migratory melanocytes), found generally in the lumbosacral region, are present in 80% of Asian infants at birth. They can often be mistaken for bruises (Jacobs & Walton, 1976; Overfield, 1995). Other areas of the skin, such as nipples, areolae, scrotum, and labia majora, are affected by hormones and as a result are often darker in Asian groups than in Whites (Overfield, 1995). Keloid formation varies among Japanese Americans but is greater in this group than in White

Americans. Keloid formations can be cause for concern in highly visible areas.

Eye Shape, Mouth, and Teeth

Japanese Americans are at higher risk for certain types of glaucoma (Aghaian, Choe, Lin, & Stamper, 2004). The central corneal thickness varies among Asian subpopulations, and Japanese Americans have significantly thinner corneas (531.7 μm) than Chinese, Filipinos, Caucasians, and Hispanics. Japanese Americans have a higher incidence of cleft lip and cleft palate than the general U.S. population (Chung & Myrianthopoulos, 1968; Erickson, 1976). When the nurse provides care for a Japanese American with these anomalies, it is essential to remember that these conditions require additional attention through culturally appropriate assessment, teaching, and risk-reduction strategies. In particular, for pregnant women or women of childbearing age, the nurse will want to counsel about the addition of folic acid to the diet to reduce the risk of these and other congenital anomalies (Eichholzer, Tonz, & Zimmermann, 2006). Endo, Ozoe, Kubota, Akiyama, and Shimooka (2006) reported a marked prevalence of hypodontia (fewer than the regular number of teeth) among the Japanese population (8.5% of the prevalence; 10.1% of the prevalence of advanced hypodontia) compared with other populations.

Enzymatic and Genetic Variations

Lactose intolerance occurs in a majority of the population of the world. In fact, it affects 94% of Asians, 74% of American Blacks, and 79% of American Indians, compared with only 17% of White Americans (Bose & Welsh, 1973; Duncan & Scott, 1972; McCracken, 1971; Overfield, 1995). The time when symptoms are first noted and the ability to consume or tolerate different amounts of milk or milk products can vary (Caskey et al., 1977; Lebenthal, Antonowicz, & Schwachman, 1975; Simoons, 1969). Some dietary strategies for individuals who have low levels of the lactase enzyme have been suggested by Jarvis and Miller (2002) to meet calcium recommendations. These include drinking milk with a meal or snack and eating yogurt and cheese low in lactose, such as cheddar, Swiss, and Parmesan.

Drug Interactions and Metabolism

In tuberculosis therapy involving isoniazid, 85% to 90% of Asians rapidly inactivate the drug, compared with 40% of White Americans and 60% of American Blacks (Overfield, 1995; Vessell, 1972). It is important to remember that the gene N-acetyltransferase 2 (NAT2), slow acetylation type, may cause adverse drug reactions in some Asian Americans (Hiratsuka et al., 2002). Asian clients must be carefully monitored while they are taking this drug to determine its

efficacy. In addition, related to tuberculosis prevention, Japanese public health policy requires bacillus Calmette-Guérin (BCG) inoculation. When screening for tuberculosis, using a purified protein derivative test may result in a heightened reaction when the individual being screened has had the BCG inoculation, and it is therefore often contraindicated. A general health check by primary health care providers or X-ray may be a preferable screen for individuals who have had BCG in the past.

Succinylcholine, a muscle relaxant used during surgery, is inactivated by the enzyme pseudocholinesterase. Asians are at risk for having pseudocholinesterase deficiency and thus may suffer prolonged muscle paralysis and inability to breathe after administration of the drug (Kalow, 1972; Overfield, 1995).

Many Japanese do not like to take medications in part because of being afraid of adverse side effects rather than the main effect. Moreover, the value for *gaman* may cause reluctance for some Japanese Americans to take pain medications. In a multiethnic cohort study of women with invasive breast cancer that included African-Americans, Caucasians, Japanese Americans, Latinas, and Native Hawaiians from Hawaii and California, Japanese American women had the lowest usage of aspirin, other nonsteroidal anti-inflammatory drugs (ibuprofen, naproxen, indomethacin), and acetaminophen (Gill et al., 2007). An analysis of data from a subset of the same sample as the multiethnic cohort study discussed previously (n = 3842) found that for women with invasive breast cancer, prediagnostic soy intake was unrelated to mortality in postmenopausal women (Conroy et al., 2013).

Genetic and physiological studies have found that Asian clients display more side effects to antipsychotic medication than their White American or Black American counterparts (Binder & Levy, 1981). In addition, they require significantly lower doses of antipsychotic medication to control symptoms (Lin & Finder, 1983; Yamamoto, Fung, Lo, & Reece, 1979). Difficulty in achieving steady-state haloperidol level–dose ratios on Japanese patients has been reported, especially among those patients who required associated antiepileptic or antiparkinsonian medication (Yukawa et al., 2003). Although lower dosages of psychotropic drugs are needed, some Japanese Americans are at risk for extrapyramidal symptoms because the drugs remain in the blood longer (Kalow, 1986; Lin & Finder, 1983; Lin et al., 1989). Factors that may be responsible are a group of drug-metabolizing enzymes called *cytochrome P-450 isozymes* that play a crucial role in psychotropic metabolism (Lin & Cheung, 1999).

Another notable finding concerns flushing after ingesting alcohol. Fifty percent of Asian Americans, including Japanese, have a deficiency of the low-K_m mitochondrial aldehyde dehydrogenase 2 (ALDH2) isoenzyme, which is responsible for metabolizing acetaldehyde. This deficiency is an inherited mutant allele that causes flushing, in particular facial flushing after alcohol ingestion (Wall et al., 1997). There is some evidence to suggest that other physiological changes among some Asian Americans after the ingestion of alcohol include faster metabolism, differences in pulse pressure, and an increase in heart rate (Sue, 1987). Because of discrepancies noted in the findings relative to the influence of genetic and physiological factors on alcohol consumption, their roles cannot be accurately assessed (Sue, 1987). These unpleasant effects tend to limit drinking and lower alcohol-related disorders for some Asian Americans.

Susceptibility to Disease

Equal incidences of blood types A, B, and O are found among Japanese Americans, with type AB found in only about 10% of Japanese Americans. Statistically, persons with type O blood are at greater risk for duodenal ulcers, whereas persons with type A blood are more likely to develop cancer of the stomach (Overfield, 1995).

Cancer of the colon and rectum occurs more frequently among Japanese Americans than among their White counterparts (Lau et al., 2013; Miller, Chu, Hankey, & Ries, 2008). The incidence of stomach cancer is higher among Japanese than any other group in the world. A possible cause of stomach cancer is believed to be chronic gastritis. In addition, salt-cured food (such as dried salty fish), diets high in nitrates and poor in vitamin C, tobacco smoking, and *Helicobacter pylori* (a problem for 80% of Japanese over the age of 40 to 50 years) are also considered possible causes (Nomura et al., 2002). In particular for Japanese Americans, younger siblings from large families appeared to be especially vulnerable to stomach cancer (Blaser, Nomura, Lee, Stemmerman, & Perez-Perez, 2007).

In recent years Japanese Americans have experienced an increased incidence of breast, prostate, and colorectal cancer (CRC) (Miller et al., 2008), which has been suggested to be related to the adoption of a more Western diet and lifestyle. Japanese Americans have significantly higher risks for colorectal diagnosis and mortality when compared to non-Hispanic Whites, yet Asian American adults have low screening adherence (Lau et al., 2013).

While having increasing rates of these cancers, both foreign and U.S.-born Japanese American women had similar morality rates and were more likely to receive diagnosis at an early stage and have better survival rates than Chinese, Filipino, Korean, South Asian, and Vietnamese women (Gomez et al., 2010). Akaza et al. (2004) found that men who have the ability to produce equol (a metabolite of soy products produced in the intestine) have a lower

incidence of prostate cancer. This finding suggests that research exploring dietary interventions based on soybean isoflavones in the prevention of prostate cancer would be useful.

In an age-specific comparison of hip fracture incidence, Japanese Americans had approximately half the rate of their White counterparts. Further research is needed to pinpoint the reasons for this significant difference (Greendale et al., 2002; Lauderdale et al., 1997; Ross et al., 1991). Despite having lower bone mineral density at most bone sites than White American women, Japanese American women had lower rates of hip and vertebral fractures (Rice, Larson, LaCroix, & Drinkwater, 2001). The risk for injury when Japanese Americans fell, however, was not less than that reported for White Americans (Davis, Ross, Nevitt, & Wasnich, 1997). There are differences in the prevalence of osteoporosis at the same skeletal region for Chinese, Japanese, and Caucasian women 50 years of age and older. The prevalence of osteoporosis in Japanese women is lower (11.6% to 16.8%) compared with the prevalence of osteoporosis in Caucasian women (13% to 20%) (Greendale et al., 2002).

Kawasaki syndrome (KS), or mucocutaneous lymph node syndrome, a disease first described in Japan and later in Hawaii, has been observed primarily in children of Japanese ancestry. Kawasaki syndrome is "an acute self-limited vasculitis of childhood that is characterized by fever, bilateral nonexudative conjunctivitis, erythema of the lips and oral mucosa, changes in the extremities, rash, and cervical lymphadenopathy" (Newburger et al., 2004). Coronary artery aneurysms or ectasia develop in approximately 15% to 25% of untreated children. It has been observed in higher rates for children younger than 1 year of age than for those 1 to 4 years of age (74.3 and 37.5 per 100,000, respectively). The KS incidence for Asian and Pacific Islander children is twice that of White children (70.9 vs. 35.3 per 100,000) and is the highest among Japanese American children living in Hawaii (197.7 per 100,000). This incidence is higher than that of children living in Japan (Holman et al., 2005). This condition has been managed by medications but is often accompanied by a variety of complications of the cardiovascular system (Newburger et al., 2004). It is the leading cause of acquired heart disease in children in North America and Japan. Although the cause remains unknown, increasing evidence has supported involvement of an infectious agent or multiple infectious agents (Freeman & Shulman, 2001; Gedalia, 2002).

Japanese Americans have a higher prevalence of type 2 diabetes than their counterparts in Japan and White Americans (McNeely & Boyko, 2004). In a study of 933 Filipino Americans, Japanese Americans, and Native Hawaiians

A1C (a blood test used to diagnose diabetes), the A1C less than 6.5% had low sensitivity (suggesting that more people had diabetes than the A1C would suggest). This may delay diagnosis of type 2 diabetes in Japanese Americans if used alone without the addition of the oral glucose tolerance test (Araneta, Grandinetti, & Chang, 2010). A study with Japanese immigrants suggests the possible interaction of gene and environment in the development of type 2 diabetes (Nemoto, Sasaki, Deeb, Fujimoto, & Tajima, 2002). Research also suggests that the causative factors may be a Westernized lifestyle (higher intake of saturated fat) and reduced activity. Impaired glucose tolerance (IGT) (Tong et al., 2007), BMI (Maskarinec et al., 2009), and visceral obesity (Wander et al., 2013) are contributing factors to the development of type 2 diabetes, but glycemic load is not (Hopping et al., 2010). Prevention strategies need to target decreased insulin sensitivity (associated with diet and activity) and beta-cell function (Torréns et al., 2004). Testosterone replacement was suggested to improve insulin sensitivity in men (Jones, 2007; Tsai, Boyko, Leonetti, & Fujimoto, 2000). Among leaner individuals, greater handgrip strength was associated with lower risk of type 2 diabetes, suggesting it may be a useful marker (Wander et al., 2011). It is interesting to note that lifestyle modifications, decreased weight, and central adiposity improved insulin sensitivity in Japanese Americans with IGT. However, Carr et al. (2005) found that such changes did not improve beta-cell function, suggesting that this degree of lifestyle modification may be limited over the long term. A Hawaiian study noted a "fat and meat" diet was a risk factor in obese and overweight men and women; a "vegetables" diet lowered diabetes risk in men, and a "fruit and milk" diet appeared to be beneficial for both men and women (Erber et al., 2010). In an intervention study with diet and endurance exercises, BMI, body composition, and body fat distribution improved. Thus, these interventions may delay or prevent type 2 diabetes in Japanese Americans with IGT (Watson et al., 2006). Furthermore, further reducing the prevalence of diabetes would significantly reduce the risk of CRC, especially among Japanese American women (He et al., 2010).

The metabolic syndrome increases the risks of cardiovascular disease and diabetes. Among the syndrome descriptors, Boyko et al. (2010) found that hypertension, dyslipidemia, and hyperglycemia were the most helpful criteria in identifying Japanese Americans vulnerable to metabolic syndrome. The prevalence of metabolic syndrome was 13.9% and 2.7% for Japanese men and women compared with 32.7% and 3.4% for Japanese American men and women, respectively (Yoneda et al., 2008). The authors indicated a Westernized lifestyle was likely the cause of the higher prevalence in the United States. It was suggested that low levels of high-density lipoprotein cholesterol play a pivotal role in a population whose total cholesterol level is not high (Oyama et al., 2006). The Honolulu Heart Project concluded that proteinuria detected at urine-dipstick screening independently predicted increased risk for incident stroke and incident coronary heart disease over 27 years in this cohort (Madison et al., 2006). In a study looking at the relationship between alcohol intake and blood pressure, 3 weeks of alcohol restriction (about one third of the amount) produced reductions in ambulatory systolic blood pressure, heart rate, and the index of sympathovagal balance and produced augmentations of parasympathetic indices of heart rate variability in Japanese young adult male drinkers (Minami et al., 2002). Another study supports the positive relationships between decreasing alcohol intake and decreasing systolic blood pressure, heart rate, and other variables (Okubo, Suwazono, Kobayashi, & Nogawa, 2001).

Cerebrovascular disease is the second leading cause of death in Japan (Ministry of Health, Labour, and Welfare, 2014). In a Hawaiian study, while stroke increased significantly with increasing age in Japanese American men, the age-related risk of thromboembolic and hemorrhagic strokes among normotensive men resulted in a decreased percentage of strokes attributable to hypertension, 50% in those aged 45 to 54 years to 18% in those aged 65 or older (Curb et al., 1996). Findings in the same project of Japanese American men revealed systolic blood pressure increases until about 59 years of age that declined when the men became older. Their diastolic blood pressure tended to decrease after reaching a peak at 60 years of age. Therefore, the findings indicate that stroke risk factors may substantially change with age (Launer, 2004). In comparing White men in the Framingham Study with Japanese Americans in the Honolulu Heart Program, White men had a 40% excess of thromboembolic stroke compared with Japanese men, although the incidence of hemorrhagic stroke was nearly identical. The difference in stroke incidence rates cannot be explained by traditional risk factors. Further studies are needed to identify factors that protect Japanese American men from thromboembolic strokes (Rodriguez et al., 2002). A large ($n = 14,464$) primary prevention study based in Japan revealed that a low dose of aspirin did not significantly reduce the risk of cardiovascular death, nonfatal stroke, or nonfatal myocardial infarction among Japanese patients 60 years or older with atherosclerotic risk factors (Ikeda et al., 2014). Although this major study was conducted in Japan, it has implications for Japanese American patients. However, because of diet and other differences between Japanese and Japanese Americans, providers should be aware of the current science but cannot generalize to their Japanese American patients.

Nutritional Preferences and Deficiencies

The Japanese place great importance on the presentation of food. For these individuals, food should be visually appealing. Color, contrast, and shapes of food are considered as important as the cooking and seasoning of a particular food. Unlike American meals that center on one main dish, Japanese meals usually consist of several small dishes (Corum, 2000; Giger & Davidhizar, 1990). A Japanese-American family that has been acculturated may serve a mixture of American and Japanese dishes.

Traditionally, food was cooked on a small grill by broiling, steaming, frying, or simmering. Food was cut so that it cooked quickly and evenly, preserving vitamins. Meat, which is expensive in Japan, is frequently eaten with vegetables. The main sources of protein have been fish and soybeans. Tofu, a soybean product, is used extensively as a dish by itself or mixed with other dishes. In a study conducted in Seattle, the soy foods most commonly consumed among Japanese-American women 65 years of age or older were tofu (soybean curd), *miso* (fermented soybean paste), and *abura-age* (fried thin soybean curd) (Rice et al., 2001). Findings from this study suggest that the mean intake of dietary soy isoflavones was approximately one quarter to one half that of previously published estimates in Japanese samples. Dietary intake of soy isoflavones was positively associated with speaking Japanese, consumption of traditional Japanese dishes (*kamaboko, manju,* and *mochi*) and low-fat or nonfat milk and yellow and red vegetables, vitamin E supplement use, and walking several blocks each day. Dietary intake of soy isoflavones was negatively associated with the consumption of butter.

The main source of carbohydrate is rice or noodles. A seasoning used extensively is soy sauce, which is high in sodium. Pickled vegetables and unsweetened green tea complete a meal. *Sake,* or rice wine, is sometimes served. Milk is often included in the diet of children but less often of adults, a finding that may be related to the high incidence of lactose intolerance in the population. The traditional diet is nutritious and low in fat but tends to be high in sodium. In Hawaii, Japanese dishes tend to be sweetened more than they are in Japan. Most Japanese Americans also consume popular American foods, such as pizza, tacos, and hamburgers. A study by Pierce et al. (2007) indicated that the *nisei* (n = 219) had higher scores associated with Japanese food and lower scores for Western food than the *sansei* (n = 277) study participants. In the *sansei,* the Western food scores were significantly associated with two risk factors for diabetes, plasma C-reactive protein, and BMI. Moreover, the scores were associated with diabetes in the *sansei* participants.

Psychological Characteristics

Cultural Values Related to Self. A study of four Asian American groups found that the Japanese Americans tended to score higher on most of the Asian value dimensions—collectivism, conformity to norms, emotional self-control, and family recognition through achievement and filial piety—than the other three groups (Kim, Yang, Atkinson, Wolfe, & Hong, 2001). Although furthest removed from immigration, this group finding suggests that generation status is not a primary factor related to adherence to Asian cultural values, which has implications for acculturation and enculturation theories (Kim et al., 2001). This supports the notion that cultural values tend to remain constant, changing only incrementally over time. The Asian sense of self is interdependent and is part of a larger social system. *Enryo* emphasizes modesty, respect, and deference toward others. *Enryo* is related to *hazukashii,* the implicit fear of being ridiculed, which results in feelings of embarrassment and reticence. *Hige* is the concept of denigration of self and others (Kitano, 1970). These concepts emphasize conformity to group norms and minimization of accomplishments (Fugita, Ito, Abe, & Takeuchi, 1991). *Gaman* refers to internalization and suppression of anger and emotion. Avoidance of confrontation and acceptance of the results of negative social interactions can be related to *gaman.* In contrast to earlier studies, ethnic identification with their traditional culture is still strong in fourth-generation (*yonsei*) Japanese Americans, similar to the levels of previous generations (Marsella, Johnson, Johnson, & Brennan, 1998). On the other hand, the more acculturated Asian American men became, the less gender-role conflict was related to restrictive emotionality (Kim, O'Neil, & Owen, 1996). These findings suggest a dynamic interplay of factors that influence ethnic identity and do not follow linear assimilation across generations for Japanese Americans.

Doutrich (2001) conducted a study of Japanese-nurse scholars working on their master's or doctoral degrees in the United States. In total, 42 interviews were completed. Interpretive analysis revealed a prevailing theme related to a change in the self. One participant described the Japanese self and touched on the changes that occur during acculturation: "The way we think is always thinking of the other person's feelings and thinking. If I cannot predict what you think, what you feel, I am lost completely." The flow of concern from the other is a foundation of self-definition in the Japanese psyche, and language and cultural values reinforce and support this notion. The Japanese-nurse scholars in this study did adapt and were able to achieve a level of bicultural fluency, but some described a new, "tougher" self unfolding in the process of acculturation. Likewise, the participants in a study of Japanese-immigrant youth in the United States described feeling conflicted living in two cultures (Yeh et al., 2003). To a lesser degree, depending on the degree of acculturation, Japanese Americans may feel this bicultural conflict and contextually shifting sense of self.

Leong (1986) found that Asian Americans have a lower tolerance for ambiguity. Findings from this study also indicate that Asian Americans are more likely to prefer structured situations. They tend to want practical and immediate solutions to their problems (Leong, 1986). This study indicates that Asian Americans are more likely to show respect for authority figures and are less likely to express their emotions.

Emotional and Behavioral Manifestations of Stress. The length of residence in a new environment and generational status of an individual are important factors in determining levels of stress perceived by an ethnic group undergoing acculturation (Padilla et al., 1985). Examining variables such as generational status, acculturation level, and personality variables, Padilla et al. (1985) found that *issei* Japanese immigrants (likely *shin-issei*) reported the most stress and were the most externally controlled. A plausible reason for acculturation stress is the disparity noted between culture and expected individual behavior. It is interesting to note that *sansei* and later-generation students scored lower on stress, higher on self-esteem, and higher on internal locus of control. Differences in scores also indicated that *nisei* individuals may be in transition from traditional values held by their parents to values held by some Japanese Americans belonging to *sansei* or later generations.

Mental Health. According to Lin and Cheung (1999), there is considerable evidence to indicate that Asian Americans use mental health services less frequently than White Americans. Those who do use mental health services drop out at a significantly higher rate than White-American clients (Sue, 1987). Kozuki and Kennedy (2004) explored the "cultural incommensurability" that results when Western models of diagnosis and treatment are applied to Japanese and Japanese American clients. Cultural incommensurability refers to the lack of a standard of common measure or fundamental cultural differences between Western and Japanese traditions in mental health. The purpose of the study was to examine how this might influence treatment outcomes. These researchers also found that the most benign consequences were ineffective treatment. The worst consequences resulted in misdiagnoses, labeling, and further damage to the patient's sense of self.

Regarding types of effective counselors, Atkinson and Matsushita (1991) found that *sansei* and *yonsei* Japanese

Americans rated Japanese American counselors as more attractive than White American counselors when portraying a directive counseling style but less attractive when portraying a nondirective counseling style. This theory supports an earlier study (Atkinson, Maruyama, & Matsui, 1978) that found that Asian Americans demonstrated a preference for an ethnically similar counselor and a directive counseling style.

Tracey, Leong, and Glidden (1986) found that Asian American students appear to find it more acceptable to react to emotional difficulties by focusing on academic and vocational concerns. When counseling was sought, Japanese American students tended to focus more on academic difficulties than on emotional conflict. Two recent Alzheimer disease studies involving Japanese American subjects, found that inflammatory mechanisms in midlife might reflect underlying processes contributing to dementia-related cognitive decline late in life (Laurin, Curb, Masaki, White, & Launer, 2009). In addition, fruit and vegetable juices might play an important role in delaying the onset of Alzheimer's disease, particularly among those who are at high risk for the disease (Dai, Borenstein, Wu, Jackson, & Larson, 2006).

Internment Trauma. For Japanese Americans, the imprisonment of more than 120,000 men, women, and children in internment camps by the U.S. government during World War II represents the most traumatic and salient episode of the past (Nagata, 1991). More than 60% of those persons incarcerated were U.S. citizens. No formal charges were ever brought against them, yet they had no opportunity for a trial. In many cases, they were given less than a week's notice to move and to sell their businesses, personal property, and other possessions. In many instances, they were unable to sell these items or were forced to sell them for much less than their actual value, which resulted in severe economic hardship. Many were forced to move twice, first to temporary assembly centers in animal stalls at horse tracks and fairgrounds and later to internment camps in isolated areas. They lived 2 to 3 years in camps enclosed by barbed wire and armed guards, with the psychological degradation associated with being accused of disloyalty (Nagata, 1991).

Yates et al. (2007) explored the verbal and art-making responses of six *nisei* Japanese American elders who experienced the trauma of internment during World War II. This qualitative study resulted in seven prominent themes identified as (1) stressful living conditions in camp, (2) art and creativity for camp survival, (3) loss and deprivation, (4) separation or division of family and communities, (5) disruption of identity, (6) resilience and reaffirmation of values, and (7) the need for legacy and social justice. The participants of the study were able to take the "shame" of being labeled "enemy aliens" and transform it into advocacy for other minority groups who were discriminated against or marginalized by war. Another study reported that the *issei* maintained a silence about their experience in the camps (Nagata & Cheng, 2003). Transgenerational effects of victimization are evident in *sansei* descendants of individuals who suffered through this ordeal (Nagata, 1991). For some *nisei*, the results were a loss of self-esteem (Nagata & Takeshita, 2002) and a heightened sense of vulnerability and fear that their rights as U.S. citizens might be violated again (Nagata, 1991). For some, the post-9/11 climate, with military tribunals and "enemy combatant status," is an all too familiar echo from the past, and, like the participants in the study conducted by Yates et al. (2007) who advocated against discrimination, some among the Japanese American community cautioned against targeting Muslim immigrants (Wood, 2005).

Somatization and Folk Traditions. According to Fujii, Fukushima, and Yamamoto (1993), folk healing is often used to treat physical ailments because Asians tend to express emotional illness or distress through physical symptoms. Being "ill" is a legitimate, socially acceptable manner of receiving care. For some Japanese Americans, complaints are usually physical (Marsella, 1993). Kitano (1969) noted that Japanese people tend to worry needlessly about body functions and are usually obsessed about a potential problem related to their blood pressure.

Cheung et al. (2013) investigated factors related to depression in Japanese Americans in the Houston area. Among 43 respondents, the depression prevalence was 11.6%. A logistic regression model revealed the overall effect of having health issues, anxiety symptoms, and a master's degree predicted depression. A perceived stigma associated with mental illness was a primary reason for rarely consulting mental health professionals. Help-seeking behaviors were mediated by the perceived stigma of seeking mental health treatment. Participants were more likely to seek help from family and friends or to talk with their physicians than with a mental health professional. The stress from expectations for high levels of achievement also had influence on the participants' symptoms. And somatization that is presenting to providers with physical problems as the chief complaint was common.

Psychopharmacology. Literature indicates Asians respond to substantially lower doses of psychotropics than Caucasians (Lin & Cheung, 1999). Several studies have suggested that Japanese Americans do well with lower dosages of psychotropic medication for depression or mania (Lin & Cheung, 1999; Yamamoto, 1982) and need significantly lower maintenance dosages (Roseblat & Tang, 1987). Evidence also indicates that Japanese Americans need lower maximum and stabilizing dosages of chlorpromazine. Although lower dosages of psychotropic drugs are needed, some Japanese Americans are at risk for extrapyramidal symptoms because the drugs remain in the blood longer (Kalow, 1986; Lin & Finder, 1983; Lin et al., 1989). Factors that may be responsible are a group of drug-metabolizing enzymes called *cytochrome P-450 isozymes* that play a crucial role in psychotropic metabolism (Lin & Cheung, 1999).

Alcohol Use. Japanese Americans appear to have lower rates of alcoholism than the rest of the U.S. population. Some researchers believe that these lower rates may be attributed to a variety of factors, such as (1) being shielded by their families, (2) seeking treatment only during the late stages of alcoholism, (3) seeking assistance from other sources rather than state mental health facilities (Kotani, 1982), and (4) being protected by *ALDH1* deficiency, the fast flushing response (Nakawatase, Yamamoto, & Toshiaki, 1993).

Lee, Han, and Gfroerer (2013) conducted a study to investigate estimates of alcohol and binge drinking among Asian American groups, to examine drinking patterns, and to explore differences in drinking between Asian American groups. The National Survey on Drug Use and Health concentrates on adult populations over 18 years; 1100 Japanese Americans participated in the 2002–2008 surveys. Korean and Japanese Americans had higher rates of alcohol use and more binge drinking than Chinese, Filipino, and East Indian Americans. Foreign-born Japanese Americans were more likely to have past-month binge alcohol use than their U.S.-born counterparts, and males were three to five times more likely to have binge alcohol use than females (Lee et al., 2013).

The effect of ethnicity and cultural identity on substance use was examined in Hawaii with 144 Japanese American and part-Japanese American high school seniors (Williams et al., 2013). Significant associations for substance use and impairment included culturally intensified events (compared to mainstream values and behaviors; e.g., avoiding family discord) and Japanese cultural identity. However, when compared with the non-Japanese American adolescents, the combined sample of Japanese and part-Japanese Americans had significantly lower scores for "sometimes drank beer or alcohol," "too much alcohol or 'pot,'" and "drinking in the morning." The authors concluded that affiliation with Japanese culture is a protective variable against substance use.

Implications for Nursing Care

It is important for the nurse to teach and counsel clients about diseases common among Japanese Americans. In addition, preventive health care techniques should be emphasized. For example, by increasing culturally relevant CRC-related knowledge, as Lau et al. (2012) were able to do in their community-based participatory intervention (i.e., using mailed educational pamphlets and family discussions), Japanese Americans could dramatically increase rates of screening. To provide culturally appropriate and competent care, the nurse must engage the support of family members.

To reduce the chronicity and severity of hypertension, the nurse must stress to the client and the family the importance of limiting the use of soy sauce, salt-cured fish, and pickles. Because somatization is used among some Japanese Americans, the nurse must recognize that frequent physical ailments may be possible signs of underlying stress. Meaning must be attached to behavior if the client is to receive optimal care. It is also essential to identify previous successful strategies in order to help the client develop and refine coping strategies. To reduce stress, the nurse might suggest exercise because it may be perceived by the client as a nonconfrontational form of release. Health promotion should also include reminding women of childbearing age to add folic acid to their diets.

It is essential for the nurse to remember that Japanese Americans generally do not seek or delay seeking professional help for mental health problems. Of those individuals who do seek treatment, many do not complete treatment (Leong, 1986). Kitano (1969) speculated that the reluctance to seek treatment may be a result of several factors, including (1) strength of the family and community and the family's ability to control and hide problem behaviors, (2) different cultural styles of expressing problems, (3) inappropriateness of current therapeutic organizations, and (4) lack of relevant connections to the therapeutic community. Another factor may be related to the inability of the therapist to provide culturally responsive forms of treatment (Kozuki & Kennedy, 2004; Sue, 1987). In addition, some Japanese Americans will look first to their families when they have emotional problems in order to maintain family honor (Atkinson & Matsushita, 1991; Leong, 1986). Therefore, the major goal of nursing care should be aimed at developing a trusting relationship between the nurse and the client by using a more structured and directive approach that emphasizes collectivism, harmony, and acceptance over individualistic ascendancy (Marsella, 1993).

SUMMARY

Japanese Americans vary in their degree of acculturation. Because of this variability, Japanese Americans may present in the clinical setting with a variety of behaviors, depending on factors such as generational, regional, and individual differences. The nurse must assess the unique needs of each individual and the extent to which the information presented applies to that person or family. The importance of establishing a trusting relationship based on respect and open communication with the client and the family cannot be underestimated.

CASE STUDY

Mr. Robert Kiyoshi Yamamoto, a 71-year-old retired *nisei* electrician, was admitted to the hospital with complaints of nausea and difficulty keeping food down that were related to recurrent colon cancer with liver metastasis. For the past few weeks, Mr. Yamamoto's appetite has been steadily decreasing. His wife of 50 years states that he has been unable to keep any solid foods down but has been able to drink some fluids. After a few days of nasogastric decompression, Mr. Yamamoto's bowel function begins to return. He is able to eat small amounts of soft foods. Because the tumor has spread despite chemotherapy, Mr. Yamamoto has decided against further chemotherapy. As he becomes weaker and weaker, Mr. Yamamoto insists that his wife remain at his bedside so that he "doesn't have to bother the nurses for little things." Mrs. Yamamoto has kept a bedside vigil and rarely leaves except to go home to shower while one of their three daughters stays with her father. The nurse notices that Mrs. Yamamoto is looking tired and appears to be losing weight. Her daughters have tried to relieve their mother at night so that she can rest at home, but she insists that "Dad is restless and calls out in the night for me." Mr. Yamamoto insists that she bathe him and assist him to the bathroom. One daughter flew in from out of town to assist indefinitely if needed. All daughters take turns in keeping their mother company or relieving her when she goes home to shower or cook special foods for her husband. Although

Continued

CASE STUDY—cont'd

he never says he is having pain, Mr. Yamamoto has family members constantly massaging his back and legs. He moves cautiously and winces with each movement. Mr. Yamamoto does not talk much to the staff. He lets his family talk for him. He denies pain when asked by the nurse but tells his family otherwise. He does not sleep well. Mr. Yamamoto's current treatment is primarily supportive care. He is constantly requesting special Japanese foods such as sushi and miso soup, which the family brings in daily. Generally, he just tastes it. The hospital staff has brought up the possibility of hospice care. A family meeting to discuss discharge plans was called by his son. Mr. Yamamoto has stated he wants to go home.

◎ CARE PLAN

Nursing Diagnosis: Altered family processes, related to situational crisis

Client Outcomes	Nursing Interventions
1. Family will devise a specific rotation plan to meet each other's need for rest and caring for their father. 2. Family will demonstrate mutual support and cohesion.	1. Provide empathy and support for the immediate family members who need to be at the bedside by providing family with liberal visitation, adequate space for members who stay overnight, and privacy. 2. Keep family abreast of current treatments and nature of illness to dispel any misunderstandings and to keep lines of communication open between family and staff. 3. Assess family members for signs of fatigue or overextension. 4. Explore with family members other possible family members or friends who would be willing and be accepted by client to keep him company or support his wife.

Nursing Diagnosis: Pain, related to cancer metastasis

Client Outcomes	Nursing Interventions
1. Client will indicate to family that the pain is tolerable. 2. Client will be able to sleep 4 hours at a time at night.	1. Observe nonverbal behaviors that indicate pain, such as wincing with movement and restlessness at night. 2. Check with family about how much pain client is having with the current treatment. 3. Give analgesic on a regular schedule without waiting for him to ask (unless refused), especially before sleep.

Nursing Diagnosis: Risk for ineffective family coping, related to deteriorating course of disease of a family member

Client Outcomes	Nursing Interventions
1. Family unit will use own resources and explore outside resources. 2. Family will devise realistic expectations of roles of members. 3. Open communication will be maintained among family members. 4. Family members will perform care without compromising their own physical and emotional health.	1. Develop trusting and respectful relationships with client and family. 2. Encourage the son to call family meetings as needed to discuss realistic plans and expectations of members, using health care providers as needed. 3. Assist and encourage family to explore outside resources as well as family resources to assist in dealing with the crisis. 4. Assess if basic physical and emotional needs of client and family members are being met.

CARE PLAN—cont'd

5. Encourage family members to support each other, especially Mrs. Yamamoto, and devise a schedule that does not compromise their physical and emotional health.
6. Continue to monitor ability of family members to carry out treatment regimen and care.
7. Discuss management of emotional outbursts, personality changes, and mood swings with family members or those providing care.
8. Encourage realistic expectations of role performance, especially by Mrs. Yamamoto.
9. Teach coping strategies to manage tension and strain if previous techniques are no longer effective.
10. Help with identification of current stressors and strain.

Nursing Diagnoses—Definitions and Classifications 2012–2014. Copyright © 2012, 1994–2012 by NANDA International. Used by arrangement with Wiley-Blackwell Publishing, a company of John Wiley and Sons, Inc. In order to make safe and effective judgments using NANDA-I nursing diagnoses it is essential that nurses refer to the definitions and defining characteristics of the diagnoses listed in the work.

CLINICAL DECISION MAKING

1. List the important cultural values that determine health-seeking and health-practice behaviors in this cultural group.
2. Identify three interventions that incorporate these values in treating the Japanese American client.
3. Analyze different strategies useful in communicating with the Japanese American family.
4. Discuss the importance of understanding generational, geographical, and acculturation issues in working with the Japanese American client.
5. Describe appropriate interventions by health care providers for clients who do not verbally express pain, discomfort, or stress.

REVIEW QUESTIONS

1. In the treatment of hypertension for a Japanese client, the nurse needs to stress to the family and client the importance of limiting which of the following?
   a. Pepper
   b. Soy sauce
   c. Tofu
   d. Milk
2. When seeking counseling, in assessing a Japanese-American student in the mental health center, the nurse is aware that this client is more apt to seek counseling for which of the following?
   a. Academic difficulties
   b. Emotional conflict
   c. Family problems
   d. Loss of self-esteem
3. The majority of communication of feelings and attitudes among Japanese Americans is primarily which of the following?
   a. Verbal
   b. Vocal
   c. Facial expression
   d. Touch

REFERENCES

Adler, S. M. (1998). *Mothering, education, and ethnicity: the transformation of Japanese American culture.* New York: Garland.

Aghaian, E., Choe, J. E., Lin, S., & Stamper, R. L. (2004). Central corneal thickness of Caucasians, Chinese, Hispanics, Filipinos, African Americans, and Japanese in a glaucoma clinic [abstract]. *Ophthalmology, 111*(12), 2211–2219.

Akaza, H., et al. (2004). Comparisons of percent equol producers between prostate cancer patients and controls: case-controlled studies of isoflavones in Japanese, Korean and American residents [abstract]. *Japanese Journal of Clinical Oncology, 34*(2), 86–89.

Akimoto, S. A., & Sanbonmatsu, D. M. (1999). Differences in self-effacing behavior between European and Japanese Americans: effect on competence evaluations. *Journal of Cross-Cultural Psychology, 30*(2), 159–177.

Akiyama, C. (2008). Bridging the gap between two cultures: an analysis on identity attitudes and attachment of Asian Americans. *Brief Treatment and Crisis Intervention, 8*(3), 251–263.

Albright, C. L., et al. (2012). Differences by race/ethnicity in older adults' beliefs about the relative importance of dietary supplements vs prescription medications: results from the SURE study. *Journal of the Academy of Nutrition and Dietetics, 112*(8), 1223–1229.

Araneta, M. R. G., Grandinetti, A., & Chang, H. K. (2010). A_{1C} and diabetes diagnosis among Filipino Americans, Japanese Americans, and Native Hawaiians. *Diabetes Care, 33*(12), 2626–2628.

Asian American Federation of New York. (2003). *Asian American elders in New York City*. New York: Brookdage Center on Aging, Hunter College.

Atkinson, D. R., Maruyama, M., & Matsui, S. (1978). The effects of counselor race and counseling approach on Asian Americans' perceptions of counselor credibility and utility. *Journal of Counseling Psychology, 25,* 76–83.

Atkinson, D. R., & Matsushita, Y. (1991). Japanese American acculturation, counseling style, counselor ethnicity, and perceived counselor credibility. *Journal of Counseling Psychology, 38,* 473–478.

Baker, J. (1993). Perceptions of privacy in Japan and America. Paper presented at the East West Center, Honolulu, Hawaii.

Barnlund, D. C. (1989). Public-private self in communication with Japan. *Business Horizons, 32,* 32–35.

Binder, R. L., & Levy, R. (1981). Extrapyramidal reactions in Asians. *American Journal of Psychiatry, 138*(9), 1234–1244.

Bito, S., Matsumura, S., Kagawa-Singer, M., Meredith, L. S., Fukuhara, S., & Wenger, N. S. (2007). Acculturation and end-of-life decision making: comparison of Japanese and Japanese-American focus groups. *Bioethics, 21*(5), 251–262.

Blaser, M. J., Nomura, A., Lee, J., Stemmerman, G. N., & Perez-Perez, G. I. (2007). Early-life family structure and microbially induced cancer risk. *PLoSMed, 4*(1), e7.

Bose, D., & Welsh, J. (1973). Lactose malabsorption in Oklahoma Indians. *American Journal of Clinical Nutrition, 26,* 1320–1322.

Bowman, K. W., & Singer, P. A. (2001). Chinese seniors' perspectives on end-of-life decisions. *Social Science & Medicine, 53*(4), 455–464.

Boyko, E. J., Doheny, R. A., McNeely, M. J., Kahn, S. E., Leonetti, D. L., & Fujimoto, W. Y. (2010). Latent class analysis of the metabolic syndrome. *Diabetes Research and Clinical Practice, 89*(1), 88–93.

Braun, K. L., & Nichols, R. (1997). Death and dying in four Asian American cultures: a descriptive study. *Death Studies, 21*(4), 327–359.

Burris, J. (1993). 442nd vets "shared a tent" in battle, in politics. *The Honolulu Advertiser,* B-1.

Carr, D. B., et al. (2005). A reduced-fat diet and aerobic exercise in Japanese Americans with impaired glucose tolerance decreases intra-abdominal fat and improves insulin sensitivity but not beta-cell function [abstract]. *Diabetes, 54*(2), 340–347.

Caskey, D. A., Payne-Bose, D., Welsh, J. D., Gearhart, H. L., Nance, M. K., & Morrison, R. D. (1977). Effects of age on lactose malabsorption in Oklahoma Native Americans as determined by breath H_2 analysis. *American Journal of Digestive Disease, 22*(2), 113–116.

Caudill, W., & Frost, L. (1974). A comparison of maternal care and infant behavior in Japanese American, American, and Japanese families. In W. P. Lebra (Ed.), *Youth, socialization and mental health; mental health research in Asia and the Pacific* (vol. 3). Honolulu: University of Hawaii Press.

Central Intelligence Agency (2015). *The CIA world fact book.* New York: Skyhorse Publishing.

Chan, S. (1991). *Asian Americans: an interpretive history.* Boston: Twayne Publishers.

Chang, B. (1981). Asian American patient care. In G. Henderson, & M. Primeaux (Eds.), *Transcultural health care.* Menlo Park, CA: Addison-Wesley.

Chang, T. (1993). A legacy of bravery: the 442nd comes home. *The Honolulu Advertiser* 442nd Special Section.

Cheung, M., Leung, P., & Tsui, V. (2013). Japanese Americans' health concerns and depressive symptoms: implications for disaster counseling. *Social Work, 58*(3), 201–211.

Ching, J. W. J., McDermott, J. F., Fukunaga, C., Yanagida, E., Mann, E., & Waldron, J. A. (1995). Perceptions of family values and roles among Japanese Americans: clinical considerations. *American Journal of Orthopsychiatry, 65*(2), 216–224.

Chung, C. S., & Myrianthopoulos, N. C. (1968). Racial and prenatal factors in major congenital malformations. *American Journal of Human Genetics, 20,* 44–60.

Colclough, Y. Y. (2005). An exploration of end-of-life decision making within Japanese-American families (Unpublished doctoral dissertation). Oregon Health & Science University, Portland.

Colclough, Y. Y., & Young, H. (2007). Decision making at end of life among Japanese American families. *Journal of Family Nursing, 13*(2), 201–225.

Connor, J. (1974). Acculturation and family continuity in three generations of Japanese Americans. *Journal of Marriage and Family, 36,* 159–168.

Conroy, S. M., Maskarinec, G., Park, S.-Y., Wilkens, L. R., Henderson, B. E., & Kolonel, L. N. (2013). The effects of soy consumption before diagnosis on breast cancer survival: The Multiethnic Cohort study. *Nutrition & Cancer, 65*(4), 527–537.

Corum, A. K. (2000). *Ethnic foods of Hawaii* (revised ed.). Honolulu: Bess Press.

Curb, J. D., et al. (1996). Age-related changes in stroke risk in men with hypertension and normal blood pressure. *Stroke, 27*(5), 819–824.

Dai, Q., Borenstein, A. R., Wu, T., Jackson, J. C., & Larson, E. B. (2006). Fruit and vegetable juices and Alzheimer's disease: the Kame Project. *American Journal of Medicine, 119*(9), 751–759.

Daniels, R. (1991). Redress achieved, 1983–1990. In R. Daniels, S. C. Taylor, & H. H. L. Kitano (Eds.), *Japanese Americans: from relocation to redress* (pp. 219–223). Seattle: University of Washington Press.

Daniels, R., Taylor, S. C., & Kitano, H. H. L. (Eds.) (1991). *Japanese Americans: from relocation to redress*. Seattle: University of Washington Press.

Davis, J. W., Ross, P. D., Nevitt, M. C., & Wasnich, R. D. (1997). Incidence rates of falls among Japanese men and women living in Hawaii. *Journal of Clinical Epidemiology, 50*(5), 589–594.

Dickerson, J. L. (2010). *Inside America's concentration camps: two centuries of internment and torture*. Chicago, IL: Lawrence Hill Books.

Doi, L. T. (1962). Amae: a key concept for understanding Japanese personality structure. In R. J. Smith & R. K. Beardsley (Eds.), *Japanese culture: its development and characteristics*. Chicago: Aldine Publishing.

Doi, L. T. (1973). *The anatomy of dependence*. New York: Kodansha International.

Dornbusch, S. M., Ritter, P. L., Leiderman, P. H., Roberts, D. F., & Fraleigh, M. J. (1987). The relation of parenting style to adolescent school performance. *Child Development, 55*, 1244–1257.

Doutrich, D. (2000). Cultural fluency, marginality, and the sense of self. In H. Riggenbach (Ed.), *Perspectives on fluency* (pp. 141–159). Ann Arbor: University of Michigan Press.

Doutrich, D. (2001). Experience of Japanese nurse scholars: insights for U.S. faculty. *Journal of Nursing Education, 40*(5), 210–215.

Duncan, I., & Scott, E. (1972). Lactose intolerance in Alaskan Indians and Eskimos. *American Journal of Clinical Nutrition, 25*, 867–868.

Eichholzer, M., Tonz, O., & Zimmermann, R. (2006). Folic acid: a public health challenge. *The Lancet, 367*(9519), 1352–1362.

Endo, T., Ozoe, R., Kubota, M., Akiyama, M., & Shimooka, S. (2006). A survey of hypodontia in Japanese orthodontic patients [abstract]. *American Journal of Orthodontics and Dentofacial Orthopedics, 129*(1), 29–35.

Engle, M. (1993). Japanese New Year's customs demystified. *Star-Bulletin*, A-4.

Erber, E., Hopping, B. N., Grandinetti, A., Park, S. Y., Kolonel, L. N., & Maskarinec, G. (2010). Dietary patterns and risk for diabetes: the multiethnic cohort. *Diabetes Care, 33*(3), 532–538.

Erickson, J. D. (1976). Racial variations in the incidence of congenital malformations. *Annals of Human Genetics, 39*, 315–320.

Evans, G. W., Lepore, S. J., & Allen, K. M. (2000). Cross-cultural differences in tolerance for crowding: fact or fiction? *Journal of Personality and Social Psychology, 79*(2), 204–210.

Fisher, N. (1996). *Cultural and ethnic diversity: a guide for genetic professionals*. Baltimore: Johns Hopkins University Press.

Freeman, A. F., & Shulman, S. T. (2001). Recent developments in Kawasaki disease. *Current Opinion in Infectious Diseases, 14*(3), 357–361.

Fugita, S., Ito, K. L., Abe, J., & Takeuchi, D. T. (1991). Japanese Americans. In N. Mokuau (Ed.), *Handbook of social services for Asian and Pacific Islanders* (pp. 61–77). New York: Greenwood.

Fugita, S. S., & O'Brien, D. J. (1991). *Japanese American ethnicity: the persistence of community*. Seattle: University of Washington Press.

Fujii, J., Fukushima, S., & Yamamoto, J. (1993). Psychiatric care of Japanese Americans. In A. C. Gaw (Ed.), *Culture, ethnicity and mental illness* (pp. 305–346). Washington, DC: American Psychiatric Press.

Galanti, G. A. (1997). *Caring for patients from different cultures: case studies from American hospitals* (2nd ed.). Philadelphia: University of Pennsylvania Press.

Gedalia, A. (2002). Kawasaki disease: an update. *Current Rheumatology Report, 4*(1), 25–29.

Giger, J. N., & Davidhizar, R. E. (1990). Transcultural nursing: a method for advancing nursing care and practices. *International Congress of Nursing Review, 37*(1), 199–202.

Gill, J. K., Maskarinec, G., Wilkens, L. R., Pike, M. C., Henderson, B. E., & Kolonel, L. N. (2007). Nonsteroidal antiinflammatory drugs and breast cancer risk: the multiethnic cohort. *American Journal of Epidemiology, 166*, 1150–1158.

Gomez, S. L., Clarke, C. A., Shema, S. J., Chang, E. T., Keegan, T. H., & Glaser, S. L. (2010). Disparities in breast cancer survival among Asian women by ethnicity and immigrant status: a population-based study. *American Journal of Public Health, 100*(5), 861–869.

Gotay, C. C., Shimizu, H., Muraoka, M., Ishihara, Y., Tsuboi, K., & Ogawa, H. (2004). Health attitudes and behaviors: comparison of Japanese and Americans of Japanese and European Ancestry. *Health & Place, 10*(2), 153–161.

Greendale, G. A., et al. (2002). Soy products may help preserve bone density in Japanese women [abstract]. *American Journal of Epidemiology, 155*, 746–754.

Gudykunst, W. B., & Nishida, T. (1994). *Bridging Japanese/North American differences*. Thousand Oaks, CA: Sage.

Güngör, D., Bornstein, M. H., De Lyeersnyder, J., Cote, L., & Mesquita, B. (2012). Acculturation of personality: a three culture study of Japanese, Japanese Americans, and European Americans. *Journal of Cross-Cultural Psychology, 44*(5), 701–718.

Hall, E. T. (1976). *Beyond culture*. New York: Doubleday.

Hamaguchi, E. (1977). *Nihonrashiga N. Saihaken. (Rediscovery of Japaneseness). Nihon Keizai Shaimbun-sha*.

Hashizume, S., & Takano, J. (1983). Nursing care of Japanese American patients. In M. S. Orque, B. Bloch, & L. S. A. Monrroy (Eds.), *Ethnic nursing care: a multicultural approach* (pp. 219–243). St. Louis: Mosby.

Hattori, K., & Ishida, D. N. (2012). Ethnographic study of a good death among elderly Japanese Americans. *Nursing and Health Sciences, 14*, 488–494.

He, J., Stram, D. O., Kolonel, L. N., Henderson, B. E., Le Marchand, L., & Haiman, C. A. (2010). The association of diabetes with colorectal cancer risk: the multiethnic cohort. *British Journal of Cancer, 103*, 120–126.

Hiratsuka, M., et al. (2002). Geno-typing of the N-acetyltransferase2 polymorphism in the prediction of adverse drug reactions to isoniazid in Japanese patients [abstract]. *Drug Metabolism and Pharmacokinetics, 17*(4), 357–362.

Hofstede, G. (1984). *Culture's consequences: international differences in work related values.* Beverly Hills: Sage.

Holman, R. C., et al. (2005). Kawasaki syndrome in Hawaii. *Pediatric Infectious Disease Journal, 24*(5), 429–433.

Hopping, B. N., Erber, E., Grandinetti, A., Verheus, M., Kolonel, L. N., & Maskarinec, G. (2010). Dietary fiber, magnesium, and glycemic load alter risk of type 2 diabetes in a multiethnic cohort in Hawaii. *Journal of Nutrition, 140,* 68–74.

Hosokawa, G. (2002). *Nisei: the quiet Americans* (revised ed.). Boulder, CO: University Press of Colorado.

Houston, J. W., & Houston, J. D. (2002). *Farewell to Manzanar.* Boston: Houghton Mifflin.

Hsu, J., Tseng, W.-S., Ashton, G., McDermott, J. F., & Char, W. (1985). Family interaction patterns among Japanese-American and Caucasian families in Hawaii. *American Journal of Psychiatry, 142,* 577–581.

Ikeda, Y., et al. (2014). Low-dose aspirin for primary prevention of cardiovascular events in Japanese patients 60 years or older with atherosclerotic risk factors: a randomized clinical trial. *Journal of the American Medical Association, 312*(23), 2510–2520.

Immigration Bureau of Japan. (2014). *Immigration control of Japanese and foreign nationals.* Retrieved from http://www.moj.go.jp/ENGLISH/IB/ib-01.html. Accessed December 8, 2014.

Ishihara, A. (1962). Kampo: Japan's traditional medicine. *Japan Quarterly, 9,* 429–437.

Ishii, S. (1987). *Nonverbal communication in Japan (Orientation Seminars on Japan, No. 28).* Tokyo: Office for the Japanese Studies Center.

Iwasaki, S. (2006). Japan: language situation. *Encyclopedia of Language & Linguistics,* 93–95.

Jacobs, A. H., & Walton, R. G. (1976). Incidence of birthmarks in the neonate. *Pediatrics, 58,* 218–222.

Jarvis, J. K., & Miller, G. D. (2002). Overcoming the barrier of lactose intolerance to reduce health disparities. *Journal of the National Medical Association, 94*(2), 55–66.

Jeong, Y. J., & You, H. K. (2008). Different historical trajectories and family diversity among Chinese, Japanese, and Koreans in the United States. *Journal of Family History, 33,* 346–356.

Jih, J., et al. (2014). Using appropriate body mass index cut points for overweight and obesity among Asian Americans. *Preventive Medicine, 65,* 1–6.

Johnson, F. A., Marsella, A. J., & Johnson, C. L. (1974). Social and psychological aspects of verbal behavior in Japanese Americans. *American Journal of Psychiatry, 131,* 580–583.

Jones, T. H. (2007). Testosterone replacement therapy. *British Journal of Hospital Medicine (London), 68,* 547–553.

Kakesako, G. K. (1993). Nisei proved their loyalty on the war front. *The Honolulu Star-Bulletin,* A-1.

Kalow, W. (1972). Pharmacogenetics of drugs used in anesthesia. *Human Genetics, 60,* 415–427.

Kalow, W. (1986). Conjugation reactions. In W. Kalow, H. W. Goedde, & D. P. Agarwal (Eds.), *Ethnic differences in reactions to drugs and xenobiotics.* New York: Alan R. Liss.

Katada, N. (1991). Gaman as a preschooler's method of coping during hospitalization (Unpublished doctoral dissertation). San Francisco, CA: University of California.

Kataoka-Yahiro, M., Ceria, C., & Caulfield, R. (2004). Grandparent caregiving role in ethnically diverse families. *Journal of Pediatric Nursing, 19*(5), 315–328.

Kim, E. J., O'Neil, J. M., & Owen, S. V. (1996). Asian-American men's acculturation and gender-role conflict. *Psychological Reports, 79,* 95–104.

Kim, B. S., Yang, P. H., Atkinson, D. R., Wolfe, M. M., & Hong, S. (2001). Cultural value similarities and differences among Asian American ethnic groups. *Cultural Diversity and Ethnic Minority Psychology, 7,* 343–361.

Kinoshita, L. M. & Gallagher-Thompson, D. (2004). Japanese-American caregivers of individuals with dementia: an examination of Japanese cultural values and dementia caregiving. *Clinical Gerontologist, 27*(1/2), 87–102.

Kitano, H. H. L. (1969). Japanese-American mental illness. In S. C. Plot & R. B. Edgerton (Eds.), *Changing perspectives in mental illness.* New York: Holt, Rinehart & Winston.

Kitano, H. H. L. (1970). Mental illness in four cultures. *Journal of Social Psychology, 80,* 121–134.

Kitano, H. H. L. (1976). *Japanese Americans: the evolution of a subculture* (2nd ed.). Englewood Cliffs, NJ: Prentice-Hall.

Kitano, H. H. L., & Daniels, R. (2001). *Asian Americans: emerging minorities* (3rd ed.). Englewood Cliffs, NJ: Prentice-Hall.

Klopf, D., Cambra, R., & Ishii, S. (1981). A comparison of communication styles of Japanese and American college students. *Current English Studies, 53,* 22–26.

Klopf, D., & Ishii, S. (1976). A comparison of communication activities of Japanese and American adults. *ELEC Bulletin, 20,* 66–71.

Kobata, F. (1979). The influence of culture on family relations: the Asian American experience. In P. K. Ragan (Ed.), *Aging parents.* Los Angeles: Ethel Percy Andrus Gerontology Foundation, University of Southern California.

Kobayashi-Winata, H., & Powers, T. (1989). Child rearing and compliance: Japanese and American families in Houston. *Journal of Cross-Cultural Psychology, 20,* 333–356.

Kotani, R. (1982). AJA's and alcohol abuse. *Hawaii Herald, 3*(13), 4.

Kozuki, Y., & Kennedy, M. (2004). Cultural incommensurability in psychodynamic psychotherapy in Western and Japanese traditions. *Journal of Nursing Scholarship, 36*(1), 30–38.

Lau, D. T., et al. (2013). Colorectal cancer knowledge, attitudes, screening, and intergenerational communication among Japanese American families: an exploratory, community-based participatory study. *Journal of Cross-Cultural Gerontology, 28*(1), 89–101.

Lau, D. T., Machizawa, S., & Doi, M. (2012). Informal and formal support among community-dwelling Japanese American elders living alone in Chicagoland: an in-depth qualitative study. *Journal of Cross Cultural Gerontology, 27,* 149–161.

Lauderdale, D. S., Jacobsen, S. J., Furner, S. E., Levy, P. S., Brody, J. A., & Goldberg, J. (1997). Hip fracture incidence among elderly Asian-American populations. *American Journal of Epidemiology, 146*(6), 502–509.

Lauderdale, D. S., & Rathouz, P. J. (2000). Body mass index in a US national sample of Asian Americans: effects of nativity, years since immigration and socioeconomic status. *International Journal of Obesity and Related Metabolic Disorders, 24*(9), 1188–1194.

Launer, L. (2004). *Epidemiology of Alzheimer's disease: lessons from cardiovascular studies.* Program and abstracts of the 9th International Conference on Alzheimer's Disease and Related Disorders, Philadelphia, PA.

Laurin, D., Curb, J. D., Masaki, K. H., White, L. R., & Launer, L. J. (2009). Midlife C-reactive protein and risk of cognitive decline: a 31-year follow-up. *Neurobiology of Aging, 30*(11), 1724–1727.

Lebenthal, E., Antonowicz, I., & Schwachman, H. (1975). Correlation of lactase activity, lactose tolerance, and milk consumption in different age groups. *American Journal of Clinical Nutrition, 28,* 595–600.

Lebra, T. S. (1976). *Japanese patterns of behavior.* Honolulu: University of Hawaii Press.

Lee, H. K., Han, B., & Gfroerer, J. C. (2013). Differences in the prevalence rates and correlates of alcohol use and binge alcohol use among five Asian American subpopulations. *Addictive Behaviors, 38*(3), 1816–1823.

Leong, F. T. L. (1986). Counseling and psychotherapy with Asian Americans: review of the literature. *Journal of Counseling Psychology, 33,* 196–206.

Lin, K. M., & Cheung, F. (1999). Mental health issues for Asian Americans. *Psychiatric Services, 50*(6), 774–780.

Lin, K. M., & Finder, E. (1983). Neuroleptic dosage for Asians. *American Journal of Psychiatry, 140*(4), 490–491.

Lin, K. M., et al. (1989). Longitudinal assessment of haloperidol doses and serous concentrations in Asian and Caucasian schizophrenic patients. *American Journal of Psychiatry, 146*(10), 1307–1311.

Lyman, S. M. (1994). *Color, culture, civilization: race and minority issues in American society.* Urbana, IL: University of Illinois.

Machizawa, S., & Lau, D. T. (2010). Psychological needs of Japanese American elders: implications for culturally competent interventions. *Journal of Cross Cultural Gerontology, 25,* 183–197.

Madison, J. R., et al. (2006). Proteinuria and risk for stroke and coronary heart disease during 27 years of follow-up: the Honolulu Heart Program [Abstract]. *Archives of Internal Medicine, 166*(8), 884–889.

Marsella, A. J. (1993). Counseling and psychotherapy with Japanese Americans: cross-cultural considerations. *American Journal of Orthopsychiatry, 63*(2), 200–208.

Marsella, A. J., Johnson, F. A., Johnson, C. L., & Brennan, J. (1998). Ethnic identity in second-(Nisei), third-(Sansei), and fourth-(Yonsei) generation Japanese-Americans in Hawaii. *Asian American and Pacific Islander Journal of Health, 6*(1), 46–52.

Maskarinec, G., et al. (2009). Diabetes incidence based on linkages with health plans: the multiethnic cohort. *Diabetes, 58*(8), 1732–1738.

Matsui, M., & Braun, K. L. (2009). Japanese Americans' death attitudes and preferences for end-of-life care. *Journal of Hospice & Palliative Nursing, 11*(6), 353–361.

Matsumoto, D. (1989). Cultural influences on the perception of emotion. *Journal of Cross-Cultural Psychology, 20,* 92–105.

Maxwell, A., Crespi, C., Alano, R., Sudan, M., & Bastani, R. (2012). Health risk behaviors among five Asian American subgroups in California: identifying intervention priorities. *Journal of Immigrant and Minority Health, 14*(5), 890–894.

McCormick, W. C., Imai, Y., & Rubenstein, L. Z. (1995). International common denominators in geriatric rehabilitation and long-term care. *Journal of the American Geriatric Society, 42,* 714–715.

McCormick, W. C., et al. (1996). Attitudes toward use of nursing homes and home care in older Japanese Americans. *Journal of the American Geriatrics Society, 44,* 769–777.

McCracken, R. (1971). Lactase deficiency: an example of dietary evolution. *Current Anthropology, 12*(4–5), 479–517.

McDermott, J. F., Jr., Tseng, W. S., & Maretzki, T. W. (1980). *People and cultures of Hawaii: a psychocultural profile.* Honolulu: John A. Burns School of Medicine and the University of Hawaii Press.

McNeely, M. J., & Boyko, E. J. (2004). Type 2 diabetes prevalence in Asian Americans: Results of a national health survey. *Diabetes Care, 27*(1), 66–69.

McNeill, D. (2006). The doomsday doctor: Japan's worsening population crisis. *The Japan Times.* <http://www.japantimes.co.jp/community/2006/03/21/issues/the-doomsday-doctor/#.VgueJpd9X9s>. Available at Lexis/Nexis Academic Universe Database. Retrieved May 24, 2006.

Mehrabian, A. (1968). Communication without words. *Psychology Today, 53.*

Miller, B. A., Chu, K. C., Hankey, B. F., & Ries, L. A. G. (2008). Cancer incidence and mortality patterns among specific Asian and Pacific Islander populations in the U.S. *Cancer Causes Control, 19,* 227–256.

Minami, H. (1985). East meets West: some ethical considerations. *International Journal of Nursing Studies, 4,* 311–318.

Minami, J., et al. (2002). Effects of alcohol restriction on ambulatory blood pressure, heart rate, and heart rate variability in Japanese men [Abstract]. *American Journal of Hypertension, 15*(2 Pt 1), 125–129.

Ministry of Health, Labour, and Welfare. (2014). *Annual health, labour and welfare report.* Retrieved from <http://www.mhlw.go.jp/english/wp/wp-hw8/dl/summary.pdf> Accessed December 8, 2014.

Miyawaki, C. (2013). Generational differences in Japanese Americans' preferred social services environments. *Journal of Gerontological Social Work, 56*(5), 388–406.

Morris, T. M. (1990). Culturally sensitive family assessment: an evaluation of the family assessment device used with Hawaiian American and Japanese American families. *Family Process, 29,* 105–116.

Nagata, D. (1991). Transgenerational impact of the Japanese American internment: clinical issues in working with children of former internees. *Psychotherapy, 28,* 121–128.

Nagata, D. K., & Cheng, W. J. Y. (2003). Intergenerational communication of race-related trauma by Japanese American former internees. *American Journal of Orthopsychiatry, 73*(3), 266–278.

Nagata, D. N., & Takeshita, Y. J. (2002). Psychological reactions to redress: diversity among Japanese Americans interned during World War II. *Cultural Diversity and Ethnic Minority Psychology, 8*(1), 41–59.

Nakamura, A. (2005). Migration expert makes case for helping foreign workers. *The Japan Times.* Available at Lexis/Nexis Academic Universe database. Accessed May 24, 2005.

Nakao, A. (2005). East Bay: Obon season means "people can put on their summer kimono and celebrate." *San Francisco Chronicle.* <http://www.sfgate.com/bayarea/article/East-Bay-Obon-season-means-people-can-put-on-2623606.php> Available at Lexis/Nexis Academic Universe database. Accessed May 30, 2006.

Nakawatase, T. V., Yamamoto, J., & Toshiaki, S. (1993). The association between fast-flushing response and alcohol use among Japanese Americans. *Journal of Studies on Alcohol, 54*(1), 48–53.

National Center for Health Statistics. (2014). *Health, United States, 2014: with special feature on death and dying.* Hyattsville, MD.

National Police Agency. (2014). *Damage situation and police countermeasures.* Retrieved from <http://www.npa.go.jp/archive/keibi/biki/higaijokyo_e.pdf> Accessed December 8, 2014.

Nemoto, M., Sasaki, T., Deeb, S. S., Fujimoto, W. Y., & Tajima, N. (2002). Differential effect of PPARgamma2 variants in the development of type 2 diabetes between native Japanese and Japanese Americans [Abstract]. *Diabetes Research and Clinical Practice, 57*(2), 131–137.

Newburger, J. W., et al. (2004). Diagnosis, treatment, and long-term management of Kawasaki disease: a statement for health professionals from the Committee on Rheumatic Fever, Endocarditis and Kawasaki Disease, Council on Cardiovascular Disease in the Young, American Heart Association. *Circulation, 110,* 2747–2771.

Ngo-Metzger, Q., Phillips, R. S., & McCarthy, E. P. (2008). Ethnic disparities in hospice use among Asian-American and Pacific Islander patients dying with cancer. *Journal of the American Geriatrics Society, 56*(1), 139–144.

Nomura, A. M., Lee, J., Stemmermann, G. N., Nomura, R. Y., Perez-Perez, G. I., & Blaser, M. J. (2002). *Helicobacter pylori* CagA seropositivity and gastric carcinoma risk in a Japanese American population [Abstract]. *The Journal of Infectious Diseases, 186*(8), 1138–1144.

Ogden, C. L., Carroll, M. D., Kit, B. K., & Flegal, K. M. (2014). Prevalence of childhood and adult obesity in the United States, 2011–2012. *Journal of the American Medical Association, 311*(8), 806–814.

Ohara, S. (2000). We-consciousness and terminal patients: some biomedical reflection on Japanese civil religion. In G. K.

Becker (Ed.), *The moral status of persons: perspectives on bioethics* (vol. 96, pp. 119–127). Amsterdam and Atlanta, GA: Rodopi.

Okamura, J. Y. (2014). *From race to ethnicity: interpreting Japanese American experiences in Hawaii.* Honolulu, HI: University of Hawaii Press.

Okubo, Y., Suwazono, Y., Kobayashi, E., & Nogawa, K. (2001). Alcohol consumption and blood pressure change: 5-year follow-up study of the association in normotensive workers [Abstract]. *Journal of Human Hypertension, 15*(6), 367–372.

Onishi, N. (2005). Japan's population fell this year, sooner than expected. *New York Times,* Tokyo (p. 8). Available at Lexis Nexis Academic Universe Database. <http://www.nytimes.com/2005/12/24/world/asia/japans-population-fell-this-year-sooner-than-expected.html?_r=0>. Accessed May 24, 2006.

Osaka, M. N. (1979). Aging and family among Japanese Americans: the role of ethnic tradition in the adjustment to old age. *Gerontologist, 19,* 448–455.

Overfield, T. (1995). *Biologic variation in health and illness.* Menlo Park, CA: Addison-Wesley.

Oyama, N., et al. (2006). Low HDL-cholesterol, hypertension and impaired glucose tolerance as predictors of acute myocardial infarction in northern area of Japan [Abstract]. *Hokkaido Igaku Zasshi, 81*(1), 25–30.

Padilla, A. M., Wagatsuma, Y., & Lindholm, K. J. (1985). Acculturation and personality as predictors of stress in Japanese and Japanese Americans. *Journal of Social Psychology, 125,* 295–305.

Petersen, W. (1966). Success story, Japanese American style. *New York Times Magazine.*

Pew Research Center. (2012). *The rise of the Asian Americans.* Retrieved from <http://www.pewsocialtrends.org/2012/06/19/chapter-1-portrait-of-asian-americans/>.

Phua, V. C., & Kaufman, G. (2008). Grandparenting responsibility among elderly Asian Americans: the effects of householder status, ethnicity, and immigration. *Journal of Intergenerational Relationships, 6*(1), 41–59.

Pierce, B. L., et al. (2007). Measuring dietary acculturation in Japanese Americans with the use of confirmatory factor analysis of food-frequency data. *The American Journal of Clinical Nutrition, 86*(2), 496–503.

Rice, M. M., Larson, E. B., LaCroix, A. Z., & Drinkwater, B. L. (2001). Diagnosing osteoporosis in Japanese American women. *American Journal of Medicine, 110,* 241–242.

Rodriguez, B. L., et al. (2002). Risk of hospitalized stroke in men enrolled in the Honolulu Heart Program and the Framingham Study: a comparison of incidence and risk factor effects. *Stroke, 33*(1), 236–246.

Rogers, T., & Izutsu, S. (1980). The Japanese. In J. F. McDermott Jr., W. S. Tseng, & T. W. Maretzki (Eds.), *People and cultures of Hawaii: a psychocultural profile.* Honolulu: University of Hawaii Press.

Roseblat, R., & Tang, S. W. (1987). Do Oriental psychiatric patients receive different dosages of psychotropic medication when compared with Occidentals? *Canadian Journal of Psychiatry, 32,* 270–274.

Ross, P. D., et al. (1991). A comparison of hip fracture incidence among native Japanese, Japanese Americans, and American Caucasians. *American Journal of Epidemiology, 133*(8), 801–809.

Ryan, C. (2013). *Language use in the United States: 2011.* American Community Survey Reports. U.S. Bureau of the Census.

Sato, H., & Takano, J. (1983). Nursing care of Japanese American patients. In M. S. Orque, B. Bloch, & L. S. A. Monrroy (Eds.), *Ethnic nursing care: a multicultural approach* (pp. 219–243). St. Louis: Mosby.

Schon, S. P., & Ja, D. A. (2005). Asian families. In M. McGoldrick, J. K. Pearce, & J. Giordano (Eds.), *Ethnicity and family therapy.* New York: Guilford Press.

Simoons, F. (1969). Primary adult lactose intolerance and the milking habit: a problem in biological and cultural interrelations. *American Journal of Digestive Diseases, 14*(12), 819–836.

Statistics Japan Bureau (2014). *Statistics Bureau, Ministry of Internal Affairs and Communication.* <http://www.stat.go.jp/english/data/index.htm> Accessed December 12, 2016.

Storry, R. (1993). *Japan—history up to 1952. The Far East and Australasia* (24th ed., pp. 372–375). London: Europa Publishers.

Strazar, M., & Fisher, N. (1996). Traditional Japanese culture. In N. Fisher (Ed.), *Cultural and ethnic diversity: a guide for genetic professionals.* Baltimore: The Johns Hopkins University Press.

Sue, D. W. (1987). Use and abuse of alcohol by Asian Americans. *Journal of Psychoactive Drugs, 19,* 57–66.

Sue, D. W. (2004). Ethnic identity: the impact of two cultures on the psychological development of Asians in America. In D. R. Atkinson, G. Morton, & D. W. Sue (Eds.), *Counseling American minorities: a cross cultural perspective* (6th ed., pp. 85–96). Boston: McGraw-Hill.

Sue, S., & Okazaki, S. (1990). Asian American educational achievement. *American Psychologist, 45,* 913–920.

Suzuki, S., Kirschling, J., & Inoue, I. (1993). Hospice care in Japan. *American Journal of Hospice and Palliative Care, 10*(4), 35–40.

Tahara, Y., Moji, K., Muraki, S., Honda, S., & Aoyagi, K. (2003). Comparison of body size and composition between young adult Japanese-American and native Japanese in 1980's. *Annals of Human Biology, 30*(4), 392–401.

Takemura, K. (2007). Institutions and psychological mechanisms behind Japanese collectivism. In T. Irimoto, N. Takahashi, & T. Yamagishi (Eds.), *Logics and practices of social groups: psychological and anthropological approaches to reciprocity* (pp. 156–170). Sapporo: Hokkaido University Press (in Japanese).

Tarn, D. M., et al. (2005). Trust in ones' physician: the role of ethnic match, autonomy, acculturation, and religiosity among Japanese and Japanese Americans. *Annals of Family Medicine, 3,* 339–447.

Time Almanac. (2013). Chicago: Time Home Entertainment, Incorporated.

Tong, J., et al. (2007). Impaired glucose tolerance is a more important risk factor for the development of diabetes than impaired fasting glucose in Japanese Americans. *Diabetes, 56*(Suppl. 1), A248.

Torréns, J. I., et al. (2004). Ethnic differences in insulin sensitivity and beta-cell function in premenopausal or early perimenopausal women without diabetes: the Study of Women's Health Across the Nation (SWAN) [Abstract]. *Diabetes Care, 27*(2), 354–361.

Tracey, T. J., Leong, F. T. L., & Glidden, C. (1986). Help seeking and problem perception among Asian Americans. *Journal of Counseling Psychology, 33,* 331–336.

Tsai, E. C., Boyko, E. J., Leonetti, D. L., & Fujimoto, W. Y. (2000). Low serum testosterone level as a predictor of increased visceral fat in Japanese-American men. *International Journal of Obesity, 24,* 485–491.

Tsuchida, T. (2007). A differing perspective on advance directives. In H. M. Sass, R. M. Veatch, & R. Kimura (Eds.), *Advance directives and surrogate decision making in health care: United States, Germany and Japan* (pp. 175–186). Baltimore: Johns Hopkins University Press.

Tsuda, T. (2014). "I'm American, not Japanese!": the struggle for racial citizenship among later-generation Japanese Americans. *Ethnic and Racial Studies, 37*(3), 405–424.

Unger, J. M. (2006). Japan: writing system. *Encyclopedia of Language & Linguistics, 6,* 95–102.

United Nations. (2014). *World urbanization prospects: the 2014 revision.* Highlights. Population Database. Retrieved from <http://esa.un.org/unup/> Accessed on December 8, 2014.

U.S. Department of Commerce, Bureau of the Census. (2012). *The foreign born from Asia: 2011.* Washington, DC: U.S. Government Printing Office.

Vessell, E. (1972). Therapy—pharmacogenetics. *New England Journal of Medicine, 287*(18), 904–909.

Wall, T. L., et al. (1997). Alcohol metabolism in Asian-American men with genetic polymorphisms of aldehyde dehydrogenase. *Annals of Internal Medicine, 127*(5), 376–379.

Wander, P. L., Boyko, E. J., Leonetti, D. L., McNeely, M. J., Kahn, S. E., & Fujimoto, W. Y. (2013). Change in visceral adiposity independently predicts a greater risk of developing type 2 tiabetes over 10 years in Japanese Americans. *Diabetes Care, 36*(2), 289–293.

Watson, G. S., et al. (2006). Effects of exercise and nutrition on memory in Japanese Americans with impaired glucose tolerance. *Diabetes Care, 29*(1), 135–136.

Watson, O. M. (1980). *Proxemic behavior: a cross-cultural study.* The Hague, the Netherlands: Mouton.

Wenger, A. F. (2007). The role of context in culture-specific care. In P. Chinn (Ed.), *Anthology on caring* (pp. 95–110). New York: NLN.

Williams, J. K. Y., Else, I. R. N., Goebert, D. A., Nishimura, S. T., Hishinuma, E. S., & Andrade, N. N. (2013). A confirmatory model for substance use among Japanese American and part-Japanese American adolescents. *Journal of Ethnicity in Substance Abuse, 12*(1), 82–105.

Wood, K. (2005). Record of a community destroyed. *The Daily Yomuri.* Available at Lexis/Nexis Academic Universe database. Retrieved on May 31, 2006.

World Almanac. (2015). *Infobase Learning.* New York, New York.

World Health Organization. (2004). Appropriate body mass index for Asian populations and its implications for policy and intervention strategies. *Lancet, 363,* 157–163.

World Population Review. (2014). Retrieved from <http://worldpopulationreview.com/countries/japan-population/> Accessed on December 8, 2014.

Wros, P., Doutrich, D., & Izumi, S. (2004). Ethical concerns: a comparison of values from two cultures. *Nursing and Health Science, 6,* 131–140.

Yamamoto, J. (1982). Japanese Americans. In A. Gaw (Ed.), *Cross-cultural psychiatry.* Littleton, MA: John Wright–PSG Publishing.

Yamamoto, J., Fung, D., Lo, S., & Reece, S. (1979). Psychopharmacology for Asian Americans and Pacific Islanders. *Psychopharmacology Bulletin, 15*(4), 29–34.

Yamamura, E. (2008). The effects of inequality, fragmentation, and social capital on collective action in a homogeneous society: analyzing responses to the 2005 Japan census. *The Journal of Socio-Economics, 37,* 2054–2058.

Yates, C., Kuwada. K, Potter, P., Cameron, D. & Hoshino, J. (2007). Image making and person narratives with Japanese-American survivors of World War II internment camps. *Art Therapy: Journal of the American Art Therapy Association, 24*(3), 111–118.

Yeh, C. J., Arora, A. K., Inose, M., Okubo, Y., Li, R. H., & Greene, P. (2003). The cultural adjustment and mental health of Japanese immigrant youth. *Adolescence, 38*(151), 481–501.

Yeh, C. J., & Huang, K. (1996). The collectivistic nature of ethnic identity development among Asian-American college students. *Adolescence, 31*(123), 645–661.

Yoneda, M., et al. (2008). Prevalence of metabolic syndrome compared between native Japanese and Japanese-Americans. *Diabetes Research and Clinical Practice, 79*(3), 518–522.

Yoo, D. K. (2000). *Growing up Nisei: race, generation, and culture among Japanese Americans of California, 1924–49.* Urbana, IL: University of Illinois Press.

Yoshishige, J. (1993). Wartime heroics: a nisei history. *The Honolulu Advertiser* 5–442nd special section.

Young, H. M., McCormick, W. M., & Vitaliano, P. P. (2002). Evolving values in community-based long-term care services for Japanese Americans. *ANS Advances in Nursing Science, 25*(2), 40–56.

Yukawa, E., et al. (2003). Interindividual variation of serum haloperidol concentrations in Japanese patients—clinical considerations on steady-state serum level–dose ratios. *Journal of Clinical Pharmacy & Therapeutics, 28*(2), 97–101.

Afghans and Afghan Americans

Razia Askaryar Iqbal and Juliene G. Lipson

BEHAVIORAL OBJECTIVES

After reading this chapter, the nurse will be able to:

1. Describe differences between the national languages of Afghanistan.
2. Identify topics of conversation that may be considered private by Afghans.
3. Discuss situations in which variations of time are utilized by Afghans.
4. Describe how Afghan beliefs about health and illness and practices affect risk reduction.
5. Describe generational differences that may be observed among Afghans in the United States.
6. List several potential health risks associated with the Afghan refugee experience.

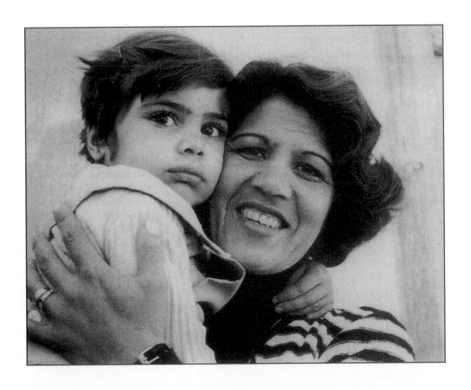

OVERVIEW OF AFGHANISTAN

Afghanistan, a poor, underdeveloped, and landlocked country of approximately 251,825 square miles, is slightly smaller than Texas. It is located in south-central Asia. Afghanistan is bordered by Iran on the west, Pakistan on the east and south, and Turkmenistan, Uzbekistan, and Tajikistan on the north; a narrow finger, the Vakhan (Wakhan) Corridor, extends in the northeast along Pakistan to the Xinjiang Uygur Autonomous Region of China (Central Intelligence Agency [CIA], 2015). Afghanistan is split east and west by the Hindu Kush mountain range that rises in the east to a height of 24,000 feet (7314 m). With the exception of the southwest, most of the country is covered by snow-capped mountains and traversed by deep valleys. It was invaded and colonized for millennia by the Persians, Alexander the Great, the Arabs, Genghis Khan, Tamerlane, and the Moguls of India, all of whom influenced language and religion and created an ethnically diverse population. The largest and most lasting impact on the region that includes the Middle East was the introduction of Islam in the seventh century. There is no census, and no one knows exactly how many people live in the largest cities—some estimates are the capital of Kabul (4,436,260), Kandahar (459,000), Herat (249,000), and Mazar-I-Sharif (183,000).

Modern Afghanistan emerged in 1921, but the last Afghan king was deposed in 1973. The invasion of Union of Soviet Socialist Republics (USSR) troops in 1979, intended to shore up the Communist faction of the government, precipitated one of the largest migrations of people in modern history. Afghanistan's population was reduced from 15.5 million to 8 or 9 million people between 1979 and 1992. More than 1 million Afghans have been killed, and more than 80% of the population has had to move at least once to avoid war or conflict since the late 1970s. The country has been devastated by war and littered with more landmines and unexploded ordinance than there are people in the country. What the war did not destroy, 10 years of the worst drought in modern history devastated. In 2010, the population of Afghanistan was 28,395,716, with an average annual rate of natural increase of 2.58%. Ethnic groups in Afghanistan are Pashtun (42%), Tajik (27%), Uzbek (9%), Hazara (9%), and smaller groups, including Aimaks, Turkmen, and Baloch (CIA, 2015).

For almost two decades, Afghans were the largest refugee population—at its peak, more than 6 million people—in the world. Of the 4 million refugees in October 2001, 2.3 million returned to Afghanistan. Although Afghans were coming to the United States for education well into the 1970s, the situation changed dramatically when the United States began processing refugee claims as it fought a proxy war against the USSR on Afghan soil. Between 1980 and 1988, when the USSR withdrew from Afghanistan, between 50,000 and 100,000 Afghan refugees came to the United States. Since 1989, most Afghans have been admitted to the United States under the family reunification classification (immigrants) rather than as refugees.

The first arrivals in the early 1980s were the urban, formerly wealthy, and highly educated elite, and later family reunification brought middle-class relatives who were less educated. The majority were from Kabul and other cities and came through Pakistan and India. Many families spent time in Europe, especially Germany, before coming to the United States. Relatively few people came directly from refugee camps. There is a small group of Afghans from rural areas who had little previous contact with Westerners; they maintain a traditional lifestyle and are illiterate in their own languages.

Although many Afghans in the United States talked about repatriating to Afghanistan, very few did so because of war, food and energy shortages, earthquakes, drought, and famine. Then, despite some peace that followed the takeover of most of the country by the fundamentalist Taliban, repression of women's and human rights further discouraged people from returning. With the demise of the Taliban and a newly elected government in 2004, young Afghan Americans in particular are returning to help rebuild the country (Lipson & Omidian, 1996). Those who have returned usually leave their families in the country where they resettled. Very few have returned permanently; most of those hold positions of power and are over 45 to 50 years of age. Younger Afghans, such as those from the San Francisco Bay Area, return to Afghanistan for short-term contracts, bringing with them vitally needed expertise and skills, but at a price. Most demand high expatriate salaries and prefer to live with other expatriates. They form a small but very tight community in Kabul because they are not really trusted by Afghans who never left the region and because they do not share the values or experiences of those who stayed behind. Many find it difficult to live with family members, preferring the international community or their own group of returnees. They return to Western countries for medical care and for a break from the harsh conditions of working in a war-torn country.

During the recent U.S. economic and unemployment crises, some Afghans have taken translator positions with the U.S. government in Afghanistan because of lucrative pay ($150,000 to $250,000 yearly salary if they are fluent and literate in the national languages, Dari and Pashto).

In Afghanistan, both men's and women's life expectancy is about 50.49 years. In the United States, they appear to be living at least a decade longer, but the population does not yet reflect national U.S. norms in longevity. Life span is shortened by stressors associated with migrating to a foreign land with no English language skills or expectations for the future. Elderly men tend to suffer from heart disease related to expectations of being breadwinners in the context of lack of jobs and lost status—for example, a CEO of a company in Afghanistan now working in a fast-food restaurant. Women tend to suffer from depression, dealt with by constantly visiting physicians to complain of physical symptoms based on psychological difficulties.

LIFE TODAY FOR AFGHANS IN THE UNITED STATES

Afghans are one of the newer U.S. refugee populations, having fled a war that began in 1978 and has continued on and off to the present. Afghans have been mistakenly called *Afghanis* in the media; in actuality, the unit of money is the afghani. The term *Afghan(s)* is used as a noun, whereas *Afghan* (not plural) is used as an adjective.

Accurate estimation of the Afghan population in the United States is notoriously difficult (Yollin, 2002). The 2010 U.S. census listed 95,453 persons of Afghan descent residing in the United States (U.S. Department of Commerce, Bureau of the Census, American Community Survey, 2013). This is likely an undercount because many Afghans reported their ethnicity to census takers rather than their national origin. In 2010, there was a concerted community effort to increase Afghan participation in the U.S. Census. Community estimates range from 30,000 to 60,000. The Afghan Coalition estimates that the largest population, in the San Francisco Bay Area, numbers 30,000 to 40,000 people, many of whom are second generation. There are eight mosques and many cultural organizations and Afghan-owned businesses.

The city of Fremont, California, in Alameda County, is known as "Little Kabul." Many families live in large apartment complexes that are heavily Afghan. After the Fremont/Union City/Hayward area, the largest Afghan populations, in order of magnitude, are the New York City suburbs, especially Flushing and Queens; Los Angeles; and the Alexandria, Virginia/Washington, DC, area. However, Afghan programs on satellite TV have callers from all over the United States. Many who lived in Europe for a few years resettled on the East Coast. There are some variations in economics and ethnic clustering in different communities; for example, Afghans in Los Angeles are spread throughout the city and are wealthier overall than Afghans in the San Francisco Bay area.

Afghans are a young population, the median age being 29.8 years. There are far more younger- than older-generation Afghans and very few elderly in comparison to the number of children. Families are large, with an average of four children. Most of the 25- to 35-year-olds are the children of the many families that arrived in the United States with young children in the late 1970s or early 1980s (U.S. Department of Commerce, Bureau of the Census, American Community Survey, 2015).

In 2011, the median household income of Afghans and Afghan Americans was $49,217 (U.S. Department of Commerce, Bureau of the Census, American Community Survey, 2015). The largest group, including the formerly wealthy, has a middle-class income; very few are currently wealthy, and a significant number depend on public assistance. In 1994, community leaders estimated that 90% of San Francisco Bay Area Afghan families were supported by Aid to Families with Dependent Children. The percentage of people on public assistance in the Bay Area reportedly dropped to about 55% in 2006 because of welfare reform and the young adults who have graduated and moved into the job market. Current estimates are more than 50% among the immigrant/refugee adult generation and 25% in the second generation, most of whom are working or in school. The number of families using public assistance is lower in other areas of the country.

Occupational issues are most difficult for middle-aged men educated in Afghanistan. Although those from middle-class backgrounds have been more willing to accept entry-level jobs, well-educated professionals and former government officials are rarely able to obtain the kind of work they did in Afghanistan. They lack experience perceived as relevant and "connections," face discrimination because of an accent or being Muslim, and are unfamiliar with job interview expectations and multiple-choice tests. Most physicians, for example, are unable to pass the licensure exam because of finances, English-language problems, or outdated medical training.

In Islam, education is more highly valued than wealth. However, war, poverty, and the recent fundamentalist emphasis on teaching only Islam have ruined the educational system of Afghanistan. In 2000, 43% of men could read and write but only 13% of the women were literate (CIA, 2015). In the rural areas today, the literacy rate for women is below 2%. It is hard to find women who can write their names, much less read. Afghanistan also experienced a "brain drain" in which many of the best educated people fled to other countries.

In the 1980s, the refugees who fled from urban areas became one of the most highly educated refugee populations in the United States, with an average education level of 15 years among men and 14 years among women and a literacy rate of about 90%. Later refugees and immigrants had less education. However, there is an extremely wide range of educational levels, from no formal education among some women and many elderly to doctoral and professional preparation, especially among Afghan Americans.

Education is very important to the young generation, illustrated by their high enrollments in San Francisco Bay Area universities and community colleges, which have increased markedly over the past 3 to 5 years. During this time, even older men have entered college. However, the children of the first arrivals in the early 1980s, who then ranged in age from 3 to 15 years, have been unable to pursue higher education because they must work full time to help support their families. A number of young men with high school diplomas or less work in blue-collar jobs, running restaurants or car repair shops, because the older son or sons in the family are responsible for providing family income, even if they desire a college education. Afghan women are by far more college educated; the ratio of women to men earning their bachelor's degrees or equivalent is 3:1. Women are also attending graduate school more than men are. They more often have the luxury of attending college because their income is not an essential source for the family (Lipson & Omidian, 1992, 1997). The U.S. Bureau of the Census now has fairly reliable educational attainment data on Afghans. In fact, according to these data, 20.2% of Afghans have less than a high school diploma; 20.8% are high school graduates or its equivalent; 27.3% have some college or an associate's degree; 21.9% have a bachelor's degree; and 9.7% hold a graduate or a professional degree (U.S. Department of Commerce, Bureau of the Census, American Community Survey, 2015).

When the value of real estate and demands for mortgages burgeoned in 2003, some younger men delayed college when they could make a six-figure income buying and selling homes or becoming mortgage brokers. The economic and real estate collapse beginning in 2007 devastated many families who regret that their children did not pursue their education.

The Afghan Coalition of Fremont has developed a number of programs to meet the needs of the Afghan population, especially the first generation. The first program, aimed to reduce elderly women's isolation and depression, has been hugely successful (see the "Mental Health Issues" section). There are several children's programs. Women's programs include support groups, English, health education, and small business training to learn and market such handcrafts as jewelry and embroidered traditional clothing. The mental health program cooperates with local agencies, although first-generation men are reluctant to participate.

COMMUNICATION

Afghanistan has two national languages: Dari, a dialect of Persian (50%), and Pashto (35%). Other languages are Turkmen and Uzbek (11%) and 30 minor languages (primarily Balochi and Pashai) (4%), and there is considerable bilingualism (CIA, 2015). Both Dari and Pashto are derived from Persian and are part of the Indo-Iranian branch of the Indo-European language family, but they are mutually unintelligible. In the United States, most Afghans speak either Dari or Pashto with regional variations, or another local mother tongue, and many speak two or three other languages in addition to English, such as Urdu, Hindi, or German. Many educated Afghans also speak Russian.

Afghans tend to speak in stories rich in context, rather than providing brief answers to specific questions. Generally, people are reluctant to share personal and family issues with people other than family members, including health care professionals, but women may discuss their problems with friends, including non-Afghans. Men do not discuss their personal problems with others.

Afghan women tend to speak loudly. Westerners observing two women engaging in a conversation tend to interpret this as high-volume speech. Afghan women tend to be very affectionate and, in public settings, speak loudly to express their affection. In private settings, the mother's voice symbolizes power and control of the children at home. Men, on the other hand, tend to speak in soft tones in private or public settings, which denotes being in control of the situation in a relaxed and comfortable manner. Showing aggression or speaking loudly means that men are losing control, and it is seen as disrespectful in public.

There may also be ethnic differences. Those who speak Pashto may sound like they are arguing when they are talking, but this is a style of speech that does not reflect emotional content. Dari speakers tend to speak softly and use polite tones and words, even when they feel strongly about a topic or issue. In some contexts, particularly when one wants to convey respect, silence may mean disagreement.

Afghans generally call elderly persons by respectful terms, such as *uncle, aunt,* or *mother.* Most people have several names: their legal name, which is rarely used, and a familiar name by which family and other Afghans will identify the person. Strangers are never given the legal or familiar name of an adult woman but refer to her by a title, such as *Bibi* or *auntie.* Because of the U.S. system of demanding the legal name on documents, this pattern is changing, and health care providers can call a woman by her legal name without causing insult. But Afghans value politeness, and an honorific or title should also be used.

Determinants of touch are family relationships and gender. Among extended family members and close friends, people often touch each other on the shoulder or leg when conversing. They greet with a kiss on each cheek, a hug, or both. However, couples do not show affection in public. Traditional men and women who are not related do not touch each other at all. They do not socialize or even remain in the same room. Unrelated men and women who are from urban backgrounds or who are more acculturated mix socially and may even greet each other with a kiss. Children and young adults raised in the United States use touch much like those in the dominant culture, although they may not do so at home in respect of their parents' values. However, families strongly disapprove of dating and touch in public.

Greetings between people who are not family members or close friends may be a simple nod or a handshake, but a man should wait for a woman to extend her hand first. However, women often greet each other with a kiss on each cheek, alternating three times or more for special friends or family members. Young or older men may accompany a verbal greeting or farewell with placing the right hand over the heart, which is a sign of respect. This is common when men greet women who are not immediate family members. Men will greet other men with hugs and kisses but greet unrelated women without touch or eye contact.

Gestures in younger Afghan Americans tend to be similar to those in the dominant society, except when they are with their family or in Afghan social gatherings, where they use typical Afghan gestures and body language. In general, youth do not look elders directly in the eyes, but stand turned slightly to the side, with their heads slightly down to convey proper respect. A young person should not correct an elder, although this is changing in American society and can vary from family to family. When an elderly person or the head of a family enters the room, people show their respect by standing. People kiss the back of an elderly person's hand as a sign of respect and acknowledgment of his or her wisdom, which comes with age (Lipson & Askaryar, 2005).

Sustained eye contact varies by acculturation and generation. More traditional unrelated men and women do not sustain eye contact nor do they "insult" someone they perceive to be of higher status by making direct eye contact. In general, health providers should avoid winking at or touching a person of the opposite gender. Winking is seen as flirting and should be avoided.

Implications for Nursing Care

An appropriate interpreter may be needed for patients who speak little or no English. A considerable number of Afghans who speak English may not read or write it; thus, it is important to check for English literacy before asking them to read forms or instructions. Ideally, the interpreter is trained, respected in the community, of the same gender as the patient, and around the same age or older. It is important to translate health education and training materials into both national languages, even though most Afghans read Dari. Be careful not to inadvertently be swept into a political faction, which can be based on language usage. People often insist that Pashto translations are unnecessary, but this plays into the politics of the country and sends a message of favoritism to the whole community. Also, it is important to use Dari or Pashto interpreters and written materials rather than using more available Farsi (Iranian Persian)–written materials (for mental health providers), despite the similarity of Dari and Farsi. The subtle differences in language usage are great enough to create major misunderstandings in treatment and follow-up. The differences between Dari and Farsi are analogous to those between Spanish and Portuguese.

Smith (2009) conducted a study of the information needs of Afghan women that resulted in a detailed guide for service providers. She found that Afghan refugee women can more successfully adjust to their new country if they develop a trusting interpersonal relationship with one or more "point persons" as the primary source of information for all their needs, learn to speak English fluently, gain understanding of how they themselves can navigate the U.S. government and social service information systems, and practice asking questions of strangers in public and customer service so they can advocate for themselves and their families. Smith listed the areas of informational needs as family reunification; immigration, migration, and mobility; education and schooling; employment; health; mental health; transportation; human rights; and community information.

SPACE

In Afghanistan, extended families live in large houses or compounds, and women socialize as they cook and do household chores together. Afghans in the United States miss the daily proximity of other family members. For example, despite having a four-bedroom house, the four teenage children in one family who has lived in the United States for many years often end up in their parents' bedroom, sleeping on mats on the floor, because "we like to be together."

As with other cultural characteristics, space varies with relationship, gender, and acculturation. Physical space between close friends and family engaged in conversation is closer than that between those of northern European heritage, often 1 to 1.5 feet. On the other hand, unrelated men and women who are more traditional keep more distance from each other, often socializing in separate rooms or separate areas of one room.

Spatial comfort depends on the activity and relationship of the people involved and on the setting, such as among all Afghans or with others present. Afghans are extremely modest people who are used to thick walls between rooms. In strictly private activities, such as using the toilet and having sexual relations, people may fear that other family members may "hear" such activities through the thin walls of the typical U.S. apartment or house; a couple may avoid sexual relations because a daughter's or mother's bedroom is next door.

Implications for Nursing Care

The topics of sexuality, birth control, and vaginal or breast examinations are considered very private and extremely embarrassing for women; older women may have minimal knowledge of how their bodies work. There is no formal education for these women in terms of sexuality, birth control, and the like. Women prefer to be seen by female gynecologists. If only a male is available, the woman's husband will accompany her to appointments and stay in the room during the examination.

The situation is somewhat different among young adults and teens educated in the United States, although some parents forbid their middle school– and high school–aged children to take sex education classes.

Traditional women avoid being touched by male nurses or physicians. For example, one couple had been promised that their baby would be delivered by a female physician, but when they arrived at the hospital in advanced labor, only a male physician was available. As they were leaving the hospital, an enterprising nurse suggested that she deliver the baby, although by law, the physician had to be in the room; the couple remained for the birth. More acculturated men and women and Afghan Americans are willing to be cared for by nurses of the opposite gender, but they may not be comfortable with the situation.

It is uncommon to leave one's children with babysitters because of language and custom. When children cannot accompany their parents to appointments, they stay with other family members who do not work. However, children usually accompany their parents to most health appointments and all social activities. Expect children and provide art materials or other diversions.

Numerous family members and friends gather at the bedside of a patient who is hospitalized and remain until asked to leave. Visiting a sick person is a very important value, and the room will seem crowded. If an Afghan is crying, it is important just to sit beside him or her, without touching or hugging or calling further attention to him or her.

SOCIAL ORGANIZATION

Family System and Roles

Family life is the core of Afghan culture and psychological well-being. People maintain close ties with extended family, and most spend almost all their free time socializing with family and old friends. New friendships are slow to develop because of distrust of those outside the family circle. Lack of social support is a problem for many Afghans in the United States, particularly homebound women and the elderly. In one study, only 7% stated that they had American friends (Lipson, Omidian, & Paul, 1995). Homebound women are isolated and lonely when they speak insufficient English to talk with American neighbors or are culturally restrained from moving outside their family circle. They miss the constant visiting of their life in Afghanistan, which is now limited by distance, transportation problems, and the fast pace of American life. Many elderly, who rarely speak English, experience severe isolation, depression, and numerous physical symptoms, and sometimes they feel they are a burden to their families (Omidian & Lipson, 1992).

Impact of Immigration and Acculturation

Afghan culture in the United States is in transition. Families range from quite traditional to more cosmopolitan, based on their background and personal choice. The intense family focus can cause culture conflict in the United States. What Western psychiatrists call *enmeshment* is normal family behavior for Afghans, and extended family obligations, especially to parents and older siblings, often supersede other responsibilities, including allegiance to one's spouse, one's job, and certainly one's own needs (Lipson & Omidian, 1997).

Women in the United States experience some role conflict in the context of divided community opinions. Traditional men expect their wives to stay home and cook for the family, take care of the children, clean house, and socialize only with Afghan female friends. More cosmopolitan women enjoy their freedom and the opportunity to be active in the community. However, all Afghan women are expected to maintain modest behavior over their lifetimes; once a woman's reputation is tarnished, she is no longer respected. Gossip, both positive and negative, is common and frequent, which is how community members know about each other and their reputations.

Given the centrality of marriage and children to Afghan women's identity, remaining single is viewed as unnatural. However, because women acculturate more quickly than men do, it may be difficult for Afghan women to find a spouse when many Afghan men perceive women who have lived in the United States for a long time as not being properly naïve or submissive. Although being married by the late teens is common in Afghanistan, most Afghan American women prefer to finish their educations, despite fears of being an "old maid" at the age of 26. Most single women live with parents or siblings, and it is rare for an Afghan woman to live alone or with peers (Lipson & Miller, 1994).

Adults work very hard but also do extensive visiting or entertaining during weekends and sometimes weeknights as well. Women with small children may prefer to remain at home, but they are also very busy with household responsibilities and entertaining relatives and friends. Hospitality, one of the most important Afghan values, requires elaborate food preparation and a very clean house. But many Afghan women work outside the home to provide or contribute to the family income, and essentially they work a double day.

Husbands tend to experience their wives' earnings as a loss of their paternal leadership as breadwinner, a source of stress and often depression. The traditional husband's power and role as head of the family is further damaged when children learn English quickly and become their parents' translators and spokespersons. While women generally like more independence, even educated and cosmopolitan men who have been in the United States for two decades maintain a tribal consciousness that supports women's submission to their husbands. Islam, however, promotes gender equality and mutual respect between husband and wife (Robson, Lipson, Younos, & Mehdi, 2002).

Children are expected to work hard in school and to come home after school to do homework; strict parents do not allow their children to engage in after-school activities. Some children and teens resort to truancy to spend time with their friends when their parents do not allow them to go out with or visit friends at their homes. Boys, however, have much more freedom than girls do. Teenagers tend to rebel against their parents up until high school (Robson et al., 2002). Children acculturate quickly to resemble their American peers, whom their parents see as "having no respect" for their parents. Their independence and assertiveness contradict the cultural values of family interdependence and strict obedience to elder family members, particularly the father's authority. Younger Afghans with strict families tend to attend colleges and universities that are sufficiently far away from home so that they must live in dormitories. They view this as an opportunity for freedom and some space to "breathe." Their parents allow them to live on campus because they so strongly value

higher education, but most students must compromise by coming home on the weekends. Men have less trouble convincing their parents to allow them to go to a university out of the area than women do.

Religion

Afghans are staunch Muslims, with 84% following the Sunni branch. Shi'a Muslims comprise 15%, and 1% practice other forms of Islam. Sunni Afghans are of the Hanafi school, the most liberal of the four schools of thought. Muslims believe in one God (Allah), and Muhammad is believed to be God's final messenger. They pray directly to God privately or in a *jumat* (congregation) where an imam leads the prayers. They must act in accordance with God's commands, as described in the Qur'an (Koran), which includes rules of cleanliness, diet (e.g., avoidance of pork and alcohol), and prayer (facing Kaaba, in Mecca). Observant Muslims plan to visit Mecca (make a *hajj*) at least once in their lives (Younos, 2002).

The majority of Afghans adhere to Islamic principles of hygiene, modest behavior, and moral values, even though most dress like other Americans. However, individuals and families vary in their adherence to traditional rituals. People vary from being very strict (prayer five times a day; *halal* and *haram* food practices; dressing to cover hair, arms, and legs) to more relaxed, such as praying to oneself rather than at specific times. In the past two decades, many Afghans in the United States have strengthened their beliefs and practices because of the availability of Islamic mosques, classes, and libraries. As part of gaining or maintaining an Islamic identity, some children and young adults have become more orthodox than their parents.

Islam expects modest dress and behavior, including female chastity until marriage. Families are concerned that children will pick up immodest behavior from their non-Muslim classmates, as well as from school itself (e.g., through sex education, being served pork, and participating in teen drinking). However, even when young people appear to be completely American in their speech and activities, most still maintain an Islamic outlook.

Implications for Nursing Care

Assess for how long the family has been in the United States, acculturation level, urban or rural origin, and whether the family is more cosmopolitan or traditional. Ask who makes decisions for the family: father, mother, or joint decisions? Nurses must recognize that family obligations and traditional hierarchy may interfere with getting to appointments or compliance. Be especially aware of Afghans' strong aversion to "interference" in family affairs, which they see as private. Most people perceive school and social service agency intervention as undermining parental authority, responsibility, and control: "What right do strangers have to intrude in our family and judge our discipline? Our children are our responsibility."

In the context of abuse education in the schools, children may tell teachers about physical discipline, which may result in a report of "child abuse" and removal of children from the home. However, teachers rarely understand Afghan methods of discipline in cultural context, assuming that when a child says, "My mom hits me," it means "beating" rather than a slap on the back or a pinch (Lipson & Omidian, 1997). Some parents are so frightened that their children might be taken away that they are afraid to discipline their children. However, some children use the system to manipulate their parents by threatening to call the police if their parents do not give them the freedom they desire.

TIME

Afghans have different orientations to time, depending on the situation. Past orientation is evident in tradition and family lineage, present orientation is observable in social interactions, and future orientation is observable in hard work and commitment to children's education. Other commitments or values may conflict with being "on time" for appointments. For example, given the central value of hospitality, if a family has guests, they would be extremely reluctant to indicate that someone has another obligation and that it may be time for the guests to leave. Instead, finishing an interpersonal encounter gracefully and naturally is more important than the ticking clock or being on time for an appointment elsewhere. Acculturation influences stricter use of clock time in business, school, or health care. Some Afghans overcompensate by coming very early for an appointment to make sure they will not be late. However, transportation problems or other family matters that come up may keep someone from coming to an appointment.

Implications for Nursing Care

Awareness of the importance of hospitality and smooth social interactions should help nurses anticipate whether Afghans may miss appointments. A reminder phone call the day before and asking if the person will have any difficulty with transportation (and if an interpreter will be needed) would be appreciated and may help. With regard to health risks, Afghans rarely tend to be future oriented, which has implications for teaching prevention and health risk reduction. It is more the case that they are unfamiliar with risk reduction than that they are not interested, however. They had little previous experience in Afghani-

stan, where prevention (except for immunizations) and screening were not done.

ENVIRONMENTAL CONTROL

Most Dari words for the concept of *health* mean "wholeness" or "completeness" (Shorish-Shamley, 1991). Afghans are very concerned about their health, as illustrated by a woman who said, "If you have health the key to the whole city is in your hand, but if you are sick, what are you going to do with riches?" (Lipson & Omidian, 1992, p. 273). Afghans combine internal and external loci of control, as well as natural and supernatural concepts of health and illness beliefs and behavior.

Individual responsibility is evident in the belief that health is maintained through regular exercise, eating fresh food and a balanced diet, staying warm, and getting enough rest. Natural illnesses are believed to be caused by things that exist in nature, such as "germs," dirt, cold, or wind; one such belief is that people are more vulnerable to colds or flu during the change of seasons (Shorish-Shamley, 1991). One cause of illness is not taking proper care of one's body; for example, a nurse might hear, "When we eat lamb and rice for lunch, it is not digestible here because we don't have time to walk and exercise after, so the amount of cholesterol goes up and blood pressure goes up, creating the possibility of heart disease" (Lipson & Omidian, 1992, p. 273).

Illness is also interpreted as the "will of God" and should be "borne with patience as it cleanses one of individual sins, and God will have mercy on a sick person." This view does not mean that a sick person should not seek treatment, however. Illness is also perceived as a result of not adhering to the principles of Islam. For example, an elderly woman who became acutely ill after someone told her that she had inadvertently eaten pork on pizza said, "I was very stupid. It is against Islam to eat pork, it is forbidden to us by our Book [Qur'an]. If we eat it, it means we are against our religion" (Lipson & Omidian, 1992, p. 273). Islam strongly emphasizes personal hygiene; for example, "Afghans are obsessive about cleanliness, we keep our bodies, our houses and our children clean." Ablution before prayer includes washing hands and arms, feet, face, nose, and inside the throat. If a person urinates, defecates, passes gas, falls asleep, vomits, or bleeds, he becomes impure and must wash again. After sexual intercourse, the entire body, head to toe, must be washed before the person is fit to pray, and women are prohibited from prayer or fasting during menstruation, until they perform a full purification ritual at 7 days.

Supernatural illnesses are caused by *jinns,* the evil eye, or punishment from God. The Qur'an mentions *jinns,* and some describe them as ghosts or spirits; "some are good and some are bad, but people don't like them." Epilepsy is believed to be caused by a *jinn*. The evil eye, *nazar*, is the belief that someone can cause illness by looking at another person, with a particularly powerful "gaze" emanating from green-eyed, impure, or ill people. Unintentional *nazar* comes from expressing excessive admiration for someone without remembering to say a preventive phrase. Intentional *nazar* is based on envy or anger and is meant to hurt another person or his property (Shorish-Shamley, 1991). *Nazar* illness is distinguished by its sudden onset and prevented by saying, "In the Name of God" or "With the power of God" when giving a compliment. Susceptible people (e.g., children, beautiful young women, brides, rich or fortunate people) are protected by wearing charms or amulets, such as blue stones or beads. *Espand* (wild rue) is burned in the fireplace for prevention, which is explained as "forcing the evil spirits out; the sounds of the seeds popping are like the sounds of eyes popping" (1992).

The choice of treatment depends to some extent on the perception of the cause of illness, although both folk-traditional and Western biomedical treatments are valued and often used at the same time. Biomedical treatment cannot cure a supernatural illness, but natural illness may also be treated by religious means. Prayer in general or verses of the Qur'an may be used for specific illnesses. A healer may select and write a specific verse on a piece of paper and administer it via *ta'wiz* (wrapped in cloth and worn like a necklace), *shuist* (soaked in water and drunk), or *dudi* (burning it with *rue* near the patient so the smoke kills germs and wards off evil spirits) (Shorish-Shamley, 1991). Natural illnesses, if mild, are treated with home remedies and dietary means alone or, if severe, by seeking biomedical care. In most families, an older woman, having been taught by her mother and grandmothers, knows how to prepare herbal remedies. Examples are *zirk* (arnica) dissolved in hot milk for broken bones or internal injuries, *zuf* (ribwort) for colds, and *sirin buya* (anise) for stomach complaints. (Cimetidine [Tagamet] is made from the latter.) These plant remedies are available in Afghan, Iranian, and Indian food stores (Lipson & Omidian, 1992). Traditional medical beliefs are also based on Arabic-Persian humoral concepts brought to Central Asia with the spread of Islam (Penkala, 1980). "Hot" and "cold" imbalances cause sickness, and hot or cold qualities describe food, drink, and medicinal herbs; individual human nature; and specific illnesses. Hot illnesses, such as fever and measles, are treated with a diet emphasizing cold foods and medicines; cold illnesses, such as arthritis, malaria, and chickenpox, are treated with hot foods and herbs.

Illness and Wellness Behaviors and Access to Health Care

Barriers to care are lack of health insurance and almost no culturally specific services. Very few hospitals or clinics employ trained interpreters of both genders. There is an enormous need for health education materials in Pashto and Dari, written and via the radio, TV, or videos for illiterate elderly women. Afghans are responsive to and enthusiastic about health education.

Conditions for which people seek health care differ for new immigrants and longer established Afghans. Newly arrived refugees in the early 1980s had dental caries (41%), dermatologic disorders (39%), intestinal parasites (36%), gastrointestinal disorders (23%), and musculoskeletal pain (joints, back, 12%) (McCaw & DeLay, 1985). Those arriving now also have tuberculosis, nutritional deficiencies, intestinal parasites, chronic hepatitis B virus infection, lack of immunization, and depression. In addition to a complete history and physical examination, tests for tuberculosis, hepatitis B surface antigen, and ova and parasites, as well as a hemoglobin measurement, are advised for most groups (Ackerman, 1997).

Afghans who have been in the United States a decade or more have diabetes, asthma, and motor vehicle injuries (because of a lack of urban driving experience and, until recently, not wearing seat belts). Public health nurses and interpreters have also noted active tuberculosis, diabetes, hypertension, and positive cultures for ova and parasites; one said, "Birth control is a problem and women don't want Pap smears and breast exams" (Lipson & Omidian, 1992, p. 273). The women need education about women's health issues and someone to talk to about them.

Mental Health Issues

Refugees experienced multiple losses. Relatives were killed or left behind; they lost their status, language, and vocational competencies, as well as their country, for which they mourn. The primary problems of one Afghan physician's patients, 75% of whom are Afghan, are depression and psychosomatic illness; their major complaints are headaches and musculoskeletal problems, such as joint and back pain. A community mental health psychiatrist described "lots and lots of depression, we establish them on meds and see some improvement, but they get stuck and never become fully functioning." Afghans themselves comment on the prevalence of "mental problems" in their community: "Afghans are sick because of thinking too much" and "Sadness is the sickness Afghans are faced with" (Lipson & Omidian, 1992, p. 273).

Although there seems to be relatively little serious mental disease, such as schizophrenia or other psychotic disorders, many people experience chronic post-traumatic stress disorder (PTSD) related to horrific experiences in Afghanistan and in transit. PTSD is expressed as sleep disorders and nightmares, re-experiencing the traumatic event, numbed or heightened responses to external stimuli, depression, and persecution reactions. Mghir and Raskin (1999) found ethnic differences in young Afghan refugees in the United States. Those with Tajik parents had significantly less evidence of PTSD and depression than those with Pashtun parents. Their socioeconomic and cultural backgrounds were quite different: Tajik parents are wealthier, more likely to speak English at home, and less religious than the Pashtun parents. Pashtun parents and their children spent more time in Afghanistan during the war, and they experienced or saw more traumatic events.

But Afghans also acknowledge current stressors in the United States: "The things they got from Afghanistan—murder, bombs—and the things they got here—children's freedom and not obeying, fear for children's future—all together makes them mentally sick" (Lipson, 1993). Iqbal (2005) conducted a survey of 60 female Afghan refugees between the ages of 25 and 65, who were born in Afghanistan and migrated to the San Francisco Bay Area after the Soviet invasion. She explored the relationship between somatization and depression as they relate to acculturation, finding that these Afghan women had high levels of somatization and depression and that the higher the depression score, the more they tended to somatize their depression. Iqbal's current clients observed that Afghans in Afghanistan are not the same as they used to be; they feel helpless and defeated. Mental health issues are more prevalent than earlier. Preliminary findings of Stempel's current study (2010) of resettlement and acculturation impacts on emotional distress show that it is mediated by gender and gender ideology. For example, gender traditionalist men and gender egalitarian women experience greater distress. Men's levels of distress are more associated with concerns about the younger generation becoming Americanized. Women's levels of distress are much more associated with social and cultural isolation than men's are. Men's and women's distress levels are equally associated with perceived discrimination and post-9/11 fears of being the target of harm (Stempel, personal communication, 2010).

Although Afghans agree that mental health is a problem in the community, families tend to seek psychiatric care only as a last resort because it is perceived as shaming the family. As one person noted, "We don't believe in psychiatry, although after 22 years of war, more than 50% of us have some mental health problems." Fears include gossip, losing face, and that a therapist may share "personal" information about the family. Many would prefer a medication (a quick cure) to "talk therapy." However, interviews revealed that Afghan women would go to a female psychologist for services if one were available in their community (Iqbal, 2005).

There are almost no available culturally sensitive mental health services, and mainstream counselors tend to treat Afghans like mainstream Americans. For example, an isolated and depressed elderly woman was told to "get a boyfriend," which so insulted her that she cried. Instead, the counselor could have suggested that she pray and increase her reading of the Qur'an (Robson et al., 2002). Group approaches with time for socializing are preferable to individual counseling. Other methods of stress reduction, such as physical activity (walking groups), are often effective in reducing depression. For example, an excellent program for the elderly in Fremont was started 15 years ago by taking seven isolated and depressed elderly women to the park so that they could socialize with each other. After a few months, these women began to organize the "Tuesdays" themselves. The group grew, and many of the women showed striking improvement in their mental health (Omidian, 1996). There are more than 100 people who attend the Fremont Senior Center weekly, aided by Dari- or Pashto-speaking staff, where they socialize and are provided with health education and other services.

Death Beliefs and Customs

While Afghans grieve expressively and strongly over the death of a loved one, death is seen not as the termination of life but as the beginning of a new and better life, a spiritual existence and a cherished state in which one solidifies one's relationship with God. Muslims believe that they are on earth to be tested; praying five times a day helps them think about God and avoid committing bad deeds. As God's children, they believe that when their time comes to go, they have no choice but to go to the other world where God is calling upon them. The belief in the power of God over all His creation makes "letting go" easier for some families. However, Afghans may oppose stopping life support, viewing it as "playing God," although they may view beginning life support as a gift of medical technology.

After the death, the body is washed in a ritual manner, only by another Muslim. Although the sooner the better, the time of washing may be delayed if family members must travel from a different state or country. The body is washed by a mullah and an immediate family member, who prays during the washing. The body is wrapped in a white cotton shroud and placed in a coffin. If the deceased is a woman, only close female family members are allowed to see her face. Not even her husband is allowed to see it.

If the deceased is a man, only close male friends and family are allowed to see his face, with the exception of his wife. Islam does not permit embalming of the dead; in Afghanistan, people are buried directly into the earth to facilitate the transition from "dust to dust." In the United States, the body is not embalmed but placed in a coffin and taken to a mosque, where men (not women) pray over the body (*Jinaza*).

The coffin is then taken to the chapel for burial. Until recently, only men were allowed to attend the burial, but now women attend as well. A cloth covering with Qur'anic verses written on it is placed on the coffin, but it is removed when the coffin is buried. Then everyone goes to the deceased's home or a local mosque for prayer (*fatya*). Men and women sit separately for the *fatya*.

Close family members gather together to mourn at specified intervals. Following the *fatya*, close family members gather every Thursday to read a chapter of the Qur'an for the first 40 days (*chil*). *Chil* ends on the fortieth day if the deceased had no children. Otherwise, one day is subtracted for each child, determining the length of *chil*. For example, the last gathering for prayer would be the thirty-fourth day if the person had six children.

For the first 40 days after the death, women in the immediate family do not wear makeup and must wear the chador. After 40 days, they can wear light makeup. Immediate family members mourn for a full year, after which they resume their customary lives. Until a year from the day the family member died, they may not attend any social (happy) gatherings such as weddings or birthday parties where there is music and laughter. If the deceased was elderly, the family finds it easier for life to go on than after the death of a young person.

Implications for Nursing Care

It is essential for the culturally competent nurse to be sensitive to values and beliefs that may be held by Afghans and the effects of such beliefs on health care practices and on behavior related to achieving an optimal state of health. For example, the nurse should enable the client to carry out beliefs related to washing before prayer and other religious practices. It is important for the nurse to appreciate that while the client may believe that illness is the "will of Allah," the client is also likely to value and seek Western medical care.

BIOLOGICAL VARIATIONS

Afghans are a mixture of original tribes and foreigners who invaded the area throughout history, including Greeks, Kushans (Caucasian nomads), Indians from the south, Huns from the north, Arabs, Turks, and Mongols.

Indo-European genetics are evident in Pashtuns and Tajiks, whose skin tones and facial features resemble those of other Mediterranean groups, with coloring ranging from blue or green eyes, light brown hair, and fair skin to nearly black eyes, black hair, and brown skin. Mongolian heritage is evident in such northern groups as Turkmen, Uzbek, and Aimaks, as well as Hazara, in high cheekbones, narrow slanted eyes, and lighter or yellow-toned skin (Ansary, 1991). Because of the variations in skin color, health care professionals may need to assess jaundice and anemia by examining the sclerae and oral mucosa rather than by relying solely on skin assessments.

Cross-cousin marriage used to be common in Afghanistan, resulting in such diseases and birth defects as epilepsy, blindness, several forms of anemia, and hemophilia. Diabetes is common, but the majority of those who have it are not aware of it, despite clear symptoms. Thalassemia is also common. Glucose-6-phosphate dehydrogenase (G-6-PD) deficiency surveys in Afghan refugees show that this trait was more common among Pashtun and Uzbek refugees (15.8% and 9.1%, respectively) than Pakistani Pashtuns (7%) who live in the same area; the prevalence in Tajik and Turkmen refugees was 2.9% and 2.1%, respectively. Hospital studies showed that the type of G-6-PD deficiency in Pashtuns could cause hemolytic crises when they eat fava beans. G-6-PD deficiency affects drug metabolism, such as increasing sensitivity to primaquine, used to prevent malaria (Bouma et al., 1995).

The Afghan diet is generally healthy, based mainly on rice seasoned with herbs, vegetables, and small amounts of meat or poultry. People enjoy fresh fruit, raisins, and nuts as snacks, although some serve cake. Unhealthy practices include cooking food with a large amount of oil, sometimes fatty meats, and loss of nutrients in vegetables that are "cooked to death," except for lettuce, cucumbers, and tomatoes in fresh salads. Since tea is always offered to guests and accompanies meals, some people may ingest too much caffeine. A nurse or nutritionist could teach people to cook traditional Afghan food with unsaturated oil and less of it and to emphasize fresh fruit over cake. Teens and children are becoming addicted to fast food, which upsets their parents and places them at risk.

Implications for Nursing Care

The nurse should be aware that major public health concerns for most Afghans include trauma related to motor vehicle accidents, maternal and child health, and control of communicable diseases. Concerns related to maternal and child health and communicable diseases may be of more concern to newly immigrated Afghans. The nurse should be aware that the gene–environment interaction of coronary heart disease and that conditions such as diabetes and hypertension, which are emerging as a major problem in Afghanistan, may also be more prevalent among Afghan Americans in the United States.

SUMMARY

Afghans and Afghan Americans are culturally unique individuals with their own customs, norms, beliefs, and practices. In the United States, Afghans are a very young population of people as compared with the median age. These young Afghans tend to highly value education. Many

Afghans come to the United States speaking either both or one of the two national languages of Afghanistan. Many Afghans believe that optimal health is an individual responsibility, and this belief is illuminated further by their desire to maintain regular exercise habits, eat appropriate foods, stay warm, and get adequate rest to sustain the body. In contrast, many Afghans believe that illness is the "Will of God," and thus illness should be borne with patience as it cleanses sin. Some Afghans believe that treatment may depend on the cause of the illness. In some cases, both folk-traditional and Western biomedical treatment are not only valued but are often used at the same time.

CASE STUDY

Mrs. Hafiza Ahmadi, 45 years old, was taken to the emergency room after she fainted. Blood tests led to a diagnosis of type 2 diabetes. She also has had hypertension for several years but does not take medication because she has no primary health care provider or health insurance. Mrs. Ahmadi, who lives with her husband and young adult son, has three sisters and a brother who live in the area, and they visit each other frequently. As part of the strong Afghan value placed on hospitality, food is always involved—black tea with accompaniments like raisins, sugared almonds, or cake and fruit between meals or lunch or dinner. The women socialize while preparing the food and cleaning up.

Mrs. Ahmadi tells an American friend about her diagnosis. The friend helps her make contact with the local public health center, and a public health nurse is assigned to her case. The nurse first helps her to reapply for Medicaid, which she was denied when she applied a few

years ago because she had trouble with and made errors on the complex application.

Mrs. Ahmadi is 62 inches tall and weighs 160 lb. She does not drive, so she walks to the market and used to walk 3 miles to her job at the local community college. She is college educated and speaks accented but fairly good English, and she reads English well. However, she has little knowledge of medical terminology and almost no knowledge of how the body works. She is concerned about her health and motivated to learn. She loves sweets and fatty foods, such as cheesecake, butter, and jam on bread. She cooks typical Afghan food with a lot of oil, large portions of rice at lunch and dinner, traditional wheat bread, and fruit. She is aware that her weight is partially causing her hypertension. She has tried to lose weight in the past, but she explains, "I can't help myself. I can't stop eating the food I love."

CARE PLAN

Nursing Diagnosis: Health maintenance, impaired, related to lack of knowledge about diabetes and hypertension

Client Outcomes

1. Client asks to learn more about food and diabetes.
2. Client will learn to balance carbohydrate intake to lower blood sugar to safe levels.
3. Client will ask her sisters to support diet.
4. Client will learn to test blood sugar and take oral medication on a schedule.

Nursing Interventions

1. Identify family health beliefs that would support proper diet.
2. Assess Afghan diet for diabetic balance; suggest exchanges.
3. Assess meaning of food and hospitality in the family.
4. Discuss with family group risks of diabetes and dietary changes to manage it. Provide simple information in English or work with a medical interpreter.
5. Teach blood sugar measurement and how the medication works.

◎ CARE PLAN—cont'd

Nursing Diagnosis: Nutrition, altered, unbalanced: more than body requirements (fat, carbohydrates)

Client Outcomes	Nursing Interventions
1. Client will learn to alter cooking methods to reduce fat and sugar and use substitutes.	1. Engage culturally competent nutritionist to work with client in altering Afghan food preparation.
2. Client will walk 3 miles at least three times a week.	2. Provide support and structure for walking program; invite sisters to join.
3. Client will lose 3 to 4 lb a month.	3. Measure blood pressure and record weekly blood sugar levels; provide feedback to encourage client and support her progress.

Nursing Diagnoses—Definitions and Classifications 2012–2014. Copyright © 2012, 1994–2012 by NANDA International. Used by arrangement with Wiley-Blackwell Publishing, a company of John Wiley and Sons, Inc. In order to make safe and effective judgments using NANDA-I nursing diagnoses it is essential that nurses refer to the definitions and defining characteristics of the diagnoses listed in the work.

CLINICAL DECISION MAKING

1. Describe the importance of family in Afghan culture and how the family can contribute to an individual's maintenance of health.
2. Discuss gender roles and how they would affect health teaching and individual or group teaching.
3. How can Afghan beliefs about causes of illness and promotion of health be used in teaching someone how to care for oneself in chronic disease?
4. What role would present orientation play in prevention and health promotion in an "invisible" disease like hypertension?
5. Describe alternative ways of providing health education materials in English, Dari, and Pashto to aid in teaching about diabetes and hypertension.

REVIEW QUESTIONS

1. Although the Afghan or Afghan-American client might believe that illness is the "will of Allah," it is important for the nurse to remember which of the following?
   a. Afghans are likely to value and seek Western medical care.
   b. Afghans, in general, refuse all but traditional folk treatment.
   c. Afghans are a genetically homogeneous group with numerous genetically linked diseases.
   d. The traditional Afghan diet is very unhealthy, providing poor nutrition.
2. Afghan or Afghan Americans' death beliefs and customs center on which of the following?
   a. Muslim practices
   b. Christian practices
   c. Buddhist practices
   d. Zoroastrian practices
3. Determinants of the use of touch among Afghans and Afghan Americans are based on which of the following?
   a. Family relationships and gender
   b. Age and social position
   c. Gender and social position
   d. Eye contact and tribe

REFERENCES

Ackerman, L. (1997). Health problems of refugees. *Journal of the American Board of Family Practice, 10,* 337–348.

Ansary, M. T. (1991). *Afghanistan: fighting for freedom.* New York: Dillon Press.

Bouma, M., Goris, M., Akhtar, T., Khan, N., Khan, N., & Kita, E. (1995). Prevalence and clinical presentation of glucose-6-phosphate dehydrogenase deficiency in Pakistani Pathan and Afghan refugee communities in Pakistan: implications for the use of primaquine in regional malaria control programmes. *Transactions of the Royal Society of Tropical Medicine and Hygiene, 89,* 62–64.

Central Intelligence Agency (CIA). (2015). *Central Intelligence Agency 2015 world factbook: Afghanistan.*

Iqbal, R. (2005). Somatization underlying depression as related to acculturation among Afghan women in the San Francisco Bay area (Unpublished dissertation). The California School of Professional Psychology, Alliant International University, San Francisco.

Lipson, J. (1993). Afghan refugees in California: mental health issues. *Issues in Mental Health Nursing, 14,* 411–423.

Lipson, J., & Askaryar, R. (2005). Afghans. In J. Lipson & S. Dibble (Eds.), *Culture and clinical care.* San Francisco: UCSF Nursing Press.

Lipson, J., & Miller, S. (1994). Changing roles of Afghan refugee women in the U.S. *Health Care for Women International, 15,* 171–180.

Lipson, J., & Omidian, P. (1992). Afghan refugees: health issues in the United States. *Western Journal of Medicine, 157,* 271–275.

Lipson, J., & Omidian, P. (1996). Health and the transnational connection: Afghan refugees in the United States. Council of Refugee Issues, American Anthropological Association. *Refugee Issues Papers, 4,* 2–17.

Lipson, J., & Omidian, P. (1997). Afghan refugee issues in the U.S. social environment. *Western Journal of Nursing Research, 19,* 110–126.

Lipson, J., Omidian, P., & Paul, S. (1995). Afghan health education project: a community survey. *Public Health Nursing, 12,* 143–150.

McCaw, B., & DeLay, P. (1985). Demographics and disease prevention of two new refugee groups in San Francisco: the Ethiopian and Afghan refugees. *Western Journal of Medicine, 143,* 271–275.

Mghir, R., & Raskin, A. (1999). The psychological effects of the war in Afghanistan on young Afghan refugees from different ethnic backgrounds. *International Journal of Social Psychiatry, 45,* 29–36.

Omidian, P. (1996). *Aging and family in an Afghan refugee community.* New York: Garland.

Omidian, P., & Lipson, J. (1992). Elderly Afghan refugees: tradition and transition in northern California. In P. DeVoe (Ed.), *Refugee issues papers* (Vol. 1, pp. 27–39). Arlington, VA: American Anthropological Association.

Penkala, D. (1980). "Hot" and "cold" in the traditional medicine of Afghanistan. *Ethnomedicine, 6,* 201–228.

Robson, B., Lipson, J., Younos, F., & Mehdi, M. (2002). *The Afghans: their history and culture. Fact sheet.* Washington, DC: U.S. Center for Applied Linguistics.

Shorish-Shamley, Z. (1991). The self and other in Afghan cosmology: concepts of health and illness among Afghan refugees (Unpublished dissertation). University of Wisconsin, Madison.

Smith, V. (2009). The information needs and associated communicative behaviors of female Afghan refugees in the San Francisco Bay Area. *Dissertation Abstracts International, 70*(02), 398A. (UMI No. 3346402.). Available from California State University East Bay's Digital Repository at <http://csueastbay-dspace.calstate.edu/handle/10211.5/9> Retrieved August 21, 2011.

U.S. Department of Commerce, Bureau of the Census. (2013). *American community survey: 2011–2013.* Washington, DC: U.S. Government Printing Office.

U.S. Department of Commerce, Bureau of the Census. (2015). American Community Survey. Washington, DC: U.S. Government Printing Office.

Yollin, P. (2002). Wide array of estimates of Bay Area Afghans. Little Kabul gets even littler. Counting Afghans is an inexact science. *San Francisco Chronicle,* A-15.

Younos, F. (2002). *Gender equity in Islam, published with Afghan community support.* Retrieved from <http://www.1stbooks.com>.

Russian Americans

Linda S. Smith

BEHAVIORAL OBJECTIVES

After reading this chapter, the nurse will be able to:

1. Describe how health care practices and perceptions in Russia may have affected the health of Russian Americans.
2. Identify at least two health problems specific to Russian Americans.
3. Explain how Russian American people use space and gestures as communication mechanisms.
4. Enumerate at least two future-oriented values for Russian Americans.
5. Relate the importance of family to Russian Americans.
6. Describe specific characteristics of the Russian language.
7. Formulate and implement a patient plan of care with clients self-reporting as Russian American.

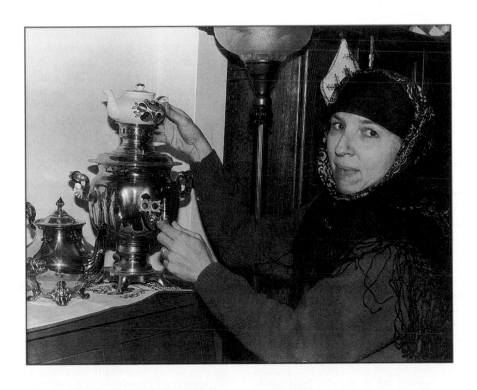

OVERVIEW OF RUSSIA

Russia (Russian Federation) is the largest (by landmass) country in the world, the largest of the 15 republics once known as the Soviet Union, and the largest country within the Commonwealth of Independent States (Central Intelligence Agency, 2014; Commonwealth of Independent States [CIS], 2014). Russia (conventional name, short form) was known as the *Russian Empire* during and after the reign of Peter I (ruled 1682–1725) and as the *Russian Soviet Federative Socialist Republic* prior to the collapse of the Soviet Union. Russia, occupying much of easternmost Europe and northern Asia, stretches from Norway to the North Pacific Ocean and from the Arctic Ocean to the Black Sea with a climate ranging from warm and humid to frigid (Central Intelligence Agency, 2014).

At approximately 1.8 times the size of the United States, Russia occupies 17,098,242 square kilometers and is, therefore, the largest country in the world (the United States is third with 9,826,675 square kilometers). This Russian landmass includes 11 standard time zones (an increase from 9 to 11) (Russia time zones, 2015). Of the 142,470,272 people in Russia, 77.7% are Russian, 1.4% are Ukrainian, 3.7% are Tartar, 1.1% Bashkar, 1% Chuvash, 1% Chechan, and 10.2% other. Within Russia's most recent census, over 190 ethnic groups were represented (Central Intelligence Agency, 2014). Although the official language is Russian (96.3% claim Russian as their language), nearly 100 minority languages are spoken (British Broadcasting Company [BBC], 2015; Central Intelligence Agency, 2014). It is important to understand that Russian-born nonethnic Russians living inside and outside Russia have unique cultural traditions and insist on Russian identities.

Russia's enormous land area is divided by the Urals (a mountain system constituting the traditional boundary between European and Asian Russia) into two land localities: European Russia and Siberia. European Russia is smaller in size but includes the greatest number of people, as well as Russia's two largest cities, St. Petersburg (named *Leningrad* until September 1991) and Moscow, Russia's capital.

Russia is the largest country in the world, yet much of Russia is sparsely populated and much of Russia's landmass is inhospitable for agriculture (too dry or too cold) (Central Intelligence Agency, 2014). The Russian National Constitution of 1993, as amended, established three government branches: executive, legislative, and judicial, but of the three branches, the executive has the greatest powers (Central Intelligence Agency, 2014; Russia, 2015). Russia's border countries include Azerbaijan, Belarus, China, Estonia, Finland, Georgia, Kazakhstan, North Korea, Latvia, Lithuania, Mongolia, Norway, Poland, and the Ukraine (Central Intelligence Agency, 2014). Russian land can be plain and grassy, forested, mountainous, frigid, and marshy; despite its size, large portions of Russia lack proper soil and climate for agriculture. Only 7.11% of the land is considered arable. Oil, natural gas, coal, metals, and wood are Russia's main exports, and income from these natural resources has helped Russia recover from its 1998 economic collapse (BBC, 2015; Central Intelligence Agency 2014). Regarding world production of agricultural and industrial products, Russia ranks first in sugar beets; second in crude oil and natural gas; third in electric power, iron, and potatoes; fifth in steel; and sixth in coal (Russian Federation Federal State Statistics Service [RSSS], 2014).

However, despite these natural resources, 11% of Russia's population falls below the poverty line. Russia has a 5.8% unemployment rate, not including a large underemployed labor force (Central Intelligence Agency, 2014). With a 6.8% inflation rate, it now takes 65.3 Russian rubles (the currency of the Russian Federation) to equal 1 U.S. dollar and nearly 76 rubles to equal 1 euro (Money converter, 2015). This compares with about 27 rubles per U.S. dollar in 2006.

Long-range economic concerns include a decreasing workforce, widespread corruption, and a poorly maintained infrastructure. In the 5-year post-Soviet period (1992–1996) Russia's gross domestic product (GDP) fell 37%; however, an economic recovery followed in 1999. Unfortunately, economic problems persist and organized crime continues to play a role in many initiatives. Because Russia depends so heavily on commodity exports, especially fossil fuels and timber, the nation is vulnerable to shifts in world prices that hit Russia hard in 2014 (Central Intelligence Agency, 2014; Library of Congress [LOC], 2011). In Russia, there are eight persons per kilometer, and 74% of the Russian population is urban. Median age is just 38, compared with 36.5 in 2000. Russia has experienced a troubling negative yearly percent change in population of −0.26% between 2010 to 2014, and this negative change is predicted to continue into 2050 (World Meters, 2015). This is influenced by the following (Central Intelligence Agency, 2014):

- Low birthrates (11.8 births per 1000 population) and low life expectancies (just 64 years for males)
- Low but improving fertility rates (current fertility rate is 1.5 births per woman, compared with 1.25 in 2000; the rate needs to be above 2.1 to ensure a stable population)
- Death rates at 14 deaths per 1000 population
- An impaired health care system, including a human immunodeficiency virus (HIV)/acquired immunodeficiency syndrome (AIDS) epidemic (health care expenditures include 6.2% of the country's GDP)

Russian industry, accounting for 37% of its GDP, has a limited ability to sustain industrial growth. Agriculture accounts for 4.2% of the GDP, with 9.7 % of the labor force; service industries make up the remaining 62.5% of the labor force and 58% of Russia's GDP (Central Intelligence Agency, 2014). Most Russians are well educated; Russia has a 99.7% literacy rate and a school life expectancy of 14 years. However, the average Russian enjoys few luxuries. Widespread, pervasive corruption (Friedman, 2012) and unemployment have increased Russia's economic problems. In 1992, the unemployment rate was 3,889,000, which has increased to 4,137,000 (RSSS, 2014).

Moscow is Russia's largest city (nearly 10.6 million people) and also its capital. St. Petersburg, to the north and west of Moscow, has 4.86 million people. In 2014, following Russia's military interventions in the border neighboring country of Ukraine (including international economic sanctions), as well as the dramatic international fall in oil prices, expectations of Russia's GDP growth were near zero (Central Intelligence Agency, 2014). Nearly three fourths of Russia's mineral wealth is located in the Siberian regions. Harsh obstacles of climate (e.g., permafrost, which covers much of Siberia), distance, and geography thwart exploration and exploitation of these Russian resources (Central Intelligence Agency, 2014).

Russia declared independence from the Soviet Union on August 24, 1991. After the fall of the Soviet Union in December 1991, Russia and other former Soviet republics joined in the Commonwealth of Independent States. In early 1992, Russia made radical changes that had enormous implications for Russians, including privatization programs and lifting of price freezes, which had stifled free enterprise for decades. Russia became a federation and a United Nations member and adopted a constitution on December 12, 1993, that includes a multiparty system and scheduled elections. All citizens 18 years and older may vote. Presidents are elected by popular vote for a 6-year term (extended from 4 to 6 in 2008) and are eligible for a second term. Since May 7, 2012, with a 64% vote, the Chief of State of the Executive Branch has been President Vladimir Putin. His term will end in March 2018. Russia has no vice president (Central Intelligence Agency, 2014).

Life Today in Russia

Today in Russia, life continues to be difficult and frustrating. Anti-Semitism escalates. Railroad stations are crowded with homeless, begging adults and children because of unemployment and underemployment, chemical addictions, mental illness, and lost pensions. Since 1992, a positive downward trend has occurred in Russia's recorded poverty levels. In 1992, nearly 34% of Russia's total population had incomes below the subsistence minimum level. This number dropped to 11% in 2013 (RSSS, 2014). Still, the total unemployment levels for Russian youth have reached 15% (Central Intelligence Agency, 2014). An estimated, though largely ignored, 1 to 4.5 million Russian children are homeless (doubled in the last decade), related

to three categories of social problems and family dysfunction. First (41%) is that one or both parents have chemical dependency problems. The second is the loss of a mother, a father, or both (e.g., through death, prison, abandonment), and the third is domestic violence. Approximately 2 million Russian children suffer abuse (Khovostunova, 2012). An estimated 5 million Russians (3.4% of the population) are homeless, and most are men trying to reintegrate into society (Loft, 2015). Hundreds freeze to death on the streets each winter (Radia & Stukalova, 2012). They have been forced into the streets by cruelty, alcoholism, neglect, and abandonment. They are beggars, thieves, substance abusers, and prostitutes; many have been viciously attacked or are suffering from hypothermia, malnutrition, and depression and are illiterate. The vast majority of street children have attempted suicide at least once. Suicide rates by Russian children and teens are the highest in Europe with a 36% increase over the past few years and three times the world average. Homeless children and boarding school and orphanage graduates are more likely than others to commit suicide (Alexandrova, 2013). Crime and fraud are everywhere fueled by a normalized sense of injustice, insecurity, and mistrust (Friedman, 2012). After the dissolution of the Soviet Union, few if any controls enforced homelessness as well as law and order within the country. Thus, crime exploded. Theft and gangs proliferated, along with weapons and explosives. Without Soviet control, murder and crime rates doubled during the early 1990s. Russia's police force is plagued by low pay, low prestige, and high levels of corruption (Frye, 2014). Crimes against women (domestic violence, prostitution, and trafficking) are pervasive and severely underreported (Novosti, 2010). Trafficking of girls and young women as foreign brides is pervasive. A Google search using the keywords "Russian women" listed 197,000,000 sites; when the words "mail order" were added, 21,000,000 sites appeared. Although Russian criminal code has laws that protect women from interpartner violence, no clear mechanisms are in place to support the women or enforce these laws (ANNA, 2010; Novosti, 2010). According to Kristjanson et al. (2007), most Russian pregnant women decreased their drinking while pregnant, but a full third of the pregnant women studied did not stop drinking.

Russia's economy and infrastructure have recently shown signs of improvement. After more than a decade of steady decline, Russia is moving to a more market-based and globally integrated economy. Russia's GDP grew last year by 1.3% (Central Intelligence Agency, 2014). The telecommunications industry has expanded (over 40.9 million Russians use the Internet), airports and airlines are being enhanced, and road construction and maintenance are improving. Importantly, governmental control over the economy and media has been reasserted by the Putin administration (Central Intelligence Agency, 2014; Russia, 2015).

Small economic gains have done little to improve Russians' health. Health indicators are good social barometers when evaluating the success of any social or political reform. This is especially true during this transition time for Russians. For Russia, population decline and homelessness pose a clear threat to national and economic security as well as the human potential and viability of the nation. In 2014, Russian women of childbearing age had an average of 1.6 children, which means there are about two more deaths than births per 1000 (Central Intelligence Agency, 2014) By the year 2050, Russia's population will have fallen by 28%. Male life expectancy in Russia dropped from 64 to 57 years between 1989 and 1994 and is currently again at 64 years for men and 76 years for women. Men and women with less education, who are homeless, and who have higher unemployment rates have higher death rates; alcohol plays an ever-increasing role in Russian mortality rates (Central Intelligence Agency, 2014; Leon, Shkolnikov, & McKee, 2009; World Health Organization [WHO], 2015). Interestingly, the total population includes just 0.86 males for each female (Central Intelligence Agency, 2014). Men, and very troubling, working men, die far sooner than women because of cardiovascular disease, poisonings, respiratory disorders (60% of Russian men and 22% of women smoke), traffic and industrial accidents, alcoholism, and suicide (Central Intelligence Agency, 2014; WHO, 2015). The infant mortality rate is 7.08 per 1000 live births (Central Intelligence Agency, 2014). Externally caused deaths in Russia are increasing and have been described as an epidemic of injury and violence. Rates of transport-related injury, poisoning, falls, burns, and drownings, as well as intentional injuries such as self- and other-inflicted violence have more than doubled since the mid-1980s (WHO, 2006).

Tuberculosis (TB) is a major concern, killing more than 18,400 per year. In 2013, TB prevalence was 160,000. Significantly, over 19% of TB cases (50,000) are multidrug resistant (MDR), 36% of newly identified cases are drug resistant, and 4% of all new cases are for children under the age of 15 (National Center for Biotechnology Information [NCBI], 2011; WHO, 2015; Wong, 2009). Poverty, unemployment, crime, and homelessness contribute to TB's spread to 320 new TB cases each day. Importantly, children from these groups contract TB 10 to 20 times more frequently; among all TB cases in Russia, 12% occur in prisoners (NCBI, 2011). Russian prisons are filled with TB-afflicted and HIV-infected persons, in part because of severe overcrowding, and when released, they spread these infectious diseases to the general population (NCBI, 2011). HIV/AIDS is also a growing but often secret epidemic, with the number of infected Russians doubling within the past decade (Wong, 2009). Among world populations, Russia and the Ukraine are believed to have the greatest HIV growth rates, with prevalence doubling every year (Russia, 2015). More than half (60%) of all new HIV-positive cases in Russia are among injection drug users (IDUs), with 83,118 IDUs in St. Petersburg alone (Szalavitz, 2011). Since 1990, the number of IDUs has increased 20-fold (Gore-Felton et al., 2003; Heimer & White, 2010). Unfortunately, many, perhaps most, IDUs have not been tested or treated for HIV status (Szalavitz, 2011). The main infected persons are drug users and sex workers. By 2005, sex workers became a leading cause of HIV transmission (partly due to the government's unwillingness to address and document the problem), and the international sex industry's use of Russian women makes Russia's rapidly rising HIV rates an international problem. In addition to prison transmission, HIV and TB infections have spread rapidly among young male Russian populations. The number of Russians infected with HIV has more than doubled since 2001 (LOC, 2011; Wong, 2009). On December 8, 2005, thousands of Russian hospital patients learned that they may have been treated with HIV-infected blood. Hospitals are incredibly understaffed, with as few as 3 nurses to 40 surgical patients. Nearly all supplies are reused, including suture needles, gloves, drapes, basins, urinals and bedpans, and intravenous (IV) bottles (Tashlein-Van Heuveln, 2009). Medications are expensive and access is tenuous. For example, use of modern, efficient, and effective forms of contraception among sexually active Russian women did not increase between 1994 and 2003 (Perlman & McKee, 2008).

For every 1000 people, Russia has 4.9 physicians, 8 nurses (an increase of 0.3% since 2000 and totaling 1.9 nurses per physician), 0.3 dentist, and 0.1 pharmacist. Russia has 62,000 hospitals (down from 126,000) and 9.3 hospital beds per 1000 population (down from 13.1 in 1992), with an average hospital stay of 11 days. Importantly, in 1992 Russia had 207,000 outpatient facilities; this number has dropped to 165,000 (RSSS, 2014; WHO, 2008). Compare these health care worker numbers with those in the United States, which has 2.5 physicians, 11.1 nurses, 1.6 dentists, and 4 hospital beds (with an average length of stay of 6 days) for every 1000 people (Organisation for Economic Co-operation and Development [OECD], 2013; WHO, 2008). Despite a negative population growth, the morbidity rate from all diseases increased from 106,328 in 2000 to 113,688 in 2012 (RSSS, 2014). The general health status of Russians is complex and fluctuates based on political and economic variables. Since 2000, morbidity levels of injuries and poisonings, respiratory and cardiovascular disorders, obesity, cancer, diabetes, and all other recorded parameters are increasing, yet deaths from all causes have, since 1992, increased only marginally; external causes of mortality such as homicides and transport injuries are in decline. Life expectancy for men in 2005 was 58.9 years, which increased to 64.6 years in 2012. Between ages 0 and 4, there are only 949 females for every 1000 males. This ratio dramatically changes by the age of 30 when there are more females than males; between ages 35 and 39, there are 1048 females for every 1000 males; by ages 60 to 64, there are 1424 females per 1000 males. Thus, the current difference in life expectancy for women and men is 11.3 years, down from 13.6 years in 2005 (RSSS, 2014). Russia's health care system remains mostly public supported via a nationalized budget and, on record, is free. It does, however, suffer from the problems of inefficiency, incompetence, low salaries, and bribery (LOC, 2011; Wong, 2009). Hospital staff often expect extra payment for medications, disposable needles, and extra services. Quality medical care depends on the patient's ability to pay for these extras. Hospitals hope for additional government reforms that would improve care and system-wide efficiency, and visitors to Russia are warned of long waiting lines for care and strongly encouraged to obtain insurance coverage for medical evaluations prior to their arrival (Konovalov, 2013). Hospitals and clinics are poorly managed, equipped, and maintained. Most physicians and nurses are paid low salaries (LOC, 2011). Thus, there is a steady shortage of skilled and specialized nurses as well as other health care personnel. There is also a shortage of medical supplies and updated equipment (Balmforth & Feifer, 2011; LOC, 2011). In a study of the fragmented Russian health care system, Danishevski, Balabanova, McKee, and Atkinson (2006) confirm the absence of processes that Russia could use to bring about additional change. As evidence of poor health outcomes, the number of surgical site infections in St. Petersburg hospitals is 3.5 times the rates in the United States, much greater than expected or reported. Possible contributors to these high rates include inadequate antibiotic prophylaxis as well as poor or ineffective infection control practices (Brown et al., 2007).

Preventive health care is a low priority, but the Russian Ministry of Health wants to change that by raising the bar for who qualifies for hospital admission, decreasing the number of hospital beds in Russia, and encouraging more doctors to specialize in preventative medicine (Davydov & Shepin, 2010; Osborn, 2004). As evidence of these changes, the total GDP spent on health care has risen from just over 3% to 6.2% (Central Intelligence Agency, 2014).

Many of the old Soviet-era system-wide health care challenges remain. Russian health care consists of outpatient clinics and emergency and in-patient care services. The need for primary care by the Russian population far outweighs the current system's treatment abilities. Although primary care strategies are getting government attention, disorganization of district-level physicians, ineffective epidemiological monitoring, and poor payment structures actually prevent primary care providers from preventing disease. Instead, patients use expensive emergency care for their outpatient care needs. Rural areas have also seen dramatic shortages of skilled health care professionals, including nurses. Importantly, Russia has not developed a system by which highly skilled, community-based nurses would provide primary care services. If primary care is indeed a national priority and the need to reduce expensive inpatient and emergency care is addressed, community-based nursing care is essential to the improvement of health and health care in Russia (Davydov & Shepin, 2010).

Russian children, when compared to their U.S. counterparts, begin drinking and smoking earlier, receive fewer prevention messages, and have fewer prevention programs available to them (Lally, 2013; Wong, 2009). Nearly 60% of Russians smoke, with a dramatic increase among women under age 30 to nearly 30% (Wong, 2009). New government efforts recently passed may help curb this trend with a bill passed in 2013 to ban smoking in public places and a new law identifying beer as an alcoholic drink rather than a food and banning the sale of beer in curbside booths (Lally, 2013).

Russian nurses are learning to expand their roles as independent practitioners into community health areas (Russian Nurses Association [RNA], 2015; Smith, 2006) with the help of the RNA, established in 1992. The RNA became a member of the International Council of Nurses in 2005 and has over 180,000 members in 56 Russian regions. Nurses' goals include role advancement, professional development, economic and professional protection, and important health care system influence. The mission of this hugely important nursing association includes "Assisting the growth of the quality and accessibility of nursing care in Russia and improving the criteria indicating the health of the nation" (Russian Nurses Association, 2015). Accomplishment of these goals will be essential if the steady increase in tobacco, IV drugs, and alcohol use in Russia is to change course, and Russian nurses express hope that, although the Russian health care system struggles, the life of a Russian nurse is better than it was 10 years ago. They express hope that modern advances will move Russian health care forward (Tashlein-Van Heuveln, 2009). For example, in 2012 the RNA received a $149,946 grant to upgrade the quality of care received by cancer patients experiencing chemotherapy at different care settings. The organization will help develop a nursing education curriculum to educate 60 nurses who in turn will educate an additional 1200 nurses within inpatient, outpatient, ambulatory, and home care settings. Evidence-based practice standards will also be implemented and evaluated (Egenolf, 2012).

History

Historically, Slavic tribes began migrating into Russia around the fifth century, and the first Russian state was established in the ninth century by Scandinavians. Mongols overran the country until 1480, and Ivan the Terrible became the first tsar in 1547. Peter the Great (1682–1725) tried to Westernize Russia, but the pace was slow. Russia had no universities until 1755. In 1917, after Tsar Nicholas II abdicated (and during the October Revolution), Lenin and the Bolsheviks overthrew the government. Between 1918 and 1924, the tsar and his family were murdered, the Bolsheviks declared ideological war on Europe, Joseph Stalin (Josif V. Dzhugashvili) became general secretary, and the Union of Soviet Socialist Republics (USSR) was established.

Further political change in Russia has been dramatic and historic. The current political situation began on March 11, 1985, when the former USSR KGB chief, Secretary Konstantin Chernenko, died and was replaced by Mikhail Gorbachev.

Between 1985 and 1990, the Gorbachev–Shevardnadze team created a new human rights movement within the USSR. Gorbachev's reforms, identified as *perestroika* (restructuring) and *glasnost* (openness), swept the country with promises of a modern democracy and freedom. However, Gorbachev inherited an inefficient, centralized, and decaying empire (Anderson, 1992; Curtis, 1996). Gorbachev believed that free enterprise and a carefully controlled form of democracy could be the overhaul needed for communism. To help him with this plan, he heralded a known reformer, Boris Yeltsin.

Yeltsin proved to be forceful, authoritarian, proud, chaotic, and critical of Gorbachev's leadership. Therefore, in a powerful control move, Gorbachev publicly humiliated and fired his former protégé. This embarrassing termination triggered Yeltsin to campaign against the Communist Party and to run as a candidate for a parliamentary seat as the people's deputy from Moscow. Yeltsin achieved enormous popularity among the people, 90% of the vote, and leadership of a growing group of people who opposed communism (Anderson, 1992).

In February 1990, the USSR's Central Committee eliminated a constitutional clause that guaranteed the leading role of the Communist Party. Independence from the Soviet Union is identified as occurring on August 24, 1991 (Central Intelligence Agency, 2014). Yeltsin left the Communist Party in 1990. After confrontations with the Baltic republics, Gorbachev began discussions that would lead to the creation of a "voluntary" union of the republics.

In May 1991, Soviet citizens were given the right to emigrate. The law titled "On the Procedure for the Exit from the USSR and Entry into the USSR of Citizens of the USSR" came into full effect in January 1993. This law was heralded as one of the most significant steps toward an open Russian society and marked the end of Communist-enforced isolation (Burlatsky, 1991). This law restored the rights of the Russian people to travel freely.

In a historic move and by democratic vote, the citizens of the Russian Republic (highest population and most wealthy republic) elected Boris Yeltsin (June 12, 1991) as its first president, with a 57% vote (Curtis, 1996; Kostikov, 1991). However, shortly thereafter, Gorbachev was overpowered in a dramatic conspiracy coup. After that time, there were ongoing struggles over rulership of this land as power passed back and forth between Yeltsin and coup forces. Yeltsin had great power but failed to use this power to make immediate and necessary reforms. Yeltsin's popularity declined dramatically as a result of internal fighting among the 1033-member parliament (also called *Congress of People's Deputies*).

The Congress (or Duma), Russia's highest legislative body, was formerly dominated by an anti-Yeltsin majority of ex-Communists (Yeltsin rival, 1993). During Yeltsin's tenure, his economic policies received much criticism, and by the spring of 1993, eight attempts on his life had been reported (Eight attempts, 1993). However, Yeltsin continued to push for democratic reform (Witt, 1993), including opening classified Soviet archives, allowing Russians the right to own property and businesses, and attempting to stabilize the unit of Russian currency, the ruble. Other reforms included increasing social care for the needy, formalizing a system of granting benefits and privileges (Yeltsin: Main points, 1993), enforcing public disclosure of environmental accidents, dismantling state economic controls, and cutting the military by half, including dramatic nuclear arms cuts, to invest resources in other areas. Vladimir Putin (Yeltsin's hand-picked successor) was president from 2000 to 2008 and again took office on May 7, 2012. Putin has inherited the conflict in Chechnya, which continues to draw international and national criticism. Universal suffrage occurs at age 18 (Central Intelligence Agency, 2014). The military draft in Russia includes males ages 18 to 27, and the length of required service is 1 year. In 2013, only 65% of the Russian men called up for military service were healthy enough to serve (Central Intelligence Agency, 2014).

For many years following the Soviet collapse, the Russian military experienced disregard. Now, under Vladimir Putin, a shift toward Russian military supremacy and power internally and beyond its borders has occurred. Putin is implementing military reforms to establish a crisis-reaction force and special operations force as well as professionalized and better organized ground forces. As evidence, its military budget has more than doubled within just 10 years. (However, because over half of Russia's federal budget income is based on oil and gas products, as these commodity prices fall, defense spending will likely follow.) As seen recently in the Crimea, Ukraine, and Georgia, Putin's administration is using military force to preserve Russia's hold on border nations. Western sanctions against these military efforts have, however, imposed economic hardships for Russian banks and businesses (Masters, 2014).

In contrast to continued military restructuring, Russia's democratic reforms have slowed and in some cases reversed. Today, the greatest danger in Russia is the widespread disregard for democracy and the repression of free speech, such as unbiased radio, television, and newspaper coverage of political issues (BBC, 2010; Russia, 2015).

IMMIGRATION TO THE UNITED STATES

As Russia has undergone rapid changes over the years, with dramatic economic fluctuations, life in Russia has been unbearable for some, and immigration to the United States has increased. Since the fall of the Soviet Union, many in Russia have chosen to leave in order to improve their own lives but, more important, to improve the lives of their children. Thus, the likelihood has significantly increased that a nurse in the United States may care for Russian clients and their families and that the nurse herself or himself may be Russian. Although collectively referred to as *Russians* as a group, Russian immigrants are diverse with diverse ethnic identities. For example, Russian Americans may self-report as Jews, Pentecostals, Muslims, or Orthodox and come from vastly different political, religious, social, and economic spheres (Aroian & Vander Wal, 2007; Magocsi, 2015).

Since the late 1800s, there have been five significant waves of Russian immigration to the United States: 1880s to 1914, 1920 through 1939, 1945 through 1955, 1970s through 1992, and the post-Soviet era to now (U.S. Department of Homeland Security [DOHS], 2014; Magocsi, 2015). They arrived in the United States after facing severe economic hardship and political and religious persecution. In many ways, immigrants have come from two Russian homelands. One includes Russia as it exists today, a land inhabited by ethnic Russians. The second includes territories in addition to Russia, once claimed by the Russian Empire and the Soviet Union. This diversity has blurred U.S. census reports, making actual census numbers difficult to interpret, and has diversified descriptions of Russian American cultural groups. Importantly, Soviet and Tsarist governments severely restricted emigration. Imperial Russia forbade emigration for everyone except Jews, which relates directly to the small numbers of non-Jewish Russian Americans prior to 1920 (Magocsi, 2015).

Immigrants from the pre-1914 Russian Empire escaped from a country economically far behind its European neighbors. They were poor and often desperate. Importantly, Russian Jews were only allowed to live in Russian Empire areas outside of mainland Russia (e.g., Lithuania, Moldova, Poland, Ukraine) (Magocsi, 2015).

From the late 1800s to 1914, more than 3.2 million Russian Empire immigrants arrived; just 65,000 were ethnic Russians (1.6 million were Jews). Many of the arriving Jews left the Russian Empire to escape Jewish persecution. Many chose not to identify themselves as Russian (Magocsi, 2015). The second wave of Russian immigration occurred as a direct result of the political chaos of the Bolshevik Revolution and civil war. All were opposed to the Communist regime.

More than 2,000,000 persons fled Russia in the early 1920s. The third wave took place following World War II. Immigrants in the second and third waves were considered traitors by the Soviet government. In contrast, in the fourth wave, beginning in 1970, immigration was legal although severely limited for Jews who were allowed to travel only to Israel; many chose to continue migrating on to the United States. Immigration policies were relaxed in the mid-1980s under Mikhail Gorbachev. The policies allowed Jews and non-Jews to leave the Soviet Union. Now, however, Russian immigrants can no longer claim political or religious persecution as they enter the United States (Magocsi, 2015). Therefore, numbers have slowed, although anti-Semitism has flourished in post-Soviet Russia. Actual recorded numbers of persons obtaining lawful permanent U.S. resident status from Russia by year (U.S. Department of Homeland Security, 2014) include 2,608,299 between 1900 and 1919, 28,132 between 1970 and 1979, 33,311 between 1980 and 1989, 433,427 between 1990 and 1999, 167,152 between 2000 and 2009, and 43,820 between 2010 and 2013. Since 2000, 203,470 Russians have immigrated to the United States. Most Russian Americans are living in the northeastern part of the United States (36%) with 17% in the Midwest, 21% in the South, and 25% in the West (U.S. Bureau of the Census, 2014).

Russian immigrant Jews were and are well educated (all high school graduates go on to college), with approximately 14 years of education (with an approximate equal number of births to deaths). Most entered the United States as refugees because of emerging and ever-increasing anti-Semitism. For many Russian Jews, the Jewish communities in which they settle provide tremendous social, religious, and economic support. Russian-speaking Jews are highly likely to be members of Jewish community centers (Berger, 2011; Kliger, 2012). For most Russian immigrants to the United States, their sphere of family and friends rests primarily with other Russian Americans; this is partly due to

U.S. immigration laws that offer the right to U.S. immigration based on family preference. Therefore, most new Russian Americans are related in some way to earlier Russian immigrants.

From 1971 to 2009, approximately 410,000 Russian Jews entered the United States (Berger, 2011). Russian Jews make up 10% of the population of American Jews, with a current estimate of approximately 700,000 to 750,000 Russian-speaking Jews in the United States. About half live in New York areas, and large numbers are located in Boston, Chicago, San Francisco, and south Florida (Berger, 2011; Kliger, 2012). Furthermore, 70% of Russian-speaking immigrants from the former Soviet Union self-identify as Jewish, and most of the remaining 30% belong to Russian-Jewish households (Berger, 2011; Kliger, 2012). Prior to the 1990s, Russian-speaking Jewish immigrants assimilated into American culture fairly well. As refugees, they entered the United States with an identity and a level of preparation called *anticipatory socialization.* Since 1990, that has changed. Recent non-Soviet Russian immigrants did not endure the long delays and confusion that earlier immigrants endured. Some recent immigrants were processed and arrived in the United States within a year or less. Immigration was more economic than political, and immigrants were less well prepared for American life (Kliger, 2012).

Historically, Soviet Jews were the most oppressed ethnic group in the USSR. In addition, policies of the former USSR encouraged, even mandated, the immigration of the family as a unit (Larkin, 2000). Therefore, when younger family members wished to leave Russia, older parents also had to leave. Yet despite the numerous challenges they have faced, 64% of Russian-speaking Jews (those having lived in the United States 9 or more years) report they are completely (or mostly) satisfied with life in the United States (Kliger, 2012). Nearly 81% of Russian-speaking Jews in the United States have relatives or friends in Israel. Thus, they retain strong political and emotional ties with Israel.

The number of Russian-speaking Jews in the United States outnumber all those living in Russia and Ukraine combined, and more Russian Jews live in New York City than in any other place worldwide (Kliger, 2012). Now, the official religion in Russia, Russian Orthodox, has a unique relationship with the Russian government (LOC, 2011). Thus, the Russian Orthodox church has resumed its privileged place at the heart of Russian culture (Jarvik, 2006; LOC, 2011) and has powerfully dictated policies relative to religious freedom. Violence, hate crimes, and overt sentiments of ethnic cleansing against Jews, Muslims, and other religious and ethnic minorities have dramatically increased (LOC, 2011), with little interference from police or government officials.

According to the U.S. Bureau of the Census, of those persons speaking a language other than English at home, 1.5% spoke Russian; this number equates to 905,843 persons. Of those persons, 52.3% say they spoke English very well, 25.6% spoke English well, 16.8% did not speak English well, and 5.3% spoke no English (Ryan, 2013). For the most part, Russians who immigrate to the United States are well educated (most having college or technical degrees and holding careers as health care professionals, economists, teachers, engineers, and skilled craftsmen and technicians) and speak at least some English. Russian Americans are courageous people who are voracious readers and passionately devoted to music, philosophy, art, and science (Kliger, 2012; Magocsi, 2015; StratisHealth, 2009).

Despite years of hardship, Russian immigrants are proud, forward-thinking people with a strong internal locus of control. Russian immigrants come to a specific location because they have relatives or other contacts in these locations, meaning that large pocket populations of Russian Americans have emerged in various regions in the United States.

Starting in 1992, immigration from Russia was reported separately, not as part of the "former Soviet Union" statistical group. Immigration numbers also include a seldom reported yet important number of Russian children adopted by U.S. citizens. Since 1992, Russia, with its limited resources to care for orphaned children, has become a major source of foreign children adopted by U.S. citizens, with a total of 6270 children adopted by American adults between 1996 and 1997. In 2009, 1580 immigrant orphans from Russia were adopted by U.S. citizens. These children were 56% male; 77% were between 1 and 4 years old (U.S. Department of Homeland Security, 2010). Importantly, these children are Russian-speaking, and many have physical or psychological health problems related to congenital malformations and maternal substance abuse problems (Tashlein-Van Heuveln, 2009). Many children living in Russian orphanages have been abandoned by parents and relatives. Importantly, with a resurgence in Russian nationalism, the Russian people and government are becoming more protective of their children, and adoption has dropped to less than 20% of former levels. As evidence, the total number of adoptions between 1999 and 2011 was 45,112 (an average of about 3400 per year. In 2011, just 962 adoptions took place (Ortman & Shin, 2011).

Life Today for Russians in the United States

Russian Americans report new and much welcomed freedoms in the United States. For example, Russian American Jews and Pentecostal Christians are often able to fully practice their faith for the first time upon arriving in the United States, and Russian parents commend the skills their children learn in schools. They report no longer feeling like persecuted members of minority groups. Russian Americans especially appreciate creative skills of thinking, analysis, and discussion. Russian women are familiar with working outside the home in well-paying professional positions. In Russia, most health care professionals are women. They are also used to doing the work of the home and are expected to do all or most of the household chores such as cooking and cleaning (Magocsi, 2015).

Russian Americans try hard to maintain strong social networks, family stability, and a self-identity that includes their Russian heritage (Sagy, Shani, & Leibovich, 2009). Within the family, Russian American women have been responsible for nurturing the Russian culture identity among family members, and Russian women counsel strong values of philanthropy and community (Magocsi, 2015). Therefore, Russian immigrant communities often provide supportive services such as career and employment guidance, housing assistance, professional networking, technical training programs, classes in English as a second language, and health care. Importantly, Russian Americans have high levels of social participation and interactions within Russian communities.

Americans should understand that in Russia, medical treatment, although limited (at least on record), remains free. Education, including postsecondary university and professional studies, is also often provided at low or no cost, although teachers and university instructors are poorly paid. Therefore, many Russian immigrants, including women, have had some form of technical training or advanced education. Nevertheless, Russian immigrants may have difficulty understanding the concepts of insurance, private pay, medical malpractice, health maintenance organizations, medical referrals, diagnostic-related groups, and reimbursement coding. The large and growing Russian-American population, when compared with other immigrant groups, is better educated and enjoys higher levels of discretionary income. For example, of the number of foreign-born Russian immigrants, 54.7% have attained at least a bachelor's degree, and 16.5% are self-employed. Russian Americans are also more likely to own their own homes and have health insurance. Almost half of foreign-born Russians (47.4%) own their own home and, along with their U.S.-born children, nearly 80% have health insurance coverage (CIS, 2014). Over 44% of Russian Americans are over the age of 55, and just 8.6% are between 0 and 24 years old (compared with 21% of all foreign-born U.S. residents). Thus, the age composition of the Russian-born U.S. population is skewed toward elders. Clearly, this group of well-educated people is keenly interested in health promotion; illness prevention; and skillful,

culturally competent, health care professionals (CIS, 2014; Orlando Russian Culture Society [ORCS], 2009).

COMMUNICATION

Dialect, Style, and Volume

The official language of Russia, and the most widely spoken of the Slavic languages, is Russian. This language has a 33-character Cyrillic alphabet (reduced to 33 characters with the 1917 Soviet revolution) named after the ninth-century apostle to the Slavs, St. Cyril. St. Cyril created the alphabet so that the Bible could be translated for liturgy use in the Slavic countries (Moore, 1988). In the tenth century, the Cyrillic alphabet was adopted by Russians, simultaneously with Christianity. The Cyrillic alphabet was last renovated in 1918. Russian belongs to the eastern branch of the Slavic linguistic family. More than 250,000,000 people speak Russian worldwide. For most Russian American newcomers, Russian is the language used to connect with family and friends. Additionally, the Russian language helps maintain Russian heritage and identity for Russian Americans. Evidence of this trend is the continued large number of Russian speakers and dramatic increase in Russian-based media (e.g., newspapers, books, television stations, Web sites) (Magocsi, 2015).

For most Russians, English is the most popular of all the Western languages. This newfound popularity of English on the part of the Russian people is related to media broadcasts, movies, rock video television programs, and Western business opportunities. In addition, professional literature (including health and medicine) is often in English, and medical students are frequently required to read English-language medical journals. There are 261,900,000 cell phones, 40,853,000 Internet users, 14,865,000 Internet hosts, and 3300 television stations (most controlled by federal or local governments) (Central Intelligence Agency, 2014). Although information is hard to suppress and English is widely used, government-controlled media and propaganda broadcasts flourish under Putin's grip.

Russian is sometimes referred to as a "house green" language because articles (such as *the*) and verbs (such as *is*) are often unnecessary. The Russian language is a flexible, beautifully rich language. Paralanguage qualities, such as tone, inflection, speed, vowel emphasis, and verbal pauses, contribute to the variety and meaning of Russian words and sounds. Russians freely use paralanguage and other nonverbal indicators to denote the value being placed on what is said. The spirit of the Russian people, their warmth and love, come through clearly in this dialect (Binyon, 1983). Importantly, just as in the United States, the Russian language carries geographic variances and vernaculars.

Russian Americans' first language may not be Russian but may instead be from the region where they grew up. Many Russian Americans studied some English while in Russia. However, the English they memorized was boring and often British English, which is significantly different in sound, spelling, and pronunciation from American English, making language comprehension difficult. In addition, American vernacular variances and geographical accents can cause problems.

Although many well-educated Russians studied English at some point in their education, English proficiency is not easy, especially for older Russian American immigrants. However, many elderly Russian Americans speak a mix of Russian and English, using both simultaneously (Leigh, 2006). In the United States, Russian speakers rank fifteenth of total speakers of various languages. Using self-report information, there are about 3.13 million Russian Americans (Norton, 2011); in 2015, 981,000 people aged five and older speak Russian at home. This number is expected to jump to 1,048,000 by 2020 (Ortman & Shin, 2011). However, younger Russian immigrants have made the adjustment to English with less difficulty. For younger Russian immigrants, the first priority on arrival in the United States is to learn conversational English, the second priority is to enroll children in school, and the third priority is to find good employment. Nearly half of all Russian speakers are over age 44 (Ortman & Shin, 2011). Most Russian Americans maintain a bicultural identity that varies based on age, employment, newcomer status, and levels of acculturation. Acculturation differences among family members may produce conflict and stress. Compounding this stress is that Russian American parents and elders expect youth to obey authority, bow to parental controls, and perform interdependently with family members. Russian children, by contrast, have absorbed American values of autonomy and independence (Jurcik, Chentsova-Dutton, Solopieieva-Jurcikova, & Ryder, 2013).

Additional stress occurs when Russian youth are frequently required to act as culture brokers for their older parents and grandparents. Brokering duties, especially prevalent among recent immigrants, such as acting as language and information interpreters for education, government, and health care institutions, are common. For Russian American teens, these brokering tasks have created increased levels of stress and relationship problems with family and friends (Jurcik et al., 2013). Using skilled language interpreters, not friends or family, is important because of potential language barriers, impediments to free and clear communication, and confidentiality and ethics violations. Family, especially younger family members, may be embarrassed and anxious during the crisis of an illness or problem. Elderly Russian Americans with English

competence enjoy better mental and physical health and, according to Aroian and Vander Wal (2007), language was not a significant predictor of health service use among elderly Russian immigrants in Boston. Notably, interpreters translate more than just words. They must also convey paralanguage, nonverbal, and subtle meanings. Thus, an additional advantage to using trained Russian interpreters is that, even when Russian Americans speak English well, they express emotions more fluently and use greater numbers of active verbs (versus adjectives) than when speaking of the same situation in English (Jurcik et al., 2013). Fortunately, many medical, chemical, and scientific terms are cognates, and although the written appearance of the word is different between Russian and English, the sound is similar. A few medical cognates are *organ(ism)*, *appetite*, *function*, *pulse*, *doctor*, *hospital*, *physical*, *diagnosis*, *normal*, and *problem*.

The volume of speech used by Russian Americans is not significantly different from that used by some Irish Americans. In Russia, because loud, aggressive demands were often necessary to receive medical care, some Russians became loud when attempting to be understood or get attention. Thus, even normal conversation may seem loud and boisterous.

Touch

Russians often use touch freely with intimate and close friends. It is not unusual to see Russian women embracing and kissing other women, as well as Russian men embracing and kissing other men. Friends who have been separated often greet each other, in public or in private, in this fashion. The technique of kissing each cheek three times seems to be a cultural trait adopted from the Middle East. The gentle kiss of a man on a woman's hand is a gesture of respect and admiration. Also, a handshake of agreement from a Russian is often more binding than a signed document. Handshakes are welcome when accompanied by direct eye contact, and gloves must not be worn. Prior to any touching, Russians may ask for and need the health care provider to explain what will be done and why (Communicating, 2007).

Context

Russian people are commonly perceived as kind, caring, and generous. When trust has been established, they express these feelings willingly and publicly. They are by nature and experience, however, cautious. Some Russians evaluate situations and people with great care. Emotions are also freely expressed. Russians have a quick appreciation for jokes and satire, often venting their feelings in this form of expression. It has been said that Russian people cry and laugh easily and that genuine expression of emotions is valued. Russians also tend to exhibit less control over negative emotions, especially with strangers (Jurcik et al., 2013).

Russian people who learned English in Russian schools may have learned from a non-native speaker. Therefore, the sound of English will be different. Native Russians who are eager to practice conversational English with a native English speaker often approach tourists traveling in Russia. However, for most new Russian immigrants, conversational English is likely to be unrecognizable.

Russian people have learned through years of government rule to look and act neutrally. With strangers and in crowded places, eye contact is avoided, affect is flat, posture is not erect, and eyes are diverted. Upon arriving in the United States, Russian Americans often express great wonder at the freedom with which Americans make nonverbal connections with strangers. However, Americans tend to be cooler and more distant with close friends and family, avoiding unsolicited advice-giving, than Russians. Historically, a distrust of authority and subsequent reliance on family and friends for help, advice, and care were survival mechanisms. Thus, for Russians, it is common to visit friends and neighbors on a whim, bringing food and gifts without notice, whereas in the United States this practice is uncommon (Jurcik et al., 2013). As interesting evidence, the Russian language includes two ways of saying the plural "you," one for only the closest of friends and family and a second, more generic, term when speaking with colleagues or strangers.

Kinesics

Russians understand that public behavior needs to be respectful. Disrespect is shown when persons fold their arms across their chest, stand with hands in their pockets, slouch, cross legs so as to expose the sole of the shoe, and walk into a house with shoes on (Minnesota Department of Employment and Economic Development [MDEED], 2006). Smiling at another person must be sincere (Resick, 2008). Until trust and comfort have been established, Russian Americans' nonverbal communication style is subtle and with few gestures. They do, however, feel free to maintain eye contact, and they do allow and expect nurses to use touch and gestures freely during the implementation of nursing procedures. Older Russian American immigrants are more entrenched in social amenities, often preferring to express themselves verbally. "Please" and "thank you" are integral to their speech, and they use these words at every possible opportunity. Russian men will courteously open doors for women. Nodding one's head is a gesture of approval; outstretching one's hand is a gesture of salute. When compliments are given, they are sincere. Gifts and flowers are presented during important meetings

as a gesture of tribute. The person seated first in a room is the one with the most authority or prestige. Nurses should not use the common American-based "OK" sign when speaking with a Russian because this is considered rude. Russian Orthodox followers will cross themselves from the forehead to the upper chest, then the right to the left shoulder (Leigh, 2006).

Implications for Nursing Care

Russian Americans expect the nurse to be warm and caring, to demonstrate empathy, and to help them cope with physical and emotional problems. An often expressed expectation of the nurse by the Russian American is that the nurse be friendly. This expectation is demonstrated by an "inviting," open posture; a smile; and a low and calm voice. As health care professionals, nurses are expected to show support in word and deed, suggest specific interventions that will improve the patient's situation, and begin these interventions immediately. Nurses should also anticipate patient needs, even when not expressed directly (Jurcik et al., 2013). Appropriate touch is considered a sign of friendliness and caring. Russian Americans do not appreciate a light, "chatty" approach to health care; they believe appearance and demeanor must always remain professional. Russian Americans want to be certain that the nurse understands them. They can easily become very shy; this is especially true of recent immigrants. Because their English may be tenuous, Russian Americans may hesitate to ask for clarification.

Russian American patients need to be assessed for their level of acculturation, English language skills, and education and social status. When doing histories or intake screenings on Russian Americans with English literacy, nurses need to understand that if they are speaking and thinking in English, they will describe symptoms and events differently than when speaking and thinking in Russian. (Jurcik et al., 2013). Even if a Russian American is fluent in English, communicating in English during times of pain, stress, and anxiety will be difficult. Knowledge of this difficulty is especially important when working with elder Russian Americans. Nurses must always avoid using family and friends as language interpreters and culture brokers.

Russian Americans expect the nurse to speak slowly and clearly and to choose simple words when needed. Russian Americans may demonstrate limited listening skills, perhaps because of language barriers, and may be unwilling to make independent health care decisions. Russians may assume the nurse and physician will tell them everything they need to know about their health problem and often prefer a more direct, versus indirect, approach to their care needs. However, gestures and demonstrations, to clarify and promote understanding, are expected and appreciated. "Look at my eyes," explained one Russian American. "My eyes will tell you that I do not understand because I will have a stupid expression!"

In most instances, Russian Americans will comply with medical directives and teachings if they believe that the nurse is trustworthy, honest, caring, sincere, and competent. Nurses will not be believed or trusted by Russian Americans if they are perceived to be mask-like, robotic, insincere, or phony in their caring behaviors. Nurses should address Russian American clients by "Mr." or "Mrs." followed by the family name. However, use of the first name, followed by the patronymic (their father's first name plus a feminine or masculine ending, depending on the person's sex) may be an acceptable alternative. Well-educated and professional Russian American women often retain their maiden names. Using this formal method of address will convey the nurse's respect. To address a Russian by his or her first name only is improper and presents a grave social error. Russians also object strongly to terms of endearment, such as "dear," "hon," "sweetie," "darlin'," "dude," and "hi, guy," when used by health care workers (Smith, 1996). As explained by one Russian American, "I want you to believe me when I tell you I have a problem. Here the nurses are perfect. We will respect them and listen to them. They know their job, and they know what they are supposed to do."

Russian Americans tend to speak freely regarding physical problems. Once language is no longer a concern, the nurse will find that clients respond warmly. However, Russian Americans may be uncomfortable using gestures when speaking to the nurse. The nurse must be aware that although younger Russian immigrants adapt well to English, older Russian immigrants may not. Often, elderly Russian immigrants choose to associate only with Russian-speaking friends and relatives, which presents a difficult problem if an interpreter is unavailable. To add to this difficulty, Russian Americans may allow only Russian to be spoken at home. Because many Russian Americans are multilingual (Yiddish, German, French, Polish, etc.), it is an advantage if the nurse understands another language familiar to the client. One way to convey respect and an understanding of Russian culture is to provide avenues for client teaching through Russian literature. Health literature written in Russian, in addition to Russian-language audio and video presentations, may prove to be great teaching aids. Additionally, cognate words and trained interpreters should be used at all times. Kravitz et al. (2000) found that Russian Americans occupied an additional 5.6 minutes of physician time for each visit. These authors believed this time was spent because of the extra demands for interpreting health information. Therefore, nurse managers will

need to adjust workload requirements for nurses working with Russian American clients.

The challenge for nurses is to expand their own culture to care effectively for members of the Russian American ethnic group. These skills can strengthen the nurse as a person and as a culturally competent health care professional.

SPACE

The Russian culture exists on two very different levels. To strangers and new acquaintances, a Russian may remain aloof, preferring to speak and work in the social or public zone. However, once friendship and familiarity have been established, Russian people are comfortable within a personal zone and will stand up close to that person when speaking or listening. The intimate zone is reserved for spouse or children, except for health care workers performing within a professional capacity. When hospitalized, Russians are extremely compliant and are generally able to tolerate the loss of privacy.

Individuals are perceived according to the boundaries they maintain, which include the degree of permeability and flexibility. Permeability is defined as the degree to which a boundary is open or closed; for the most part, permeability varies from closed to open. When an individual has closed boundaries, very little exchange occurs between this person's internal and external environments, and the person may be perceived as being quiet, withdrawn, and set in his or her ways. On the other hand, if boundaries are open, much exchange occurs between the person's internal and external environments, and this individual may be perceived as being talkative and social and as one who enjoys taking risks. Russian Americans may be very superstitious. Death or other potentially negative events should not be spoken of in the abstract. Joking, teasing, or play-acting is not appropriate in a serious or potentially serious situation.

Flexibility is defined as the ability of a person to move along a permeability continuum. A person who is sometimes closed and sometimes open and who thereby uses the entire permeability continuum is considered flexible. On the other hand, a person who always gravitates toward the closed end of the continuum, which is indicative of a low degree of flexibility, is described as a rigid, closed person. A person who is always open and never closed is described as an open individual. People who are perceived as rigid and closed may be quiet and withdrawn and seldom if ever share intimate secrets, dreams, or thoughts, even with best friends or a spouse (Scott, 1988).

Some Russian persons are perceived as rigid and closed because they remain aloof and distant. However, the word *friend* is not a casual term to Russians. Friendship is taken very seriously by Russian Americans, with specific terms in Russian reserved for this special relationship. Close Russian friends may embrace, but mere acquaintances may not even shake hands. Russians may prefer to greet and meet acquaintances on a verbal level only.

Implications for Nursing Care

The nurse who cares for Russian American clients will generally find that health-assessment procedures done in the intimate areas such as the genitalia are accepted without argument or problem, provided that adequate information and justification have been given before the procedure, the nurse is perceived as a trusted health care professional, and permission from the client has been professionally requested and provided. The nurse should be aware that, for the most part, Russians prefer to remain at a social distance rather than an intimate distance with caregivers. If personal distance must be invaded to provide therapeutic assistance, the nurse should provide a careful explanation before the intervention to alleviate the stress and anxiety created by the violation of space. As with all aspects of care, it is important for the nurse to modify approaches based on a careful assessment of the individual client and family.

SOCIAL ORGANIZATION

Family

Russian American people are very family-oriented, and family relations and roles have a significant influence on them. In both Russia and the United States, extended family members often live together, relying on each other for financial and emotional support, child care, physical care, and completion of household tasks.

For the Russian American immigrant who may have left loved ones to come to America, family members in the United States become even more significant, and their U.S.-based family attachments become ever more important. Therefore, Russian Americans are a very close-knit group, often living together and caring for each other. Elders help raise grandchildren and expect to stay with their children as long as possible, and they may consider that children who place parents into a nursing home do not care about them. Within a few years after immigrating to the United States, Russian children tend to become assimilated into the American culture, leave home, and may even leave the geographic area. Remaining family members are often elderly and lack employment or language skills. They may isolate themselves from American contacts (Jurcik et al., 2013; Leigh, 2006; St. Elizabeth Medical Center [STEMC], 2006).

One Russian American explained that her children were also her best friends. Because she had so few other contacts, her son had become enormously important to her. In Russia, even in one- or two-room apartments, parents often live with married children and grandchildren, which may be one reason why Russian couples choose to have just one child.

Also related to family size in Russia is the very large number of abortions performed each year. Although abortion rates are decreasing, Russian women continue to use abortion as the most common method of birth control. Recently, a resurgence of Russian Orthodox religious influences; better, more available forms of contraception; and governmental efforts to curb abortion rates have decreased abortions to approximately 73 abortions for every 100 births. Yet these abortion declines have done little to improve Russia's population decline (School of Russian and Asian Studies [SRAS], 2010). Surprisingly, the majority of abortions in 2009 took place with married women, between 20 and 32 years of age, who already had one child. Teenage girls also frequently have abortions because very few sexually active teens practice safe sex (Kononova, 2010). Reasons for continued reliance on abortion include poverty and low living standards and little or no knowledge of modern family planning methods. In 1955, abortions were legalized in the Soviet Union, and soon after the USSR had the highest abortion rates worldwide, mostly because other methods of contraception were unavailable. A single Russian woman may have had as many as 25 abortions in her lifetime. Because abortion complications may include hemorrhage, inflammation, infection, and infertility, as well as a huge emotional burden, a history of multiple abortions may severely impact the mental and physical health status of Russian American women (Arnold & Kurmasheva, 2008; Kononova, 2010).

Within the Russian family structure, the father/patriarch tends to have the greatest influence (although in some families this role may be delegated to an older female). Children, especially male children, look up to the father and absorb his values and beliefs. In addition, the husband of the household makes decisions on behalf of the family, although he does consult with his wife, especially when the wife is well educated. Children must show respect for elders by addressing them as *Mr.* or *Mrs.*, *Aunt* or *Uncle*, and *Grandmother* or *Grandfather*. Women primarily care for children and complete all or most household tasks. Arguing and dish throwing may occur during family disagreements.

Education, family, and cultural activities are learned values that begin when children are infants. During social gatherings, children are often seen dancing with their parents. Fathers often walk arm in arm with a child through an art museum in an effort to instill an appreciation of philosophy, history, and culture. Children as young as 5 years of age learn to read classic literature and attend the ballet, opera, museums, and concerts. Russian American men are expected to financially provide for the family and respect and show courtesy toward women (Jurcik et al., 2013). Russian women are expected to maintain family, language, and cultural heritage. Russian Americans place great value on education; girls and boys are strongly encouraged toward academic excellence and college studies. Russian parents demonstrate high levels of involvement in their children's education. Russian Jews come to the United States with a powerful and centuries-long tradition of learning (Magocsi, 2015). Better school performance for Russian American youth is positively related to degree of acculturation (personal and family), English language skills, family involvement and stability, and an interdependent family environment (Jurcik et al., 2013). Conversely, Jeltova, Fish, and Revenson (2005) found that recent young Russian immigrants had higher levels of risky sexual behavior (risks for unplanned pregnancy and HIV infection) with higher levels of American culture acculturation.

Most Russians are life-hardened people and come to the United States with few possessions, but they come full of hope and the joy of life, which contribute to their success (Gromov, 2004–2005). Other factors contributing to success is that they are future oriented and have made immigration to the United States a family endeavor. Russian Americans complain of having felt stifled, oppressed, and desperate in Russia. A "group" and "ethnic" identity has been reinforced by the Russian problems they were forced to endure. Russians proudly express their unresolved questions of the meaning of personal existence and the reasons for their suffering. Theirs is a priority of spiritual and moral values over material ones— the most cherished of all gifts are gifts of the spirit. Thus, Russians enjoy lengthy discussions about their attitudes toward material values and often repeat a famous phrase, "you can understand Russia by your mind" (Leigh, 2006). The Russian cultural identity and love of wisdom and learning have been sustained and even renewed (Jurcik et al., 2013). Therefore, a strong bond develops in Russian-American families and communities because of similar backgrounds, culture, language, lifestyles, educational levels, and geographical core. Despite the ethnic bond found in many Russian-American communities, Russian Jews have historically felt isolated from dominant Russian life and culture, and this heritage has helped to maintain a strong ethnic identity. Thus, Russian Americans are dependent on and rely on person-to-person networks and referrals.

Life satisfaction levels for Russian Americans depend on the length of time since immigration. For the first 2 or 3 years, 72% report partial or complete dissatisfaction with life in the United States. Reasons provided include poor language skills, lack of employment stability, financial setbacks, and family conflicts. Importantly, life satisfaction levels improve yearly until, within just 8 or 9 years since immigrating, Russian Americans report satisfaction levels similar to those of the average American. By then, they have experienced employment, housing, and financial stability; their children are or have committed to a university education, and they have personally experienced the benefits of American life (Reklama, 2007).

The life of the elderly Russian immigrant can be difficult. In Russia, elders found important roles by helping support their children with child care and household duties, and, in return, Russian adult children cared for their parents. Once in the United States, parents and children may experience conflicts. Elders may represent the "old" and "mother" country, or the culture that no longer applies, and parents may lose their authority and dominant family status This is especially difficult when elders believe that children should do what they are told, without question. If Russian American children become the means for contact and communication because of their English competence, they will, paradoxically, sense a reversal of power and authority over their parents. For the elderly, fears may increase because of concerns over the acculturation of their children and grandchildren. Because of language barriers, certification requirements, regulatory criteria (such as for Russian physicians and nurses), and age, they may be unwilling or unable to restart their careers (Jurcik et al., 2013; Magocsi, 2015; Tran et al., 2000).

One Russian American explained,

> In Russia, we gathered together many, many people at my house. We could talk endlessly about politics. Russians love to come together with friends and neighbors, forming a very close connection with each person we live and work with. But in the United States, everyone is very busy. They drive in separate cars, have separate houses, and separate neighborhoods. Americans watch television at home rather than go out to the theater or see friends. Here in America I am less social and my friends are few.

Individualism

Russian Americans are hardworking and have very little tolerance for people who do not have the wish to work, stay active, and contribute to their family's well-being. They are self-reliant and independent. Russian Americans who become ill will use home care, hospitalization, or both as much as possible rather than become a burden to their families. They have a strong desire to stay in their own homes and will remain independent until the last possible moment. Caring for aging and elderly parents is considered the duty and responsibility of all children. To place one's parent into a "home" is considered socially and morally shameful.

This strong individualism and autonomy, with a pervasive sense of self-help, contradicts the former Russian social structure. Being a product of a society in which free choice was punished, Russian Americans may appreciate yet find themselves underprepared for a life that depends on initiative, independence, creativity, critical thinking, and personal decision making (Jurcik et al., 2013). One Russian American nurse explained, "Teamwork was the biggest change in terms of the work system. Here, I'm part of a team, but I still have independence. In the Russian system, you have the doctor … making all the decisions but here I can decide the proper care until the point when I need to call the doctor" (Alaniz, 2001, p. 20).

Problems occur when the nurse or physician expects the Russian American to make independent decisions regarding self-care and self-help, especially when those decisions exclude concepts of holistic care. Many expect health care professionals and older family members to tell them what to do. Furthermore, care regimens will most likely be successful if the nurse includes client and family and presents positive health outcomes as family goals. Using both directive and nondirective approaches and explaining the rationale behind nondirective strategies will improve health outcomes for Russian Americans (Jurcik et al., 2013). One elderly Russian American explained, "You ask me to tell you all about my health problems. I shouldn't have to tell you—you are supposed to know what they are and then give me medicine to fix them."

Position of Women in the Family and Society

Russian American women are not liberated at home. Although both husband and wife have full-time employment outside the home, most Russian men prefer to have their wives do the cooking, shopping, housework, and childrearing. Russian women spend hundreds of hours a month on household responsibilities.

In Russia, although jobs for women are considered equal (unemployment rates are nearly identical), salary and authority are not. Because Russian men die younger than women, for working-age Russians between 25 and 54 years, there are about 1.4 million more women than men; for every 100 women in that age group, there are about 95 men. Within the age bracket of 55 to 64, there are only 74 males for every 100 females (Central Intelligence Agency, 2014). The good news is that Russian women are well educated; schooling is higher for women, with a 15-year average (14 years for males), and literacy levels are near equal for both genders, with a 99.7% overall rate (Central Intelligence Agency, 2014).

The 1917 Russian Revolution demanded that women and men hold legal status as equals. Because violence against women was a crime against the state (disabled, impaired women could no longer contribute to the Communist goals), these crimes were hidden and even denied. With the fall of Communism, the percentage of women in government fell sharply (as a result of the change in government-forced quotas), and domestic violence denial continues. Besides unequal wages for Russian women, sex discrimination and violence against women permeate current Russian society. Male unemployment, poverty, and chemical addiction may fuel these problems (Jurcik et al., 2013). Hence, most Russian women need to learn assertiveness, positive self-esteem, relationship communication skills, and a new vision of their important societal role. It is interesting to note that the Russian language has no phrase for sexual harassment and that Russian American men and women experiencing domestic violence continue to consider the issue private (ANNA, 2010; Jurcik et al., 2013). They feel (and are often treated as such by law enforcement) responsible for the abuse and believe that keeping the family together at all costs is their burden (ANNA, 2010; Crandall, Senturia, Sullivan, & Shiu-Thornton, 2005).

There has been a rapid increase in prostitution among young women in Russia. A recent search on Google using "Russian women" as keywords yielded 163,000,000 listed sites, and when "mail order" was added, 15,100,000 sites were displayed. Many escort agencies and personal massage services for men opened within the first 6 months of 1992. With the relaxing of puritanical Communist mores, beautiful, obedient women have become status symbols for Russian men, and the Moscow newspapers are full of advertisements for these kinds of services. Russian women are also exploited via numerous Web sites that promote Russian brides and escorts. Tens of thousands of women from Russia are trafficked yearly all over the world, notably to the United States. They are attractive, well educated, and desperate to leave Russia due to poverty and unemployment. Nearly 44% are victims of dysfunctional, abusive families. Profit margins are high, and without resources or government intervention, these women are easily victimized (ANNA, 2010). Following research on the problem of domestic violence among Russian American women, Crandall et al. (2005) reported that these so-called mail-order brides reported experiencing many forms of domestic violence including isolation, financial restrictions, and verbal and physical abuse. Of the Russian American women in their sample, 77% had experienced abuse by their partner, and 23% had been abused by someone in their extended family. These women emphasized that women brought to the United States as mail-order brides are especially isolated and focused on the real need for culturally competent outreach and protective services.

Spirituality and Religious Beliefs

Between 15% and 20% of Russians practicing religion are Russian Orthodox, closely followed by Muslim (10%–15%) and other Christian groups at 2%. However, as a carry-over of more than seven decades of antireligion Soviet rule, Russia has a large nonpracticing population (Central Intelligence Agency, 2014). Until the eighteenth and nineteenth centuries in Russia, literacy was traditionally associated with the Russian Orthodox Church. Historically, the church was highly regarded by the people, mostly uneducated peasants, as a source of power and salvation. This undoubtedly contributed to the manner in which Russians surrendered to authority. One Russian American explained, "We were not raised with God; we made fun of the religious." Thus, many non-Jewish Russian Americans understand spirituality only in terms of artistic and literary endeavors. This causes them bewilderment when 90% of U.S. residents believe in God and donate nearly $300 billion to charities (Reklama, 2007).

In Russia, traditionally, Russian Jews could not own property or land, which may explain why many became merchants. As a result of this role, other Russian ethnic groups developed resentment and anti-Semitic feelings. With the relaxation of censorship and a new emphasis on Russian nationalism, there has been a resurgence of anti-Semitism and ethnic cleansing sentiments.

Russian Jews immigrated to the United States and other countries in a greater percentage than non-Jewish Russian people. The greater the Jewish oppression and anti-Semitism in Russia, the greater was the rate of immigration, even when severe hardships occurred, related to that immigration. The immigration has led to further discrimination. New freedoms of speech and expression have brought out old, otherwise buried, prejudices. In this newfound climate, Russian Jews feel persecuted and often fear for their children.

Perestroika and *glasnost* changes, along with the dramatic fall of Communism in Russia, witnessed a resurgence of religious freedoms. Christianity has had a remarkable revival. The Russian Orthodox Church is well respected by both believers and nonbelievers, who consider it an important part of their Russian heritage. As evidence of this renewed respect, Orthodox churches that had been abused and abandoned during Soviet rule are being meticulously restored. This religion requires followers to observe fast days as well as a "no-meat" rule on Wednesdays and Fridays.

During Lent, all animal products, including butter and other dairy products, are forbidden. Fasting also occurs during Advent. It is believed that God is served in a more powerful way during periods of fasting. However, even if fasting is strictly observed, special allowances are made for illness and pregnancy. Fear, sin, and punishment have been major themes for the Russian Orthodox Church.

After more than 70 years of war against religion, most Russians hope that the Orthodox Church will be able to positively influence the people's family, moral, and social values and consequently decrease the rate of divorce, crime, and abortion. As the Russian Orthodox Church attempts to reclaim state-confiscated churches and land, more and more Russians are returning to their once-hidden faith. Before *perestroika* and *glasnost*, religious expressions were prohibited in Russia. However, some churches did remain open. As a result, some people believed that Russian Orthodox Church leaders were obliged to report to the Secret Service and that confessions were not confidential. In addition, the training of Russian Orthodox priests was poor because of the general absence of good academic education programs. Today in Russia the church holds power over the people and government. This power is strong and desperate because of the hardship of Russian life, especially for the elderly. However, relevant to this history, just 25% of Russian Americans report having trust in religious figures such as rabbis and priests (Reklama, 2007).

Implications for Nursing Care

In all human societies, actions that are done for survival, such as eating, elimination, sexual intercourse, and health practices, although physical, take on cultural and social regulations. Cultural functions and norms dictate behavior patterns in a profound way. It is essential for nurses to understand the role culture plays to provide safe, compassionate, and effective nursing care.

Despite persecution and hardships, Russian Americans maintain a significant degree of individualism. Russian American parents teach their children an appreciation for Russian land and country. One Russian immigrant explained, "Whether good or bad, it is still mine. I still love my homeland." Another Russian American said it this way: "I miss everything—my home, my language, my friends. Here, I am another personality. I am not me. I cannot say what I want because I don't know the right words. This makes me tired and frustrated. I want so much to visit Russia, my country." It is important for the nurse to understand that strong feelings of national pride are experienced by many Russian immigrants. Russian Americans remain staunchly loyal to the Russian culture and do not fully embrace U.S. culture, perhaps because of their belief in Russian supremacy. Soviet prejudices against

Westernization remain (Reklama, 2007). However, although the Russian American does not or did not practice a religion while in Russia, this does not mean that, as this person ages, religious expression will remain unimportant (Leigh, 2006).

Because Russian Americans have strong family ties and values, the nurse must remember to involve the entire family (especially important for teens), including extended family members, in the formulation and intervention of care. Because the father and grandfather are often perceived as having a paramount role and function in the Russian family, the astute nurse will solicit the opinions and advice of this patriarch before presenting a treatment and intervention plan to the rest of the family. In this instance, if the patriarch's opinions and advice are solicited before the presentation to the rest of the family, the father may be of particular assistance in getting the family's cooperation and support. Because the entire Russian family becomes the client, time, respect, and information must be presented carefully to the entire family.

Some Russian Americans hold particular beliefs in regard to religion, death, and dying. Therefore, it is important for the nurse to respect these beliefs and practices and incorporate them into a therapeutic plan of care that will assist the client in returning to a high level of wellness. Because of a belief that the human body is sacred, Russian Americans will be reluctant to donate organs. More important, the nurse needs to keep imminent death topics away from the terminally ill. Tell the head of the family first. Family members believe they must "take on" the burden of illness on behalf of their loved one. "We choose to give mercy to the person; that person must not know that he or she will soon die. We don't need time to prepare a will because we have so few possessions to write wills about," replied one Russian woman.

Russian Americans, especially elders and mail-order brides, tend to feel displaced and isolated. Nurses need to be extremely thorough in gathering data in the psychosocial and physical assessment. The nurse must also remember to expect visitors to Russian American clients. Russian Americans are accustomed to long discussions with friends, which they find socially and spiritually rewarding. Therefore, unless visitors become potentially harmful toward client outcomes, they should generally be permitted and supported.

TIME

Some Russian Americans hold a perspective of time that is past-, present-, and future-oriented. For these people, there is a future within the present and a present within the past. On the other hand, some Russian Americans, particularly the well educated, hold only a future orientation. One example of this cultural attitude is seen in immigration.

Although the study of history and heritage is important to Russian Americans, most look to the future more than to the past, a characteristic related to socialism and Marxism. "Not now," such ideology preaches, "the future!" "Work hard now and have patience; suffer now so that the future will be better." Because living conditions in Russia for most immigrants were desperate, now they feel hope for themselves and their children. Many endure the hardships of leaving Russia so that a better life is available for their children and grandchildren.

Russian Americans believe the U.S. system of free elections to be a future-oriented, meaningful, and significant way toward change. They enthusiastically vote in even primary elections and serve as jurors within the judicial system. Although imperfect, most believe the legal system works fairly well (Reklama, 2007).

Another important example of future orientation is seen in the Russian people's almost universal belief in education for themselves and their children. Education begins early and is reinforced in the home. For Russian Americans who espouse a belief in future orientation, education is viewed as an awakening or a light. Lack of education is viewed as a void or darkness. Self-learning and lifelong learning are valued and practiced. On immigration to the United States, Russian children are encouraged to attend school immediately, even before they have any knowledge of English. In fact, Russian children learn English very easily. It is obvious that present efforts are vehicles for future achievements.

Implications for Nursing Care

For the Russian American, the United States offers opportunities for goal establishment and attainment impossible in Russia. For some Russian immigrants who hold a time orientation that is a combination of past, present, and future beliefs, it is important for the nurse to remember that such an individual may be reluctant to seek preventive therapeutic interventions. For example, the topic of contraception and safe sex, as well as antismoking and drinking strategies, may be challenging topics for past- and present-oriented Russian Americans. The nurse must design and implement teaching strategies that will assist the client in developing an understanding about the implications of past and present behavior on future wellness and quality of life.

On the other hand, Russian immigrants who hold a future orientation value preventive therapeutic techniques that have long-range future benefits on wellness and wellness behavior. Because these individuals have a future orientation, the nurse will find it easier to encourage preventive screening techniques than with past-oriented individuals. In fact, the client may even request information on preventive techniques and their benefits.

To a Russian American, punctuality is important, and arriving late for an appointment is considered rude. Therefore, the nurse must remember to keep appointments and be punctual because this will help build rapport and trust with the Russian American client. One Russian explained that to have been late for work under the former Soviet regime meant death; tardiness was considered a sabotage of social goals.

ENVIRONMENTAL CONTROL

Locus of Control and Effect on Wellness and Illness Behaviors

The Russian culture instills in its members a belief that man has little control over nature. This external control is especially apparent in health care activities. Spiritually, however, Russian Americans with Russian Orthodox beliefs may have difficulty with current self-help practices. These beliefs center on ideas of Christ's teachings. It is believed that Christ will give as much help as is deserved in relation to the strength of the beliefs, which means that an ill person who is not recovering may somehow not have had enough faith. Illness in this sense is perceived as punishment. Russian Americans who espouse these beliefs have an external locus of control.

In contrast, some Russian Americans believe that one can control both internal and external forces in the environment, thereby creating opportunities for high levels of wellness. This perception is regarded as an internal locus of control.

When Russian Americans have an internal locus-of-control orientation, they are likely to have a unique self-care approach to wellness, illness, and hospitalization. Resick (2008) found that Russian American research participants placed great importance on their ability to trust themselves and self-manage their health. One participant explained that in Russia, "We did not trust anybody" (Resick, 2008, p. 251), but they did trust natural herbs and roots as well as their own plan of care. Certainly, these Russian Americans believed in their own personal control over at least some aspects of their own health.

Russian Methods of Health Treatment

In Russia, *feldshers* deliver a great deal of primary health care. After 3 years of medical school, the feldsher is trained in basic preventive medicine, with a special focus on mothers and preschool children, in suturing, and in emergency care techniques. Some consider feldshers to be similarly placed in Russia as physician's assistants are placed in the United States. When Russians are ill, they are expected to stay in bed and call the clinic. The physician or feldsher may make a house call that same day, determine the severity of the problem, and make a recommendation. Russians expect to be hospitalized.

Although the Russian health care system may lag behind that of the United States, preventive health care has recently been identified as important. Russians believe that physical screening is the answer to good health care and is widely accepted among Russian immigrants. Female Russian Americans are quite familiar with frequent and routine pelvic and Pap screenings, gastric acid tests, sedimentation rates, and prothrombin times. In contrast, however, they are unfamiliar or unaccepting of mammograms, routine breast examinations, and cholesterol screenings and state that the cholesterol findings are inconclusive and of little or no value. Other Russian health care alternatives sometimes used are charm men and barbershops. In the past, barbershops and other clinics were equipped to do a procedure called "cupping" or "bonki," which was used primarily for the treatment of colds, flu, and respiratory disorders. In this procedure, cups with the approximate appearance of a large bulging shot glass are heated, placed up and down the back, and left in place for about 10 minutes. Believed to extract evil humors from the body, the cups leave ecchymosis-like marks that may last for days. Cupping is a technique currently taught to Russian nursing students and still practiced in some Russian-American communities. In addition to cupping, Russian Americans often turn to alternative systems of care: Russian holistic healers, Russian physicians unable to practice in the United States, Russian medications, fresh air and sun exposure, oil rubs, mud or steam baths, Russian-based herbal remedies, and U.S. over-the-counter remedies (Aroian & Vander Wal, 2007; STEMC, 2006; StratisHealth, 2014).

One concern Russian Americans have is that the U.S. medical system lacks a powerful emphasis on prevention. One Russian American responded:

Too many pills—pills for everything without a clear reason. In Russia, physicians make house calls. If I have a fever, I will stay home, and the doctor will come. This is why United States doctors consider Russians as crying too much and complaining too much. We are used to less intensive medicine. Here, I need to call for an appointment, and it's one month away. In Russia we have more alternative medical therapies—the whole cleansing of the body of toxins, massages, acupressure, and acupuncture. In our hospitals, we have prescribed massages. Here, the doctors don't even consider alternative medicine or any Oriental medical practice.

Russian Americans may doubt the ability of their nurses and physicians to understand their troubles. They may criticize American medical treatment systems. Russian Americans do not trust nor appreciate the U.S. health care system of (in their view) expensive insurance, Medicare and Medicaid fraud, incompetent health care providers, multiple medical mistakes, rude health care staff, and endless waiting in offices and emergency departments. Conversely, they do appreciate the excellent care provided when patients are critically ill (Reklama, 2007; StratisHealth, 2014).

Somatization of emotional problems is widespread. Russian Americans may describe emotional disorders as physical symptoms such as headaches, stomach pain, and exhaustion. Therefore, although screenings for most physical problems are widely accepted, screenings for domestic violence, depression, and post-traumatic stress disorder are not.

Folk Medicine

Russian Americans describe health as highly appreciated and cherished and as more than just the absence of disease. They are generally knowledgeable about health treatments, often self-diagnose, seek health advice from family members, and actively participate in self-care practices (Resick, 2008; StratisHealth, 2009). Russian immigrants, especially the elderly, believe in an almost unlimited power of therapeutics and may still practice some form of homeopathic or folk medicine. For example, one client had an amber necklace from Riga and stated that the necklace would cure her thyroid disease. Besides being worn as jewelry, amber is ground into a powder, added to hot water, and used as a kind of medicinal potion.

Other home remedies include herbs, which are prepared as drinks or enemas, and charcoal in water, which is ingested for the treatment of stomach acidity. Mud and hot steam baths are considered healthful for pneumonia and upper respiratory tract infections. Mineral water and plasters are also used, as is exposure to clean air and sunlight. Because of their belief in the healing qualities of mineral water, emerging Russian health care providers are using products that are rich in these properties.

Russian Americans strongly believe in the usefulness of massage (with or without contact) and oil rubs. This philosophy seems to stem from a kind of somatic idealism. In addition, orthopedic shoes for foot or leg pain are commonly used.

Some Russian Americans use dry heat for the treatment of back pain. Others use a raw dough of dark rye flour and honey that is placed on the spinal column. Another back remedy is a loosely knit or compacted pad made of rough, coarse wool or animal hair, which is placed directly on the bare skin in the lower back region.

Headaches are often treated with a strong ointment placed behind the ears and temples and along the back of the neck. For the treatment of rhinitis, Russian Americans may extract raw onion juice and place several drops in each naris with a medicine dropper. A cold may be treated by immersion of both legs in hot water containing strong salts. Sore throats are said to be relieved by a salt and baking soda gargle. Leech therapy is still widely taught and practiced in Russia. Leeches are particularly useful because of the anesthetic, vasodilatation, and anticoagulant properties of leech saliva. Leeches are successfully used to treat angina, migraine headaches, and poor circulation to digits or limbs.

Health is seen as the greatest of all gifts and goals. Russians will define health as a mental, physical, and spiritual harmony, the greatest of which is spiritual; they will also wish for good health to all loved ones. One religious requirement is that male Russian Jews be circumcised. Illness, in contrast, is defined as a painful disharmony among body systems. Body systems are blended and functioning as God created them to be, with each part doing its job in perfect interrelatedness. When the mind is troubled, the body will respond negatively. Holistic medicine is a way of life for Russians, through the use of cosmic energy work. Spirituality carries an important place in Russian medicine. Russians believe that bad news must be shielded from the client and that a terminally ill person should not be informed of imminent death. They believe such disclosure would increase anxiety, decrease hope, and hasten death. This may be changing. The first hospice in Russia opened in Moscow in 1997, and palliative care for cancer patients is being promoted throughout Russia. Tashlein-Van Heuveln (2009) described an understaffed 100-bed hospice in Russia that included 60 pediatric beds. Of the 40 adult beds, 10 were occupied by HIV patients. Although grief counseling was available upon request, no formal training was available for physicians who implemented it. As death approaches, family, loved ones, and the spiritual advisor gather at the bedside. Still, Russian Americans often do not sign living wills or agree to organ donations. As an ill person worsens, family members pay continuous watch; all members seek a presence with their loved one who may, if able, place a hand on their heads as a symbolic gesture of blessing. Because Russian soil is linked to home and heritage, containers of dirt—soil obtained from the Russian homeland—may be brought in by family members (Patient & Family, 2007).

Practices at the Time of Death

Russian families with members who have recently died often keep vigil over the coffin for hours. For Russians, the body is sacred and must be treated with dignity and respect. The family members wear black. The deceased person is carefully washed, dressed, and placed in the coffin before the wake and funeral. Using a rolled cloth placed under the chin, mouths are closed and eyelids shut with coins; all mirrors are covered. Mourners pool their money to make sure men are dressed in suits and women have fine dresses. Families must bear the weight of every aspect of the funeral. A black wreath may be placed on the door of the deceased person's home. At the funeral, a priest (if the family is Catholic or Russian Orthodox) places holy oil on the forehead while making the sign of the cross. A paper band is placed on the forehead with this prayer: "Oh God, Father, be merciful to thy servant (name) and accept into thy fold (name)." Each member of the grieving family places a few symbolic grains of soil onto the coffin. Mourners carry carnations, often placing them on the body prior to burial. Russian Orthodox beliefs dictate that friends and family pray for the deceased from the ninth to the fortieth day after death because until the ninth postmortem day, the soul remains with the body. On the ninth day, it begins its journey either to heaven or hell, depending on the consideration given to all the sins committed (Lally, 2000). Regardless of the temperature, Russians, especially Russian Jews, generally believe in rapid burial. However, prior to burial, the coffin may be driven past the home of the deceased, allowing the body to see home one last time. Following burial, friends and family return to the host home and enjoy food and liquor in honor of the deceased. One traditional dish is rice with raisins. Loud expressions of grief, such as wailing, are generally reserved for this home setting (Patient & Family, 2007).

Implications for Nursing Care

The nurse should be aware that Russian American clients find the way in which health professionals relate somewhat different from that to which they are accustomed. Traditionally, American physicians and nurses have been taught to have a nondirective, listening approach to client interactions. This approach is unsatisfactory for many Russian immigrants, who seem to need almost immediate information and answers. Subjective symptoms may be difficult to assess because of lack of information presented by the client and the tendency to somatize emotional problems. Psychological disorders were rarely appropriately attended to by the Russian health care system.

Russian Americans are nearly 100% compliant with follow-up medical appointments, if they fully understand, trust, and believe in the health care instructions. Generally, Russian Americans are respectful and admire their physicians and nurses. They ask appropriate questions and accept what they are told. Russian Americans are not familiar with medical gatekeepers and appreciate choosing their own providers. Upon experiencing illness and pain, Russians may believe that these problems were caused by something they did or did not do (e.g., poor eating habits). Russians' health-seeking behavior is most likely related to high, not low, personal health responsibility, since they view themselves as responsible for getting needed care, and improving their own health (Aroian & Vander Wal, 2007; StratisHealth, 2014). To know Russian American clients is to admire, respect, and validate their courage, intelligence, and unique cultural backgrounds and experiences.

Russian Americans tend to comply with most medical directives, doing what is needed to get well and stay independent. However, nurses need to understand and accept that Russian Americans will seek out that which is familiar to them. For example, in addition to following Western medial protocols, Russian Americans will often combine these with home therapies and treatments. In contrast, some Russian Americans may stop taking medications with any sign of a side effect, even if the side effect is unrelated. This is particularly noted with psychotropic drugs. The nurse may also notice a kind of cancer phobia among elderly Russian immigrants, who seem to have an "if it isn't broken, don't fix it" philosophy in relation to cancer screenings. In a study by Ivanov, Hu, and Leak (2010), younger, better educated, well-insured, English-competent, Russian American women were more likely to have cancer screenings such as Pap smears and mammograms. Helping clients understand the value of these screenings is important. Notably, the concept of "do not resuscitate" or hospice care can be a significant problem for Russian family members who cannot understand not doing everything possible for a loved one.

Unless directly harmful, nurses need to remain open to alternative therapies and medications. It is important that nurses ask for information regarding alternative health care practices that may be practiced. Many traditional Russian medications are available and frequently purchased through the Internet. Several large pharmaceutical firms in New York cater to Russian clients in Russian. Nurses can encourage self-directed learning via trusted, accepted Web sites. As evidence that Russian Americans use the Internet, new sites have surfaced that list directories for *family, children, health/wellness,* and many other topics important to Russian Americans. These sites can be accessed in English or Russian, and culturally appropriate, free patient education information resources are available. Importantly, a number of well-written Web sites offer information for nurses and physicians working with Russian Americans. In addition, Russian Americans are able to locate Russian-speaking dentists and physicians by using Web-based search tools. The health magazine *Zdorovie,* written in Russian and available online, claims a strong commitment to increasing the medical awareness of the Russian-speaking population in the United States. Furthermore, the Russian American Medical Association (members include physicians, nurses, dentists, and students) also has a Web site with news and education articles.

BIOLOGICAL VARIATIONS

Body Size

In Russia, nearly 58% of the women and 51% of the men are considered obese or overweight. This Russian obesity epidemic places a great strain on health care services. Obesity-linked diseases such as cancer and diabetes are on the rise (Rtveladze et al., 2012). Obesity is even more common among elderly Russian women. This problem is attributed to the lack of fresh fruits and vegetables in Russia; many culturally preferred foods are high in saturated fats and salt, and a sedentary lifestyle is growing more common. Many Russian Americans retain their traditional dietary preferences, and as a result, overuse of meat, saturated fats, carbohydrates, and salt and underuse of healthy fruits and vegetables often continue after immigration.

Stature and skin color among Russian Americans are quite similar to those of other White American clients seen by the health care provider because most Russians are White. Even the Russians of Tartar descent have a Europoid appearance, with any Mongoloid elements being mostly diluted (Hurwitz, 2005). Kulikov, Buzhilova, and Poltaraus (2004) studied 47 individual mitochondrial DNA samples isolated from bones taken from graves in northern Russia and found that these ethnic groups may be assigned to the European population group.

Enzymatic Variations

Incidence of cardiovascular disorders and the related cholesterol levels of Russian Americans are generally high (StratisHealth, 2014), and excessive alcohol use is a national embarrassment. The prevalence of alcohol use disorder among Russian men is 31% and among Russian women 6.2% (compared with 7.5% average for other European regions) (WHO, 2015). In Russia, morbidity rates for diabetes and other endocrine, digestive, and metabolic disorders are on a steady and dangerous rise (RSSS, 2014), and with a 30% obesity rate for women and 18.4% for men, these numbers are projected to increase dramatically (WHO, 2015). About 10.6% of Russians over 24 years old

have raised blood glucose levels, and 37.2% of men and 31.8% of women have raised blood pressures. Tobacco use rates are even more startling. For Russian men over 14, the tobacco use rate is 59% (for women it is 25%). Although some proposals for smoke-free legislation have occurred, there is currently no smoke-free legislation anywhere, not even in hospitals. Interestingly, there are tobacco-related taxes (WHO, 2015).

In contrast to their Russian counterparts, the prevalence of diabetes among Russian American adults is 5%. However, with a 55% obesity rate, these numbers are projected to increase (Oza-Frank & Naraya, 2010). The prevalence of type 2 diabetes among Russian Americans is higher than that for non-Hispanic Whites (Perlman & McKee, 2008).

Susceptibility to Disease

Hypertension. Mortality rates from noncommunicable diseases account for 86% of total deaths in Russia. Cardiovascular diseases alone account for 60% of the mortality rate and are the major causes of death in Russia (WHO, 2015). Blood pressure screening is routine in Russia, so Russian Americans are keenly aware of the causes and effects of hypertension and will identify themselves as either hypertensive or borderline hypertensive. Unfortunately, because Russian Americans often equate pain with illness, hypertension can be ignored as a health problem. Diet, tobacco use, and lifestyle are major risk factors; therefore, for Russian Americans, especially those arriving within the past 3 years, these cardiovascular mortality rates continue.

Tuberculosis. Incidences of HIV/AIDS and TB have risen together. Russia has the eleventh highest TB burden in the world and the third highest of MDR TB. The WHO classifies Russia as a high-burden TB, HIV, and MDR TB nation with TB prevalence rates at 160,000 (Shpilko, 2006; WHO, 2015). Tuberculosis is rapidly spreading across Russia (including in the wealthier and more stable middle and upper classes) because of an inefficient health system, a significant HIV/AIDS infection rate, poverty and unemployment, prophylaxis resistance, sex workers, alcoholism, and infected prison populations spilling into communities. Two areas of real concern are cases of MDR TB cases, at 19% of all new cases and 49% of retreatment cases (WHO, 2015) and incidence rates among prison inmates. Russia ranks seventh in the world for the number of prison inmates and a significant number are TB and HIV positive. Over 10,160 inmates have TB and 18.7% of these inmates have both TB and HIV. Out of the total HIV incidence in Russia, the prison share is over 13%. Importantly, the effectiveness of treatment for newly diagnosed TB patients in prisons is less than in the Russian civilian sector (56.5% versus 66.6%) partly due to release dates that occur prior to the end of treatment (Mikhaylova, 2013).

Cancer. Because Russians (especially Russian men) die young, the overall deaths resulting from all cancers is 16% (WHO, 2015). As noted, smoking and tobacco use is a major public health issue in Russia, particularly affecting low-income, underemployed, and vulnerable men and young women living in urbanized areas. These high rates of smoking have implications for increased morbidity and mortality cancer rates. A dramatic increase in smoking rates among women seems related to transnational tobacco company advertising. Stickley and Carlson (2009) reported that smoking among Russian women was also related to age (teens had higher rates), binge drinking, an external locus of control, and poor economic status. With regard to Russian Americans, Baker (2008) found an alarmingly high smoking rate (53%–63%) among male immigrants of the former Soviet Unions now living in Ohio.

After studying the differences in somatic mutation, based on an analysis of peripheral blood lymphocytes, Jones et al. (1995) found that because of chronic exposure to environmental toxins, including smoking, dichlorodiphenyltrichloroethane-like pesticides, and the Chernobyl nuclear power plant accident, the mutation frequency in Russians was higher; in addition, Russians have a higher risk of health consequences because of accumulated genetic damage. The population of adult Russian accumulated genetic damage is at a 250% higher rate than that of Americans. The research work of Vadlamani et al. (2001) seems to concur with these findings. These researchers found a high rate of colorectal neoplasms, much higher than control groups or U.S. national averages, for their Russian American study subjects. They recommend greater care and vigilance, with more aggressive cancer screening, for this population group. These findings are supported by Resick (2008), who found that immigrant study participants associated newly diagnosed cancers with former exposures to industry-based air and water pollution, and chemical and nuclear waste. These perceptions were related to participants' avoidance of routine cancer screenings.

Genetic Diseases. For Russian Americans from Eastern European Jewish descent, genetically linked disorders are a real concern. Approximately one in four is a carrier of one or more genetically linked disorders. These disorders include Tay-Sachs, Canavan, Niemann-Pick, and Gaucher disease, familial dysautonomia; Bloom syndrome; Fanconi anemia; cystic fibrosis; and mucolipidosis IV (Victor Center, 2015).

Dental Needs. Most Russian Americans value healthy teeth and gums and seek regular dental care because traditionally they have had access to dental care and often have bridges and removable plates. Russian American youth learn early oral hygiene self-care practices. Unfortunately, there are just three dentists for every 10,000 people in Russia (WHO, 2008). Older Russian Americans may be edentulous related to the severe hardships of post–World War II Russia.

Eye Care Needs. Because eye care and eye surgery received a great deal of Russian money and attention, most Russians have had access to eye care.

Nutritional Preferences and Deficiencies. The Russian immigrant who has come from a rural district will prefer to eat cabbage, buckwheat, millet, barley, and bread, along with sour milk and salted pork (if the person is non-Jewish). Russian bread is a kind of heavy rye bread that can weigh as much as 12 lb per loaf. Salted meats are usually kept in a barrel and stored all winter in a kind of fruit cellar. Meat, as a delicacy, may be severely rationed. Thus, most Russians respect food and handle it with great care. Not a single morsel of food, especially meat, is wasted.

Russian Americans value good nutrition as a way to achieve good health. In Russia, one reason attributed to high death rates is poor nutrition, since diets typically contain inadequate amounts of water-soluble vitamins. Calcium, iron, and iodine are also often lacking (Shpilko, 2006). Just 6% of Russian households consume adequate amounts of iodized salt (WHO, 2015). The poorest families in Russia have the least amount of iron in their diets, since these Russians cannot afford the foods they need. Consumption of iron inhibitors (e.g., grains) results in additional iron loss. In rural Russia, people grow their own vegetables, carrots, beets, and potatoes. Therefore, many Russian Americans express concern over America's use of fertilizers and pesticides to grow produce. Russian American women love to cook food from scratch, especially soups, and dairy products are considered important meal components (STEMC, 2006). Lunch is often the main meal of the day.

Psychological Characteristics

Illness and Wellness Behaviors. Many Russian Americans believe that American medicine is the best in the world but only for the most seriously ill. Russian Americans, accustomed to home visits by health care workers in Russia, would like to have U.S. physicians and nurses provide home care when possible. In emergency departments, some Russian Americans may become frustrated by the voluminous paperwork required to establish financial competence, including private insurance as well as Medicaid and Medicare sources. Older Russian Americans may consider the medical system a natural place for seeking the help they believe they need. For these immigrants, the clinic and its staff are viewed in a social context. Russian Americans, familiar with making loud demands to receive care in Russia, may appear pushy and excessive.

Having endured years of poor medical care, poor nutrition, and continued frustration, Russian Americans also have a higher number of somatic complaints than other groups the nurse may encounter (Jurcik et al., 2013). These complaints may be caused partially by the cultural stigma of psychiatric illness and treatment by "just talking." Mental illness is considered to be a character defect. Thus, Russian Americans are ashamed of psychiatric diagnoses and often will not provide answers regarding any family or past history of psychiatric illness (McKee, Dugan, & Levenson, 2014). Because in Russia any diagnosis of a mental illness included legal and social consequences, Russian Americans do not trust psychiatrists, psychologists, or other counseling services. Thus, they may magnify aches and pains disproportionately to their primary care providers rather than describe an emotional problem. Expression of psychosocial problems, such as depression, through somatic complaints, is common since many diseases and illness are considered to be related to emotional stress.

Russian Americans tend to perceive health care professionals as high-status people. Feelings of poor self-concept are lifted when attention is received; for example, "I must have some worth if a high-status person pays attention to me." Russian Americans may thus seek health care as a social exercise to increase feelings of worth. They want and need the nurse to demonstrate care, empathy, competence, and attention.

Russian Americans generally have many important health-promoting behaviors. Having been accustomed to media portrayals of average people doing extraordinary deeds, Russian Americans long for high-quality newspapers and television programs that provide enthusiasm and inspiration for them. Russian Americans are familiar with hard work and difficulties, but most enjoy American freedoms and believe in the future.

Mental Health. In Russia, citizens with mental disorders could expect years of prison-like hospitalization under the influence of potent, mind-numbing drugs. Psychiatric wards contained many who had refused military service or disagreed with political policies. Psychiatric diagnoses were applied to those practicing political dissent. Russian citizens who tried to criticize political bosses, organize labor unions, or speak out against Communist dogma were perceived as state enemies, labeled as insane, and hospitalized in prison-like psychiatric facilities. This medicalized system of power and control was scorned by the rest of the world's psychiatric community, who found the diagnosis of "sluggish schizophrenia" used in Russia to describe these persons objectionable. Hospitalization occurred despite Soviet law, which stated that citizens could be forcibly hospitalized only if they displayed signs of deep depression, were suicidal, or threatened the lives of others.

There are indications that such psychiatric practices changed after the mid-1980s. In 1987, the May 1 issue of *Psychiatric News* carried a report of a change in policy in the USSR regarding psychiatric treatment and treatment of the homeless (APA representatives, 1987). Perhaps Soviet psychiatrists were trying to improve their tarnished image by releasing political prisoners and placing psychiatry under the governance of the Ministry of Health rather than the Ministry of Internal Affairs (police). Traditional Russian psychiatric therapies included pharmacotherapy, hydrotherapy, physiotherapy, insulin therapy, inhalation therapy, work therapy, and drug therapy (Hess, 1971). Further evidence of this shift has been the exchange of training and information with Russian psychiatric nurses. Although Russian psychiatric institutions are underfunded, goals to improve services, deinstitutionalization, and move into more holistic care for the mentally ill have been established.

Russian Americans who are not English competent may endure isolation and loneliness. Hence, in the United States, the most common mental health problem diagnosed in Russian Americans is depression. Conversely, Sagy, Shani, and Leibovich (2009) use the term *stress resilience* to describe young Russian immigrants' ability to adapt to their new environment and ward off drug and alcohol abuse. This resilience, a kind of healthy immigrant effect, was attributed to a sense of family coherence as well as coherence with their new peer group.

Although relocating to a new nation and unfamiliar culture is enormously stressful for any immigrant group, this problem is identified primarily in elderly Russian immigrants who traveled with their children to the United States. They are unfamiliar with the language and customs, have left home and family, and often can get only minimum-wage jobs because of their age. Even after a mental diagnosis is given, they may remain reluctant to adhere to antidepressant drugs because of a fear of such medications in general and a reluctance to experience any side effects. Because of decreased emotional, physical, and financial resources and the realities of illnesses that may accompany aging—including impaired mobility, obesity, diabetes, and heart disease—older Russian American immigrants are at great risk for depression. Many Russian immigrants experienced a lifetime of stress, including wars, political turmoil and fear, religious and political persecution, poor health care, financial instability, and nutritional deficits. Often dependent on family or themselves for the first time in their lives, older Russian Americans may feel noncontributive, depressed, helpless, isolated, and demoralized (Jurcik et al., 2013; McKee et al., 2014).

Alcoholism. In Russia, alcoholism is a major and growing national health problem. Genetic ancestry bears consideration. One possible relationship to high alcoholism rates is the Russian inheritance of a particular Mongolian gene (Mongol occupation took place in the thirteenth century) that generates within its host an inability to process ethanol derived from fruit or potatoes, creating greater susceptibility to alcoholism (Gabriel, 2005).

Alcoholism, since the Soviet Union breakup, is worsening because of the chronic stress of unstable prices, inflation, crime rates, unsafe living and working conditions, and social upheavals. The morbidity and mortality resulting from alcohol consumption are greater for persons less well educated, unemployed, and living in poverty. Since the collapse of the Soviet Union, alcoholism has taken a severe toll on the nation's productivity and health. Alcohol addiction contributes to traffic fatalities, domestic violence, and industrial accidents (Marquez, 2005). Although alcoholism is an enormous problem in Russia, it has not emerged as a significant mental health problem among Russian American immigrants. A plausible explanation is that Russian immigrants often have an internal locus of control or a future orientation. They want to survive in the United States. Pessimistic Russian alcoholics stay in Russia. "Why shouldn't I drink and smoke?" one Russian explained. "There is nothing else to live for here." Another reason for the low rate of alcoholism in Russian Americans is the religious sanctions on alcohol consumption among Jewish and Christian Pentecostal groups. In addition, Russian Americans do not generally use illegal drugs, which might lead to promiscuous sexual behavior. Perhaps the lack of these self-abuse problems is attributable to attitudes and values, an internal locus of control, high levels of education, future orientation, and the cohesiveness of this skewed Russian population. Unfortunately, because Russian Jews did not drink in the homeland, they were often ridiculed and further ostracized by Russian society.

Radiation Accidents and Toxic Pollution

Environmental pollution in Russia is a growing concern for its European and Asian neighbors. Polluted air and contaminated soil, food, and water have been major health problems for Russians. Unfortunately, Communism and an indiscriminate industrialization policy left Russia and the

other former Soviet republics too poor and disorganized to fix the massive pollution problems. Much of Russia's air pollution has been caused by industrial waste, and motor vehicle emissions are becoming an increasing problem. With few regulations, lead, carbon monoxide, carbon emissions, and nitrogen oxide are entering the environment. As more and more vehicles are on Russian roads, this problem will worsen. More than 6 million people were exposed to the radiation fallout after the 1986 Chernobyl disaster. Russian nuclear reactors are considered old, huge time bombs. The disastrous results of Soviet industrialization policies have been realized, and awareness regarding the need for environmental protections have yielded some important policy changes. This is due to international pressure, especially from the European Union, as well as the hope of the Russian people to reduce or eliminate existing problems (Henry & Douhovnikoff, 2008).

Implications for Nursing Care

American nurses quickly recognize that Russian Americans are friendly, approachable, generous, interesting, likable, intelligent, and well educated. The nurse should be aware, however, that Russian immigrants might be skeptical of psychiatric-related assessments, questions, and services because psychiatric treatment often appears similar to oppression. Education about psychiatric symptoms and the modalities of treatment available in the United States are an essential part of a psychosocial intervention strategy. The client and the family should believe that they are participants and decision makers in treatment selections and strategies.

The nurse who cares for Russian Americans needs to be aware of possible nutritional implications for nursing care. Because very recent immigrants may be unable to accept American foods, the nurse would be wise to introduce new foods slowly. Religious dietary restrictions may also be a concern. In addition, nutritional deficits such as anemia and goiter must be identified and immediately treated with dietary and medical supplements.

Although alcoholism is not a reported problem among Russian Americans, residual effects of alcoholism, whether physiological or psychological, must be looked for in individuals, families, and adopted orphans. In addition, the nurse should assist Russian American clients in identifying culturally sanctioned coping strategies that will reduce anxiety and tension, depression, and low self-worth, thereby reducing the potential for mental health disorders.

Large numbers of Russian Americans are hypertensive. The nurse should use motivational strategies to devise teaching techniques that emphasize the benefits of dietary restraints, weight control, and adequate exercise. In addition, the Russian American client who is treated for hypertension needs to appreciate the importance of medication adherence and timely reporting of all unusual and untoward signs and symptoms.

Although not well researched, Russian Americans may be suffering physically and psychologically from the ill effects of water, air, and land pollution. The nurse should be keenly alert to these possible effects and assess clients accordingly.

For Russian Americans, U.S. nurses and primary care physicians represent the frontline liaison to a whole array of social and medical benefits. Russian immigrants tend to expect the health care professional to provide social and financial as well as medical services for them. If medical benefits are financially available, as in many Russian Jewish immigrant groups, this may not be a severe problem. However, many Russian Americans arrive without the ability to access appropriate health care services. If they are underpaid or unemployed, Russian immigrants may not have insurance coverage. The nurse also needs to understand that Russian Americans are a very proud and noble people, perhaps too proud to seek needed help or go on public assistance. One response offered by the Russian immigrant may be, "If I am sick, I'll have to go back to Russia to get care." Therefore, as a resource liaison, the nurse should identify and facilitate access to all possible health and assistance programs, keeping vigilance over possible exploitation.

SUMMARY

As nurses transcend their own cultural mindset, they learn to celebrate and use cultural uniqueness as an indicator for nursing interventions. Among experiences that are assisting nurses in gaining transcultural perspectives are transcultural educational experiences, such as learning about additional cultural groups from a current as well as a historical perspective.

In addition to gaining an understanding of persons from other cultures, the nurse needs to gain knowledge and competence that empowers culturally appropriate care to immigrant clients. Complexity, multiplicity, and cultural diversity contribute to the nurse's challenge, responsibility, and enjoyment while caring for Russian Americans.

CASE STUDY

Victor and Vera have immigrated to Milwaukee, Wisconsin, from St. Petersburg, the second largest city in Russia. They are Jewish and believe that the strong anti-Semitism as well as the economic instability they felt in Russia had become unbearable. Their only alternative, they decided, was to leave the country and join relatives in Milwaukee. Aurora Sinai Medical Center offered 1 year of free primary health care to them when they arrived. Now, 3 years later, Victor and Vera continue to seek services at this large teaching hospital and clinic. Victor and Vera are both 58 years old, and Vera speaks very little English. Victor has found a new peer group at the local brewery, his place of employment. However, Vera has been unable to find work and prefers to stay near family and friends. Jewish Family Services of Milwaukee has been minimally successful in involving Vera in social and mental wellness activities. Vera reads and sits in her chair most of the day. Recently, she has become more withdrawn, with an overwhelming feeling of sadness and loneliness for her native land. She states she regrets immigrating and has focused her bitter feelings inward.

A painful venous occlusion brings Vera to the health clinic, where the nurse examines her lower extremities and finds swelling, tenderness, edema, and a positive Homan's sign on Vera's left leg. A health history is difficult because of the language barrier, but with the help of a professional health care interpreter, the nurse learns about Vera's sedentary lifestyle, high-fat and high-cholesterol diet, and recent episodes of sadness. Victor is supportive but impatient for his wife to "get back on her feet again." Vera says very little.

On laboratory examination, Vera's plasma low-density lipoprotein cholesterol level is 240 mg/dL. Left ventricular hypertrophy is noted on the electrocardiogram. Vera is obese and has a blood pressure of 180/116 mm Hg. Slight hemorrhages of the retinas are also noted.

Vera is presented with two medical diagnoses: symptomatic hypertension and clinical depression. The nurse realizes that Vera's dietary instructions need to be presented with great care and attention given to cultural habits and beliefs. The nurse shows Vera an extensive list of "good" foods (written in Russian) and asks her to identify her favorites. With Vera's help and the help of the culturally competent dietitian, the nurse works out a weekly menu. The nurse must also teach Vera specific techniques for controlling her hypertension. Vera is

Continued

CASE STUDY—cont'd

instructed to take her own weight and blood pressure every morning, record them on a graph, and bring the graphs with her for her every-other-week clinic visits. Vera learns that she will need to diligently follow medication, dietary, and exercise regimens to decrease her risk of further disability. Vera is especially motivated to help herself because of her fear of losing her eyesight and thus being unable to read (her favorite pastime). Walking is encouraged after Vera's leg becomes asymptomatic.

After all instructions are repeated carefully and slowly several times (Russian and English), Vera is escorted into a private office. The nurse, who has known Vera for 3 years, asks her about her sadness and isolating behaviors. Vera adamantly rejects the nurse's suggestion that she see a psychiatric consultant.

The nurse understands that a few important psychosocial questions could include: Who do (did) you turn to for help and hope? How is that different (the same) now that you are in the United States? What part in your life does religion play? What was life like in Russia? How is your life different now? What is the most significant difference? What do you miss (not miss) the most about Russia? What were the decisions that brought you to the United States? Help us understand what it's like to leave everything you have ever known—language, culture, friends, family—to come to the United States. I know a great deal about medicine and being a nurse, but I do not know all that you know about getting healthy. From your perspective, what important information do I need to best help you help yourself?

CARE PLAN

Nursing Diagnosis: Imbalanced nutrition: more than body requirements (animal fat, salt), related to excessive intake in relation to metabolic need

Client Outcomes	Nursing Interventions
1. Client will decrease her weight by 4 lb per month. 2. Client will walk 2 miles per day (after leg has healed). 3. Client will learn to swim and will swim twice weekly at the Jewish Activity Center.	1. Teach client about importance of exercise. 2. Teach client about menu planning in relation to avoidance of high-salt, high-fat foods. 3. Encourage and support compliance with medications, exercise, diet, and follow-up care.

Nursing Diagnosis: Individual coping, ineffective, related to chronic feelings of loneliness and isolation

Client Outcomes	Nursing Interventions
1. Client will attend social activities at Jewish Family Services twice a week. 2. Client will enroll in English at the Milwaukee Area Technical College (MATC).	1. Familiarize client with Jewish Family Services and staff and involve Victor and other family members in relation to therapeutic adherence. 2. Arrange for client to visit the library of Russian books and journals located at Jewish Family Services. 3. Help client make initial contacts for classes in English as a second language held at MATC. (MATC is a short two-block walk from the clinic and hospital.) 4. Arrange transportation for client for all activities and clinic visits.

CARE PLAN—cont'd

Nursing Diagnosis: Social isolation: related to inadequate personal resources

Client Outcome	Nursing Interventions
Client will network with other Russian immigrants.	1. Encourage and support social networking (via Jewish Family Services of Milwaukee); with Vera's permission, set up appointments with Russian-based self-help and social groups. 2. Respect and honor client's cultural needs and preferences. 3. Provide Russian-language reading and patient teaching materials for client. 4. Introduce client to other Russian immigrants outside her family, and follow up with kindness, caring, and honest concern. 5. Explore employment or volunteer opportunities with Vera, connecting her with available services at the Jewish Family Services Center.

Nursing Diagnoses—Definitions and Classifications 2012–2014. Copyright © 2012, 1994–2012 by NANDA International. Used by arrangement with Wiley-Blackwell Publishing, a company of John Wiley and Sons, Inc. In order to make safe and effective judgments using NANDA-I nursing diagnoses it is essential that nurses refer to the definitions and defining characteristics of the diagnoses listed in the work.

CLINICAL DECISION MAKING

1. Why is it important that Vera's own list of foods be used when the nurse is creating a weekly menu?
2. How will the nurse keep Vera motivated toward self-help and self-care?
3. What role will Vera's family play in her recovery?
4. During client teaching, how much space should be between the nurse and Vera?
5. How may the nurse use Vera's spiritual values and beliefs to the best advantage?
6. What role does language play in this nurse–client relationship?
7. In addition to what is listed in the care plan, how else might the nurse increase Vera's self-esteem and decision-making potential?
8. When talking with Vera, what should the nurse be careful not to do?
9. How may Vera's attitudes toward self-learning and life-long learning enhance nursing care strategies?
10. Why did Vera adamantly refuse psychiatric consultation? What should the nurse do now?

REVIEW QUESTIONS

1. When communicating with Russian American clients, it is important for the nurse to address the client by which of the following?
   a. Mr. or Mrs. followed by last name
   b. First name only
   c. Terms of endearment
   d. Using a friendly outgoing manner
2. When caring for a Russian American client, the nurse should be aware that, for the most part, Russians prefer which of the following?
   a. To remain at an intimate distance rather than a social distance with caregivers
   b. To remain at a social distance rather than an intimate distance with caregivers
   c. That health assessment procedures be done in the intimate zone
   d. That boundaries are open between internal and external environments
3. When assessing Russian American clients, the nurse should use a direct approach to client interaction because the Russian American client is likely to have which belief or value?
   a. Is used to home care by nurses and physicians
   b. Values the American medical system
   c. Believes in being direct
   d. Has a tendency for somatization of emotional problems

REFERENCES

Alaniz, J. (2001). Crossing cultures: Russian nurses navigate the unfamiliar US health care system, finding career advantages and obstacles. *Nurseweek, 6*(18), 20–21.

Alexandrova, L. (2013, March 16). *Russia & India Report: Russia. Russia's child, teenage suicide rates highest in Europe. ITAR-TASS.* Available at <http://in.rbth.com/society/2013/03/16/russias_child_teenage_suicide_rates_highest_in_europe_22979.html>. Retrieved January 19, 2015.

Anderson, J. (1992). Two men clashed and a nation rose. *Parade Magazine*, 10.

ANNA National Centre for the Prevention of Violence. (2010, July). *Violence against women in the Russian Federation.* Available at <http://www2.ohchr.org/english/bodies/cedaw/docs/ngos/ANNANCPV_RussianFederation46.pdf>. Retrieved January 19, 2015.

APA representatives meet with Soviets to discuss abuse of psychiatry in USSR. (1987). *Psychiatric News*, 37.

Arnold, C., & Kurmasheva, A. (2008, June 28). Abortion remains top birth-control option in Russia. *Radio Free Europe/Radio Liberty*, Available at <http://www.rferl.org/articleprintview/1145849.html>. Retrieved September 22, 2010.

Aroian, K. J., & Vander Wal, J. S. (2007). Health service use in Russian immigrants and nonimmigrants older persons. *Family and Community Health, 30*(3), 213–223.

Baker, C. J. (2008). Smoking behavior among immigrants from the former Soviet Union (Unpublished dissertation). Columbus, Ohio: Ohio State University.

Balmforth, T., & Feifer, G. (2011, August 14). *Radio Free Europe. Radio Liberty. RFE/RL., Inc.* Accessed at <www.rferl.org/content/russian_healt_car_provides_no_real_safety_net/24296527.html>. Retrieved January 20, 2015.

Berger, P. (2011, November 25). How many Russian speakers are in U.S.? Experts spare over numbers and ponder who is a Jew. *The Jewish Daily Forward*. Available at <http://forward.com/articles/146812/how-many-russian-speakers-are-in-us/?p=1&p=1&p=1>. Retrieved January 22, 2015.

Binyon, M. (1983). *Life in Russia*. New York: Berkley.

British Broadcasting Company (BBC). (2010). *Russia country profile*. Available at <http://newsvote.bbc.co.uk>. Retrieved August 30, 2010.

British Broadcasting Company (BBC). (2015). *Languages across Europe: Russia. BBC news online; country profile—Russia.* Accessed at <http://www.bbc.co.uk/languages/european_languages/countries/russia.shtml>. Retrieved January 18, 2015.

Brown, S. M., et al. (2007). Prospective surveillance for surgical site infection in St. Petersburg, Russian Federation. *Infection Control & Hospital Epidemiology, 28*(3), 319–325.

Burlatsky, F. (1991). Coming and going in the USSR. *Soviet Life, 7*(418), 14–45.

Central Intelligence Agency (CIA). (2014). *The world factbook: Russia.* Accessed at <https://www.cia.gov/library/publications/the-world-factbook/geos/rs.html>. Retrieved January 18, 2015.

Commonwealth of Independent States (CIS). (2014). *CIS indicators. Interstate Statistical Committee of the Commonwealth of Independent States.* Accessed at <http://www.cisstat.com/eng/frame_cis.htm>. Retrieved January 18, 2015.

Communicating with Your Russian Patient (2007). *Culture clues.* Seattle: Patient and Family Education Services, University of Washington Medical Center. Available at: <http://depts.washington.edu/pfes/PDFs/RussianCultureClue.pdf> Retrieved August 30, 2010.

Crandall, M., Senturia, K., Sullivan, M., & Shiu-Thornton, S. (2005). "No way out": Russian-speaking women's experiences with domestic violence. *Journal of Interpersonal Violence, 20*(8), 941–958.

Curtis, G. E. (Ed.). (1996). *Russia: a country study*. Washington, DC: GPO for the Library of Congress. Accessed at: <http://countrystudies.us/russia/> Retrieved January 22, 2015.

Danishevski, K., Balabanova, D., McKee, M., & Atkinson, S. (2006). The fragmentary federation: experiences with the decentralized health system in Russia. *Health Policy and Planning, 21*(3), 183–194.

Davydov, M. I., & Shepin, O. P. (2010, September). The Russian healthcare system. *Medical Solutions* (Siemens), pp. 74–78.

Egenolf, F. (2012, September 11). *Philanthropy news: Bristol-Myers Squibb Foundation announces five new grants to advance cancer nursing skills in central and Eastern Europe.* Press Release. Accessed at <http://news.bms.com/press-release/philanthropy-news/bristol-myers-squibb-foundation-announces-five-new-grants-advance-ca&t=634829736664117945>. Retrieved January 21, 2015.

Eight attempts reported on Yeltsin's life. (1993). *The Journal Times*, 4A.

Friedman, M. (2012). For Russians, corruption is just a way of life. *New York Times Sunday Review*. Accessed at <http://www.nytimes.com/2012/08/19/opinion/sunday/for-russians-corruption-is-just-a-way-of-life.html?_r=0>. Retrieved January 19, 2015.

Frye, T. (2014, February 17). The culture of corruption: Russians pay, but don't like it. *Washington Post*. Accessed at <http://www.washingtonpost.com/blogs/monkey-cage/wp/2014/02/17/the-culture-of-corruption-russians-pay-but-they-dont-like-it-2/>. Retrieved January 19, 2015.

Gabriel, R. (2005, March). A commentary of pharmacogenomics: what can it do? *Medical Laboratory Observer*, Farmington Hills, MI: Nelson. Available at <http://findarticles.com/p/articles>. Retrieved January 28, 2007.

Gore-Felton, A. M., Somlai, E. G., Benotsch, J. A., Kelly, J. A., Ostrovski, D., & Kozlov, A. (2003). The influence of gender on factors associated with HIV transmission risk among young Russian injection drug users. *American Journal of Drug and Alcohol Abuse, 29*(4), 881–894.

Gromov, M. N. (2004–2005). The eternal values of Russian culture: on the interpretation of our fatherland's philosophy. *Russian Studies in Philosophy, 43*(3), 90–100.

Heimer, R., & White, E. (2010). Estimation of the number of injection drug users in St. Petersburg, Russia. *Drug & Alcohol Dependence, 109*(1–3), 79–83.

Henry, L. A., & Douhovnikoff, V. (2008). Environmental issues in Russia. *Annual Review of Environmental Resources, 33,* 437–460.

Hess, G. (1971). Impressions of mental health service delivery systems in Finland, Poland, Soviet Russia, and Czechoslovakia. *International Journal of Nursing Studies, 8*(4), 223–235.

Hurwitz, P. (2005). Readers letters: scratching Tartars. *Russian Life, 48*(6), 5.

Ivanov, L. L., Hu, J., & Leak, A. (2010). Immigrant women's cancer screening behaviors. *Journal of Community Health Nursing, 27*(1), 32–45.

Jarvik, L. (2006). Cultural challenges to democratization in Russia. *Orbis, 50*(1), 167–186.

Jeltova, I., Fish, M. C., & Revenson, T. A. (2005). Risky sexual behaviors in immigrant adolescent girls from the former Soviet Union: role of natal and host culture. *Journal of School Psychology, 43*(1), 3–22.

Jones, I., et al. (1995). Impact of age and environment on somatic mutation at the hprt gene of T lymphocytes in humans. *Mutation Research, 338*(1–6), 129–139.

Jurcik, T., Chentsova-Dutton, Y. E., Solopieieva-Jurcikova, I., & Ryder, A. G. (2013). Russians in treatment: the evidence base supporting cultural adaptations. *Journal of Clinical Psychology, 69*(7), 774–791.

Khovostunova, O. (2012, May 31). *Russia's invisible children: the unrelieved plight of Russia's invisible youth. IMR: Institute of Modern Russia.* Accessed at <http://imrussia.org/en/society/245-besprizorniki?start=2>. Retrieved January 19, 2015.

Kliger, S. (2012, January 23). *Russian-Jewish immigrants in the U.S.: social portrait, challenges, and AJC involvement.* Paper prepared for the American Jewish Committee (AJC) Commission on Contemporary Jewish Life. Accessed at <http://www.ajcrussian.org/site/apps/nlnet/content2.aspx?c=chLMK3PKLsF&b=7718799&ct=11713359>. Retrieved January 22, 2015.

Kononova, S. (2010, July 27). *A harmful tradition. Unwrapping the mystery inside the enigma.* Available at <http://www.russiaprofile.org>. Retrieved September 22, 2010.

Konovalov, A. (Ed.). (2013). *To Russia with ease: healthcare in Russia.* Accessed at <http://torussia.org/health_care_in_russia>. Retrieved January 20, 2015.

Kostikov, V. (1991). Boris Yeltsin's political victory. *Soviet Life, 7*(418), 2–5.

Kravitz, R. L., Helms, L. J., Azari, R., Antonius, D., & Melnikow, J. (2000). Comparing the use of physician time and health care resources among patients speaking English, Spanish, and Russian. *Medical Care, 38*(7), 728–738.

Kristjanson, A. F., Wilsnack, S. C., Zvartau, E., Tsoy, M., & Novikov, B. (2007). Alcohol use in pregnant and nonpregnant Russian women. *Alcoholism, Clinical and Experimental Research, 31*(2), 299–307.

Kulikov, E. E., Buzhilova, A. P., & Poltaraus, A. B. (2004). Molecular genetic characteristics of medieval populations of the Russian North. *Russian Journal of Genetics, 40*(1), 1–9.

Lally, K. (2000). Death offers no relief for woes of Russians. *Baltimore Sun,* 1A.

Lally, K. (2013, February 21). Europe: Russia tries to improve life expectancy with laws curbing drinking, smoking. *Washington Post,* Accessed at <http://www.washingtonpost.com/world/europe/russia-tries-to-improve-life-expectancy-with-laws-curbing-drinking-smoking/2013/02/20/7ad5c290-77ab-11e2-95e4-6148e45d7adb_story.html>. Retrieved January 21, 2015.

Larkin, M. (2000). Russian biomedical science survives against all odds. *Lancet, 355*(9200), 294.

Leigh, J. (Ed.), (2006). *Russian culture profile.* Queensland, Australia: DC Diversicare.

Leon, D. A., Shkolnikov, V. M., & McKee, M. (2009). Alcohol and Russian mortality: a continuing crisis. *Addiction (Abingdon, England), 104,* 1630–1636.

Library of Congress (LOC). (2011). *A country study: Russia. Federal Research Division, Library of Congress.* Accessed at <http://lcweb2.loc.gov/frd/cs/rutoc.html>. Retrieved January 18, 2015.

Loft. (2015). *Homeless world cup: Russia.* Accessed at <http://www.homelessworldcup.org/content/homelessness-statistics>. Retrieved January 19, 2015.

Magocsi, P. R. (2015). *Countries and their cultures: Russian Americans. Adrameg, Inc.* Accessed at <http://www.everyculture.com/multi/Pa-Sp/Russian-Americans.html>. Retrieved January 22, 2015.

Marquez, P. V. (2005). *Dying too young: addressing premature mortality and ill health due to non-communicable diseases and injuries in the Russian Federation.* Europe and Central Asia Human Development Department: The World Bank. Available at: <http://siteresources.worldbank.org/INTECA/Resources/DTY-Final.pdf> Retrieved June 24, 2006.

Masters, J. (2014, November 17). *The Russian military. Council on Foreign Relations.* Accessed at <http://www.cfr.org/russian-federation/russian-military/p33758>. Retrieved January 21, 2015.

McKee, K., Dugan, T., & Levenson, R. (2014, November 10). *Cultural profile: Russian Americans. Center of Excellence for Culturally Competent Mental Health.* Accessed at <http://ssrdqst.rfmh.org/sites/ssrdqst.rfmh.org.cecc/userfiles/profiles/Russian%20Profile.pdf>. Retrieved January 22, 2015.

Mikhaylova, Y. (2013, November 28). *TB and HIV in Russian prison system. Federal Research Institute for Health Organization and Informatics of Ministry of Health of the Russian Federation.* Report submitted to the conference, Helsinki, Finland: Combating HIV and TB through a joint regional action NDPHS PAC-10 side-event. Accessed at <http://www.ndphs.org///documents/3878/TB_and_HIV_in_Russian_prison_system.pdf>. Retrieved January 26, 2015.

Minnesota Department of Employment and Economic Development (MDEED). (2006). *Cultural diversity information: Russian immigrants in Minnesota.* Available at <http://www.mnssb.org/rcb/moc/russian.htm>. Retrieved January 21, 2007.

Money converter. (2015). *Convert Russian rouble to US dollar and euro. The money converter.* Accessed at <http://themoneyconverter.com/RUB/USD.aspx>. Retrieved January 18, 2015.

Moore, R. (Ed.). (1988). *Fodor's 89 Soviet Union.* New York: Fodor's Travel Publications.

National Center for Biotechnology Information (NCBI). (2011). *Drug resistant tuberculosis in the Russian Federation. The new profile of drug resistant tuberculosis in Russia: a global and local perspective: summary of a joint workshop.* National Library of Medicine; National Academy of Sciences. Accessed: <http://www.ncbi.nlm.nih.gov/books/NBK62453/> Retrieved January 19, 2015.

Norton, W. P. (2011, October 19). *Rediscovering Russian America. Institute of Modern Russia [IMR].* Accessed at <http://www.imrussia.org/en/?option=com_content&view=article&id=133:rediscovering-russian-america&catid=56:society-a-trends&Itemid=99&lang=en>. Retrieved January 23, 2015.

Novosti, R. (2010). Russia: Russian authorities should take more measures to prevent violence against women, Amnesty International said in its latest annual report issued on Thursday. *Sputnik News.* Accessed at <http://sputniknews.com/russia/20100527/159178795.html>. Retrieved January 19, 2015.

Organisation for Economic Co-operation and Development (OECD) (2013, November 21). *Health at a glance 2013.* OECD Indicators. OECD Publishing. OECD iLibrary. Accessed at: <http://dx.doi.org/10.1787/health_glance-2013-en>. Retrieved January 19, 2015.

Orlando Russian Culture Society (ORCS) (2009). *Demographics of Russian speakers in USA.* Orlando, FL: Aurous, in partnership with the Russian-American Community Center of Florida. Accessed at: <http://www.orlandorussians.com/research-data/demographics-of-russian-speakers-in-usa/> Retrieved January 22, 2015.

Ortman, J. M., & Shin, H. B. (2011, August 20–23). *Language projections: 2010–2010.* Presented at the annual meeting of the American Sociological Association, Las Vegas, NV. U.S. Bureau of the Census. Washington, DC. Accessed <http://www.census.gov/hhes/socdemo/language/data/acs/Ortman_Shin_ASA2011_paper.pdf>. Retrieved January 24, 2015.

Osborn, A. (2004). Half of Russia's doctors face sack in healthcare reforms. *British Medical Journal, 328*(7448), 1092.

Oza-Frank, R., & Narayan, K. M. V. (2010). Overweight and diabetes among US immigrants. *American Journal of Public Health, 100*(4), 661–668.

Patient and Family Education Committee (2007). *Culture clues: end-of-life care: the Russian culture. Seattle: Patient and Family Education Services.* University of Washington Medical Center. Accessed at: <http://depts.washington.edu/pfes/PDFs/End%20of%20Life%20Care-Russian.pdf>. Retrieved January 25, 2015.

Perlman, F., & McKee, M. (2008). Diabetes during the Russian transition. *Diabetes Research and Clinical Practice, 80,* 305–313.

Radia, K., & Stukalova, T. (2012, December 24). *Moscow's homeless walk all night to avoid freezing to death.* ABC News: World News Network. Accessed at <http://abcnews.go.com/International/moscows-homeless-walk-night-avoid-freezing-death/story?id=18057192>. Retrieved January 19, 2015.

Reklama, R. (2007, July 18). *How happy Russian immigrants are in U.S.? Voices that must be heard, Edition 280.* Accessed at <http://www.ajcrussian.org/site/apps/nlnet/content2.aspx?c=cHLMK3PKLsF&b=7718799&ct=11208009>.

Resick, L. K. (2008). The meaning of health among midlife Russian-speaking women. *Journal of Nursing Scholarship, 40*(3), 248–253.

Rtveladze, K., Marsh, T., et al. (2012). Obesity trends in Russia: the impact on health and healthcare costs. *Health, 4*(12a), 1471–1484.

Russia. (2015). *Infoplease.* Accessed at <http://www.infoplease.com/encyclopedia/world/russia-land-people.html>. Retrieved January 18, 2015.

Russia time zones. (2015). Russia current times. *Time, temperature@@@com.* Accessed at <http://www.timetemperature.com/europe/russia_time_zones.shtml>. Retrieved January 18, 2015.

Russian Federation Federal State Statistics Service (RSSS). (2014). *Russia in figures 2014.* Accessed at <http://www.gks.ru/bgd/regl/b14_12/Main.htm>. Retrieved January 20, 2015.

Russian Nurses Association (RNA). (2015, January). *Russian Nurses Association:* <www.medsestre.ru>. V. Sarkisova, President. (Written in Russian). Limited English version available on the Infusion Nurses Society Web site at <http://www.ins1.org/m/pages.cfm?pageID=3727>.

Ryan, C. (2013). *Language use in the United States: 2011.* American community survey reports. U.S. Department of Commerce, U.S. Bureau of the Census. Census.gov. Accessed at: <http://www.census.gov/prod/2013pubs/acs-22.pdf>. Retrieved January 22, 2015.

Sagy, S., Shani, E., & Leibovich, E. (2009). Factors related to attitudes towards drug use and alcohol drinking: comparing immigrants from the former Soviet Union and Israeli-born adolescents. *Journal of Substance Use, 14*(1), 10–18.

School of Russian and Asian Studies (SRAS). (2010, January 20). *Number of abortions in Russia comparable to births. Itar-Tas.* Accessed at <http://www.sras.org/number_of_abortions_in_russia_comparable_to_births>. Retrieved January 24, 2015.

Scott, A. (1988). Human interaction and personal boundaries. *Journal of Psychosocial Nursing, 26*(8), 23–27.

Shpilko, I. (2006). Russian-American health care: bridging the communication gap between physicians and patients. *Patient Education and Counseling, 64,* 331–341.

Smith, L. S. (1996). New Russian immigrants: health problems, practices, and values. *Journal of Cultural Diversity, 3*(3), 68–73.

Smith, L. S. (2006). Nursing in Russia: an overview of healthcare, nursing education, and practice. In P. S. Cowen & S. Moorhead (Eds.), *Current issues in nursing* (7th ed., pp. 828–842). St. Louis: Mosby.

St. Elizabeth Medical Center (STEMC). (2006). *Cultural diversity: Russians*. Available at <www.stemc.org/about_stemc/cultural_diversity/russians>. Retrieved September 23, 2010.

Stickley, A., & Carlson, P. (2009). The social and economic determinants of smoking in Moscow, Russia. *Scandinavian Journal of Public Health, 37*(6), 632–639.

StratisHealth (2009). *Fact sheet: Russian Americans in Minnesota.* Bloomington, MN: Stratis Health. Available at: <www.stratishealth.org> Retrieved August 30, 2010.

StratisHealth. (2014). *Russians in Minnesota: common medical issues and cultural concerns of Russian patients. Culture care connection.* Accessed at from <http://culturecareconnection.org/matters/diversity/russian.html>. Retrieved January 25, 2015.

Szalavitz, M. (2011, January 18). Perspective: to prevent AIDS in Russia, drug addicts need care. *Time*. Accessed <http://healthland.time.com/2011/01/18/perspective-to-prevent-aids-in-russia-drug-addicts-need-care/>. Retrieved January 19, 2011.

Tashlein-Van Heuveln, D. (2009, August 3). Russian healthcare: observing nurses a world away. *Carolina Nursing News.* Available at <http://carolinanursingnews.com/2009/08/03/russian-healthcare-observing-nurses-a-world-away/>. Retrieved July 21, 2010.

Tran, T. V., Khatutsky, G., Aroian, K., Balsam, A., & Conway, M. A. (2000). Living arrangements, depression, and health status among elderly Russian-speaking immigrants. *Journal of Gerontological Social Work, 33*(2), 63–77.

U.S. Bureau of the Census. (2014, May 28). *Russian ancestry. U.S. Census Bureau Statistical Abstracts of the United States: 2012.* Accessed at <http://www.census.gov/prod/www/statistical_abstract.html>. Retrieved January 22, 2015.

U.S. Department of Homeland Security (DOHS) (2010). *Immigrant orphans adopted by US citizens by gender, age, and region and country of birth: fiscal year 2009* Table 12. 2009 Yearbook of Immigration Statistics. Office of Immigration Statistics.

U.S. Department of Homeland Security (DOHS). (2014, June 16). *Yearbook of Immigration Statistics, 2013. Table 2: Persons obtaining lawful permanent resident status by region and selected country.* Accessed at <http://www.dhs.gov/yearbook-immigration-statistics-2013-lawful-permanent-residents>. Retrieved January 22, 2015.

Vadlamani, A., et al. (2001). Colorectal cancer in Russian-speaking Jewish emigres: community-based screening. *American Journal of Gastroenterology, 96*(9), 2755–2760.

Victor Center for Jewish Genetic Diseases. (2015). *Judaism: Ashkenazi Jewish genetic diseases. American-Israeli Cooperative Enterprise.* Accessed at <http://www.jewishvirtuallibrary.org/jsource/Health/genetics.html>. Retrieved January 26, 2015.

Witt, H. (1993). Inside the Russian court. *Chicago Tribune,* 1–13.

Wong, G. (2009, May 19). Russia's bleak picture of health. *CNN,* Accessed at <http://edition.cnn.com/2009/health/05/russia.health/index.html>; Retrieved January 19, 2015.

World Health Organization (WHO). (2006). *Highlights on health in the Russian Federation 2005. Highlights on Health.* WHO Regional Office for Europe. Available at: <http://www.euro.who.int/highlights>. Retrieved August 30, 2010.

World Health Organization (WHO). (2008). *Core health indicators: United States of America; Russian Federation. WHOSIS database.* Available at <http://apps.who.int/whosis/database>. Retrieved August 30, 2010.

World Health Organization (WHO). (2015). *Countries: Russian Federation.* Accessed at <http://www.who.int/countries/rus/en/>. Retrieved January 19, 2015.

World Meters. (2015). *Population by country: Russia population. World meters@@@info.* Accessed at <http://www.worldometers.info/>. Retrieved January 19, 2015.

Yeltsin rival backs down. (1993). *The Journal Times,* 3A.

Yeltsin: Main points. (1993). *The Journal Times,* 11A.

Chinese Americans

Chyi-Kong (Karen) Chang

After reading this chapter, the nurse will be able to:

1. Describe Chinese philosophy, beliefs, and values.
2. Explain the ways that Chinese Americans communicate.
3. Describe the influences of the family system on Chinese Americans.
4. Explain the time concept of Chinese Americans.
5. Describe the illness behaviors of Chinese Americans.
6. Identify the biological variations of Chinese Americans.
7. Articulate the implications of providing effective nursing care for Chinese Americans.

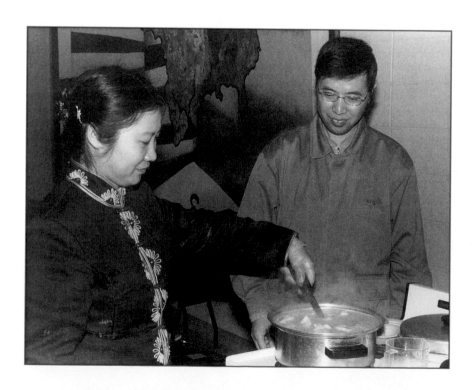

OVERVIEW OF CHINA

China (the People's Republic of China), literally "Central Kingdom," occupies the eastern portion of Asia and is slightly larger in area than the United States (*World Almanac*, 2015). In fact, China occupies roughly 3,705,386 square miles (9,596,960 square kilometers) (Central Intelligence Agency, 2015). The coastline of China is roughly a semicircle. The topography and climate of China are extremely varied. The greater part of China is mountainous; it is only in the lower portions of the Yellow and Yangtze rivers that there are any extensive low plains. The principal mountain ranges include the Tien Shan (translates as "Celestial Mountains") in the northwest part of the country; the Kunlun chain, which runs south of the Takla Makan and Gobi deserts; the Tanggula mountain range, which connects the Kunlun chain with Tibet (*World Almanac*, 2015); and the Da Xing, a mountain range in northeast China. Mount Everest on the border with Nepal is the world's tallest peak. The major plains in China include the Northeast Plain, the Inner Mongolia Plain, the Central Plain, the lower Yangtze Plain, and the Pearl River Delta Plain.

In July of 2014, the total population of China was estimated at 1,355,692,576 (Central Intelligence Agency, 2015; *World Almanac*, 2015). The average annual growth was 12.79 million, or an average rate of natural increase of 0.44% (Central Intelligence Agency, 2015). The birth rate in China is 12.17 per 1000, compared with 16.3 per 1000 for the United States (Central Intelligence Agency, 2015). In 2014, the infant mortality rate in China was 14.79 per 1000, compared with 9.8 per 1000 for the United States (Central Intelligence Agency, 2015; National Center for Health Statistics, *Health, United States*, 2013). The population of China makes it one of the densest countries in the world (353 people per square mile).

China has some of the largest cities in the world by population. The capital city of China is Beijing (translates as "northern capital" and was previously known as *Peking*), which has an estimated population of 11,106,000. The largest city in China is Shanghai (translates as "on-the-sea"), which has an estimated population of 14,987,000. Other large cities include Tianjin (7,180,000 metro area), Guangzhou (8,829,000), Wuhan (7,243,000), and Xi'anguan (4,528,000) (Central Intelligence Agency, 2015; *World Almanac*, 2015).

The principal agricultural products of China include rice, wheat, potatoes, grains, tea, and cotton. In 1998, the makeup of the labor force by occupation sector was as follows: agriculture, 50%; industry, 24%; and services, 26% (Central Intelligence Agency, 2015; *World Almanac*, 2015). Major exports are machinery and equipment, textiles and clothing, footwear, toys and sporting goods, and mineral fuels (Central Intelligence Agency, 2015; *World Almanac*, 2015). In 2010, China overtook Japan as the world's second largest economy (Central Intelligence Agency, 2015).

The president of China is Xi Jinping (2013–), and the premier is Li Keqiang (2013–). The ruling governmental authority in China is the Communist Party. The National People's Congress is the chief legislative organ. Within the governmental hierarchy, the State Council has the executive authority. It is the Congress that elects the premier and the deputy premiers. In China, the ministries are under the auspices of the State Council headed by the premier.

According to incomplete statistics, China has 300 million religious believers. Among them, there are 14 million Christians (10 million Protestants, 4 million Catholics) and 18 million Muslims. In addition, there are 13,000 Buddhist and 1500 Taoist temples (Central Intelligence Agency, 2015).

OVERVIEW OF CHINESE AMERICANS

The majority of Chinese Americans are immigrants from Taiwan, Hong Kong, and mainland China. Today, the 3,535,382 Chinese Americans constitute the largest group of Asian Americans (U.S. Department of Commerce, Bureau of the Census, *The Asian Population*, 2012). This new figure represents a 37.9% growth rate from 1990 to 2010. This figure compares with 104.1% from 1980 to 1990. Chinese Americans residing in the United States represent 0.7% of the total U.S. population (U.S. Department of Commerce, Bureau of the Census, *The Asian Population*, 2012). Of the number of Chinese Americans residing in this country, 52.4% live in the West, 27.0% live in the Northeast, 12.4% live in the South, and 8.1% live in the Midwest (U.S. Department of Commerce, Bureau of the Census, *The Asian Population*, 2012). The states with the largest populations of Chinese Americans are California (704,850), New York (284,144), and Hawaii (68,804). A total of 66% of Chinese Americans live in five states: California, New York, Hawaii, Illinois, and Texas (*World Almanac*, 2015; U.S. Department of Commerce, Bureau of the Census, *The Asian Population*, 2012).

Of the Chinese Americans residing in the United States before 1975, 18.5% were foreign born; of the number residing in the United States between 1975 and 1979, 11.4% were foreign born; and of those entering in 2000 or later, 29.3% were foreign born. Immigration has definitely contributed to the growth in the Chinese-American population over the past two decades. It is interesting to note, however, that the percentage of Chinese Americans who are foreign born differs considerably across time periods. The median age of Chinese Americans residing in the United States is 35.5 years, compared with 36.7 years for the general U.S. population. In addition, only 11.0% of all Asian Americans are 65 years of age or older, compared with 12.7% of the general U.S. population (U.S. Department of Commerce, Bureau of the Census, *American Community Survey,* 2013; *World Almanac,* 2015).

Chinese Americans are noted for maintaining high educational standards. For example, in 2009, 81.2% of Chinese-American males and 82.8% of Chinese-American females 25 years of age or older held a high school diploma; 45.2% of Chinese American males and 49.3% of Chinese-American females held a bachelor's degree (U.S. Department of Commerce, Bureau of the Census, *American Community Survey,* 2013; *World Almanac,* 2015).

Of the number of Chinese Americans in the United States, 65.1% participate in the workforce. Chinese Americans have lower labor force participation rates than Filipinos (71.0%) and Asian Indians (72.3%). The poverty rate for Chinese Americans is 9.5%, compared with 14.3% for the general U.S. population (*World Almanac,* 2015. This lower rate represents the first time in a decade that the poverty rate is lower than that of the general U.S. population.

There is a bimodal distribution with regard to socioeconomic status and educational attainment in the U.S. Asian and Pacific Islander population, including Chinese Americans (U.S. Department of Commerce, Bureau of the Census, *American Community Survey,* 2015; U.S. Department of Commerce, Bureau of the Census, *Asian Population, 2012*). The median family income for Chinese Americans is $81,323 compared with $62,367 for the rest of the general U.S. population (U.S. Department of Commerce, Bureau of the Census, *American Community Survey,* 2013). As a subgroup, the socioeconomic status and educational attainment of Chinese Americans are comparable to those of Asian Indians, Japanese, and Korean Americans but higher than those of other Asian subgroups, such as Filipinos, Vietnamese, Laotians, Cambodians, and Thais. In other words, there is a significant segment of Chinese Americans who are college-educated professionals with high income. At the same time, there are a large number of barely literate individuals of Chinese descent working in low-paying occupations (Wong, 2006).

The contrasting socioeconomic characteristics of the Chinese immigrants in different historical periods determined, to a large extent, their educational attainment and their occupations. Before 1965, most Chinese immigrants had little or no education, and many were alone because their families were not allowed to immigrate with them. They were forced to immigrate for political, social, or economic reasons. The majority of them came from Guangdong Province and took up occupations such as mining, railroad construction, and farming or engaged in small family businesses, such as restaurants, laundries, and groceries. After 1965, when immigration laws changed in the United States to seek skilled labor, better educated professionals and specialists began to immigrate. Now families were also allowed to immigrate together. These immigrants came from Taiwan, mainland China, and Hong Kong. As a result, a wide cultural and linguistic diversity exists among Chinese Americans.

Chinese culture is dominated by Confucianism, which encourages individuals to pursue reciprocity, benevolence, respect for authority, self-improvement, filial piety, righteousness, modesty, integrity, and wisdom. A harmonious relationship with nature and other people is stressed, and a person is expected to accommodate rather than confront. If individual interests conflict with community interests, a person is expected to submit to the interest of the group. Public debating of conflicting views is perceived as socially unacceptable. A person is expected to be sensitive to what other people perceive and think and to be gracious toward others so as not to make them "lose face." Self-expression and individualism are discouraged, whereas showing filial piety to parents and loyalty to family, friends, and government is highly valued. Modesty, self-control, self-reliance, self-restraint, and face-saving are taught at home and school and are indicators for maturity and consistency with the cultural norms. When they fail to follow these cultural practices and meet these expectations, many Chinese may feel shame or guilt (Li, 2004). In fact, shame is such an important concept and its influence is so prevailing in the Chinese society, Chinese culture has been termed as a "shame-oriented culture" by some scholars (Li, 2004). Consequently, the Chinese appear to be quiet, polite, pleasant, and unassertive and often suppress personal feelings such as frustration, disagreement, anger, or pain.

Reciprocation, or treating others as one would wish to be treated, is often practiced and expected in interpersonal relationships. Interpersonal interactions have a hierarchical structure, so that older or higher-status people have authority over younger or lower-status people. A person's status is always referred to during interactions. For example, brothers address each other as "older brother" and "younger brother" in addition to the first name. Educational achievement and professional success are highly valued because pride and honor are brought to the family and the community as a result. Therefore, Chinese parents not only willingly support their children who pursue education but also frequently sacrifice, at almost any cost, to ensure a good education for their children.

The sharp contrasts between the Chinese and American cultures often cause a high level of stress among

Chinese Americans during the acculturation process. Some may hold onto traditional Chinese culture, observe holidays according to the lunar calendar, and maintain Chinese customs; some may reject their traditional heritage; and some may assimilate both the Chinese culture and the American culture. Poorly adjusted individuals may not be able to perform work productively, may have low self-esteem, and may exhibit some lawless behaviors. Second- and third-generation Chinese Americans, who are already well acculturated into Western culture, may not be influenced much by traditional Chinese culture. However, they may experience an identity issue of being culturally and linguistically American, even though others perceive them as Chinese (Wong, 2006). Of the number of Chinese Americans 5 years of age or older residing in the United States, 82.7% speak a language at home other than English; 46.4% speak English less than very well; and 17.3% speak only English at home (U.S. Department of Commerce, Bureau of the Census, *American Community Survey*, 2013).

COMMUNICATION

Dialect

A wide cultural and linguistic diversity exists among Chinese Americans. Linguistic diversity may cause communication problems among Chinese people. Although the official Chinese language is Mandarin (Putonghūa), there are many dialects spoken that are not understood by other groups of Chinese. However, all the dialects have the same written characters and grammatical structures, which have been relatively stable for 3000 years despite having undergone great changes. This stability in the language permits all literate Chinese to be able to communicate in writing. Each Chinese character (or logogram) consists of only one syllable. Each character has its own meaning, but if one character is combined with one or more characters, the combination produces words or phrases with different concepts. There are four tones in Mandarin (as well as a neutral tone), and changes of tone produce complete changes in the meaning of a syllable or a word. For instance, *ma* may mean "mother" with the flat tone, "numbness" with the rising tone, "horse" with the curving tone, and "scold" or "curse" in the falling tone. Undoubtedly, the complexity arising from toning is one of the toughest challenges for any non-Chinese trying to master the spoken language. On the other hand, the Chinese language generally does not use copulas and plurals (although both exist) and has no tenses.

Style, Volume, and Touch

The Chinese value silence and avoid disagreeing or criticizing, especially in public. Disagreements are not verbalized so that harmonious relationships will be maintained, at least outwardly. To raise one's voice to make a point, a common behavior for some Americans, is viewed by many Chinese as being associated with anger and a sign of loss of self-control. To avoid confrontation and subsequent "loss of face," a direct "no" is rarely used. On the other hand, the word "yes" with or without nodding may merely mean "I heard you" and may not indicate agreement or consent. In some circumstances, "yes" can even mean "no" or "perhaps." Hesitancy, ambiguity, subtlety, and implicitness are dominant features in Chinese communication (Liu, 2005). Understanding nonverbal cues and contextual meanings is also necessary to communicate effectively with some Chinese Americans.

Touching and touching different parts of the body have different meanings that are largely defined culturally. Chinese people do not ordinarily touch each other during conversation (Millet, 2010). Touching someone's head indicates a serious breach of etiquette, particularly when the involved person is elderly or of higher social status. Touching during an argument indicates shameful loss of self-control. In the same respect, putting one's feet on a desk, table, or chair is regarded as impolite and disrespectful. On the other hand, public displays of affection toward a person of the same sex are quite permissible in the Chinese culture. Unlike the American culture, however, public displays between the opposite sexes are considered socially unacceptable (Burkett, 1995). The Chinese are often viewed as polite but reserved, shy, cold, unassertive, or uninterested (Chen & Yang, 1986; Fisher, 1996; Watson, 1970).

Context

Communication among the Chinese is high-context, in contrast to communication among mainstream Americans. A high-context communication is one in which most of the information is either in the physical context or internalized in the persons involved, whereas very little is in the coded, explicit, transmitted message. A low-context communication is just the opposite; that is, the mass of the information is vested in the explicit code (Hall, 1981, 1989).

The Chinese people tend to perceive, value, and rely on nonverbal and contextual cues during communication and do not communicate explicitly (Millet, 2010). For example, facial expressions, tensions, movements, pace of speech, and location of interactions are perceived during interactions to formulate specific meanings. They expect others to figure out the underlying meanings of communicated words (Gudykunst, 2001; Liu, 2005). Again, it cannot be overemphasized that understanding nonverbal cues and contextual meaning is necessary for effective communication with the Chinese people.

Kinesics

In the past, Chinese people greeted others by bowing. It is more commonplace now to greet people with "Have you had your breakfast [lunch, dinner]?" The greeting person is not really interested in the question literally. Instead, it is merely a culturally determined format of greeting other people. Nodding the head may indicate "yes," whereas shaking the head may indicate "no." To answer a question such as "Haven't you had anything to eat?" is problematic for many Chinese Americans. They may be confused about whether to answer affirmatively or negatively: "Yes, I haven't had anything," or "No, I would like something."

Many Chinese Americans experience feelings of shame and embarrassment when they cannot communicate well. Some apologize frequently and repeatedly for their linguistic inadequacies because they think they are inconveniencing others. Although most Chinese Americans will often refrain from expressing their emotions openly, some may narrow their eyes to express anger and disgust (Chin, 2005). In general, Chinese Americans tend to have less eye contact than other Americans have because, in the Chinese culture, excessive eye contact may indicate impoliteness and rudeness (Watson, 1970); it may also be perceived as threatening (Chin, 2005).

Chinese Americans, like other immigrants, experience a great amount of stress when they are in health care facilities. The language barrier and their different cultural background often cause confusion, depression, frustration, helplessness, and powerlessness (Barrett, 2006; Shih-Yu, 2009). However, they tend not to discuss their concerns or express their emotional problems with health care professionals (Cheung, Nelson, Advincula, Young Cureton, & Canham, 2005; Liu, 2005; Mortenson, 2009; Shih-Yu, 2009). Some Chinese Americans believe that emotional problems are personal issues and are often embarrassed to ask questions when no health care workers speak their language. These emotional experiences are often not orally expressed but may be indicated by nonverbal cues. Frequently, observing nonverbal behaviors and encouraging clients to verbalize will help identify these psychological problems.

Implications for Nursing Care

It is important for the nurse to remember that there are diverse Chinese dialects that are not comprehensible to other Chinese groups. If the client needs a translator in the health care setting, the nurse must first find out which dialect the client speaks and then find a translator who can speak that dialect.

Because the Chinese language is quite different from English, the nurse must remember that when Chinese Americans communicate in English, they often experience a high level of stress (Barrett, 2006; Liu, 2005; Mortenson, 2009; Shih-Yu, 2009). The nurse may observe and validate its associated symptoms and help the client control and lower the stress level. Because Chinese Americans tend to be "good patients"—quiet and polite, with few requests, with a tendency to suppress feelings such as anxiety, fear, depression, or pain—it is important for the nurse to recognize nonverbal cues and their cultural meanings to develop culturally appropriate nursing care plans. The nurse can never assume that a Chinese patient has no unmet need if he or she does not request anything.

Some Chinese Americans hesitate to ask questions when they do not understand; therefore, after rapport has been established, the nurse should elicit and encourage Chinese Americans to verbalize their feelings and ask questions. Because of culturally determined communication patterns, the nurse would do best to validate the patient's understanding by asking questions or having the patient do a return demonstration, instead of relying solely on the patient's verbal and nonverbal responses. In addition, the nurse should avoid using negative questions to elicit responses because negative questions are comprehended differently in the Chinese language.

In addition, because some Chinese Americans do not ordinarily touch another person during conversation, it is important for the nurse to explain the necessity of touching for therapeutic purposes. Showing respect, demonstrating empathy, and being nonjudgmental can help establish rapport with Chinese-American patients. The nurse can communicate better with Chinese Americans by understanding their cultural norms, values, and practices and unique communication styles. Therapeutic communication techniques can also be used to promote conversations to help Chinese-American patients express thoughts and feelings and to ensure mutual understanding, especially when the nurse believes that the patient is experiencing anxiety, fear, depression, or pain.

SPACE

In studying human spatial relationships, Hall (1981) divided humans into two groups: contact and noncontact. People from a contact group interact with each other by facing each other more directly, being closer, touching more, making more eye contact, and speaking more loudly than members of a noncontact group. People from a contact group may perceive people from a noncontact group as being shy, uninterested, cold, and impolite. Conversely, people from a noncontact group may view people from a contact group as being pushy, aggressive, obnoxious, and impolite (Hall, 1981). Both Chinese Americans and most middle-class mainstream Americans are categorized as noncontact individuals. However, from the Asian person's point of view, Americans face each other more, touch more, and have more visual contact than Asians do. Chinese people feel more comfortable in a side-by-side or right-angle arrangement and may feel uncomfortable when placed in a face-to-face situation. Americans prefer to sit face to face or at right angles to each other. In the Asian culture, the person of higher status has the prerogative of sitting as proximally as desired; thus the burden of correct behavior is on the person of lesser status (Samovar & Porter, 2003; Watson, 1970).

Implications for Nursing Care

Because Chinese Americans are categorized as noncontact, it is important for the nurse to remember that some Chinese Americans may be erroneously perceived as being extremely shy or withdrawn. It is equally important for the nurse to remember that some Chinese Americans may view tasks that are associated with closeness, increased eye contact, and touch as being impolite or offensive. The nurse can reduce these misunderstandings by providing explanations when performing these tasks. Because some Chinese Americans feel uncomfortable with face-to-face arrangements, the nurse may seek the client's input in terms of comfortable seating arrangements and remain alert and sensitive to the patient's comfort level of personal space.

SOCIAL ORGANIZATION

Effect of Immigration on Social Organization

Many early Chinese immigrants came to this country as contract laborers or with money that was borrowed from various Chinese-American organizations. These organizations assumed a supervisory role for these early immigrants once they arrived in the United States. The Chinese immigrants were similar to immigrants from other ethnic and cultural groups in that most of them were unfamiliar with the language and the culture of the United States. Therefore, many of the early Chinese immigrants worked as laborers in gangs. Although many of these individuals were physically smaller than those in other ethnic or cultural groups in the United States, they were hard workers. Historically, Chinese Americans helped build the United States by constructing railroads and working at other equally taxing jobs. Early Chinese immigrants worked cheaply and saved money by living frugally. These virtues made many of the early Chinese immigrants employable, but they were feared and hated as competitors by American workers (Lyman, 1974; Wong, 2006).

By 1851, there were 25,000 Chinese Americans living in California alone (Sung, 1967). By 1870, the number of Chinese immigrants in the United States had increased to 63,000. In 1880, approximately 6000 Chinese persons entered the United States. Nearly twice as many entered the United States in 1881, and nearly five times as many entered in 1882 (Sung, 1967). However, in 1882 an exclusionary immigration law reduced the inflow of Chinese immigrants to less than 1000 until the year 1890. Because of this law, the initial Chinese immigration was almost exclusively male. The immigration of Chinese men to the United States was believed to be a tentative rather than a permanent move, and during the 1880s the number of Chinese persons leaving the United States was greater than the number entering.

In addition to the Chinese Exclusion Act of 1882, other laws that severely curtailed not only immigration but also the possibility of a Chinese person's becoming a naturalized citizen were enacted in the United States. Furthermore, some of these laws were specific enough to require citizenship as a prerequisite for entering many occupations and for owning land (Sowell, 1981). From 1854 to 1874, there were laws that prevented Chinese people from testifying in court against White men (Lyman, 1974). Some historians believe that such laws in effect made it possible to declare "open season" on Chinese Americans because many of these individuals had no legal recourse when robbed or assaulted. The almost total exclusion of Chinese immigration from 1882 to 1890 had devastating long-range effects on Chinese Americans that are still evident. Because the early Chinese immigrants were almost exclusively male, there was little hope for a normal social or family life. Many of these early male immigrants had wives and children in China, whom they would not see for many years, if at all. Because of the severe restrictions on economic opportunities, it was impossible to earn enough money to book passage to China.

Over the years, the few Chinese women who had managed to immigrate to the United States were able to produce a small number of first-generation children. When these children grew up, there was a slight ease in the serious shortage of women that remained characteristic of Chinese Americans from the early immigration period until World War II. In addition, an unknown number of Chinese women were smuggled into the United States for the specific purpose of prostitution (Lyman, 1974). As recently as the 1960s, many illegal aliens from China entered the United States to pursue a better life. As a result, many Chinese residents deliberately avoided census takers.

Despite the fact that economic opportunities for early Chinese immigrants were highly restricted, many Chinatown communities took care of their own indigents. This fact may explain why even during such disasters as the San Francisco earthquake in 1906 and the Great Depression of the 1930s, many Chinese Americans did not seek or receive federal aid.

In 1943, the Chinese Exclusion Act of 1882 was repealed, and that repeal did help ease the imbalance of the male-to-female ratio and permitted a more normal family life to develop among a very family-oriented people. After the repeal of the Chinese Exclusion Act of 1882, the bulk of the new Chinese immigrants were female (Sung, 1967). The labor shortages of World War II opened many new job opportunities that were not previously available to Chinese Americans. Thus many Chinese Americans abandoned traditional Chinatown occupations to move into these new jobs (Sowell, 1981).

In 1940, only 3% of Chinese Americans in California had jobs that were considered "professional," compared with 8% of the White population. By 1950, the percentage of Chinese Americans in professional fields had doubled to 6%. Over the next decade the percentage of Chinese Americans working in professional fields tripled and for the first time passed the percentage of Whites working in professional fields. By 1970 it was reported that Chinese Americans in general had a higher income or higher occupational status than most other Americans. In 1970 at least one fourth of all employed Chinese Americans were working in scientific or professional fields. Many Chinese Americans are in the science and engineering fields (National Science Foundation, 2009). The Chinese Student Protection Act in 1992 allowed many students from the People's Republic of China to apply for permanent resident visas, which led to an increased number of Chinese Americans in the science and engineering fields.

Family

The Chinese family can be classified into five categories: old immigrant families, professional immigrant families, American-born Chinese families, new working-class immigrant families, and biracial/bicultural Chinese families (Wong, 2006). The socioeconomic, educational, or acculturation status of these families varies. The old immigrant families may own small grocery stores or restaurants, speak limited English, and hold onto traditional Chinese values. The parents of professional immigrant families mostly came to the United States as international students and have professional jobs after graduation. They may sponsor their parents for immigration to the United States and form an extended family. The American-born Chinese families may have children ranging from first generation to fifth generation. The children of these families may be well acculturated, receive college degrees, and have high occupational status and income. However, the children of the working-class immigrant families may not acculturate well. Both parents may be employed in the labor-intensive market (such as tourist shops, restaurants, and garment sweatshops) with an enclave economy. Because of their work schedule, they have little time with their children. The biracial Chinese families happen mostly among the U.S.-born population. The children of these families may identify themselves as Chinese and another race.

Chinese, like other Asian Americans, have a culture of collectivism. This culture of collectivism emphasizes loyalty to family and devotion to tradition and de-emphasizes individual feelings (Gudykunst, 2001). The Chinese are willing to submit individual interests to those of the family to maintain a strong and cohesive bond. In return, the family is expected to take care of its members, both immediate and extended. Doing so brings honor to the family; not doing so brings shame.

The Chinese family generally has a hierarchical structure. The older children have authority over the younger children, and the younger children must show deference to authority figures, usually the elderly male in the household (Chin, 2005). Boys may be more valued than girls. Husbands may have more authority over their wives. Wives may be expected to be obedient to parents and parents-in-law (Cheung et al., 2005); failure to do so causes shame for the family. The authority figure has more influence on decision making. In most cases, decisions are made on the basis of consensus rather than majority rule. The individual learns to submit to prevailing opinion rather than disagree (Gudykunst, Stewart, & Toomey, 1985). However, the values of the Chinese-American family erode in the acculturation process. Many youngsters do not show respect to the elderly. Youngsters who embrace individualism are more likely to engage in misconduct (Le & Stockdale, 2005). On the other hand, youngsters who hold traditional Chinese family values (filial piety) and do not exert early individualism have less misconduct (Juang, 2009). Elderly Chinese Americans who are dissatisfied with support from family members have a high risk of depression (Mui & Kang, 2006).

Marital Status

Because of the early Chinese Exclusion Act in the United States, there was a disproportionately large number of Chinese men compared with Chinese women. Many of the early unmarried Chinese men who came to the United States had virtually no opportunity to marry; thus in 1890 only 26.1% of the total number of Chinese-American men were married. The percentage of married Chinese-American women from 1890 to 1950 ranged from 57.4% to 69.1%. During this time there appeared to be a lower percentage of single Chinese women who immigrated, which was partially accounted for by the Chinese tradition of females marrying at a younger age. Chinese Americans divorce less frequently than their American counterparts (Sung, 1967).

Today, Chinese Americans remain family-oriented. Married couples may experience conflicts but will avoid divorce or separation, which may be viewed as a shame. According to the 2000 census, 60.1% of Chinese Americans are married, 29.7% have never married, 1.1% are separated, 4.6% are widowed, and 4.5% are divorced (Reeves & Bennet, 2004; U.S. Department of Commerce, Bureau of the Census, *American Community Survey,* 2015).

Religion

There are four primary religions in China: Buddhism, Taoism, Islam, and Christianity (Catholicism and Protestantism). Of these four primary religions, Buddhism has the largest number of professed followers while Taoism has the smallest number. Among Chinese and Chinese Americans, Christianity is regarded as a newcomer; nevertheless, its effects are pronounced. Christianity is viewed as being partially responsible for the introduction of Western culture into China as well as to Chinese Americans. Many Chinese Americans convert to Christianity after they come to the United States (Yang, Fenggang, & Tamney, 2006). The number of Chinese Roman Catholics has increased rapidly, particularly among foreign-born Chinese Americans (Central Intelligence Agency, 2015; Fisher, 1996; Sowell, 1981).

Implications for Nursing Care

It is important for the nurse to remember that Chinese Americans are a family-oriented people who normally put family commitments before personal interests. In addition, the Chinese-American family has traditionally had a hierarchical structure. By assessing the client's kinship relationship and identifying the authoritative family member, the nurse can effectively use the influential family members to achieve the therapeutic goals. Chinese Americans believe that they have a major responsibility in taking care of family members and relatives. Therefore, family members may view the hospitalization or health care needs of a family member as a personal concern. The nurse needs to understand this sense of responsibility and be sensitive to the family's needs. Opinions and ideas of the family members should be incorporated into the plan of care. Also, it is important to provide health care education to all family members, not just the client, when procedures are to be done. However, parents of the ill child may not want the siblings to know about the illness to avoid unnecessary worry. The nurse should assess the family situation to avoid disclosing information to inappropriate family members (Cheung et al., 2005). A rule of thumb with regard to caring for Chinese Americans is to involve the family to the highest possible extent. Otherwise, the family may take away the health professional's access to the patient. The notion that an individual has rights independent of his or her family is alien to many Chinese and Chinese Americans. In addition, Chinese-American women may be very uncomfortable and uneasy when examined by male health professionals. Therefore, a female nurse should be present and assist in the examination.

Chinese Americans vary widely in educational background and socioeconomic status, have varied cultural and religious values and practices, and have different levels of acculturation. For example, some Chinese Americans speak English very poorly, whereas others can communicate in English without any problem. Some have medical insurance, whereas others do not. Some use herbal medicine, whereas others do not. Language deficiency is one of the primary barriers to health care access and utilization for Chinese Americans (Smedley, Stith, & Nelson, 2003). If the client has a language barrier, a translator is needed and can usually be found in the local Chinese community. Visual displays, flip charts, or exhibits can be used to facilitate the client's understanding. Recently, more credible and reliable patient education materials in Chinese are available (e.g., National Diabetes Education Program: http://ndep.nih.gov/index.aspx, MedlinePlus' Health Information in Chinese: http://www.nlm.nih.gov/medlineplus/languages/chinesetraditional.html, and National Library of Medicine's Materials in Asian Languages—Chinese: http://asianamericanhealth.nlm.nih.gov/Alchinese.html). The nurse can refer the patient to these Web sites and use information in these Web sites to provide patient education.

TIME

The Chinese have a different perception and experience regarding time; it is not past, present, or future oriented. Some Chinese Americans perceive time as a dynamic wheel with circular movements and the present as a reflection of the eternal. This metaphoric wheel continually turns in an unforeseeable direction, and individuals are expected to adjust to the present, which surrounds the rotating wheel, and seek a harmonious relationship with their surroundings (Kim, 2015).

Hall (1981) has described the time concept of Asians as polychronic and that of Westerners as monochronic. An individual with a polychronic time orientation adheres less rigidly to time as a distinct and linear entity, focuses on the completion of the present, and often implements more than one activity simultaneously. On the other hand, an individual with a monochronic orientation to time emphasizes schedules, promptness, standardization of activities, and synchronization with clocks.

When making decisions regarding current and future events, some Chinese people may be affected by traditions and customs. Before making decisions, they may seek symbols, correlations, and intuitive understanding, as well as consider significance, consequences, future situations, and present factors. They do not make decisions according to an individual's own benefit (Gudykunst et al., 1985).

Implications for Nursing Care

Because Chinese Americans are perceived as being polychronic, it is important for the nurse to remember that some Chinese Americans may not adhere to fixed schedules. Polychronic individuals may arrive late for appointments; may insist on completing a task before moving on to a new one, even though the new task may be time sensitive and more urgent; and may implement more than one task at a time. It is important for the nurse to recognize that when some Chinese Americans make important decisions related to current events, they may appear hesitant and request time for deliberation because of the need to consider as many variables as possible, including consultation with family members.

ENVIRONMENTAL CONTROL

Many Chinese Americans, especially the first generation, may not believe that they have control over nature because they subscribe to a belief in fatalism and may view people as adjusting to the physical world, not controlling or changing the environment (McBride, Morioka-Douglas, & Yeo, 2003). In traditional Chinese philosophy, a harmonious relationship with nature is stressed (Chen, 2001). Ancient Chinese philosophers believed that *qi* (or *chi*) was the vital life energy flowing around the universe and differentiated *qi* into two forces, *yin* and *yang*. While *yin* and *yang* are opposites, they exist only by virtue of each other. *Yin* and *yang* regulate the universe, including the body and food. *Yang* represents the positive, active, or "male" force, and *yin* represents the negative, inactive, or "female" force. Accordingly, body organs are categorized into *yin* and *yang* groups. For example, the liver, heart, spleen, lungs, and kidneys are *yin,* whereas the gallbladder, stomach, large intestine, small intestine, bladder, and lymphatic system are *yang*. The *yin* forces store the strength of life, while the *yang* forces protect the body from outside invasions. Many Chinese Americans believe that an imbalance between *yin* and *yang* will result in illness, whereas a balance between the two maintains and enhances health (Chen, 2001).

Likewise, food is divided into *yin* (cold) and *yang* (hot) groups and is considered to be either the cause or the treatment of illnesses. A person with leukemia may believe that too many "cold" foods have been consumed. Diseases with excessive *yin* forces, such as cancer, postpartum psychosis, menstruation, or lactation, are treated with foods with *yang* qualities, such as beef, chicken, eggs, fried foods, spicy foods, hot foods, vinegar, and wine. Diseases or conditions with excessive *yang* forces, such as infection, fever, hypertension, sore throat, or toothache, require foods with *yin* properties, such as bean curd, honey, carrots, turnips, green vegetables, fruits, cold foods, and duck (Ludman & Newman, 1984). In addition, Chinese Americans often use tea, honey, prunes, or vegetables such as bok choy to treat constipation; they use chrysanthemum, crystal (preserved ginger), ginseng, or other herbal decoctions to treat indigestion (Hess, 1986).

Feng shui (translated literally to mean "wind [and] water"), which some Chinese Americans subscribe to, is the art of spatial arrangement of physical structures to achieve proper harmony and balance with nature (Fisher, 1996). Positive *feng shui* is believed to ward off evil spirits and promote good health and prosperity. Shapes of objects, buildings, and so on take on significance for some Chinese Americans and are thought to be correlated with good or bad luck. For example, a triangular building is considered to lead to bad luck and would not usually be used by Chinese Americans for house construction. Likewise, it is believed that doors should not open to direct traffic because this would allow evil spirits ready access into the home. Similarly, it is believed that the best location for a building is directly facing water while its rear is backed by mountains. Such an arrangement encourages prosperity while offering protection.

Some Chinese Americans hold beliefs related to colors and numbers that may take on significance to health and health care. For example, the number 4 (*sì*), because it is pronounced the same as the word for "death" in Mandarin, is considered bad luck (Pan, 2004), whereas the number 8 (*ba*), which sounds like the word for "prosperity" in Cantonese, is considered good luck. On the other hand, the color white is considered bad luck because it is a color of mourning, whereas the color red is considered good luck and is associated with happiness and celebration. Thus a person born on 8/8/88 would be considered to be extremely fortunate or lucky, whereas a person born on 4/4/44 would be considered to be extremely unlucky. It is conceivable that a Chinese American subscribing to these beliefs might have considerable difficulty going for diagnostic testing in a triangular building that was located at 444 Fourth Street, where all the personnel wear white laboratory coats (Fisher, 1996).

Illness and Wellness Behaviors

Cultural differences, language barriers, and financial status play a major role in the utilization of health services by

Chinese Americans. Jang, Lee, and Woo (1998) found that income, language ability, and citizenship status are associated with health care access and utilization in Chinese Americans. In addition, cultural norms and social stigma are major barriers associated with low utilization of mental health services (Du, Kramer, Juthani, & Kim, 2009).

Many Chinese Americans underutilize health services because of their socioeconomic status, associated high cost, and perceived cultural insensitivity of the health care system (Chen & Kazanjian, 2005). Although unemployment rates for Chinese Americans are lower than for the general U.S. population, underemployment rate among Chinese Americans is much higher; underemployment is evidenced by a shorter work week, a mismatch between education and employment, and longer working hours for the same pay. In addition, at least 14.0% of Chinese Americans live at or below the poverty level. Many elderly Chinese Americans live alone with a fixed income, and this may be a direct result of early discriminatory immigration laws that barred reunion with wives. Chinese immigrant families may have no health insurance because they may not believe in insuring health or may be unable to afford it (Fisher, 1996). In fact, factors such as marital status, length of residence in the United States, education, employment, and average household income were associated with health insurance coverage among Chinese Americans (Takeuchi, Chung, & Shen, 1998). In addition, income, language ability, and citizenship are associated with health care access and utilization among Chinese Americans (Jang, Lee, & Woo, 1998). Chinese Americans may fear medical institutions because of language barriers and unfamiliarity with the U.S. health care system. As a result, some Chinese Americans may not access or comply with medical treatments. Cultural beliefs and practices such as those regarding mental health also underscore such underutilization.

Many diagnostic tests, such as amniocentesis, glucose tolerance testing, ultrasonography, or drawing blood, are often perceived as being dangerous and unnecessary (Minkler, 1983). For instance, the invasive procedure of drawing blood on a daily basis not only is perceived as unnecessary but also is tolerated poorly by Chinese Americans because blood is believed to be part of the irreplaceable vital energy of the body and the belief in the intactness of the body (wholism) (Pan, 2004). There was a report that a department store in Beijing had to resort to a lottery to determine whose turn it was to give blood "voluntarily," even with a bonus equivalent to a 2-month salary and 15 days of vacation (Fang, 1998). In addition, many Chinese Americans have a tendency to self-medicate with over-the-counter drugs, herbal remedies, tranquilizers, and antibiotics (Zhan & Chen, 2004). In this regard, some Chinese

Americans may save part of a prescribed medicine and take it at their own discretion at a later time (Campbell & Chang, 1973).

Many Chinese Americans use Western and Chinese health providers simultaneously (Chen, 1995; Zhan & Chen, 2004), often failing to inform either. The failure to inform either Chinese or Western health providers when using both Chinese medicines and Western medicines at the same time can lead to unnecessarily increased safety risks and even tragedies (Tsai, 2007; Zhan & Chen, 2004). Because some herbal and Western medicines have similar effects, using both can create problems. For example, ginseng is a tonic stimulant and an antihypertensive medicine. A client may overmedicate by taking antihypertensive drugs and ginseng at the same time.

Typically, Chinese Americans seek opinions and treatments of minor or chronic illnesses first within the informal health care system (family members, relatives, and friends) and try to manage on their own. If unsuccessful, they tend to consult with and seek treatment from Chinese medical providers. Western physicians tend to be the last option. However, Western physicians may be the first choice if the conditions are acute or serious (Liu, 1986). The delay for treatment is especially common among Chinese-American psychiatric clients because of the sociocultural stigma associated with mental illnesses (Zhan, 2004). This practice also accounts for the observed phenomenon that admitted Chinese patients tend to be sicker and more symptomatic (Chen & Kazanjian, 2005).

The preparation and administration of Chinese medicines are unique. Chinese herbal medicines are boiled in a specified amount of water over low heat for an extended time until the desired concentration is reached. The medicines are then taken as a single dose. If the client does not feel better after the initial dose, the client may need to return to the herbalist. Because of this tradition, some Chinese Americans are unfamiliar with the Western practice of continuing to take medications such as antibiotics over the entire prescribed duration even when feeling better (Zhan & Chen, 2004). In addition, the Western practice of taking multiple drugs in tablet or capsule form at various times and over several days or weeks is inconvenient and can be confusing.

Traditionally, Chinese Americans as a group are health-conscious and believe in preventive health practices, frequently incorporating health promotion activities such as walking into their daily lives. Confucianism mandates that one should treat one's own physical well-being as an expression and duty of filial piety (Hui, 1999). For this reason, many Chinese Americans are reluctant to take medications unless absolutely necessary because they believe every medication has side effects. Some Chinese people respond to pain stoically because they fear addiction to analgesics and because of the cultural value on self-control and the belief that suffering is inherent in life (Hui, 1999).

Death and Dying Issues and Practices

Like birth, death is an important life event. However, it is a cultural taboo for Chinese Americans to talk about death and related issues for fear of bringing bad luck or even jinxing their lives (Pan, 2004; Yick & Gupta, 2002; Zheng, 1999). Euphemisms are used when death or dying has to be dealt with (Yick & Gupta, 2002). Therefore, it is unlikely that Chinese Americans will have a living will and power of attorney at hospital admission, especially for first-generation Chinese immigrants. Talk or even mention of death is to be avoided during daily conversation, especially when illness strikes (Pan, 2004). Although life is mortal, Chinese Americans believe in "natural and peaceful death" (*shou zhong zheng qin*). It is essential for the health care professional to remember that for most Chinese Americans, dying at home surrounded by family members is more desirable than dying at a health care facility (Chen, 2001). It is also important to remember that euthanasia and suicide in general are inconsistent with Chinese bioethics. In addition, according to traditional Chinese teaching, life is given by one's parents, and, moreover, it is the extension of one's family life (Zheng, 1999); therefore, one has no right to take it away. This belief may serve as a protective factor against suicide at the cultural level.

For Chinese Americans, the rituals surrounding death can be very elaborate, with the primary purpose to help the dead live a comfortable and rich afterlife. Upon death, the body is washed and clean clothes are put on. Among Chinese Americans, burial in the ground is preferred, signifying that the body returns to where it came from (nature). Food offerings and burning of fake paper money at burial time, as well as annual visitations in the spring at the Qing Ming Festival, are commonly practiced so that the dead will not be hungry and poor in the afterlife (Zheng, 1999). Many of these rituals are symbolic, with no practical reasons for the dead, but they serve the important purpose of comforting and relieving the burden of the living. Organ donation is inconsistent with the Chinese belief in wholism, which mandates that the body must remain intact, even after death (Yick & Gupta, 2002).

Folklore and Folk Practices

Maintaining the balance of *yin* and *yang* is the fundamental principle of Chinese medicine (Chen, 2001). Chinese medical practice includes acupuncture, herbal medicines, moxibustion, massage, coining, cupping, and so forth. Acupuncture involves the insertion of fine, sterile, metal needles through specific body points to treat or cure illnesses such as pain, stroke, or asthma. Herbal medicines are also categorized according to their *yin-yang* properties and their therapeutic functions and are prescribed on the basis of the *yin-yang* nature of the particular illness. Moxibustion involves heat treatment of illnesses such as mumps or convulsions. When moxibustion is used as a modality, the ignited moxa plants are placed near specific areas of the body. After moxibustion, tiny craters about 1 cm in diameter can be observed on the skin. Massage is used to stimulate the circulation, increase the flexibility of the joints, and improve the body's resistance to illnesses. Massage is a useful technique to relieve tension and stress. Coining involves applying a special oil to a symptomatic area and rubbing the area with the edge of a coin in a firm, downward motion. This treatment is used to treat cold, heatstroke, headache, and indigestion. Linear multiple bruises may be observed on the skin as a result of this process. Cupping is used to treat headaches, arthritis, and abdominal pain. A vacuum is created inside a glass jar by burning a special material. Then the inverted jar is placed immediately on the selected area and kept there over a designated duration until it is removed. Circular, ecchymotic marks 2 inches in diameter can be observed on the skin after this treatment (Andrews & Boyle, 2003; Spector, 2004).

Implications for Nursing Care

Because Chinese Americans often believe that they do not have control over nature and maintain a fatalistic outlook on life, they may be hesitant about seeking health care treatment. In addition, because some Chinese Americans subscribe to the theory of *yin* and *yang,* such individuals are more likely to engage in self-treatment. Therefore, the nurse must be able to distinguish between practices that could be harmful, neutral, or beneficial to the client's particular medical problem. For example, some Chinese Americans from Southeast Asia or rural areas in China may practice native healing processes in which they may tie a string around the wrist, burn incense, or make food offerings to the spirits. As long as these practices are not harmful and pose no safety hazards, the nurse should respect them and allow them to continue. In addition, the nurse who observes that a Chinese American client is taking herbal medicine concurrently with prescribed Western medications should inform the attending physician and caution the client about the possibility of overmedicating and the possible side effects of drug interactions. For those Chinese Americans who subscribe to the theory of *yin* and *yang* and believe that food has *yin* and *yang* qualities, the nurse should assist the clients to select the appropriate foods accordingly. Finally, the nurse should encourage the family of a Chinese-American client to bring familiar and more tasteful foods from home if (1) the client wishes and

(2) there is no contraindication. For dying Chinese-American patients, home hospice is more culturally congruent because the dying is often surrounded by family members in a familiar and intimate environment to achieve a dignified death. The nurse should allow and make adaptation to the request for death rituals if safety and health risks are nonissues or can be minimized. Being empathetic, sensitive, and supportive is the key to meeting the family needs at this critical and trying time.

BIOLOGICAL VARIATIONS

Physical variations among races have been the subject of study for physical anthropologists. People are the product of both genetic factors and environmental influences. For example, it has been hypothesized that the epicanthic fold that gives the Chinese a slant-eyed look may have evolved as a protection against blinding blizzards of snow or sand (Bleibtreu & Downs, 1971). Others have theorized that Chinese people may have a thickened corneum, creating the yellowish skin color (Molnar, 2006). Most Chinese have thick, straight hair. Chinese men tend to have less facial hair compared with Whites.

Body Size and Structure

Chinese Americans tend to be shorter compared with Whites at all ages, with long trunks and short legs, and tend to complete their growth earlier (Molnar, 2006). On the standard growth charts, the mean height and weight of Chinese American children fall in the 10th percentile, whereas the mean height and weight of mainstream American children fall in the 50th percentile (Andrews & Boyle, 2003). The children of Chinese immigrants are generally taller than native Chinese children, perhaps because of better nutrition in a large part, but their sitting and standing height ratios do not change. On the average, Asians have smaller chest volumes than Whites. The average forced expiratory volume for Chinese Americans is 2.53 L, compared with 3.22 L for White Americans; average forced vital capacity is 3.27 L for Chinese Americans, compared with 4.3 L for White Americans (Overfield, 1995).

Skin Color

The "yellow" color of the Chinese skin is believed to be caused by a smaller amount of melanin in the skin than in the skin of Black people (Race and ability, 1967). Others have theorized that Chinese people may have a thickened corneum, creating the yellowish skin color (Molnar, 2006). The majority of Chinese infants have mongolian spots (irregular areas of deep blue pigmentation observed primarily in the sacral and gluteal regions and occasionally in other areas of the body). Neonatal jaundice is seen in 50%

of Chinese infants. The bilirubin level peaks on the fifth and sixth days of life, compared with the second and third days for other races. Bilirubin levels higher than 12 mg/dL occur in 25% to 40% of Chinese infants. Breastfeeding is more acceptable and common compared with Whites. Yet breastfeeding may elevate the bilirubin level. The physician may suggest that the mother stop breastfeeding until the baby's bilirubin levels return to normal (Andrews & Boyle, 2003; Overfield, 1995).

Enzymatic and Genetic Variations

A majority of Chinese Americans have a lactase deficiency and are unable to tolerate fresh milk. Lactase splits milk sugar (lactose) into simple glucose and galactose. Lactase deficiency may cause a person who drinks fresh milk to have flatus, abdominal cramps, diarrhea, or vomiting. However, the person can often eat cheese to relieve or avoid the effects of this deficiency because bacteria do the work of lactase. This enzyme may also be induced by long-term consumption of fresh milk.

Chinese people have relatively higher incidences of thalassemia and glucose-6-phosphate dehydrogenase (G-6-PD) deficiency (Molnar, 2006). Thalassemia is a type of hemoglobin abnormality characterized by a high rate of red blood cell destruction, necessitating frequent blood transfusions. The G-6-PD deficiency is another red blood cell defect, causing fragility of the red blood cells. Persons with G-6-PD deficiency are prone to anemia when exposed to certain drugs, such as analgesics (aspirin, phenacetin), sulfonamides and sulfones, antimalarials (primaquine, quinacrine), antibacterials (nitrofurantoin, chloramphenicol, para-aminosalicylic acid), vitamin K, probenecid, and quinidine (Molnar, 2006; Overfield, 1995). Another genetic difference is that Chinese people usually experience noticeable facial flushing and vasomotor symptoms after drinking alcohol.

Research has confirmed different reactions to the same prescribed pharmacological agents among different racial and ethnic groups caused by drug polymorphisms during metabolism. After reviewing research and clinical evidence, Kudzma (1999, 2001) reported that Asian Americans, including Chinese Americans, respond differently to some psychotropic and antihypertensive agents. Specifically, Asian-American patients need lower doses of haloperidol (Haldol), diazepam (Valium), and propranolol (Inderal) to achieve the same therapeutic effect, even after body weight and stature (surface area) have been taken into consideration. Recent empirical research has also revealed that Asian Americans require lower dosages than Whites for psychotropic medications, such as lithium, antidepressants, and neuroleptics. The plasma levels of desipramine (Norpramin) are higher and peak earlier for Asian

Americans than for Whites. Asian Americans experience extrapyramidal effects at lower neuroleptic doses than Whites. The plasma levels of diazepam of the same oral dose are higher in Asian Americans than in Whites. Asian Americans are reported to tolerate the sedating effects of diphenhydramine (Benadryl) better. The causes for such differences are considered to be both genetic and environmental and need to be further investigated to ensure patient safety. Another plausible explanation is that the standard dosage is based on clinical trials in which Asian Americans and other ethnic minorities were either underrepresented or not represented at all. The National Institutes of Health, the primary health research agency in the United States, took steps to correct the problem (National Institutes of Health, 1994, 2007). One major action implemented was mandating that all federally funded studies include minority subjects and women, unless strong explanations were offered, to ensure that the research findings can be generalized to the entire population.

Susceptibility to Disease

There is a lack of national health statistics on Chinese Americans, primarily because existing census and health databases contain only aggregate data on Asian Americans and Pacific Islanders (AAPIs) (Ghosh, 2003). In other words, the data on Chinese Americans have been dispersed in the lump sum data. Although Census 2000 created "Asians" as a stand-alone category, there will be continuing methodological and statistical challenges to separate data (often impossible) to study Chinese Americans, 1 among about 50 ethnic subgroups of Asian Americans in the United States. Moreover, the compatibility of the current and future data categories with the existing ones remains an issue.

Infectious Diseases. Immigrants from Indochina and mainland China share many increased health risks, such as tuberculosis (TB), intestinal parasites, malaria, malnutrition, anemia, and hepatitis. Most Southeast Asians received vaccinations (bacillus Calmette-Guérin [BCG]) against TB in their childhood (Overfield, 1995). However, the exposure to BCG vaccinations tends to produce false-positive results on the Mantoux test. This situation makes it harder to differentiate an authentic TB case from a false-positive one (Overfield, 1995).

Cancer. The burden of cancer for Asian Americans and Pacific Islanders (AAPIs), including Chinese Americans, is "unusual," "unequal," and "unnecessary" (Chen, 2000). The burden of cancer is unusual in that cancer is and has been the leading cause of death for AAPI females since 1980, when these statistics were first collected. No other racial or

ethnic gender group has experienced this. Cancer is also the leading cause of death for AAPIs ages 25 to 64; by comparison, cancer does not become the leading cause of death for Whites until they reach the 45- to 64-year age bracket (Chen, 2000).

The burden of cancer for AAPIs is also unequal. Cancer death rates for AAPIs have increased at higher rates than for any other racial or ethnic group. Between 1980 and 1996, the number of cancer deaths for AAPI females increased 323.6%, compared with 132.6% for White females. In addition, the number of cancer deaths for AAPI males increased 276.8%, compared with 123.1% for White males (Chen, 2000). The incidence of liver cancer in Chinese, Filipino, Japanese, Korean, and Vietnamese populations is 1.7 to 11.3 times higher than rates among White Americans (Miller et al., 1996). In fact, Asian-American men have the highest age-adjusted incidence rates of liver cancer in the United States (Pan, 2004), primarily caused by chronic hepatitis infection.

Finally, the burden of cancer for AAPIs is unnecessary in many respects. Smoking is the single most important preventable cause of death. AAPI men smoke at rates higher than most other racial and ethnic groups (Lew, 2009). Studies (Chen, Unger, Cruz, & Johnson, 1999; Chen, Unger, & Johnson, 1999) demonstrated that smoking patterns of Asian-American youth, including Chinese youth, are different from those of their White peers in California. Although Asian-American youth have lower smoking rates and later age of smoking onset, high levels of acculturation are associated with higher smoking prevalence rates and earlier age of smoking onset. In a more recent study on smoking among Chinese Americans in Chicago's Chinatown, Yu, Abdulrahim, Chen, and Kim (2002) found that the smoking rate for Chinese men was 34%, significantly higher than for the U.S. general population. Low education, use of a non-Western physician or clinic for health care, and no knowledge of early cancer warning signs and symptoms were significantly associated with smoking. Lam, Ho, Hedley, Mak, and Peto (2001) noted that the proportion of male deaths between 35 and 65 years of age attributable to tobacco will jump from 13% in 1998 to about 33% over the next few decades in mainland China, which has 20% of the world's population and consumes 30% of the world's tobacco. What impact these data will have on Chinese Americans and smoking behaviors remains to be studied.

East and Southeast Asian women, including Chinese-American women, have the lowest rates of breast cancer screening (Carey Jackson et al., 2000; Juon, Choi, & Kim, 2000). General findings from those studies reveal that because of cultural, educational, institutional, and logistical barriers, East and Southeast Asian women as a group tend to underuse existing cancer screening and early detection programs, thus putting them at increased risks for cancer. The identified contributing factors include, among others, language barriers, lack of knowledge of biomedicine, unfamiliarity with the U.S. health care system, distrust in Western physicians, poverty, and lack of health insurance.

Recognizing the disproportionate cancer risks, the National Cancer Institute launched two multisite studies to increase the awareness, training, and research on cancer control in Asian Americans (Chen, 2000). The two major studies have evolved into two major networks (one headquartered at the University of California at Davis and the other one based at Temple University in Philadelphia) that intend to build and provide the infrastructure to study cancer control in Asian Americans (Chen, 2000). The outcomes of the two networks are impressive in terms of the populations impacted, number of new Asian-American researchers trained, and new knowledge discovered and disseminated (Trinh-Shevrin, Islam, & Rey, 2009).

Chinese people are also known to be at higher risk for cancers of the nasopharynx, esophagus, stomach, liver, and cervix. The intake of fermented and moldy foods and of the nitrosamines contained in corn, bran, millet, and pickled vegetables is believed to be a possible contributing factor for esophageal and liver cancers. In addition, salted fish has been linked with stomach cancer in East and Southeast Asians, including Chinese. Recent studies have revealed a downward trend for these cancers among Chinese Americans. On the other hand, cancers that were of low risk in the past (such as cancers of the colon, rectum, lung, and female breast and leukemia) are gradually increasing among Chinese Americans (King & Locke, 1988; Overfield, 1995). One significant study (Ziegler et al., 1993) confirmed that increased acculturation is linked with increased risks for breast cancer in Asian-American women. Acculturation is also increasing eating disorders in Chinese college students in the United States (Davis & Katzman, 1999), along with fat-related dietary behavior (Liou & Contento, 2001).

Mortality and Leading Causes of Death

In 2007, mortality data revealed the four leading causes of death for Chinese Americans to be identical to those for White Americans: heart disease, cerebrovascular disease, cancer, and chronic respiratory disorders (National Center for Health Statistics, *Health, United States,* 2014). However, the proportional mortalities are different. Chinese Americans have a lower mortality from heart disease (32%) than White Americans (39%) and a higher mortality from cancer (27%) than White Americans (21%). The fifth leading causes of death for Chinese Americans are pneumonia and influenza. Suicide ranks ninth as a cause of death for Chinese Americans compared with eleventh for White Americans. Chinese women have a higher suicide rate than White women (National Center for Health Statistics, *Health, United States,* 2014). The specific causes of the higher suicide rate warrant further investigation.

Psychological Characteristics

There is a deeply entrenched sociocultural stigma associated with mental illnesses among Chinese and Chinese Americans (Du et al., 2009; Zhan, 2004). For instance, mental hospitals in China recently were renamed "brain hospitals" to translate literally. Many Chinese Americans believe that psychiatric illnesses indicate an inability to exert control of one's behavior, bringing shame to the individual client as well as the family. Therefore, the family will often attempt to manage the sick family member on their own for as long as possible. As a result, hospitalized Chinese psychiatric clients tend to appear more symptomatic (Chen, 1995). Research cited by Chen (1995) identified five phases regarding family help-seeking behaviors with mentally ill family members for Chinese individuals residing in Vancouver, Canada. The five phases included (1) exclusive intrafamilial coping; (2) inclusion of certain trusted outsiders in the intrafamilial attempt at coping; (3) consultation with outside helping agencies, physicians, and finally a psychiatrist while keeping the patient at home; (4) the labeling of mental illness and a subsequent series of hospitalizations; and (5) scapegoating and rejection.

Chinese Americans, like other immigrants, experience multiple psychosocial stresses while adapting to the new culture and environment, including cultural conflicts, language difficulties, poverty, and discrimination. Many Chinese Americans experience depression and loneliness (Casado & Leung, 2001), but few seek help until associated psychosomatic symptoms are more severe (Chen, 1995). In addition, Asian Americans, including Chinese Americans, are disproportionately affected by problem gambling because historically gambling was not seen as an issue in many Asian cultures. For instance, according to the Chinese Community Health Study, about 70% of the 1808 respondents indicated that gambling was the number one social problem in the San Francisco Chinese community (Fong, 2009). Another epidemiological study conducted by the University of California at Los Angeles in 2006 revealed that about 30% of the casino patrons identified themselves as Asian American or Pacific Islander; this figure is much higher than the 12% combined share of these two groups in California (Fong, 2009).

Chinese Americans tend to seek help from other physicians rather than psychiatrists or related mental health professionals for psychosomatic complaints. Somatization is the most common form of symptom manifestation, frequently caused by mental issues such as experienced shame with no pathological etiology (Chen, 1995). Studies are needed to differentiate whether the low admission rate of Chinese Americans to psychiatric units across the country should be attributed to the "protective factors" offered by the Chinese family and social network or to the social pressure to confine the mentally ill to closely guarded family circles, or to both.

Implications for Nursing Care

It is important for the nurse to know that growth and development norms for Chinese Americans may be different from standards for White Americans. A standard growth chart for healthy Chinese children and adolescents is available (Wong & Hockenberry-Eaton, 2001). However, the nurse should not rely on the growth chart alone. A comprehensive assessment of general health status is necessary to identify malnutrition, anemia, or growth retardation (Gallo, Edwards, & Vessey, 1980).

The nurse should reassure the Chinese American mother that it is normal for her newborn to exhibit more jaundice than other American babies. Otherwise, the mother may feel guilty and believe that the jaundice is caused by something she ate. The observed mongolian spots in Chinese-American infants should not be interpreted as lesions.

When working with a Chinese-American family that has a family member with a physical or mental problem, the astute nurse can make use of general or mental health facilities easier by providing information regarding available services, encouraging the family to seek help early, and arranging for follow-up care. Rather than waiting until the symptoms are advanced, the nurse should assist the family in getting appropriate care for their family member as soon as possible.

The following case report illustrates the profound effect of the Chinese culture on a client with a medical problem and psychotic symptoms. An 83-year-old Chinese woman exhibited psychotic symptoms at home for 15 months until the family could not handle the situation any longer and admitted her to a hospital. The family members felt guilty and ashamed because they could not take care of their mother. After admission, a health history revealed that the client had had a gastrectomy about 13 years earlier, and her blood level of vitamin B_{12} was 91 mg/dL (normal is 180–900 mg/dL). She was treated with vitamin B_{12}, and the psychotic symptoms disappeared. If the family had brought the patient to the hospital earlier, perhaps they could have avoided 15 months of agony (Binder, 1983).

Patient and family teaching are important in providing care for the Chinese-American client and family. Lack of knowledge related to illnesses and treatments is a common

problem and causes fear and anxiety. The nurse can assess the family's understanding of illnesses and treatments and provide education accordingly. If the patient takes herbal medicines (not currently regulated by the government), the nurse should provide education to increase the awareness of the patient and family regarding possible synergistic and antagonistic effects of Western and herbal medicines taken together.

Because Asians are known to require lower dosages of psychotropic medications, the nurse should provide education about these medications and keep a watchful eye on their possible side effects. The nurse needs to remain alert to possible adverse effects from one-size-fits-all prescriptions. The nurse should also emphasize the importance of taking medications as prescribed and discourage the practice of taking them only when symptoms are present. In addition, the nurse should keep in mind that Chinese Americans have a relatively high incidence of G-6-PD deficiency; therefore, it is essential to urge the patient to seek help early when any side effects of medications are experienced.

The need for teaching about medications is illustrated by the following example. A Chinese-American man took captopril (Capoten) at home as prescribed for 1 week and developed severe thirst and hyponatremia, leading to irreversible neurological damage (Al-Mufti & Arieff, 1985). He was polydipsic and drank about 7 L daily. If he had been taught the side effects of captopril and encouraged to seek help when he experienced this side effect, his death could possibly have been avoided.

Although many Chinese women breastfeed their babies, recently many Chinese-American women who are more acculturated into Western culture have changed to bottle-feeding. The nurse should provide information regarding the benefits of breastfeeding and encourage mothers to breastfeed for at least 6 weeks (Minkler, 1983). If the mother has to stop breastfeeding because of jaundice, the nurse can teach the mother to express milk to continue breastfeeding when the baby is ready to be breastfed again.

Dietary education is also very important in providing care to the Chinese American patient and family (Kolonel, 1988). Some Chinese Americans believe in the theory of *yin* and *yang* and eat foods accordingly when they are sick. For example, postpartum and after surgery, some Chinese Americans will not drink or eat anything with *yin* qualities, such as cold drinks, vegetables, salad, or cold meat; they will eat only chicken, beef, or fried foods. The nurse should help the client select foods and encourage the family to bring the desired foods from home.

Chinese foods are usually cooked with soy sauce and monosodium glutamate (MSG). The nurse must remember that many preserved foods are also high in salt content.

Therefore, the nurse should advise patients who require a salt-restricted diet to reduce their sodium intake gradually by reducing the use of soy sauce, MSG, and preserved foods and to discourage high intake of fermented and moldy foods, which are thought to contribute to the high incidence of esophageal and liver cancer. Because many Chinese Americans may be unable to tolerate fresh milk because of a lactase deficiency, the nurse should encourage the use of tofu (bean curd) and other protein- and calcium-rich foods to provide the needed nutrients.

SUMMARY

Chinese Americans are one of the fastest growing ethnic groups in the United States. As numbers of Chinese immigrants continue to increase, the nurse will encounter more Chinese Americans in daily practice. Because of the complex cultural values and beliefs, diverse degrees of acculturation, and various educational levels among Chinese Americans, the nurse needs to work with individuals to assess their unique values, communication styles, social organization, time concepts, illness behaviors, and biological variations in order to provide effective and individualized care. For example, the health beliefs, attitudes, and health-seeking behaviors of the second or third generation of Chinese Americans are different in important ways from those of their parents and grandparents (Willgerodt, Miller, & McElmurry, 2002; Yick & Gupta, 2002), although some of the core values remain unchanged. As a general rule for caring for Chinese Americans, the nurse should involve the family, convey respect for the patient, encourage pride in the Chinese culture, reduce feelings of shame, and facilitate adaptation to the Western culture. One successful example is provided by Hsueh, Hu, and Clarke-Ekong (2008), who found that all of their participants—filial caregivers—had acculturated filial practices into the American mainstream while preserving their heritage to meet the challenges of parental care.

CASE STUDY

A 40-year-old Chinese American woman is admitted to a local hospital with the diagnosis of uremia. Her blood urea nitrogen (BUN) level is 168 mg/dL (normal is 8–18 mg/dL). She has a history of hypertension and was previously given a prescription for hydrochlorothiazide (HCTZ), which she stopped taking because of increasing dizziness, dry mouth, and weakness. She is single, lives alone, has no immediate family nearby, has a temporary job, and has no medical insurance. Her physician prescribes peritoneal dialysis and HCTZ. The following are noted by the nurse on assessment: blood pressure, 180/100 mm Hg; respirations, 20 per minute; pulse, 110 per minute; height, 5 feet, 1 inch; weight, 100 lb; dry skin with multiple scratching marks; no urine output; and complaints of blurred vision, itchiness, weakness, and insomnia. Her gait is slightly unsteady. She talks with a soft and low voice and speaks English slowly but not fluently. She sometimes asks questions that have already been discussed. Although she smiles frequently during conversation, she appears tense and restless. The nurse notices some hand tremors, a shaky voice, and twisting fingers. Although she has limited information about peritoneal dialysis, the woman changes the subject as the nurse explains the procedure.

CARE PLAN

Nursing Diagnosis: Pain related to pruritus

Client Outcome	Nursing Interventions
Client will verbalize discomfort to others when it exists and will relate relief with therapeutic measures.	1. Explain that pruritus will be decreased when client's BUN level is down.
	2. Keep client's room cool and avoid excessive warmth from clothes or blankets because warmth will increase itchiness.
	3. Apply cool lotions to dry and itchy areas.
	4. Apply cool, wet soaks to reduce itchiness if client desires.
	5. Ask client's doctor if any medicines can be used to decrease itchiness.
	6. Encourage client to engage in diversional activities.
	7. Advise client to keep her fingernails short to avoid injury to her skin when she scratches.

Continued

⊙ **CARE PLAN—cont'd**

Nursing Diagnosis: Anxiety related to peritoneal dialysis

Client Outcome	Nursing Interventions
Client will verbalize her understanding of peritoneal dialysis and will experience less anxiety after teaching.	1. Assess client's understanding of peritoneal dialysis. 2. Present information to client related to peritoneal dialysis by using pamphlets and drawings. 3. Explain rationale for peritoneal dialysis. 4. Describe feelings the client may have during dialysis. 5. Contact dialysis nurses to obtain some audiovisual aids to help client understand.

Nursing Diagnosis: Noncompliance related to side effects of HCTZ

Client Outcome	Nursing Interventions
Client will describe the experience that caused her to stop taking HCTZ, describe appropriate treatment of side effects, and demonstrate appropriate alternatives to the previous plan.	1. Assess any other contributing factors for stopping HCTZ (such as cost—refer to social worker to seek any financial help). 2. Identify current effects and side effects of HCTZ on client. 3. Teach effects and side effects of HCTZ. 4. Assist client in reducing discomfort (such as dizziness—change positions slowly; dry mouth—ice chips, hard candy; weakness—get plenty of sleep and ask for help for what she is limited in doing). 5. Explain client's dizziness; weakness could be improved when her BUN level is down. 6. Ask client to verbalize what she understands.

Nursing Diagnosis: Communication, impaired verbal, related to foreign-language barrier

Client Outcome	Nursing Interventions
Client will be able to communicate basic needs and relate feelings of acceptance.	1. Talk slowly and clearly to client. 2. Write down important information. 3. Use gestures, actions, pictures, and drawings to facilitate client's understanding. 4. Encourage client to teach others some Chinese words. 5. Seek a translator to discuss important matters.

Nursing Diagnoses—Definitions and Classifications 2012–2014. Copyright © 2012, 1994–2012 by NANDA International. Used by arrangement with Wiley-Blackwell Publishing, a company of John Wiley and Sons, Inc. In order to make safe and effective judgments using NANDA-I nursing diagnoses it is essential that nurses refer to the definitions and defining characteristics of the diagnoses listed in the work.

CLINICAL DECISION MAKING

1. List at least three contributing factors for hypertension among Chinese Americans.
2. Delineate at least two things that the nurse can do to facilitate the communication process between the nurse and the Chinese-American client.
3. Identify at least two factors about lack of family structure and its significance to the Chinese culture that may contribute to the difficulties of hospitalization for the Chinese-American client.
4. Describe factors regarding the time concept that may hinder health care services for a Chinese-American client.
5. Describe health and illness practices that may augment problems associated with the treatment of hypertension for Chinese-American clients.

REVIEW QUESTIONS

1. Mr. Chan, an 81-year-old Chinese-American man, has been admitted to the hospital for abdominal pain. His oldest son answers questions for him and expresses his needs. Mr. Chan's wife, who does speak English although not fluently, defers to the son when asked to participate in discussions. This is an example of which of the following?

a. The cultural value of male–female hierarchy
b. The cultural value of giving authority for decision making to the young
c. An attempt by the son to gain control of the situation
d. The need for family members to participate in caregiving decisions
2. A Chinese American who is experiencing a symptom such as diarrhea (which is felt to be "yin") is likely to try to treat it with which of the following?
a. High doses of medicines thought to be "cold"
b. No treatment at all, since diarrhea is an expected part of life
c. Foods that are "hot" or "yang"
d. Readings and Eastern medicine medications
3. People from Chinese American cultures, although valuing family, are generally more often inclined toward individualistic behavior. This statement is

_____.

a. True
b. False

REFERENCES

Al-Mufti, H. I., & Arieff, A. I. (1985). Captopril-induced hyponatremia with irreversible neurologic damage. *American Journal of Medicine, 79*, 769–770.

Andrews, M., & Boyle, J. (2003). *Transcultural concepts in nursing care* (4th ed.). Philadelphia: Lippincott Williams & Wilkins.

Barrett, S. (2006). Interviewing techniques for the Asian-American population. *Journal of Psychosocial Nursing and Mental Health Services, 44*(5), 29–34.

Binder, R. L. (1983). Cultural factors complicating the treatment of psychosis caused by B_{12} deficiency. *Hospital and Community Psychiatry, 34*(1), 67–69.

Bleibtreu, H. K., & Downs, J. F. (1971). *Human variations: readings in physical anthropology* (revised ed). Beverly Hills, CA: Glencoe.

Burkett, H. (1995). Being culturally correct. *Health Traveler, 2*(4), 4–46.

Campbell, T., & Chang, B. (1973). Health care of the Chinese in America. *Nursing Outlook, 21*(4), 245–249.

Carey Jackson, J., et al. (2000). Development of a cervical cancer control intervention program for Cambodian American women. *Journal of Community Health, 25*(5), 359–375.

Casado, B. L., & Leung, P. L. (2001). Migratory grief and depression among elderly Chinese American immigrants. In N. G. Choi (Ed.), *Social work practice with the Asian American elderly* (pp. 5–26). New York: The Haworth Social Work Practice Press.

Central Intelligence Agency (2015). *The CIA world factbook.* New York: Skyhorse Publishing.

Chen, D. (1995). Cultural and psychological influences on mental health issues for Chinese Americans. In L. L. Adler & B. R. Mukherji (Eds.), *Spirit versus scalpel: traditional healing and modern psychotherapy* (pp. 186–196). Westport, CT: Bergin & Garvey.

Chen, M. S., Jr. (2000). Launching of the Asian American Network for Cancer Awareness Research and Training (AANCART). *Asian American and Pacific Islander Journal of Health, 8*(1), 1–3.

Chen, Y. (2001). Chinese values, health and nursing. *Journal of Advanced Nursing, 36*(2), 270–273.

Chen, A. W., & Kazanjian, A. (2005). Rate of mental health service utilization by Chinese immigrants in British Columbia. *Canadian Journal of Public Health, 96*(1), 49–51.

Chen, X., Unger, J. B., Cruz, T. B., & Johnson, C. A. (1999). Smoking patterns of Asian-American youth in California and their relationship with acculturation. *Journal of Adolescent Health, 24*(5), 321–328.

Chen, X., Unger, J. B., & Johnson, C. A. (1999). Is acculturation a risk factor for early smoking initiation among Chinese American minors? A comparative perspective. *Tobacco Control, 8*, 402–410.

Chen, C. L., & Yang, D. C. V. (1986). The self-image of Chinese-American adolescents: a cross-cultural comparison. *International Journal of Social Psychiatry, 32*(4), 19–26.

Cheung, R., Nelson, W., Advincula, L., Young Cureton, V., & Canham, D. L. (2005). Understanding the culture of Chinese children and families. *The Journal of School Nursing, 21*(1), 3–9.

Chin, P. (2005). Chinese. In J. G. Lipson & S. L. Dibble (Eds.), *Culture & clinical care* (pp. 98–108). San Francisco: USCF Nursing Press.

Davis, C., & Katzman, M. A. (1999). Perfection as acculturation: psychological correlates of eating problems in Chinese male and female students living in the United States. *International Journal of Eating Disorders, 25*, 65–70.

Du, N., Kramer, E. J., Juthani, N., & Kim, L. (2009). The cultural context of mental illness in Asian Americans. In W. B. Bateman, N. Abesamis-Mendoza, & H. Ho-Asjoe (Eds.), *Praeger handbook of Asian American health: taking notice and taking action* (pp. 283–299). Santa Barbara, CA: Praeger.

Fang, B. (1998). Why it's really hard to draw blood in China. *U.S. News & World Report, 4*, 4.

Fisher, N. L. (1996). *Culture and ethnic diversity: a guide for genetic professionals.* Baltimore: Johns Hopkins University Press.

Fong, T. W. (2009). Gambling addiction. In C. Trinh-Shevrin, N. S. Islam, & M. J. Rey (Eds.), *Asian American communities and health: context, research, policy, and action* (pp. 627–631). San Francisco: Jossey-Bass.

Gallo, A. M., Edwards, J., & Vessey, J. (1980). Indochina moves to Main Street: little refugees with big needs (part 4). *RN, 43*, 45–48.

Ghosh, C. (2003). *Healthy People 2010* and Asian Americans/Pacific Islanders: defining a baseline of information. *American Journal of Public Health, 93*(12), 2093–2098.

Gudykunst, W. B. (2001). *Asian American ethnicity and communication*. Thousand Oaks, CA: Sage.

Gudykunst, W. B., Stewart, L. P., & Toomey, S. T. (1985). *Communication, culture, and organizational process*. Newbury Park, CA: Sage.

Hall, E. T. (1981). A system for the notation of proxemic behavior. *American Anthropologist*, 65, 1003–1026.

Hall, E. T. (1989). *Beyond culture*. New York: Anchor Books.

Hess, P. (1986). Chinese and Hispanic elders and OTC drugs. *Geriatric Nursing*, 7(6), 314–318.

Hsueh, K. H., Hu, J., & Clarke-Ekong, S. (2008). Acculturation in filial practices among U.S. Chinese caregivers. *Qualitative Health Research*, 18(6), 775–785.

Hui, E. (1999). A Confucian ethic of medical futility. In R. Fan (Ed.), *Confucian bioethics* (pp. 127–163). Boston: Kluwer Academic Publishers.

Jang, M., Lee, E., & Woo, K. (1998). Income, language, and citizenship status: factors affecting the health care access and utilization of Chinese Americans. *Health and Social Work*, 23(2), 136–145.

Juang, L. P. (2009). Misconduct among Chinese American adolescents: the role of acculturation, family obligation, and autonomy expectations. *Journal of Cross-Cultural Psychology*, 40(4), 649–666.

Juon, H. S., Choi, Y., & Kim, M. T. (2000). Cancer screening behaviors among Korean American women. *Cancer Detection and Prevention*, 24(6), 589–601.

Kim, Y. Y. (2015). Intercultural personhood: an integration of Eastern and Western perspectives. In L. A. Samovar, R. E. Porter, E. R. McDaniel, & C. S. Roy (Eds.), *Intercultural communication: a reader* (14th ed.). Belmont, CA: Cengage Learning.

King, H., & Locke, F. B. (1988). The national mortality survey of China: implications for cancer control and prevention. *Cancer Detection and Prevention*, 13(3–4), 157–166.

Kolonel, L. N. (1988). Variability in diet and its relation to risk in ethnic and migrant groups. *Basic Life Science*, 43, 129–135.

Kudzma, E. C. (1999). Culturally competent drug administration. *American Journal of Nursing*, 99(8), 46–51.

Kudzma, E. C. (2001). Cultural competence: cardiovascular medications. *Progress in Cardiovascular Nursing*, 16(4), 152–160, 169.

Lam, T. H., Ho, S. Y., Hedley, A. J., Mak, K. H., & Peto, R. (2001). Mortality and smoking in Hong Kong: case-control study of all adult deaths in 1998. *British Medical Journal*, 323, 1–6.

Le, T. N., & Stockdale, G. D. (2005). Individualism, collectivism, and delinquency in Asian American adolescents. *Journal of Clinical Child and Adolescent Psychology*, 34, 681–691.

Lew, R. (2009). Addressing the impact of tobacco on Asian Americans: a model for change. In W. B. Bateman, N. Abesamis-Mendoza, & H. Ho-Asjoe (Eds.), *Praeger handbook of Asian American health: taking notice and taking action* (pp. 729–749). Santa Barbara, CA: Praeger.

Li, J. (2004). The organization of Chinese shame concepts. *Cognition and Emotion*, 18(6), 767–797.

Liou, D., & Contento, I. R. (2001). Usefulness of psychosocial theory variables in explaining fat-related dietary behavior in Chinese Americans: association with degree of acculturation. *Journal of Nutrition Education*, 33(6), 322–331.

Liu, J. E. (2005). Perceptions of supportive communication in Chinese patients with cancer: experiences and expectations. *Journal of Advanced Nursing*, 52(3), 262–270.

Liu, W. T. (1986). Health services for Asian elderly. *Research on Aging*, 8(1), 156–175.

Ludman, E. K., & Newman, J. M. (1984). The health-related food practices of three Chinese groups. *Journal of Nutrition Education*, 16, 4.

Lyman, S. (1974). *Chinese Americans*. New York: Random House.

McBride, M., Morioka-Douglas, N., & Yeo, G. (2003). Aging and health: Asian and Pacific Islander American elders. In *Ethnographic reviews working paper series 3* (2nd ed.). Palo Alto, CA: Stanford Geriatric Education Center.

Miller, B. A., et al. (1996). *Racial/ethnic patterns of cancer in the United States 1988–1992*. Available at <http://seer.cancer.gov/publications/ethnicity/index.html> Retrieved July 25, 2002.

Millet, J. (2010). *Chinese etiquette and protocol*. Retrieved from <http://www.culturalsavvy.com/chinese_culture.htm>.

Minkler, D. H. (1983). The role of community-based satellite clinics in the perinatal care of non-English speaking immigrants. *Western Journal of Medicine*, 139(6), 905–909.

Molnar, S. (2006). *Human variation: races, types, and ethnic groups* (6th ed.). Upper Saddle River, NJ: Pearson Prentice Hall.

Mortenson, S. T. (2009). Interpersonal trust and social skill in seeking social support among Chinese and Americans. *Communication Research*, 36(1), 32–53.

Mui, A. C., & Kang, S. (2006). Acculturation stress and depression among Asian immigrant elders. *Social Work*, 51(3), 243–255.

National Center for Health Statistics (2013). *Health, United States, 2013. Urban and rural chartbook*. Hyattsville, MD: National Center for Health Statistics.

National Institutes of Health (1994). *NIH guidelines on the inclusion of women and minorities as subjects in clinical research*, NIH Guide. Bethesda, MD: National Institutes of Health.

National Institutes of Health. Office of Extramural Research. (2007). *Monitoring adherence to the NIH policy on the including of women and minorities as subjects in clinical research*. Available at <http://report.nih.gov/biennialreportfy0607/pdf/NIH_BR_Ch5_appendixE.pdf> Retrieved July 25, 2002.

National Science Foundation. (2009). *Women, minorities, and persons with disabilities in science and engineering (NSF 09-305)*. Arlington, VA. Available at <http://www.nsf.gov/statistics/wmpd/> Retrieved August 26, 2011.

Overfield, T. (1995). *Biological variations in health and illness*. Reading, MA: Addison-Wesley.

Pan, C. X. (2004). Older Chinese Americans. In R. N. Adler & H. K. Kamel (Eds.), *Doorway thoughts: cross-cultural health care for older adults* (pp. 95–107). Sudbury, MA: Jones and Bartlett.

Race and ability. (1967, September 29). *Time*, 46–47.

Reeves, T. J., & Bennett, C. E. (2004). *We the people: Asians in the United States.* Available at <http://www.census.gov/prod/2004pubs/censr-17.pdf> Retrieved June 2, 2006.

Samovar, L. A., & Porter, R. E. (2003). *Intercultural communication: a reader* (10th ed.). Belmont, CA: Wadsworth/Thomson Learning.

Shih-Yu, L. (2009). When East meets West: intensive care unit experiences among first-generation Chinese American parents. *Journal of Nursing Scholarship, 41*(3), 268–275.

Smedley, B. D., Stith, A. Y., & Nelson, A. R. (2003). *Unequal treatment: confronting racial and ethnic disparities in health care.* Washington, DC: National Academy Press.

Sowell, T. (1981). *Ethnic America.* New York: Basic Books.

Spector, R. E. (2004). *Cultural diversity in health and illness* (6th ed.). Upper Saddle River, NJ: Pearson Prentice Hall.

Sung, B. (1967). *Mountain of gold: a story of Chinese in America.* New York: Macmillan.

Takeuchi, D. T., Chung, R. C. Y., & Shen, H. K. (1998). Health insurance coverage among Chinese Americans in Los Angeles County. *American Journal of Public Health, 88*(3), 451–453.

Trinh-Shevrin, C., Islam, N. S., & Rey, M. J. (Eds.), (2009). *Asian American communities and health: context, research, policy, and action.* San Francisco: Jossey-Bass.

Tsai, P. (2007). Use of complementary and alternative medicine by Chinese American women: herbs and health care resources (Unpublished dissertation). University of Illinois at Chicago.

U.S. Department of Commerce, Bureau of the Census (2012). *The Asian Population, 2012.* Hyattsville, MD: U.S. Government Printing Office.

U.S. Department of Commerce, Bureau of the Census (2013). *American Community Survey.* Washington, DC: U.S. Government Printing Office.

Watson, O. M. (1970). *Proxemic behavior: a cross-cultural study.* Mouton: The Hague, the Netherlands.

Willgerodt, M. A., Miller, A. M., & McElmurry, B. J. (2002). Becoming bicultural: Chinese American women and their development. *Health Care for Women International, 23,* 467–480.

Wong, B. P. (2006). *The Chinese in Silicon Valley: globalization, social networks, and ethnic identity.* Lanham, MD: Rowman & Littlefield.

Wong, D., & Hockenberry-Eaton, M. (2001). *Wong's essentials of pediatric nursing* (6th ed.). St. Louis: Mosby.

World Almanac. (2015). Mahwah, NJ: World Almanac Books.

Yang, D. C. V., Fenggang, Y., & Tamney, J. (Eds.), (2006). *Conversion to Christianity among the Chinese: a special issue of the* Sociology of Religion: A Quarterly Review, *67*(2).

Yick, A. G., & Gupta, R. (2002). Chinese cultural dimensions of death, dying, and bereavement: focus group findings. *Journal of Cultural Diversity, 9*(2), 32–42.

Yu, E. S. H., Abdulrahim, S., Chen, E. H., & Kim, K. K. (2002). Smoking among Chinese Americans: behavior, knowledge, and beliefs. *American Journal of Public Health, 92*(6), 1007–1012.

Zhan, L. (2004). Caring for family members with Alzheimer's disease: perspectives from Chinese caregivers. *Journal of Gerontological Nursing, 30*(8), 19–29.

Zhan, L., & Chen, J. (2004). Medication practices among Chinese American older adults: a study of cultural influences. *Journal of Gerontological Nursing, 30*(4), 24–33.

Zheng, X. J. (1999). *Good death: the Chinese philosophy on death.* Kunming, Yunnan: Yunnan People's Press (in Chinese).

Ziegler, R. C., et al. (1993). Migration patterns and breast cancer risk in Asian-American women. *Journal of the National Cancer Institute, 86,* 1819–1827.

Filipino Americans

Marilyn Uvero

After reading this chapter, the nurse will be able to:

1. Describe the problems encountered regarding communication when giving culturally appropriate nursing care to Filipino-American clients.
2. Explain the Filipino-American orientation to time and space and the relevance to culturally appropriate nursing care.
3. Describe how health care beliefs, values, behaviors, medical and folk practices, and attitudes affect health-seeking behaviors of Filipino-American clients.
4. Identify how beliefs of Filipino Americans affect the internal locus of control and subsequently the environmental control variable.
5. Describe biological variations that may be found in the Filipino-American client.

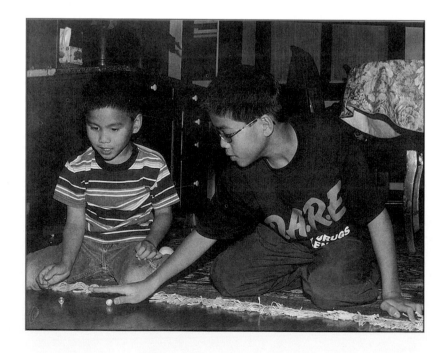

OVERVIEW OF THE PHILIPPINES

The Philippine Islands constitute an independent nation located in the Pacific Ocean approximately 450 miles off the southeastern coast of China. Taiwan is the nearest neighbor, approximately 65 miles to the north; Indonesia is 150 miles to the south.

More than 7000 islands compose the Philippine Archipelago; however, the largest islands, Luzon (40,420 square miles) and Mindanao (36,537 square miles), account for 94% of the country's total land area. All the remaining islands are less than 6000 square miles in area. Most of the Philippine Islands are hilly and mountainous, with very little level land. The principal island, Luzon, has several mountains that run from the north to the south of the island. The range, known as the *Sierra Madre*, runs parallel with the northeastern coast combined with the central Cordillera to form the spine of the Philippines. The highest mountain is Mount Apo (6690 feet) on Mindanao. The islands are of volcanic origin (*World Almanac*, 2015).

The Philippine Islands enjoy warm, even temperatures throughout the year. The average monthly temperature in the Philippines ranges from 76° to 84° F. Cooler temperatures are found at higher altitudes; however, temperatures below 60° F are a rare occurrence. Typhoons usually strike the Philippines at least once a year. The average rainfall for most of the islands is at least 60 inches of rain per year, with some areas receiving up to 125 inches of rain.

The population of the Philippines in 2014 was estimated at 107,668,231 people, with a birth rate of 24.24 live births per 1000 persons and an infant mortality rate of 17.64 per 1000, down from 35.2 per 1000 in 1997. Similarly in 2014, the life expectancy at birth was 72.48 years for the total population: 69.52 years for men and 75.59 for women (Central Intelligence Agency, 2015). The population density is 935.2 per square mile, with the Philippines ranking the thirteenth most populous country (*World Almanac*, 2015). The median age of the population is 23.5 years in the aggregate. Likewise, the median age is 23.0 for males and 24.0 years for females (Central Intelligence Agency, 2015). Of the population, 35% is under age 15 and 4.1% is 65 or older. The life expectancy is 69.52 years for males and 75.59 years for females. Most of the people in the Philippines are of Malaysian (that is, Austronesian) descent, with the two major ethnic groups being Christian Malay (91.5%) and Muslim Malay (4%) (*World Almanac*, 2015). More specifically, 28.1% are Tagalog, 13.1% are Cebuano, and 9.0% are Ilocano (Central Intelligence Agency, 2015). However, people of Chinese, American, and Spanish origin are also native to the Philippines. The population is unevenly distributed, with Luzon, Cebu, Negros, Bohol, Leyte, and Panay being the most heavily populated islands. Education on the islands is free and compulsory for ages 7 to 12, resulting in a literacy rate of 92.6% (Central Intelligence Agency, 2015; *World Almanac*, 2015).

The economy of the Philippines is based on agriculture. One of the principal crops is rice, which occupies about half the farmed land in the Philippines. Corn and coconuts are also very important crops, and other significant crops include root crops, fruits, nuts, sugarcane, abaca, tobacco, ramie, kapok, and rubber. Although agriculture is the principal industry, the yields per crop per acre are among the lowest in Asia (Central Intelligence Agency, 2015). Causes of low productivity of agriculture in the Philippines include poor farm management, inadequate use of fertilizers, poor seeds, and lack of incentive on the part of the farmers because many are tenant farmers (Central Intelligence Agency, 2015). The lack of agricultural productivity has resulted in a variety of dietary deficiencies among the people, including insufficient iron and vitamins (Cheong, Kuizon, & Tajaon, 1991; Solon et al., 1996). The living environment also results in the prevalence of *Ascaris lumbricoides* worm populations in Filipino children in both urban and rural areas (Monzon, 1991). Fishing is also a major industry in the Philippines, with the number of persons engaged in fishing being second only to those in agriculture, and it provides one of the primary dietary mainstays, second only to rice. Major industries include textiles, pharmaceuticals, chemicals, food processing, and electronics assembly. Natural resources include forests, crude oil, and metallic and nonmetallic minerals. Approximately 36% of the labor force is agricultural. The rest of the work force is divided between industry (16%) and services (48%) (*World Almanac*, 2015). The gross domestic product (2014) was $453.2 billion, which was $4700 per capita, up from $2530 in 1997 (*World Almanac*, 2015). The unemployment rate was 7.0% in 2010 (Central Intelligence Agency, 2015; *World Almanac*, 2015).

More than 40% of the country is covered by forest. Resources found in the forest include Philippine mahogany and pine. Minerals mined in the Philippines include gold, copper ore, and chromite. The country continues to lack adequate supplies of mineral fuels, although coal is mined on the islands of Cebu and Mindanao.

The ancestors of the Malay people probably migrated from Southeast Asia and were undoubtedly hunters, fishers, and unsettled cultivators (*World Almanac*, 2015). Magellan first visited the archipelago in 1521. Twenty-one years later, the islands were named in honor of King Philip II of Spain, and Spain retained possession of the islands for 350 years. Following the Spanish-American War in 1898, Spain ceded the islands to the United States for $20 million. However, the Filipinos declared their independence and initiated guerrilla warfare against the troops from the

United States until peace was established in 1902 and a civilian governor-general from the United States assumed control. Throughout the early 1900s, a Philippine legislature was established and steps set in motion to establish a commonwealth (*World Almanac,* 2015).

When Japan attacked the Philippines in 1941 and occupied the islands in World War II, enormous destruction occurred (McKay, Hill, & Buckler, 2007). During the war, the United States extended economic aid to the Philippines as compensation for the large military bases established on the island, and following the war, the Philippines were granted independence. The Republic of the Philippines was established in 1946. From 1946 to 1965, the Philippines pursued an American-style, two-party government. However, in 1965 President Ferdinand Marcos subverted the constitution and ruled as a lifetime dictator. Marcos abolished martial law in 1981 but retained most of his own power. From 1981 to 1986 there was a growing resistance to Marcos's rule. In 1986, Corazón Aquino, whose politically involved husband had been assassinated, possibly by Marcos' supporters, won a spectacular electoral victory over Marcos and forced him to flee the country (McKay et al., 2007). In the year that followed, the Aquino government survived coup attempts by Marcos's supporters. Negotiations on renewal of leases for U.S. military bases threatened to sour relations between the two countries. However, when volcanic eruptions from Mount Pinatubo severely damaged Clark Air Base in July 1991, the United States simply abandoned the base. In 1992, General Fidel Ramos, who had the support of outgoing President Corazón Aquino, won the presidency, and the opposition gained control of Congress. In 1992, the U.S. Navy officially ended a long U.S. military presence and turned over Subic Bay Naval Base to the Philippines. A cease-fire agreement was signed between the government and Muslim separatist guerrillas in 1994, but the rebels did not abide by the accord. A new treaty providing for the development of an autonomous Muslim region on Mindanao was signed in 1996. This treaty formally ended the 24-year rebellion, which had claimed more than 120,000 lives.

Joseph Estrada won the presidential election in 1998 but was impeached in 2000 for bribery. In 2000, the government repeatedly clashed with the Moro Islamic Liberation Front, which abducted several groups of hostages, including tourists, while demanding money for their release (*World Almanac,* 2015). In the spring of 2001, Vice President Gloria Macapagal-Arroyo became president (*World Almanac,* 2015). After battles with an Islamic guerrilla group and assistance from the United States, the insurgents were suppressed and President Arroyo won reelection in 2004. Tropical storms and flooding in 2004 displaced

880,000 and left 1060 dead and 560 missing (Central Intelligence Agency, 2015; *World Almanac,* 2015).

IMMIGRATION TO THE UNITED STATES

Three different waves of Filipino immigrants have come to the United States: the first-wave, or pioneer, group; the second-wave group; and the third-wave, or new immigrant, group (Palaniappan et al., 2010). Although "Philipino American" is the correct spelling because there is no F in the Philipino alphabet, "Filipino American" is the accepted English spelling (Cantos & Rivera, 1996). The feminine form, "Filipina," is acceptable usage, although it does not appear often. Today, Filipinos are the second largest Asian-American subpopulation in the United States and represent 4.4% of all foreign-born U.S. residents.

First-Wave Immigrants

The first-wave, or pioneer, group is diverse, particularly because of the different times of arrival of its members in the United States and their reasons for immigrating. The first-wave Filipino immigrants were originally drafted to work on trade ships that were traveling from China to the United States (Bartlett, 1977). From 1565 to 1815, hundreds of Filipinos escaped from the trading ships and went first to Mexico and finally to Louisiana and other regions throughout the United States. In 1907, with the passage of the gentleman's agreement that restricted Japanese immigration, Filipinos were recruited to work in Hawaii on sugar plantations (Van Horn & Schaffner, 2003). Many of the first-wave Filipino immigrants worked on California farms or in Alaskan canneries, and still others worked as cooks or domestic helpers. From 1907 to 1930, Filipinos provided inexpensive and unskilled labor, such as housekeepers, janitors, farmhands, and cooks. In 1934, the United States passed what was known as the Tydings-McDuffie Act, which held Filipino immigration to an annual quota of no more than 50 persons. This act established a Philippine commonwealth and changed the legal status of Filipinos from "nationals" to "aliens" in the United States. When Filipinos were labeled "nationals," they had the rights of citizenship except the rights to vote, own property, or marry. However, with the new alien status, the technical rights of limited citizenship were abolished (Parreno, 1977).

Second-Wave Immigrants

The second wave of immigration began after the Philippine Islands won independence from the United States in 1946, when the annual quota was raised to 100 persons. Many Filipinos who served in the U.S. Armed Forces immigrated to the United States with their families after World War II. Lott (1976) noted that during this period many of the Filipino men were physically separated from their immediate kin and denied full participation in the larger American society. Therefore, many of the second-wave group, particularly the men, relied on communal arrangements as their social group.

Third-Wave Immigrants

The new immigration group, or the third wave of immigrants, is composed of those Filipinos who have immigrated to the United States since 1965 as a result of the liberalization of the immigration quota. In 1974, Urban Associates reported that in the 10-year period from 1960 to 1970, the Filipino population residing in the United States doubled, from 343,000 to 774,652. From 1965 to 2009, the population of Filipino Americans almost doubled again, to 2,475,754 (U.S. Department of Commerce, Bureau of the Census, *American Community Survey,* 2013). In 2010, a total of 2,628,168 Filipinos called the United States home (U.S. Department of Commerce, Bureau of the Census, *American Community Survey,* 2013). Today, Filipinos represent approximately 0.7% of the total U.S. population. This number represents a 30.3% increase in the Filipino population since the 1990 census (U.S. Department of Commerce, Bureau of the Census, *American Community Survey,* 2013). Currently, Filipino Americans are the largest Asian group in California, where more than half of the Filipinos in the United States reside. By geographical location, 52.4% of Filipino Americans reside in the West, 27.0% reside in the Northeast, 8.1% in the Midwest, and 12.4% in the South (U.S. Department of Commerce, Bureau of the Census, *American Community Survey,* 2013). In 2010, Filipino Americans again constituted the third largest group of Asians in the United States, outnumbered in terms of population only by Chinese Americans (U.S. Department of Commerce, Bureau of the Census, *The Asian Population,* 2013).

Of the number of Filipino Americans residing in the United States before 1975, 21.7% were foreign born. Of the number residing in this country between 1975 and 1979, 11.1% were foreign born; between 1980 and 1990, 31.6% were foreign born; and between 2000 and the present, of the number of adults 18 years of age and older, 73.5% were foreign-born (U.S. Department of Commerce, Bureau of the Census, *American Community Survey,* 2013). The median age of Filipino-American people residing in the United States is 38.3 years, compared with 33.0 years for other Asian Americans and 36.7 years for the general U.S. population. In addition, only 6% of all Asian Americans are 65 years of age or older, compared with 13% of the general U.S. population (U.S. Department of Commerce, Bureau of the Census, *American Community Survey,* 2013).

Among Filipino Americans, third-wave immigrants appear to be better educated than members of the first and second waves; however, some of these people still experienced discrimination. In general, Filipino Americans are noted for high educational standards, with parents placing high value on education (Champeau, 1998). In 2010, 91.8% of Filipino-American males and 93.5% of Filipino-American females 25 years of age or older held a high school diploma, and 43.4% of males and 50.7% of females held a bachelor's degree (U.S. Department of Commerce, Bureau of the Census, *American Community Survey,* 2013).

The median family earnings in 2009 for Filipino Americans ranges from slightly lower to higher than that for the general U.S. population, depending on whether it is the median per capita individual income or median family income being analyzed. The median family income for Filipino Americans was $75,000 compared with $49,800 for the general U.S. population (U.S. Department of Commerce, Bureau of the Census, *American Community Survey,* 2013). The median per capita income for Filipino-American males was $44,416 compared with $45,320 for the U.S. population. For Filipino-American women it was $42,258 as compared with $35,549 for women in the general U.S. population (U.S. Department of Commerce, Bureau of the Census, *American Community Survey,* 2013). It is interesting to note that the opposite is true for the poverty rate among Filipino Americans, which is slightly lower than that among their White counterparts (7% vs. 8%) (U.S. Department of Commerce, Bureau of the Census, *American Community Survey,* 2013).

Takaki (1998) reports in *Strangers from a Different Shore* that for many Filipinos, although they toil in America, they still experience an "unfinished dream," with a society unwilling to embrace its own diversity. On the other hand, many Filipino Americans are being recognized across the United States for excellence, including achievement in academia (Champeau, 1999), in theater (De Leon, 1999), in higher education (De La Cruz, 1999), in medicine (Bofill, 1999), in politics (Pilapil, 1999), and in poetry (Gloria, 1999). Unlike other Asian Americans, recent Filipino immigrants tend not to stand out as much; they speak English fluently, are highly educated, have economic well-being, and are Christians (Agbayani-Siewert, 2004). The label of "invisible minority" also extends to the relative lack of political power and representation of, by, and for Filipino Americans. Congress has established 2 months in celebration of Filipino-American culture in the United States. "Asian Pacific American Heritage Month" is celebrated in May. Upon Filipinos' becoming the largest Asian-American group, "Filipino American History Month" was established for October, commemorating the first landing of Filipinos on October 18, 1587, in Morro Bay, California.

Since the 1960s, there has been an exodus of nurses from the Philippines to the United States (Cantore, 2001). Nurses educated in the Philippines have been attracted to the United States because of job opportunities, which have become especially attractive in the present nursing shortage. Although most nurses coming from the Philippines have a bachelor of science in nursing and graduate education offers additional opportunities to advance, many continue to work in staff positions, often with a second job, in order to maintain a steady financial support for family members still living in the Philippines (Cantore, 2001). Filipino nurses have had to make many adjustments to deliver nursing care in the United States, including learning new technologies and the American work ethic and value system. Cantore (2001) noted that cultural attributes common in the Philippines that may be retained by the Filipino nurse working in the United States can be negative but may also be positive—for example, showing deference to elders and persons who outrank them, thus appearing timid, and working very hard and not complaining. Although Filipino-American nurses have their own unique ethnic identity and rich cultural heritage, Filipino nurses are often lumped into the general category of "Asian nurses." Because they are not given a separate ethnic grouping in statistics collected by the Health Resources and Services Administration's National Sample Survey of Registered Nurses, Cantore (2001) noted that Filipino nurses are, for the most part, a "hidden minority." Berg, Rodriguez, Kading, and De Guzman (2004) noted that a significant number of nurses who have emigrated from the Philippines and have enjoyed full-time employment and high job satisfaction are now at retirement age, which will negatively affect the registered nurse population in the United States.

COMMUNICATION

Dialect and Language

One of the greatest difficulties that faced Filipinos during the 1960s was the task of forming a more integrated national community. This task was made even more difficult because of sociological diversity and because more than 93 dialects were spoken in the Philippines at the time (Voegelin & Voegelin, 1997). The boundary between "language" and "dialect" in the Philippines is blurred. The most common languages are Tagalog, Ilocano, Cebuano, Bicolano, Pampangan, and Chabacano (Cantos & Rivera, 1996). Although 86% of Filipinos speak one of eight major languages as their mother tongue, the fact remains that many diverse languages and dialects are spoken across the country. Filipinos have long recognized the problem with dialect and language, and in 1930 the government

adopted a policy to develop a national language based on Tagalog. In addition to Tagalog, English and Spanish were also adopted as official languages of the Philippines. However, adoption of a national language by the people was slow, and by 1960 only 44.5% of Filipinos spoke Tagalog, 39.5% spoke English, and 2% spoke Spanish (Corpuz, 1965). At that time more than 93 Filipino languages were being spoken in the country (Melendy, 1977). Today most Filipinos speak the national language, Tagalog (also known as Filipino) but use English for business, legal transactions, and school instruction beyond the third grade. A hybrid of Tagalog and English (Taglish) is used commonly in business and social interactions as well as in health interactions (Pacquiao, 2003).

In the United States, Filipino immigrants have been willing to undergo discomfort and cultural alienation with the hope that their children might improve the economic status of the people through education. However, one tragic flaw in this scheme is the language barrier encountered by the children in the public school systems in the United States (Melendy, 1977). Even today, the public schools are not able to cope with the problem of bilingual education in languages other than Spanish and English. In 2009, 61% of Filipino Americans spoke a language other than English at home. Even today, Filipino Americans continue to have the fourth largest percentage (22.1%) of linguistically isolated people among all of the Asian groups residing in the United States. Some 20% of Filipino Americans live in linguistically isolated households (Asian and Pacific Islander American Health Forum (APIAHF), 2005; U.S. Department of Commerce, Bureau of the Census, *American Community Survey,* 2013). A great number of Filipinos speak Tagalog, Visayan, Taglish, and Ilokano at home. Tagalog is the sixth most spoken language in the United States (APIAHF, 2005; U.S. Department of Commerce, Bureau of the Census, *American Community Survey,* 2013).

Style

Shimamoto (1977) noted that the elderly Filipino man is generally concrete in thinking and pragmatic in problem solving. Shimamoto also noted that when a Filipino man acknowledges emotions in a verbal manner, this may be interpreted as a sign of unmanliness or weakness. Cultural values emphasize group harmony and smooth interpersonal relationships; decision making may be shared among family members according to a patient's needs. A clinician could develop a family decision tree or algorithm. Decisions may be referred to family members living outside the United States, or birth order may be used to designate decisions (McBride & Parreno, 2006; Tompar-Tiu & Sustento-Sereniches, 1995).

Tone

Filipino Americans tend to use tone of voice to emote or to romanticize the language (Cantos & Rivera, 1996). An individual may get loud in the presence of a group of family members or may become agitated or emotional when nervous or frightened. Typically, however, Filipinos are soft spoken and will say nothing rather than disagree.

Context

Filipino Americans are "laid-back, easy-going, serene people" (Santiago, 2001). Thus, there is a tendency for Filipinos to avoid direct expression of disagreement. This protects them from losing face or respect. For example, it was noted in a Midwestern psychiatric hospital that a Filipino male physician, who was a family practitioner, would not disagree directly with a female psychiatrist. In areas of disagreement, the physician would communicate information to the psychiatrist by telling the nursing staff to relay the message (Davidhizar, personal communication, 1997). In this scenario, the difficulties were encountered because Filipinos are a polite people who do not like to disagree, particularly with people in authority, and because some Filipino men experience discomfort with women as authority figures.

Some Filipino people experience difficulties when discussing topics that are considered personal, including sex, tuberculosis, and socioeconomic status. The issues of sex and sex education are considered so sensitive that Filipino parents generally do not openly or deliberately discuss them with their children (Guthrie & Jacobs, 1966). Because tuberculosis is a dreaded and feared disease among Filipino people—in the Philippines the morbidity and mortality for this disease remains high as a result of unsanitary living conditions—some Filipino people may also avoid discussion about tuberculosis (Hooper, 1958; Orque, 1983; Wooley, 1972).

Some Filipinos have an expressed need for modesty, privacy, and confidentiality. Therefore, it is often difficult for the nurse to begin interventions immediately without a period of small talk on topics considered safe conversation, such as the weather, the condition of family members, or sports events. It is also important for the nurse to remember that Filipino-American clients may be hesitant to express feelings and emotions in a group setting. Filipinos are sensitive to the concept of shame or saving face. It may be only out of strong respect for the health care professional that they will disclose personal information that is needed to plan adequately for health care (Orque, 1983).

Kinesics

Nonverbal language is important for Filipino persons. For example, direct eye contact in the Filipino culture between an older man and a younger woman may be indicative of either seduction or anger. Little eye contact is likely to be used with superiors and authority figures. Another situation in which a nurse may encounter nonverbal communication on the part of a Filipino-American client is in a group setting. Because some Filipino people fear losing face in public situations, the Filipino-American client may be hesitant to express personal feelings in a group setting and may resort to remaining silent. It is important to assess the meaning of silence and to determine if it means approval or not.

Filipinos tend to be very polite and therefore tend to behave agreeably even to the extent of personal inconvenience (Cantos & Rivera, 1996). The term for this form of agreement is *pakikisama,* which means "getting along with others at all costs." Some Filipino nurses have difficulty giving commands to staff but rather prefer to request politely that they do an assignment. Another trait for which some Filipinos are known is *amor propio,* which is actually a Spanish term adapted to the Filipino language, meaning "self-esteem." Therefore, when a Filipino's *amor propio* is wounded, there is a tendency to preserve personal dignity by silence or aloofness to demonstrate self-pride. Filipinos will tend to agree even when they mistrust the physician or nurse because they do not want to risk hurting the other person's feelings. Therefore, for some Filipinos a hesitant "yes" could be indicative of a positive "no" because they wish to avoid a direct, blunt "no." In the Filipino language, there are hierarchical terms for "yes" and "no." The term used depends on whether one is speaking to a person of lower, equal, or superior status. When uncertain as to the status of the person with whom they are conversing, some Filipino Americans will use a silent nod to avoid giving possible offense. Also, a Filipino-American client will commonly address a physician or nurse as "Doctor" or "Mrs."; however, if the name is unknown, this same individual may only nod (DeGracia, 1979).

Touching is not uncommon, although handshakes are not commonly practiced by Filipino Americans. Elderly people are shown respect by being kissed on the hand, forehead, or cheeks (Wilson & Billones, 1994).

Implications for Nursing Care

It is important for the nurse to remember that a large majority of first-wave Filipino immigrants came to this country with little or no education and may have extreme difficulty comprehending English, especially English spoken in medical jargon (Vance & Davidhizar, 1999). Therefore, the nurse should use interpretive aids such as pictures and interpreters. It is also important for the nurse to remember that if an interpreter is used, the interpreter should speak the same language and same dialect as the client. The nurse should be aware that many Filipinos use a nonverbal response, such as a smile or a raised eyebrow, as an acknowledgment to what has been said, rather than giving a verbal response (Espíritu, 1995). It is important for the nurse to watch the Filipino client when speaking rather than waiting for a verbal response.

Regardless of immigration-wave status, the Filipino-American client may view the nurse as an authority figure and therefore relate to the nurse with formality and modesty. Because gender and age differences also have particular significance in the Filipino culture, it would be wise for the nurse to consider both gender and age when communicating with the client. For example, because an elderly person is highly revered in the Filipino culture, it would be inappropriate as well as disrespectful for the nurse to address the elderly Filipino-American client by a first name. The nurse might try using such Tagalog designations as *opo* or *oho,* which are used to show respect and honor to the person being addressed (Orque, 1983). The Tagalog designation *po* should be inserted when an elderly Filipino American is addressed because it conveys respect and is similar to designations in the English language such as "madam" or "sir" (Guthrie & Jacobs, 1966).

It is important for the nurse to remember that direct eye contact for Filipinos has various connotations. A young female nurse who is assigned to an elderly Filipino-American male client may encounter difficulties when communicating with this client, who may remain aloof and reserved and avoid eye contact altogether (Bush & Babich, 1986).

Because Filipino men, regardless of age, have great difficulty acknowledging emotions verbally, Shimamoto (1977) recommended that the nurse assume an authority-figure role during the development of the nurse–client relationship. Because of the Filipino trait of deference toward authority figures, Filipino-American men, regardless of age, are likely to respect the nurse's position and to listen and adhere to the nurse's suggestions because of the position. It is important for the nurse to appear knowledgeable and competent when communicating with a Filipino-American client and to avoid talking down to the client. It is also important for the nurse to remember that because some Filipino men experience discomfort with women as authority figures, difficulties may arise even in nurse–physician relationships. For example, when a female nurse is communicating with a Filipino-American male doctor, the nurse should use sensitivity in offering suggestions or criticism. Some Filipino Americans encounter difficulties in group settings, particularly in situations where both men and women are present. Therefore, one-on-one encounters may be best, so that the client or professional

with whom the nurse is talking feels free to express true feelings and emotions (Orque, 1983).

Because Filipino-American clients tend to be modest, it is important to offer female clients not only a gown but also a robe. Male clients should be offered pants as well as a gown (Cantos & Rivera, 1996).

Because Filipinos have arrived in the United States in different groups and have adapted to the culture at different levels, it is important for the nurse to recognize that different acculturation patterns will be present and to assess for level of acculturation. Dela Cruz, Padilla, and Agustin (2000) have adapted for use with Filipino Americans an acculturation tool first developed for Hispanics. The 12-item instrument, Acculturation Scale for Filipino Americans (ASASFA), has been validated with experts and psychometric testing and is available in two versions, English and Tagalog. Use of the ASASFA can provide a measure for comparing the acculturation patterns of individuals and lead to broader cross-cultural knowledge and understanding.

SPACE

Some Filipino Americans tend to collapse their space inward and limit the amount of personal space available. This is caused in part by the Filipinos' strong feeling for family (Cantore, 2001). On immigration to the United States, the personal space of Filipino Americans also collapsed inward because some of the people lived in urban ghettos, or "little Manilas," that were vastly overpopulated (Burma, 1974).

Implications for Nursing Care

Filipino Americans are perceived as a family-oriented cultural group. Therefore, it is not uncommon for a Filipino client to have the entire family, which includes nuclear and extended family members, hovering at the bedside. Even an adult who is unmarried with no relatives in the vicinity is likely to have a number of Filipino-American visitors because they are sensitive to the loneliness that illness can provoke. The astute nurse will use family members to the advantage of the client. Rather than viewing their presence as an overcrowding of space in the hospital for both the health care professionals and the client, the nurse should capitalize on these customs and traditions by involving family members in educational training programs that will assist the client in returning to an optimal level of functioning. In addition, it is important to solicit family and client input to develop shared goals.

It is also important for the nurse to remember that Filipino Americans are familiar with a limited personal space because it is always shared with other family members.

Therefore, the space provided in a hospital setting may appear to be overextended, thus leading the client to collapse personal space inward even more. While hospitalized, Filipino Americans may be reluctant to venture out of the personal space that is allocated or leave their room for any reason (DeGracia, 1979).

In response to illness, Filipino elders may often follow a pathway to seeking professional health care that begins with self-monitoring of symptoms to ascertain possible cause, severity, threat to one's functional capacity, and economic and emotional inconvenience to the family. The extended trajectory from symptom onset to medical treatment may also be affected by sociopolitical and historical experiences of injustice, by racial or gender discrimination felt by the elders themselves, or by attitudes passed on to them by family members who had difficult experiences (Yeo et al., 1998).

SOCIAL ORGANIZATION

Family

Most of the first-wave immigrants who came to the United States were not allowed to immigrate with their wives. This immigration pattern was responsible for a disproportionate ratio of males to females. The male-to-female ratio in 1930 for Filipinos residing in the United States was 14 to 1, compared with 1.1 to 1 for the rest of the population (Melendy, 1977). Lott (1976) noted that because Filipino men were separated from their families, they tended to rely on communal arrangements with other Filipino immigrants, who often came from the same island in the Philippines. Most of the first-wave immigrants had little or no education and, because of discriminatory practices that existed throughout the United States, did not receive more education or a better job.

After World War II, when the immigration policies became more relaxed in the United States, more Filipino women began to enter the country, and a more normal family pattern followed. Despite the fact that more women were able to immigrate during the second and third waves, it has been noted that the age of Filipino-American husbands continues to exceed that of their wives. Because of their disproportionate ages, many young Filipino-American women have been widowed early, thus leading to the establishment of the Filipino matriarchal system. In 1974, 69% of Filipino-American families were matriarchal with young children, and at least 23% of all Filipino-American families were extended (Urban Associates, 1974). Wagner (1973) noted that the ratio of extended families to nuclear families was at least twice that of the rest of the U.S. population. Today, however, married couples represent approximately 59.7% of all Filipino-American households, whereas female-headed households (matriarchal) make up only 13.6% of Filipino-American families (U.S. Department of Commerce, Bureau of the Census, *American Community Survey*, 2013).

In 1974, 38% of all Filipino-American families had five or more members (Urban Associates, 1974). In 2009, this number decreased somewhat, and the average Filipino-American family now has 4.0 persons, compared with the national average of 3.2 (U.S. Department of Commerce, Bureau of the Census, *American Community Survey*, 2013). Pollard (1995) studied ethnic groups in relation to twinning rates in California. Numbers of Filipino twins were similar to those of Chinese and Japanese but higher than those of Koreans, Thai, and Vietnamese, an indication that twinning rates are modified by both migration and interethnic mixing.

Although the number of matrifocal families has decreased, the matriarchal system remains an integral part of Filipino cultural values. The matriarchal system may be the reason that the family has taken on paramount importance for Filipino Americans. This is evidenced even during times of illness. When a member of a Filipino-American family becomes ill, family members often keep a bedside vigil and participate in client care. Burr and Mutchler (1993) noted that Filipino-born women who are less acculturated are more likely than women from some other ethnic groups to move in with others who are more acculturated.

Family Systems and the Relationship to Culture

The Filipino culture is a blend of various heritages, although there are some basic traits that most Filipino people manifest. Individualization is a key to understanding the Filipino culture and an individual of Filipino descent. As a result of the Chinese influence on family solidarity, Filipinos on the Philippine Islands tend to socialize with people from the same region. This same clannishness is evident in the United States among the many organizations in the Filipino communities. Persons in the younger generations may have values that are in direct opposition to the traditional values held by older persons. In the Philippine Islands, many youths resemble their Western counterparts, particularly in areas of social values, dress, and music (DeGracia, 1979). Although these same similarities exist among adolescents in the mainstream United States and Filipino-American adolescents, many Filipino-American youths still observe such traditional values as respect for elders, love of family, and preservation of self-esteem.

In the Filipino culture there is a strong feeling for family, which is a result of the Chinese influence. Today, these strong feelings for family continue and may be manifested by old-fashioned patterns imposed by the family patriarch or the equally authoritarian matriarch. Lee (2004) noted Filipino-American men traditionally have positions of power, dominance, and privilege and are concerned about challenges to their family leadership and to "losing face." The Filipino child is taught always to give deference to an elder and never to question the decision of an elder. In return for such obedience, the Filipino child receives solicitous protection from elders. In the absence of both parents, the eldest Filipino child becomes the ruling authority and must be obeyed. Kataoka-Yahiro, Ceria, and Yoder (2004) conducted qualitative research with Filipino-American grandparents and noted that, rather than viewing grandparenting as a burden, it is viewed as an integral part of the role and part of the "give and take" of family responsibility.

Parent–adolescent communication about sex has been found to be sometimes limited, resulting in limited sex education (Chung et al., 2005). On the other hand, a study by Lantican and Corona (1992) noted that social support for pregnant women was extensive and included a network size of 5.74. For the most part, in the Filipinos studied, immediate family members provided the support. Filipinos also reported that sisters were most likely to be the first to receive information about the pregnancy, with husbands listed third. This was in contrast to the Mexican Americans studied, who reported discussing the pregnancy first with their husbands.

Religion

Filipinos are predominantly Roman Catholic, which has been attributed to the influence of the Spanish missionaries in the Philippines as early as 1520. In 2006, chief religions included Roman Catholic, 81%, and Muslim, 5% (*World Almanac*, 2015). The remaining religious groups include Evangelical, Aglipayan, Iglesia ni Kristo, other Christian, and other (Central Intelligence Agency, 2015).

Birth Rituals

Filipino mothers are encouraged to eat well and to get plenty of sleep at night. In the last few months of pregnancy, they are discouraged from staying in a dependent position, such as sitting or sleeping during the day, for fear of water retention. Sexual intercourse during the last 2 months of pregnancy is considered taboo. Eating prunes, sweet foods, or squid is also considered taboo for a pregnant woman (Kittler & Sucher, 2001; White, Linhart, & Medley, 1996). It is believed that such foods will, respectively, make the baby wrinkled, lead to a large baby and difficult delivery, and tangle the baby's cord inside the mother. If a physician is not available, a midwife may be called on to assist in the delivery. Fathers are usually not present but rather are with male friends for support while their wives deliver. A pregnant Filipino woman may walk around the room to promote dilatation. Most Filipino women will moan or grunt during labor. Others may become loud and almost hysterical (Weber, 1996). A symbolic unlocking ritual may be performed during labor. Traditionally, showers and bathing were prohibited for 10 days postpartum (Spector, 2004a).

Traditionally, it was an expectation of all Filipino mothers to breastfeed. This tradition is changing. In a study by Adair and Popkin (1996), Filipino women who ceased breastfeeding early or did not breastfeed were studied. It was found that a low birth weight reduced the likelihood of breastfeeding. This is significant because there are already high risks related to low birth weight and proved benefits of breastfeeding. Thus, these researchers noted that nurses should give special emphasis to promoting breastfeeding. For example, a working mother may have the baby fed formula while she is at work or may have breast milk left for the baby.

Traditionally, male circumcision was not done at birth. Today it is more common for a male baby to be circumcised before discharge from the hospital.

Rituals Related to Death and Dying

If a client has a diagnosis of terminal disease, the client should not be told before the family is consulted. The family will usually want to disclose the prognosis to the client and in some cases will prefer to protect the client from knowing the diagnosis (Geissler, 1998). The health care professional should generally continue to communicate with the head of the family outside of the patient's presence regarding the health status. If the family is Catholic, the family will usually want the Catholic priest to give the sacrament of the sick, in which the client is anointed with holy oil. A Filipino client given a terminal diagnosis will probably prefer to die at home with dignity. A decision to not resuscitate is usually very difficult and will be determined by the entire family. Death is given very high regard by Filipino Americans. Death is a spiritual event, and the client and family may ask for religious medallions, rosary beads, and other objects of spiritual significance to be near the client. The family may pray at the bedside of a dying family member. If a client dies in a hospital room, the family members will usually want to say goodbye before having the body taken out of the room and may want to wash the body. Muslims will want Muslim rites performed (Geissler, 1998). McAdam, Stotts, Padilla, and Puntillo (2005) investigated attitudes of critically ill Filipino-American patients and their families toward advance directives and noted that the overall attitude was positive. However, the completion rate and knowledge of advance directives were low, which suggested to the researchers that participants may have wished to avoid disagreement. Terminally ill Filipino-American patients usually prefer to die at home, and Becker (2002) noted that in a study of 78 Filipino Americans contemplating death, many expressed a desire to die in their homelands. Becker noted that the preoccupation of respondents with where to die apparently reflects the desire to reconcile issues of continuity, as well as cultural meanings surrounding memory, ritual, and family.

Funerals in the Philippines can be simple or elaborate, with a band accompaniment, several priests officiating, and a large group of mourners. Rituals generally include a wake, novenas, and establishing a burial site acceptable to all the members of the family. A first-year anniversary of the death event in which the family unites draws closure to the mourning. For the traditional Filipino, women related to the deceased may wear white during this period, and weddings and other celebrations may be delayed as a show of respect. Most Filipinos believe in life after death and believe that caring for the spiritual needs of the dying is necessary for peaceful transition of the soul to the afterlife (Pacquiao, 2003).

Implications for Nursing Care

In the Philippine Islands, the family unit is the basic unit of social organization. Several generations of Filipinos are linked by descent and marriage. For some Filipinos, family relationships are so important that many of the kinfolk live under the same roof or as close to each other as possible. Furthermore, membership in a family union is perceived by some Filipinos as being more important than membership in a trade union (Caringer, 1977). Therefore, many nursing implications are based on family structure and organization. Because Filipino-American clients are very family oriented, the nurse must remember that these clients may always have their families hovering about them. The sick Filipino child may feel lost without the mother constantly at the bedside, and when grandparents are ill, the entire family may keep vigil at the bedside out of respect for the elderly. Whenever it is possible, the nurse should arrange for family members to stay at the client's bedside during a hospital stay. Family members will want to bring food from home that is soothing for the body, such as rice soup, and in most cases clients will expect that this will occur.

It is important for the nurse to remember that the family structure of first- and second-wave immigrants may be significantly different from that of third-wave immigrants in that more matriarchal family structures may be found in the earlier generations. Thus the varying family structures may present the need for unique and varying approaches to health care needs. Another implication for

nursing care is associated with the fact that some first- and second-wave immigrants have a limited education compared with third-wave immigrants, who were better educated when they came to the United States. When a Filipino-American client from the first- or second-wave group is hospitalized, it is important that the nurse not only involve families but also recognize the need to modify educational approaches to the family's and client's level of understanding.

It is helpful for the nurse to be aware that throughout the United States and particularly in California, Filipino-American centers are being established (Manila, 1999). Filipino student organizations are available at some universities (Suzara, 1999), and the location of Filipino organizations, including the Web site of the Philippine Nurses Association (http://pna-ph.org), are available online.

TIME

Filipino Americans appear to have both a past- and a present-time orientation. According to Kluckhohn and Strodtbeck (1973), human nature has a postulated range of variations, including evil, good and evil, and good. People react to these value orientations by virtue of a time frame of reference. For example, past-time–oriented people view human nature as being basically evil, and so control and discipline of the self are continuously required if any real good is to be achieved. On the other hand, present-time–oriented people view human nature as a mixture of good and evil, and so although control and effort are needed, lapses in control and effort can be understood and need not always be severely condemned. For some Filipino Americans there is a prevailing attitude that one should unquestionably accept what life and death bring because, regardless of human effort, supernatural forces are mitigating and control the world. It is this attitude that influences some Filipino-Americans' time orientation.

Because Filipino Americans are both past- and present-time oriented, they distinguish between social and business time. They tend not to become too aggravated when social functions do not start on time, and so they operate on "Filipino time." This trait results in part from their past-time orientation, which values human relationships and human nature over current events. However, Filipino Americans do equate success in business in Western society with a prompt observation of business time, which is perceived as being both present- and future-time oriented (Orque, 1983). Nevertheless, for some Filipino Americans there is a prevailing attitude that time and providence will solve all (Corpuz, 1965).

Implications for Nursing Care

Because Filipino Americans are both past- and present-time oriented, it is important for the nurse to remember that often a Filipino-American client may ignore health-related issues, preferring to leave these things in the hands of God (*bahala na*). Some Filipino Americans may use the term *talaga*, which means "destined" or "inevitable." When some Filipino Americans are ill, past-time orientation becomes obvious because of a tendency to attribute conditions to the will of God and to cope with illness by praying and hoping that whatever God's will is, it is best for the individual.

Because of their past-time orientation, there is a tendency among some Filipino Americans toward noncompliance regarding medical regimens. In addition, these same individuals may not adhere to appointments or scheduled deadlines for health-related matters. Filipino immigrants are considered at risk for hypertension, coronary heart disease, and diabetes at midlife and at old age, along with other metabolic conditions.

ENVIRONMENTAL CONTROL

As indicated, Filipino Americans are perceived as being both past- and present-time oriented and have a tendency to believe that events, particularly illnesses, are related to supernatural forces. As a result of this belief, some Filipino Americans have a value orientation that is perceived as fatalistic. Thus some Filipino Americans have an external locus of control that is evidenced by a belief in supernatural forces and by the treatment methods of illness.

Physical and mental health and illness are viewed holistically as an equilibrium model. Explanatory models may include mystical, personalistic, or naturalistic causes. The basic logic of health and illness consists of prevention and curing; it is a system oriented to moderation. Parallel to this holistic belief system is the understanding of modern medicine, with its own basic logic and principles, that treats certain types of diseases. Filipino elders use a dual system of health care: avoiding inappropriate behavior that leads to imbalance and restoring balance (Pacquiao, 2003).

Folk Medicine

Filipinos and Filipino Americans support at least two, often competing, medical systems. A Filipino individual who becomes ill might consult both a folk healer and a Western-trained physician. Filipino Americans are like other ethnic groups in that they continue to practice folk medicine simply because it works (McKenzie & Chrisman, 1977). In some situations, folk remedies may be the only treatments available for Filipino Americans, whereas in other situations some Filipino Americans will combine folk remedies with the therapy prescribed by Western health professionals. It is important for the nurse to remember that folk beliefs are an important part of some Filipino Americans' lives and therefore may significantly influence health practices. In a study of ethnic reactions to chronic illness in African-Americans, Latinos, and Filipino Americans, Becker, Beyene, Newson, and Rodgers (1998) noted that while the illness patterns were similar, responses to and management of the illnesses varied among the groups and was related to self-care practices and knowledge about the illness.

Folk medicine has enjoyed a long history; in fact, folk medicine is believed to be older than contemporary scientific medicine. Some anthropologists believe that folk beliefs have persisted through the generations because they are so closely interwoven with other aspects of culture. Moreover, the therapeutic value of many of the health practices has been verified scientifically (McKenzie & Chrisman, 1977). The Filipino folk medicine system is based primarily on the Malaysian culture but may also be based on the Bisayan culture. The Filipino culture has been influenced by Indian, Chinese, Arabian, Spanish, Mexican, and American belief systems. It is believed that many of the elements of the health practices found in the Philippines may actually have been borrowed from these cultures.

In the Filipino culture, certain illnesses may be assigned to natural causes, such as overeating, poor diet, or excessive drinking. These illnesses would normally be treated with home remedies, including herbal preparations, decoctions, massage, sleep, and exercise.

Illnesses are believed to be caused by supernatural agents. Some Filipino people associate disease with the total life situation, with the result that disease can have both natural and supernatural causes. Some Filipinos believe that there are invisible spirits that replicate the life of the individual and possess supernatural powers that are generally denied to most humans (Hart, 1966; McNall, 1989).

Individuals who subscribe to supernatural causes of disease may feel protected from harmful supernatural influences by such things as talismans, amulets, prayer, and seeking advice from a folk healer. Sickness and death are believed by some Filipinos to be the result of actions of angry ancestral spirits or witches, evil eyes, or the lethal bite or power of a supernatural animal. In such cases, if the client does not recover or if the illness worsens, the client will generally seek the advice of various folk medicine specialists. The client may also seek the advice of a conventional medical practitioner if resources are available. In the Philippine Islands, it is not uncommon for a physician to incorporate certain aspects of the folk medicine belief system, such as the theory of hot and cold, when implementing the treatment plan (Hart, Rajadhon, & Coughlin, 1965).

Filipino culture has a variety of folk medicine healers, including shamans and curers. A shaman is a priest or priestess who practices folk remedies. A curer diagnoses illness by palpating the pulse. Many Filipino curers believe that the pulse is the best place to detect an illness because the pulse is an outlet, or a substation, of the heart. They believe that, if the pulse lies, the heart lies (Lieban, 1967). An ill person's pulse may be either "hot" or "cold," depending on the type of illness. Some Filipinos believe that a healthy person has a balance regarding hot and cold air elements in the body; however, if the body becomes too hot or subsequently too cold, the circulation of the blood will be increased or decreased and the person will experience a loss of appetite and fatigue that will ultimately lower the body's natural defenses against the illness. It is believed by some Filipinos that both metaphysical and real hot and cold temperatures will cause an illness if absorbed by the body in excessive amounts.

Many Filipino individuals also believe in the theory of the four humors. The body humors include phlegm or mucus, air or vapors, bile, and blood. Filipinos who subscribe to this theory accept one overriding theme that involves health in relationship to air or wind (*mal aire*). For these Filipinos, there are two ways in which one can become ill. One way is related to air and includes exposure to a normal draft or breeze that results in an illness such as a cold. The other way is by absorbing excessive amounts of hot or cold air, which ultimately will cause an imbalance of these principles in the body. A Filipino mother may wrap the navel of her baby with a cloth to prevent air from entering the body through the navel cord. Some Filipinos use coconut oil to soak or rub the skin in order to prevent wind from entering the pores. Some Filipinos believe that air circulates in the veins and, if hot air is absorbed through the pores, the blood will carry it to the brain, resulting in mental illness (Hart, 1981). Another *mal aire* illness includes the means by which the spirits penetrate the body by magically propelling thorns, pebbles, bones, and other foreign objects into the body.

Illness and Wellness Behaviors

Three concepts underlie Filipino health beliefs and practices: flushing, heating, and protection. Flushing is believed to keep the body free from debris, heating is believed to maintain a balanced internal temperature, and protection is believed to guard the body from outside influences. Flushing is based on the premise that the body is a container that can collect impurities. Heating involves the belief that hot and cold qualities must be in balance in the body. Protection involves safeguarding the natural boundaries of the body from supernatural as well as natural forces. Among Filipinos who subscribe to the theory of

flushing, there is a complex system of beliefs based on the theory that flushing is a complex system of stimulating perspiration, vomiting, flatulence, or menstrual bleeding for the sole purpose of removing evil forces from the body. A common home remedy used to promote flushing is vinegar. Vinegar may be used to flush the body to cure an ailment such as a fever or a chest cold. In such cases the vinegar is mixed with water, salt, or hot pepper. Drinking this mixture will stimulate perspiration and subsequently remove all the evil or bad things from the body. It must be remembered that such practices are not all that unorthodox when compared with the Western medical system (McKenzie & Chrisman, 1977).

Because Filipinos are deeply religious and a God-fearing people, they believe that many diseases and illnesses are the will of God. When a Filipino client is given a poor prognosis, the client may continue to hope for a cure, despite the severity of the problem. This attitude may help to explain why some Filipino clients are uncomplaining and frequently suffer in silence.

Implications for Nursing Care

It is important for the nurse to remember that Filipino folk-related health practices may be beneficial, neutral, or harmful. Folk practices that are beneficial or neutral should be incorporated into the plan of care. However, the nurse should develop educational training programs that will help the client and family identify and eliminate folk practices that are harmful.

Some Filipino Americans have an external locus of control that is based on the belief that illness is caused by external forces, which may be either natural or supernatural. Therefore, it is important for the nurse to remember that the client's noncompliance with medical regimens may be based on a fatalism-oriented system. It is important for the nurse to ascertain whether the client's noncompliance is based on fatalistic beliefs or a lack of understanding.

The nurse should be aware that many Filipino Americans relate health to food. For example, eating healthful food such as vegetables, meat, chicken, and fruits is related to maintaining health. Eating pigeon soup is related to protecting health or preventing illness. Eating chicken soup is related to restoring health. In addition, some Filipino Americans believe actions taken relate to health. For example, praying relates to maintaining health. Soaking one's feet in salted water after working in the fields and avoiding too much sun or rain protect health and prevent illness. Herbal medicines and special home remedies, such as pounding ginger with coconut oil and massaging painful joints, are cures that will restore health. Another home remedy is toasting uncooked rice until brown, adding water, and drinking the resulting mix for stomachache.

Wounds may be treated by boiling guava leaves and drinking the fluid (Spector, 2004b).

BIOLOGICAL VARIATIONS

Body Size and Structure

In the United States, prematurity is defined as a birth weight of less than 2500 g (5 lb, 8 oz). When controls for income, maternal age, parity, and smoking were done, Filipino Americans tended to have a lower mean birth weight than their White counterparts (Morton, 1977). Morton suggested that the birth-weight requirement for maturity should be lowered for some ethnic groups, including Filipino Americans, and recommended that prematurity be redefined as less than 2200 g (4 lb, 14 oz) for Filipino Americans and Blacks.

Filipinos are short and tend to have very small frames. Some Filipinos have short limbs in comparison with the trunk size. At 3 years of age, the mean standing height is 85.7 cm (33.7 inches) for Filipino boys and 84.8 cm (33.4 inches) for Filipino girls. Thus Filipino children are considerably shorter than White children, for whom the mean standing height is 95 cm (37.4 inches) for boys and 93.9 cm (37 inches) for girls (Meredith, 1978). However, the average height and weight of Filipinos are quite similar to those of Thais and Vietnamese persons. Filipinos tend to lag behind Japanese persons in both height and weight. The height of Japanese boys and girls from birth to 1 year of age exceeds the height of Filipinos (Matawaran & Gervasio, 1971). It is believed, however, that Filipinos overcome this difference by 21 years of age and that their growth increments are quite similar to those of Japanese persons.

In a classic 1958 study, José and Salcedo observed that Filipino-American women tended to be leaner and slimmer than their White counterparts. Anchacosa-Angala and Márquez-Sumabat (1964) noted that body weight for Filipino Americans increased significantly when an increase in skinfold thickness occurred. Based on data, they concluded that skinfold thickness could be used as an index of leanness and fatness for Filipino Americans.

Kusumoto, Suzuki, Kumakura, and Ashizawa (1996) compared foot morphology between Filipino and Japanese women and found that Filipino women showed pronounced deformity of the great toe laterally, "like a hallux valgus," without any complaints (p. 373). A pathological deformity of the hallux valgus appears to be related to the Filipino genetic structure.

Skin Color

Mongolian spots are commonly found at birth on Filipino infants. Normal pigmentation among Filipinos ranges from brown to peach brown, and it is extremely difficult to detect conditions such as cyanosis in darker-pigmented skin. In addition, some darker-skinned Filipinos may also have heavy deposits of subconjunctival fat, which contains high levels of carotene in sufficient quantities to mimic conditions similar to jaundice. If the nurse is to distinguish between carotenemia and jaundice, it is necessary for the nurse to inspect the posterior portions of the hard palate of the client in an extremely good light or in bright daylight (Roach, 1977).

Other Visible Physical Characteristics

Filipinos are classified as members of the Mongoloid race because of very common racial characteristics, including brown skin color, almond-shaped inner-eye folds, and extremely sparse body hair, particularly in men, on whom chest hair is often absent. Hair on the head is typically coarse and also either straight or wavy (Garn, 1971). In addition, male pattern baldness appears to be a rarity among Filipino Americans (Garn, 1971).

Chung and Kau (1985) noted that the tendency for cleft lip or cleft palate was higher for Japanese, Chinese, and Filipinos than for Whites and Hawaiians. These researchers also noted that the high-risk groups had smaller dimensions than Whites and Hawaiians in regard to cranial-base measurement, facial height, palatal length, and mandibular length, which might be contributing factors to the higher incidence of cleft lip and cleft palate.

Enzymatic and Genetic Variations

Motulsky, Stransky, and Fraser (1964) found a high prevalence of glucose-6-phosphate dehydrogenase (G-6-PD) deficiency among Filipinos. Since that time, this finding has been supported by a meta-analysis performed by Nakoma, Poole, Vannappagari, Hall, and Beutler (2009). It would appear that G-6-PD deficiency affects Filipinos as severely and as quantitatively as it affects persons in the Mediterranean group. In addition, alpha-thalassemia, a form of which is known as *hemoglobin H disease*, is prevalent in Filipinos, Chinese, Thais, and Greeks (Knapp, Metterville, Kemper, & Perrin, 2010).

Susceptibility to Disease

Cardiovascular Disease.   Gerber (1980) noted that White mortalities for coronary artery disease are higher than those for either Japanese Americans or Filipino Americans. Gerber's study also suggested that mortalities for coronary artery disease are higher in urban areas than in rural areas and that differences in mortality noted among races are probably not attributable to genetic factors but rather to environmental ones. This conclusion was based on the fact that when Japanese Americans or Filipino Americans moved from rural to urban areas, their mortality for coronary artery disease rose, which was believed to be directly related to changes in lifestyle, diet, and work patterns. Ryan et al. (2000) investigated 527 Filipino-American patients and 3176 Caucasian patients from a center treating coronary artery disease in California. The researchers concluded that Filipino Americans have a higher prevalence of hypertension and diabetes and a lower prevalence of smoking and obesity than Caucasians. Ethnicity was an independent predictor of higher mortality after catheterization intervention and increased need for late reintervention. These data suggested that Filipino-American patients need to be followed closely after percutaneous intervention or cardiac surgery procedures. Brown, James, and Nordloh (1998) evaluated Filipino-American and Caucasian female health care workers, relating ethnicity to blood pressure variation. They concluded that cultural background and emotional state influence the extent of blood pressure variation in daily life.

Among Filipino Americans, heart disease is the leading cause of death, cancer is the second leading cause of death, and stroke is the third leading cause of death (National Center for Health Statistics, *Health, United States*, 2014). In addition, relatively higher rates of hypertension have been reported, with a prevalence rate of 79% as compared with 61% for their White counterparts (National Center for Health Statistics, *Health, United States,* 2014; Ryan et al., 2000).

Hypertension. In a classic study, Stavig, Igra, and Leonard (1988) found that the prevalence of controlled and uncontrolled hypertension in the United States is lower for persons of Asian descent, except for Filipinos. In fact, the California Department of Health Services hypertension study found that Filipino Americans have one of the highest prevalences of hypertension, second only to that of Blacks (Requiro, 1981). The analysis of the data from the study by Stavig et al. (1988) indicated that Asians and Pacific Islanders with hypertension are less likely to be aware of the condition, to seek treatment or take medication for the condition, or to control the condition through diet. In addition, these ethnic groups recorded lower frequencies of hospital stays for the condition, fewer days of bed disability, and fewer days of not feeling well as a result of hypertension than all other ethnic groups. The study concluded that because of their high levels of poverty and lack of education and the relationship of these factors to health-seeking behavior for hypertension, additional study is needed to improve health care for Filipino Americans.

Klatsky and Armstrong (1991) reported a study in which 4211 Filipino men and women were compared with Japanese, Chinese, and other Asians for incidence of hypertension. This study noted that the Filipino men and

women had the highest rate of hypertension of any of the groups.

In another classic study, Young, Lichton, Hamilton, Dorrough, and Alford (1987) noted a high positive relationship between sodium intake and the prevalence of hypertensive disease. This study examined the relationship between ethnicity and blood pressure in young adults of six ethnic groups residing in Hawaii. The findings suggested that body weights and heights of Whites and Hawaiians tended to exceed those of Chinese, Filipinos, Japanese, and Koreans. The study noted that both systolic and diastolic pressures were significantly higher in men than in women across all races. The study also found no significant differences between sexes or across races regarding urinary excretion of sodium and potassium.

Stavig, Igra, Leonard, McCullough, and Oreglia (1986) conducted a study to determine the death rates in California for hypertension-related diseases for the periods 1969 to 1971 and 1979 to 1981. The data indicated that during both periods, age-standardized rates for composite hypertension-related mortality were highest for Blacks, followed by Whites, and lowest for Asians and Pacific Islanders. Filipinos, who were noted to have high prevalence rates of hypertension, tended to have a lower rate of hypertension-related mortality. Findings from this study suggest that the possible reasons for the decline in hypertension-related mortality may include population awareness, level of treatment, control of hypertension, knowledge of cardiovascular risk factors, improved medical technology, and modification of behavior. A study by Klatsky and Armstrong (1991) also found that Filipino men and women had the highest prevalence of hypertension when Chinese, Japanese, other Asians, and Filipinos were studied.

Diabetes Mellitus. There is an increased incidence of diabetes mellitus among Filipino Americans (Araneta & Barrett-Connor, 2005; National Center for Health Statistics, *Health, United States*, 2014). Sloan (1963) concluded that diabetes mellitus occurs three times more often among Filipino Americans than it does among White Americans. Cuasay, Lee, Orlander, Steffen-Batey, and Hanis (2001) studied 831 Filipino Americans and noted an overall prevalence for type 2 diabetes of 16.1%, supporting earlier studies that Filipinos are at higher risk than the U.S. non-Hispanic White population.

Cancer. Among Filipino Americans, it is interesting to note that they have the highest incidence rate for prostate and thyroid cancers compared with all other Asians. In addition, mortality rates for breast cancer, prostate cancer, and thyroid cancer are the highest among all Asian Americans (Kwong, Chen, Snipes, Bal, & Wright, 2005). Filipinos also have the second poorest 5-year survival rates for cancers such as colon and rectal compared with all other ethnic groups in the United States (Cooper, Yuan, & Rimm, 1997).

In a classic study, Kolonel (1985) compared the cancer incidence rates for Filipinos in Hawaii. Filipino women in Hawaii had the highest incidence of thyroid cancer among all ethnic groups in Hawaii. In addition, the data indicated a lack of increase in female breast cancer rates among Filipinos in Hawaii and a lower than expected increase in colon cancer rates. In contrast to this study, Goodman, Yoshizawa, and Kolonel (1988) noted that the incidence rates for thyroid cancer remained relatively stable from 1960 to 1984. However, this study also concluded that when Filipinos in Hawaii were compared with other ethnic groups in Hawaii, Filipinos were found to have the highest reported incidence rates for thyroid cancer. The conclusion of this study was that environmental influences may be responsible for the unusually high rate of thyroid cancer among Filipinos in Hawaii.

Young, Ries, and Pollach (1984) found that the rates of gallbladder and urinary bladder cancer for women exceeded those for men among the Filipino population. The primary site of cancer associated with the highest survival rate for both Filipino men and women was found to be the thyroid gland. The 5-year relative survival rate for cancer of the thyroid gland was 91%, whereas the survival rate for other primary sites of cancer, including the esophagus and the pancreas, was found to be uniformly low. Rosenblatt, Weiss, and Schwartz (1996) compared the incidence of primary liver cancer among ethnic groups and found Filipino males born in the United States to be 6.5 per 100,000 compared with Whites at 3.4 per 100,000, and Filipino women at 0 per 100,000 compared with 1.1 for Whites. The incidence of liver cancer was lower for Filipinos born in the United States than for those born in the Philippines.

Gallbladder Disease. Yamase and McNamara (1977) in a classic study examined the hospital admission rates for gallbladder disease in Chinese, Japanese, Koreans, Filipinos, Hawaiians, Portuguese, Puerto Ricans, and Whites. This study found that although differences in admission rates among races were statistically significant, they were not clinically significant.

Amyotrophic Lateral Sclerosis. Studies have indicated that the prevalence for amyotrophic lateral sclerosis (ALS) among Filipino Hawaiians exceeds that found among Whites and Japanese Hawaiians (Matsumoto, Worth, Kurland, & Okazaki, 1972; Pobutsky, Hirokawa, & Reyes-Salvail, 2003). However, the findings from other studies suggest that the excess in regard to ALS found among

Filipinos in Hawaii is more or less a function of population and age distribution, rather than a true racial or ethnic difference (Kurtzke, 1982).

Palatal Mucosal Changes. The habit of reverse smoking is practiced in various parts of the world, including the Philippines (Ortiz, Pierce, & Wilson, 1996). A study of reverse smokers compared with conventional smokers in Cabanatuan City in the Philippines found that 96.7% of reverse smokers exhibited palatal mucosal changes, including leukoplakia, mucosal thickening, fissuring, pigmentation, nodularity, erythema, and ulceration, compared with only 26.7% of conventional smokers (Mercado-Ortiz, Wilson, & Jiang, 1996). This study provides a basis for classification of the palatal mucosal changes among reverse smokers and has implications for nurses in terms of health care teaching with Filipino women.

Patterns of smoking differ from one cultural group to the next, with the Filipino rate at 24%, higher than the 19% rate of non-Hispanic whites, the 20% rate of Hispanics, and the 14% rate of Chinese Americans and lower than that of American Indians/Alaska Natives (29%) and Pacific Islanders (32%). In a study by Chen and Unger (1999), 20,482 subjects between 12 and 17 years of age were randomly sampled in California. The investigators concluded that Filipino Americans showed the highest risk of smoking initiation, Japanese and Korean were in between, and Chinese Americans were at the lowest risk.

AIDS. Research by Woo, Rutherford, Payne, Barnhart, and Lemp (1988) in San Francisco indicated that the number of acquired immunodeficiency syndrome (AIDS) cases had disproportionately increased among Asians and Pacific Islanders (177%), compared with increases among Blacks, Whites, Hispanics, Native Americans, and Alaska Natives (54%). The incidence of AIDS among Filipinos was reported to be 92 per 100,000. Longitudinal studies were done with children born to human immunodeficiency virus–1 antibody–positive Filipino women (Manaloto et al., 1996). Maxwell, Bastani, and Warda (2000) interviewed 211 Filipino American adolescents and young adults in Los Angeles to assess AIDS-related knowledge and behaviors. More than half reported condom use at last intercourse. Statistically significant correlates with condom use were higher self-efficacy and the practice of carrying condoms.

Hepatitis B. Chronic carrier rates of hepatitis B virus infection and tuberculosis range from 5% to 15% in Chinese, Koreans, Filipinos, and Southeast Asians, compared with the 0.2% rate found in the total U.S. population (Franks et al., 1989).

Glaucoma. Aghaian, Choe, Lin, and Stamper (2004) investigated central corneal thickness of various ethnic groups. Chinese, Hispanics, and Filipinos were all found to have similar central corneal thickness; in comparison, central corneal thickness in African Americans was thinner. Other parameters also differed among these ethnic groups.

Nutritional Preferences

Some Filipino Americans reflect their culture through their preparation and consumption of specific foods. Because some Filipino Americans subscribe to a theory of hot and cold, foods with these properties are incorporated into their dietary regimen. For example, it is customary to include both "hot" and "cold" foods in cooking, such as mixing beans, which are considered hot foods, with green vegetables, which are considered cold foods, regardless of how they are prepared. In addition, Filipino Americans who practice imitative magic may incorporate the concept of magic into the preparation and consumption of foods. For example, a pregnant Filipino woman may believe that eating dark foods such as prunes will produce a dark-complected baby (Affonso, 1978; Pimentel, 1968).

For some Filipino Americans, religious or family customs also dictate the foods that are prepared and consumed. For example, Filipino Catholics may abstain from eating meat during Lent, particularly on Ash Wednesday and Good Friday. Zaide (1961) concluded that Filipino beliefs and customs are so entrenched in the culture that some Filipinos may even refrain from eating meat during the burial of a relative.

The traditional foods for Filipinos include rice, fish, and vegetables. For Filipino Americans, typical dishes include *adobo, pancit,* and *lupia. Adobo* is a method of preparation that includes cooking certain meats, such as pork, chicken, or beef, that have been marinated in vinegar, garlic, and other typical Filipino condiments. The meat is simmered slowly until it becomes tender and brown (Day, 1974). *Pancit* is pasta made of rice or wheat noodles that is cooked with chicken, ham, shrimp, or pork in a soy- and garlic-flavored sauce. *Lupia* is similar to the Chinese egg roll and is either deep-fried or prepared fresh with selected vegetables (Day, 1974). Although Filipino Americans have changed their diets to reflect customs traditionally found in the United States, they also tend to retain ethnic food habits (Lewis & Glasby, 1975). Althaus (1999) notes that dietary patterns are related to degree of acculturation; in particular, the immigrants in the "first wave" tend to eat a more traditional diet, while "second and third wavers" are much different, eating primarily American fare with "just a sprinkling" of Filipino foods.

Psychological Characteristics

Flaskerud (1984) conducted a classic study to determine whether there was a difference in perspective placed on problematic behaviors exhibited by six minority groups: African-Americans, Native Americans, Chinese Americans, Mexican Americans, Filipino Americans, and Appalachians. The findings of the study indicated that there are differences in perceptions of problematic behavior and its management between mental health professionals and minority groups. Flaskerud also concluded that although these differences are related to different levels of education and expertise, they are also likely to be related to cultural influences on conceptual explanations of problematic behavior and appropriate management. Cultural groups that were considered dominant viewed problematic behavior as mental illness and recommended psychiatric treatment, whereas cultural groups that were considered ethnic minority groups (including Filipino Americans, Chinese Americans, Mexican Americans, African-Americans, Native Americans, and Appalachians) viewed the behavior from a broader perspective that encompassed spiritual, moral, social, economic, vocational, recreational, personal, physical, and psychological assessments. Bjorck, Cuthbertson, Thurman, and Lee (2001) examined appraisal, coping, and distress among Korean American, Filipino American, and White American Protestants. Filipino Americans reported more problem-solving strategies than White Americans, and both Asian American groups reported using more strategies of accepting responsibility, religious coping, distancing, and escape avoidance than the White Americans.

Psychological defenses vary by culture and thus result in a different configuration of depression (Rosenbaum, 1989). Marsella (1997), who studied depression in various cultural settings, reported that depression occurred infrequently in Filipinos.

A culture-bound syndrome, *amok,* was first reported among persons from Malaysia. A similar behavior pattern has been found in the Philippines, Polynesia, Laos, New Guinea, and Puerto Rico and among the Navajo (Bonder, Martin, & Miracle, 2002). This is classified as a dissociative episode, characterized by a period of brooding, followed by an outburst of violent, aggressive, or homicidal behavior directed at people and objects (American Psychiatric Association, 2000). Instances of *amok* may occur during a brief psychotic episode or at the onset of an exacerbation of a chronic psychotic process.

Alcohol and Drug Use. A classic study by Danko et al. (1988) found that although Filipinos and Hawaiians who drink have substantial alcohol usage, a large proportion of Filipino Americans are abstainers. Lubben, Chi, and Kitano (1988) found that approximately 50% of the women in a population sample of 298 Filipinos were abstainers, whereas approximately 80% of the men in the sample were drinkers, an indication that heavy drinking is almost exclusively a male activity among Filipinos. The study concluded that the only significant variable found among Filipino men and women in regard to drinking was regular participation in religious services.

Gee, Delva, and Takeuchi (2007) conducted a secondary analysis to determine associations between self-reported unfair treatment and prescription medication use, illicit drug use, and alcohol dependence. The American Community Epidemiological Survey, a cross-sectional investigation involving 2217 Filipino Americans interviewed between 1998 and 1999, was used to gather information for this sample population. Findings from this study indicated that among these Filipino respondents, self-reports of unfair treatment were associated with prescription drug use, illicit drug use, and alcohol dependence even after control was performed for age, gender, location of residence, employment status, educational level, ethnic identity level, nativity, language spoken, marital status, and several health conditions. Further findings from this study also suggested that unfair treatment among some Filipino Americans may contribute to illness and subsequent use of prescription medications.

Implications for Nursing Care

Because Filipino Americans tend to have darker-pigmented skin than White Americans, the nurse must be able to distinguish between the norm and carotenemia, jaundice, or cyanosis. When the nurse is inspecting the skin of a Filipino American, it is important to inspect the buccal mucosa for petechiae. When looking for evidence of carotenemia, the nurse can substantiate this finding if a yellow tint is absent in the palate when the sclerae are yellow (Roach, 1977). If the nurse is unable to determine the presence of carotenemia, the client's stool may be observed to determine if it is light or clay-colored, and the urine may be examined to determine if it is a dark golden color.

Because some Filipino Americans have a prevalence for enzymatic conditions, such as G-6-PD deficiency, lactose intolerance, or thalassemia, it is important for the nurse to encourage the client to eat meals that are high in protein and to replace whole milk with high-calcium substitutes such as buttermilk, yogurt, and sharp cheese or to add lactic aids to foods or other dairy products.

Filipino Americans are essentially very gentle and mild and have passive temperaments. It is believed that the reason for the passive temperament is the desire of Filipinos to maintain a harmonious balance between people and nature. These people generally are neither assertive nor aggressive and may often appear guarded or reticent. The nurse may often misunderstand this need for passivity and misconstrue and mislabel this behavior as an inferiority complex. Very often Filipino Americans are erroneously labeled as passive-aggressive and as having a personality disorder with anger as the underlying cause. When angry, Filipino Americans do have a temperament that is passive-aggressive, and this anger often produces anxiety, which is usually handled through covert and passive means. Behavioral manifestations of passive-aggressive behavior are evidenced through procrastination, stubbornness, intense craving for acceptance, and varying demands for attention (DeGracia, 1979).

The nurse should be cognizant that some Filipino foods are high in purine, such as *dinuguan* (from *dugu,* "blood"), which is a food prepared from the small intestines, liver, heart, kidney, and blood of pork. Because *dinuguan* is extremely high in purine, a client who is following a purine-restricted diet should be instructed to modify the diet with leaner meats than pork organs. Because Filipinos, particularly men, have been reported to be hypertensive, the nurse should instruct these clients to modify traditional high-sodium Filipino diets. Foods that are considered high in sodium include traditional Filipino condiments such as soy sauce. For the client following a diet moderately restricted in sodium, the nurse may suggest brands of soy sauce that have a lower or reduced sodium content. The client who is following a diet totally restricted in sodium can be taught to prepare certain dishes, such as *adobo,* by marinating the meat overnight in a mixture of lemon juice, onions, garlic, sugar, and crushed peppercorns (Orque, 1983).

The nurse should also be aware that intercultural differences in expression of depression may be the result of differences in social structure and worldview. The concept of *self* is culture specific and must be considered in transcultural care of depressed people (Rosenbaum, 1989).

SUMMARY

The literature dealing with Filipino Americans has sometimes been confusing because Filipinos have been lumped together in the literature with Asians, Spanish-speaking people, and "other" categories (Orque, 1983); therefore, the nurse must carefully apply data from the literature to Filipino-American clients who receive care. In addition, the nurse should be careful to notice the dates on research studies of Filipino Americans because many studies in the literature are old and may not reflect current needs. It is important for the nurse to assess the Filipino American client carefully and to keep in mind what is known about the client's cultural background so that culturally appropriate care can be provided.

CASE STUDY

Mr. Rom Recio, a 46-year-old Filipino American, is admitted to the hospital with a diagnosis of hypertension. Mr. Recio has lived in an urban area in Los Angeles since coming from the Philippines 2 years earlier. This is Mr. Recio's third admission to the hospital because his hypertension is uncontrolled. Mr. Recio has repeatedly refused to comply and take the Aldomet (methyldopa) the physician prescribed for him during the initial diagnostic hospitalization. The nurse notes on examination that Mr. Recio's blood pressure is 140/104 mm Hg, his pulse is 88, his respirations are 16, and his temperature is 98.6° F.

Although Mr. Recio speaks English, occasionally he has difficulty understanding what is being communicated in English terminology. Mr. Recio has a wife and three children, ages 10, 12, and 15. Mr. Recio's wife speaks very little English; however, all the children are proficient in English. When Mr. Recio is examined by the nurse, he states that he believes the problem with his blood has occurred because of disfavor with God.

CARE PLAN

Nursing Diagnosis: Ineffective health maintenance, related to ineffective coping

Client Outcomes	Nursing Interventions
1. Client and family will verbalize desire to learn more about the condition and preventive techniques to reduce symptoms. 2. Client and family will verbalize a willingness to comply with prescribed medical regimen. 3. Client will verbalize an understanding of the need to comply with routine schedule for antihypertensive drugs.	1. Identify with client and family sociocultural factors that influence health-seeking behavior. 2. Determine with client and family knowledge of hypertension and severity of illness. 3. Determine with client and family knowledge and level of adaptation to news about condition of hypertension. 4. Identify with client and family necessity for adherence to prescribed time limits for taking antihypertensive drugs.

Nursing Diagnosis: Communication, impaired verbal, related to cultural difference (ineffective health, recent immigration, and the use of English as a second language)

Client Outcome	Nursing Interventions
Client and family will be able to communicate basic needs to health personnel.	1. Use visual aids that will aid client in understanding the condition. 2. Use gestures or actions that communicate various tasks and procedures to be done. 3. Write down messages to provide visual stimulation about procedures to be accomplished. 4. Encourage client and family to express their needs to health personnel.

Nursing Diagnosis: Interrupted family processes related to shift in health status of family member

Client Outcomes	Nursing Interventions
1. Family will participate in care of the ill family member. 2. Family will assist nurse in assisting client in returning to a high level of wellness.	1. Determine family's understanding of client's condition. 2. Determine support systems available to family. 3. Determine with family a supportive network with friends available. 4. Involve family in care and scheduling of client-centered activities (such as taking Aldomet on time).

Nursing Diagnoses—Definitions and Classifications 2012–2014. Copyright © 2012, 1994–2012 by NANDA International. Used by arrangement with Wiley-Blackwell Publishing, a company of John Wiley and Sons, Inc. In order to make safe and effective judgments using NANDA-I nursing diagnoses it is essential that nurses refer to the definitions and defining characteristics of the diagnoses listed in the work.

CLINICAL DECISION MAKING

1. What factors related to culture are most likely to influence the noncompliance exhibited by Mr. Recio?
2. Explain how the Filipino-American orientation to time may influence Mr. Recio's health-seeking behavior and his adherence to specific schedules.
3. Describe the locus-of-control variable that some Filipino Americans have that may influence health-seeking behavior.
4. Describe at least three other nursing interventions that can be implemented to facilitate communication between Mr. Recio, his family, and the health care team.
5. Describe the structure of some Filipino-American families and the relationship the family may have on health-seeking behavior.

REVIEW QUESTIONS

1. Filipinos tend to have a higher incidence of which of the following?
   a. G-6-PD and alpha-thalassemia
   b. Metabolic syndrome and Tay-Sachs disease
   c. G-6-PD and Mediterranean spotted fever
   d. Mediterranean spotted fever and Rocky Mountain spotted fever
2. The official language of the Philippines is which of the following?
   a. English
   b. Patois
   c. Tagalog
   d. Spanish
3. The universal language spoken in the Philippines is which of the following?
   a. Patois
   b. Spanish
   c. English
   d. Arabic

REFERENCES

Adair, L. S., & Popkin, B. M. (1996). Low birth weight reduces the likelihood of breast-feeding among Filipino infants. *Journal of Nutrition, 126*(1), 103–112.

Affonso, D. (1978). The Filipino American. In D. Clark (Ed.), *Culture, childbearing, health professionals* (pp. 128–153). Philadelphia: F. A. Davis.

Agbayani-Siewert, P. (2004). Assumptions of Asian American similarity: the case of Filipino and Chinese American students. *Social Work, 49*(1), 39–51.

Aghaian, E., Choe, J., Lin, S., & Stamper, R. (2004). Central corneal thickness of Caucasians, Chinese, Hispanics, Filipinos, African Americans, and Japanese in the glaucoma clinic. *Ophthalmology, 111*(12), 2211–2219.

Althaus, C. (1999). Food: multi-cultural mix shifts diet patterns. *Food Service Director, 12*(7), 50.

American Psychiatric Association. (2000). *Diagnostic and statistical manual of mental disorders* (4th ed., rev.). Washington, DC: American Psychiatric Association.

Anchacosa-Angala, S., & Márquez-Sumabat, L. (1964). Skinfold thickness as indication of leanness-fatness in some female college students. *Philippine Journal of Nutrition, 17*, 176–197.

Araneta, M., & Barrett-Connor, E. (2005). Ethnic differences in visceral adipose tissue and type 2 diabetes: Filipino, African-American, and white women. *Obesity Research, 13*(8), 1458–1465.

Asian and Pacific Islander American Health Forum (APIAHF). (2005). *Health brief: Filipinos in the United States.* San Francisco: Asian and Pacific Islander American Health Forum.

Bartlett, L. (1977). The Filipino "Cajuns." *Dixie*, 9.

Becker, G. (2002). Dying away from home: quandaries of migration for elders in two ethnic groups. *Journals of Gerontology. Series B, Psychological Sciences and Social Sciences, 57*(2), S79–S95.

Becker, G., Beyene, Y., Newson, E., & Rodgers, D. (1998). Knowledge and care of chronic illness in three ethnic minority groups. *Family Medicine, 125*, 173–178.

Berg, J. A., Rodriguez, D., Kading, V., & De Guzman, C. (2004). Demographic survey of Filipino American nurses. *Nursing Administration Quarterly, 28*(3), 199–206.

Bjorck, J., Cuthbertson, W., Thurman, J., & Lee, Y. (2001). Ethnicity, coping, and distress among Korean Americans, Filipino Americans, and Caucasian Americans. *Journal of Social Psychology, 141*(4), 421–442.

Bofill, M. (1999). Dr. Rano S. Bofill, the music man. *Heritage, 13*(2), 33.

Bonder, B., Martin, L., & Miracle, A. (2002). *Culture in clinical care.* Thorofare, NJ: Slack.

Brown, D., James, G., & Nordloh, L. (1998). Comparison of factors affecting daily variation of blood pressure in Filipino-American and Caucasian nurses in Hawaii. *American Journal of Physical Anthropology, 106*(3), 373–383.

Burma, J. (1974). *Spanish-speaking groups in the United States.* Detroit: Blaine Ethridge Books.

Burr, J., & Mutchler, J. (1993). Nativity, acculturation, and economic status: explanations of Asian American living arrangements in later life. *Journal of Gerontology, 48*(2), 55–63.

Bush, M., & Babich, K. (1986). Cultural variation. In D. Longo & R. Williams (Eds.), *Clinical practice in psychosocial nursing: assessment and intervention* (2nd ed.). Norwalk, CT: Appleton-Century-Crofts.

Cantore, J. (2001). Giving voice to the "invisible minority." *Minority Nurse*, 26–30.

Cantos, A., & Rivera, E. (1996). Filipinos. In J. Lipson, S. Dibble, & P. Minarik (Eds.), *Culture and nursing care.* San Francisco: UCSF Nursing Press.

Caringer, B. (1977). Caring for the institutionalized Filipino. *Journal of Gerontological Nursing, 3*(7), 33–37.

Central Intelligence Agency (CIA). (2015). *The world factbook.* New York: Skyhorse.

Champeau, A. (1998). Indiana's bountiful crop of Filipino American graduates. *Heritage, 12*(3), 19.

Champeau, A. (1999). Gallery of Filipino American graduates in Indiana. *Heritage, 13*(3), 32.

Chen, X., & Unger, J. (1999). Hazards of smoking initiation among Asian American and non-Asian adolescents in California: a survival model analysis. *Preventive Medicine, 28*(6), 589–599.

Cheong, R., Kuizon, M., & Tajaon, R. (1991). Menstrual blood loss and iron nutrition in Filipino women. *Southeast Asian Journal of Tropical Medicine in Public Health, 22*(12), 595–604.

Chung, C. S., & Kau, M. C. (1985). Racial differences in cephalometric measurements and incidence of cleft lip with or without cleft palate. *Journal of Craniofacial Genetic Development and Biology, 5*(4), 341–349.

Chung, P., et al. (2005). Parent-adolescent communication about sex in Filipino American families: a demonstration of community based participatory research. *Ambulatory Pediatrics, 5*(10), 50–55.

Cooper, G. S., Yuan, Z., & Rimm, A. A. (1997). Racial disparity in the incidence and case-fatality of colorectal cancer: analysis of 329 United States counties. *Cancer Epidemiology Biomarkers Prevention, 6*(4), 283–285.

Corpuz, O. (1965). *The Philippines.* Englewood Cliffs, NJ: Prentice-Hall.

Cuasay, L., Lee, E., Orlander, P., Steffen-Batey, L., & Hanis, C. L. (2001). Prevalence and determinants of type 2 diabetes among Filipino-Americans in the Houston, Texas metropolitan statistical area. *Diabetes Care, 24*(12), 2054–2058.

Danko, G. P., Johnson, R. C., Nagoshi, C. T., Yuen, S. H., Gidley, J. E., & Ahn, M. (1988). Judgments of "normal" and "problem" alcohol use as related to reported alcohol consumption. *Alcoholism, 12*(6), 760–768.

Day, B. (1974). Philippine fare. *Gourmet,* 25.

DeGracia, R. T. (1979). Cultural influences on Filipino patients. *American Journal of Nursing,* 1412–1414.

De La Cruz, E. (1999). De La Cruz honored as 1999 outstanding teacher. *Heritage, 13*(3), 8.

Dela Cruz, F., Padilla, G., & Agustin, E. (2000). Adapting a measure of acculturation for cross-cultural research. *Journal of Transcultural Nursing, 11*(3), 191–198.

De Leon, R. (1999). Conversations with actor Fran de Leon. *Heritage, 13*(3), 9.

Espíritu, Y. L. (1995). *Filipino American lives.* Philadelphia: Temple University Press.

Flaskerud, J. (1984). A comparison of perceptions of problematic behavior by six minority groups and mental health professionals. *Nursing Research, 33*(4), 190–197.

Franks, A., et al. (1989). Hepatitis B virus infection among children born in the United States to Southeast Asian refugees. *New England Journal of Medicine, 321,* 1301–1305.

Garn, S. (1971). *Human races* (3rd ed.). Springfield, IL: Thomas.

Gee, G. C., Delva, J., & Takeuchi, D. T. (2007). Perceived unfair treatment and the use of prescription medications, illicit drugs, and alcohol dependence among Filipino Americans. *American Journal of Public Health, 97*(5), 933–940.

Geissler, E. (1998). *Pocket guide: cultural assessment.* St. Louis: Mosby.

Gerber, L. M. (1980). The influence of environmental factors on mortality from coronary heart disease among Filipinos in Hawaii. *Human Biology, 52*(2), 269–278.

Gloria, E. (1999). Gloria honored with poetry awards. *Heritage, 13,* 3–41.

Goodman, M. T., Yoshizawa, C. N., & Kolonel, L. N. (1988). Descriptive epidemiology of thyroid cancer in Hawaii. *Cancer, 61*(6), 1272–1281.

Guthrie, G., & Jacobs, P. (1966). *Childrearing and personality development in the Philippines.* University Park, PA: Pennsylvania State University Press.

Hart, D. V. (1966). The Filipino villager and his spirits. *Solidarity, 1,* 66.

Hart, D. V. (1981). Bisayan Filipino and Malagan folk medicine. In D. V. Henderson & M. Primeaux (Eds.), *Transcultural health care.* Reading, MA: Addison-Wesley.

Hart, D. V., Rajadhon, P. A., & Coughlin, R. J. (1965). *Southeast Asian birth customs: three studies in human reproduction.* New Haven, CT: Human Relations Area Files.

Hooper, H. (1958). A Filipino in California copes with anxiety. In G. Seward (Ed.), *Clinical studies in cultural conflict.* New York: Ronald Press.

José, F., & Salcedo, J. (1958). Subcutaneous fat distribution and body form of Filipino women. *Acta Medica Phillippina, 14,* 161.

Kataoka-Yahiro, M., Ceria, C., & Yoder, M. (2004). Grandparent caregiving role in Filipino American families. *Journal of Cultural Diversity, 11*(3), 110–117.

Kittler, P., & Sucher, K. (2001). *Food and culture in America* (3rd ed.). Belmont, CA: Wadsworth/Thomson Learning.

Klatsky, A. L., & Armstrong, M. A. (1991). Cardiovascular risk factors among Asian Americans living in northern California. *American Journal of Public Health, 81*(11), 1423–1428.

Kluckhohn, F., & Strodtbeck, F. (1973). *Variations in value orientations.* Westport, CT: Freeport.

Knapp, A. A., Metterville, D. R., Kemper, A. R., & Perrin, J. M. (2010). *Evidence review: hemoglobin H disease.* Rockville, MD: Maternal and Child Health Bureau. Available at <http://www.hrsa.gov/heritabledisorderscommittee/reports/hemoglobinh.pdf>.

Kolonel, L. N. (1985). Cancer incidence among Filipinos in Hawaii and the Philippines. *National Cancer Institute Monogram, 69,* 93–98.

Kurtzke, J. F. (1982). Epidemiology of amyotrophic lateral sclerosis. *Advances in Neurology, 36,* 281–302.

Kusumoto, A., Suzuki, T., Kumakura, C., & Ashizawa, K. (1996). A comparative study of foot morphology between Filipino and Japanese women, with reference to the significance of a deformity like hallux valgus as a normal variation. *Annals of Human Biology, 23*(5), 373–385.

Kwong, S. L., Chen, M. S., Snipes, K. P., Bal, D. G., & Wright, W. E. (2005). Asian subgroups and cancer incidence and mortality rates in California. *Cancer, 104*(12), S2975–S2981.

Lantican, L. S., & Corona, D. F. (1992). Comparison of the social support networks of Filipino and Mexican-American primigravidas. *Health Care of Women International, 13*(4), 329–338.

Lee, R. (2004). Filipino men's familial roles and domestic violence: implications and strategies for community-based intervention. *Health and Social Care in the Community, 12*(5), 422–429.

Lewis, J., & Glasby, M. (1975). Food habits and nutrient intakes of Filipino women in Los Angeles. *Journal of American Dietetic Association, 67*, 122–125.

Lieban, R. W. (1967). *Cebuano sorcery: malign magic in the Philippines.* Berkeley: University of California Press.

Lott, J. (1976). Migration of a mentality: the Filipino community. *Social Casework, 57*, 165–172.

Lubben, J. E., Chi, I., & Kitano, H. H. (1988). Exploring Filipino American drinking behavior. *Journal of Studies of Alcohol, 49*(1), 26–29.

Manaloto, C., et al. (1996). Longitudinal studies of children born to HIV-1 antibody positive Filipino commercial sex workers (CSW): diagnostic dilemmas. *International Journal of the Study of AIDS, 7*(3), 212–220.

Manila, E. (1999). The Filipino American center. *Heritage, 13*(3), 7.

Marsella, A. (1997). Depressive experience and disorder across cultures. In H. Triandis & J. Draguns (Eds.), *Handbook of cross-cultural psychology* (2nd ed.). Boston: Allyn & Bacon.

Matawaran, A. J., & Gervasio, C. C. (1971). Preliminary report on the average heights and weights of some Filipinos. *Philippine Journal of Nutrition, 24*, 74–92.

Matsumoto, N., Worth, R. M., Kurland, L. T., & Okazaki, H. (1972). Epidemiology study of amyotrophic lateral sclerosis in Hawaii: identification of high incidence among Filipino men. *Neurology, 22*, 934–940.

Maxwell, A., Bastani, R., & Warda, U. (2000). Knowledge and attitudes toward condom use—do they predict behavior among Filipino Americans? *Ethnicity and Disease, 19*(1), 113–124.

McAdam, J., Stotts, N., Padilla, G., & Puntillo, K. (2005). Attitudes of critically ill Filipino patients and their families toward advance directives. *American Journal of Critical Care, 14*(1), 17–25.

McBride, M., & Parreno, H. (2006). Filipino American families and caregiving. In G. Yeo & D. Gallagher-Thompson (Eds.), *Ethnicity and the dementias* (2nd ed.). New York: Routledge.

McKay, J., Hill, B., & Buckler, J. (2007). *A history of world societies* (7th ed.). Boston: Houghton Mifflin.

McKenzie, J., & Chrisman, N. (1977). Healing herbs, gods, and magics. *Nursing Outlook, 25*, 326–328.

McNall, C. (1989). Healing we cannot explain. *American Journal of Nursing, 89*(9), 1162–1164.

Melendy, H. (1977). *Asians in America: Filipinos, Koreans, and East Indians.* Boston: Twayne.

Mercado-Ortiz, G., Wilson, D., & Jiang, D. (1996). Reverse smoking and palatal mucosal changes in Filipino women. Epidemiological features. *Australian Dental Journal, 41*(10), 300–303.

Meredith, H. (1978). Research between 1960 and 1970 on the standing heights of young children in different parts of the world. In H. Reese & L. Lipsitt (Eds.), *Advances in child development and behavior* (pp. 1–59). New York: Academic Press.

Monzon, R. B. (1991). Replacement patterns of *Ascaris lumbricoides* populations in Filipino children. *Southeast Asian Journal of Tropical Medicine in Public Health, 22*(4), 605–610.

Morton, N. E. (1977). Genetic aspects of prematurity. In D. M. Reed & F. J. Stanley (Eds.), *The epidemiology of prematurity.* Baltimore: Urban & Schwartzenberg.

Motulsky, A. G., Stransky, E., & Fraser, G. R. (1964). Glucose-6-phosphate dehydrogenase (G6PD) deficiency, thalassaemia, and abnormal haemoglobins in the Philippines. *Journal of Medical Genetics, 1*, 102–106.

Nakoma, E., Poole, C., Vannappagari, V., Hall, S. A., & Beutler, E. (2009). The global prevalence of glucose-6-phosphate dehydrogenase deficiency: a systematic review and meta-analysis. *Blood Cells, Molecules and Diseases, 42*, 267–278.

National Center for Health Statistics. (2014). *Health, United States with chartbook.* Hyattsville, MD: National Center for Health Statistics.

Orque, M. (1983). Nursing care of Filipino American patients. In M. Orque, M. S. Block, & B. Monroy (Eds.), *Ethnic nursing care: a multicultural approach.* St. Louis: Mosby.

Ortiz, G., Pierce, A., & Wilson, D. (1996). Palatal changes associated with reverse smoking in Filipino women. *Oral Disease, 2*(9), 232–237.

Pacquiao, D. (2003). People of Filipino heritage. In L. Purnell & B. Paulanka (Eds.), *Transcultural health care* (2nd ed.). Philadelphia: F. A. Davis.

Palaniappan, L., et al. (2010). Call to action: cardiovascular disease in Asian Americans: a science advisory from the American Heart Association. *Circulation, 122*, 1242–1252.

Parreno, H. (1977). How Filipinos deal with stress. *Washington State Journal of Nursing, 49*, 3–6.

Pilapil, V. (1999). The truth about the first Pinoy in the U.S. Congress. *Heritage, 13*(2), 34.

Pimentel, L. (1968). The perception of illness among the immigrant Filipinos in Sacramento Valley. Master's thesis. Sacramento, CA: Sacramento State College.

Pobutsky, A., Hirokawa, R., & Reyes-Salvail, F. (2003). Estimates of disability among ethnic groups in Hawaii. *Californian Journal of Health Promotion, 1*(Special Issue: Hawaii), 65–82.

Pollard, R. (1995). Ethnic comparison of twinning rates in California. *Human Biology, 67*(6), 921–931.

Requiro, R. (1981). Filipino hypertension rate leads Asian-Pacific group. *Philippine News, 20*, 12.

Roach, L. (1977). Color changes in dark skin. *Nursing, 7*, 48–51.

Rosenbaum, J. (1989). Depression: viewed from a transcultural nursing theoretical perspective. *Journal of Advanced Nursing*, 14, 7–12.

Rosenblatt, K. A., Weiss, N. S., & Schwartz, S. M. (1996). Liver cancer in Asian migrants to the United States and their descendants. *Cancer Causes and Control*, 7(3), 345–350.

Ryan, C., et al. (2000). Coronary heart disease in Filipino and Filipino-American patients: prevalence of risk factors and outcomes of treatment. *Journal of Invasive Cardiology*, 12(3), 134–139.

Santiago, M. (2001). Personal conversation with Jean Ann Contore in giving voice to the "invisible minority." *Minority Nurse*, 27.

Shimamoto, Y. (1977). Health care to the elderly Filipino in Hawaii: its cultural aspects. In M. Leininger & K. Carbol (Eds.), *Transcultural nursing care of the elderly*. Proceedings from the second National Transcultural Nursing Conference. Salt Lake City: University of Utah College of Nursing.

Sloan, N. (1963). Ethnic distribution of diabetes mellitus in Hawaii. *Journal of the American Medical Association*, 183, 419–424.

Solon, F., et al. (1996). Evaluation of the effect of vitamin A-fortified margarine on the vitamin A status of preschool Filipino children. *Europe Journal of Clinical Nutrition*, 50(11), 720–723.

Spector, R. (2004a). *Cultural diversity in health and illness* (6th ed.). Upper Saddle River, NJ: Pearson Prentice Hall.

Spector, R. (2004b). *Culture care: guide to heritage assessment and health tradition* (3rd ed.). Upper Saddle River, NJ: Pearson Prentice Hall.

Stavig, G. R., Igra, A., & Leonard, A. R. (1988). Hypertension and related health issues among Asians and Pacific Islanders in California. *Public Health Reports*, 103(1), 28–37.

Stavig, G. R., Igra, A., Leonard, A. R., McCullough, J., & Oreglia, A. (1986). Hypertension-related mortality in California. *Public Health Reports*, 101(1), 39–49.

Suzara, A. (1999). Suzara named director of student cultural center. *Heritage*, 13(3), 5.

Takaki, R. (1998). *Strangers from a different shore* (revised ed.). Boston: Little, Brown & Co.

Tompar-Tiu, A., & Sustento-Seneriches, J. (1995). *Depression and other mental health issues: the Filipino American experience*. San Francisco: Jossey-Bass.

Urban Associates, Inc. (1974). *A study of selected socioeconomic characteristics of ethnic minorities based on the 1970 census* (HEW Pub. No. 5). Arlington, VA: U.S. Department of Health, Education, and Welfare.

U.S. Department of Commerce, Bureau of the Census. (2013). *American community survey*. Washington, DC: U.S. Government Printing Office.

U.S. Department of Commerce, Bureau of the Census. (2013). *The Asian Population 2013*. Hyattsville, MD: U.S. Government Printing Office.

Vance, A., & Davidhizar, R. (1999). Developing cultural sensitivity: when your client is Filipino American. *Journal of Practical Nursing*, 49(4), 16–20.

Van Horn, C., & Schaffner, H. (2003). *Work in America: an encyclopedia of history, policy, and society*. Santa Barbara, CA: Authors.

Voegelin, C. F., & Voegelin, F. M. (1997). *Classification and index of the world's languages*. New York: Elsevier.

Wagner, N. (1973). Filipinos: a minority within a minority. In S. Stanley & N. Wagner (Eds.), *Asian-Americans: psychological perspectives*. Palo Alto, CA: Science & Behavior Books.

Weber, S. E. (1996). Cultural aspects of pain in childbearing women. *Journal of Obstetric, Gynecologic, and Neonatal Nursing*, 25(1), 67–72.

White, J., Linhart, J., & Medley, L. (1996). Culture, diet, and the maternity. *Advances for Nurse Practitioners*, 26–28.

Wilson, S., & Billones, H. (1994). The Filipino elder: implications for nursing practice. *Journal of Gerontological Nursing*, 20(8), 31–36.

Woo, J. M., Rutherford, G. W., Payne, S. F., Barnhart, J. L., & Lemp, G. F. (1988). The epidemiology of AIDS in Asian and Pacific Islander populations in San Francisco. *AIDS (London, England)*, 2(6), 473–475.

Wooley, P. (1972). *Syncrisis: the dynamics of health—an analytic series on the interactions of health and socioeconomic development. The Philippines* (Vol. 4). Washington, DC: U.S. Department of Health, Education, and Welfare.

World almanac. (2015). New York: World Almanac Books.

Yamase, H., & McNamara, J. (1977). Geographic differences in the incidence of gallbladder disease: influence of environment and ethnic background. *American Journal of Surgery*, 123, 667–670.

Yeo, G., Hikoyeda, N., McBride, M., Chin, S. Y., Edmonds, M., & Hendrix, L. (1998). Cohort analysis as a tool in ethnogeriatrics: historical profiles of elders from eight ethnic populations in the United States. In *SGEC working papers series 12* (2nd ed.). Stanford, CA: Stanford Geriatric Education Center.

Young, F., Lichton, I. J., Hamilton, R. M., Dorrough, S. A., & Alford, E. J. (1987). Body weight, blood pressure, and electrolyte excretion of young adults from six ethnic groups in Hawaii. *American Journal of Clinical Nutrition*, 45(1), 126–130.

Young, J. L., Ries, L. G., & Pollach, E. S. (1984). Cancer patient survival among ethnic groups in the United States. *Journal of National Cancer Institute*, 73(2), 341–352.

Zaide, G. (1961). *Philippine history: developing our nation*. Manila: Bookman.

Vietnamese Americans

Susan J. Appel

BEHAVIORAL OBJECTIVES

After reading this chapter, the nurse will be able to:

1. Identify communication barriers a Vietnamese American may encounter when using the U.S. health care system.
2. Identify beliefs about space that may influence how Vietnamese people feel about care given to females.
3. Describe the organization of the Vietnamese family.
4. Articulate ways the nurse might modify instructions to a Vietnamese-American client based on differences in time perception.

5. Discuss briefly the basic *yin* and *yang* theory of Chinese medicine and how it is expressed in the cause and treatment of disease.
6. Articulate at least three explanations for the causes of illness that influence traditional Vietnamese thinking.
7. Discuss implications for care of the small body size of many Vietnamese Americans.

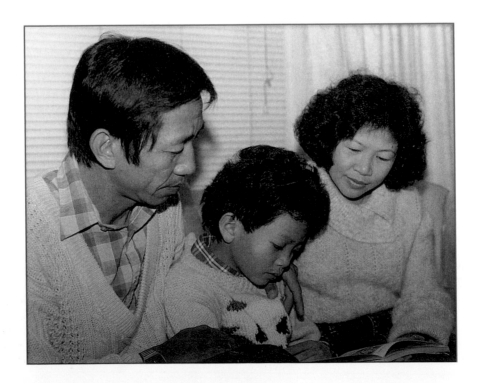

OVERVIEW OF VIETNAM

Vietnam is situated on the eastern coast of the Indochina peninsula, bordered on the north by China, with the Gulf of Thailand surrounding the Mekong Delta on the south. On the west, Vietnam is bordered by Cambodia (Kampuchea) and Laos and on the east by the South China Sea. The country is slightly smaller than Japan, with 127,000 square miles. Vietnam, along with Laos and Cambodia, is often referred to as *Indochina* or *Southeast Asia*. These three countries are strikingly dissimilar, with different languages, unrelated social roots, long histories of unique development, and varying sources of strife.

The northern part of Vietnam is mountainous, with deep valleys and the industrial Red River Delta. The central ribbon is a long, narrow corridor with a mountain range, coastal plain, and miles of beautiful white sand beaches. The southern part of Vietnam is mostly the flat Mekong Delta, the agricultural area where most of the rice for the country and for export is grown. Vietnam is considered a tropical country, although the north has four distinct seasons and the south has two seasons: rainy and dry.

The population of Vietnam is 93,423,835 (2014 estimate) (Central Intelligence Agency, 2015; *World Almanac*, 2015), which includes lowland people (often urban and more educated), rural village people (with varying degrees of sophistication and education), and mountain people (made up of at least 30 different groups or tribes with a culture all their own). Ethnic groups include Kinh (Viet), 85.7%; Tay, 1.9%; Thai, 1.8%; Muong, 1.5%; Khmer, 1.5%; Nun, 1.1%; Hmong, 1.2%; and others, 4.1% (2014 census) (Central Intelligence Agency, 2015). The mountain people number approximately 1 million (*World Almanac*, 2015). The life expectancy is 72.91 years (2014 estimate), with an infant mortality rate of 18.99 deaths per live births. The literacy rate is 93.4% (Central Intelligence Agency, 2015; *World Almanac*, 2015).

Vietnam has a recorded history of more than 2000 years, with legends that cover an additional 2000 years. Earliest records are of dynasty rule and domination by the Chinese (111 B.C. to 938 A.D.). There were 900 years of independence until the French came in 1858. Throughout the French domination (until 1954), the Vietnamese continued to work toward independence.

The country was divided into the Communist north and the non-Communist south by the Geneva Accords in 1954, when it became clear that the "nationalist" movement in the north had been monopolized by leaders leaning toward Communist ideology. The struggle between the Soviet-assisted North Vietnam and the United States–assisted South Vietnam ended in 1975, when Vietnam was reunited under the victorious Socialist Republic of Vietnam. More than 30 years of war had physically, economically, and socially devastated the country. There was a great deal of turmoil and isolation during the next 15 years, as the Communists attempted to rebuild the country under a new philosophy. Floods and drought added to the crises and poverty. Thousands of people left the country for hope in the outside world, especially France, the United States, Canada, and Australia. By the late 1980s, however, the need and opportunity for economic exchange helped ease restrictions, and there was a pronounced influx of economic interests and business with countries around the world. By 1993, the country had a trade surplus and was the world's third largest exporter of rice (Hiebert, 1993). The years-long trade embargoes from the United States were lifted in 1994, and in 1995 the United States extended Vietnam full diplomatic recognition. The 25% unemployment rate of 1995 has decreased to an estimated 5.5% in 2012, and the Vietnamese have become less anxious to leave the country (Central Intelligence Agency, 2015). The 2013 estimate of the gross domestic product was $358.9 billion, with a per capita income of $4000 (Central Intelligence Agency, 2015). Some 12.3% of the people live below the poverty line (2013 estimate). Today, 56.8% of the labor force is agricultural, 37% is industrial, and 6.2% is service oriented. By 2002, "going back" to visit Vietnam was a common occurrence in most U.S. Vietnamese communities. Dollars carried in by friends still provide welcome help for improving the quality of life for many Vietnamese. Today, tourism provides many jobs for the people of Vietnam. The United States has become Vietnam's top export market, with an annual trade totaling over $6 billion (*World Almanac*, 2015).

IMMIGRATION TO THE UNITED STATES

In 2009, 1,471,509 people (0.37% of the population of the United States) identified Vietnam as their country of origin. The Vietnamese population ranked as the fourth largest Asian American group, preceded only by Chinese, Filipinos, and Asian Indians (U.S. Department of Commerce, Bureau of the Census, *American Community Survey*, 2013). Vietnamese make up approximately 11.0% of the total Asian American population.

Of the Asian Americans residing in the United States, 20.7% reside in the Northeast, 11.7% in the Midwest, 18.8% in the South, and 48.8% in the West (U.S. Department of Commerce, Bureau of the Census, *The Asian Population*, 2013). The highest concentrations of Vietnamese Americans are in California, Virginia, Texas, and Florida. Approximately 84.0% of Vietnamese persons in the United States today were born in a foreign country (U.S. Department of Commerce, Bureau of the Census,

The Asian Population, 2013). Between 1980 and 1990, 69.7% of all Vietnamese residing in the United States were immigrants, compared with 27.1% between 1975 and 1979. The number of Vietnamese immigrants slowed somewhat between 1991 and 2009. In fact, while the Vietnamese population grew by 134.8% from 1980 to 1990, it was only 35.1% from 1991 to 2009 (U.S. Department of Commerce, Bureau of the Census, *American Community Survey*, 2015; U.S. Department of Commerce, Bureau of the Census, *The Asian Population*, 2013). The median age for Vietnamese Americans is 37.5 years, compared with 35.7 years for the rest of the U.S. population (Central Intelligence Agency, 2015; U.S. Department of Commerce, Bureau of the Census, *American Community Survey*, 2013; U.S. Department of Commerce, Bureau of the Census, *The Asian Population*, 2013). Approximately 48.8% of Vietnamese Americans are females, compared with 51% for the total nation (U.S. Department of Commerce, Bureau of the Census, *The Asian Population*, 2013).

First-Wave Immigrants

The first group of refugees, who began arriving in 1975, included lowlanders, professionals, ranking South Vietnamese military personnel, and those with close U.S. connections. This group also included those who had the means to get out of the country and those who stood to lose the most under the new regime. A high percentage of these immigrants were educated in Vietnam or abroad, and some spoke English. Many were young and single or married with small children. The children moved into the school systems and could soon speak English more fluently than their parents and in some cases more fluently than they could speak Vietnamese.

Some of these immigrants had been exposed to European cultures or to the American culture for years and had economic or vocational assets. They generally did not go through a long, stressful period of economic and psychological deprivation affecting their health. Of the 145,000 Vietnamese persons who came to the United States in 1975, 14% lived in single-family households, 42% were under 18 years of age, and 11.6% were over 44 years of age. Approximately 90% were employed 1 year after arrival (Coelho & Stein, 1980).

Second-Wave Immigrants

A higher percentage of the second-wave refugees (1979–1980) were Chinese-Vietnamese extended family groups who left Vietnam under duress and pressure from the government. These immigrants were educated and part of the business community in or near Saigon and had as much social status as was permitted under the existing regime. For many persons in the second wave of refugees, however,

Vietnamese was a second language, and fewer spoke English than in the earlier group. These immigrants also included elderly persons and other extended family members who often had health needs.

Third-Wave Immigrants

Most of the Vietnamese refugees during the 1980s were "boat people," who in many cases had lived through not only economic struggles but also political and social change while at home. In addition, the boat people had survived life-threatening situations for days at sea. Persons in the third wave often spent months or even years in refugee camps along the way, and these earlier experiences caused turmoil that needed to be dealt with once they arrived and got settled in the United States. Third-wave immigrants were even more diversified than those in the two former groups. Many were in poorer physical condition than those arriving earlier, and generally the adjustment was more difficult and more complex. Although many refugee education programs and school systems had organized programs to absorb the newly arrived children and adults in the first and second waves, these programs were not as effective with persons in the third wave. Life in camps did not encourage rigorous study habits or academic excellence, and many children in the third wave were not able to read or write well in either Vietnamese or English. For the boat people, education to assist in adjustment to the new environment needed to be much more comprehensive.

By 1986, nations surrounding Vietnam, Cambodia, and Laos had tightened laws for illegal travelers to their shores, and the traffic of boat people slowed down. At the same time, the government of Vietnam gave new economic life to the country by allowing the people some private marketing and land use. In 1989, the government agreed to voluntary repatriation of Vietnamese who had left the country, and during the next 3 years, with the United Nations' help, more than 32,000 boat people returned from camps, especially from where they had been held in Hong Kong (Balfour, 1993). Foreign-born Vietnamese usually represent one of the three waves of immigration. In addition, it is helpful to know if the individual is first, second, or third generation in the United States, since these factors will influence adherence to cultural behaviors that are practiced (Bonder, Martin, & Miracle, 2002).

COMMUNICATION

Language

In the United States, Vietnamese is the language of most of the 1,687,951 people who call or have called Vietnam their home. In 2013, 53.1% of all Vietnamese 5 years of age or older could not speak English well; 87.5% spoke a language other than English at home; and 12.5% spoke only English (U.S. Department of Commerce, Bureau of the Census, *American Community Survey, 2013*).

Vietnamese is not mutually intelligible with any other Asian language. It is monosyllabic and disyllabic and polytonal (five to six tones), and so a syllable when spoken with different tones has an entirely different meaning. The language is flowing and musical, and for the most part, pronunciation is consistent and the grammar simple.

Until the 1960s, French was the language of educated Vietnamese people, along with Vietnamese; therefore, much of the scientific and technical vocabulary was borrowed from French or, more recently, English. After 1975 in Vietnam, English was more common as the choice for a second language in high schools and colleges. Three distinct dialects of Vietnamese separate the northern, central, and southern regions of Vietnam. Dialects identify the speaker's origins and are understood by others regardless of region.

For many years before the Vietnam War, Vietnam had a large Chinese minority who had their own schools with classes conducted in Chinese. In the Chinese suburb of Saigon called Cholon, many older Chinese persons spoke only Chinese, and the children learned Vietnamese as a second language. This explains why many persons in the large Chinese–Vietnamese refugee group can speak both Chinese and Vietnamese or only Chinese. In contrast to this, the ethnic mountain people, or *Montagnards,* have their own tribal languages (usually of Austronesian type and, in the north, Miao-Yao type) and often do not understand Vietnamese.

Style

Respect is very evident in communication and is a cornerstone of Vietnamese society (Huynh, 1987). The proliferation of titles in the Vietnamese language is evidence of the cultural focus on respect. For example, when describing family relationships, English users have titles reserved for family members that include *mother, father, sister, brother, uncle, aunt, cousin, grandmother,* and *grandfather.* However, the language and style of the Vietnamese not only encompass family descriptors such as *uncle* but also designate which side of the family a family member represents (mother's or father's) and further indicate whether that relative is the eldest brother or sister. Grandparent titles also reflect paternal or maternal side. When a sister or brother is being described, the term used indicates if the sister or brother is younger (*em*) or older (*chi* or *anh*).

Context

The word *yes* is used in English to express agreement and does not reflect an attitude of respect or disrespect. For Vietnamese people, *ya* indicates respect and not necessarily agreement. Therefore, a troubling verbal communication between health workers and Vietnamese-American clients is the polite "*Ya, ya, Thua bà, ya, ya,*" response, which Americans interpret as "Yes, yes, I understand, and I'll do it." For the Vietnamese, the "yes" of *ya* is simply being respectful, indicating "I'm listening, and I respect what you're saying" (even though the request may not be within the realm of possibility). Nurses often reflect later, "But he said, 'Yes, yes,' and agreed to . . . ." Noncompliance by Vietnamese Americans can often be traced to this misinterpretation of *ya.*

Vietnamese people often use personal pronouns to describe various roles held. For example, the speaker may refer to the self as *con* (referring to a child) when addressing parents and as *em* to the nurse or to any superior. However, the same individual may refer to himself or herself as *thầy* (teacher) when addressing students. It is common for Vietnamese persons to use only the title of a person, such as "Uncle" or "Teacher" except with family and close friends. Especially when there is considerable distance between the speaker and the listener, the title alone is most correct. This custom is practiced even in the United States. For example, people often say "Madam Chair" or "Mr. President," indicating that the title is more important than the name.

Two distinct features of the Vietnamese culture and consequently the language are moderation and caution (Huynh, 1987). Vietnamese people are taught from childhood to think before speaking. High value is placed on modesty of action and speech. A Vietnamese proverb suggests that "bragging reflects an empty soul." There is also concern that a slip of the tongue may bring discord and be disruptive to harmony and respect. Ethnic Vietnamese lowlanders, as well as those from the mountain tribes, place high value on showing respect: communication should always be in a formal, polite manner (Rairdan & Higgs, 1992). Table 18-1 highlights some differences between Asian and American communication styles.

Touch

Traditionally, the high value of emotional self-control and the general esteem for correct behavior have limited touch as a form of communication. Physical behavior, including backslapping, is not considered proper by the well-bred. The young people have been less formal, and in Vietnam in the 1970s it was not uncommon to see groups of Vietnamese boys jostling each other in the street or girls walking arm in arm on the sidewalk. Today in the United States, many Vietnamese youths are taking cues from their American counterparts. For some Vietnamese people, the head is considered the "seat," and touching it, even in the process

TABLE 18-1　Communication Style and Expression of Emotion

Asian	American
Nonverbal	Verbal
Subtle, indirect	Open, direct
Serene, stoic, suppress negative emotions	Expressive, spontaneous
Indirect expression of affection by fulfilling obligations, needs	Direct verbal and physical expression of affection

From Nilchaikovit, K., Hill, J., & Holland, J. (1993). The effects of culture on illness behavior and medical care. *General Hospital Psychiatry, 15,* 41–50.

of giving care, may cause some vital force to escape (Hoang & Erickson, 1982).

Kinesics

In the Vietnamese culture, respect is also conveyed by non-verbal communication. By the time standing is possible, the child is taught to cross the arms over the chest, lower the head, and bend the upper torso slightly forward when greeting an elder or a guest coming into the house. Non-verbal methods to communicate respect continue to be used throughout life. Deference to others shows a Confucian and Buddhist influence in that how something is done is often more important than what is done. Posture and manner of walking can be used to indicate self-concept (Sideleau, 1992). Respect is also shown by avoiding eye contact when talking with someone who does not have equal standing in education, social standing, age, or gender. A student avoids eye contact with a teacher, an employee with the boss, a younger member of the family with the elders, and so on. Direct eye contact in these settings generally means a challenge or an expression of deep passion. Bowing the head slightly when entering the presence of an elderly person conveys respect. Using both hands to give something to or receive something from an adult, especially an elder, or person of higher status shows respect. The head may be considered sacred, and care should be taken in touching and patting. Feet are the lowliest body parts and should be kept on the floor.

A silent form of communication may also be used that relies heavily on implied understanding between people of the culture. Because of cultural norms, sometimes implicit concerns are not allowed to be discussed verbally. For example, it may be very unusual or could be considered improper for a son or daughter to discuss issues of death and dying with parents, yet concern by either of them may be expressed by nonverbal cues, such as bowing of the head

or direct eye contact. When dealing with Western health care professionals, these understandings are not overtly stated. Unless the health care professional knows the culture well enough to address the unspoken, this valuable information is lost and often leads to misunderstanding of family–patient dynamics or lack of agreement with the plan of care (McLaughlin & Braun, 1998).

In contrast to the usual palm-up position used by persons in the dominant culture in the United States, Vietnamese persons beckon for someone to come by turning the palm downward and waving the fingers. The upturned palm is used to call a dog or other animal or as an insult. It is never proper to snap one's fingers or wave violently to gain someone's attention.

Except in private circumstances, open expression of emotions is considered in bad taste. Emotions interfere with self-control and can be considered weaknesses. Romantic overtures and demonstrative joyous expressions are reserved for home or other private settings. One exception to the usual restraint is the expected behavior of a widow at the grave for the burial of her husband, when she may wail or attempt to throw herself into the grave.

Implications for Nursing Care

Because respect and harmony are highly valued in relationships, there is a great desire in the Vietnamese culture not to disappoint, upset, embarrass, or cause another person to lose face. The desire to maintain harmony takes precedence over what the actual truth of a situation may be. When a Vietnamese-American client is confronted with a difficult or delicate question, particularly if the answer is negative, such as "Did you take your medication?" the client may choose not to give a direct answer in favor of the higher good of keeping peace with the nurse. In the Western culture, this avoidance might be considered an attempt to avoid the truth; however, in the Vietnamese culture the answer would be considered the correct way to handle a delicate situation.

The nurse should recognize that negative emotions or expressions of disagreement are usually conveyed by silence or a reluctant smile. For the Vietnamese a smile may express joy, but more often it is used to convey many other messages, such as stoicism in the face of difficulty or an apology for a minor social offense. A smile may be a proper response to a scolding to show sincere acknowledgment for the wrongdoing, as well as to convey that there are no ill feelings. A smile is also a way to respond when it is improper to say "thank you" or "I'm sorry" because of age or status. A smile is often present, regardless of the situation. Even if angry, feeling neglected, or in need, the Vietnamese-American client will rarely express this to the health care professional but rather will speak quietly and smile. Instead of asking questions that allow an answer, such as "Are you having pain?" or "Do you want something for pain?" the nurse should acknowledge the likelihood of pain and state, "Please let me get you something for pain."

The nurse may experience difficulty with gathering information from Vietnamese-American clients. Vietnamese-American clients tend to be discreet and passive, quietly understanding problems and rarely expressing feelings. Usually there is even more difficulty obtaining information in the area of emotional problems or sexual difficulties because these topics are considered private and to be avoided in public (Nilchaikovit, Hill, & Holland, 1993). In short-term relationships, it is crucial to have a same-sex Vietnamese interpreter; for the long term, the health professional should work toward a trusting relationship. For the Vietnamese client, a caring, accepting attitude helps bridge the gap to true understanding.

Because most Vietnamese American clients entering the health care system in the United States do not speak English, with many medical terms, an interpreter or bicultural medical translator can assist in accurate communication. It is important that the translator be culturally aware and conscientious to bridge the gap between the culture of the client and members of the health care team. Accurate translation can be assisted if the interpreter is Vietnamese because of the built-in cultural awareness. However, the Vietnamese interpreter may be hesitant to translate certain complaints that are unacceptable to Western practitioners, such as symptoms the client states are "caused by the wind," a common expression. Other important factors are the effect of differences in social class between interpreter and client, the possible effect of a male interpreter with a female client, and the need for a female interpreter or companion when a physical examination is done on a female client. When an interpreter is unavailable, it is important for the nurse to choose vocabulary carefully, to keep instructions simple and brief, and to avoid medical jargon (Tran, 1980) (Box 18-1).

The nurse should be aware that English phonetic practices applied to Vietnamese names often result in pronunciations that are unintelligible to the Vietnamese. Nguyên Thi Hồng, who has been responding to approximately/Wee-un/Tee-hung/ for 23 years, can hardly be expected to appear at the clinic desk when she is summoned as /Hung Thigh Nugooen/. (In Vietnam, the family name—for example, Nguyên—is spoken first and always appears first on listings. In the United States the family name is always spoken last, although it appears first on listings.) In a clinic where clients must be called, it may be useful to have the clients take numbers because numbers are more readily understood. It is important for the nurse to appreciate that pronunciation may also cause difficulties with questions regarding addresses and phone numbers. It may be easier for the client to write answers to such questions. Such a client should be encouraged to carry instructions in written form.

A question about age may also be difficult for the Vietnamese-American client. A Vietnamese mother may be able to indicate the year a child was born but may not be able to state the child's exact age. In Vietnam individual birthdays are not usually celebrated; rather, everyone becomes a year older at the beginning of each new year (Tết). Thus a newborn who arrives during the week before New Year would be considered 1 year old following the first Tết celebration. Another reason for confusion about age, especially for persons who immigrated as teenagers, is that new birth certificates may show an age adjustment of 2 or 3 years earlier. This adjustment may have been done in Vietnam to avoid the draft or in the United States to facilitate entrance into high school. (After 18 years of age, the student was not usually accepted into high school regardless of educational level attained in Vietnam.) The slight build of many Vietnamese persons facilitates this age adjustment. Elderly Vietnamese persons without birth certificates usually know the year of their birth and are officially assigned, on arrival in the United States, a birthday of January 1. Finally, the nurse should be cognizant of the fact that for many Vietnamese Americans the numerous questions asked by health professionals in the United States raise doubt about the competency of the health professionals. The nurse should attempt to communicate both acceptance of varying cultural practices and genuine concern in order to bridge the gap between the cultures and to increase the client's trust in the caregivers.

SPACE

Intimate Zone

Beliefs about space are rooted deep in Vietnamese culture. For traditional Vietnamese persons, intimate-zone activities are confined to private settings. Holding hands in public, especially with members of the opposite sex, is considered in poor taste, and hugging or emotionally touching in public, even by close friends or family members, is embarrassing to the traditional Vietnamese.

Beliefs about space also influence how Vietnamese people feel about care given to females. Until the early 1900s, traditional practitioners were not to touch the bodies of their female clients except to take their pulse. Figurines were used for the female client to indicate where she was having problems. Today, many Vietnamese persons still emphasize virginity at the time of marriage, especially for the woman, and have strong feelings about unmarried young women having pelvic examinations.

BOX 18-1   Using an Interpreter

Unless there are large numbers of a specific cultural group, most hospitals or medical centers cannot afford professional interpreters. But with careful selection and guidance, good interpreters can be home grown.

1. Find a good bilingual person in the Vietnamese community who lives near enough to be called upon to help, either in person or on the phone, when needed. Often Vietnamese can suggest suitable candidates. Except in real emergencies, avoid using the family's 10-year-old daughter, friends, or "the cleaning lady."

2. Get to know the interpreter beforehand and practice saying the Vietnamese name correctly. Usually a title should be used.

3. Be sure the interpreter understands the idea of confidentiality, "a commitment of all members on the health team."

4. Impress on the interpreter that you consider him or her a bridge between the two groups of people involved, the family and the health team, and in a special way an important member of both teams.

5. If the terminology for the anticipated causes, symptoms, suspected diagnosis, and other matters is not routine or familiar, review it briefly with the interpreter so these can be looked up or clarified before the interview.

During the Interview

1. The interpreter's seat should be about halfway between you and the patient group. This helps communicate that the interpreter is a bridge, not a member of only the health team or of only the family.

2. Greet the family, and then introduce the interpreter by name to the patient. If the patient is elderly, show respect by introducing the interpreter to the patient, but then also include the accompanying family, who likely will be doing much of the communicating.

3. Always look and talk directly to the patient family group, not at or to the interpreter. Remember, the interpreter is the bridge, not the original messenger. (An exception is when you and the interpreter need to clarify something with each other.)

4. To make it easier: Use short, direct sentences.
   • Plan questions carefully. Do not use double negatives. Focus on one item for yes–no questions.
   • Avoid technical jargon, idioms, and metaphors.
   • Avoid humor or jokes, which are often difficult to translate.
   • Be aware that questions related to the reproductive system or sexual behavior are sensitive areas.

5. Be prepared to hear new names for familiar symptoms without showing surprise or scorn. One way of handling unfamiliar diagnoses can be to ask, "Can you tell me what I need to know about [the specific diagnosis mentioned]?" (McPhee, 2002, p. 499).

6. At the end of the interview, thank the family and specifically thank the interpreter.

The interpreter is not only bilingual but also bicultural. With sensitivity and respect in working together, the professional will be fortunate to come to depend on him or her not only to translate words but also to translate culture, raising the caution flag when the culture is being inadvertently violated in some way. Often the interpreter can come up with a good solution to the situation if the professional can be depended on for respect and understanding.

After the Interview

1. Document the interpreter's name on the medical record.

2. Discuss any part of the interview that was problematic, and attempt to learn the cause and find possible options for the solutions.

3. Validate any information or important decisions the professional understood had been made, including the plan of action.

4. Thank the interpreter and check that the institutional plan for reimbursement is clear.

Personal, Social, and Public Zones

Vietnamese individuals are likely to feel more comfortable with more distance during personal and social relationships than that required by persons in the dominant culture. Social exchanges generally do not involve physical contact other than handshaking, which may be practiced between men.

Living Space

In Vietnam, extended families live comfortably in relatively small areas. The moderate or warm climate allows many family activities to be carried on outside. Often the kitchen is separate from the rest of the house, and the two or three main rooms double as living rooms and bedrooms, with the mosquito nets neatly tied back during the day. Even in spacious homes, family members often prefer to spend much of their time in proximity to each other. In rural Vietnam, homes are typically arranged in communities and villages with several homes near each other.

Although many Vietnamese persons were used to living in close proximity, refugee camps brought a new kind of cramped and confined closeness. As refugees, many Vietnamese persons lived for several months or years with 8 to 10 persons occupying a one-room space, sometimes enclosed only by a blanket curtain. Special adjustment was required by most refugees when they received housing in the United States because many well-intentioned sponsors made an effort to provide single-home dwellings for the refugees because "they've been so crowded so long." Unfortunately, this space lacked the familiar sounds, smells, and people and soon brought feelings of loneliness. Today, many Vietnamese Americans have homes with room for parents and additional family members and desire to have relatives and friends in close proximity.

Implications for Nursing Care

When caring for Vietnamese American clients, the nurse should be cognizant of the effect space may have on client care. For example, the nurse should be aware that if a pelvic examination is to be conducted, it is important for a female translator to explain carefully why it is necessary and what will be done and to remain with the client during the examination.

The nurse should also be aware that a back rub from a stranger could cause feelings of uneasiness. The nurse should use discretion in including a back rub as a routine part of nursing care.

SOCIAL ORGANIZATION

Family

In Vietnam, the family is the basic institution of society and provides lifelong protection and guidance for the individual members. The roles and structure are well defined, with extensive terminology designating kinship relationships. The lineage is patriarchal, with the father considered the head of the household. The mother often handles much of the household responsibilities and management.

The immediate family includes the parents, unmarried children, daughters, sometimes the husband's parents, and sons with their wives and children. In addition, the extended family includes other close relatives (usually with the same family name and ancestors) who live in the same community (Box 18-2). The oldest son has the heavy responsibility of carrying on the family name, of taking over for the parents when they become elderly, of seeing to their care, and of following through with the religious and ancestral

observances. The oldest daughter takes responsibility for the care of the household in the absence of the mother.

The family has been the chief source of cohesion and continuity for the Vietnamese for hundreds of years. In comparison with Chinese and other Southeast Asian groups, the Vietnamese family is seen "as the backbone of tradition and heritage" (Davis, 2000, p. 137), the center around which ancient traditions, customs, and ways of life continue (Fong & Mokuau, 1994).

The crux of family loyalty is "filial piety," which commands children to obey and honor their parents. According to Huynh (1987), the worst insult a Vietnamese can receive is to be accused of failure to fulfill the obligation of filial piety. Along with the three major historical religions of Vietnam, "Honor your father and mother" is also commanded in the Christian faith (Exodus 20:12).

Parents consider it important to train their children, and this responsibility is usually shared by members of the extended family living in the household. Obedience and honor are shown in several ways: obedient behavior and attitudes, using the detailed kinship terminology for each person, and contributing to the family name through outstanding achievements. Personal interests and destiny are seldom considered outside the framework of the immediate and extended family. Behavior or misbehavior (juvenile delinquency, academic failure, mental disorders, and so on) reflects on the entire family and has great significance beyond the person involved. It has often served to curb antisocial behavior, especially among the young.

If personal feelings or ambitions do not contribute to the good of the family or cause disharmony, the individual is expected to bend toward the family and give up personal wishes. In a study using open interviews to understand Vietnamese culture, Laura, a 26-year-old, reflected on how parents or other older members of the family direct children in making life decisions:

Actually my older brother he really wanted to become a doctor. But my uncle said, "You can't do that. You know that, you have to bring them (rest of the family) here, so you have to study something that take a short time. Engineering, something like that." And my brother, he listened to my uncle. (Davis, 2000, p. 142)

As Vietnamese point out, Vietnamese family traditions began to change decades before immigration to the United States. With the years of war, the prescribed gender roles and decision making had to be taken on by the females of the family. Large extended families were less common or more scattered, or family homes were located in inaccessible territory. The intergenerational households in the United States create stress in the family, with young family

BOX 18-2   Names

Many Vietnamese family names originated during the various dynasties that ruled in Indochina during the past 3000 years. There were about 100 family names for more than 56 million people, and of those 100 names, "only a score" are in common usage today (Huynh, 1987). *Nguyên* (near pronunciation is /Nwee-un/) is the family name for more than 25% of the Vietnamese family units in the United States and Canada. With so many persons having the same family name, it has limited usefulness in identification; therefore, given names are used.

Names in Vietnam are always written family name first, middle name (or names) second, and given name last—for example, "Nguyên Thi Hồng" or "Trần Văn Hai." The same names may be used for males and females, and the middle name can be a clue as to gender. "Văn" used as a middle name usually indicates male gender ("Trần Văn Hai") compared with "Thị" (pronounced /Tee/), which is used for females (Nguyên Thị Hồng). Sometimes several middle names are used, and therefore there is no gender indicator.

After marriage, a woman keeps her maiden name and does not combine it with her husband's name. Informally she may be called by her given name or her husband's given name ("Mrs. Hai"), but formally she uses her full maiden name preceded by "*Bà,*" which can be used as a respectful "Mrs." Children take their father's family name. Customs are changing in the United States, but to avoid confusion, many Vietnamese-American wives are adopting their husband's family name. Either name may

be used, depending on the setting, and children have interesting choices when asked for "mother's name."

Given names usually have special meanings, often describing the baby or expressing the hopes of the parents for the baby. Names can be chosen from virtues or from nature or music; for example, "Hồng" means "rose" and "Xuân" means "spring." At home or in the village, people may be called by their number in the sibling ranking, rather than by their given names, which explains the nicknames of Nam (fifth) or "Bảy" (seventh).

Today, many babies born in the United States are given both an American name and a Vietnamese name. This is not a new practice for the Vietnamese. During the past half-century, for example, the Chinese Vietnamese were commanded by law to change their Chinese given names to Vietnamese names. These persons may also have taken a Christian name when they converted to Christianity. In this resettlement period, almost every Vietnamese child who has an English first name can also give a Vietnamese name if asked.

Except for close friends and coworkers, Vietnamese custom dictates that a person's name is used with a title, never alone. An example of this in English would be "Mr. Bill," "Mrs. Mary," "Director James," or "Uncle John." Titles are important and therefore should be selected carefully by the speaker to convey appropriate respect as well as sometimes to place emotional distance between the speaker and the listener.

members becoming acculturated into the American way of life, while parents and grandparents retain more traditional values (Tran, 1991).

The Vietnamese concept of family and extended family that has existed across generations as a "super organic unit" is profoundly different from the individualism of the nuclear family in the United States in the beginning of the twenty-first century. And this disparity continues to strongly affect the stress levels of Vietnamese communities in the many pressures toward acculturation. Every culture has particular characteristics that help a member of the culture meet everyday life situations. When a cornerstone of the cultural structure is attacked, the cost of the resulting anxiety cannot be overestimated.

Socialized Role of Children

Children are socialized to their roles in the family at an early age. Children are to obey and respect all elders,

address them by correct titles, and correctly cross their arms over the chest and bow slightly from the hips when introduced or coming into the presence of elders.

There is increasing concern noted in the literature with the practice in the West of equating the Asian concept of "training" with the Western ideas of "authoritarian" and "control" types of child rearing. Chao (1994) noted that these terms may have entirely different implications for Asians because they are from a different cultural system, an American-European cultural tradition Asians do not necessarily share. The Asian concept of "training" describes the responsibility of parents to be highly involved, caring, and concerned. The mother as the central caretaker has major responsibility for promoting the success of the child, having the child physically near her, even through the night. Chao notes that Asian immigrant children do well in U.S. schools, often not true for the U.S. "authoritarian-type"–parented offspring.

Rudy and Grusec (2001) examined "authoritarian" Asian parenting and the transmission of values. Again, control seemed to be less the determinant; rather the warmth, involvement, and kindness perceived by the child make the difference. Also, the importance of whether the culture is an individualistic or collectivistic culture and the dilemma of the immigrant parents (and African-American parents) raising children as minorities in a culture seen as a high-risk environment for the child personally and for the group. "Best values" may be best values for the whole group rather than simply the individual.

Although not mentioning Vietnamese specifically, in the article, "Understanding Context and Culture in the Parenting Approaches of Immigrant South Asian Mothers," Maiter and George (2003) caution social workers against counseling these parents to accept Western culture, but rather establish support groups where parents support each other while finding their way as they "train" their children to survive in their new culture—and also survive in their old one.

Vietnamese children in the United States who are in school and learning English at a faster rate than their seniors at home are often placed in the role of translator. This situation, continued over a period of time, gives the child a sense of power in the family hierarchy that is difficult for both the child and the family.

Education

Before 1954, Hanoi was the educational center for Vietnam and contained most of the medical and dental schools. After the Geneva Accords, South Vietnam had its own educational centers in Saigon, Hue, and Can Tho, but the demand far exceeded the supply. The high demand and limited seats in the high schools and universities caused many students to delay their education, go abroad, or, for the men, be drafted.

Today in the United States, education continues to be highly valued in the Vietnamese community. The Vietnamese, like their other Asian-American counterparts, continue to excel in educational attainment. These data illuminate some interesting trends. For example, in 2013, among Vietnamese-American men 25 years of age and older, 73.3% were high school graduates, and 29.9% held a bachelor's degree or higher. Similarly, among Vietnamese women 25 years of age and older, 69.7% were high school graduates and 27.0% held a bachelor's degree or higher (U.S. Department of Commerce, Bureau of the Census, *American Community Survey*, 2013).

Religion

Vietnam has a history of religious tolerance except for the period immediately before the French takeover, when Christians were suspected of being spies. More recently, the official government position is religious tolerance, with much of the governance being left to the local officials.

Three major religions from China have combined to strongly influence Vietnamese thought and practice and become an ingrained part of the culture during the past centuries: Buddhism, Confucianism, and Taoism. Buddhism is considered less an organized orthodoxy than a state of mind, using the Four Noble Truths taught by Buddha: (1) life is suffering, (2) suffering is caused by desire, (3) suffering can be eliminated by eliminating desire, and (4) to eliminate desire, one must follow the eightfold path.

Confucianism is a code of ethics and emphasizes hierarchy of society, worship of ancestors, and respect for age, customs, teacher, and family. Taoism from Tao, or "The Way," originated in the sixth century B.C. and is a creative principle that governs the physical universe. When things are allowed to take their natural course, they move toward harmony and perfection. Therefore, individuals should attempt to blend into the natural world rather than try to conquer it (U.S. Department of Commerce, Bureau of the Census, *The Asian Population*, 2015).

Two minor religious sects, Cao Dai and Hoa Hao (harmony), began in Vietnam during the past century, with a present combined following of about 3 million. Another belief system, Animism, continues to have a strong influence among the mountain tribal groups. It includes practices to deal with demons, evil spirits, angry gods, and elements of the natural world.

The first Catholic missionary arrived in Vietnam in 1513, and Jesuits arrived in the early 1600s. The Protestants came in the early 1900s. Today Christians number over 2 million. Buddhists (along with many Vietnamese who consider themselves Buddhists because of their practices relating to their ancestors) claim approximately two thirds of the country's 79 million people. Many Vietnamese have turned to both Eastern and Western religions following the 1975 change of government.

Values

Respect and harmony are the two most important values in the Vietnamese culture and are based on the three major religious belief systems that have dominated the country. The strength of filial piety in the culture expresses the first value in many ways and throughout the life cycle.

Preserving harmony affects the lifestyle of a culture, from the highest government echelons to the most remote villages, from handling information to dealing with world conflicts. Specifically, it can affect health care decision making. Families may be less willing to share bad news with the group. Family members tend to be more likely to accept

TABLE 18-2 Comparison of Eastern and Western Value Systems

Eastern System	Western System
Harmony with nature	Mastery of nature (skyscraper)
Tradition	Change, innovation
Hierarchy	Mobility, upward or downward movement
Age	Youth
Extended family (few family names)	Nuclear family, small, individualistic
Convergent thinking	Divergent thinking
Cyclical concept of time	Specific point, schedules, clocks
Group orientation and reward	Self-concept and self-actualization
Rote learning	Discovery learning
Conformity	Competition

From Cao, A. Q. (1986). Linguistic and cultural issues in refugees. In *The next decade: the 1986 Conference on Refugee Health Care Issues and Management*. 1986 Refugee Health Care Conference Proceedings (pp. 70–75), University of Miami; Nguyen, D. (1988). Culture shock: a study of Vietnamese culture and the concept of health and disease. *Journal of the Association of Vietnamese Medical Professionals in Canada, 98*, 26–30.

decisions made by the family, feeling the decisions were made for the overall good. Clients may be more willing to endure hardship or pain quietly to avoid causing problems or inconvenience for the family. When the belief values common to the Oriental or Eastern system found in Vietnam and those of the Occidental or Western system found in the United States are compared (Table 18-2), the nature and extent of the tasks of acculturation faced by the Vietnamese who must mesh two systems are apparent.

The Asian and Pacific Islanders as a Group

Although many surveys handle Asian and Pacific Islanders (APIs) as a single group, it is imperative to keep in mind that the 2010 U.S. Census identified 30 Asian and 21 Pacific Islands groups in the API (U.S. Department of Commerce, Bureau of the Census, *American Community Survey*, 2015). The label includes more than 30 distinct ethnocentric entities, each with its own languages and customs. With this diversity, unless the specific ethnicity of the individual is known, generalizations must be avoided.

The "model minority" is a good example of the extreme unevenness within the API designation. In 2009, there were many API immigrants with an annual income above $50,000, but even greater numbers had income at or below the poverty level. In education, the API group could boast the highest percentage of women age 23 years and older who had completed college in 2004 (U.S. Department of Commerce, Bureau of the Census, *The Asian Population*, Census Brief, 2013). The disparity has been referred to as the "bipolar nature" of the API status, in which the successes of some API groups mask the severe problems of other API groups (Braun & Browne, 1998). For example, McPhee (2002) noted that Asian immigrants as a whole are healthier than their U.S. counterparts; however, the pattern is not uniform, and data used to estimate the whole API population are deceptive. To ensure accurate research data, it is important to ascertain the specific ethnic identity of the test group and not to mix populations (Fong & Mokuau, 1994).

In 2013, 66.1% of Vietnamese Americans participated in the labor force. Among Vietnamese Americans participating in the labor force, 32.6% held jobs in management, professional, or related occupations; 29.4% held jobs in service occupations; 16.5% held jobs in sales or office occupations, and 16.5% held jobs in production, transportation, or material-moving occupations (U.S. Department of Commerce, Bureau of the Census, *American Community Survey*, 2013). In 2013, the median family income for Vietnamese Americans was $58,289 as compared with the rest of the general population at $52,250. Unlike other Asian Americans, the median family income and the median per capita income are both somewhat lower than the rest of the general population and are significantly lower especially for the median family income for other Asian Americans. The median per capita income for Vietnamese men was $40,940 as compared with $45,320 for the rest of the general population. Similarly for Vietnamese American women, the median per capita income was $30,924 as compared with $35,299 for the rest of the general population (U.S. Department of Commerce, Bureau of the Census, *American Community Survey*, 2013).

Implications for Nursing Care

Because of the high priority placed on respect, harmony, filial piety, and material sharing found in most Vietnamese family systems, both immediate and extended family serve a significant role in providing emotional, physical, and economic support for the Vietnamese patient. A restriction to two visitors per patient in a hospital is incomprehensible to many Vietnamese, who may be used to large family gatherings in the home during illness. The feeling of support from the family outweighs any extra burden from the presence of additional family members and friends.

The culturally competent nurse will include family members in planning care and assisting with care whenever possible. If the client cannot speak English, the family will usually be appreciative if the nurse asks someone to stay with the client to serve as translator.

In most cases, communication about plan of care, legal documents needed, or preference of treatment options should be handled with a person designated by the family. Depending on the English proficiency within the family, the person speaking with the staff may be an interpreter. When an interpreter is used, adequate time should be given for the family to clearly understand treatment options. The value of respect and harmony can cause reluctance to tell family members of the client the true diagnosis or prognosis, especially if they are elderly. For example, a family may ask that the client not be told of a terminal diagnosis.

In addition to the potential to upset harmony in the group, it is sometimes believed that the diagnosis will hasten the death and cause the patient to give up prematurely. For many Buddhists, karma determines when death comes. This orientation makes the signing of informed consent and advance directives at best puzzling and, at worst, totally irrelevant. The nurse should appreciate that an elderly patient may delay signing papers until a designated family member arrives. Understanding the values of each individual client and family is essential to providing culturally competent care.

TIME

The Vietnamese culture dates back thousands of years, and this antiquity is reflected in time orientation. Emphasis is placed on ancestors and their wishes, memories, and graves. Most Vietnamese people have been oriented to think of time in terms of cycles, events, or occurrences (Hoang & Erickson, 1982). Since many Vietnamese individuals, even those who are not Buddhist, have some belief in reincarnation, time is less of a fixed point (here and gone) and more of a recurring reality. In other words, there was yesterday, there is today, and there will be tomorrow . . . which will in fact be today, followed by tomorrow . . . and so on. This belief results in a less stressful and less time-conscious pace than that commonly experienced in the West. Being late or early is not considered a problem.

As refugees, Vietnamese people practiced a present- and future-time orientation as they struggled to survive and focused on food, housing, employment, transportation, child care, and education. Today, Vietnamese Americans have goals and save for the future, and for many the motivation to live wisely may not only be to please the ancestors (past) but may also be connected with "the good life" (present) or the anticipation of heaven or reincarnation (future).

Implications for Nursing Care

The nurse should be aware that the concept of illness prevention requires both a future- and a present-time orientation. Illness prevention is a difficult concept if a person lacks a scientific understanding of disease processes. The nurse should also be aware that Vietnamese-American clients may believe that luck and fate play a significant role in suffering and that illness may easily be considered a result of spiritual failure or punishment. Agreeing to vaccinations for children, having a Pap smear or a mammogram, or even just the act of seeking medical care, is influenced by many factors, including time orientation.

Noncompliance with keeping appointments is often a result of factors other than time orientation. Some noncompliance can be traced to not understanding oral or appointment card communications or not being able to read the instructions. The nurse needs to review carefully the appointment card and any instructions given to be certain the client understands what is written. When a client is given a phone number to call for an appointment or for assistance, it is important to determine for sure that the client has a telephone available, knows how to use it, and has the correct clinic telephone number. Arriving at a clinic appointment on time can be a complex assignment for a Vietnamese American client, considering the usual work schedule of Vietnamese households, transportation by bus or subway, child care for those left at home, and the translation and challenges along the way.

Time orientation also contributes to the frustration of the nurse attempting to obtain a chronological sequence of the history of an illness. Especially rural Vietnamese may use life events such as births, marriages, or deaths rather than a specific date on the calendar to mark points of time. Sometimes the nurse can clarify historic events by referring to one of these events: "Did you start having these stomach pains before your husband died or since then?"

ENVIRONMENTAL CONTROL

Concepts of Illness

The medical system in Vietnam is a complex one, providing various options for health care from which the Vietnamese person may choose. Many traditional Vietnamese individuals tend to combine Chinese medicine with scientific techniques brought in from the West (Tran, 1972, 1980; personal communication, 1989). For most, the choice is usually deliberate and purposeful but rarely rigid or restricted in any single direction. "The baseline is often a set of time-honored beliefs, customs, and usages that are faithfully followed by some, fiercely contested by others, but more or less consciously incorporated by the majority".

Tran (1980; personal communication, 1989) divided the explanations of cause of illness into three types: naturalistic (folk medicine), supernaturalistic (animistic beliefs), and metaphysical (the theory of hot and cold). None of these theories excludes the others, and a client may explain illness by aspects of all three. A fourth explanation of germs as a cause of illness is gaining an increased following as Vietnamese interact with persons in Western cultures.

Natural Causes. The naturalistic explanation for illness encourages a search for a natural or obvious cause of the symptoms, such as bad food or contaminated water or an obvious cause-and-effect relationship. To counteract the effects of these natural elements, an informal body of knowledge has been collected about indigenous medicinal herbs, therapeutic diets, and simple medical and hygienic measures. The information is usually transmitted orally and often treated with secrecy, remaining inside the clan or extended family. Vietnamese folk medicine may fall into the category of either *thu c nam* (southern medicine) or *thu c b c* (northern medicine), which more closely resembles Chinese medicine (Box 18-3).

Supernatural Causes. The supernaturalistic explanation for disease lays the blame on supernatural powers, such as gods, demons, or spirits. The illness is considered a punishment for a fault, for a violation of religious or ethical codes, or for an act of omission causing displeasure to a deity. In the supernaturalistic theory, disease may be caused by black magic or the evil incantation of an enemy who has bought the services of a sorcerer (Westermeyer & Winthrop, 1979).

The supernatural explanation for illness is the more likely choice of the mountain tribespeople or peasants from the rural areas. The Hmong (meaning "free"), for example, believe the individual's spirit is the guardian of the person's well-being. If the spirit is happy, the person is happy and well. A severe shock or scare may cause the individual's spirit to leave, and the individual will become ill. The shaman then must come and call the spirit to return. Copper or silver bracelets, necklaces, or anklets lock the soul to oneself so that it cannot leave.

Metaphysical Causes. A metaphysical explanation for illness may be found in areas of Vietnam heavily influenced by the Chinese (Box 18-4). The metaphysical explanation is built on the theory that nature and the body operate within a delicate balance between two opposite elements: the *Am* and *Duong* (Vietnamese) or the *yin* and *yang* (Chinese), such as female and male, dark and light, or hard and soft. In medicine the opposites are expressed as "hot" and "cold," and health is the result of a balance between hot and cold elements, which results in harmonious functioning of the viscera and harmony with the environment. An excess or shortage in either direction causes discomfort and illness.

All illnesses, foods, medications, and herbs are classified along a continuum according to their "hot" and "cold" qualities. Hot medications and food are used to balance the need in cold diseases and vice versa. Fever, ulcers, and infections are usually hot, although some febrile illnesses are cold. Severity, cause, and duration can influence where diseases are placed. Hot usually includes strong, rough, spicy, and oily foods. Beef, eggs, cheese, and chocolates are usually hot; chicken, fish, honey, and fresh vegetables are cold. Some fruits are hot; tropical fruits are cold. The source and how food is prepared can be significant. Almost all Western medicines are considered hot and Oriental herbs are cold. Water is usually cold but is not always advised for treatment.

Different countries and locales develop their own version of the Chinese system, and there is considerable variation in application. Knowledgeable practitioners seem reluctant to construct "lists" of hot and cold specifics, possibly because of the complexities involved in correct use. Laypeople, on the other hand, often seem quite certain of what should be used and when, probably because of what their family has practiced for generations. These ideas are strongly integrated into the thought systems of many Vietnamese and can cause major stress and conflict for the client and family in the Western setting.

Germs. There is widespread understanding that disease can come from contaminants (germs) in the environment. The basic sciences were studied in the upper levels in the schools, and through decades of French occupation and more recently the American influence, even the most rural Vietnamese have become acquainted with the healing power of antibiotics in eye ointments, oral medications, and injections.

Death Beliefs and Practices

Many of the beliefs and practices about death are so woven into the fabric of Vietnamese life that it is difficult to separate them into either religious or cultural concepts (Table 18-3). An important aspect of filial piety and family loyalty is an obligation that extends beyond death: observing the anniversary day of the death, gathering at the family home and altar, and cleaning the ancestral tombs. For Buddhists, typically there are special observances, usually with elaborate rites at 100 days, and 1 and 2 years after the death.

Remembrance of deceased elders is culminated during Memory Day, a day set aside annually in homage of the person on the anniversary of the day on which the family

BOX 18-3 Common Folk Practices

1. **Cạo gió** ("rub-wind": skin rubbing with a coin) is a folk practice used for diseases caused by wind entering the body, such as a common cold or flulike symptoms. A layer of balm or ointment is spread on the skin over the affected area—often the chest, upper back, or shoulders. A coin (preferably the size of a nickel or quarter) is pressed on the skin and drawn in one direction, and the coin is moved a short distance on the skin without breaking the skin. This is repeated several times, and if dark blood appears under the skin, the treatment is considered to be working. Often these ecchymotic stripes are continued in symmetrical rows down the back or chest. The purpose is to create areas where the offending wind or air may escape from the body. It is usually not a painful procedure for children or adults, and most report feeling improved by the procedure (Lan, 1988).

2. **Bắtgió** ("catch-wind": skin pinching) is a folk practice used for a headache. Fingers and thumbs are pressed on both temples in an attempt to move the blood across the forehead toward a spot between the eyes. After this has been repeated several times, the area on the forehead between the eyes is pinched between the thumb and forefinger and twisted slightly. If petechiae or ecchymoses appear, the treatment is considered successful. Skin pinching is also used on the neck for sore throat.

3. **Xông** is a folk practice in which Vicks VapoRub or a similar agent or herb is stirred into scalding water. Depending on the reason for the treatment, the patient may simply inhale the vapor or may be treated under a blanket as in a steam tent.

4. **Inhalation of aromatic oils** or liniments, such as menthol, eucalyptus, or mint-based aromatic oils, is used as a folk practice for symptoms such as motion sickness, indigestion, or cold or wind illness. The oils and liniments may be carried in vials in a pocket or purse for ready access and may be smelled when necessary; rubbed on the temple, under the nose, or on the abdomen; or taken internally in small amounts.

5. **Balm and medicated plasters** are a folk practice involving direct application to the skin. Many common balms, such as Red Tiger Balm, *Cù-Là-Mác-Su*, or *Nhị*. Thiên-Dường oil, are available in Asian shops, with certain balms obtainable only from an Asian pharmacy. *Salonpas* is a Japanese preparation (Hisamitsu Pharmaceutical Co., Tosu Sagu, Japan) with widespread availability and use. Many of the ointments have a mild "deep heat" quality on application and are used for bone and muscle problems as well as a variety of other ills.

6. **Herbal decoctions, soups, and condiments** are used as a folk practice for a variety of symptoms and to maintain health (Spector, 2004). The more complex, involving a variety of ingredients and combinations, are prepared by a pharmacist, whereas the simpler ones are prepared at home. The recipes may be generations old and have a mystical or secret quality about them. Many medicines are prepared to be given as soups. A familiar treatment is the use of garlic for hypertension. There is increasing interest and experimental evaluation of Eastern herbs in Western pharmaceutical firms.

7. **Giác hơi** ("cup-vapor": cup suction) is a folk practice in which small, heated, cuplike forms applied to the skin cause a suction on the skin as the cups cool. The suction is used to remove unwanted wind or other elements from the body and is a favorite remedy for joint and muscle pains.

8. **String tying** is a folk practice to control spirits. This practice is more common among the mountain people. Although the string, which stays on the arm, on the leg, or around the neck for long periods, may become dirty, it is relatively harmless and is a source of security for the wearer and significant others. Usually it can be left on without difficulty for anyone except health care workers, who may not understand the possible significance of this practice.

---

member died. Memory Day is more important in most families in Vietnam than birthdays. In the United States, a 48-year-old mother of two had a large portrait of her late father-in-law displayed in her living room. She said, "I do in Vietnam the same as I do here. Memory Day. Like my husband . . . the day his father died is June 30, that day my kids, never mind about where they are, they have to come home to celebrate that day, the Memory Day for your grandfather dead. . . . The only one I do the same thing in Vietnam" (Davis, 2000, p. 143). Although most of the ancestors are buried in Vietnam and the custom of gathering in the family home around the family altar and ancestral graves is not possible, many Vietnamese in the United States continue to observe Memory Day.

White or black is the color of mourning, and at the time of death and for a period following, black clothing may be worn by family members (Dinh, Kemp, & Rasbridge, 2000). Traditionally in Vietnam and somewhat in the United

BOX 18-4 Chinese Medicine

Any attempt at probing into the nature of Asian health practices must begin with a search into the age-old philosophy from which they—and indeed all Eastern concepts of health and illness, cure, and death—evolved (Branch & Paxton, 1976).

Chinese medicine is a 5000-year-old system of medicine in which an 81-volume classic on the philosophy of life became the primary medical textbook. Body, mind, and soul are integrated and never separated. Man is seen in relationship to the environment. The system encompasses all of the following (in order of their importance as preventive concepts): philosophy, meditation, nutrition, martial arts, herbology, acumassage, acupressure, moxibustion, acupuncture, and spiritual healing (Branch & Paxton, 1976; Huard & Wong, 1968).

Part of the theoretical and philosophical basis for Chinese medicine comes from the Taoist concept that nature maintains a balance in all things and that as part of the universe, man interacts with this balance. The balance is measured in terms of energy and is articulated by the principle of *yin* and *yang* (negative–positive, dark–light, cold–hot, feminine–masculine, etc.).

An important difference between Chinese and Western medicine is the emphasis on prevention rather than disease and crisis intervention. This difference can be illustrated by the Chinese story of the "old days," when people would go to their physician to have their energy balanced. The physician, knowing the client well, would prescribe the specific approach to life, type of meditation, exercise, diet, and occasional herbs to keep the client healthy. For this service the doctor would be paid regularly. If the client became ill, however, the client stopped paying, and the treatment was free of charge. This may not be as true for Chinese medicine today, but it does underline a major difference in approach from Western medicine.

Disease theory and "germs" are two other areas where the basic approach separates the two systems. Western medicine has spent the past 200 years identifying disease-causing organisms under the microscope and finding ways of destroying them, in many cases with dramatic success. The goal of the treatment is to destroy the microorganisms causing the illness.

In Chinese medicine, when illness results in an imbalance caused by faulty diet or strong emotional feelings, body harmony can be restored through self-restraint and the use of a corrective diet, often aided by herbs. Action is taken not to kill organisms but to restore a balanced state, countering the effects of unwise lifestyles or food. When the *yin–yang* balance is disturbed, the body is more likely to become ill. Use of massage, steam baths, and the application of Tiger Oil are methods to protect health and prevent illness (Spector, 2004).

TABLE 18-3 The Meaning of Life, Illness, and Death

Asian	American
Life	
Life = suffering	Life = happiness, health, opportunity
One's life is determined by various factors out of one's control	One has control over one's own life
Your life is not yours	Your life is your own
Death and Illness	
Part of normal life cycle	Disruption of normal life cycle
Bad luck, result of former deeds, and so forth	Personal failure
Something to be accepted and dealt with calmly	Something to be beaten
Response to Illness	
Ideal response: serenity, stoicism	Seeking control, fighting (beating) illness, heroic self-healing
Possible Problems	
Helplessness	The burden of having to be positive
Denial	Sense of personal failure
Depression	Anger, depression, difficulty letting go
Sick Role	
Permission for regression and dependency	Little permission for regression and dependency
Cooperation	Participation
Conflicts over unmet expectations and dependency needs	Conflicts over losing independence and control

From Nilchaikovit, K., Hill, J., & Holland, J. (1993). The effects of culture on illness behavior and medical care. *General Hospital Psychiatry, 15,* 41–50.

States, for a specified period of time some family members wear a black armband or a small piece of black cloth pinned on the shirt or blouse.

Burial in Vietnam is preferred, although cremation is also practiced. Especially for older people, cremation is chosen so the ashes can be taken back to Vietnam and buried near the family, a very important promise to fulfill. For some, only through the proper observance of age-old traditions is the soul of the loved one set free; thus traditions after death are the ultimate familial duty and sign of respect.

Implications for Nursing Care

Vietnamese American clients who are oriented to Eastern beliefs and practices regarding illness may explain their illness by entities totally unfamiliar to Western practitioners. The nurse should not be surprised by complaints of being hit by the wind, bad karma problems, "the evil eye," or problems with the spirits (Box 18-5).

If the disease is understood to be a problem of hot and cold balance, the nurse should attempt to learn which the patient understands to be lacking and what corrective plan has been used. If fever or diarrhea, which are both "cold" diseases, is the problem, then the Eastern system of treatment would restrict fluids. On the other hand, Western-style treatment would consider fluids to be very important. A brief explanation should be given. For example, if the patient is losing fluids from the body through perspiring or through diarrhea, to restore the balance, it must be replaced. Promptly giving medication to lower the temperature and stop the diarrhea will also help. Since verbal disagreement with the caregiver is rare, and if the situation involves an elderly person or a baby, it may be wise to keep the family in the care area for a period to demonstrate and see that fluids are given. Fluids may need to be given intravenously.

Serious problems may result during longer-term illness when food is restricted to correct an imbalance. Fresh fruits and vegetables (considered cold) are often banned in the case of pregnancy. Pork or chicken, but not beef, is added to the diet slowly. Maternity clients who eat a very salty diet with almost no fruits or vegetables may acquire a nutritional deficiency. Since the theory of hot and cold has been used by many people for generations with some success, it is important to understand that these beliefs will not be discarded immediately just because Western health care providers do not approve. The nurse should try to work with the family in combining approaches to facilitate a high level of wellness.

Probably the most serious problem in the use of Eastern remedies as the first line of treatment is the delay in getting help. Fatalism, denial, acceptance of illness as part of one's destiny, or identification of the cause as non-Western may all be reasons for delay in seeking medical care. Usually Vietnamese have had no or very little preventive care experience and tend to go for help when they have symptoms. When the symptoms disappear, often medications are stopped until the next episode.

The nurse who does physical assessments of Vietnamese-American patients should be aware that ecchymotic areas may be the result of "coin rubbing" on the skin to rid the body of harmful substances. After years of blaming Vietnamese parents or caregivers for child abuse and the like, Western practitioners are at last being told to accept the practice as a nurturant and not a harmful folk practice (Yeatman & Dang, 1980).

The Vietnamese use of herbal medicines in soups and teas is not surprising since herbal medicine has official government sanction through the Institute of Popular and Traditional Medicine and is taught in the medical school curriculum in Vietnam. Imported medications are expensive and less familiar.

Although the benefits of folk medicine are likely to outweigh the risks, the nurse relating to Vietnamese-American clients should be aware of possible risks:

1. Toxicity may result from the use of remedies containing heavy metals (lead, mercury, arsenic). On several occasions, high blood lead levels among Vietnamese and Hmong children were tentatively blamed on folk medicine; however, a well-controlled study of all under-7, newly arrived refugee children in Massachusetts in a 4-year period indicated that 27% of the Vietnamese group had elevated blood lead levels. Country of origin was the chief predictor, and the cause is not certain (Geltman, Brown, & Cochran, 2001).
2. Inadequate labeling of Chinese medicines may result in excessive use of chemicals, such as phenylbutazone or aminopyrine, neither of which is listed as an ingredient. Agranulocytosis cases are blamed on this.
3. Human error. Many herbs and plants such as mushrooms and seeds found in the United States are new to Southeast Asians. Some have been mistaken, resulting in poisonings.

As Vietnamese-American clients experience success with Western medicine and develop positive relationships with health care providers and the system, and as children move through the school systems, new understandings will emerge for both the Eastern clients and the Western health care givers.

It is interesting to note that, while for many Vietnamese Western medicine is foreign, the growth of the Vietnam drug market has been considered the most promising in the world. Some 400 drug companies operate in the country. Drug advertising from manufacturers to prescribers, dispensers, and consumers is intensive and not always

BOX 18-5   Common Misunderstandings about Illness and Diagnostic or Treatment Procedures

1. **Drawing blood** for diagnostic purposes may cause a crisis for a Vietnamese-American patient. The patient may complain, although often not to the health care worker, of feeling weak and tired for varying periods after the procedure. Such symptoms may last for months. A Vietnamese-American client may feel that any body tissue or fluid removed cannot be replaced, and that once it is removed, the body will continue to suffer the loss, not only in this life but also in the next life.

2. **Donating blood** may be a major decision for the Vietnamese. In one rural hospital in Vietnam, Western staff members made an effort not only to teach the Vietnamese staff the "facts" about donating blood but also to have the Vietnamese staff assist as the Western staff donated blood and, after a short recovery time, rejoined the medical team. Vietnamese staff members were invited to have their blood typed and to place their names on a possible donor list for emergency situations. Some did donate blood when the need arose (although, because Vietnamese often weigh less than 100 lb, only one half or three fourths of a unit was drawn).

3. **Donation of body parts**, such as the donation of an eye after death, is an act that is often viewed with much skepticism by many Vietnamese individuals, who have been heavily influenced by Buddhist beliefs that a body part cannot be replaced once it is removed and that the body may suffer in the next life. Even those who have been Christians for several generations may be very serious about care given to the body after death and are unlikely to feel comfortable with such practices.

4. **Hospitalization and surgery** were often considered a last resort in Vietnam. Unless insurance considerations are important, outpatient care for the refugee is likely to cause much less anxiety and should be offered as an option when possible.

5. **Clergy visitation** is usually associated with "last rites" by the Vietnamese, especially those who have been influenced by the Catholic religion. A visit by the clergy may be considered an indication that the situation is grave, and the common practice of priests and ministers visiting clients in hospitals in the United States can be quite upsetting for Vietnamese-American clients. It is important to provide the client with a careful explanation of a visit by the hospital clergy.

6. **Giving flowers** to the sick is a practice that may surprise and upset a Vietnamese-American client who has not been given an explanation of this practice. In Vietnam, flowers are usually reserved for the rites of the dead.

7. **American medicines** are considered by the Vietnamese to be much more concentrated than Eastern medicines. American medicine is likely to be given in tablet form, rather than in tea or soups. Also, Americans are often much larger than the average Vietnamese; therefore, medication needs to be carefully titrated so that it will not harm the Vietnamese-American client. It is important for the professional to let the client know that small stature has been considered when the dosage was calculated, which can be done by either weighing the client or by orally discussing this when the prescription is written. It is not an uncommon practice for some Vietnamese-American clients to take only half of their prescribed dosage.

8. **The germ theory** can be very confusing to some of the mountain tribes people who may have had less exposure to Western ideas. Clients with animistic beliefs have a supernatural or spirit-world disease-cause orientation. In an effort to move the client's understanding into the scientific, or natural, world, germs are presented as the cause of disease because they are a component of the real Western world. For all practical purposes, however, germs also cannot be seen and are far less real to the refugee with animistic beliefs than the spirits and demons that the client knows can cause trouble.

accurate or within ethical guidelines. David Finer, a Swedish medical reporter, has published documentaries warning both the Vietnamese and the world that lack of regulation can have critical effects. However, despite the efforts of the World Health Organization (WHO) and the Swedish International Development Agency to develop the national drug policy in 1996, the drug market in Vietnam is "effectively unregulated" (Finer, 1999, p. 21).

BIOLOGICAL VARIATIONS

Body Size and Structure

Vietnamese people generally have small frames and build, with average body weights between 80 and 130 lb. An overweight Vietnamese person is uncommon, except among the Vietnamese-Chinese population (Williams & Westermeyer, 1986).

Blood Type

Approximately 30% of the Vietnamese have the type B blood group, which is present in only 11% of White people. Fortunately, the availability of type O (including O+) red blood cells from the "universal donor" group as well as good transportation systems have helped keep the ratio (more than 30% of Vietnamese Americans) from becoming a concern in the areas of high Vietnamese concentration throughout the United States (Bloodbook .com, 2011).

Skin Color

The skin coloring is usually light to medium with yellow tones. Newborns are usually fair skinned. In the United States there appears to be a higher-than-average incidence of newborn icterus among Vietnamese Americans, as compared with the rest of the general population.

Other Visible Physical Characteristics

Noses may be small and "classically Asian" or larger with a less-defined bridge. The eyelids usually have an epicanthic fold and a slight droop over the cartilage plate. Both variations are common to Asians.

Teeth are usually proportionately large, with a high incidence of mandibular torus (lump on the inner side of the mandible near the second molar). Some dentists who have treated Vietnamese clients estimate that at least 40% of Vietnamese Americans have these tori, compared with 7% of the White U.S. population (Nguyen, personal communication, 1988).

Enzymatic and Genetic Variations

Although some Vietnamese people enjoy milk, cheese, and ice cream, an unknown percentage, possibly as high as 50%, have some congenital lactase deficiency. For most Vietnamese people, the intolerance is not a total one, and many Vietnamese persons can digest some milk in small amounts without incidence. For some Vietnamese individuals, a glass of milk can simply be an inexpensive solution for constipation. Vietnamese babies show a lesser degree of the deficiency by their ability to accept the usual formula preparations without difficulty.

Alcohol is broken down in the body by two enzymes: one converts the alcohol to acetaldehyde, which the other enzyme then breaks down to acetate. Several genes code for the second enzyme, aldehyde dehydrogenase, and a variant of one of these produces an inactive enzyme, which then allows the buildup of acetaldehyde in the body. Depending on the combination of genes inherited, the accumulated acetaldehyde causes the "flushing" reaction—various amounts of facial flushing, nausea, headache, dizziness, or rapid heartbeat (Makimoto, 1998).

This unpleasantness may discourage people from drinking, even casually, and was thought to possibly lower the likelihood of alcoholism among the Vietnamese. However, studies over the years suggest that drinking norms and the availability of alcoholic beverages probably have at least as great an impact on alcohol consumption in Asian populations as do genetic factors (Makimoto, 1998).

Medical Problems among Vietnamese Refugees

In a classic study, Hoang and Erickson (1982) reported on a survey identifying the major medical problems of 594 Vietnamese refugees (see following list). The present health care literature indicates numbers 1, 5, 7, and 9 have all but disappeared. Numbers 2, 3, and 6 are present but not in dangerous percentages. However, numbers 4, 8, and 10 continue and are of even more concern than they were in the original survey.

1. Skin: superficial fungal infections and scabies, 10% to 15%
2. Teeth: moderate to severe dental problems, 90%
3. Endocrine system: thyroid diseases, especially goiters, 10% in the group of 400 and 6% in the group of 194
4. Cardiovascular system: mitral valve prolapse, 1.7%; hypertension, 7% of adults over 30 years of age; rheumatic heart disease, 1%
5. Renal system: microscopic hematuria may be present with no specific cause
6. Blood: anemia, 16%
7. Parasites: ascariasis, hookworm infestation, giardiasis, trichuriasis (most common), and amebiasis
8. Hepatitis B surface antigen: 13%
9. Malaria: 2.5% of the sample of 194 persons had a history of malaria, and 1% of this number developed an acute episode
10. Psyche: 5% in the sample of 194 persons had "significant" psychiatric problems

Hypertension. In a classic but relevant study, Hoang and Erickson (1982) found that only 7% of the Vietnamese adult immigrants over age 30 had hypertension. However, risk factors were brought from Vietnam. The universal use of fish sauce daily in food preparation and seasoning produces a built-in high-sodium diet, and smoking among the men was common, especially in the military. In Vietnam, a diet normally low in red meats and fat and higher in fruits and green leafy vegetables, as well as the physical exercise of walking, biking, and working, made obesity and hypertension uncommon problems for the average villager, except for the Chinese or Chinese-Vietnamese.

However, newly arrived refugees faced stressors with communication and language problems; a diet high in red meats and fats and lower in fish, fruits, and vegetables; and, often, work that requires less physical exercise. In a classic and culturally sensitive work, Duong, Bohannon, and Ross (2001) interacted with 201 Vietnamese in two Gulf Coast communities. For this study, one of the meeting places was the only Vietnamese market in a 50-mile radius on a weekend shopping day. Findings from this study suggested that 88 (43%) had a blood pressure over 139 mm Hg systolic, over 89 mm Hg diastolic, or both. Of the 88 participants, 24 of them had blood pressures in excess of 179/100, and 13 were referred for a blood pressure of 180/110 or higher. One was sent for immediate attention for a blood pressure over 210/120. More than 75% of the sample had never been hospitalized or had surgery, 52% paid for their own medical care, and 59% did not see a medical provider regularly. About half were middle-aged, and 47% worked full-time. Risk factors identified include a "profound" need for health education related to cardiovascular disease, smoking, and alcohol use, as well as increased understanding of the need and ways to control diet, weight gain, and stress in their new setting and way of life. The research team began the final discussion of the report by stating "hypertension is likely to be a significant health risk in Vietnamese people and screening should be a part of all interaction between Vietnamese-Americans and care providers" (Duong et al., 2001, p. 10).

Hepatitis B.   Hepatitis B is the leading cause of liver cancer worldwide. Each year in the United States, 5000 people die of cirrhosis of the liver related to hepatitis B, another 1500 succumb because of hepatitis B itself, and another 1500 die of hepatitis B–related cancer of the liver (Wiecha, 1999). Hepatitis B virus (HBV) is endemic in South Asian populations, including the Vietnamese. Studies of Vietnamese adults in the United States verify rates from 7% to 14% (Hoang & Erickson, 1982; McPhee et al., 2003). The high rate of chronic infection is almost certainly linked with the high rates of liver and intrahepatic bile duct cancers among Vietnamese-American males (41.8 per 100,000 compared with 3 per 100,000 for U.S. White males). About two thirds of these cancers are hepatocellular carcinomas associated with hepatitis B and C virus infection (McPhee, 2002).

Hepatitis B can be transmitted horizontally through contact with blood products, through sexual contact, and through casual contact in the household. It can also be transmitted vertically in the newborn child. A neonatal infection often persists in a carrier state with significant risk of cirrhosis and hepatocellular carcinoma in early childhood. It is estimated that 25% of those chronically infected as infants or young children and 5% of adolescents and adults who become chronically infected die prematurely from chronic liver disease (McPhee et al., 2003). Infection during adolescence or adulthood presents a lower risk to the individual but can become a serious public health problem.

In the United States, HBV is already a national public health priority. A study near Boston assessed knowledge of the definition and risk factors of hepatitis B among 2816 middle- and high-school students in five ethnic groups, including 226 Vietnamese adolescents. The Vietnamese students (who had been tested for hepatitis B at three times the percentages in other groups) responded with the most correct definition (35.3% versus 22.6%). However, sexual contact with an infected person was correctly identified as a risk for infection by 880 (31.3%) of all the respondents, compared with 13.7% of the Vietnamese, the group with the highest seroprevalence of hepatitis B (Wiecha, 1999).

In transcultural studies, when there are unusual correlations, it is imperative to check for contributing factors. For example, when a disease is sexually transmitted and the traditional culture does not discuss sex openly or value sexual permissiveness, Vietnamese sons and daughters would be expected to simply avoid the subject—and the problem, taking their cues from their family, at least for the present. The result is that surveys report seemingly low concern and low-risk behaviors, despite incidence statistics relative to the cultural group.

To respond to the needs of this high-risk population, it is imperative that the facts of the disease be known and that cultural constraints alone not be counted on to provide the critical protection needed in the future. Noninfected persons can be protected against HBV and the sequelae by having three doses of human papillomavirus vaccine. The Centers for Disease Control and Prevention (CDC) recommends universal vaccination of all children ages 0 to 18 years. As of 2003, 42 states require protection to enter middle school (McPhee et al., 2003). Progress is being made, and data from the 1996 National Immunization Survey report that 88% of API (not specifically Vietnamese but including Vietnamese) children age 19 to 35 months had received three doses of the hepatitis B vaccine (McPhee et al., 2003). But beyond these covered groups are many unknowing and unprotected persons.

Dr. Stephen McPhee and his group, working with Suc Khoe La Vang (Health Is Gold), the Vietnamese Community Health Promotion Project of the University of California, San Francisco, Department of Medicine, designed and led a 3-year experiment on several ways to change this. The goal was to improve Vietnamese-American parents' awareness and knowledge about HBV, and the need for their children to get the available free vaccinations. They also organized a media education campaign in the large Houston, Texas, community (over 58,000) and a community mobilization strategy in Dallas (41,000), with 38,000 from the Washington, DC, area serving as a control group. Success was measured by the proportion of parents responding correctly to various knowledge questions as well as the vaccinations recommended. In Houston, a 2-year media blitz involved print and electronic media, billboards, calendars, and a 26-page, four-color booklet completed entirely in the Vietnamese language to showcase a campaign titled "Immunize Against Hepatitis B to Protect Future Generations," and more. For Dallas, a local Vietnamese-American community-based group contracted to plan and execute the community mobilization strategy. The 19-member coalition consisted of medical, public health, and education professionals; business leaders; editors; seniors; and homemakers, who worked together over a 3-year period to get the word out to get the vaccinations "caught up." The pre- and postcampaign contacts with the parents in both locations were encouraging and confirmed the good potential of these culturally appropriate efforts. According to McPhee et al. (2003), "In every community where Vietnamese Americans have settled in large numbers, they have established vibrant Vietnamese-language print, radio and television media. These media have flourished because [they] . . . are avid consumers of news, community information and advertising."

Economic considerations are also important for public policy, and an economic analysis of the preceding study by a group working with the CDC demonstrates in detail the advantages of hepatitis B prevention (Zhou et al., 2000). Longitudinal studies are needed to tell the story about how preventive medicine can affect the Vietnamese.

Tuberculosis Risk. Although the bacillus Calmette-Guérin (BCG) vaccine was widely used in Vietnam during the 1960s and was given to babies shortly after birth in hospitals across the country, the living conditions and general upheaval during the next 25 years affected the long-term effectiveness of any preventive effort. Between 1968 and 1974, the movement of people from the less secure countryside to the cities, with the accompanying overcrowding and poor nutritional status, simply exacerbated an already precarious situation.

BCG vaccination often produces a positive skin test, and there is no reliable way to distinguish a skin test reaction to BCG from that caused by tuberculosis (TB). Furthermore, people with latent infection have no symptoms of the illness and cannot spread TB to others. In their work with refugees from Vietnam, Hoang and Erickson (1982) recommended the use of isoniazid prophylactically for 1 year for all refugees under 35 years of age with positive skin tests, and that children with negative skin readings on arrival in the United States be checked in 3 to 6 months to single out false-negative readings. This practice continues in various forms in much of the country today.

According to a CDC report in 2005, there were 14,093 cases of active TB in the United States, and of these, 7656 (54.3%) were foreign born, with Vietnam as the third highest contributor with 576 of these cases (CDC, 2005). Similarly, according to the American Lung Association in 2010, there were more than 12,904 cases of active TB in the United States. Of that number, approximately one third of the cases were in foreign-born persons; of 7563 cases, 869 (11.4%) were from Vietnamese (American Lung Association, 2010).

Effective medications are available, but improper and sporadic use of the medicines often contributes to the emergence of multidrug-resistant (MDR) strains, an increasing problem worldwide (Lindsay, Narayan, & Rea, 1998). In the United States there was an MDR increase to 128 cases for 2004, 10 of them from Vietnam (CDC, 2005). For the first time in 50 years, six new TB drugs have been tested by humans. The hope is that the new medications will reduce the length of therapy time by 30% to 70%, making completion of the treatment more likely and, if effective, give more options in the treatment of persons with MDR bacilli.

Directly observed therapy (DOT) is a plan in which health care workers observe or assist TB patients as they take their medications. The plan can be clinic or field-based in the home, school, workplace, park, or any other convenient location. The average cost of a 6-month TB DOT program is approximately $1000 more than a non-DOT program, which compares favorably with the cost of treating MDR TB, with an average cost of over $200,000 (Mac, Doordan, & Carr, 1999).

During the early 1990s, the number of TB cases steadily rose in Santa Clara County, California, to 18.2 cases per 100,000 population in 1996. The county health department made the DOT plan an option for the Vietnamese and did a study among 30 of the patients (5 in the DOT program and 25 on the usual regimens) to check effectiveness. Results of the comparisons between the two groups showed that among the DOT group, all completed therapy, there were no relapses, and the sputum conversion rate was 2 to 7 weeks. On the other hand, among the non-DOT group, only 21 patients completed the course, 2 patients relapsed, and sputum conversion rates ranged from 4 to 16 weeks. These data suggest that DOT programs can effectively control TB (Mac et al., 1999).

Cancer. Records from the Cancer Hospital in Ho Chi Minh City (Saigon) from 1976 to 1981 showed that cervical cancer accounted for 53.3% of all cancers diagnosed among their female patients (Phipps, Cohen, Sorn, & Braitman, 1999). During the years following that finding in Saigon, thousands of women left Vietnam and settled in the United

States, surrounded by people speaking a different language, in a culture very different in many ways, with differing ways of accessing a strange medical system and help. These factors, coupled with the stresses of resettlement, would surely affect the cancer statistics that accompanied them to their new home.

Compared with breast cancer, cervical cancer is a disease of the "developing world," with 80% of over 470,000 cases worldwide as reported by the WHO. Until the 1970s, 75% to 80% of cervical cancer in the United States was in the invasive stage at the time of diagnosis. Today with Pap smears and vaginal examinations, 78% of cervical cancers are instead diagnosed in the *in situ* stage, reducing the mortality of cervical cancer by approximately 40% (Phipps et al., 1999). Stage of disease at time of diagnosis appears to be a major predictor of survival. Present mortality rates in Vietnam are twice those in the United States, and it is hoped that recent Vietnamese arrivals will have chances of lowering the risks the longer they are in the United States (Ho et al., 2005).

In the 1980s, breast cancer was reported as the leading cancer among Vietnamese females in the United States. But by 1996, the National Cancer Institute released its findings on cancer incidence and mortality in 11 U.S. racial and ethnic groups, and cervical cancer (43 per 100,000) was the most commonly diagnosed cancer among Vietnamese women, even though breast cancer was the most common for the other 10 groups. The rate was more than 2.5 times the rate for any of the other groups and nearly 5 times higher than that of American White women (Schulmeister & Lifsey, 1999).

Because of the urgency of early diagnosis of cervical cancer, there is frequent documentation of efforts (Ho et al., 2005) to "get the word out" to Vietnamese communities regarding the importance of screening programs. This is also true in other countries, such as Canada and Australia (Taylor et al., 2003), where screening use is also 10% to 12% lower than use by the local non-Vietnamese populations, but survey results present similar findings. As was true of White women in the United States 30 years ago, high percentages of Vietnamese females over 65 have never had a Pap test or a vaginal examination as a preventive measure. This was true for 10 of the 11 eldest women in one study of 96 women (Schulmeister & Lifsey, 1999) and may explain why this age group contained 25% of the patients with cervical cancer but 40% of the deaths—too many with advanced invasive cancer at diagnosis. Some common reasons given by women for not having the tests were feeling their risk was low because of no family history of cancer (29%) and not being sick (24%). Other common barriers were having no female doctor, the cost (lack of insurance), fear of the embarrassing procedures, and time.

Knowledge, attitudes, and beliefs about cancer are important in determining behavior, but as is also true for the dominant culture population, these do not explain all behavior. The natural reticence of Vietnamese to openly discuss sexual problems, disease, or activity, especially with a new doctor and in a different language, makes a Pap smear, vaginal examination, or mammogram a troubling request indeed. To complicate the request, the patient is expected to do this when feeling healthy.

Worldwide, cervical cancer is second only to breast cancer as the most common female malignancy in both incidence and mortality. Breast cancer claims over 1 million cases a year worldwide. In fact, 55% of these cases occur in "more developed" countries. It is interesting to note that the age-adjusted mortality rate for cervical cancer is much the same throughout the world (Ho et al., 2005). The incidence of breast cancer in Vietnam as reported is 3% lower than that in the United States, with a mortality rate of 6% (Ho et al., 2005). These findings may suggest that Vietnamese women are at a lower risk of both developing and dying of breast cancer (in Vietnam) than are women in the United States.

In a survey study done to determine predictors in a breast and cervical screening program in a large Vietnamese community near Houston, Texas, one surprise result was that the Vietnamese women were far more worried about breast cancer (52%) than they were about cervical cancer (2%). Although unexplainable, the information was helpful in planning approaches to breast self-examination (BSE) and medical self-examination (MSE) and mammography screening. Further findings from this study assisted in the creation of lists of beliefs about the barriers and benefits as reported by the 209 participants in the study. The findings indicate the most significant predictors of the use of the Pap test, BSE, MSE, and mammography were being married, high education level, lack of barriers, a family history of cancer, older age, and increased concern about cancer (Ho et al., 2005). In "Differences in Breast Cancer, Stage, Treatment, and Survival by Race and Ethnicity," Li, Malone, and Daling (2003) observed that across races and ethnicities, the differences in the treatment received are likely to be "solely the result of socioeconomic and cultural factors." For health care providers this means that targeting women with low socioeconomic status and improving their treatment programs may be the means not only toward early detection but also improved survival rates in these populations.

It is imperative for the nurse to be understanding of the cultural beliefs that Vietnamese women face in order to decrease their risk for cervical cancer during the period of resettlement (Labun, 2000, 2001). By building positive relationships with clients and appreciating a common humanity, health teaching can be effective. Behaviors that can address this high risk include the following:

- Determine the adequacy of the patient's understanding of cancer, risk factors, and hope of treatment. Use translation if at all needed and possible; brochures may be available (McPhee, 2002).
- Encourage and prepare the Vietnamese client by explaining the procedures, draping well, granting that there may be some discomfort, practicing relaxation breathing, and always staying with the client throughout the procedure. Assist after the procedure as needed.
- Give an estimate about how soon and in what way the client will be told of the results.
- Discuss strategies for reminders of upcoming routine examinations in the future.
- Keep alert for opportunities to share the information with all Vietnamese females as situations arise, remembering that older Vietnamese (who do not speak English) are at especially high risk for having advanced cervical cancer at the time of diagnosis.

Perhaps the most significant information about lung cancer and the Vietnamese is the findings from one study done in 1995. The study was conducted with face-to-face interviews with men and women 18 years of age and older in Hanoi, a rural community in North Vietnam, in Ho Chi Minh City, and a rural community in South Vietnam. Approximately 500 interviews were done at each site for a total of 2001 participants. Findings from this study suggested that smoking prevalence was 72.8% among the men and 4.3% among the women. Males had smoked a mean of 15 years beginning at a median age of 19. Vietnam had the highest reported male smoking prevalence in the world (Jenkins et al., 1997). For the men, smoking seemed an integral part of the serious business, social, and cultural landscape, from top government negotiations on down to family functions. In fact, the offering of cigarettes was found to be a common courtesy. Foreign cigarettes especially were often given as gifts to one's boss, or those in high places. Smoking rates for the younger women are among the lowest in the world because smoking is considered unfeminine and unattractive socially and culturally and thus is a taboo, especially for older women.

Smoking is a habit among the Vietnamese, and as such is not easily given up because it also serves social or cultural purpose (hospitality, maleness). Jochelson, Hua, and Rissel (2003) reported from Australia that the Vietnamese and Lebanese immigrant communities have the highest and next-to-highest smoking prevalences in Australia, respectively. The level of knowledge and type of attitudes and behaviors of the Vietnamese and Arabic communities were very similar to the research previously done in the English-speaking community. The major difference was the fact that the English-speaking group did not associate the problem of environmental tobacco smoke with the problem of sociability and hospitality and asked, "How can we ask our friends not to smoke in our homes?" (Jochelson et al., 2003).

In "Cancer Risk Factors of Vietnamese Americans in Rural South Alabama," Xu, Ross, Ryan, and Wang (2005) surveyed 284 Vietnamese, most of whom lived in a semi-isolated fishing village, had spent most of their lives in Vietnam, and had had fewer education and acculturation experiences in the United States than Vietnamese Americans who participated in urban health surveys. A total of 73.8% of the current smokers began smoking in their teens, and 41.5% of the sample currently live with a family member who smokes. The statement was made that a "culture of smoking" is believed to be the primary culprit for the high smoking rate. For many of the men smoking was a way of life to "initiate rapport, strengthen bonding, and maintain relationships" (Xu et al., 2005, p. 237).

It is an understatement to suggest that the challenge to reduce smoking calls for the best efforts of health care providers. All the multidisciplinary team members must collaborate to bring changes in social, political, and economic arenas to discourage smoking (such as banning smoking in public places, cigarette taxes, and restraining the tobacco industry's aggressive foreign marketing). Nurses know that smoking is the single most preventable cause of premature death, increasing the risk of lung cancer, emphysema, heart disease, stroke, and other diseases. Nurses also understand the powerful cultural components that help determine habits. The implications for nursing care are to use health status promoters to discourage "the culture of smoking," and help patients—and friends—to find more healthful ways to take care of themselves (Levy, Bales, Lan, & Nikolayex, 2006; Morrow & Barraclough, 2003, p. 376).

HIV/AIDS. A study used a random sample of 319 students attending four community colleges in Orange County, California, to determine human immunodeficiency virus (HIV) and acquired immunodeficiency syndrome (AIDS) knowledge and past and present sexual behavior. The Vietnamese appeared to have low knowledge of the disease, little concern about AIDS, reluctance to be tested, and the lowest incidence of high-risk behavior. Most of the survey sample had been born in Vietnam, had lived in the United States for 5 to 10 years, and probably were still taking cues from family rather than from non-Vietnamese peers. The main concern of the research team was what will happen if and when that allegiance changes and they join the dominant culture in their sexual practices (Shapiro, Radecki, Charchian, & Josephson, 1999).

Nutritional Preferences

The common food staple in Vietnam is rice, eaten from a large bowl with chopsticks two or three times a day. One way a client may describe a medical problem to the doctor is to hold a hand up in the form of a bowl and say, "Now I eat only one bowl of rice instead of three the way I used to do." During the French occupation, bread was introduced and widely consumed in the form of small tasty French rolls, available fresh daily on the street corners everywhere. Today many Vietnamese in the United States replace some of their rice with fresh white bread.

In Vietnam, brown unpolished grains were considered the food of the mountain people and were almost never eaten by the more sophisticated lowlanders. In the United States, except for those Vietnamese Americans who take nutrition facts seriously, polished rice and white bread continue to be favorites among the Vietnamese people.

Rice and many other cooked dishes are seasoned with the unique condiment *nuoc mam*, a "fish sauce" made by marinating small fish in salt in kegs for a month or more. Depending on use, some sugar, fresh lime juice, garlic, chili peppers, and water are added. Fish sauce is a serious, continuing, major source of salt in the Vietnamese diet.

Fish is usually readily available, and meats served are cut into bite-size pieces and served with rice and vegetables. Chicken and duck eggs are often available. Tofu is served in many vegetable dishes, but dry bean dishes are uncommon.

In Vietnam, green leafy vines or plants are gathered from gardens or the countryside and brought to the local markets in truckloads each morning. Although they are not served in large quantities, the regular presence of these greens, raw or lightly stir-fried and served with rice, contributes to a diet unusually high in vegetable nutrients.

In 1988, the U.S. Department of Agriculture described the traditional Vietnamese diet as "low in fat and sugar, high in complex carbohydrates and moderate in fiber," comparing very favorably with the best U.S. dietary guidelines (Burtis, Davis, & Martin, 1988). About 59% of the more than 1 million Southeast Asians who had immigrated to the United States since 1975 were Vietnamese, and 25% of those were children. What effect has acculturation had on this diet, which, except for the present emphasis on calcium consumption, was flawed only by its lack of dairy products?

In 2001, a survey team (Wiecha, Fink, Wiecha, & Herbert) used a simple questionnaire ("How many servings of fruits, vegetables, and dairy foods do you eat each day?") for 2618 adolescents in two middle schools and two high schools near Boston. Vietnamese, White, African-American, and Hispanic students were involved. There were 226 Vietnamese, 64 of whom had either been born in the United States or had lived here more than 10 years, and 162 had been here 10 years or less. Compared with the Whites, the Vietnamese were much more likely to eat five servings of fruits and vegetables (35.5% and 15.3%, respectively), but more than 44% were less likely to take in three or more dairy servings. Younger Vietnamese students were more likely than the older students to eat the five servings of fruits and vegetables (Wiecha et al., 2001).

When other aspects of the diet such as fat and sugar intake are considered, indications are that Southeast Asians tend to adopt a less healthy diet in the United States. This study indicates that at least preference for fruits and vegetables seems to persist during the acculturation period. This practice is protective against disease and should definitely be encouraged.

Milk and dairy foods have not traditionally been staples of Vietnamese rural or urban diets. Some canned evaporated milk may be used in cooking or sweetened condensed milk used to prepare *sinto* (vitamin), a delicious drink made by blending a small amount of the milk with ice and fresh chopped fruit, sold along the sidewalks in towns and cities. Too often the sweetened milk was placed in a baby bottle and warm water added to make formula, especially during travel. But milk and ice cream were not common or valued tastes or consistencies to the Vietnamese palates.

While a low calcium intake has always been a feature of traditional Asian diets, the effects of it may have been offset by an active lifestyle. Osteoporosis, apparently associated with low calcium intake, is a major public health concern in the United States at present, with the highest risk group being Asian women—and Vietnamese women presenting as the fastest growing group numerically.

In Louisiana, five focus group discussions were held with 34 Vietnamese mothers, ages 25 to 47, with incomes up to $30,000 a year, to learn what they knew about calcium intake and what barriers there may be to increasing it (Reed, Meeks, Nguyen, Cross, & Garrison, 1998). For these study participants, a perceived negative taste of dairy products was the most common problem with including these foods in the regular diet. Only two mothers stated that milk was a desirable dietary component, and only one felt that drinking milk would improve her diet. Unfamiliarity with milk foods, cost, time, and, to a lesser degree, problems with lactose intolerance were also given as reasons.

The study participants were not aware of how serious the lack of calcium could be for their future and were open to trying high-calcium recipes using both American and Vietnamese foods, adding milk to Vietnamese pancakes, and using milk in drinks and puddings (Reed et al., 1998). Their children with school cafeteria experience may find these tastes familiar.

Thirty years into their "new life in a new country," many Vietnamese are joining their American friends struggling to control weight gain as they watch their blood pressure, glucose, and cholesterol readings rise to dangerously high levels. Understandably, those without insurance (often 50% or more) do not see a doctor regularly, and one study identified as a risk factor a profound need for increased understanding of the need and ways to control diet and weight gain in their new setting and way of life (Duong et al., 2001). It is suggested that those Vietnamese Americans with average adult weights of 80 to 130 lb are more oriented to attaining or maintaining weight rather than to concern with grams of fat. Their children, however, are having many opportunities to become sensitized to the problems of weight as their peers are targeted in schools and community preventive programs today.

Dioxin

More than 40 years ago in Operation Ranch Hand (1962–1971) during the Vietnam conflict, some 19 million gallons of Agent Orange were sprayed as a defoliant over selected areas of Vietnam and Laos to remove cover on Viet Cong supply routes and to reveal troop movements from the North. The herbicide, named from the color-coded drums it was shipped in, contained minute amounts (3 parts per million, but 1000 times more powerful than domestic weed killers) of 2,3,7,8-tetrachlorodibenzo-*p*-dioxin (TCDD), or dioxin, a persistent organic pollutant with a half-life of 8.7 years. In the time since, dioxin has become linked to health problems such as immune system suppression, birth defects, and soft tissue sarcomas (Satchell, 1999).

The Air Force Health Study (Pavuk et al., 2005) is a 20-year longitudinal study (1982–2003) detailing the health, mortality, and reproductive outcomes in the U.S. Air Force veterans of Operation Ranch Hand, the unit responsible for 85% of all Agent Orange sprayed in Vietnam. Included in the study was a comparison Air Force group of veterans matched for age, race, and military occupation who flew or serviced aircraft in Southeast Asia (SEA) but did not handle or spray the herbicides as did the Ranch Hand veterans. Previous studies after 5 and 15 years showed no increases in Ranch Hand morbidity or mortality. But more recent comparisons with the U.S. general White male population to December 1999 showed increases in prostate cancer and melanoma in Ranch Hand veterans. However, the comparison Air Force veterans also reported an increase in prostate cancer. The final results reported in a 2005 article were that "TCDD and years of SEA service interacted with all sites of cancer, but the risk was greatest in those with the highest TCDD levels and the longest time served in Southeast Asia" (Pavuk et al., 2005).

Dioxin enters the body primarily through food, possibly animal fat. The U.S. military base at Bien Hoa, about 20 miles north of Saigon, was the location of the Ranch Hand spraying operations, the Agent Orange storage facility, and in 1971, a substantial leak of more than 5000 gallons of Agent Orange (Dalton, 2001). In the early 1970s, some dioxin levels of human breast milk in areas of the spraying were recorded at over 300 times the usual accepted range of 5 ppt, which correlated with the extremely high levels found in certain local fish, a main source of food for the mothers.

Now more than 30 years later, in 5 years of following the dioxin content in blood samples of 43 Vietnamese residents of Bien Hoa, approximately 95% proved to be above the 5 ppt level (Schecter et al., 2003). This study was done to determine if food is the current route of intake in the dioxin "hot spots" in Vietnam today. The highest levels were in free-ranging duck fat (over 20 ppt) and certain fish. Researchers caution that significant studies of Agent Orange alone do not explain all the dioxin-like toxicity measured in the Vietnamese people or their food (Schecter et al., 2003).

In January 2001, the National Toxicology Program added TCDD to the Report on Carcinogens as a known human carcinogen (Booker, 2001). All 2.6 million U.S. military personnel who served in Vietnam are eligible to apply for benefits for themselves and their children if they suffer from any of 10 proven or suspected dioxin-related conditions (Satchell, 1999).

Epidemiologists, toxicologists, and environmental scientists gathered for 4 days of meetings in Hanoi in March 2001, after which Vietnam and the United States formally established a joint research program. Although the passing of time has been helpful, several significant handicaps inherent in the situation indicate that it will take wisdom and commitment to follow through on the plans; those handicaps include, for the United States, concern about exposing the damage and, for the Vietnamese, protecting their fishing and food export industries (Cyranoski, 2002).

It is hoped that the results of these joint research efforts will not only add to the worldwide state of the science regarding the health effects of dioxin but also be helpful for the Vietnamese in Vietnam. Although the long-term picture is not yet clear, it is important that the nurse understand the dioxin event and its possible significance in the "history of the present illness" of Vietnamese clients currently and for some years to come.

Psychological Characteristics

Mental Health. The Vietnamese believe the nervous system to be the source of all mental and physical activities.

Therefore, when there is a disturbance in mental or physical activity, the nervous system is considered central to the malfunction. Neuroses are called "weakness of the nerves," a term used to describe many kinds of anxiety, depression, weariness, mental deterioration, or retardation. Psychoses are known as "turmoil of the nerves," more accurately reflecting the client's behavior or feelings. The two possible sources of mental disease are the organic model, which considers damaged nerves or brain, and the inorganic model, which may attribute bizarre behavior to various causes, such as disobedience, sin, or demons (more common in tribal groups).

The terms *psychiatrist* and *mental doctor* have no direct Vietnamese translation. *Nerve doctor* is slightly better, but the best comprehension comes with an explanation of "a specialist who treats crazy people". The following are some Vietnamese words that may be helpful to health care givers to identify what could be causing symptoms:

- *Lu lan:* confusion related to retardation
- *Lang tri* and *dang tri:* slipping away of memory, loss of memory caused by the absence of the mind
- *Mat tri nho:* the mind is already lost
- *Lmat tri giac:* the mind is lost quickly (as in multi-infarct dementia)
- *Binh tam than:* indicates mental illness or high anxiety
- *Dien:* usual lay term for "crazy" (Braun & Browne, 1998, p. 268)

In Vietnam, often there was some optimism regarding most illness affecting the nerves, with the possibility of using folk remedies, a nerve tonic to restore strength to weak nerves, or a calming medicine to quiet inner turmoil. In the United States, some feel medication is the logical answer, although there is some concern about oversedation or dependency.

Probably the most important single factor in accessing mental health care for Vietnamese Americans is the cultural pattern of keeping psychiatric problems within the family and solving them there if at all possible. The value of "face saving" in the tradition continues, and discussing or expressing emotions, especially with a stranger, is avoided unless absolutely necessary. Working with traditional doctors and healers when possible can be an effective treatment plan when this kind of cooperation is available and the illness is not of a psychotic nature (Bernier, 1999). Otherwise, persons with mental health problems may not enter the health care system until their problems have become critical. Evaluation of severity and decisions on treatment of refugee psychiatric problems by Western professionals are extremely difficult.

Emotional and Behavioral Manifestations of Distress in Refugees. The Vietnamese are used to dealing with the problems of life within the family as a unit. However, in the refugee/immigrant situation, the family is often incomplete, with few or no elderly to give balance and stability because many of the ancestors are far away in a very different setting. On the one hand is the anticipated freedom for the middle-aged and younger in the group to make independent decisions, but on the other hand are the unexpected uncertainty and loneliness of that independence. Anxiety and depression are not uncommon in Vietnamese immigrant communities, sometimes handicapping their best efforts to embrace their new home.

It is easy to assume acculturation challenges lessen as time in the new setting passes. And with concentrated effort, this is usually true for the language. Bernier (1999) observed that among the Vietnamese Americans with repeated failures and frustrations over time, the psychological stresses of change may accumulate. Families go through acculturation together but each member reacts individually. With the growing family with children in school, learning the language in "fast forward" and interacting daily with new ideas are challenging. In addition, for some Vietnamese-American families, children moving into the teenage years rarely decrease the stress in American families as the teens "acculturate" into the current peer culture. This is especially true for the "strong" Vietnamese family with "two-culture" children. Among the understandably concerned elder members in the home, the value conflicts can become even more focused as the children grow older and move toward the values of the host culture. With much change, and without help, the family ties can deteriorate, and the family conflicts unfortunately may lead to disruptive family crises (Nguyen, personal communication, 1988).

By the early 2000s, longitudinal studies were attempting to examine the complex phenomenon of depression in Vietnamese communities. Especially for the middle-aged and elders, the societal cornerstone values of self-control, harmony, and respect continued largely intact (if not more appreciated and cherished) against the 30-year backdrop of war, boats, refugee camps, and settling into a very different culture, all with a relatively small family or community support group.

Earlier research has shown mixed results for the role of social support in psychological distress. As expected, persons with a strong support network do better in a crisis than those with a weak support system. However, the immigration experience, by definition, involves disruption of the immigrant's social support systems, and successful acculturation is accomplished when new reference points and networks are integrated into or alongside the old. This may explain why other studies find that immigrants with strong ties only to their ethnic group tend to have more psychological distress than those with additional nonethnic social supports. Strong and meaningful emotional commitments to personal relationships and networks provide good mental health, but that does not mean that change will be easy or painless, especially if it involves major life adjustments.

In 2003, Gellis reported a study on the relationship of social support and depression and the effect of "kin" and "nonkin" support groups, as experienced by a sample of 79 Vietnamese immigrant men and women receiving mental health services in a psychiatric hospital. These study participants had immigrated between the ages of 26 and 35 and had lived in the United States an average of 14 years. Most were diagnosed with major depressive disorder and had an average hospital stay of almost 2 months. Their kin group averaged five people to whom they could turn for advice and discussion of personal problems, and with whom they had disagreements. The nonkin group averaged four people who were friends, coworkers, or mental health service providers.

A common problem during the acculturation years for families is the different rates and patterns of change, which easily become sources of conflict causing strained relations within the entire family. The strong Vietnamese family will likely continue to try to support its own, sometimes increasing the psychological stress for everyone. Depending on the severity of the problems and the management options, medical services may be required. With this history and a diagnosis of major depressive disorder, the client may be unable to translate the efforts of a family support group (kin) into evidence of their efforts to help in recovery. In this event, perhaps the nonkin support team can be perceived to be more helpful. Gellis (2003) calls for caregivers who can assess therapeutic support networks, social workers who understand cultural family dynamics, and appropriate follow-up services.

General Patterns of Coping and Adaptation. A general pattern of coping and adaptation is experienced by many persons in their cultural adjustment to immigration (Cook & Timberlake, 1984).

Stage I. For the first few months, there is a positive attitude with high expectations; energy is focused toward language, employment, and meeting basic needs. The excitement of a new physical environment and "things" helps suppress the pain of the multiple losses.

Stage II. The period of "psychological arrival" occurs 6 to 18 months after immigration, when the person becomes more aware of losses and "the past" becomes idealized. This agrees with Hoang and Erickson (1982), who noted that psychiatric problems may become more obvious 6 to 12 months after immigration. Survivor's guilt (e.g., "Why did

I survive and my child did not?") must be faced. Post-traumatic stress disorder (PTSD) is common, and the normal tensions of close family life are magnified. Interpersonal conflict is common. Other symptoms may be feelings of hopelessness, acute distress and grief, fatigue, and mood instability. The period may be transitory or long-lasting, mild or severe, and it seems to occur regardless of how much help or support has been given. It is usually a very frustrating time for sponsors and "helping persons," who feel inadequate to help. During this period somatization is common. Somatization is not new among Southeast Asian refugees. In a culture where overt expression of anxiety, disappointment, or anger is considered failure, a high value is placed on suppressing negative feelings; then, expressing mental distress through various physical ailments is a preferred and acceptable option. It is less worrisome to see a physician for a physical problem (Eyton & Neuwirth, 1984).

Stage III. After roughly 18 to 24 months, the person is able to reformulate the grief and get involved with the tasks at hand. There is less idealizing of the past, and helping those left behind becomes important. Adaptation moves ahead at a more rapid rate as former ways of coping are given up for more effective ones. A new self-identity emerges.

A Vietnamese nurse on a Canadian university nursing faculty, Tan Truong Donnelly (2002), examined the Western approach to coping with stress as a personality style or trait, especially as it informs health care professionals in their understanding and counseling of clients. She makes the case that "coping" theories should emphasize the contextual nature of stress and that coping should be viewed as a dynamic process that varies under different social, cultural, political, economic, and historical conditions. The author refers specifically to the needs of the recent Vietnamese immigrants entering Canada. Using the dominant view of coping as a personality trait leads to unfairly categorizing and understanding these clients whose culture, perception of power structures, history, ethnicity, and personal place in their group influence their response to "stress." Traditional Vietnamese women are taught and expected to be the caretakers of their children, spouses, and elderly members of their extended family. They accept these responsibilities and hardships as a part of life, to be handled in the best way possible. These methods of coping are supported by their community and the high regard given to "good mothers" and "good daughters." This "passive coping" is considered successful in the context of the collectivist society. But it becomes an important source of stress when judged by an individualistic Western society, which applauds self-assertiveness and grieves the "unsuccessful coping" they observe. Coping happens contextually, and how the challenge is met depends on many factors in the situation. The factors vary at any given time and influence the "coping response."

Cook and Timberlake (1984) list denial as the defense mechanism most often used by Vietnamese refugees. The authors believe that denial is congruent with the values of the culture: submission to the common good (and to fate), harmony, and self-sacrifice. Denial is needed to lessen the profound effect of losses and to allow the refugees to go on with the task of survival. When denial fails, facing the hard realities without the needed support systems may encourage withdrawal or the turn to alcohol, drugs, or medication abuse (Cook & Timberlake, 1984).

Alcohol and Drug Abuse. Few well-controlled longitudinal studies are available on substance abuse among the Vietnamese. However, evidence suggests that pockets of trouble have emerged in the communities, and these appear to be directly related to a host of psychosocial stressors (O'Hare & Tran, 1998). Some of the Vietnamese have come to the United States following a refugee and immigration experience that was among the more traumatic in recent memory (see discussion of PTSD), resulting in significant stress in many areas. This may well place them and their children at increased risk for alcohol and substance abuse (Makimoto, 1998).

Depression seriously slows the ability of the sufferer to successfully meet the daily challenges without being overwhelmed and discouraged. One Vietnamese immigrant study reported that 14% of the study group had trouble with other drugs "some of the time," a much higher percentage (40%) reported using alcohol as a means of "coping with sorrow," and almost 12% reported using drugs for the same purpose (O'Hare & Tran, 1998).

Women rarely drank in Vietnam, and the effect of men drinking a bottle of "33" (*Ba Muoi Ba*) beer at the village café with friends in the evening seems to have little in common with "drinking" in the United States. Here, wine and liquor are readily available, and drinking is more acceptable in the dominant culture. Drinks were served at weddings in Vietnam, but guests rarely became drunk, a not uncommon occurrence at Vietnamese weddings in the United States at the present time. The effects of the increased drinking on the persons, their families, and community can be expected to become more apparent in the coming years as acculturation continues.

In working with Vietnamese clients in abuse problems, it is wise to remember the cultural importance of "face saving" and of not openly disagreeing with or confronting another. Also helpful will be sensitivity to the guilt and shame to the family, especially for the older Vietnamese clients.

Insight-oriented therapies or pressuring clients to admit "alcoholism" or "addiction," for example, may seem so rude and unprofessional, especially to older clients, and be such a foreign approach to handling a problem that it may only call into question the competence of the caregiver. Cognitive-behavioral therapies (CBTs) appear to have more promise for effective intervention (O'Hare & Tran, 1998).

CBT for persons with addiction problems typically include some combination of the following: (1) self-monitoring thoughts, feelings, and events likely to "trigger" the impulse to abuse; (2) teaching more effective social skills to deal with situations in which the client is pressured to use drugs; and (3) teaching stress management skills to lower anxiety and deal with somatic complaints (O'Hare & Tran, 1998). These skills can also be helpful with depression and anxiety, which often co-occur with substance abuse.

Cognitive-behavioral therapies may feel more comfortable to Vietnamese clients because they are easily adapted to family- and community-based approaches. They feel less personally intrusive, often complement Asian values, and use stress management techniques that clients may find familiar. More work is being done using CBT, which may provide insight into other helpful approaches. For valid statistics on drug abuse in Vietnamese, more studies using Vietnamese are needed, rather than Southeast Asian, Asian-American, or API.

Post-traumatic Stress Disorder. The exact relationship between premigration and postmigration experiences and adaptation challenges continues to be debated. Nicholson (1997) noted that current stressors best predicted mental health outcomes. However, experienced events better predicted PTSD than did either anxiety or depression.

The exact causes of the increased number of mental health disorders in the Vietnamese resettlement communities are often evasive and are difficult to isolate, identify, or even test; possibilities include language, the high value of communicating only positive feelings, the somatization option, or the cultural practice of handling psychiatric problems within the family if at all possible.

The stresses of immigration have been found to be particularly difficult for women. Fox, Cowell, and Johnson (1995) identified the chief role of Southeast Asian women as meeting the needs of husband, children, and extended family. They had the responsibility of home and children while husbands were in the army for years and then in re-education camps. They were with their children; were abused as "boat people"; and lost family members through sickness, exposure, drowning, and killing. Men were also traumatized for years, and it is not clear how much these premigration experiences have continued to produce great emotional stress and handicap years into the resettlement period (Fox et al., 1995).

Although first described in war veterans, PTSD is now being recognized by health professionals in other settings, and the definition is broadening to include more than "exposure to actual or threatened death or injury." Not only did Vietnamese immigrants have war and violence in their history, but they also had the added difficulty of upheaval inherent in the refugee immigration experience, which affected every area of life for the individual, family, and "village." In "Contextual Analysis of Coping: Implications for Immigrants' Mental Health Care," a Vietnamese nurse named Tan Truong Donnelly (2002) used Vietnamese immigrant experiences to make the case that "coping theories should emphasize the contextual nature of stress and coping, and that coping should be viewed as a dynamic process that varies under different social, cultural, political, economic, and historical conditions."

One way of categorizing symptoms of PTSD can be to consider three groupings: intrusion (nightmares, flashbacks, memories with intense emotional and physical distress), avoidance (avoiding people, activities, thoughts connected with the trauma, becoming numb to all emotions, positive or negative), and arousal (being constantly on guard, resulting in problems concentrating, insomnia, emotional outbursts, and instability) (Harvard Women's Health Watch, 2005).

Many of these symptoms are normal experiences after trauma, but if after a month the symptoms are getting worse or interfering with ability to function, the diagnosis may be an acute stress disorder. After 3 months, chronic PTSD can be considered and sometimes requires treatment over an extended period of time. As of 1990, 15 years after the Vietnam conflict ended, over 9% of Vietnam veterans still suffered from PTSD, and 15 years beyond that, in 2005, many continued to be compensated for PTSD-like symptoms (McNally, 2006). PTSD can occur with other stressors, such as an unexpected death or mental illness, making diagnosis and recovery more difficult. Also, treatment for substance abuse will likely be unsuccessful in the presence of underlying PTSD (Harvard Women's Health Watch, 2005).

Exposure therapy, a CBT approach, is a type of psychotherapy that is a good fit culturally for Vietnamese adults and elders. Often, antianxiety and antidepressant medications are part of the regimen. The selective serotonin reuptake inhibitors paroxetine (Paxil) and sertraline (Zoloft) have been approved by the Food and Drug Administration for the treatment of PTSD.

The Indochinese Psychiatry Clinic near Boston served many Vietnamese who came as refugees under the 1989 Released Reeducation Center Detainees Resettlement Program. These refugees were former South Vietnamese political prisoners who had worked for the United States and came with their spouses and unmarried children. All of them had experienced suffering. Men averaged 7 to 8 years of brainwashing and hard labor in the camps; the women and children were at home, were unable to get jobs or buy food, and were ostracized in their villages in many areas. Both men and women were diagnosed with PTSD, and half also experienced a major depressive disorder (Allden, 1998).

Although the Boston setting is not a typical Vietnamese resettlement community, most Vietnamese communities have some common history with this group in their premigration experiences. PTSD and the accompanying or resulting anxiety and depression are becoming more recognized in the communities, and efforts are being made to work with those who are suffering. Without help, adjustment and adaptation to a new culture are slow and extremely taxing, learning a new language is very difficult, and people understandably become emotionally and physically isolated and increasingly discouraged.

Drug Interactions and Metabolism

Caffeine, a component of many drugs as well as coffee, tea, and colas, appears to be metabolized and excreted faster by Whites than by Asians (Grant, 1983). Alcohol is also metabolized differently (see "Enzymatic and Genetic Variations" earlier in this chapter).

Many Chinese herbs and medicines are given as soups or teas. Most Vietnamese believe that Western medicines in tablets, capsules, or injections are "too strong" or "hot" and upset their internal balance, and unfortunately there is poor understanding of the possible serious effects of underdosage, sudden withdrawal, or, for antibiotics, short-term usage. Immediate results are anticipated, and often the medication is discontinued when the patient feels better or there is no improvement, behavior similar to that in many of their American counterparts.

Many Vietnamese believe that they have a different physical constitution from Americans so that Western drug dosages may not be appropriate for them. It is true that many Vietnamese weigh less than Americans, and, especially in the case of sedative or psychiatric medications, many of their experiences have been very troubling and encouraged the practice of "halving the dosage" (experience of the author). Current research into ethnopharmacology indicates that, indeed, the Vietnamese do have a pharmacodynamic difference in therapeutic response to psychotropics. For example, the Asian clients' mean required dose for haloperidol is significantly lower than the average for optimal therapeutic response, and extrapyramidal symptoms emerged (Helm, Quan, Herfindal, &

Gourley, 2006; Lin et al., 1989). Many researchers and practitioners suggest that Asian clients also generally respond to substantially lower doses of neuroleptics (Helm et al., 2006; Murphy, 1969; Rosenblat & Tang, 1987). Wise and kind practitioners make an obvious effort to take these factors (weight, ethnicity, increased sensitivity) into account when prescribing medication for Vietnamese clients by checking the weight and asking about previous experience with medications. Vietnamese want to please those trying to help them—and also want to be healthy.

Implications for Nursing Care

The small body size of many Vietnamese-American clients has an important implication in terms of nursing treatment. Some nurses have delayed giving pain medication to a Vietnamese-American client in pain "because the client is so tiny" (Tien-Hyatt, 1989). Because Vietnamese-American clients may be stoic, it is important for the nurse to evaluate carefully the need for pain medication and to provide sufficient medication without delay (Lin & Finder, 1983; Tien, 1984; Tien-Hyatt, 1989). Offering medication for pain rather than asking if it is needed may result in a more accurate response.

Smither and Rodríguez-Giegling (1979) have noted that within the first 5 years after leaving Vietnam, personality and coping are the more important determinants of which acculturation patterns develop. Other significant factors are level of income and social class (Smither & Rodríguez-Giegling, 1979). Allden (1998), however, in her work with persons who had undergone very traumatic premigration experiences in Vietnam and Cambodia, has treated a number of clients with PTSD diagnoses and sees these premigration stresses as continuing to slow down adaptation for years into the resettlement period. It will take time and more studies to resolve the differences in these and other similar findings.

In the difficult everyday situations that require translations in psychiatric evaluation and counseling, the use of bilingual paraprofessionals has gained increasing attention (Leung, 1988). Professionals and clients readily recognize that the person communicating between them is indeed a key person in determining the outcome of this effort. When the inherent potential of the "translator" is recognized, persons should be selected and trained in techniques of information gathering, importance of not reinterpreting the report, confidentiality, and so on (McPhee, 2002). When this interpreter is welcomed as a colleague on the team, the client also comes to see this person not only as a member of "my" team, the only possibility of communicating the problem, but also as a respected member of "their" team who is trying to help. Trained or untrained, the paraprofessional often becomes the first source of help

Vietnamese-American clients turn to because they are hesitant to contact the professional with personal or family matters.

The nurse should also recognize that for many Vietnamese-American clients, food is medicine. Many Vietnamese Americans are able to practice their food beliefs without difficulty. However, if a client develops a health problem and encounters Western medical practitioners, the need to adopt Western food practices may be considered necessary for survival, such as the need for fluids, the restriction of salt, the need for specific medications (such as cardiac medications), and the need for specific nutrients in the diet. Helping the client to understand why dietary restrictions have been recommended is essential. A client may be willing to limit the amount of *nuoc mam* in the diet when health care professionals carefully explain the reason for this request. For many Vietnamese Americans, eating habits are changing. Children are learning to eat hamburgers, french fries, pizza, spaghetti, and tacos in school lunch programs. Vietnamese Americans are pragmatists, and teaching about dietary practices in relation to Western medicine can result in changed behavior (Reed et al., 1998).

Another important health care issue for the nurse who provides care for Vietnamese-American clients is utilization of health care resources. Tran (1980) suggested that utilization of health care services is related to the identification of a problem and the availability of an appropriate service. A study by Strand and Jones (1983) found that health services utilization is not directly correlated with education and English-language skills but is related to a variety of factors. For example, working two jobs makes it difficult to make time for a clinic appointment. The person who speaks English best and those persons who should accompany the client to the health facility are usually at work or at school. A car or a babysitter may be unavailable. Choosing health care may be difficult. The options for health care are fewer than they were in Vietnam, and even wealthy Vietnamese persons may have problems finding health care providers who understand the Vietnamese language. Phan (1996) reported how taking the clinic to the community and working with individual families in their own environment helped eliminate many of the utilization problems.

The importance of the nurse in teaching, modeling, and encouraging health promotion and illness prevention practices among the children cannot be overemphasized. As Nguyen (1988, personal communication) observes, "Children can learn to make positive health behaviors an integral part of their lives." Understandably for parents, ideas of illness and treatment are deeply ingrained. Vietnamese-American children are immersed in new ideas and change, understand the new language, and will make important health decisions that will influence their lives, the lives of their children, and the lives of their parents.

The majority of health care problems does not occur or at least is not reported by Vietnamese refugees during the initial settlement period. This may result from the fact that immediately before or after arrival, the refugees are routinely screened and treated for existing problems. After the excitement of arriving and getting settled, however, previously untreated health problems often become evident, and eventually the patient finds the way into the health system.

Another deterrent for a few Vietnamese Americans in the utilization of health services is integration into ethnic subcommunities. For a small group of persons, especially the elderly, who have found learning English and the process of adaptation too difficult, surrounding themselves with familiar lifestyles, language, friends, and family has made loneliness less of a problem. In these subcommunities, traditional beliefs and superstitions survive more comfortably than in the "outside world." Health care givers should keep in mind that these sometimes are the persons being admitted to the hospital for emergency care by a concerned family. It is crucial and helpful that the nurse have some cultural awareness and sensitivity.

SUMMARY

The initial arrival of large groups of Vietnamese to the United States began some 36 years ago. It is important for the nurse to recognize that the present Vietnamese-American clients are a diverse group, moving through differing stages of acculturation to life in a new setting and a different health care system. The Vietnamese are survivors, and how rapidly this is happening depends on many factors in their past as well as many experiences in their day-to-day life here: length of time, group support, language proficiency, place in the family and community, economic stability, general mental health, and the quality of the contacts with the host culture. Encouraging the children toward healthy lifestyles and illness prevention is a key to the future.

The customs, values, health beliefs, and practices the Vietnamese-American clients have brought with them are an important consideration for the Western health care provider. The nurse who develops an appreciation of these will promote more effective health care delivery and will encourage use of, and comfort in, the new health care system.

Age, sex, and individual idiosyncrasies also contribute to variations in response to the American health care system. The customs, values, and health beliefs and practices of Vietnamese-American clients are important considerations for the Western health care professional (Tripp-Reimer & Thieman, 1981). Most adult Vietnamese Americans have retained some folk medicine beliefs that affect not only explanations for causes of symptoms but also the type of treatment that will be selected. The nurse who develops a knowledge and understanding of these beliefs will promote more effective health care delivery and will ease the adjustment and comfort in the new health care system.

CASE STUDY

Mr. Yen Van Nguyen is a 26-year-old man who has recently arrived in the United States from Vietnam with his wife and 2-year-old son, Tran. Yen arrives at a local emergency room one evening carrying his son, Tran, and gesturing that his son needs medical attention because he has been running a low-grade fever, sneezing, and coughing for the past 2 days. Yen speaks very poor English and appears to be somewhat excited.

The emergency room nurse takes Tran back to an examination room, where she can get him undressed and into a gown for examination by the physician. While undressing Tran, the nurse notices bruising over the sternum and along the spine and immediately summons the physician. On examination, the physician notices that the bruised areas do not appear tender but nevertheless suspects child abuse. The child's father, Yen, is escorted back to the child's room by a hospital security officer, where he is questioned by the physician. Yen speaks very poor English, and communication is difficult. The harder the physician tries to communicate with Yen, the more frustrated both the physician and Yen become.

A young Vietnamese woman who works in housekeeping is requested to report to the emergency department to help with the communication problem between the emergency room staff and Yen. After a short discussion with Yen, the young Vietnamese woman explains the custom of c o gió (rub-wind), or "coin rubbing," to the emergency room staff. On further examination, the physician can find no other evidence of child abuse. The emergency staff realize that the bruising is from the coin rubbing and not from child abuse, as initially suspected. The child is given an injection of an antibiotic and discharged.

◎ CARE PLAN

Nursing Diagnosis: Communication, impaired verbal, related to foreign-language barrier

Client Outcome	Nursing Interventions
Parent will be able to communicate more effectively about customs and beliefs used in treating illnesses, and nurse will better understand these customs.	1. Determine parent's understanding and ability to communicate in English. 2. Talk slowly, enunciating words. 3. Face parent and speak in a slow, clear voice. 4. Use gestures to convey meanings, but do not use excessive "touching." 5. Attempt to locate a translator for assistance. 6. Provide parent adequate space to communicate without "crowding." 7. Keep language simple.

Nursing Diagnosis: Fear related to Americans' misunderstanding of Vietnamese culture with a potential for prosecution for child abuse

Client Outcome	Nursing Interventions
Parent will experience reduced fear with awareness of nurse's understanding of Vietnamese cultural folk medicine.	1. Allow parent to explain Vietnamese traditional folk medicine. 2. Provide parent with a quiet area to help reduce fears. 3. Attempt to communicate in a nonthreatening manner. 4. Recruit others familiar with Vietnamese culture to help parent explain. 5. Remove persons perceived as threatening to parent.

Nursing Diagnosis: Knowledge deficit related to modern medical practices secondary to cultural differences

Client Outcome	Nursing Interventions
Parent will demonstrate an understanding of the importance of modern medical treatment in conjunction with traditional folk medicine.	1. Explain to parent the importance of modern medical care in conjunction with cultural folk medicine. 2. Determine parent's perception of medical model of treatment. 3. Keep language simple; avoid long medical terms. 4. Explain importance of compliance with medical treatment ordered. 5. Keep instructions simple and brief. 6. Arrange for an interpreter to help explain importance of seeking medical attention for illness or injury.

Nursing Diagnosis: Parental role conflict related to child's present illness and need to seek "foreign" medical attention

Client Outcome	Nursing Interventions
Parent will demonstrate an understanding of the importance of seeking qualified medical attention for the betterment of the child's well-being.	1. Educate parent on importance of seeking medical attention to treat illnesses. 2. Provide parent the opportunity to describe how similar situations were handled. 3. Assess past medical practices and folklore that the parent normally uses in similar situations. 4. Allow parent time to ask questions related to child's health care. 5. Provide information in a clear, concise, easy-to-understand manner.

Continued

CARE PLAN—cont'd

Nursing Diagnosis: Noncompliance (risk for) related to misunderstanding of the prescribed treatment as a result of the belief that medications in the Western world are much stronger than those found in the Far East

Client Outcome	Nursing Interventions
Parent will demonstrate an understanding of prescribed treatment and importance of following prescribed medical regimen.	1. Assess parent's fear of prescribed treatment. 2. Promote health teaching to educate parent on the effects, desired outcome, and side effects of prescribed medicine. 3. Warn parent that some medications may make the client sleepy and that this is an expected occurrence. 4. Teach parent about importance of adhering to prescribed medical treatment. 5. Reassure parent that prescribed medication is appropriate and safe for client. 6. Review medication, dosage, and proper administration technique to help parent feel more comfortable with the treatment.

Nursing Diagnosis: Coping, ineffective family: compromised, related to illness of a family member and the necessity to seek culturally unfamiliar medical treatment

Client Outcome	Nursing Interventions
Family members will be better able to cope with illness-related problems after obtaining information on prescribed medical treatment.	1. Reassure parent of appropriateness of prescribed medical treatment. 2. Provide parent the opportunity to express fears and concerns. 3. Encourage parent to verbalize familiar treatments that family sought in Vietnam, including customs and folk medicine. 4. Direct parent to areas of potential help (such as churches, Vietnamese communities, social workers). 5. Instruct parent how to perform prescribed treatment to increase feelings of being needed.

Nursing Diagnosis: Role performance, altered (risk for), related to undue stress of an ill family member in an unfamiliar culture

Client Outcome	Nursing Interventions
Parent will discuss feelings of altered role performance and identify areas of undue stress.	1. Encourage parent to talk openly about actual or potential areas of stress. 2. Provide quiet area for parent to gather thoughts. 3. Help parent to understand what resources are available in the community (such as self-help groups). 4. Reassure client. 5. Avoid negative criticism. 6. Encourage parent to openly discuss concerns about the health of child and about the care that child will receive.

CLINICAL DECISION MAKING

1. List several ways that the nurse and the emergency room staff might better communicate with the Vietnamese-American client.
2. Should the client be told that his folk medicine treatment is foolish and that he should abandon it? Why or why not?
3. How could the nurse effectively teach the client about the benefits of seeking conventional medical treatment in the United States?
4. When asked questions, Yen answers, "Yes." Does this always indicate that he necessarily means "yes"?
5. List some strategies and techniques to help the nurse communicate more effectively with the Vietnamese-American family.
6. Describe the misconceptions that Vietnamese Americans have concerning Western medical practices and medications.
7. In American society, hospitalization and visitation by clergy is a common, almost expected, act by some. How do the Vietnamese view hospitalization and clergy visitation?
8. Describe the importance of folk medicine and folk healers to Vietnamese Americans.

REVIEW QUESTIONS

1. A nurse in a doctor's office explains to a Vietnamese female client the medication regimen for the prescription the client has been given. The client nods her head and smiles as the explanation is given. However, in 2 weeks she returns. Her condition has deteriorated, and the nurse discovers that she has not taken any medication. Initially, the nurse should do which of the following?
   a. Find out if she understood the instructions as they were provided in English.
   b. Firmly explain that she needs this medication to improve.
   c. Call in the client's husband and explain the schedule again.
   d. Provide her with printed directions in Vietnamese on how to take the medication.
2. Mrs. Nguyen, a Vietnamese client, is to undergo cancer surgery. She seems frightened. The best way for the nurse to initiate a therapeutic relationship is to do which of the following?
   a. Give Mrs. Nguyen a hug and pray with her.
   b. Ask Mrs. Nguyen how she is feeling.
   c. Tell Mrs. Nguyen that the outcome of the surgery should be favorable.

   d. Tell Mrs. Nguyen the nurse will call the hospital chaplain.
3. A Vietnamese resident in a nursing home does not want to follow the nursing care plan regarding diet. The best course of action for the nursing staff would be to do which of the following?
   a. Insist the resident accept the diet as ordered.
   b. Document the stubbornness of this resident.
   c. Avoid making an issue of his noncompliance.
   d. Consider the possibility of cultural differences.

REFERENCES

Allden, K. (1998). The Indochinese Psychiatry Clinic: trauma and refugee mental health treatment in the 1990s. *Journal of Ambulatory Care Management, 21*(2), 30–38.

American Lung Association, Research and Program Services, Epidemiology and Statistics Unit (2010). *Trends in tuberculosis morbidity and mortality*. Washington, DC: American Lung Association.

Balfour, F. (1993). Return of the boat people. *World Press Review, 40*(7), 10–12.

Bernier, D. (1999). The Indochinese refugees: a perspective from various stress theories. *Journal of Multicultural Social Work, 2*(1), 15–30.

Bloodbook.com (2011). *Racial & ethnic distribution of ABO blood types*. Available at: <http://www.bloodbook.com/world-abo.html> Retrieved September 11, 2011.

Bonder, B., Martin, L., & Miracle, A. (2002). *Culture in clinical care*. Thorofare, NJ: Slack.

Booker, S. (2001). Dioxin in Vietnam: fighting a legacy of war. *Environmental Health Perspectives, 109*(3), A116. 2P, IBW.

Branch, M., & Paxton, P. (1976). *Providing safe nursing care for ethnic people of color*. East Norwalk, CT: Appleton-Century-Croft.

Braun, K., & Browne, C. (1998). Perceptions of dementia, caregiving, and help seeking among Asians and Pacific Islander Americans. *National Association of Social Workers, 23*(4), 262–274.

Burtis, G., Davis, J., & Martin, S. (1988). *Applied nutrition and diet therapy*. Philadelphia: Saunders.

Cao, A. Q. (1986). Linguistic and cultural issues in refugees. In the next decade: the 1986 Conference on Refugee Health Care Issues and Management (70–75). 1986 Refugee Health Care Conference Proceedings. Miami, FL: University of Miami.

Centers for Disease Control and Prevention (CDC) (2005). *Trends in tuberculosis—United States*. Atlanta, GA: Centers for Disease Control and Prevention.

Central Intelligence Agency (CIA) (2015). *The world factbook: Vietnam*. New York: Skyhorse.

Chao, R. (1994). Beyond parental control and authoritarian parenting style: understanding Chinese parenting through the cultural notion of training. *Child Development, 65,* 1111–1119.

Coelho, G., & Stein, J. (1980). Change, vulnerability, and coping: stresses of uprooting and overcrowding. In G. Coelho & P.

Ahmed (Eds.), *Uprooting and development*. New York: Plenum.

Cook, K., & Timberlake, E. (1984). Working with Vietnamese refugees. *Social Work, 29*(2), 108–113.

Cyranoski, D. (2002). U.S. and Vietnam join forces to count cost of Agent Orange. *Nature, 416*(21), 252.

Dalton, R. (2001). Bilateral Vietnam study plans to assess war fallout of dioxin. *Nature, 413*(6855), 442.

Davis, R. (2000). The convergence of health and family in the Vietnamese culture. *Journal of Family Nursing, 6*(2), 136–156.

Dinh, A., Kemp, C., & Rasbridge, L. (2000). Culture and the end of life: Vietnamese health beliefs and practices related to the end of life. *Journal of Hospice and Palliative Nursing, 2*(3), 111–117.

Donnelly, T. (2002). Contextual analysis of coping: implications for immigrants' mental health care. *Issues in Mental Health Nursing, 23*, 715–732.

Duong, D., Bohannon, A., & Ross, M. (2001). A descriptive study of hypertension in Vietnamese Americans. *Journal of Community Health Nursing, 18*(1), 1–11.

Eyton, J., & Neuwirth, G. (1984). Cross-cultural validity: ethnocentrism in health studies with special reference to the Vietnamese. *Social Science and Medicine, 18*(5), 447–453.

Finer, D. (1999). *Pressing priorities. Consumer drug information in the Vietnamese marketplace*. Stockholm: IHCAR, Karolinska Institute.

Fong, R., & Mokuau, N. (1994). Not simply "Asian Americans": periodical literature review on Asians and Pacific Islanders. *Social Work, 39*(3), 298–305.

Fox, P. G., Cowell, J. M., & Johnson, M. M. (1995). Effects of family disruption on Southeast Asian refugee women. *International Nursing Review, 42*(1), 27–30.

Gellis, Z. (2003). Kin and nonkin social supports in a community sample of Vietnamese immigrants. *Social Work, 48*(2), 248–258.

Geltman, P., Brown, M., & Cochran, J. (2001). Lead poisoning among refugee children resettled in Massachusetts, 1995–1999. *Pediatrics, 108*(1), 158–162.

Grant, D. M. (1983). Variability in caffeine metabolism. *Clinical Pharmacology Therapy, 33*, 591–602.

Harvard Women's Health Watch (2005). *Not getting over it: post-traumatic stress disorder*. Boston, MA: Harvard Publications, Harvard University.

Helm, R., Quan, D., Herfindal, E. T., & Gourley, D. (2006). *Textbook of therapeutics: drug and disease management* (8th ed.). Philadelphia: Lippincott, Williams & Wilkins.

Hiebert, M. (1993). Miles to go. *Far Eastern Economic Review, 156*(30), 24–26.

Ho, V., Amal, J., Atkinson, E., Basen-Engquist, K., Tortolero-Luna, G., & Follen, M. (2005). Predictors of breast and cervical screening in Vietnamese women in Harris County, Houston, Texas. *Cancer Nursing, 28*(2), 119–129.

Hoang, G., & Erickson, R. (1982). Guidelines for providing medical care for Southeast Asian refugees. *Journal of the American Medical Association, 248*(6), 710–714.

Huard, P., & Wong, M. (1968). *Chinese medicine*. New York: McGraw-Hill.

Huynh, T. D. (1987). *Introduction to Vietnamese culture*. Multifunctional Resource Center. San Diego, CA: San Diego State University.

Jenkins, C., et al. (1997). Tobacco use in Vietnam prevalence, predictors, and the role of transnational tobacco companies. *Journal of the American Medical Association, 277*(21), 1726–1731.

Jochelson, T., Hua, M., & Rissel, C. (2003). Knowledge, attitudes and behaviors of caregivers regarding children's exposure to environmental tobacco smoke among Arabic and Vietnamese-speaking communities in Sydney, Australia. *Ethnicity and Health, 8*(4), 339–351.

Labun, E. (2000). Discovering our common humanity: developing partnerships in a Vietnamese community. *Journal of Christian Nursing, 17*(3), 8–11, 39.

Labun, E. (2001). Cultural discovery in nursing practice with Vietnamese clients. *Journal of Advanced Nursing, 35*(6), 874–881.

Lan, L. V. (1988). Folk medicine among the Southeast Asian refugees in the U.S.A.: risks, benefits, and uncertainties. *Journal of the Association of Vietnamese Medical Professionals in Canada, 98*, 31–36.

Leung, L. (1988). Training bilingual paraprofessionals for counseling services. *Hawaii Journal of Counseling and Development, 4*(1), 16–22.

Levy, D. T., Bales, S., Lan, N. T., & Nikolayex, L. (2006). The role of public policies in reducing smoking and deaths caused by smoking in Vietnam: results from the Vietnam tobacco policy simulation model. *Social Science and Medicine, 62*, 1819–1830.

Li, C., Malone, K., & Daling, J. (2003). Differences in breast cancer stage, treatment, and survival by race and ethnicity. *Archives of Internal Medicine, 163*, 49–56.

Lin, K. M., & Finder, E. (1983). Neuroleptic dosage for Asians. *American Journal of Psychiatry, 140*, 490–491.

Lin, K. M., et al. (1989). Longitudinal assessment of haloperidol doses and serous concentrations in Asian and Caucasian schizophrenic patients. *American Journal of Psychiatry, 146*(10), 1307–1311.

Lindsay, J., Narayan, M., & Rea, K. (1998). Nursing across cultures: the Vietnamese client. *Home Healthcare Nurse, 16*(10), 693–700.

Mac, J., Doordan, A., & Carr, C. (1999). Evaluation of the effectiveness of a directly observed therapy program with Vietnamese tuberculosis patients. *Public Health Nursing, 16*(6), 426–431.

Maiter, S., & George, U. (2003). Understanding context and culture in the parenting approaches of immigrant South Asian mothers. *Affilia, 18*(4), 411–428.

Makimoto, K. (1998). Spotlight on special populations. Drinking patterns and drinking problems among Asian-Americans and Pacific Islanders. *Alcohol Health and Research World, 22*(4), 270–275.

McLaughlin, L., & Braun, K. (1998). Asian and Pacific Islander cultural values: considerations for health care decision making. *Health and Social Work, 24*(2), 116–126.

McNally, R. J. (2006). Psychiatric casualties of war. *Science, 313,* 923–924.

McPhee, S. (2002). Caring for a 70-year-old Vietnamese woman. *Journal of the American Medical Association, 287*(4), 495–505.

McPhee, S. J., et al. (2003). Successful promotion of hepatitis B vaccinations among Vietnamese-American children ages 3–18: results of a controlled trial. *Pediatrics, 111*(6), 1278–1288.

Morrow, M., & Barraclough, S. (2003). Tobacco control and gender in South-East Asia. Part II: Singapore and Vietnam. *Health Promotion International, 18*(4), 373–380.

Murphy, H. B. (1969). Ethnic variations in drug responses. *Transcultural Psychiatric Research Review, 6,* 6–23.

Nguyen, D. (1988). Culture shock: a study of Vietnamese culture and the concept of health and disease. *Journal of the Association of Vietnamese Medical Professionals in Canada, 98,* 26–30.

Nicholson, B. (1997). The influence of pre-emigration and postmigration stressors on mental health: a study of SEA refugees. *Social Work Research, 21*(1), 12–15.

Nilchaikovit, K., Hill, J., & Holland, J. (1993). The effects of culture on illness behavior and medical care. *General Hospital Psychiatry, 15,* 41–50.

O'Hare, T., & Tran, T. (1998). Substance abuse among Southeast Asians in the U.S.: implications for practice and research. *Social Work in Health, 26*(3), 69–80.

Pavuk, M., Michalak, J., Schecter, A., Ketchum, N. S., Akhtar, F. Z., & Fox, K. A. (2005). Did TCDD exposure or service in Southeast Asia increase the risk of cancer in Air Force Vietnam Veterans who did not spray Agent Orange? *Journal of Occupational Environmental Medicine, 47*(4), 335–342.

Phan, T. (1996). Ethnic and cultural specificities of domestic violence: a research and clinical discourse with references to the Vietnamese emigrant community. *International Journal of Psychiatric Nursing Research, 2*(2), 187–197.

Phipps, E., Cohen, M., Sorn, S., & Braitman, L. (1999). A pilot study of cancer knowledge and screening behaviors of Vietnamese and Cambodian women. *Health Care for Women International, 20*(2), 195–207.

Rairdan, B., & Higgs, Z. R. (1992). When your patient is a Hmong refugee. *American Journal of Nursing, 92*(3), 52–55.

Reed, D. B., Meeks, P. M., Nguyen, L., Cross, E. W., & Garrison, M. E. B. (1998). Assessment of nutrition education needs related to increasing dietary calcium intake in low-income Vietnamese mothers using focus group discussions. *Journal of Nutrition Education, 30*(3), 155–163.

Rosenblat, H., & Tang, S. W. (1987). Do Asian patients receive different dosages of psychotropic medication when compared to Occidentals? *Canadian Journal of Psychiatry, 32,* 270–274.

Rudy, D., & Grusec, J. (2001). Correlates of authoritarian parenting in individualist and collectivist cultures and implications for understanding the transmission of values. *Journal of Cross-Cultural Psychology, 32*(2), 202–212.

Satchell, M. (1999). Questions in a village: did Agent Orange cause Vietnamese birth defects? *U.S. News and World Report, 126*(16), 62.

Schecter, A., Hoang, Q., Pavuk, M., Päpke, O., Malisch, R., & Constable, J. D. (2003). Food as a source of dioxin exposure in the residents of Bien Hoa City, Vietnam. *Journal of Environmental Medicine, 45*(8), 781–788.

Schulmeister, L., & Lifsey, D. S. (1999). Cervical cancer screening knowledge, behaviors, and beliefs of Vietnamese women. *Oncology Nursing Forum, 26*(5), 879–887.

Shapiro, J., Radecki, S., Charchian, A., & Josephson, V. (1999). Sexual behavior and AIDS-related knowledge among community college students in Orange County, California. *Journal of Community Health, 24*(1), 29–43.

Sideleau, B. (1992). Space and time. In J. Haber, A. Leach McMahon, P. Price-Hoskins, & B. Sidleau (Eds.), *Comprehensive psychiatric nursing* (4th ed., pp. 193–209). St. Louis: Mosby.

Smither, R., & Rodríguez-Giegling, R. (1979). Marginality, modernity, and anxiety in Indochinese refugees. *Journal of Cross-Cultural Psychiatry, 10,* 469–478.

Spector, R. (2004). *Cultural diversity in health and illness* (6th ed.). Upper Saddle River, NJ: Pearson Prentice Hall.

Strand, P., & Jones, W. (1983). Health service utilization by Indochinese refugees. *Medical Care, 21*(11), 1089–1098.

Taylor, R., Morrel, S., Mamoon, H., Macansh, S., Ross, J., & Wain, G. V. (2003). Cervical cancer screening in a Vietnamese nominal cohort. *Ethnicity & Health, 8*(3), 251–261.

Tien, J. L. (1984). Do Asians need less medication? Issues in clinical assessment and psychopharmacology. *Journal of Psychosocial Nursing and Mental Health Services, 22,* 19–22.

Tien-Hyatt, J. (1989). Keying in on the unique care needs of Asian clients. *Nursing and Health Care, 11,* 269–271.

Tran, T. (1991). Family living arrangements and social adjustments among three ethnic groups of elderly Indochinese refugees. *International Journal of Aging and Human Development, 32*(2), 91–102.

Tran, T. M. (1972). The family and the management of mental health problems in Vietnam. In W. P. Lebra (Ed.), *Transcultural research in mental health.* Honolulu: University of Hawaii Press.

Tran, T. M. (1980). *Indochinese patients.* Falls Church, VA: Action for Southeast Asians.

Tripp-Reimer, T., & Thieman, K. (1981). Traditional health beliefs/practices of Vietnamese refugees. *Journal of Iowa Medical Society, 71*(12), 533–535.

U.S. Department of Commerce, Bureau of the Census (2013). *The Asian population 2004: census 2004 brief.* Washington, DC: U.S. Government Printing Office.

U.S. Department of Commerce, Bureau of the Census (2013). *American Community Survey.* Hyattsville, MD: U.S. Government Printing Office.

U.S. Department of Commerce, Bureau of the Census (2015). *American Community Survey.* Washington, DC: U.S. Government Printing Office.

Westermeyer, J., & Winthrop, R. (1979). Folk criteria for the diagnosis of mental illness in rural Laos. *American Journal of Psychiatry, 136,* 136–161.

Wiecha, J. (1999). Differences in knowledge of hepatitis B among Vietnamese, African-American, Hispanic and White adolescents in Worcester, Massachusetts. *Pediatrics*, *104*(5 Pt. 2), 1212–1216.

Wiecha, J. M., Fink, A. K., Wiecha, J., & Herbert, J. (2001). Differences in dietary patterns of Vietnamese, White, African-American, and Hispanic adolescents in Worcester, Mass. *Journal of the American Dietetic Association*, *101*(2), 248–251.

Williams, C., & Westermeyer, J. (1986). *Refugee mental health in resettlement countries*. New York: Hemisphere.

World almanac. (2015). New York: World Almanac Books.

Xu, Y., Ross, C., Ryan, R., & Wang, B. (2005). Cancer risk factors of Vietnamese-Americans in rural south Alabama. *Journal of Nursing Scholarship*, *37*(3), 237–244.

Yeatman, G. W., & Dang, V. V. (1980). C o gió (coin rubbing). Vietnamese attitudes toward health care. *Journal of the American Medical Association*, *244*(24), 2748–2749.

Zhou, F., et al. (2000). Economic analysis of promotion of hepatitis B vaccinations among Vietnamese-American children and adolescents in Houston and Dallas. *Pediatrics*, *111*(6), 1289–1296.

East Indian Hindu Americans

Scott Wilson Miller and Kira Ann Lass

After reading this chapter, the nurse will be able to:

1. Identify two important East Indian Hindu cultural values that influence the behavior of East Indian Hindus living in the United States and Canada.
2. Describe concepts of health and illness influencing East Indian Hindus in relation to illness and health-seeking behaviors.
3. Outline the characteristics of the three waves of immigrants who have come to the United States and Canada from India.
4. Describe the effect culture has had on symptoms of mental illness experienced by the East Indian Hindu in India and after immigration.
5. Understand the unique beliefs about touch held by East Indian Hindus and explain how these beliefs may influence attitudes and reactions of East Indian Hindu Americans to caregivers.
6. Describe the beliefs and values held by East Indian Hindus concerning the family.
7. Explain the past-, present-, and future-time orientation held by East Indian Hindus.
8. Describe the Ayurvedic system and the way this system explains illness.

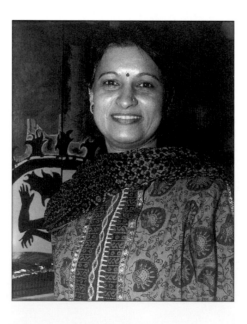

OVERVIEW OF INDIA AND HINDUISM

The Republic of India is a subcontinent that is a vast, wedge-shaped triangular peninsula jutting from the south mainland of Asia into the Indian Ocean. India includes an area of about 1,269,338 square miles and stretches about 2000 miles from north to south. It has three major land regions: the Himalayas and associated mountain ranges to the north, the Indus-Ganges-Brahmaputra Plain in the north central, and the Deccan Plateau in the south. The country contains a large part of the great Indo-Gangetic plain, extending from the Bay of Bengal on the east to the Afghan frontier and the Arabian Sea on the west. This plain is the richest and most densely populated part of the subcontinent.

The climate of India varies according to region. The Himalayas shield the Indian subcontinent from the main body of the Eurasian landmass, resulting in a unique climate. High-pressure winds moving down the Gangetic Plain into the Bay of Bengal result in winters that are generally dry on most of the continent. The Ganges Valley is noted for summer monsoons and rain, although rainfall may vary considerably. In the Ganges-Brahmaputra delta and surrounding areas, rainfall may exceed 80 inches per year, whereas in the northeastern portions of the Deccan region and along the southeastern coast, the total rainfall ranges from 40 to 80 inches per year. In the areas around the western half of the Deccan region, the annual rainfall is 20 to 40 inches per year. In the southern half of the country, temperatures are tropical and vary little from month to month. In northern India, however, the annual range is considerable, and in January the average temperature in the north may be 30°F lower than in the south (Simons, 1976).

About 70% of India's working population is engaged in agriculture. The average Indian farmer, living in small villages, working farms that average 2 acres per family, and using age-old cultivation techniques based on human or animal power, lacks efficiency and is seldom able to provide more than the bare subsistence for the family. Rice, wheat, peanuts, corn, and millet are traditional crops. Cash crops include sugarcane, tea, tobacco, jute, and cotton (Central Intelligence Agency, 2015). Cultivation potential is further handicapped by lack of water, allowing only 50% of the land to be cultivated. About 49% of the land is suitable for crop production, and only 3% of that contains permanent crops (Central Intelligence Agency, 2015; McKay, Hill, & Buckler, 2007; Simons, 1976). The Indian constitution prohibits the slaughter of cattle. India has one of the largest livestock populations in the world, yet most of the animals are undernourished and diseased.

While the majority of the country is involved in agricultural activities, the urban areas of India are indeed heavily industrialized. The textile industry is an important area. Other industry includes iron and steel as well as machine tools, transportation equipment, and chemicals (Central Intelligence Agency, 2015).

India is a federal republic with a parliamentary system of government. The head of state is a president who is elected for a 5-year term by members of the national and state legislatures. Effective executive power is exercised by a prime minister who is normally the leader of the majority political party. Prime ministers have included Jawaharlal Nehru (1984–1989), Chandra Shekhar (1989–1991), and P. V. Narasimha Rao (1991–1996). In 1991, Prime Minister Shekhar resigned. Two months after Shekhar's resignation (May 22, 1991), former Prime Minister Rajiv Gandhi was assassinated (*World Almanac*, 2015). In November 1991, an election was held and P. V. Narasimha Rao was chosen to form a new government. In May 1996, the ruling Congress Party lost the parliamentary elections. At that time, Atal Bihari Vajpayee of the Hindu nationalist Bharatiya Janata Party became prime minister for 13 days. After this short regime, Deve Gowda of the United Front Coalition became prime minister. However, Prime Minister Gowda lost a confidence vote in April 1997. At that time Foreign Minister Gujral was sworn in as Prime Minister. In 1998, Atal Bihari Vajpayee once again became Prime Minister. On July 25, 1997, Kocheril Raman Narayanan was elected president. In 2002, A. P. J. Abdul Kalam was elected president, a position he currently still holds. In 2004, the Indian National Congress Party led by Sonia Gandhi prevailed in the parliamentary elections, thus prompting Prime Minister Atal Bihari Vajpayee to resign. Because of a variety of reasons, the Congress Party ultimately chose to elect former finance minister Manmohan Singh as the new Prime Minister in 2004 (Central Intelligence Agency, 2015; *World Almanac*, 2015).

Despite a large landmass, India is overpopulated. The most densely populated state is West Bengal, with 767 people per 274 square kilometers. The most densely populated union territory is Delhi, with 6352 people per 274 square kilometers. The most densely populated district is Calcutta, with 23,783 people per 274 square kilometers (Central Intelligence Agency, 2015).

Most of the population, crowded into the Ganges River Valley and the eastern and western coastal regions, is of diverse racial genotypes. The people of India speak approximately 200 different languages, including 1652 dialects. Some of the languages spoken include Hindi (41%), Bengali (8.1%), Telugu (7.2%), Marathi (7.0%), and Tamil (5.9%) (Central Intelligence Agency, 2015).

In 2004 the population increased to 1,095,351,995; likewise, the population continued to increase in 2014 and now numbers 1,236,344,631 (Central Intelligence Agency, 2015).

Based upon 2014 statistics, the birth rate in India was 19.89 births per 1000 persons, showing a slight decrease; for example, in 2002 the birth rate was 23.8 per 1000 persons, and in 2006 the birth rate was 22.01 births per 1000. Infant mortality for 2010 was 49.13 per 1000 live births, which is significantly down from 2002 when it was 61.5 per 1000. In 2006, the infant mortality was 54.63 deaths per 1000. In 2010, the death rate was 7.53 deaths per 1000. The Hindu population is increasing at the rate of 1.8%, or almost 13 million people each year. The median age of the population is currently 27.0 years. Life expectancy for the general population is 67.08 years (Central Intelligence Agency, 2015).

In the slums of Calcutta, Mumbai (formerly Bombay), and other large cities, thousands die yearly from malnutrition and disease. Some of these diseases include bacterial diarrhea, hepatitis, typhoid fever, dengue fever, and malaria. The prevalence of human immunodeficiency virus (HIV) in adults is 0.9%, and it is estimated that 5.1 million people live with HIV or acquired immunodeficiency syndrome (Central Intelligence Agency, 2015; *Information Please Almanac, 2007*). Under the pressure of population increases, the economic, political, and social aspects of life are strained (Warshaw, 1988).

Today the situation in the region is further complicated by the forces of religion and nationalism. The people of the subcontinent are deeply divided by the Hindu and Muslim faiths. Their loyalties are divided between the nation-states of India, Pakistan, and Bangladesh, which share the subcontinent. Indian society is composed of many separate fragments coexisting through mutual tolerance and general agreement on the states and functions of various groups. The regions vary considerably in their historic traditions, cultural patterns, and complement of castes. Within each region, contrasts in customs and traditions parallel class and caste differences. Cutting across linguistic and class divisions are the "communities," which are large aggregates of people defined by some common denominator, such as religion, ethnic affiliation, or area of origin (Melendy, 1977). Some Indians believe that there is no need for people in these diverse groups to conform to a single set of practices and beliefs. The underlying unity of the country is derived from the larger arena of cultural traditions shared by most groups and from the dominance of certain national elites.

Hinduism is the title given for convenience to the religion of most of the population of the Indian subcontinent (Warshaw, 1988). Consequently, approximately 82% to 85% of the population is classified as Hindu (Central Intelligence Agency, 2015). Other religions include Islam (13%), Christianity (2%), and Sikhism (2%) (Central Intelligence Agency, 2015).

Hinduism is a culture as much as it is a religion, and the balance of culture and religion forms the social structure of the Hindu society. Social and religious mores are so predominant that if an Orthodox Hindu were to abandon Hindu belief for another religion, this individual, like the Orthodox Jew, would become an outcast from the people.

Hindus agree on a philosophy rather than doctrine (Thrane, 2010). Although Hindus built magnificent temples, they developed no church. The priesthood is hereditary and can be achieved only through reincarnation. Of the few beliefs shared by all Hindus, respect for a priest is among the foremost. Hinduism evolved over the past 4000 years and has no single founder or creed; rather, it consists of a vast variety of beliefs and spiritually based health practices and customs. Formal organization is minimal, and a religious hierarchy is nonexistent.

A common belief shared by most Hindus is veneration of life, especially regarding the cow, which is believed to embody fertility. Although rivers, trees, and other forms of life are also regarded as sacred, the cow is considered the holiest life form.

Early Hindus were united in other philosophical respects. The transmigration of the soul represented one essential element of faith. In the backward or forward movement of the soul, there existed an underlying moral responsibility (*dharma*, which may be translated as law, religion, virtue, morality, or custom). It was *dharma* that obliged each member of society to maintain the role that was assigned at birth. On the individual level, *dharma* required the pursuit of *nirvana* in ways that were defined by the priests (Warshaw, 1988).

The doctrine of reincarnation, of which transmigration is an integral part, provided a vital link between the religion of Brahmanism and the social order in which it was practiced. The religion claimed a divine mandate to separate people by castes, otherwise known as the *vara* (color) system. At the same time, it suggested to members of the toiling lower castes that they might become reincarnated at a higher level in another life. To attain advancement in the other life, the individual must fulfill moral obligations in the present one. Thus the doctrine of reincarnation was an incentive for members of the lower caste to be dutiful. The ultimate bliss of final union with Brahma, although dim and distant, was a realizable goal. Although this union might be achieved through correct actions, the nature of action was limited by each caste (Warshaw, 1988).

The relationship between the people's beliefs concerning the causes of illness and attempts to seek relief from its effects is learned from local folk practitioners. Illness and its treatment are perceived as biological as well as social phenomena (Kakar, 1977).

Many health professionals do not recognize that the health beliefs and practices of Hindus evolved over the centuries and that every cultural trait has direct relevance to the environment. Although beliefs concerning the causes of prevalent disease may appear illogical, they are difficult to dismiss or substitute with Western medical practices. Adequate knowledge about these beliefs can assist nurses in the formulation of nursing diagnoses and nursing interventions and guard against undue conflicts with the practice of folk medicine.

IMMIGRATION TO THE UNITED STATES AND CANADA

First-Wave Immigrants

The arrival of East Indians from the Indian subcontinent during the first two decades of the twentieth century caused considerable uproar along the Pacific Coast of Canada and the United States (Melendy, 1977). Although East Indians immigrated to these countries in very small numbers, their immigration coincided with increasing American hostility toward the Japanese. Before the nineteenth century, very few Hindu Indians migrated overseas from the Indian subcontinent because most Hindu Indians believed that crossing the "black waters" was dangerous to the Hindu soul. By 1900, the U.S. Bureau of the Census reported that 2050 East Indian residents had immigrated to the United States. Many of the immigrants in this group were non-Indians who were born in India, some were Indian students, and some were Indian businessmen (Melendy, 1977).

In 1901, East Indian students began arriving in the United States to enroll in various colleges and universities throughout the East Coast area. Many of these students enrolled in such prestigious institutions as Cornell University. It was not until 1904 or 1905 that East Indian students began to immigrate to the western portion of the United States to enroll in such universities as the University of California and the California Polytechnic Institute. Students were not the only immigrants who were included in this first major wave of Hindu Indians. During this period, U.S. ports of entry began to register major increases in East Indian immigrants; from 1904 to 1906, 674 East Indians immigrated, compared with only 9 in 1900. The majority of the East Indian immigrants were unskilled agriculturalists and small entrepreneurs from the arid lands of the Punjab, the United provinces, Bengal, and Gujarat (Melendy, 1977).

From the onset of the first wave of East Indian immigrants, these people were classified as Hindus (or Hindoos) regardless of their home, culture, or religion. The U.S. Immigration Commission in 1911 mandated that any native of India was to be considered a Hindu for immigration purposes (Divine, 1972; U.S. Immigration Commission, 1911). In 1917 Congress passed, over President Wilson's veto, an immigration restriction act for East

Indians. This new law required a literacy test and also encompassed a barred zone for immigration. All Asians who resided in India, Southeast Asia, the Indonesian islands, New Guinea, or regions of Arabia, Afghanistan, or Siberia were excluded by the new immigration law (Melendy, 1977).

Second-Wave Immigrants

In 1909, Canada closed its doors to East Indian immigrants; however, immigration of East Indians to the United States continued for another 5 years. The Immigration Exclusion Act of 1917, which excluded most persons of East Indian descent, including Hindu Indians, severely curtailed the number of Hindus in the United States. The number of East Indian immigrants residing in the United States began to decline sharply in 1910. In that year, the U.S. Commission reported that there were some 5000 East Indians residing in the United States, but in 1930 this number was disputed by the U.S. Bureau of the Census, which reported that there were only 2544 East Indians residing in the United States, most in California. In 1946, President Harry Truman signed into law a bill that allowed East Indian immigration on a quota basis and allowed naturalization of East Indians. This law is credited with beginning the second wave of immigration of East Indian Hindus to the United States.

These new immigrants, who arrived after World War II and before 1965, were mostly professional Hindu people and their families. These immigrants came mostly from large cities of Mumbai (formerly called Bombay) and Calcutta (Ramakrishna & Weiss, 1992).

Third-Wave Immigrants

In 1965, an immigration law marking the beginning of a third wave of immigrants to the United States was enacted. The Immigration Act raised quotas for Asians to the same level as Europeans, facilitating entry to the United States (Koshy, 2001). Although the first-wave immigrants were primarily agriculturists with some students and the second-wave immigrants were primarily university-educated professionals and their families, the third-wave immigrants were entirely different (Bhungalia & Kemp, 2002). These new generations of immigrants were very young, with 3 out of 5 under 30 years of age and 1 out of 7 less than 10 years of age. In 1974 approximately 12,777 East Indians resided in the United States; by 2009 this number significantly increased to more than 2.5 million people (U.S. Department of Commerce, Bureau of the Census, *American Community Survey*, 2013).

Initially these immigrants were predominantly male, coming to the United States for graduate education in the science and business fields. Eventually, in the 1980s, women who wanted an education started arriving. Among

Asian Indian males, 91.0% have at least a high school education compared with 93.4% of Asian Indian females; 74.6% of males and 64.8% of females have at least a bachelor's degree (U.S. Department of Commerce, Bureau of the Census, *American Community Survey*, 2013). In addition, these new immigrants may not be coming directly from India. Many have emigrated from other countries in Asia and Europe before coming to the United States (Korom, 2001).

It is essential to distinguish who are the East Indian Americans. Indian Americans are of Asian descent and either were born in or native to India or have ancestors who were born in or native to India (U.S. Department of Commerce, Bureau of the Census, *American Community Survey*, 2013). To make a clear distinction and difference between Indians of Asian origin and Indians who are indigenous peoples of the Americas, the U.S. Census Bureau popularized the term "Asian Indians" to avoid confusion with the term "American Indian" (U.S. Department of Commerce, Bureau of the Census, *American Community Survey*, 2013). In 2010, there were 2,578,978 people of East Indian descent or from the Indian diaspora (Asian Indians) residing in the United States (U.S. Department of Commerce, Bureau of the Census, *American Community Survey*, 2013). The median age of Asian Indians in 2010 was 32.0, compared with 36.7 for the rest of the general U.S. population. The number of married-couple East Indian Hindu Americans (Asian Indians) represented 71.9% of that population, compared with 49.3% of the general U.S. population. In 2009, the median per capita income of Asian Indian males was $71,605, compared with $45,320 for the rest of the general U.S. population. Similarly, for Asian Indian women, the median per capita income was $51,316, compared with $35,299 for the rest of their female counterparts. The median family income was also higher for Asian Indians. In 2009, the median family income for Asian Indians was $98,508, compared with $62,367 for the general U.S. population (U.S. Department of Commerce, Bureau of the Census, *American Community Survey*, 2013).

COMMUNICATION

Origins of Hindustani Dialect

Language is a means of communication, and it disseminates new ideas. It is the storehouse of tradition and literature that provides a people with a sense of pride, self-confidence, and emotional unity. The national elite groups of a culture emphasize the value of a common language as a unifying force and the necessity for the development of language and literature. The study of linguistic heritage not only is an end in itself but also serves to establish the conditions for nationhood (Pye, 1976).

Hindustani (the name given by Europeans to an Indo-Aryan dialect), as a result of political causes, has become the great *lingua franca* of modern India. The name is not used by natives of India, except as an imitation of the English nomenclature. Hindustani is by origin a Hindi dialect of western India. Hindustani has been called a mongrel pidgin form of speech composed of contributions from the various languages spoken in a Delhi bazaar. This theory has not been disproved because of the discovery that the language is the actual living dialect of western India, which has existed for centuries in its present form (Singh, 1966).

Hindustani is the natural language of the people of Delhi. Because the origin of Hindustani began with the people in the Delhi bazaar, it became known as "bazaar language." From the inception of Hindustani, this language became the *lingua franca* of the mongrel camp and was transported everywhere in India by the lieutenants of the empire. Several recognized forms of the dialect exists, such as Dakhini, Urdu, Rekhta, and Hindi. Dakhini, or "southern," is the form in current use in southern India and the first to be used in the literature. It contains many archaic expressions now extinct in the standard dialect. Urdu, "the language of the camp," is the name usually used for the Hindustani by natives and is now the standard form of speech used by Muslims. All the early Hindustani literature was written as poetry, and this literary form of speech was named Rekhta, or "scattered," from the way in which words borrowed from Persia were scattered through it. Hindustani is the dialect used in poetry, with Urdu being the dialect of prose and conversation (Singh, 1966).

There are approximately 18 languages spoken in India, with Hindi being the most prevalent (40.2%). Bengali is spoken by 8.3% of the population, Telugu by 7.9%, Marathi by 7.5%, Tamil by 6.32%, Urdu by 5.2%, Gujarati by 4.8%, Kannada by 3.9%, Malayalam by 3.6%, Oriya by 3.4%, Punjabi by 2.8%, Assamese by 1.6%, Sindhi by 0.3%, Nepali by 0.3%, Konkani by 0.2%, Manipuri by 0.2%, Kasmiri by 0.01%, and Sanskrit by 0.01%. All but Nepali, Konkani, and Manipuri are considered official languages (Census of India, 2011; Central Intelligence Agency, 2015).

Hindi is the official language of India. English is considered to be an associate official language, with some states declaring it as their official language. The use of English in India is in a fairly fluid state because of the political ideology of each state. The languages taught in the education system are variable, as is the timeframe in which the various languages are introduced. In general, the languages would be the regional dialect pertinent to the school system—Hindi because it is the national official language, and English as a means to improve social mobility and compete in the workforce (Bayer & Gupta, 2006).

Style

The term *Hindi* is ambiguous and therefore the source of much controversy because it is not easily defined. It is considered a regional dialect with a variety of common structural and interchangeable content elements. Its usage depends on both the regional affiliation and the social background of the speaker. Hindi is a highly open language closely related to other Indo-Aryan languages; therefore, the degree of stylization is determined by the degree of language-orientation consciousness in the speaker's mind (Corlett & Moore, 1980). Hindi encompasses three areas of stylization: high, medium, and low. An individual may shift between high and low stylization according to situational requirements, as in formal discourse, during conversations with equals, and in giving instruction to subordinates.

Volume and Kinetics

East Indians are generally noted for their soft-spoken manner, almost considered mumbling by some. Frequently, head movements and hand gestures accentuate conversations, adding vitality to the speaker's content. Men maintain direct eye contact with each other when conversing and may become loud and intense when addressing family members. Women usually draw their eyes downward when addressing their husband, father, or grandfather. This gesture demonstrates a sign of respect and should not be misconstrued as not caring or not listening (Purnell, 2014).

Touch

Displays of public affection are prohibited and viewed as disrespectful in the eyes of the gods. Married East Indian couples may show signs of affection in the privacy of their own home but not in view of children or elders. Affectionate touching or embracing among friends, relatives, and acquaintances is not a socially acceptable Hindu practice.

Implications for Nursing Care

The use of Hindi among East Indian Hindus is the one culturally unifying trait these people possessed after immigration to the United States or Canada. Reluctantly, East Indian Hindus have recognized the need for adoption of English as a communicative norm in the Western culture. Still, most elderly family members are unwilling to abandon the native language, which is regarded as meaningful to their cultural identity, and find it difficult to learn and communicate in English. On the other hand, younger family members, especially children, easily adapt to the Western culture and are more inclined to incorporate English into their language skills. Whenever possible, translators should be used by the nurse and other health care personnel when administering care to persons in the East Indian Hindu American population.

When obtaining a health history from an East Indian Hindu American client or family, both Hindi- and English-speaking family members should be involved. Because of uncertainty with the English language, the client may feel frustrated and not communicate conditions thoroughly. When a Hindi-speaking client becomes frustrated, the client may first attempt to translate needs by using Hindi; therefore, it may be necessary to translate Hindi responses into English. This process preserves the client's cultural identity while promoting client confidence.

When interacting with recently immigrated traditional Hindu patients, it is important for the nurse to remember that it is considered taboo for a man other than the woman's husband to extend his hand toward her in greeting. In introducing oneself to a female Hindu client, the greeting is first addressed to the husband or eldest female companion.

It is also considered taboo for a man other than a woman's husband to initiate or maintain direct eye contact with a woman. This may be perceived by the husband as a seductive gesture. The wife, as a show of respect and out of fear of reprisal, may divert her eyes downward during conversation.

In today's health care system it is imperative that practitioners incorporate cultural competency. In terms of the East Indian client, practitioners must consider and include complementary and alternative medications used by the patients; the way medical advice, instruction, and education has been understood or filtered by the prevailing cultural norms; and the impact of such on adherence of medication regimens and treatments. In addition, in terms of disability and death, practitioners must incorporate religious beliefs such as karma that help the patient in coping (Gupta, 2010).

SPACE

In countries that are vastly overpopulated, such as India, the time lag between a decline in death rate and the acceptance and practice of rational control of fertility presents a serious strain on the economy of the country. India made positive efforts to reduce the birth rate and thus reduced the phenomenon of overcrowding that existed (Moore, 1963). The automobile has been poorly adapted in India because the cities are so physically crowded, and the Indian society has buildings with elaborate architectural designs (Hall, 1990). Most Hindu Americans are surprised to find that internal ornaments such as ceiling fixtures do not fit into American houses because the ceilings are too low, the rooms are too small, and privacy from the outside is viewed as inadequate (Hall, 1990).

Implications for Nursing Care

East Indian Hindus are a family-oriented people who do not view family as intrusive in personal space parameters. When an East Indian Hindu American becomes ill and is hospitalized, the entire family may gather at the bedside. Health care decisions are often made communally with the senior family member or the eldest son as the final authority (Thrane, 2010). Also, an important, highly valued role for grandparents is raising the grandchildren (Bhungalia & Kemp, 2002). It is important for the nurse to remember that the client may feel that the space in the hospital is overextended and that the family's presence is essential to collapse the space inward. In this case it is important for the nurse to involve family members in the plan of care and to ascertain which family members will provide personal care.

SOCIAL ORGANIZATION

Family

In a traditional East Indian Hindu household, married sons live with the family under the parental roof and are subject to parental authority. Frequently the joint family includes approximately 25 individuals and may include up to 200 people. The average joint family is composed of six or seven family members, and the family may comprise several generations. It is of note that the average household size of the East Indian family residing in the United States is 3.0 (U.S. Department of Commerce, Bureau of the Census, *American Community Survey*, 2013).

The patriarch controls the finances of the group, giving the sons allowances from their earnings. With globalization and the impact of the growing middle class, men are still considered the primary provider for the family. Thus, the primary role of men in these households is to provide financial income to support the family (Larson, Verma, & Dworkin, 2001). The matriarch is the autocrat of the home, and her daughters-in-law are subject to her rule. Although this system provides the members of the family with security and sustenance, it has been suggested that it encourages dependence and lack of initiative among many family members (Bhungalia & Kemp, 2002; Reddy, 1986). In the past, East Indian Hindu girls have wept at the prospect of marriage, not because of objections to little-known bridegrooms but in fear of their future mothers-in-law (Reddy, 1986). The joint family is a powerful social unit, whose pressures on the individual are greater than most Westerners can imagine. It has also been suggested that the East Indian family demands much sacrifice and devotion and consequently fosters timidity and lassitude in its members (Reddy, 1986).

The hierarchy of the joint family places the father or eldest brother at the highest level. However, the family relies heavily on a democratic system of governance, and decisions of prime importance are determined by a vote in which heads of family may be overruled. Although the head of the family (the patriarch) is the undisputed overseer of other male members of the household, the matriarch is responsible for the family's female members and is instrumental in determining other domestic concerns. Modern East Indian women continue to be the dominant force in home life activities even if they enter the workforce and also provide income for the family (Larson et al., 2001). Recent efforts to promote family planning to reduce the burden of the mushrooming population for the most part has resulted in action by women. Indian men appear to reject sterilization for both psychological and religious reasons, fearing it will destroy their male power or will interfere with God's will (McKay et al., 2007; Nossiter, 1970).

The East Indian Hindu father is perceived as being distant from his children, who prefer to bond closely with their mother (Kurian & Ghosh, 1983). The eldest son is destined to continue the family name and perform the holy death rites that will ensure peace for his father's soul. This expectation places the eldest son in the position of being one of the closest family members to the patriarch. Throughout his life the eldest son, even when fully mature, rises when his father enters a room or is near him and greets his father with the *pranām*, the sign of deference in which one touches the feet of a highly respected figure. East Indian Hindus tend to be respectful of authority figures but are more distant with male superiors than with their female counterparts. These people cherish courtesy, which is reflected in the traditional greeting, wherein the head is bowed, the hands are clasped, as if in prayer, and the Hindu word *namaste* ("I bow to thee") is uttered softly.

It is the family, above all other institutions, that is responsible for the implantation of social mores and values in the Hindu culture. Ancient traditions that are suggestive of the existence of external rituals are strictly practiced, and it is the adherence to these ancient traditions that determines whether young East Indians become conservative or rebellious (Warshaw, 1988).

Marriage

In India, marriages of Hindu Indians have always been arranged by parents or other intermediaries. Because marriage was regarded as a union of families rather than of individuals, the marriage traditionally took place when the husband and wife were only children. In 1955 in India, it became illegal to arrange for the marriage of girls under 15 and boys under 18 years of age. This law has been amended in subsequent years to reflect the current legal age for marriage to be 18 years of age for girls and 21 years of age for boys (UNICEF, 2011). However, this law is not easily enforced, and almost 60% of girls are married before they reach 18 years of age. Poverty is a major risk factor in the practice of child marriages. The National Family Health Survey from 1988 to 1999 found that up to 60% of girls were already married by the time they reached 18 years of age. Marriage at a young age brings about difficult challenges, such as financial responsibility, early and frequent pregnancies, and poor health (UNICEF, 2011).

The long-standing practice of courtship rituals, which is primarily a Western phenomenon, is beginning to gain wide acceptance as traditional arranged marriages are being displaced. Now only the educated elite are able to personally arrange marriages, and these marriages account for less than 10% of the total marriages in India (Warshaw, 1988).

The nuclear family, at 38.74%, is the predominant household classification type in India. Couples with married children and relatives residing in the home, termed *extended* and *supplemented* nuclear families, are also common. Males are overwhelmingly (91.2%) considered the head of household (Census of India, 2011).

East Indians have long considered marriage a financial and social arrangement designed to strengthen the position of the whole family, and traditionally one of the most important factors determining the choice of a bride has been the size of the dowry, that is, the property a woman brings to her husband at marriage (Warshaw, 1988). In India, marriage proposals traditionally have been elicited through a third party who may or may not be a member of the immediate or extended family. In contrast to this, today in the United States, East Indian Hindus frequently place a classified advertisement in their search for a suitable candidate for a prospective bride or groom (Warshaw, 1988).

According to Singh and Unnithan (1999), "The divorce rate is one of the lowest in the world" (p. 642). Because of societal pressures, the majority of married couples stay together even when there is dissatisfaction with their partner. Women are especially vulnerable to miserable, imbalanced, constricting, and even violent relationships. Fernandez (1997) states that "it is not just the husband but also members of his family, especially the mother-in-law, who abuses directly as an oppressor or indirectly as an instigator" (p. 445). In Indian society oppression of women was considered the norm, and continued use of this oppression in a different social setting, such as in the United States, is thought to be "one way of recapturing a familiar primordial order in an alien setting" (Singh & Unnithan, 1999, p. 653). Thereby, acceptance of violence against women can be traced back to cultural beliefs.

Position of Women in the Family and in Society

In the past, East Indian women ranked far below men in social status. Marriage became obligatory because the unmarried woman was believed to have no place in heaven. Traditionally the belief has been held by East Indian Hindus that the role of a woman is faithfulness and servility to her husband. Because women were deprived of inheritance, a male descendent was essential (Reddy, 1986).

Traditionally, the wife had few legal rights and could not publicly contradict or challenge her husband. Mentioning her husband's name in public was also not permitted. This taboo proved particularly confusing when she was required to identify herself for legal purposes (Warshaw, 1988). Among the upper class in the Hindu communities of the northern regions of India and in some areas of southern India, many wives practice *purdah,* the anglicized form of Hindi *parda,* meaning "veil." This tradition decrees that in public a wife hides her face behind a veil to ensure that she will be seen only by her husband. This custom is intended to protect her husband's rights over her (Warshaw, 1988).

Mahātma Gandhi was one of the first champions for women's political and social rights in India. In addition, the Women's Indian Association (1917) and the All-India Women's Conference (1927) were organized to unite women in their quest for status attainment through education, social reform, and politics. The association and conference included political picketing and voluntary social work. Although the Indian women's organizations provided tremendous support for the independence movement, it has been reported that they were unable to promote the essential issues related to women's emancipation. It has even been alleged that these organizations were means of maintaining and gaining status to move into higher echelons of power and that only upper- and middle-class women benefited from them (Reddy, 1986). Cumulatively, change in the status of women in postindependence Indian society has been moderate and not far reaching in its influence; for example, the issues of marriage (particularly regarding the remarriage of widows), divorce, and property inheritance serve to illustrate the inequities still occurring in India where women are concerned (Mukherjee, 1983; Sinha, 1977).

In concurrence with modern feminist movements throughout the world, a "sisterhood of women" hoping to establish "a global female community" is flourishing in the Indian province of the Madras presidency (Raman, 2001, p. 131). The goals of these women include improving literacy, abolishing caste traditions, and the option to delay marriage.

Caste Systems in India

For centuries East Indians have divided themselves by caste, by language, and by religion (Spear, 1972). The Hindu

BOX 19-1   Caste System in India

1. *Brahmins.* The Brahmins ("possessing sacred knowledge") were the priests and occupied a position of prestige and influence. These priests performed scholarly pursuits. The distinguishing color of the Brahmins was white.
2. *Kshatriyas.* The *Kshatriyas* were the warriors who in ancient times had been the head of society and later were ranked second to the priests. The color of their dress was red to symbolize their work of providing military and political leadership. Warfare was considered a duty of the Kshatriyas, and any hesitancy to fight, even against one's own kin, was considered a violation of the *dharma,* or "law," of the caste.
3. *Vaisyas.* The *Vaisyas* ("community men settled on soil"), who made up the largest caste, were involved in commerce. The ritual color of this caste was yellow. The members of this caste had the more mundane

tasks of raising cattle, tilling the soil, shopkeeping, and lending money. Although the *Vaisyas* lacked the social, ritualistic, and political privileges associated with *Brahmins* and the *Kshatriyas,* they ultimately gained great power and wealth as a mercantile order.
4. *Śūdras.* The function of the *Śūdras* was to perform menial tasks for the higher groups. Most members of this caste were poor tenant farmers and artisans. The most the *Śūdras* could hope for was that they would be reborn in a higher caste. The ritual color of this lower caste was black.
5. *Untouchables. Untouchables* were not allowed to live within the boundaries of a community or to have access to the village water well. They had to perform those duties that were considered unclean, such as tanning leather, cremating the dead, and executing criminals.

From Spear, P. (1972). *India: a modern history.* Ann Arbor, MI: University of Michigan Press.

population was divided into four *váras* (colors), which became castes (Box 19-1). These segregated castes were the *Brahmin,* or priestly caste; the *Kshatriya,* or warrior caste; the *Vaisyas,* or trading and farming caste; and the *Aasādra,* or artisan caste. Approximately 60% of the population held membership in one of these four castes. Outside the caste system, another group of people were referred to as *untouchables.* Gandhi renamed the untouchables the *Harijans* or "children of God." These people were the handlers of slaughtered animals, garbage, and the dead. Whereas the members of the highest caste, the Brahmins, were regarded as pure, Harijans were thought of as polluted and defiled (Spear, 1972; Thrane, 2010). See Box 19-1 for a description of each caste's or noncaste's role in Hindu society.

An individual became a member of a caste at birth, and it was believed that only death could release an individual. Individuals were expected not to marry outside of caste. The exception to this rule was when a man took a bride from a lower caste. Work, acquisition of property, and education could not enable an individual from a lower caste to move to a higher caste.

Historically in India, an intricate system of subcastes known as *jātis,* interlaced with the four main *váras.* The members of a *jāti* ("caste, lineage") were closely united by family, village, and region. A *jāti* had more prestige and gained greater rewards for services than other people had. Often the members of a *jāti* would claim to have descended from a common ancestor, whether they had or not, to proclaim kinship with one another. These people shared customs, traditions, and usually a dialect. Based

on an occupation or a set of related occupations, the *jāti* did not encourage members to seek social relationships outside of the group. Tailors, sweepers, or moneylenders (some of the occupations included in the *jātis*) did business with one another but maintained a social distance (Spear, 1972).

The caste system was officially abolished by the Indian constitution in 1950 (Warshaw, 1988). Today, in most large cities, educated workers and professionals of many castes intermingle. Caste taboos on eating and drinking with others tend to be ignored. Schools, public transportation, facilities, restaurants, and apartment houses have been almost entirely desegregated. Caste lines in major cities are so blurred that a person of the merchant caste may be an officer in the army, whereas a person of the military caste may be a prosperous business executive. However, although commercial practices are forcing East Indians to abandon old castes, family life continues to use them.

Religion

The Hindu religion may be the oldest religion in the world (Eshleman, 1992). In India, Hindu (80.5%) is the most prevalent religion. Other religions practiced are Islam (13.4%), Christianity (2.3%), Sikhism (1.9%), Buddhism (0.8%), and Jainism (0.4%) (Central Intelligence Agency, 2015).

There are at least 1.5 million practicing Hindus in the United States, including those of East Indian descent, and there are over 400 Hindu temples (Central Intelligence Agency, 2015; *World Almanac,* 2015). Hinduism, especially as learned and practiced in the United States, is a religion of disciplined acts, or karma yoga ("the path of deeds") (Miller, 1995). Major Hindu scriptures are the *Vedas,* the *Upanishads,* and the *Bhagavad-Gita.* Early Hindu scriptures are collections of writings by seers or prophets; the *Bhagavad-Gita* is a dialogue between Lord Krishna and Prince Arjuna (Bhungalia & Kemp, 2002; Thrane, 2010). Key teachings of Hinduism emphasize the importance of *satya* ("truthfulness, reality"), self-control, and respect for others. Many practicing Hindus engage in meditation, *pranāyamā* ("breathing exercises"), singing of *bhajans* ("sacred hymns"), yoga, and daily prayer.

The Hindu religion is polytheistic in the sense that there are numerous gods and goddesses, but there is an overriding sense of a supreme spirit. The origin of Hinduism is based on the Vedas, the sacred written scriptures. In Hinduism, the belief is that Brahma is the principle and source of the universe and the center from which all things proceed and to which all things return. Reincarnation is a central belief in Hinduism. Life is determined by the law of karma, which states that rebirth is dependent on moral behavior in a previous stage of existence. In Hinduism, life on earth is transient and a burden. The goal of existence is liberation from the cycle of rebirth and redeath and entrance into *nirvāna* (literally, "outblowing"), a state of extinction of passion.

Religion continues to play a part in assimilation into a new culture and of preserving one's native culture and identity. As East Indians assimilate into the American culture, their religious customs may have changed. Hindu religious leaders in the United States and India are returning to classic texts and turning away from certain modern adaptations in an effort to unify the practitioners of the religion. Also, the World Hindu Council is in the process of completing a code of conduct manuscript based on Hindu beliefs and traditions. This return to the classics is a way of combining different views, beliefs, and attitudes to one common goal. Hindus are protective of their religion, especially in the United States, where pressures come from the mainstream Christian culture. The challenge of preserving ethnic identity in light of cultural assimilation may have made many East Indians present a "model minority image of themselves and their culture" (Kurien, 1999; Yang & Edbaugh, 2001).

Hinduism is a common part of life for most Hindu Indians. Religious shrines are prevalent within many Hindu households and are located in various parts of the home, based on family preference. Each family has a set of specific gods and goddesses to whom they pray, and by popular account the Hindu pantheon numbers some 33 million gods. The shrines contain statues and pictures of the chosen gods, candles, incense, and offering of milk, flowers, and fruits. Times for prayer and meditation is reserved for the early morning (after bathing) and early evening, as time permits.

The common Hindu custom of fasting is observed on specific days of the week, depending on which god the individual worships. This practice is predominant among the women of the family, and children are not allowed to participate. Based on the family's degree of compliance to orthodox Hindu laws, fasting rituals may vary from abstinence to consuming only one meal a day. This practice may span over a 1-month time period or merely an observance of a holy day. Pittsburgh is a major center of Hindu cultural and religious strength. The first major Hindu temple in the United States, the Śri Venkatewars Temple in Penn Hills (a suburb of Pittsburgh), is an internationally known pilgrimage site for Hindus. Other major temples have been established in Washington, DC, Chicago, Austin, Berkeley, Los Angeles, and Boston. Temples serve as the centers of community, promoting the retention of Hindu values and instruction in the scriptures and key teaching, such as *ahimsā* ("nonviolence"), vegetarianism, and self-control. The temples often sponsor cultural events, language classes, and secular activities (Miller, 1995). There is a World Hindu Council of America, a subset of the international organization, which seeks to promote the Hindu religion in the United States by offering information via a wide variety of formats (World Hindu Council of America, 2015).

Effect of Immigration to the United States on Social Organization

The restricted immigration policies that were in place before 1965 in the United States created fear for many East Indian Hindu Americans because it appeared that the culture was losing its significance. Before 1965, there were so few East Indian Hindus residing in the United States that the few who did reside there chose to remain culturally isolated. Those Hindu Indians who did choose to assimilate believed that there was no free access to the White community and therefore chose to assimilate the Mexican-American culture, particularly because there were so few East Indian Hindu women residing in the United States before 1865. Some sociologists concluded that the assimilation between East Indians and Mexicans occurred as a result of their similarities in physical characteristics. In addition, some sociologists believe that East Indian Hindus may have lost their ethnicity entirely in the Mexican subculture, but others regard the fact of intermarriage between East Indian Hindu Americans and Mexican Americans as evidence of mutual acceptance (Melendy, 1977). In a classic study of 50 East Indian Hindu men, 26 had wives in the United States, 22 of whom were

Mexican. Consequently, the children from these Mexican–East Indian marriages were raised predominantly in the Mexican culture (Dadabhay, 1954).

As a new wave of East Indian Hindu immigrants began to assert themselves in the 1960s, the sagging Hindu culture and traditions were revived and prospered. This was attributable in part to the fact that after 1965, more East Indian Hindu wives and families began to arrive in the United States, which facilitated a revival of the traditional culture. On arrival, these wives continued to wear saris, the traditional dress, whereas only 10% of the men continued to wear traditional garb because many of the men felt the need to conform to the business community in the United States (Wenzel, 1965). Most of the newer immigrants were more adaptable and moved more easily into the American way of life, whereas the older generation remained apart from the mainstream society. Although the older groups of East Indian Hindus, who continued to live in rural areas, managed to adjust to economic demands, the social acculturation of this group remained significantly behind that of the newer generation of immigrants (Melendy, 1977). Some East Indian Hindu wives in the United States continued to practice *bindī* ("forehead dots," also called *tilak*) as a sign of the husband's well-being and prosperity.

Urbanization, industrialization, and education are major interacting forces disrupting the framework of the joint family system traditionally found in the East Indian culture and consequently are affecting the East Indians' family value system in the United States.

The concepts of ethnic identity and acculturation are important to note. Ethnic identity is at the level of the individual and that particular person's feeling of belonging and the amount of involvement they have to a particular ethnic group. Acculturation is the process by which the individual changes, adapts, or interacts with the new culture that they are in contact with. In general, Asian Indian families have maintained their cultural identity and values such as the importance of family, traditional gender roles, and group dynamics (Farver, Narang, & Bhadha, 2002).

Education is so highly valued among East Indian Hindu culture that approximately 80.1% of East Hindu Americans 25 years of age or older have a high school education, compared with 66% for the rest of the general U.S. population. Of the U.S. population 25 years of age or older, East Indian Hindus have the highest percentage of college graduates, with approximately 68% of Hindu men and 36% of Hindu women obtaining a college education as compared with approximately 20% of men and 13% of women for the general U.S. population (U.S. Department of Commerce, Bureau of the Census, *American Community Survey*, 2013). Indian college students in the United States have

expressed a desire to improve communication between their parents and with other family members, along with improved emotional and financial independence. Conversations are typically one-sided, especially on the sensitive subjects of dating, marriage, and sexuality. Change has been slow because of societal, cultural, and financial limitations (Medora, Larson, & Dave, 2000).

Politically, the adult East Indian Hindu community in the United States tends to favor a low profile, with fewer members serving in public office. Relationships between East Indian immigrants and U.S. society vary based on the community where they reside. According to Miller (1995), "discrimination against East Indian groups can be severe, ranging from 'dot buster' violence in New Jersey (perpetrated by white racist 'skinheads') to subtle forms of job discrimination that are difficult to document statistically" (p. 80).

An increasing number of young East Indian Hindu Americans are relocating to large urban centers in New York, New Jersey, Pittsburgh, Texas, and California (Helweg & Helweg, 1990) and are living in apartments. As a result, the joint family system has been rendered impractical. In school and at work, more East Indian Hindu Americans have learned to depend on ability rather than the caste system formerly found in India. The development of individualism among family members has resulted in uncertainty about the need for elaborate rituals of the past. Some of the values learned from the family are therefore extinct, especially as more young people detach themselves from the traditions that previously controlled them.

Recent East Indian immigrants to the United States, coming predominantly from western India, continue to bring their religious and cultural beliefs with them. Some of these beliefs as stated by Singh and Unnithan (1999) include the following: "Religion, caste, and regional affiliations are important criteria for mate selection, the families of both partners play crucial roles in mate selection and choice, patriarchy is the norm, and the status of women is predominantly secondary and dependent" (p. 642). As East Indian communities flourish in the United States, the communities have strived to maintain their cultural and ethnic identity.

Implications for Nursing Care

It is important for nurses to appreciate that the traditional East Indian Hindu family is the basic unit wherein values, manners, and morals are learned as part of its social structure. The pursuit of individualism, which is so predominant in Western culture, is not the accepted norm. The nurse should appreciate that the father is highly regarded as the head of the family and is the primary spokesman concerning important family matters, including the health care of the individual members. It is unusual for the East Indian Hindu American to seek medical care outside the confines of the family because of the fear that the family will be subjected to public scrutiny by strangers.

The nurse who cares for traditional, newly immigrated East Indian Hindu American clients should expect that the wife will usually sit passively by her husband, expecting all questions and inquiries to be directed toward him. He in turn may consult with his wife regarding the health status of other family members. The nurse who ignores the husband and seeks information directly from the wife may precipitate, on the part of the husband, feelings of mutual humiliation and disrespect in the eyes of his family. The major objective in developing an effective nurse–client relationship is to develop trust by gaining the husband's confidence so that the husband no longer views the nurse as an intruder but instead as a health care advocate.

TIME

The sense of time is an important concept for East Indian Hindus, who are past, present, and future oriented. Time is seen as cyclic involving four ages, starting with the "age of perfection" and ending with the "age of degeneration" (Purnell, 2014). East Indian Hindus are perceived as past oriented because of the traditions and rituals that are inherent to the culture. On the other hand, they are perceived as present oriented because of the view that they are "beings-in-becoming" (Kluckhohn & Strodtbeck, 1973). Finally, they are perceived as future oriented because life in the present is lived with an emphasis of the hereafter.

At the highest intellectual level, Hindus seek the one reality, whether this is conceived impersonally or theistically. Once they succeed in reaching this reality, they may continue to live in the world but without emotional attachment to it. They will have passed beyond sorrow and joy, pain and pleasure, and good and evil (Warshaw, 1988). In other words, the present is transcended by concern for the future and future reward.

Hindus, through cremation of their dead, hope to release the individual's spirit for union with an all-pervading one. The act is suggestive of the existence of a timeless presence in which all Hindus may share. The doctrine of rebirth—that every living being, animal or heavenly, will again be reborn and for all eternity—is a popular Hindu belief. The precise form of each rebirth is determined by the balancing of the being's deeds, good and evil, in previous existences. Escape from the cycle of birth constitutes salvation, a state of perfect, blissful consciousness that may be gained by acquiring perfect knowledge and performing one's duty flawlessly. Most Hindus aim only to improve their condition in the next existence.

Implications for Nursing Care

Because East Indian Hindu Americans are perceived as being past, present, and future oriented, it is important for the nurse to remember that the client may place little or no value on some present things, such as being on time for appointments, but may place considerable importance on other present-oriented concepts, such as the spiritual atonement of the self. At the same time, the same client may place equal importance on past-oriented things, such as traditions and rituals, and on future-oriented concepts, such as the preparation of the soul for the life hereafter.

ENVIRONMENTAL CONTROL

According to Kluckhohn and Strodtbeck (1973), it is essential for a people to answer the question of whether humans are innately good or bad. In regard to this question, there exists a range of variabilities, including evil, good and evil, and good. Hindus believe that the goodness in the soul of man is recaptured by virtue of the process of reincarnation. In addition, they believe in the man-to-nature orientation, as proposed by Kluckhohn and Strodtbeck, that man is not only subjected to nature but also has the need to live in harmony with nature. Being a past-, present-, and future-oriented cultural group that subscribes to a multiple man-to-nature orientation, some Hindus believe that because man is a mixture of good and evil, there is a need for constant control and discipline of the self if any real goodness is to be achieved.

Hindus are viewed as having both an internal and an external locus of control, meaning that some Hindu people believe that although external forces control destiny, internal forces, such as feeling states or misuse of the body, can also control destiny. For example, Hindu Americans who subscribe to both an internal and an external locus of control believe that internal conditions are influenced by psychological factors such as anger, jealousy, envy, fright, and shame. This belief is supported by the premise that when an individual is unable to control internal conditions that are self-perpetuated, a possibility exists for a susceptibility to disease (Henderson & Primeaux, 1981). The external locus of control is evident in that illness is an external event or misfortune, the cause of which may be related to the fault of a family member or the wrath of a disease goddess against the entire family. It is not uncommon for Hindus to believe that the malevolent spirits of dead ancestors, sins committed in a previous life, or jealous living relatives are responsible for one's ill health. Such phenomena as "soul loss," "breach of taboo," and "wrath of a goddess" are viewed as symbolic expressions of internal conflict. Hindus believe that people make themselves vulnerable to such calamities through conscious or unconscious transgressions against the ghosts and spirits. Agents empowered by evildoers to precipitate illness are numerous and varied; thus, to avert the vile intentions of these demons, Hindus wear charms, make offerings to the saints and their ancestors, and avoid visiting areas in the village where spirits are believed to reside.

Perception of Illness

According to classical East Indian theory, the human body consists of five natural elements: earth (bones and muscles), water (phlegm or *kapha*), fire (gall or *pittá*), wind (*vāyú*), and space (in hollow organs) (Andrews & Boyle, 2003). Water, fire, and wind are the three elements that interact in harmony to produce wellness. Illness results from an excess or deficiency of one of these elements, which are also referred to as the *tridosha,* or the "three troubles." *Pránjá* deals not only with respiration but also with a pneumatic element circulating in channels, distributing the "humors" and body fluids (bile, blood, and phlegm) throughout the body. In addition to giving attention to the five natural elements, East Indian theory also identifies bone, flesh, marrow, fat, chyle, blood, and sperm as seven essential constituents of the body. Although the nomenclature of bones is extensive, the viscera are given less attention in East Indian theory.

A great deal of attention traditionally was devoted to the source of disease and to the hygienic prescription. The intention of medical treatment addressed not only the disease symptoms but also the diagnosis of causes. For example, the treatment of fever consisted of giving antithermic drugs in addition to prescribing medication against *pittá* or the causative element involved (Dash, 1974). Hindus believe that praying for health is the lowest form of prayer. Among East Indian Hindus, it is preferable to be stoic rather than pray for recovery (Peck, 1981).

Folk Medicine

Significance of Folk Beliefs in the Hindu Culture. Today, there is a growing sense among psychologists, sociologists, and biologists that illness and its treatment are both biological and sociological phenomena. It is believed there are at least three different types of medical systems practiced at three different cultural levels. On the first level are primitive or preliterate people, who practice a form of primitive medicine based predominantly on a supernatural theory of disease causation. These people are believed to seek treatment through magico-religious means. On the second level are people who belong to the folk culture level and practice folk medicine, which encompasses a theory of illness that involves both supernatural and physical treatments as well as causations. On the third level are people who subscribe to a modern theory of treatment and disease causation. At this level, people recognize natural rather than supernatural causes of disease. When East Indian medicine is traced back historically, there is a magico-religious mixture of theology. In early East Indian history, disease causation as attributed to gods and goddesses and was explained on the basis of a cause-and-effect relationship with these gods and goddesses or with ghosts and evil spirits. However, Indian folk beliefs have undergone centuries of transition and now include herbal medicines and the ayurvedic system (Kakar, 1977; Lynch & Braithewaite, 2005).

The belief that certain diseases have natural or physical origins does not preclude the simultaneous role of a supernatural antecedent. For example, diarrhea in a child is generally attributed to consumption of a combination of incompatible foods. However, the possibility of someone casting an "evil eye" or "evil mouth" on the child is also recognized (Kakar, 1977).

Another system of beliefs is the ayurvedic doctrine, which dictates that disease not only has a germ causation but also occurs because of an imbalance of the essential body elements.

Āyurveda is a term that is composed of two words: *āyus* and *veda.* A primary concern for East Indian Hindus is knowledge of favorable or unfavorable conditions that assist in the introduction or resistance of the growth of harmful or nonharmful germs. East Indian Hindus believe that there are three fundamental elements in the body—*dosha, dhātu,* and *mála*—which must be in balance if a state of optimal equilibrium is to exist. *Dosha* ("disease") governs the physiochemical and physiological activities of the body; *dhātu* ("layer") forms the basic structure of the body cell; *mála* ("dirt") consists of substances partly used in the body and partly excreted in modified form after their physiological function has been completed (Bhungalia & Kemp, 2002; Kakar, 1977; Ramakrishna & Weiss, 1992).

Many medications may be prescribed in the ayurvedic system of medicine. For example, drugs for rejuvenation may be prescribed by an ayurvedic physician (Dash, 1974). Another example for ayurvedic medicine is found with the treatment of amebic dysentery, which is caused by the organism *Entamoeba histolytica.* In ayurvedic medicine, the belief is that the organism is not the major etiological factor of the condition. Rather, the major cause is attributed to irregularity of diet; intake of heavy, indigestible foods; and emotional factors, such as worry, anxiety, and anger (Dash, 1974). As a folk remedy for amebic dysentery, the drug *cyávana prâsa* ("disease causer–eating") is used, but this drug is considered more a food than a medicine. Two tablespoons of this medication are taken in a glass of milk, and the client is instructed to avoid salt in excess as well as sour things. Another part of the treatment includes avoidance of anxiety, worry, and sexual indulgence (Dash, 1974; Lynch & Braithewaite, 2005; Ramakrishna & Weiss, 1992).

According to Satow, Kumar, Burke, and Inciardi (2008), in a study of East Indians living in the United States, 95% of the respondents indicated that they were aware of Āyurveda, 78% had knowledge of ayurvedic products or treatments, and 59% had used or were currently using Āyurveda. It is interesting to note that only 18% of those using Āyurveda had informed their Western medical doctors of this use. Findings from this study certainly clearly illuminate the knowledge gap between traditional ayurvedic traditions and mainstream Western medical practice.

Emphasis on the diet of a client is a unique feature of ayurvedic medicine. The popular belief is that the client does not require any medication if he or she has a wholesome diet. According to this belief system, even if errors and diagnoses are made, most of the ayurvedic herbal medicines will not produce any harmful effect; however, if a diagnosis is correct, these herbal medications will act instantaneously.

Diseases in ayurvedic medicine are considered to be psychosomatic, involving both the body and the mind. This point is always kept in mind when medicines and regimens are prescribed for the client (Bhungalia & Kemp, 2002; Dash, 1974; Lynch & Braithewaite, 2005; Ramakrishna & Weiss, 1992).

Types of Folk Practitioners. A majority of East Indians obtain their beliefs in relation to the cause, prevention, and elimination of illnesses from their families, their parents-in-law (particularly the mother-in-law), elderly women of the neighborhood, indigenous midwives, other folk practitioners, and government health care workers. Usually the decision to seek medical treatment is influenced by factors such as the client's sex, the economic condition of the family, the family's perception about the cause of the illness, and the family's relationship with the local practitioner (Kakar, 1977).

Therapeutic advice is generally obtained at five different levels: family level, *mohalla* (properly, *mahalla*) level, caste level, village level, and beyond the village level (Kakar, 1977).

1. At the family level, the mother-in-law, who is regarded as the family practitioner and is well versed in the use of home remedies, is the source of treatment for any illness. Her authority is highly regarded and usually unchallenged in the scope of maternal and child care. Acting as diagnostician and therapist, she uses such healing techniques as the purgatives, massages, and various body-stretching devices.

2. At the *mohalla* ("eunuch in palace or harem") level, there exist two or three highly respected *syānas* or *syānis* ("wise or holy men") who are readily available and consulted only for certain illnesses. Intervention by the *syānas* is decided by the mother-in-law, and it is assumed that the importance of not relinquishing the family's secrets and affairs to the community is understood.

3. At the caste level, the intervention by one or two *syānas* is often sought. The practitioners cater to people's needs, especially members of their own caste. They are highly respected members of the caste and recipients of special treatment on socially important occasions.

4. At the village level, the faith healer, the most religious member, is a popular practitioner of choice and is employed for his free services regardless of caste or creed.

5. Beyond the village level, consultation is sought with a variety of folk and indigenous practitioners, ranging from exorcists to spirit mediums. There have been instances where a simple reassurance of the client by the spirit medium, without any actual medication, had resulted in instant relief (Kakar, 1977).

Principles of Hygiene

Personal hygiene is extremely important to East Indian Hindus. As part of the religious duty, a bath is required at least once every day. Some Hindus believe that bathing after a meal is injurious and that a cold bath may prevent a blood disease, whereas a hot bath may cause an alternative effect on blood diseases. East Indian Hindus also believe that if the bath is too hot, injuries to the eyes may occur. Hot water may be added to cold water, but cold water is not to be added to hot water when one is preparing a bath. When the bath is completed, the body is to be carefully rubbed dry with a towel and properly dressed (Jee, 1981).

Perception of Death

Death, according to the Hindu belief, is perceived as a passage from one existence to another. From the scriptures and the inspiration of "seers," the Hindu learns that all creatures are in a process of spiritual evolution extending through limitless cycles of time. A person's lifetime is like a bead on a necklace whose other beads represent past and future lifetimes. Each *atman* ("basic self") strives through successful rebirths to ascend the scale of merit until, after a life of rectitude, self-control, nonviolence, charity, reverence for all living creatures, and devotion to ritual, it wins liberation from worldly existence to achieve union with Brahma (Chakravarty, 1978). Palliative care is in alignment with Hindu values. Thus, many Hindu patients prefer to die in the home, or return to India, especially the sacred city of Varanasi during their lasts days on earth (Bhungalia & Kemp, 2002; Thrane, 2010).

In India, the death rite called *antyesti* or "last rites" involves preparation of the body for cremation, bathing the remains with a milk and yogurt solution, symbolically cleansing the soul of the disease (Purnell, 2014). When a married woman dies, she is attired in a traditional white wedding sari, devoid of make-up or jewelry, the wearing of which is considered a bad omen. A man is attired in a plain, off-white, East Indian suit. Religious prayers and chanting are continually offered by friends, family members, and priests before and after death to promote safe passage of the soul. Outward displays of grief are accepted practice within the Hindu faith. Open grieving by family, friends, and acquaintances encompasses wailing, crying, and even fainting. Men are as expressive in their grief as women and do not project a stoic demeanor (Chakravarty, 1978; Thrane, 2010). The eldest son of the deceased carries the body to the funeral pyre, and a priest chants prayers while the body is cremated. The ashes are then placed in a container and transported by the eldest son to a designated holy ground and scattered.

Implications for Nursing Care

It is important for the nurse to remember when working with Hindu Americans that there may be a belief that self-control of strong feelings is one of the keys to balancing health or a wellness state. In addition, some Hindu Americans believe in a value orientation that encompasses the belief that man is subjected to nature and at the same time is expected to live in harmony with nature. Because of this belief, it is important for the astute nurse to keep in mind that the client may believe that illness has a twofold causation, which may include ill favor or overindulgence of self.

Because Hindu Americans have very strict beliefs regarding things such as bathing, it is important for the nurse to remember that the Hindu American may refuse to take a bath after breakfast, which may be a common policy in some health care facilities. In addition, because some Hindu Americans believe that it is not permissible to add cold water to hot water, if the water is too hot, the nurse should pour the water out and begin the process again rather than risk offending the Hindu client.

Because some Hindu Americans subscribe to a theory that encompasses the belief that there are three elements in the body that must be in harmony to produce wellness, it is important for the nurse to identify with the client those beliefs that are beneficial, neutral, or harmful. If the client has beliefs that are beneficial, it is important for the nurse to identify these beliefs and practices and incorporate them into the plan of care. It is equally important for the nurse to identify those beliefs and practices that are considered neutral, having no effect one way or the other on the outcome of treatment, and that therefore do not need to be eliminated from the daily rituals of the client. Finally, it is extremely important for the nurse to identify those practices that could be considered harmful and therefore need to be eliminated from the practices and daily rituals of the client.

When nearing death, ideally the patient will recite his or her *mantra* (sacred phrase) as death occurs. If none is chosen, then *aum namo narayana* or *aum nama sivaya* may be used (Bhungalia & Kemp, 2002; Thrane, 2010). When a Hindu American client dies, the priest may tie a thread around the neck or wrist to signify a blessing, and this thread should not be removed. The nurse should expect that after death, a priest will pour water into the mouth of the body, and the family will request to wash the body. Because Hindus are particular about who touches the body after death, it is essential that the nurse communicate respect and provide privacy for the family so that these rites can be carried out (Murray & Huelskoetter, 1991; Potter & Perry, 2001).

BIOLOGICAL VARIATIONS

Variations According to Racial Strain

The modern population of India can be classified into six major racial strains. Two of the six racial groups can be related to a geographical region, and the other four groups may be found throughout India. Persons in the upper classes are different in physical type from those in the lower social strata. East Indians can be regarded as a separate racial group occupying an intermediate position between the peoples of Asia on the one hand and those of Europe on the other.

1. **Mediterranean strain.** These people are characterized by a long head, moderate stature, slight build, and dark skin. The face is narrow, the nose is small and moderately broad, and the hair is wavy or curly. These are the dominant features among the Dravidian-speaking people of southern India.
2. **Broad-headed strain.** This section of the population varies in stature from short to medium and in skin color from light to dark brown. The head is broad and sometimes high. The nose is prominent, and the hair is straight and usually abundant on the face and body.
3. **Nordic strain.** A distinguishing characteristic of this people is their long head. They are tall, long-faced with a straight and narrow nose, and light-skinned. This type of strain predominates in the upper caste in northern India.

4. **Mongoloid strain.** The head on these people varies from long to medium, and the skin color varies from light to dark brown. Their stature is medium, and the hair is sparse on the face and body. The face is short, with predominant cheekbones, and the eye sockets are slanted, giving a slit-like appearance to the eye.

5. **Negritos.** These people represent earlier inhabitants of India. Their stature is less than 5 feet, and frizzy hair is among the chief distinguishing features.

6. **Proto-Australoids.** This strain is predominant with tribal people of central, western, and southern India. Features of the lowest social strata of the population include a long head; short stature; broad, short face, with strongly marked brow edges and a small, flat nose; and wavy to curly hair. The skin is dark to black. The strain is so-named because of certain resemblances of people of this type and the Australian aborigines (Guha, 1944), but genetic evidence of such a relationship is exceedingly weak (Cavalli-Sforza, Menozzi, & Piazza, 1994).

Enzymatic and Genetic Variations

Thalassemia, a genetic condition that can result in various degrees of anemia, is believed to have a high incidence in people of the Mediterranean region, the Middle East, and Southeast Asia. It is believed that thalassemia has a range of variability in occurrence of people of Indian descent (Overfield, 1995). In addition, glucose-6-phosphate dehydrogenase (G-6-PD) deficiency, which also causes anemia, is believed to have a high occurrence in high-risk malarial areas. What is believed to occur in high-risk malarial areas is that the malarial parasite attacks red blood cells that contain the G-6-PD enzyme. Therefore, cells with a deficiency are less likely to be parasitized, which lowers the parasite load and consequently lowers the G-6-PD deficiency.

Lactose intolerance is another condition that affects persons of East Indian descent. Lactose intolerance is believed to occur among African and Asian populations because of genetic selection that may lead some groups of people to have adequate levels of intestinal lactase and others to have inadequate levels (Overfield, 1995). It is believed that although lactose intolerance varies by race, at least 80% to 90% of the world's population become lactose intolerant in adult life, except for some Whites (Overfield, 1995).

Susceptibility to Disease

The average life expectancy for East Indians residing in India is 66.46 years of age. Yet for Asian Indians, the average life expectancy at birth has climbed dramatically to 76.4 years as opposed to 77.85 years of age for the rest of the general U.S. population. In addition, the infant mortality rate in India is 49.3 deaths per 1000 live births as opposed to 6.43 deaths per 1000 live births in the United States (Central Intelligence Agency, 2015).

It is believed that susceptibility to heat stress is influenced by factors such as age, race, body build, body fat, climatic experience, and possibly gender (Wagner, 1972). According to Frisancho (1981), there is a possibility that certain races have the ability to withstand heat stress better than other races do; however, the racial effect is compounded by climatic exposure. Frisancho (1981) concluded that persons brought up in hot climates, such as that in India, are better able to tolerate heat than those persons raised in cooler regions, such as certain regions of the United States. In general it is believed that Blacks, southwestern American Indians, Asian Indians, East Indians, and Australian aborigines have the ability to withstand heat better than their White counterparts (Frisancho, 1981; Riggs & Sargent, 1964). The belief is that these people have lower sweat rates than Whites but similar body temperatures and therefore may have more efficient sweat production (Dill, Yousef, & Nelson, 1983). It is believed that part of the climatic influence on heat tolerance is directly related to the effect of heat on the development of the body during childhood. Eveleth (1966) concluded that children who grew up in hot climates, such as conditions found in India, have a tendency to be more slender than their counterparts raised in more temperate areas. In addition, these children also have thinner arms and legs.

In the area of stroke, public awareness in India of signs and symptoms, as well as affected organs, is marginal, which is comparable to knowledge in other nations. There has been an identified need to improve public education regarding stroke, as the data suggest that the population is aging, thus putting them at higher risk. Current stroke prevalence in India is variable, from 40 to 270 per 100,000 people, 12% of which occur in people less than 40 years of age. Should the incidence of stroke increase, there needs to be further discussion regarding the availability of resources for caring for the acute and rehabilitative needs of this population (Pandian et al., 2005).

Nutritional Preferences and Deficiencies

Most caste Hindus are vegetarians. However, strictness in adherence to the vegetarian diet varies. In most cases, the vegetarian diet consists primarily of grains (wheat, rice, millet, and barley) and legumes (grains, beans, and pulses, the edible seeds of plants having pods). In northern and western India, baked or fried cakes made with wheat are common. *Chapātī*, a popular form of bread, is a round, flat cake made of whole wheat flour and water and baked on a convex iron plate. *Pūrī* is similar to *Chapātī* except for the addition of shortening and being fried in deep fat. *Parāthā*, a third form of bread, is cooked on a convex metal pan.

In eastern and southern India, rice is the staple food. It is usually boiled, but it can be combined with *ghee* (*ghi*, or clarified butter) and spices to become *pilau* (or pilaf). Corn, barley, and millet are served alone or as supplements to wheat and rice dishes. The primary sources of protein are the grains and pulses, which include *chanā* (chick pea) and *arhar* (pigeon pea), which when split and dried is referred to as *dāl*. Vegetables include most of the green leafy vegetables, especially spinach, mustard, and radish greens, as well as gourds, eggplant, okra, cucumbers, cabbage, turnips, and potatoes.

Most East Indians eat a very light breakfast on rising in the morning, a heavy meal at midday, and a light meal between 7 and 9 p.m. (Ashraf, 2000). Before partaking of the meal, traditional Hindus chant the name of their god of preference, as if offering food to him or her before they eat. East Indian dietary laws dictate that the right hand is used for eating, whereas the left hand is used for personal hygiene and toileting.

Psychological Characteristics

Community tolerance for mental illness is high in India, and in many cases any idiosyncrasies are channeled into occupations or lifestyles in which the behavior can be carried out. For example, a marginally schizophrenic Indian person may wander the country doing odd jobs and living off handouts. Approximately 500 years ago *ambalams* were built throughout India to house travelers. Today, these ancient buildings are used by many persons who wander through India, including the mentally ill, as places to obtain food, beg, get water, and bathe.

The growing number of East Indian female immigrants to the United States has been found to seek mental health services less often than other populations. The Hindi concept of *Shakti* (feminine spiritual power) is thought to play a role, especially as it relates to the multiple roles maintained by East Indian women living in the United States (Navsaria & Petersen, 2007).

For the East Indian Hindu, environment has a significant effect on mental illnesses that may develop (Murthy, 2010). For example, because of the strong belief in supernatural forces, when a client becomes psychotic, delusions and hallucinations are often related to possession by a god, demons, or a witch, rather than to the mind's being influenced by equipment being placed or fears that the place is "bugged," which is more often the case in Western societies. An East Indian immigrant who has difficulty with English and with understanding what is occurring in the environment and who becomes psychotic will often manifest a paranoid reaction rather than one of the other psychotic illnesses. The delusions of the new immigrant frequently relate to the supernatural and reflect the culture of India. However, as East Indians have become assimilated into the Western culture, the nature of these delusions has changed to more "Western" symptoms.

Because mental illness is consistent with the sociological beliefs of the people, the treatment is also sociologically based and must be appropriate for the beliefs about the cause of the illness, such as exorcism of a spirit, demon, or god. The most effective exorcism is dramatically performed in a room with others in the family or in front of neighbors and friends (Ali, personal communication, 1989).

Many drugs that are restricted in the United States are legal in India, such as cocaine, opium, and marijuana. Although these drugs are cheap and available, abuse is much less common than in the United States. Drugs that are commonly abused in the United States may be used in India for therapeutic purposes. For example, marijuana leaves in water may be used for a baby's cramps, and opium may be used for diarrhea. Although Judeo-Christian beliefs regarding drug use as wrong have been present in India since the British arrived and to some extent have been adopted by the upper-class people, most East Indian Hindus still retain the value that although drugs may not be "good," their use is not "wrong."

Implications for Nursing Care

The most crucial aspect for proper nutrition is to make Hindus aware of the advantage of diet in relation to the survival of children. As East Indian Hindu Americans become assimilated into Western culture, it is important for them to understand the significance of using available foods in a nutritious manner. The nurse must keep in mind that a Hindu person may be reluctant to use Western foods because of sociocultural restrictions. Therefore, because dietary considerations are of utmost importance to some Hindu Americans, the astute nurse will involve the nutritionist or dietitian in the development of a culturally appropriate plan of care. The nurse should also be aware that fasting is an important part of religious practice and that this practice may have consequences for persons on special diets or with diabetes or other diseases related to food (ElGindy, 2005; Murray & Huelskoetter, 1991).

Nurses and other health care workers must be aware that the joint family is an important characteristic of the East Indian Hindu community. In planning culturally relevant nutritional programs, the nurse must understand the nutritional patterns in relation to other aspects of the culture and to identify those elements that can be changed without disorganization of the whole cultural scheme. The nurse also needs to explore the beliefs and attitudes of not only the people but also the authorities from whom these beliefs are derived.

It is also important for the nurse to remember that , because some East Indian Hindu Americans have a genetic predisposition for G-6-PD deficiency, thalassemia, and lactose intolerance, alternative methods of supplying calcium in the adult diet may be necessary. Another consideration for the nurse is the theory that people from warmer climates have a more efficient heat production system and thus can better tolerate heat. In this case it is important to teach the client that overexposure to heat does have profound effects on the body. In addition, they should also be taught about risk factors for stroke as well as the signs and symptoms of a stroke.

Because of the concept that health results from the body's ability to help itself, the traditional East Indian Hindu American may discount Western medical practices while responding positively to traditional folk healing practices. It is important for the nurse to appreciate that these clients may believe that the treatment they receive for an illness is more likely to be effective if both a pill and a solution are prescribed. A physician who is aware of this belief may prescribe both types of medications because this is what the client believes will effect a cure.

SUMMARY

Nurses who work in a transcultural setting providing health care services to clients of East Indian descent and Hindu affiliation are challenged by the multiplicity of norms, mores, and values, all of which influence and shape the delivery of nursing care. It is essential that the professional nurse and other health care providers use a holistic approach toward the assessment, planning, intervention, and evaluation of nursing care activities.

CASE STUDY

Vaidya Chuttani is admitted to the hospital with a diagnosis of Cooley's anemia (thalassemia major). Although Vaidya is only 16 years old, she is a student at the local university. Vaidya speaks English, but she is experiencing difficulty communicating her needs to the health care team. Her family, which consists of her mother and father and five brothers and sisters, all reside in Mumbai, India. Vaidya has not seen her family or talked with them for the 3 months that she has been enrolled in the American school. She tells the nurse that it is not unusual for some Indian families to allow their children to come to the United States to study at such a young age. In addition, she relates to the nurse that after she receives her degree, she will return to her country to assist her family by working and contributing to the family's monetary resources.

On admission, Vaidya's presenting complaints include (1) cholelithiasis as revealed on radiographic examination, (2) a right leg ulcer about 1 inch in diameter, (3) jaundice, and (4) an enlarged spleen as revealed on radiographic examination. The nurse notes the following on examination: blood pressure, 140/70 mm Hg; pulse, 88; respirations, 20; and temperature, 99.2° F.

◎ CARE PLAN

Nursing Diagnosis: Communication, impaired verbal, related to cultural differences (recent arrival from India and use of English as a second language)

Client Outcomes	Nursing Interventions
1. Client will be able to communicate basic needs to health care personnel. 2. Client will relate feelings of acceptance, reduced frustration, and decreased feelings of isolation.	1. Use gestures or actions instead of words to communicate information. 2. Use visual aids that will communicate to client necessary procedures to be done. 3. Write down messages in the hope that client can understand written English better than spoken English. 4. Obtain a translator, if necessary, to communicate important information.

◎ **CARE PLAN—cont'd**

Nursing Diagnosis: Tissue perfusion, ineffective: peripheral, resulting from Cooley's anemia related to decreased hemoglobin concentration in blood

Client Outcomes	Nursing Interventions
1. Client will verbalize activities that promote vasodilatation. 2. Client will verbalize factors that inhibit circulation. 3. Client will communicate existence of pain from right leg ulceration to health care professionals.	1. Assess causative and contributing factors of right-leg ulceration as related to Cooley's anemia. 2. Promote factors that will improve arterial blood flow and explain factors to client. 3. Encourage client to keep right leg in a dependent position and explain reasons. 4. Encourage client to change position every hour when in bed and discuss rationale. 5. Assess right leg in regard to pain and sensation.

Nursing Diagnosis: Health maintenance, ineffective, related to inability to make thoughtful judgments and lack of information about Cooley's anemia (thalassemia major)

Client Outcome	Nursing Interventions
Client will verbalize a willingness to comply with treatment regimen.	1. Identify sociocultural factors that affect health-seeking behaviors. 2. Determine present knowledge of illness severity and prognosis. 3. Determine client's level and stage of adaptation to present condition (such as disbelief, denial, depression). 4. Using appropriate visual aids, describe necessity for blood transfusions to correct Cooley's anemia.

Nursing Diagnosis: Family processes, interrupted, related to separation from family because of schooling in another country

Client Outcomes	Nursing Interventions
1. Client will verbalize fears and anxiety related to separation from family. 2. Client will identify support systems available within school and community and from external resources that will facilitate return to optimal health. 3. Client will verbalize desire to be involved in health care and scheduling of client-centered activities.	1. Encourage client to express feelings related to being separated from her family. 2. Determine client's understanding of present medical condition. 3. Determine support systems available in school and community from external outside resources that will facilitate return to optimal functioning. 4. Involve client in care and scheduling of client-centered activities (such as wound care for right-leg ulceration).

CLINICAL DECISION MAKING

1. List other nursing interventions that can be implemented to facilitate communication between Vaidya and the health care team.
2. Describe the family structure of some East Indian Hindu families and the effect the family organization may have on health-seeking behavior, as well as how this may affect nursing interventions for Vaidya.
3. Describe why Cooley's anemia is perceived as a biological variation for East Indian descent.
4. Identify at least two other biological variations that are common to East Indian descent.
5. Identify how Vaidya's health-seeking behavior may be affected by time and space variables.

REVIEW QUESTIONS

1. In bathing an East Indian American client, the nurse should do which of the following?
   a. Add hot water to cold water.
   b. Add cold water to hot water.
   c. Provide a bath after breakfast.
   d. Have a family member assist with the bath.
2. When a Hindu American client dies, the nurse should prepare for the family to do which of the following?
   a. Anoint the body with oils.
   b. Cleanse the body.
   c. Celebrate the passing of their loved one.
   d. Chant Hindu prayers to the soul.
3. In providing morning care to a Hindu client, the nurse takes into consideration the very strict beliefs regarding which of the following?
   a. Bathing
   b. Medication
   c. Drinking fluids
   d. Body massage

REFERENCES

Andrews, M., & Boyle, J. (2003). *Transcultural concepts in nursing care* (4th ed.). Philadelphia: Lippincott Williams & Wilkins.
Ashraf, K. M. (2000). *Life and conditions of the people of Hindustan*. New Delhi: Gyan.
Bayer, J. M., & Gupta, A. (2006). Englishes in India. *Language in India*. Available at: <http://www.languageindia.com> Retrieved May 28, 2006.
Bhungalia, S., & Kemp, C. (2002). (Asian) Indian health beliefs and practices related to the end of life. *Journal of Hospice and Palliative Nursing*, 4(1), 54–58.
Cavalli-Sforza, L. L., Menozzi, P., & Piazza, A. (1994). *The history and geography of human genes*. Princeton, NJ: Princeton University Press.
Census of India (2011). Available at from: <http://www.censusindia.net> Retrieved May 28, 2006.
Central Intelligence Agency (CIA) (2015). *The CIA world factbook 2011*. New York: Skyhorse.
Chakravarty, A. (1978). *Quest for the universal one: great religions of the world*. Washington, DC: National Geographic Book Society.
Corlett, W., & Moore, J. (1980). *The Hindu sound*. Scarsdale, NY: Bradbury.
Dadabhay, Y. (1954). Circuitous assimilation among rural Hindustani in California. *Social Forces*, 33, 141.
Dash, V. B. (1974). *Ayurvedic treatment for common diseases*. Delhi: Delhi Diary.
Dill, E., Yousef, M., & Nelson, J. (1983). Volume and composition of hand sweat of White and Black men and women in desert walks. *American Journal of Physical Anthropology*, 61(1), 67–73.
Divine, R. (1972). *American immigration policy, 1924–1952*. New York: Da Capo.
ElGindy, G. (2005). Hindu dietary practices: feeding the body, mind and soul. *Minority Nurse*. Available at: <http://www.minoritynurse.com/features/health/10-25-05b.html> Retrieved September 11, 2011.
Eshleman, J. (1992). Death with dignity: significance of religious beliefs and practices in Hinduism, Buddhism, and Islam. *Today's OR Nurse*, 19–20.
Eveleth, P. (1966). The effects of climate on growth. *Annals of the New York Academy of Sciences*, 134(2), 750–759.
Farver, J. A. M., Narang, S. K., & Bhadha, B. R. (2002). East meets West: ethnic identity, acculturation, and conflict in Asian Indian families. *Journal of Family Psychiatry*, 16(3), 338–350.
Fernandez, M. (1997). Domestic violence by extended family members in India: interplay of gender and generation. *Journal of Interpersonal Violence*, 12, 433–455.
Frisancho, A. (1981). *Human adaptation*. Ann Arbor: University of Michigan Press.
Guha, B. S. (1944). *Racial elements in the population of India*. Milford: Oxford University Press.
Gupta, V. B. (2010). Impact of culture on healthcare seeking behaviors of Asian Indians. *Journal of Cultural Diversity*, 17(1), 13–19.
Hall, E. (1990). *The hidden dimension*. New York: Doubleday.
Helweg, A. W., & Helweg, U. M. (1990). *An immigrant success story: East Indians in America*. Philadelphia: University of Pennsylvania Press.
Henderson, G., & Primeaux, M. (1981). *Transcultural health care*. Reading, MA: Addison-Wesley.
Information Please Almanac (2007). Available at: <http://www.informationplease.com> Retrieved May 28, 2006.
Jee, H. H. (1981). *Aryan medical science: a short history*. Delhi: Maharaja of Gundal.
Kakar, D. (1977). *Folk and modern medicine*. New Delhi: New Asian Publishers.

Kluckhohn, F., & Strodtbeck, F. L. (1973). *Variations in value orientations*. Westport, CT: Freeport.

Korom, F. J. (2001). Live like the banyan tree: images of the Indian American experience. *Journal of American Folklore, 114*(451), 70–73.

Koshy, S. (2001). Morphing race into ethnicity: Asian Americans and critical transformations of whiteness. *Boundary, 228*(1), 153–194.

Kurian, G., & Ghosh, R. (1983). Child-rearing in transition in Indian immigration families in Canada. *Journal of Comparative Family Studies, 83*, 132–133.

Kurien, P. (1999). Gendered ethnicity: creating Hindu Indian identity in the United States. *The American Behavioral Scientist, 42*(4), 648–670.

Larson, R., Verma, S., & Dworkin, J. (2001). Men's work and family lives in India: the daily organization of time and emotion. *Journal of Family Psychiatry, 15*(2), 206–224.

Lynch, E., & Braithewaite, R. (2005, July). A review of the clinical and toxicological aspects of "traditional" (herbal) medicines adulterated with heavy metals. *Expert Opinions on Drug Safety, 4*(4), 769–778.

McKay, J., Hill, B., & Buckler, J. (2007). *A history of world societies* (7th ed.). Boston: Houghton Mifflin.

Medora, N. P., Larson, J. H., & Dave, P. B. (2000). East-Indian college students' perceptions of family strengths. *Journal of Comparative Family Studies, 31*(4), 407–425.

Melendy, H. (1977). *Asians in America*. Boston: G. K. Hall.

Miller, B. D. (1995). *Precepts and practices: researching identity formation among Indian Hindu adolescents in the United States: new directions for child development*. San Francisco: Jossey-Bass.

Moore, W. (1963). *Man, time and society*. New York: John Wiley & Sons.

Mukherjee, P. (1983). The image of women in Hinduism. *Woman's Studies International Forum, 6*, 375–381.

Murray, B. M., & Huelskoetter, M. M. (1991). *Psychiatric mental health nursing* (3rd ed.). San Mateo, CA: Appleton & Lange.

Murthy, S. R. (2010). From local to global: contributions of Indian psychiatry to international psychiatry. *Indian Journal of Psychiatry, 52*, 30–37.

Navsaria, N., & Petersen, S. (2007). Finding a voice in shakti: a therapeutic approach for Hindu Indian women. *Women & Therapy, 30*(3/4), 161.

Nossiter, B. (1970). *Soft state: a newspaperman's chronicle of India*. New York: Harper & Row.

Overfield, T. (1995). *Biological variation in health and illness: race, age, and sex differences* (2nd ed.). Boca Raton, FL: CRC Press.

Pandian, J. D., et al. (2005). Public awareness of warning symptoms, risk factors, and treatment of stroke in northwest India. *Stroke; a Journal of Cerebral Circulation, 36*(3), 644–648.

Peck, M. F. (1981). The therapeutic effect of faith. *Nursing Forum, 22*(2), 153.

Potter, P. A., & Perry, A. G. (2001). *Fundamentals of nursing* (5th ed.). St. Louis: Mosby.

Purnell, L. (2014). *Culturally competent health care* (3rd ed.). Philadelphia: F. A. Davis.

Pye, L. (1976). *Politics, personality, and nation building: Burma's search for identity*. Westport, CT: Greenwood.

Ramakrishna, J., & Weiss, M. (1992). Health, illness, and immigration: East Indians in the United States. *Western Journal of Medicine, 157*, 265–270.

Raman, S. A. (2001). Crossing cultural boundaries: Indian matriarchs and sisters in service. *Journal of Third World Science, 18*(2), 131–148.

Reddy, G. (1986). Women's movement: the Indian scene. *The Indian Journal of Social Work, 46*(4), 507–514.

Riggs, S., & Sargent, F. (1964). Physiological regulation in moist heat by young American Negro and White males. *Human Biology, 36*(4), 339–353.

Satow, Y. E., Kumar, P. D., Burke, A., & Inciardi, J. F. (2008). Exploring the prevalence of Ayurveda use among Asian Indians. *Journal of Alternative and Complementary Medicine, 14*(10), 1249–1253.

Simons, B. (1976). *The volume library*. Nashville, TN: Southwestern.

Singh, B. (1966). *The dialect of Delhi*. New Delhi: Lakherwal Press.

Singh, R. N., & Unnithan, N. P. (1999). Wife burning: cultural clues for lethal violence against women among Asian Indians in the United States. *Violence Against Women, 5*(6), 641–653.

Sinha, D. (1977). Ambiguity of role-models and values among youth. *Indian Journal of Social Work, 38*, 241–247.

Spear, P. (1972). *India: a modern history*. Ann Arbor, MI: University of Michigan Press.

Thrane, S. (2010). Hindu end of life: death, dying, suffering, and karma. *Journal of Hospice and Palliative Nursing, 12*(6), 337–342.

UNICEF (2011). Available at: <http://www.unicef.org/india/child_protection.html> Retrieved September 11, 2011.

U.S. Department of Commerce. Bureau of the Census (2013). *American community survey*. Washington, DC: U.S. Government Printing Office.

U.S. Immigration Commission (1911). *Dictionary of races of people*. 63rd Congress. 3rd Session, 52–54, 75–76.

Wagner, J. (1972). Heat intolerance and acclimatization to work in the heat in relation to age. *Journal of Applied Physiology, 33*(5), 616–622.

Warshaw, S. (1988). *India emerges*. Berkeley, CA: Diablo.

Wenzel, L. (1965). East Indians of Sutter County. *California Living, 17*, 3–15.

World Almanac (2011). New York: World Almanac Books.

World Hindu Council of America (2015). Available at: <http://www.vhp-america.org/aboutus> Retrieved May 28, 2006.

Yang, F., & Edbaugh, H. R. (2001). Transformations in new immigrant religions and their global implications. *American Sociological Review, 66*(2), 269–288.

Haitian Americans

Ora L. Strickland

BEHAVIORAL OBJECTIVES

After reading this chapter, the nurse will be able to:

1. Describe the etiology of the Haitian Creole language.
2. Explain the tradition of spatial behavior often found among Haitian Americans.
3. Understand the Haitian family structure and the relevance to assimilation of Haitian Americans into the Western culture.
4. Describe the relationship of time and social class in Haitian Americans.
5. Identify the beliefs regarding Voodoo commonly found in the Haitian culture and how they pertain to healing.
6. Identify diseases that are prominent in Haitian-American people.

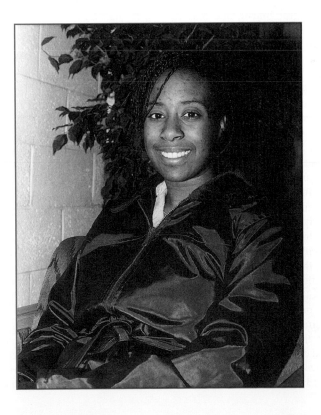

The small republic of Haiti in the West Indies has a colorful but tormented history. To provide appropriate care to Haitian-American clients, the nurse needs to have knowledge about the social and political turmoil that Haiti has experienced. In addition, the nurse should be aware of the difficulties that have surrounded migration as Haitians have sought sanctuary from their troubled homeland. It is only through an understanding of Haitian culture and health beliefs that the nurse can adequately meet the needs of Haitian-American clients. In addition to discussing the land of Haiti, the immigration process, and the influence of the six cultural phenomena on nursing care of Haitian-American clients, this chapter explores the struggles that Haitians have experienced in their attempts to assimilate the cultural traits of the dominant culture in North America.

OVERVIEW OF HAITI

Social History

Haiti (République d'Haïti) is situated in the western third of the island of Hispaniola. The other two thirds of the island is occupied by the Dominican Republic. Haiti is in the Caribbean Sea, with Cuba to the northwest, Jamaica to the southwest, and Puerto Rico to the east. Haiti, about the size of Maryland, is two thirds mountainous, and the rest of the country is characterized by great valleys, extensive plateaus, and small plains (Central Intelligence Agency, 2015; World Almanac, 2015). Columbus discovered the island of Hispaniola on Christmas Eve in 1492, when his flagship, the Santa María, ran aground and was wrecked at Cap Haitien, a historic town on Haiti's northern coast. As the French took over the island, the native Indians were either exterminated or removed to Mexican gold mines. Black slaves were imported from Africa as the French became owners of flourishing sugarcane plantations. By 1681 there were 2000 slaves in St. Domingue, the French name for Haiti. A little more than 100 years later, there were at least 500,000 African slaves, and some estimate as many as 700,000, compared with 40,000 Whites and 28,000 freemen of color—offspring of masters and slaves (Wilentz, 1989). Many slaves were newly imported because many died of overwork, beatings, disease, and undernourishment. The masters were obviously outnumbered, necessitating harsh measures to keep the slaves in line.

Interestingly, the African religions were seen as a source of resistance to the French (Thomas, 1997). Although night ceremonies and dances were often forbidden, they continued and fomented the desire for power and freedom. Legend has it that one night the slaves on half a dozen plantations rose up and burned down their masters' homes, killing their masters. This revolt spread throughout the country, continuing for some 13 years. In 1802, Napoleon's

troops landed at Cap Haitien, planning to recapture the island from the slaves and use it as a jumping-off place for an invasion of the United States. However, because of yellow fever epidemics, which assisted the Haitians in killing the French soldiers, the Haitians altered the course of world history, and the French admitted defeat. In 1804, Haiti was freed from France and became the second independent nation in the Western Hemisphere and the first independent Black republic in the world. According to Hobsbawn (1996), the failure of Napoleonic France to recapture Haiti was one of the main reasons why France liquidated its entire remaining American empire, which was sold by the Louisiana Purchase to the United States. Thus a consequence of the revolution in Haiti was to make the United States a continental world power.

Unfortunately, independence from France did not end the misery for the poor in Haiti. Although they were no longer slaves, the poor soon found that the oppressive French rulers had been almost immediately replaced by equally oppressive new Black rulers, the mulattos. With the advantage of money inherited from their French fathers, the mulattos became educated and wealthy and continued to monopolize Haiti's resources, with little regard for the social conditions of the poor (Seligman, 1977).

The American occupation, from 1915 to 1934, resulted in reorganization and improvements of the country regarding its road system, telecommunications, health care system, universities, banking system, and so on but did not effect permanent change. This assistance failed to solve the economic and social problems, and when the majority of Americans left in the 1930s, the country once again regressed.

In addition to the attempt at revitalization by the Americans, François Duvalier, who came to power in 1957 and was to become president for life (Abbott, 1991), can be credited with initiating comprehensive programs to alleviate economic and technological problems. Unfortunately, Duvalier, preoccupied with wealth and power and the programs that were initiated, failed to have long-lasting effects, and the country's money was squandered. In 1963, Duvalier murdered countless enemies and managed to incur the wrath of Haiti's neighbor, the Dominican Republic, by harboring enemies of its new president. Upon his death in 1971, his son, Jean Claude, succeeded him. A drought from 1975 to 1977 brought famine, and in 1980 Hurricane Allen destroyed most of the rice, bean, and coffee crops. In 1986, following weeks of political unrest, President Jean Claude Duvalier fled Haiti aboard a U.S. Air Force plane. Democracy was attempted, but the country was soon taken over by a military coup (Masland, 1992). In 1991, the United States joined members of the Organization of American States in a regional embargo aimed at reinstating

Haiti's first democratically elected president, Jean-Bertrand Aristide. The economic blockade led to a sharp downturn in an already poor economy. In July 1991, Aristide and the army signed an accord to return the exiled president to power. When the military leaders failed to resign, the United Nations reimposed an embargo. The embargo had a severe effect on the health of the population because it created difficulties in distributing aid and health care in Haiti. Although food and medicine are exempt from United Nations sanctions, an increase in acquired immunodeficiency syndrome (AIDS), tuberculosis, and malnourishment among children occurred (Chelala, 1994). After Aristide's return to Haiti in October 1993, he quickly replaced the police force, downsized the military, and purged the officer corps.

On May 14, 2011, Michel Martelly was sworn in as president of Haiti, with the UN Security Council remaining in the country to assist in maintaining peace. The social and political unrest in Haiti has contributed to despoliation of the land. In 1996, it was estimated that only 2% of the country is forested and more than half of the land had been destroyed by erosion (United Nations Program Development, 1996). The remaining agricultural land is capable of producing food for only half of the population. Still, Haitian farmers continue to despoil the remaining land by removal of roots and stumps for charcoal manufacture to heat their cooking stoves in order to survive. The lack of farming land in the country has resulted in dependence on food from foreign aid (Hiebert, 1997). There are at present efforts in the country by charitable groups to assist the country economically. One example of this is the Mennonite Economic Development Association, which has 20 paid staff who assist Haitians in developing their own small business by giving them small loans for start-up money. This organization has been very effective in helping hardworking Haitians have a chance to be self-supporting (Claude, 1997). The Mennonite Central Committee has also had workers doing projects, including producing seedlings in 20 community-based tree nurseries (Dening, 2001).

Recent Developments in Haiti

In the greatest tragedy in modern times impacting the country, Haiti was struck by a massive earthquake on January 12, 2010. The earthquake, striking some 15 miles southwest of Port-au-Prince, measured 7.0 on the Richter scale and was immediately followed by two aftershocks measuring 5.9 and 5.5, respectively (Central Intelligence Agency, 2015; *World Almanac*, 2015). Although the exact number of those who died during this earthquake may never be known, it is estimated that 222,570 people lost their lives and more than 1.6 million people were displaced, especially in the densely populated area around Port-au-Prince (Central Intelligence Agency, 2015; *World Almanac*, 2015). Subsequently, a significant portion of Haiti's debt was cancelled as a part of the "Poor Countries" initiative of the International Monetary Fund and the World Bank. Along with this forgiveness, and in light of the massive $1 billion debt owed to so many other creditors and a barely functioning economy and nation, the G7 countries forgave Haiti's remaining debts to them (Central Intelligence Agency, 2015; *Time Almanac*, 2015).

Life in Haiti

Today, Haiti is an independent republic with 9,996,732 inhabitants (2014 estimate) (Central Intelligence Agency, 2015; *World Almanac*, 2015). Between 90% and 95% of the population are descendants of West African slaves; 5% of the population are mulatto and White, whereas 95% are Black. Fifty-three percent live in rural settings, 37% live in urban settings, and 10% are overseas. Haiti is considered to be the poorest nation in the Western Hemisphere, with a gross domestic product of $13.4 billion (2013 U.S. dollar estimate) and a per capita income of $1300 (Central Intelligence Agency, 2015). However, other estimates of the income for most rural Haitians is probably more realistically set at $3.56 a day, with 80% living below the poverty line. Haiti's real economic growth rate is 3.4%, with an inflation rate of 5.9% (*World Almanac*, 2015); this slight growth has not dramatically increased the purchasing power of the population. In 2000, the local currency drastically declined in value, dropping from 16 to 22 gourdes per U.S. dollar (Dening, 2001) and further plummeting to 41.87 in 2009 and to 70 gourdes per U.S. dollar (*World Almanac*, 2015).

More than two thirds of the labor force do not have formal jobs, and there is widespread unemployment and underemployment (2011 estimate) (*World Almanac*, 2015). Of course, this number is a gross underestimation because of the almost nonfunctionality of the economy of Haiti because of the massive earthquake in 2010. It is postulated that the devastation and massive number of those who died or were displaced occurred because of the inadequate reinforcement of the buildings that disintegrated or imploded on the people, making recovery of some bodies nearly impossible (Central Intelligence Agency, 2015; *World Almanac*, 2015). So many people lost their lives during the earthquake that many were never properly identified and a great number were buried in mass graves (Central Intelligence Agency, 2015).

Before the earthquake, some 92% of the population lived in small, rural hamlets in small straw shacks without light, water, or windows. In sharp contrast to the destitute living conditions is the pride of the Haitians, their value of self-respect, and their strong work ethic. Although the issues and problems confronting the people of Haiti are similar to those of many other countries, they seem to be more numerous and more intensified. The country is drastically overpopulated, with a density of 890 persons per square mile (*World Almanac,* 2015). In 2013, the annual population growth rate was 1.08%. The life expectancy is 63.18 years overall, 61.77 years for males and 64.60 years for females. The birth rate is 22.8 per 1000, and the death rate is 7.9 per 1000 (not taking into account the 2010 earthquake). Infant mortality is 49.43 per 1000 live births. Haiti has a young population: 34.0% of the population is 0 to 14 years old, and the median age is 22.2 years (Central Intelligence Agency, 2015). Although these numbers have been reported as accurate, caution should nonetheless be exercised when considering their validity given the massive destruction and slow recovery of the infrastructure (Central Intelligence Agency, 2015).

Haiti has numerous unresolved obstacles to public hygiene, including an inadequate water supply for 77% of the rural population and 62% of the urban population. There is inadequate access to sanitation for 64% of the rural population and 59% of the urban population. Some 80% of the population suffers from malnutrition. Health care services are lacking throughout Haiti. A national health service is responsible for the medical care of the population, but only 50% of the population (47% of the rural population) has access to health care. There is one physician for 8800 people and one nurse for 8600 people. This is even more problematic than it appears because most of the physicians are on the government payroll and are disproportionately concentrated in the capital city, Port-au-Prince (Central Intelligence Agency, 2015).

Health care is also provided by private foundations such as the Mellon Foundation, which sponsors the Hôpital Albert Schweitzer in central Haiti. To make health care more available to the people, small medical teams go out from this hospital into the rural areas to provide village-based health services. In this program, rural farmers, both men and women, are trained in primary health skills and provide direct services to clients. Health service delivered to the natives has resulted in a significant decrease in tetanus, which formerly ranked with tuberculosis and malnutrition as one of the three major health problems (Grant, 1989; Reichman, 1989; Stauffer, 2006; Westphal, 1989). However, although this hospital operates as a charity to the local people, it is not without exposure to the unrest in Haiti. For example, administrators are sometimes threatened that their family members will be harmed if they do not hire certain Haitians who come seeking employment (Venton, 1997). A number of nursing and medical schools in the United States use Haiti for transcultural experiences in a third-world setting (Gregg, 2001). Nurses from the United States and Canada have gone to Haiti to assist with

flooding, disaster, and earthquake recovery (Barnard & Sincox, 2004; Benedict, 2004; Central Intelligence Agency, 2015; Hardcastle, 2004).

IMMIGRATION TO THE UNITED STATES

Most of the immigrating Haitians in the early years were upper-class individuals who came to the United States as resident aliens. These upper-class Haitians were able to obtain permanent residence and citizenship with little difficulty and became assimilated into the dominant culture.

In 1980, an explosion of Haitian immigration took place as a result of a short-lived (April–October 1980) change in the U.S. immigration policy. More than 14,000 Haitian refugees landed on the shores of southern Florida in 1980 (Dempsey & Gesse, 1983), which includes the Mariel boatlift from Cuba. The influx of Cuban refugees required that a special status be created by the U.S. State Department, called "Cuban-Haitian entrant, status pending." Haitian refugees were included in this status to prevent the policy from being discriminatory (Metropolitan Dade County, 1981; Walsh, 1980). The "entrant" status described a temporary status and was used rather than granting the new arrivals political asylum. However, this "entrant" status placed the Haitian immigrants in a bureaucratic limbo that cannot lead to citizenship (Wilk, 1986).

The immigration policies changed in October 1980. A maritime interdiction program was initiated to turn back Haitian refugees at sea. Haitians who arrived in the United States were not classified as entrants but as parolees and were subject to deportation. Haitians were kept in detention along with Cubans while their cases were processed in the courts. Unlike other refugees arriving at the time (such as Indochinese refugees), resettlement was not guided by the federal government. The federal government's refusal to grant asylum deprived the refugees of benefits under the new 1980 Refugee Act. Emergency aid was limited, and most of it had lapsed by 1983 (Holcomb, Parsons, Giger, & Davidhizar, 1996). Lacking either jobs or government assistance, many refugees were compelled to rely on private charity and to invent jobs in a burgeoning "informal" economy in Miami. In 1991, mass migration of Haitians led to 34,000 Haitians being held at the U.S. Naval Base in Guantánamo Bay, Cuba, while their immigration status was determined (Lillibridge, Conrad, Stinson, & Noji, 1994). Numerous health problems, including active tuberculosis and AIDS, were addressed by the uniformed service medical support personnel (Bonnlander, 1996; Granich, Sfeir, & Jacobs, 1994). In 1993, the Supreme Court of the United States ruled that repatriation was legal and that illegal aliens could be returned to Haiti (Holcomb et al., 1996). Despite this ruling, thousands of Haitians still attempt to enter the United States each year by trying to travel from Haiti to the United States by boat. Some give all their money to private entrepreneurs and board barely seaworthy crafts for a chance to escape to a better life in the United States (Portes & Stepick, 1985). Many Haitians do not survive because the conditions at sea are too harsh or the boat is too full to permit safe travel. When weather conditions are too harsh, older Haitians may be thrown into the sea to lighten the load (Veeken, 1993). Still, perilous as the journey is, many Haitians would rather try for the hope of the opportunities of living in the United States. Of those who do arrive, only a fraction (5%) is allowed to stay under the status of political refugees. The United States has steadfastly clung to a policy that makes it difficult for Haitians to meet the requirements for political refugee status. For example, since the immigration act of 1990, mandatory human immunodeficiency virus (HIV) testing with indefinite detention without treatment in HIV-positive detention camps has discriminated Haitians from other immigrants (that is, Cubans, Vietnamese, Chinese) and required that persons with HIV be held rather than "paroled" (Annas, 1993). In 1998, the Omnibus Budget Bill made changes in the Haitian Refugee Immigration Fairness Act, which allowed amnesty for some Haitian immigrants in the United States (Isgro, 1998).

These waves of immigrants have resulted in four classifications or categories of Haitians in the United States: (1) citizens, (2) residents or legal aliens, (3) entrants, and (4) illegal aliens. Illegal aliens have all the pressures and fears of discovery, which could result in sudden deportation. Entrants, on the other hand, suffer from the uncertainty of whether they will be able to remain and from being unable to make permanent plans or feel entirely settled (Wilk, 1986). Because possibly half of the Haitians in the United States are here illegally, few programs exist to provide assistance. Some Haitians are understandably reluctant to discuss their difficulty, and they attempt to maintain a low profile with government agencies that might return them to Haiti. Another effect of an uncertain status in North America is infrequent use of health care services after immigration. The nurse should be aware that the Haitian immigrant probably will not seek medical treatment until the condition is severe or has become chronic (Bryan, 1988). The nurse should also be aware that hope is related to economic factors, and lack of economic assets results in feelings of hopelessness (Holt & Reeves, 2001).

Despite these difficulties and the possibility of deportation, many, primarily poor, Haitians continue to try to enter the United States. Those who do make it to North America are in one of the most at-risk populations now living in the United States. This high risk becomes actualized in several ways; for example, a study by Moskowitz et al. (1983) reported unusual cases of death among Haitians residing in Miami and a high prevalence of opportunistic infections. The nurse should expect, when caring for a Haitian, that the client may never have had immunizations. If a client needs a tetanus immunization, it is unlikely that a tetanus booster is appropriate because the client probably has not received the series.

Adaptation of post-1980 Haitians to the dominant culture in the United States and Canada has been especially problematic because the proportion of refugees having a high school or college education and skills in English has declined. With limited education and money, many Haitians arriving in North America have been restricted to occupations such as migrant agricultural work and service industry jobs in restaurants and hotels (Eshleman & Davidhizar, 1997). Only a few of the more educated Haitians have been able to find work as mechanics and construction workers. Gaining the requirements needed to adjust to the urban, industrialized culture encountered in the United States and Canada is for most Haitians a stressful, overwhelming, and slow process because the people continue to cling to their cultural values and beliefs. Potocky (1996) noted that although many other refugees are faring moderately well in the United States, Nicaraguans and Haitians tend to be faring poorly. Assimilation to U.S. culture for Haitians has been particularly difficult. When they are compared with other groups, Potocky (1996) noted that Haitians on the average had a significantly lower economic status in regard to yearly earnings, percentage employed, and percentage never employed and living in poverty. A substantial proportion of Haitians arriving in the United States are children, who often arrive without their parents and are placed with extended family or in foster care (Office of Refugee Resettlement, 1993). Children who are with families face intergenerational problems. Children often experience a role reversal because they tend to more quickly adopt the language and culture of the United States and then must translate English for their parents. Because most of the asylum cases of Haitians are denied (U.S. Committee for Refugees, 1995), many Haitians in the United States are considered illegal aliens. Children who are denied asylum but remain in the country illegally have suffered from nonhumanitarian treatment even into their adult years. Whereas other immigrants have been welcomed, the lack of welcome experienced by many Haitians has had a negative effect (Fernández-Kelly & Schauffler, 1994). Haitians have not consistently received the same treatment as other asylum-seeking refugees. It was not until May 1995 that the Clinton administration reversed the *de facto* policy that granted virtual blanket asylum to all Cubans (Epstein, Lantigua, & Cavanaugh, 1995).

In 1975, Haitians could be found in 45 of the 50 states (Seligman, 1977). Large settlements of Haitian people are located in the southern and eastern parts of the United States, with 75% to 95% residing in Florida (Boswell, 1982; Wilk, 1986). New York City (especially Brooklyn) and Montreal have large, established Haitian communities that have mushroomed during times of revolution and political unrest in Haiti. For example, in 1960 there were reported to be 2584 Haitians living in New York City (Laguerre, 1984; Rosenwarke, 1972). It was estimated that 34,000 Haitians had arrived in the United States in 1968, and in 1970 it was estimated that 50,000 Haitians were living in New York City alone (McMorrow, 1970). According to the U.S. Census Bureau, in 2009, 1,000,000 people of Haitian descent resided in the United States (U.S. Department of Commerce, Bureau of the Census, *American Community Survey, Haitians,* 2013). This census figure may underrepresent the true numbers because of the number of illegal aliens from Haiti and particularly in light of the 2010 earthquake (Central Intelligence Agency, 2015). The Bahamas, which lie between Haiti and Florida, have been inundated with an estimated 60,000 Haitians who have failed in their attempt to cross the sea and instead have been shipwrecked on the vast Bahamian chain of some 700 islands (Fineman, 2001). Haitians report paying as much as $5000 for the privilege of the odyssey, only to land undetected on the tourist-dependent islands hoping to raise the fare to go on to Florida (Fineman, 2001).

Some Americans have been supportive of the plight of Haitians in Haiti and of the treatment of Haitians who have come to America (Barnes, 2000). In 2000, Haitian Americans marched in New York to protest policy brutality against Haitians in New York City and demanded the resignation of New York City Mayor Giuliani. Cases of mistaken identity have resulted in violence against Haitian Americans (Barstow, 2000). Others have protested deportation practices in which the Immigration and Naturalization Service has made Haitian immigrants who have received deportation orders choose between leaving their children in the United States in hopes of giving them the opportunity for a better life or taking the children back to Haiti (Bragg, 2000).

Life in the United States

As of 2013, approximately 59% of all Haitians residing in the United States were foreign-born compared with only 13% of the total U.S. population (U.S. Department of Commerce, Bureau of the Census, *American Community Survey, Haitians,* 2013). This high number of foreign-born Haitians is reflected in the 81.2% of Haitian Americans 5 years of age or older who speak a language other than English at home, compared with only 20% of the general

U.S. population. In 2009, among Haitian Americans 25 years of age and older, 18.2% of both males and females held a bachelor's degree or greater, compared with 28% of all U.S. males and 27% of all U.S. females.

In 2013, compared with the rest of the general population, slightly more Haitian Americans were actively working in the labor force. In fact, in 2013, 70.9% of Haitian Americans 16 years of age or older were in the civilian labor force, compared with only 65% of the total population (U.S. Department of Commerce, Bureau of the Census, *American Community Survey, Haitians,* 2013). Nonetheless, the yearly median per capita income for both Haitian-American women and men was lower than the general U.S. population at $32,650 for men and $28,937 for women (compared with $45,485 for all U.S. males and $35,549 for all U.S. females). Similarly, the median Haitian-American family income was significantly lower at $45,626, compared with $61,082 for the general U.S. population. Despite the number of Haitians employed in the United States in 2013, the percentage of this population who live below the poverty rate is 19.6% compared with 14.3% of the general U.S. population (U.S. Department of Commerce, Bureau of the Census, *American Community Survey, Haitians,* 2013).

COMMUNICATION

Issues related to communication present a variety of problems for Haitians living in the United States or Canada. In Haiti there are two official languages: Haitian Creole (Kreyòl) and French. French is the official national language and is understood and spoken only by the upper or wealthy class. Although Haitian Creole is the language of the rural or poor population, it is also the primary language and is understood and spoken throughout the country (Holcomb et al., 1996; Weil, 1973). Speaking only Haitian Creole, a hybrid of old French vocabulary and African grammar, is perceived as a sign of poverty and a lack of education. Both Haitian Creole and French are often spoken so fast that one word is slurred into another. Because many Haitian immigrants in the United States continue to combine Haitian Creole and French, a dialect undergoing further creolization has been created, and it creates language barriers for some Haitian immigrants because most people in the dominant U.S. society are unfamiliar with it.

Haitians frequently use hand gestures to complement their speech. Hand gesturing and tone of voice become more pronounced during communication. Primarily, hand gesturing is used as an addition to verbalizations. Touch and direct eye contact are also used in both casual and formal conversation. The Haitians' use of touch in conversation is perceived as friendship and does not violate personal space. Direct eye contact is used to gain the attention and respect of the other person during conversation. The Haitian cultural uses of touch and direct eye contact and the perception of friendship through conversation are much like those used throughout the United States.

Implications for Nursing Care

Language is often an area where problems arise between refugees and health care providers. One reason Haitians have received limited health care in the United States is the failure of many Haitians to speak either of the dominant languages: English or Spanish. Many schools in the United States have extensive bilingual programs for native Spanish speakers but have paid little attention to other non-English speakers. The problem of providing bilingual education for Haitians is complex and begins with a lack of materials for teaching English to Haitian Creole speakers. There are also varying opinions on the best way to teach literacy skills. Some persons believe that Haitians who have immigrated to the United States must be taught literacy in their native language. The view is that if Haitian Creole is used as a teaching tool, it can facilitate acquisition of reading and writing skills in English (Dejean, 1983).

The nurse should promote the Haitian-American client's interest in gaining English-language skills to facilitate the client's adjustment to the dominant culture. Although most Haitians are eager to learn English, learning to read and write as an adult is often difficult and time consuming, and support from health care professionals can encourage the Haitian individual to stick with this difficult task. Many Haitians who use French as their primary language have retained it, even though they have made a permanent move to the United States or Canada. Although many in the United States and Canada share the French-speaking Haitian's view that French is the language of the culturally elite, it should be noted that French-speaking Haitians have as much difficulty learning English as any other non-English speakers do.

If the client does not speak English, the nurse should first determine what language the client does speak. If the nurse does not know Haitian Creole or French, an interpreter may be necessary. When possible, a bilingual family member can help convey to the client and nurse information essential to health care. The nurse may find that Haitian Americans with children are more likely to speak correct English because speaking correct English is a status symbol and parents who know English will usually speak correct English in the home. The nurse caring for a Haitian-American client should be aware that Haitians value a touch or a smile by the nurse as a sign of friendship. Nonverbal communication can assist in bridging gaps between the differences in language because it can facilitate an understanding of client needs.

Haitian Americans who have newly arrived from Haiti may be unfamiliar with modern technology, including use of the telephone since Haiti has only 140,000 main lines, many of which may be down for a month after a rain (*World Almanac*, 2015). Access to the Internet is new in Haiti, with only four local servers and limited satellite links.

SPACE

Personal space to the Haitian can be defined as a public zone. Haitians as a cultural group are a sharing population. If they possess something that another person could or might benefit from, it will be shared. Another factor that tends to make the culture a public zone is the closeness of the living arrangements or dwellings. As a result, the Haitians are a public-oriented society. Haitians in the United States, for the most part, usually socialize with other immigrants arriving from their own town in Haiti and maintain primary loyalty to family members, many of whom remain in Haiti. Legal immigrants look forward to spending holidays in Haiti and regard the allowed time each year as a focal point. Illegal aliens are more isolated because they cannot maintain family contact. This represents a great change from the lifestyle led in Haiti, where extended family and the closeness of the community are emphasized.

Implications for Nursing Care

It is important for the nurse caring for a Haitian-American client to know that data from studies have indicated that Haitians find touch by caregivers to be supportive, comforting, and reassuring (Dempsey & Gesse, 1983; Holcomb et al., 1996). In a study of 10 women, Dempsey and Gesse noted that there were diverse views on whether these women preferred to be touched during childbirth and if the preference was for a man or woman to touch them. In the study, two women specified a preference for being touched by a woman, three preferred to be touched by a man, and three did not have a preference. Nine stated that the father should be present. What is implied by this is that Haitian women may be less likely than women from some cultural groups to insist on having female nurses in the delivery room.

Although Haitians and African-Americans share a heritage that extends back to Africa, the two groups do very little social mixing and tend to mistrust each other (Dempsey & Gesse, 1983). It is important for the nurse to understand that just because two clients may be Black does not mean they will share common interests or find each other suitable companions for sharing a hospital room.

Some Haitians, like people from some other social groups, are not free of social prejudice. Appreciation of these cultural socioeconomic issues by the nurse will facilitate assignment of staff to care for Haitian clients as well as room assignments of clients.

Because of the large gap in social classes, it is important for the nurse to consider the economic background of Haitian-American clients before placing them in the same area. For example, a poor client and a wealthy client with a Haitian background, although from the same country, may find a room assignment together in a hospital very distasteful.

SOCIAL ORGANIZATION

Social Class

The Haitian masses are essentially divided into two class structures: the wealthy and the poor. Statistically, 85% of the Haitian population is classified as poor, 10% as middle class, and 5% as wealthy (Bell, 1981). Class is demonstrated in many interesting ways. Wearing shoes is a requirement by law in the capital city, but many Haitians, especially in the small towns and villages, go barefoot. This is by no means a matter of choice but a mark of social standing. As an illustration of this, a Haitian physician who was enjoying a little recreation in one of the small towns was told that a client was waiting for him nearby. The physician asked if the client had shoes on. What was implied in this question was that if the client had shoes on, the physician would be obliged to go immediately. On the other hand, if the client did not, the client would be in for a wait (Jeanty, personal communication, 1989). Regardless of class, Haitians are a proud and independent people.

Education

Education in Haitian schools differs greatly from that in American schools. Until 1979, French was the only officially recognized language and the language that was required to be used in school. The educational system and schools are strict and authoritarian. Children who are financially able to attend must wear starched uniforms. The Haitian teacher has the right to use corporal punishment on a misbehaving child. Thus the lack of structure and discipline of many American schools meets with disapproval from Haitians. Much of the information given to students in the Haitian schools is memorized; memorization through repetition is the primary source of learning. Haitian children can be heard reciting multiplication tables through rhyme and song throughout the community. Sheer repetition of the same formula, problem after problem written on the blackboard, manages to register the information in the student's mind. Haitian teachers enunciate clearly when

communicating with their students (DeStefano & Miksic, 2007; Verdet, 1985).

Rather than attend the public high schools, Haitian Americans prefer to remain out of the mainstream of education and often strive to accelerate the educational process and obtain the credentials they value by seeking a high school equivalency diploma. Haitian Americans view a college education as a form of prestige and status.

Family

The commonality among Haitians in Haiti and Haitians in the United States, whether wealthy or poor, is family. The family structure or system is very different from that of the American system. The practice of common-law marriage is predominant, particularly among the poor. Most legal marriages occur among the wealthy as a result of their economic status. Common-law marriage gives the father of the family much freedom and imposes much of the responsibility of caring for and meeting the needs of the family unit on the mother. The father, perhaps dividing his time between several family units, becomes a powerful but unreliable figure. The concept of a single-parent family, primarily the single mother, is similar to that in the United States but is more prevalent in Haiti. The Haitian mother is commonly left to raise the children without the support system of the father.

The term *plaçage* may be defined as the union of a man and woman who desire to live together and who fulfill certain obligations and perform certain ceremonies at the home of the woman's parents, after which a new household is established. These unions are said to endure as long as recognized church marriages and constitute two thirds of all unions in Haiti (Herskovits, 1971; Schaedel, 1962). Haitian women involved in *plaçage* can be classified into four groups according to their relationship with Haitian men:

1. *Femme caille* (common-law): a woman who shares her home with a man in a common-law marriage situation.
2. *Mama petite* ("mother of my children"): a woman who is the mother of some of the man's children but does not share his house. This is similar to some *plaçage* unions with children, but in this situation the husband continues to live with his first wife while maintaining the second relationship.
3. *Femme plaçage* (woman whom a man "goes with" or a friend): a woman who neither lives with nor has had children by a man but who shares his bed intermittently and often maintains a garden, usually furnished by him.
4. *Femme avec* (woman who is lived with): a woman with whom the man cohabits for pleasure and without firm economic ties (Williams, Murthy, & Berggren, 1975).

Affection from both parents is readily given to children, and physical punishment is given as a form of discipline. Haitian mothers rely less on parent–child dialogue and more on physical punishment to effect changes in the child's behavior and to instill proper attitudes and values (Charles, 1979). Although Haitian mothers are extremely affectionate with their children, the children are taught from infancy that there is an unquestioned obedience to adult wishes. Haitian children do not presume to question parents or seek information concerning matters such as sex education because this would be seen as disrespectful of adult authority (Bestman, 1979). Childrearing is shared by siblings as well as by the parents.

The Haitian family is traditionally extended, with each dwelling or residence paralleling a small community. Outside the extended family, godparents play a very important role in the family organization and are generally considered part of the natural family. Rural or poor families tend to be matriarchal and child centered, with parents exercising strong influence and authority over their offspring, even when the children are grown. Haitians view their children as direct reflections of themselves and the family. If children fail to fulfill obligations or meet expectations, they are seen as having failed the family and as having brought disgrace on the parents (DeSantis & Thomas, 1987). Because of the parent–child ties, many Haitian couples separate only temporarily when immigrating. The wife usually immigrates with the younger children, and the husband remains in Haiti with the older children until the entire family can obtain authorization to relocate. One-parent families are quite common among this immigrant group in the United States. Immigrants often lack support of extended families in child rearing (Prudent, Johnson, Carroll, & Culpepper, 2005).

DeSantis and Ugarriza (1995) investigated Haitian mothers and their childrearing practices. They identified the need for psychiatric mental health nurses to assist immigrant Haitian families in handling intergenerational conflict because there are significant differences between the culture of origin and the culture encountered in the United States. Conflicts arise for children between what their parents say and what they see in the culture around them. Adolescent Haitians tend to fit the profile of high school dropouts in that they are often poor and Black and live in households with high levels of stress. Social support for education is necessary if the adolescents are to remain in school (Rosenthal, 1995).

Traditionally, Haitian parents have a strong voice in their children's selection of a mate and in their choice of a career. Haitians tend to be an extremely status-conscious group and desire marriages or careers that enhance the status of the family. For most Haitian immigrants in the United States, home ties to Haiti remain strong. Even though there may be little opportunity for travel back and forth because of cost and the illegal status of many, ties to the motherland and home remain. Letters, packages, and money are sent regularly. Because many Haitians were illiterate, at one time, sending cassettes to relatives in the United States or home to Haiti was a common form of communication (Jeanty, personal communication, 1989).

Some older Haitian immigrants have been found to depend more on the members of their social support network than other Haitian age groups (Degazon, 1994; Seabrooks, 1992). The older immigrants experienced more changes in life events and loss of network members because of age, in addition to problems associated with migration. The older Haitian immigrants also reported that they encountered hostility and stress because of their African heritage and skin color (Seabrooks, 1992). On the other hand, Robinson (1994) reported that aides in nursing homes caring for Black clients from three cultural groups were generally positive toward the elderly but negative toward the families of the elderly residents who did not take care of the elderly at home. Findings indicated the need for education for aides related to differences among people in different cultural groups.

Implications for Nursing Care

Cultural factors related to social organization have an important influence on health and health care behavior. Fundamental norms, such as the desirability of having many children and the traditional roles of men and women, affect reproductive behavior. Because the legal status of many is either questionable, as for entrants, or undesirable, as for illegal aliens, Haitians frequently use different names, giving one name at one clinic and another name at another clinic. In addition to causing confusion to health care providers, this practice leads to people "falling through the cracks" because records are not available. Consequently, there is a loss in continuity of care for some Haitian clients. In addition, because of the repeated intake procedures on the same client, health care services may be delayed (Wilk, 1986).

An astute nurse should keep in mind that because the Haitian family is traditionally extended, the opinions and ideas of the family must be incorporated into a culturally sensitive plan of care. It is also important to remember that because Haitian children are taught from infancy to be unquestioningly obedient to adult wishes, it is especially important to provide parents with adequate health education if children are to benefit from improved and knowledgeable health care.

The nurse should also be aware that bisexuality may be an occurrence among Haitian men. Even when this information is important, the client may not readily offer it. The nurse may need to elicit this information by asking if the client has ever had sex with another man, rather than using the labels of *homosexual* or *bisexual* (Laguerre, 1981; Randall-David, 1989).

Immigrant Haitian mothers have been found to believe that little can be done to avoid childhood illnesses considered medically preventable in the United States (DeSantis & Thomas, 1992). Many Haitian mothers adhere to the beliefs and practices of Haitian folk medicine because they have not been taught or do not believe in preventive health care. This has important implications for the health education of parents and children (DeSantis & Thomas, 1992). DeSantis and Thomas (1992) found that nurses were considered the best persons to do health teaching. Teaching is valuable when it is understandable, is practical, reinforces parenting abilities, and allows time for questions.

TIME

Traditionally, Haitians have not been committed to time or a schedule. It is not considered impolite to arrive late for an appointment. Everyone and anything can wait. Nelson (2002), a Haitian business consultant in Florida, describes how present-time orientation, which might include conducting a personal conversation rather than waiting on a customer, can cause Haitian-owned businesses in the United States to fail. On the other hand, some Haitian Americans have learned to compensate for lack of time orientation by manipulating the timing of activities. For example, a wedding invitation will show a starting time of 6 p.m. when the actual starting time is actually 7 or 7:30 p.m. (Colin, 2005).

The time orientation of Haitian Americans is related to social class. Poor or lower-class Haitian Americans tend to be relatively past- and present-time oriented because they find it necessary to live from day to day, looking for food and trying to sustain a meager living. Because of their economic and educational status, the future for some of these people remains bleak. If a poor Haitian American has little to no chance of getting ahead, it is unlikely that a future-time orientation will be developed.

On the other hand, wealthy Haitian Americans may perceive time from a totally different perspective. For these people, time orientation may be a combination of both present and future orientations. It would appear that as a result of adequate financial resources, upper-class Haitians and Haitian immigrants do make plans for the future. Because wealth may ensure educational attainment, which may translate into status and prestige, it is likely that a well-educated upper-class Haitian may have a future-time orientation.

Implications for Nursing Care

Because Haitians may have different orientations to time, depending on their social status and class, it is important for the nurse to adequately assess each individual client. It is also important for the nurse to remember that personal ethnocentric attitudes toward time may negatively affect planning care for clients. Persons with a present-time orientation may view future-oriented tasks as irrelevant or unimportant to present situations. Thus a present-time orientation may restrain a Haitian from gaining upward mobility because future-time orientation is required in gaining an education and planning to achieve future goals. It is also important to remember that when a Haitian immigrant does not keep an appointment or does not arrive for a clinic appointment on time, it may be a result of both a present-time orientation and economic constraints. It is important for the nurse to assess not only the time variable but also other socioeconomic variables, including the availability of transportation to and from clinic appointments. If a Haitian American is to arrive at clinic appointments on time, it is very important for the nurse to emphasize the importance of adhering to the clinic's schedule. The nurse should be aware that Haitian Americans frequently stop a treatment regimen as soon as the symptoms appear to be relieved. It is also very likely that the Haitian American will fail to follow through with a treatment regimen or preventive health care because cultural beliefs do not relate personal actions to health status.

ENVIRONMENTAL CONTROL

Although Haitians and African-Americans share a lineage that extends back to Africans who were seized from their countries and enslaved, some individuals have surmised that these two cultural groups fraternize very little socially and tend to mistrust and be suspicious of each other (Wilentz, 1989). It is believed that Haitians place a high value on personal liberty and are therefore resentful of American prejudice and at times indignant and critical of African-Americans, whom they discern as too submissive and accepting of discrimination (Wilentz, 1989). At the same time, African-American militancy and violent protest seem to be contrary to the Haitian personality and are generally regarded by Haitians with disapproval (Wilentz, 1989).

Traditionally, the upper classes in Haiti have been the lighter-skinned Blacks, whose skin color results from crossbreeding with lighter-skinned people. Light skin traditionally has been regarded as more prestigious than dark skin in Haiti (Leyburn, 1980), with the upper-class, lighter-skinned Haitians dealing with the lower-class, darker-skinned persons in an authoritarian manner. Therefore, because of indoctrination regarding the color of the skin and its perceived relationship to social status or class, some Haitians have developed a social prejudice that causes difficulty in the assimilation process in the United States. As a result of social prejudice formed by such variables as color grading and social status, some Haitians living in the United States or Canada continue to have trouble adjusting to other groups and thereby choose to remain in isolated areas, socializing only with other Haitians and family members.

Some Haitians view illness and disease as natural or unnatural events. Natural events keep balance between nature and humankind and as such are believed to be designed by God. Natural laws are believed to give life predictability (Snow, 1981). Unnatural events are believed to upset the balance of nature and at their worst represent forces of evil and the devil. Unnatural events lack predictability because they exist beyond the parameters of nature and are beyond the control of "mere mortals." This view is in sharp contrast to traditional Western medical beliefs. It is essential that the nurse remember that some Haitians believe illness is a result of witchcraft. People who supposedly possess supernatural power are believed to be able to alter the health status of others (Snow, 1981).

Voodoo Practices

The practice of Voodoo, the primary religion in Haiti, is prevalent throughout the country. Voodoo is a religious cult practice that dates back to the preslavery days in the West African homeland (Miller, 2000). Today, the term *voodoo* is commonly used both as a derogatory term by non-Haitians to describe the illogical and unexplainable and as a catchword of ethnomedical or ethnoreligious beliefs that involve magic and spirit possession (Miller, 2000).

In the 1600s, slavery was rationalized by the Code Noir, instituted by Louis XIV, by mandatory evangelization on arrival to a French colony (Thomas, 1997). Catholicism was implemented by required religious assemblies. Nevertheless, the outlawed African religious practices were loosely incorporated, as the slaves identified their deities with the saints of the Catholic church. European religious and decorative objects were also incorporated, allowing the slaves to appear nominally Catholic while still preserving the basic structure common to West African religious systems (Mena, 1996). However, when the sovereignty of the country was not recognized by the Catholic church from 1804 to 1858, the Catholic church forbade priests to enter the country, and all ordained priests were ordered to leave. During this time, Voodoo flourished and became the dominant belief practice. In 1860, partly as a result of the spread of Protestant missions on the islands, a concordat

was approved in Rome, a bishop was consecrated in Port-au-Prince, and Catholicism was once again the official religion recognized by the state. Nevertheless, the new priests sent by the church faced an ineradicable folk religion and a people who were able to reconcile living with two parallel albeit often contradictory spiritual belief systems (Laguerre, 1989; Mena, 1996; Miller, 2000). The majority of Haitians combine some degree of both Voodoo and Christianity (Mena, 1996).

Today many Haitians still believe that humanity is surrounded or enveloped by a variety of powerful, dominant spirits and that it is essential to invoke spirits. In the Haitian culture, the invoked spirits are called *loas, mystères,* or saints. Some Haitians believe that Voodoo spirits manifest and reveal themselves by possessing or "riding" the devoted believer. It is believed that the personality of the loa "mount" may change; he or she may be calm and subdued one minute and then suddenly become violent. Such transformations may be caused primarily by nervous instability under the influence of compelling drum rhythms and mass emotion (Logan, 1975). Haitians trust and depend on their Voodoo beliefs and also rely on "readers" or "diviners," who predict the future by reading cards or hands and cure by means of being possessed by the Voodoo spirit. The readers, or diviners, also considered Voodoo priests, are organized into independent cults.

Voodoo priests may be either male (*hungan*) or female (*mambo*) and are categorized into five classes: shaman (Voodoo practitioner), herbalist (*docte fey,* literally "leaf doctor"), midwife (*matronn,* or *fam saj*), bonesetter (*docte zo*), and injectionist (*pikirist*). Healers are often not well defined, and a Haitian may go to a neighbor who has "extra" medicine or a healing practice in hopes of relief. In terms of the number of practitioners and frequency of use, the herbalists constitute the most significant class of healers. Herbalists are the most generalized caregivers, and thus their role characteristics overlap to a certain extent with those of all other healer types (Coreil, 1983). Haitians often use home remedies and herbs for treating illnesses that are suggested by healers or priests. Many Haitians believe that tea made from leaves of the Bible will cure rheumatism. In this case, the Bible serves as protection against black magic, which is believed to cause rheumatism (Nida, 1954).

Magic powers may be used for purposes other than destroying enemies or healing the sick. The Voodoo sorcerers of Haiti claim to be able to change themselves into animals, to pass through locked doors, and to raise the dead and make them slaves (zombies). Almost everyone who is a native Haitian claims to know someone who has been a genuine zombie. One man requested his family to cut his corpse into two pieces to be buried in separate graves for fear that the local sorcerer, who was his enemy, would bring him to life as a wretched slave. Although the Haitian government has no valid evidence of the existence of zombies, it sanctioned the belief by passing a law against the supposed practice (Nida, 1954).

In Haiti, Voodoo is sometimes actualized as fetishes, which are shared by groups of native Haitians. For example, a Haitian might have a small bottle containing some reddish liquid and a small mirror backed by cardboard facing the bottle, and all this wrapped in coarse red cloth with yards of black thread. This object is safeguarded in the most remote part of the house, with its location kept secret from visitors. If the Haitian could be induced to talk about this, he might explain that his father, who was a kind of Voodoo priest, captured his soul when he was very young and put it in the bottle. As long as the bottle is preserved, the person will live, but once the bottle is broken, the soul will depart and the man must die. Not only would this fetish be held by this individual but also identical or similar fetishes might be shared by others in the community (Nida, 1954).

Many Haitian influences regarding Voodoo practices are evident in the mainstream of American society. For example, in some cities and towns in Louisiana, the Haitian influence is extremely prevalent and is perceived or felt by persons from other cultural groups as well. Louisiana is renowned for its Voodoo society, which is a carryover from Haitian slaves who were brought to areas such as New Orleans for various domestic duties. Even today, because of early Haitian influence, Voodoo and mystical thought remain evident regardless of ethnic or cultural background in cities such as New Orleans (Snow, 1981). Traditionally, some Haitians believed that a spell could be cast with the possession of a lock of the individual's hair (Calypso, 1999).

Although health care is a significant problem in urban Haiti, it is even more of a problem in rural Haiti, with pregnant and postpartum women being particularly vulnerable (Wiese, 1976). Many Haitians know nothing about prenatal care and do not routinely seek such care. Some may never have seen or been to a physician in their lives. Healers are related to protection, and physicians are related to sickness. Use of a midwife is culturally permissible and is much more likely among Haitian people than among other cultural groups in the United States. When a nurse is interacting with a pregnant Haitian woman or is providing care for a baby, using the phrase "We will help you have a strong baby" will often elicit cooperation. Staff who are willing to help the mother have a "strong baby" (rather than a "healthy baby") are more likely to be accepted (Jeanty, personal communication, 1989).

Some pregnant Haitian women who experience an increase in salivation do not believe they should swallow the saliva. Sometimes they carry a "spit" cup with them and are not embarrassed to use it in public (Colin, 2005). Many dietary precautions are followed by Haitian pregnant women.

Pregnant women are viewed as special and are likely to be treated with more kindness and respect than other women. Chants or sounds of a woman in labor include praying, singing, crying, and moaning in various combinations, which is done to call on their Voodoo protectors (Dempsey & Gesse, 1983).

A study conducted by Scott in 1978 identified the postpartum period as the most crucial and decisive period of childbearing for the Haitian woman. During the postpartum period of 6 to 11 weeks, the Haitian woman follows a cultural regimen of baths, teas, vapor baths (see later in this paragraph), and dressing warmly. This practice is supposed to make the client healthy and clean again after the birth. For the first 3 days, the mother bathes in hot water in which herb leaves have been boiled. She also drinks a decoction made from boiled herb leaves. (Also during the first few days after childbirth, the mother takes "vapor baths" by sitting above a pot of steaming water with leaves in it, especially orange tree leaves, and draping a cloth over her head and shoulders.) For the next 3 consecutive days, the mother takes her second series of baths, which are prepared with leaves in water warmed by the sun. At this point the mother drinks only water warmed by the sun or an infusion made with leaves steeped in water warmed by the sun. The mother takes constant special care to keep her body warm. She stays inside her dwelling for at least 3 days after the birth and keeps the doors and windows closed to keep out the cool air. She wears long sleeves, keeps her head covered, and wears heavy socks and shoes.

After 2 weeks to 1 month, the mother takes another bath. She may take a cold bath or perhaps jump into a cold stream. After this ritual, she may self-induce vomiting to cleanse her inner body. After all of this is completed, she can again resume normal activities and is considered clean (Harris, 1987).

The Miami Health Ecology Project (Scott, 1978) reported beliefs about menstruation among Haitians, a majority of whom believed the function of menstruation was to rid the body of "unclean," "waste," or "unnecessary" blood. Many Haitians also described menstruation in this manner: "It means you are a woman," with "woman" meaning that the individual has sexual feelings or needs and is not sterile. The Haitian girl reportedly learns about menstruation at a median age of 10 years. For 85% of the sample, this information was obtained from their mothers or in classes at school.

Rituals Related to Death and Dying

Laguerre (1981) has studied patterns of bereavement among Haitian-American families. Death arrangements are usually taken care of by a male kinsman of the deceased who has had experience with American bureaucracies. Death appears to mobilize the entire extended family, including matrilateral and patrilateral members. Because Haitians frequently believe that illness and death can be of a supernatural as well as natural origin (Métraux, 1953), death is often accompanied by feelings of guilt and anger. The surviving relatives may believe that the death was a result of failure to relate appropriately to the Voodoo spirit. Recurrent dreams of the deceased person, so much a part of grief work, take on a particular meaning to the Haitian. Haitians commonly evaluate illness in terms of symptoms previously experienced by close kin (Laguerre, 1981), and grief work frequently includes taking on symptoms of the deceased person's last illness (Eisenbruch, 1984).

Colin (2005) noted that health care professionals should tell the family spokesperson when death is imminent so family members can assemble at the bedside. Family members try to meet the spiritual needs of the dying person by using religious medallions, pictures of saints, or fetishes or talismans for protection or as good luck for a peaceful death and restful afterlife. A kinsman usually makes the arrangements of telling the family and making preburial arrangements, including purchase of a coffin and prayer services before the funeral. Traditional Haitians have 7 days of consecutive prayer to assist the passage of the soul to the next world. This is terminated by a mass that begins the official mourning process.

Implications for Nursing Care

The nurse should be aware that the healing systems associated with Voodoo and Haitian ethnomedicine may be seen by some health care professionals as barriers to health care and even as adversely affecting health care (Carrazana et al., 1999). If Haitian Americans do use conventional means of health care, they tend to use emergency rooms or clinics and to seek health care only when they are quite ill (Orque, Bloch, & Monrroy, 1983; Samet et al., 1994). Haitian Americans may also seek relief from their symptoms through a physician and at the same time consult a cultural healer. The client's having both a faith healer and a physician should not be perceived as incongruent (Jeanty, personal communication, 1989). A client's fear and anxiety that he or she has been "hexed" may be alleviated or reduced if the therapist combines conventional treatment with the assistance of a cultural healer who is believed to be able to remove the hex or spell. Nurses, as primary health care providers, must formulate and use a treatment plan that displays respect and understanding of the client's cultural healing system or systems and must accept that a Haitian-American client may use a variety of sources to obtain relief when sick.

It is important for the nurse to understand that for many Haitians, leaves have a special significance. When the client comes into the hospital or the clinic for an examination, leaves may be found in the clothes and on various parts of the body. Leaves are believed to have mystical power, and therefore keeping them close to the body is related to regaining or keeping health (Jeanty, personal communication, 1989). The nurse should be accepting of this practice and avoid being shocked if leaves are found in the luggage or on the body of a client being treated. The nurse should also appreciate that religious medallions, rosary beads, or figures of a saint to whom the Haitian client is devoted may have special significance and be felt to offer protection; they should be left with the client (Colin, 2005). The nurse should be cautious about forming negative judgments about a client who may have practices with Voodoo origins (Quillen, 1999).

Haitians have grown accustomed to receiving some direction from authority figures in their lives—parents as well as religious and social leaders. The nurse, as an authority figure, will usually find that Haitian Americans respond well to counseling approaches that foster self-help and independence and should consider the need for heightened self-esteem, which is manifested by the pride and willingness to work that is present in most Haitians.

Haitian Americans need to have occupational options expanded for them and need to understand the steps involved in achieving an occupational goal. Because Haitians have not traditionally had the freedom to set goals, the nurse may be of assistance in this process, as well as in problem solving, to achieve the established goals.

A variety of tools have been used to measure Haitians' beliefs about illness and wellness (Neilsen, McMillan, & Díaz, 1992). Neilsen (1989) used a semistructured interview for three Black cultures, including Haitian.

BIOLOGICAL VARIATIONS

Body Size and Structure, Skin Color, and Other Visible Physical Characteristics

Haitians and African-Americans are similar biologically. As with some other racial groups, the body size and structure of Haitians vary greatly. Haitians have no specific or distinctive size that can be linked genetically. This phenomenon may be a result of crossbreeding with other races throughout history. For this reason, Haitians can be short or tall, light skinned or dark skinned. Haitians are characterized as having shades of brown to black skin as well as brown to black eyes. The hair on the head is often tightly curled, and the body hair is sparsely distributed. The "true" Haitian is tall and exhibits an erect stature. The skull is dolichocephalic in form, being long and relatively narrow. The eyebrow ridges are scant or absent, and the forehead is moderately wide. The form of the orbits is almost square, and their margins are strongly built. The cheeks are wide and, with their supports or zygomatic arches, are bowed laterally in keeping with the powerful jaw musculature. The eyes are set widely apart by the broad and flattened nasal bones. The nose is flat, and the nostrils are widely expanded. The face is large and prominent. The jaws are prognathic and covered by full, fleshy lips, the prominent mucosae of which are reddish black or purple (Godsby, 1971).

Some years ago, anthropologists and scientists discovered that two different types of earwax are present among the human race and that the composition of the earwax determines racial origin. Haitian earwax is described as moist and adhesive (Godsby, 1971).

Susceptibility to Disease and Other Health Concerns

Several major areas of health concerns have been identified in the Haitian culture, including intestinal problems, malnutrition, venereal disease, high birth rate, tuberculosis, sickle cell anemia, hypertension, and cancer. AIDS has also become a serious and increasing health issue for Haitians since the 1970s both in Haiti and in the United States.

Intestinal Problems and Malnutrition. Intestinal problems stemming from malnutrition and ranging from stomach ailments to peptic ulcers are common. The peasant Haitian suffers more from these types of ailments than the wealthy or elite Haitian does. Typically, the Haitian diet tends to be spicy and greasy. Haitians cook almost everything in oil or grease. Even after immigration to the United States, some Haitians continue to prepare foods that are spicy and greasy.

In Haiti, the poor Haitian will consume virtually any type of food to sustain human life. Because many Haitians who have immigrated to the United States have remained at or below the poverty level, they will most likely continue to consume any type of food available. Chronic abdominal discomfort is primarily caused by parasites that are common to the Haitian population (Wilk, 1986).

Venereal Disease. Another problem is venereal disease. Haitian men tend to be more susceptible to different kinds of venereal diseases as a result of promiscuity (Jeanty, personal communication, 1989). Because most marriages are common-law, the man of the family generally lacks commitment to one woman and usually has more than one sexual partner. In addition, the venereal disease is

difficult to treat because the medication is usually taken only as long as the symptoms persist. Premature discontinuation of medication results in an incomplete cure. The problem of venereal disease is also extremely difficult to treat because Haitians do not equate venereal disease with sexual intercourse.

Because there are numerous illegal Haitian immigrants, the prevalence of venereal disease among Haitians in the United States is likely, but the extent is unknown. Testing for syphilis has been required since the Immigration Act of 1990 (Herip, 1993). When Haitians were interdicted at sea and subsequently tested, 5% of Haitians had serological evidence of past or present syphilis (Herip, 1993).

High Birth Rate. The high birth rate has many health and cultural implications for Haitians. One factor contributing to the population explosion is the lack of contraception, which is virtually nonexistent in the conventional manner. This is attributed to a lack of education and technology. An unusually large number of very young Haitian women become pregnant (Jeanty, personal communication, 1989), and Haitian women also tend to become pregnant at older ages. Pregnancy in women 35 years of age and older in Haiti is fairly common (Wilk, 1986). In a classic study, Williams et al. (1975) reported that Haitian women between 35 and 49 years of age have an average of eight pregnancies. Because of this pattern, the nurse must be aware of the high risk among Haitian women in relation to their childbearing habits. Furthermore, family spacing is not an option, and a series of pregnancies within a short time leaves the woman's body unable to fully recover or replenish iron levels.

Haitian women still suffer the highest maternal mortality ratio in the entire Western Hemisphere. Although this number may be undercounted since the massive earthquake of 2010, 670 Haitian women of 100,000 live births died of some pregnancy-related causes compared with only 11 per 100,000 live births in the United States. When compared with the Latin American and Caribbean averages, Haiti's mortality rate is five times higher. In fact, Haiti's maternal mortality rate is higher than any South Asian or Middle Eastern country (Central Intelligence Agency, 2015).

Tuberculosis. Tuberculosis is another concern to the Haitian population. As a result of the poor economic levels, which lead to poor living conditions and malnutrition, Haiti has one of the world's highest rates of tuberculosis (Wilk, 1986). Another factor is overcrowding, which results in poor sanitation. The majority of the population has no waste facilities. Garbage and human excrement are thrown into the streets or placed in community pits, and the water for drinking is contaminated, resulting in a vast number of diseases, including tuberculosis. Malnutrition complicates the situation. The poor cannot afford the cost of examination or the medication to treat the illness if it is diagnosed. Of the number of Haitians who attempted to immigrate to the United States from November 1991 to April 1992, 55% tested positive for tuberculosis on a purified protein derivative test. Chest radiographs confirmed pulmonary tuberculosis in approximately 5% of this group (Herip, 1993). Approximately one third of those testing positive had findings suggestive of active infection. In 21% of the cases, culture and sensitivities for tuberculosis isolates were found to be resistant to medication. Because there is a high incidence of tuberculosis among Haitian immigrants, assessment for symptoms of tuberculosis is an important part of health screening when the nurse is caring for Haitian clients.

Sickle Cell Disease. Sickle cell disease (anemia), or hemoglobin S (HbS) disease, is a chronic hereditary hemolytic disorder mainly affecting the Black populations of the world and is characterized by the presence of erythrocytes that primarily contain HbS instead of HbA. The red blood cell assumes a sickle shape when exposed to lower oxygen levels. Persons who are homozygous for HbS are estimated to have erythrocytes that contain 80% to 100% abnormal HbS and only up to 20% normal HbA. The erythrocytes of persons with sickle cell trait contain approximately 25% to 40% HbS and 60% to 75% HbA.

Sickle cell disease develops as a result of a genetic mutation that is transmitted from parent to child. Laboratory testing is available to determine if the sickle cell trait is present (Sorensen, Luckmann, & Bolander, 1994). It is important for the nurse to have a working knowledge of sickle cell disease when assessing Haitian-American clients and to be able to refer the client to a sickle cell association or support group. It is important to provide the client with information about this illness because most of these clients know little about it (Jeanty, personal communication, 1989).

Hypertension. Little is known about hypertension among Haitians. A pilot study was conducted with 88 Haitian clients by Preston, Materson, Yoham, and Anapol (1996). This study indicated that hypertension was highly prevalent and unusually severe in terms of blood pressure level, refractoriness to treatment, and target organ consequences.

Malaria. *Plasmodium falciparum* malaria was a major problem among displaced Haitians in temporary camps at the U.S. Naval Base, Guantánamo Bay, Cuba. From December 1991 to March 1992, 235 cases of unmixed *falciparum* malaria were diagnosed, giving a cumulative attack rate of 160 per 10,000 camp residents. Health professionals who are treating Haitian immigrants should plan for malaria, and preventive medicine measures are indicated (Bawden, Slaten, & Malone, 1995).

Cancer. Cancers reported in Haiti include cervical, hepatic, stomach, and intestinal cancer and Kaposi's sarcoma (Mitacek, St. Vallières, & Polednak, 1986). Cervical cancer accounts for 39% of all cancers among Haitian women and may be related to poor feminine hygiene as well as early sexual activity with multiple partners (Sebastian, Leeb, & See, 1978). Failure to have Pap smears, which would allow early detection, may relate to the high incidence of cervical cancer. Fruchter et al. (1985) reported that approximately 50% of Haitian women had never had a Pap smear, compared with 25% of the English-speaking Caribbean immigrants and 10% of U.S.-born Black women studied. In a study by Consedine, Magai, Spiller, Neugut, and Conway (2004), Haitian-American women were found to be least knowledgeable about breast cancer and behavior that puts them at risk. Liver, stomach, and intestinal cancers are high among Haitian males. From 1979 to 1984, cancer of the liver (23.4%) and stomach and intestines (20.5%) accounted for 43.9% of all cancers (Mitacek et al., 1986). Gastrointestinal cancer is related to the poor nutrition and low vitamin intake. Kaposi's sarcoma is found in some Haitians who are HIV positive. In a study with seven ethnic groups, American Haitian men were noted to report fewer digital rectal examinations and prostate-specific antigen tests than their counterparts. The importance of fear as a psychological determinant to male screening behavior must be considered in designing models to increase male screening frequency (Consedine, Morgenstern, Kudadjie-Gyamfi, Magai, & Neugut, 2006).

Francois, Elyseé, Shah, and Gany (2009) qualitatively evaluated the views of Haitian Americans about colorectal cancer and the influence that culture played on cancer screening among this population. Findings from this study suggested that among these subjects, many misconceptions regarding colorectal cancer and its development were held. These respondents noted that the greatest problems with seeking screening for colorectal cancer were lack of insurance and illegal immigration status.

AIDS. Cases of AIDS in Haiti are believed to date back to the late 1970s. Actual incidence is unclear, though Herip (1993) noted that 7% of Haitians interdicted at sea tested positive for HIV. Unfortunately, Haiti is the country most heavily affected by AIDS in the Caribbean and accounts for more than 50% of all cases in the region. Because of the publicity of AIDS originating in Haiti, Haitians who have immigrated to the United States face constant discrimination. Samet et al. (1994) noted that most Haitian-American clients presented for primary care with advanced immune dysfunction. Many had waited a year to initiate medical care after testing positive for HIV. The belief of the prevalence of AIDS in Haitians prompted the U.S. Centers for Disease Control and Prevention in Atlanta to list Haitians as one of the four high-risk groups for AIDS, along with homosexuals, hemophiliacs, and heroin users. Testing of Haitian immigrants for AIDS has been required since the Immigration Act of 1990 (Herip, 1993). Finally in 1991, Haitians were removed from the list. Although Haitians are no longer listed as a high-risk AIDS group, public opinion is slow to change. In 2007, the adult prevalence rate for HIV/AIDS was estimated at 2.2% in Haiti compared with 1% in the United States, and this rate is down from 5.6% in 2003, with 7200 deaths annually and 120,000 persons living with HIV/AIDS (2007 estimate) (Central Intelligence Agency, 2015). HIV/AIDS among Haitians and Haitian Americans is an illness highly related to cultural beliefs. Fitzgerald, Maxi, Marcelin, Johnson, and Pape (2004) conducted an investigation in Port-au-Prince and found that issues related to the belief that HIV can be transmitted by magic, to depression during counseling, and to female fear of economic ruin and domestic violence related to notifying sexual partners could predict a patient's future adherence to risk reduction counseling and medical referral. However, health disparities can be reduced with culturally sensitive intervention. An integrated prevention and care project in Haiti by Devieux et al. (2004) indicated that since 1993 there was a 50% drop in incidence among pregnant women. Critical to culturally sensitive care is the reduction of AIDS-related stigma. Preliminary data from research by Castro and Farmer (2005) indicated that with the introduction of quality HIV care, stigma can be reduced and willingness for testing increased.

Haitian-American women are particularly vulnerable to health disparities. Santana and Dancy (2000) investigated the long-term effects of AIDS stigmatization in Haitian-American women. This study noted effects in five categories: rejection by the dominant society, self-doubt, effect on self-esteem, effect on intimate relationships, and rejection by Haitians within the community. The damaging effect of stigma was found to permeate the lives of the women studied in myriad situations, either daily or on a frequent basis. In the study by Samet et al. (1994), women presented with significantly higher CD4 cell counts than men did.

Health–illness beliefs are highly significant in intervention strategies. Martin, Rissmiller, and Beal (1995) conducted a qualitative study of health–illness beliefs and practices of Haitian Americans with HIV disease living in Boston. Five themes were identified: (1) incorporation of traditional health–illness beliefs into beliefs about HIV

disease; (2) a perceived need to hide HIV disease to avoid rejection, humiliation, and isolation; (3) use of spirituality to help cope with HIV disease; (4) history of limited contact with doctors before diagnosis of HIV disease; and (5) use of traditional healing practices for HIV disease. Malow, Jean-Gilles, Devieux, Rosenberg, and Russell (2004) describe an HIV prevention study among Haitian youths in Florida with Haitian-American adolescents. Self-efficacy, behavioral intentions, social factors, and acculturation issues all influence the risk behavior of Haitian-American adolescents and can be influenced to reduce health disparity. Ellerbrock et al. (2004) conducted a population-based study in 1986 and 1998–2000 in a rural Florida community and found that HIV prevalence and risk factors can be changed positively with culturally sensitive interventions in the Haitian-American communities.

Nutritional Preferences and Deficiencies

There was a critical problem with malnutrition in the agricultural areas of Haiti among the poor (Rodman, 1984). Some estimate that 80% of Haitians suffer from malnutrition (Haitians in America, 1983). For the Haitian peasant, environmental, technological, and economic factors alone account for a substantial amount of poor nutrition.

Haiti's rugged topography combines with a generally limited system of mass transport to accentuate the regional and seasonal nature of many of the crops. The economic status of most Haitians confines their food expenditures to a survival level of foods chosen from among locally produced foodstuffs. In addition, the humeral medical beliefs that classify food into "hot" and "cold" categories further restrict dietary selection (Wiese, 1976). Haitian Americans often combine "cold" foods, natural sedatives and purgatives from herbal medicine, religious treatments, and Western medicine in treating illness (Prudent et al., 2005).

The nurse should be aware of food preferences customary to the Haitian culture (Box 20-1). As a result of the lack of ready availability of food items, Haitians have learned many poor nutritional habits, which have persisted even after immigration to the United States, particularly if similar economic conditions prevail.

Dietary Habits for Childbearing. Childbearing Haitian women are very particular about their dietary habits both before and after delivery. These dietary cultural habits include foods that a woman should and should not eat (Box 20-2). The nurse should assess these foods to ensure that the client maintains adequate nutrition (White, Linhart, & Medley, 1996).

Breastfeeding has traditionally been common among Haitians because bottle-feeding was considered unnatural (Jeanty, personal communication, 1989). However, as

BOX 20-1   Common Cultural Foods

Fruits and Nuts
Avocados
Cashews
Coconuts
Granadilla flesh
Mangos
Pineapples
Soursop (guanabana) fruit
Star apples (*Chrysophyllum*)
Cassava bread (manioc, tapioca)
Bananas
Limes
Grapefruit
Oranges
Tomatoes
Watermelons

Meats, Vegetables, and Other Foods
Beef
Beets

Okra
Biscuits (from imported white flour)
Cabbage
Carrots
Imported cheese
Chicken
Milled corn
Eggplant
Fish
Goat meat
Kidney beans
Lima beans
Peas
Pork
Rice
Sweet potatoes
Pumpkin
Sugarcane

BOX 20-2   Childbearing Women and Food Preferences

Foods Eaten by Childbearing Women
Cornmeal porridge with bean sauce
Rice and beans
Plantains
Vegetables
Red fruits

Foods Avoided by Childbearing Women
Lima beans
Tomatoes

Black mushrooms
White beans
Okra
Lobster
Fish
Eggplant
Black peppers
Milk
Bananas

traditional beliefs are changing among Haitian Americans, the incidence of breastfeeding is decreasing (Thomas & DeSantis, 1995).

Psychological Characteristics

Psychiatric care is also limited in Haiti. In 1956, Kline (Bordeleau & Kline, 1986) reported the presence of one psychiatrist and one psychiatric hospital in Haiti. In 1989, Gustafson reported that there were fewer than a dozen psychiatrists in Haiti, and all were located in the capital.

The first modern psychiatric hospital was opened in 1959, amid prejudice and resistance, by two psychiatrists from Canada and the United States. Because perphenazine (Trilafon) was donated by the three founding pharmaceutical companies and was used abundantly, the psychiatrists were called "Trilafon doctors." Although psychiatric treatment has improved, the frequency of mental illness in Haiti is unknown, and the psychiatric services remain undeveloped. Bordeleau and Kline (1986) have reported that psychiatric symptoms do not appear to be much different from those found in other countries. Projection has been identified as a frequent defense mechanism because paranoid delusions often appear in clients who are psychotic. Delusions are profoundly colored by Voodoo religious beliefs. Aggressiveness is seldom directed toward others, with psychomotor hyperactivity being more often noisy than destructive. Affective disorders are more often of the hypomanic or manic type than depressive, and suicide among Haitians is rare. More recently, psychiatric care has advanced with the development of outpatient clients (Azaunce, 1995; Bordeleau & Kline, 1986). However, in 1986 the Pan-American Health Organization reported no listing of psychiatric diagnoses in Haiti in a study involving the years 1981 to 1984. Rather than psychiatric care, most emotionally disturbed clients sought native healers who treat with amulets, packets of herbs and spices, liquids, baths, powders, rubbing, and massage (Gustafson, 1989). Wilson (1984) noted that disclosure of the belief in Voodoo can result in the diagnosis of psychiatric illness by a Western-trained practitioner.

Possession crisis, which has been diagnosed in some Haitian clients, is not unique to Haitian Voodoo but has also been observed in many African countries and on rare occasions among American Indians. This belief has much similarity with the early Greek Dionysian mysteries, the evil possession of the European Middle Ages, the witch possession in the New England colonies, and the contemporary African-American religious services of certain extreme groups in the South. See Box 20-3 for the conditions that must be present to have a possession crisis (Bordeleau & Kline, 1986).

Implications for Nursing Care

Because stomach ailments are a major problem for Haitians, the astute nurse will carefully assess the Haitian-American client for various stomach ailments, including worms, which may be the result of spoiled food. In fact, a nurse may assume that if a Haitian-American family has poor nutritional habits and at the same time cannot afford nutritious food, the likelihood that the family members

BOX 20-3   Possession Crisis

1. The general population of the local community must believe that a human being can communicate with the deities.
2. The person being "mounted" by the spirit (*loa*) is one of a group involved in a religious ceremony where the drums control the rhythm of the dance and the *hungan* behaves at first as a ritualistic priest.
3. Some spirits "participate" only at a certain time of the year and with a similar type of personality; that is, a gentle *loa* mounts a calm person and a fighting *loa* chooses an aggressive person.
4. The group considers being possessed to be a privilege, not a shameful event.
5. The possession crisis is stereotyped in the sense that someone mounted by a specific *loa* will talk like the *loa*, ask for the needed symbolic ornaments, and generally behave and dance in the way traditions in the region have dictated.

From Bordeleau, J. M., & Kline, N. S. (1986, July). Experience in developing psychiatric services in Haiti. *World Mental Health, 170–183.*

will have worms is increased. Garlic is considered a folk remedy for worms and is boiled and eaten to prevent and treat worms. When a Haitian-American client brings in a specimen and hands it to the clinic nurse, it is important for the nurse to understand that this may be a communication about a problem with worms and that the specimen should be analyzed with this in mind. The nurse will be better able to assist the Haitian-American client by not trying to convince the client that garlic is inappropriate. The folk remedies should be accepted and combined with Western medicine.

The nurse should appreciate that in addition to diet being important in relation to the health of pregnant women, dietary practices are generally related to health. Eating well and eating fresh foods are related to maintaining health. Drinking tea every day made with *sorosi* (mulberry juice) is believed by many Haitian Americans to increase appetite, protect health, and prevent illness. One can treat fever by mixing castor oil, alcohol, and shallot (*Allium ascalonicum*); heating the mixture; rubbing it together; and rubbing it all over the fevered body (Spector, 1996).

It is important for the nurse to know that many Haitian Americans have little information about disease or medical problems. Therefore, an illness is more commonly considered a "hex" or the result of an evil curse. The nurse should collect information from the client about the possible cause for the medical problem and should remain nonjudgmental, even when Voodoo is provided as a possible explanation. Health teaching (such as regarding diarrhea or pneumonia) is essential to help the Haitian client understand that the illness is not an evil curse imposed by a neighbor but an illness with natural physical causes.

The nurse cannot assume that all Haitian Americans will have the same beliefs. It is useful to ask Haitian-American clients how long they have been in the United States, which will provide an indication of how Americanized the client may be. The age of the client is also a consideration when health beliefs are being assessed. Younger people are more likely to have made an effective adjustment to the Western culture, whereas older people often continue to find such things as American food strange and unacceptable.

Haitian-American clients are more likely to believe that they are receiving effective treatment when a nurse is seen. In Haiti a nurse is given more authority and status than a physician, and the client will often be more cooperative with directions given by a nurse (Jeanty, personal communication, 1989). When nursing procedures are being implemented (such as taking the client's blood pressure), the nurse should tell the client orally what is being done and that this is for the client's benefit. Actions by the nurse are related to being helped.

Some Haitian Americans associate wheelchairs with being sick. Therefore, on discharge the client who is allowed to walk out of the hospital will be more likely to feel that care has been effective (Jeanty, personal communication, 1989).

Great stress has been placed on Haitians as they have attempted to adjust to life in the United States and Canada. Coming from a disadvantaged background and often arriving in the United States with a history of poor health care, Haitians have been hesitant to reach out for health care. For some of these people, a hospital is perceived as a place to go to die, which may contribute to large numbers of visitors when a Haitian is ill (Jeanty, personal communication, 1989). Health professionals at all levels must communicate a nonjudgmental attitude while trying to encourage the Haitian-American client to take advantage of available health services. Not only do Haitian Americans need to be educated regarding health care agencies but may also need information on health insurance, on how to use health benefits, and on finding a job that has medical benefits. Conway and Buchanan (1985) suggest that what is most helpful to Haitians adjusting to life in the United States is to focus on the strengths from their cultural heritage, such as attitude, perseverance in the most arduous circumstances, deep religious faith, high self-respect, reliance on the extended family, and the tradition of sharing.

SUMMARY

Haiti is an independent, underdeveloped republic that continues to face many critical issues, such as a poor economy, lack of technology, high mortality, inadequacy in food and water supplies, and lack of adequate health care. With the ever-growing Haitian population immigrating to the United States, the nurse must constantly keep these issues in mind when formulating a treatment plan for a Haitian-American client. The holistic approach must take priority when the nurse is assessing, treating, and evaluating the Haitian-American client. The Haitian cultural method of health care delivery must be included with conventional methods of treatment, and transcultural issues in nursing must be recognized before high-quality care can be rendered. Cultural behavior is meaningful and should not be ridiculed, judged negatively, or ignored. The nurse must be aware of cultural and behavioral considerations that affect the care of the Haitian immigrant and use this understanding in implementation of the nursing process. High-quality health care that is culturally sensitive to the needs of Haitian refugees is possible when knowledge of their culture and beliefs is used as a basis for intervention.

CASE STUDY

A 33-year-old Haitian man is admitted via the emergency room with symptoms of persistent coughing and spitting up small amounts of blood. Through the nursing assessment and by talking with the client and his family members, the nurse determines that the client has been experiencing a progressive lack of appetite and is visibly underweight. Radiographic examination reveals that the client has an active and communicable case of tuberculosis. Respiratory assessment reveals low partial pressure of arterial oxygen (PaO_2) and elevated partial pressure of arterial carbon dioxide ($PaCO_2$). When the client and the family are informed that the diagnosis is tuberculosis, there is little reaction. The nurse is informed by the client's family members that the client was initially diagnosed as having a positive Mantoux test in Haiti approximately 2 years previously. At that time the client was given a prescription for isoniazid (INH) by a clinic physician but was noncompliant with his medication regimen.

CARE PLAN

Nursing Diagnosis: Gas exchange, impaired, as evidenced by low PaO_2 and elevated $PaCO_2$

Client Outcome	Nursing Interventions
Client will have no further coughing or viscous secretions.	1. Maintain adequate hydration (increase fluid intake to 2 to 3 quarts per day). 2. Maintain adequate humidity of inspired air. 3. Minimize irritants in inspired air (such as dust, allergens). 4. Provide periods of uninterrupted rest. 5. Administer prescribed medication such as cough suppressant or expectorant as ordered by physician.

Nursing Diagnosis: Nutrition, imbalanced: less than body requirements, inability to ingest food because of biological factors (tuberculosis) as evidenced by anorexia and weight that is below normal for age, sex, and body stature

Client Outcome	Nursing Interventions
Client will gain weight to be within normal range for body size.	1. Maintain good oral hygiene (make sure client brushes teeth, rinses mouth) before and after ingestion of food. 2. Arrange to have foods with the most protein and calories served at times the client feels most like eating. 3. Use dietitian for meal planning.

Continued

◎ CARE PLAN—cont'd

Nursing Diagnosis: Noncompliance related to perceived beliefs of significant others as evidenced by failure of client to take isoniazid

Client Outcome	Nursing Interventions
Client will take prescribed medication as ordered.	1. Allow client an opportunity to make decisions about his own health care; assume an advisory approach when counseling, rather than one that is dictatorial. 2. Consult with an interpreter who speaks both English and Haitian Creole to provide instructions on how to take medication. 3. Consult with an interpreter who speaks both English and Haitian Creole to help client vent his feelings of anxiety and frustration.

Nursing Diagnosis: Medication noncompliance related to referral process

Client Outcome	Nursing Interventions
Client will keep scheduled follow-up appointments.	1. Whenever possible, allow client to make own appointments. 2. Shorten referral waiting time. 3. Personnel handling referral appointment should inquire about transportation, suggesting help if needed.

Nursing Diagnosis: Interrupted family processes, related to shift in health status of family members

Client Outcome	Nursing Interventions
Family will achieve functional support for client.	1. Include family members in group education sessions about tuberculosis. 2. Refer family members to support and self-help groups. 3. Obtain Haitian Creole–speaking interpreter to facilitate communication. 4. Facilitate family involvement with social supports.

Nursing Diagnoses—Definitions and Classifications 2012–2014. Copyright © 2012, 1994–2012 by NANDA International. Used by arrangement with Wiley-Blackwell Publishing, a company of John Wiley and Sons, Inc. In order to make safe and effective judgments using NANDA-I nursing diagnoses it is essential that nurses refer to the definitions and defining characteristics of the diagnoses listed in the work.

CLINICAL DECISION MAKING

1. If a Mantoux test is given incorrectly and no wheal appears (because the injection was made too deep), should the nurse repeat the test at another site that is at least 2 inches away from the first injection?
2. What does *erythema without induration* mean?
3. In tuberculosis, treatment is continued until when?
4. The physician says the client has induration. What does this mean?
5. List the possible side effects of INH.
6. What preventive steps can be taken to avoid the spread of a diagnosed case of tuberculosis?
7. Why is proper nutrition important with a client diagnosed as having tuberculosis?
8. Why is the Haitian population at high risk for being infected by tuberculosis?
9. What is the nurse's role when caring for a client with tuberculosis?
10. Compare the similarities and differences in family structure between the American and Haitian cultures.
11. What are the contributing factors that lead to the high birth rate in Haiti and among Haitian immigrants?
12. Why are Haitian women at risk during pregnancy?
13. Describe the practice of healers and their importance to the Haitian population.
14. Describe the role of the Haitian man as it pertains to family.

REVIEW QUESTIONS

1. In planning care for a pregnant Haitian-American client, the nurse needs to be alert that the most crucial and decisive cultural compliance associated with childbearing are related to which of the following?
   a. Delivery of the baby
   b. Time of labor
   c. Antepartum period
   d. Postpartum period

2. A Haitian-American client comes to the clinic and tells the nurse she has been eating garlic to cure an intestinal problem. Which of the following is the most appropriate action for the nurse to take?
   a. Convince the client that garlic is an inappropriate treatment.
   b. Accept folk remedies and combine them with Western medicine.
   c. Teach the client to seek medical help earlier.
   d. Accept that the intestinal ailment is a curse.

3. When assessing the sexuality of Haitian men, it is best for the nurse to ask the client which of the following questions?
   a. Are you bisexual?
   b. Are you homosexual?
   c. Are you heterosexual?
   d. Have you ever had sex with another man?

REFERENCES

Abbott, E. (1991). *Haiti: the Duvaliers and their legacy* (revised ed.). New York: Simon & Schuster.

Annas, G. (1993). Detention of HIV-positive Haitians at Guantánamo. *The New England Journal of Medicine, 329*, 589–592.

Azaunce, M. (1995). Is it schizophrenia or spirit possession? *Journal of Social Distress and the Homeless, 4*(3), 255–263.

Barnard, R., & Sincox, A. (2004). A call for help from across the sea. *Michigan Nurse, 9*, 16.

Barnes, J. (2000). *New York Times, 149*(51364), B3.

Barstow, D. (2000). Shooting resonates among Haitians. *New York Times, 149*(51335), B6.

Bawden, M. P., Slaten, D. D., & Malone, J. D. (1995). *Falciparum* malaria in a displaced Haitian population. *Transactions of the Royal Society of Tropical Medicine and Hygiene, 89*(6), 600–603.

Bell, I. (1981). *The Dominican Republic.* Boulder, CO: Westview.

Benedict, M. (2004). Vermont nurses venture to Haiti. *Vermont Nurse Connection, 7*(3), 5.

Bestman, E. (1979). *Cultural, linguistic and racial barriers in providing health services to Haitian refugees.* Paper presented at a workshop on improving health services to Haitian refugees, sponsored by the U.S. Metro-Dade County, FL, Health Service Administration.

Bonnlander, H. (1996). Migrant TB treatment in Haiti resulting in U.S. policy change at Guantánamo Bay, Cuba. *Bulletin of the Pan American Health Organization, 30*(3), 206–211.

Bordeleau, J. M., & Kline, N. S. (1986). Experience in developing psychiatric services in Haiti. *World Mental Health,* 170–183.

Boswell, T. (1982). The new Haitian diaspora. *Caribbean Review, 11*(1), 18–21.

Bragg, R. (2000). Haitian immigrants in U.S. face a wrenching choice. *New York Times, 149*(51342), A1.

Bryan, S. (1988). *Ethnic disease.* Paper presented at a workshop sponsored by the U.S. Metro-Dade County, FL, Health Service Administration.

Calypso, A. (1999). Tet Grenn. *Essence, 30*(7), 90.

Carrazana, E., DeToledo, J., Tatum, W., Rivas-Vasquez, R., Rey, G., & Wheeler, S. (1999). Epilepsy and religious experiences: voodoo possession. *Epilepsia, 40*, 239–241.

Castro, A., & Farmer, P. (2005). Understanding and addressing AIDS-related stigma: from anthropological theory to clinical practice in Haiti. *American Journal of Public Health, 95*(1), 53–59.

Central Intelligence Agency (CIA). (2015). *The world fact book.* New York: Skyhorse.

Charles, C. (1979). *Anthropological consideration of barriers affecting delivery of health services to Haitian refugees in Florida.* Paper presented at a workshop on improving health services to Haitian refugees, sponsored by the U.S. Metro-Dade County, FL, Health Service Administration.

Chelala, C. (1994). Fighting for survival. *British Medical Journal, 309*(6953), 525–526.

Claude, J. (1997). *Presentation on Haiti at the Mennonite Economic Development Conference.* Kansas City, MO.

Colin, J. (2005). Haitians. In J. Lipson & S. Dibble (Eds.), *Culture and clinical care.* San Francisco: UCSF Nursing Press.

Consedine, N., Magai, C., Spiller, R., Neugut, A. I., & Conway, F. (2004). Breast cancer knowledge and beliefs in subpopulations of African American and Caribbean women. *American Journal of Health Behavior, 28*(3), 260–271.

Consedine, N., Morgenstern, A., Kudadjie-Gyamfi, E., Magai, C., & Neugut, A. I. (2006). Prostate cancer screening behavior in men from seven ethnic groups: the fear factor. *Cancer Epidemiology Biomarkers Prevention, 15*(2), 228–237.

Conway, F., & Buchanan, S. (1985). Haitians. In D. Haines (Ed.), *Refugees in the United States* (pp. 95–109). Westport, CT: Greenwood.

Coreil, J. (1983). Parallel structures in professional and folk health care: a model applied to rural Haiti. *Culture, Medicine and Psychiatry, 70*, 131–151.

Degazon, C. (1994). Ethnic identification, social support and coping strategies among three groups of ethnic African elders. *Journal of Cultural Diversity, 1*(4), 79–85.

Dejean, Y. (1983). Revisiting the issues of the native language as a natural medium of instruction (Unpublished master's thesis). New York: Bank Street College of Education.

Dempsey, P. A., & Gesse, T. (1983). The childbearing Haitian refugee: cultural applications to clinical nursing. *Public Health Reports, 98*(3), 261–267.

Dening, E. (2001). Haiti. *Workbook, walking with a hurting world*. Akron, PA: Mennonite Central Committee.

DeSantis, L., & Thomas, J. (1987). Parental attitudes toward adolescent sexuality: transcultural perspectives. *Nurse Practitioner, 12*, 43–48.

DeSantis, L., & Thomas, J. (1992). Health education and the immigrant Haitian mother: cultural insights for community health nurses. *Public Health Nursing, 9*(2), 87–96.

DeSantis, L., & Ugarriza, D. (1995). Potential for intergenerational conflict in Cuban and Haitian immigrant families. *Archives of Psychiatric Nursing, 9*(6), 354–364.

DeStefano, J., & Miksic, E. (2007). *School effectiveness in Maissade, Haiti*. Washington, DC: American Institutes for Research/Equip2.

Devieux, J., et al. (2004). Reducing health disparities through culturally sensitive treatment for HIV+ adults in Haiti. *ABNF Journal, 25*(6), 109–115.

Eisenbruch, M. (1984). Cross-cultural aspects of bereavement: part 2. Ethnic and cultural variations in the development of bereavement practices. *Culture, Medicine and Psychiatry, 8*, 315–347.

Ellerbrock, T., et al. (2004). Human immunodeficiency virus infection in a rural community in the United States. *American Journal of Epidemiology, 160*(6), 582–588.

Epstein, G., Lantigua, J., & Cavanaugh, J. (1995). U.S. ship taking rafters to Cuba. *Miami Herald*, 1A.

Eshleman, J., & Davidhizar, R. (1997). Life in migrant camps for children: a hazard to health. *Journal of Cultural Diversity, 4*(1), 13–15.

Fernández-Kelly, M., & Schauffler, R. (1994). Divided fates: immigrant children in a restructured U.S. economy. *International Migration Review, 28*, 662–689.

Fineman, M. (2001). Desperate Haitians inundate Bahamas. *The Journal Gazette*, 11A.

Fitzgerald, D., Maxi, A., Marcelin, A., Johnson, W. D., & Pape, J. W. (2004). Notification of positive HIV test results in Haiti: can we better intervene at this critical crossroads in the life of HIV-infected patients in a resource-poor country? *AIDS Patient Care and STDs, 18*(11), 658–664.

Francois, F., Elyseé, G., Shah, S., & Gany, F. (2009). Colon cancer knowledge and attitudes in an immigrant Haitian community. *Journal of Immigrant Minority Health, 11*, 319–325.

Fruchter, R. G., Wright, C., Habenstreit, B., Remy, J. C., Boyce, J. G., & Imperato, P. J. (1985). Screening for cervical and breast cancer among Caribbean immigrants. *Journal of Community Health, 10*, 121–135.

Godsby, R. (1971). *A race and races*. New York: Macmillan.

Granich, R., Sfeir, M., & Jacobs, B. (1994). Detention of HIV-positive Haitians and Cubans. *The New England Journal of Medicine, 330*(5), 372.

Grant, W. (1989). *The prevalence of antibodies to HTLV-I virus in the Aribonite Valley*. Burlington, VT: Paper presented at the annual reunion of the Hospital Albert Schweitzer Alumni Association.

Gregg, V. (2001). The world in our classroom. *Emory University: A Magazine for Alumni and Friends*. Atlanta: Nell Hodgson Woodruff School of Nursing.

Gustafson, M. (1989). Western voodoo: providing mental health care to Haitian refugees. *Journal of Psychosocial Nursing, 27*, 22–25.

Haitians in America. (1983). *National Catholic Reporter*, 1.

Hardcastle, M. (2004). Reflection: lessons from Haiti. *Canadian Nurse, 100*(5), 12–13.

Harris, K. (1987). Beliefs and practices among Haitian American women in relation to childbearing. *Journal of Nurse-Midwifery, 32*(3), 149–155.

Herip, D. (1993). Health status of Haitian migrants: U.S. naval base, Guantánamo Bay, Cuba, November 1991–April 1992. *Journal of the American Medical Association, 269*, 1395.

Herskovits, M. J. (1971). *Life in a Haitian valley*. Garden City, NY: Anchor Books.

Hiebert, C. (1997). Presentation on Haiti at the Mennonite Economic Development Conference, Kansas City, MO.

Hobsbawn, E. J. (1996). *The age of revolution: 1789–1848*. New York: Vintage Books.

Holcomb, L. O., Parsons, L. C., Giger, J. N., & Davidhizar, R. E. (1996). Haitian Americans: implications for nursing care. *Journal of Community Health Nursing, 13*(4), 249–260.

Holt, J., & Reeves, J. (2001). The meaning of hope and generic caring practices to nurture hope in a rural village in the Dominican Republic. *Journal of Transcultural Nursing, 12*(2), 123–131.

Isgro, F. (1998). New law grants amnesty to Haitians. *Migration World Magazine, 26*(5), 41.

Laguerre, M. (1981). Haitian Americans. In A. Harwood (Ed.), *Ethnicity and medical care*. Cambridge, MA: Harvard University Press.

Laguerre, M. (1984). *American odyssey: Haitians in New York City*. Ithaca, NY: Cornell University Press.

Laguerre, M. (1989). *Voodoo and politics in Haiti*. New York: St. Martin's.

Leyburn, J. G. (1980). *The Haitian people*. Westport, CT: Greenwood.

Lillibridge, S., Conrad, K., Stinson, N., & Noji, E. (1994). Haitian mass migration: uniformed service medical support, May 1992. *Military Medicine, 159*(2), 149–153.

Logan, M. (1975). Selected references on the hot-cold theory of disease. *Medical Anthropology Newsletter, 6*(2), 8–11.

Malow, R., Jean-Gilles, M., Devieux, J., Rosenberg, R., & Russell, A. (2004). Increasing access to preventive health care through cultural adaptation of effective HIV prevention interventions: a brief report from the HIV prevention in Haitian youths study. *ABNF Journal, 15*(6), 127–132.

Martin, M., Rissmiller, P., & Beal, J. (1995). Health-illness beliefs and practices of Haitians with HIV disease living in Boston. *Journal of the Association of Nurses in AIDS Care, 6*(6), 45–53.

Masland, T. (1992). Haiti: "We could turn our back." *Newsweek*, 30–32.

McMorrow, T. (1970). Haitians try to adopt U.S. with three strikes on them. *Daily News*, B1.

Mena, A. (1996). Cuban Santeria, Haitian voodun, Puerto Rican spiritualism: a multiculturist inquiry into syncretism. *Journal for the Scientific Study of Religion, 37*, 15–27.

Métraux, A. (1953). Médecine et voudou en Haïti. *Acta Tropica*, *10*, 28–68.

Metropolitan Dade County (1981). *Social and economic problems among Cuban and Haitian entrant groups in Dade County, Florida: trends and implications*. Miami, FL: Metropolitan Dade County.

Miller, N. (2000). Haitian ethnomedical systems and biomedical practitioners: directions for clinicians. *Journal of Transcultural Nursing*, *11*(3), 204–211.

Mitacek, E. J., St. Vallières, D., & Polednak, A. P. (1986). Cancer in Haiti 1979–1984: distribution of various forms of cancer according to geographical area and sex. *International Journal of Cancer*, *38*, 9–16.

Moskowitz, L. B., Kory, P., Chan, J. C., Haverkos, H. W., Conley, F. K., & Hensley, G. T. (1983). Unusual causes of deaths in Haitians residing in Miami. *Journal of the American Medical Association*, *250*(9), 1187–1191.

Neilsen, B. (1989). Beliefs towards a diagnosis of cancer: a transcultural approach. In A. P. Prichard (Ed.), *Proceedings of the Fifth International Conference on Cancer Nursing* (pp. 129–132). London: Macmillan.

Neilsen, B., McMillan, S., & Díaz, E. (1992). Instruments that measure beliefs about cancer from a cultural perspective. *Cancer Nursing*, *15*(2), 109–115.

Nelson, M. (2002). *Haitian-owned businesses: why we often fail*. Available at <http://www.uhhp.com/business>. Retrieved July 25, 2002.

Nida, E. (1954). *Customs and cultures*. New York: Harper & Brothers.

Office of Refugee Resettlement (1993). *Refugee resettlement program: annual report to Congress, FY 1992*. Washington, DC: U.S. Government Printing Office.

Orque, M. S., Bloch, B., & Monrroy, L. S. A. (1983). *Ethnic nursing care: a multicultural approach*. St. Louis: Mosby.

Portes, A., & Stepick, A. (1985). Unwelcome immigrants: the labor market experiences of 1980 (Mariel) Cuban and Haitian refugees in South Florida. *American Sociological Review*, 493–515.

Potocky, M. (1996). Refugee children: how are they faring economically as adults? *Social Work Journal of the National Association of Social Workers*, *41*(4), 354–373.

Preston, R. A., Materson, B. J., Yoham, M. A., & Anapol, H. (1996). Hypertension in Haitians. *Journal of Human Hypertension*, *10*(11), 743–745.

Prudent, N., Johnson, P., Carroll, J., & Culpepper, L. (2005). Attention-deficit/hyperactivity disorder: presentation and management in the Haitian American child. *Companion Journal of Clinical Psychiatry*, *7*(4), 190–197.

Quillen, T. (1999). The voodoo religion [letter]. *Journal of Psychiatric Nursing and Mental Health*, *31*(1), 4.

Randall-David, E. (1989). *Strategies for working with culturally diverse communities and clients*. Washington, DC: U.S. Department of Health and Human Services.

Reichman, L. (1989). *Treating tuberculosis in developing countries*. Burlington, VT: Paper presented at the annual reunion of the Hospital Albert Schweitzer Alumni Association.

Robinson, A. (1994). Attitudes toward nursing home residents among aides of three cultural groups. *Journal of Cultural Diversity*, *1*(1), 16–18.

Rodman, S. (1984). *Haiti: the Black republic* (6th ed.). Old Greenwich, CT: Devin-Adair.

Rosenthal, B. (1995). The influence of social support on school completion among Haitians. *Social Work in Education*, *17*(1), 30–39.

Rosenwarke, I. (1972). *Population history of New York*. Syracuse, NY: Syracuse University Press.

Samet, J., Retondo, M., Freedberg, K. A., Stein, M. D., Heeren, T., & Libman, H. (1994). Factors associated with initiation of primary medical care for HIV-infected persons. *American Journal of Medicine*, *4*, 347–353.

Santana, M., & Dancy, B. (2000). The stigma of being named "AIDS carriers" on Haitian-American women. *Health Care for Women International*, *21*, 161–171.

Schaedel, R. (1962). The human resources of Haiti. Unpublished manuscript.

Scott, C. (1978). Health and healing practices among five ethnic groups in Miami, Florida. *Public Health Report*, *55*, 524–532.

Seabrooks, P. (1992). Social supports of older Haitians in Port-au-Prince and Miami: effects on health practices and perceived health status (Unpublished dissertation). Doctor of Nursing Services, University of California, San Francisco.

Sebastian, J. A., Leeb, B. O., & See, R. (1978). Cancer of the cervix: a sexually transmitted disease. *American Journal of Obstetrics and Gynecology*, *131*, 620–623.

Seligman, L. (1977). Haitians: a neglected minority. *Personnel and Guidance Journal*, *2*, 409–411.

Snow, L. F. (1981). Folk medical beliefs and their implications for the care of patients: a review based on studies among Black Americans. In G. Henderson & M. Primeaux (Eds.), *Transcultural health care*. Reading, MA: Addison-Wesley.

Sorensen, K., Luckmann, J., & Bolander, V. (1994). *Sorensen and Luckmann's basic nursing: a psychophysiologic approach*. Philadelphia: Saunders.

Spector, R. (1996). *Culture care: guide to heritage assessment and health traditions* (3rd ed.). Upper Saddle River, NJ: Pearson Prentice Hall.

Stauffer, R. (2006). Personal communication with the former Assistant Director of Nursing at Hôpital Albert Schweitzer. Haiti: Deschapelles.

Thomas, H. (1997). *The slave trade: the story of the Atlantic slave trade 1440–1870*. New York: Touchstone.

Thomas, J., & DeSantis, L. (1995). Feeding and weaning practices in Cuban and Haitian immigrant mothers. *Journal of Transcultural Nursing*, *6*(2), 34–42.

Time Almanac. (2015). Chicago: Encyclopedia Britannica.

United Nations Development Program (1996). *Rapport de Coopération au Développement-Haïti*. Port-Au-Prince, Haiti.

U.S. Committee for Refugees. (1995). Asylum cases filed with INS, April 1991–Sept. 1995. *Refugee Reports*, *16*(12), 12.

U.S. Department of Commerce, Bureau of the Census (2013). *American Community Survey, Haitians*. Washington, DC: U.S. Government Printing Office.

Veeken, H. (1993). Hope for Haiti. *British Medical Journal, 307,* 312–313.

Venton, D. (1997). *Report on volunteer experiences in Haiti.* Kansas City, MO: Mennonite Economic Development Association Conference.

Verdet, P. (1985). Trying times: Haitian youth in an inner city high school. *Social Work in Health Care,* 228–233.

Walsh, B. (1980). The boat people of South Florida. *America,* 420–421.

Weil, T. E. (1973). *Area handbook for Haiti.* Washington, DC: U.S. Government Printing Office.

Westphal, R. (1989). *Transfusion transmitted infectious diseases.* Burlington, VT: Paper presented at the annual reunion of the Hospital Albert Schweitzer Alumni Association.

White, J., Linhart, J., & Medley, L. (1996). Culture, diet and the maternity. *Advance for Nurse Practitioners,* 26–29.

Wiese, J. (1976). Maternal nutrition and traditional food behavior in Haiti. *Human Organization, 35*(2), 193–200.

Wilentz, A. (1989). *The rainy season.* New York: Simon & Schuster.

Wilk, R. (1986). The Haitian refugee: concern for health care providers. *Social Work in Health Care, 11,* 61–74.

Williams, S., Murthy, N., & Berggren, G. (1975). Conjugal unions among rural Haitian women. *Journal of Marriage and the Family, 37,* 1022–1031.

Wilson, M. (1984). Voodoo believers: some sociological insights. *Journal of Sociology and Social Welfare, 9,* 373–383.

World Almanac. (2015). New York: World Almanac Books.

Jewish Americans

Anita Renau Bralock and Cheryl Smythe Padgham*

BEHAVIORAL OBJECTIVES

After reading this chapter, the nurse will be able to:

1. Identify how the religion of Judaism affects the cultural behaviors of Jewish Americans.
2. Identify some of the differences between health-oriented behaviors demonstrated by various religious groups within Judaism.
3. Identify how the various ethnic backgrounds of Jewish Americans affect their cultural behaviors.
4. Describe attitudes and beliefs affecting health care within and across individuals in various Jewish groups.
5. Identify how the verbal and nonverbal communications of Jewish individuals may affect health care.
6. Identify implications or precautions for providing effective nursing care to Jewish Americans.
7. Recognize those health care practices that are mandated by Jewish law for people who are Jewish.

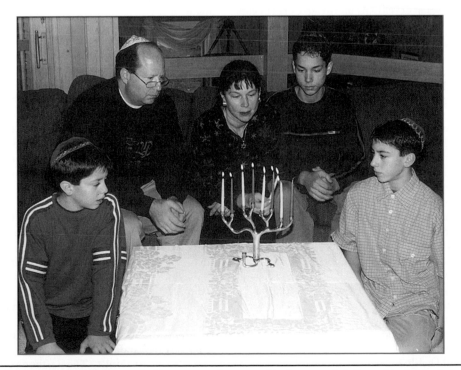

*We wish to thank Enid A. Schwartz for her nearly 30-year commitment to this chapter and dedicate this chapter in her memory.

Explaining what it means to be Jewish is not easy. It is more than just belonging to a religious organization; it is also being a part of a specific people (Glazer, 1989; Popenoe, 2000; Trepp, 1980). It is a shared feeling of "Jewishness." Jewish people are linked together by a common history, common ethical teachings, a common language of prayer (Hebrew), a vast quantity of literature, common folkways, and, above all, a sense of common destiny (Kertzer, 1993). Jewish people share centuries of history as a minority subjected to hostility wherever they go.

The Jewish-American culture has many subcultures because of the different areas of the world in which Jews live as well as a diversity of religious observances. Jews came to the United States predominantly from Spain, Portugal, Germany, and Eastern Europe. There are four main religious groups: Orthodox, Conservative, Reform, and Reconstructionist. Within the orthodox group are the Chassidic (or Hasidic) and Lubovitch subgroups, which are the largest subgroups in the United States today.

Despite differences, there are some cultural similarities that are indigenous to this group of people. To understand the culture, one must have knowledge of some of the religious dictates. Through a discussion of the six common variables found within and across cultural groups as they apply to Jewish Americans, this chapter attempts to clarify some behaviors that are commonly found among Jews in order to assist nurses in developing an effective plan of care for the Jewish-American client. Attention is also placed on Jewish rituals and the effects of assimilation on their cultural traits.

OVERVIEW OF THE JEWISH PEOPLE IN THE UNITED STATES

The history of American Judaism encompasses three distinct waves of immigration. The first wave of people, who began arriving in the middle 1600s, was relatively small. They were Sephardic Jews from Spain and Portugal, and they had little effect on the development of modern American Judaism (Sachar, 1965). The beginning of the nineteenth century saw a steady German immigration, which swelled after 1836, when Jews sought to escape persecution in Bavaria and other German states (Glazer, 1989). The last tide of immigration began slowly in 1845, when Polish Jews began arriving in the United States, but swelled to tens of thousands in 1881 as a result of a wave of pogroms and a series of new anti-Jewish decrees in Russia. This last wave, consisting of Eastern European Jews and German Jews, has had a profound effect on modern Jewish-American culture and religious practices.

To understand Jewish-American culture today, it is necessary to consider Europe during the Middle Ages. At that time, most of the internal law in European Jewish communities was strongly controlled by the Talmud (the Rabbinic code). Talmudic law governed not only the religious behavior of Jews but also almost every other aspect of life, such as birth, marriage, and death, as well as the proper foods to eat and the proper clothes to wear. The Jews were kept separate from the general population not only by persecution from others but also by the boundaries set by these laws.

In the nineteenth century, not all German Jews were isolated in their communities; some were involved in non-Jewish communities. Many of these Jews were embarrassed by the ancient laws and found them distasteful, especially if they desired the status of full members of the German nation (Glazer, 1989). To maintain their beliefs and yet not appear different from the general culture, German Jews of high social status attempted to start the Reform movement. The freedom experienced in the United States allowed the Reform movement to flourish. The German Jews who immigrated to the United States and wished to become part of the American community were willing to rid themselves of the old traditions and become increasingly "Americanized." They were insistent, however, that the Jews be maintained as a people.

The Eastern European immigrants came predominantly from Russia, Romania, Poland, and Austria. In contrast to many of the German Jewish immigrants who had lived in nonsegregated areas, most of the Eastern European Jews came from all-Jewish villages, known as *shtetls*, where a Jewish culture was created that was almost totally unaffected by the cultures of the people around them. Life was dictated by the religious traditions Eastern European Jews followed and was much the same as it had been during the Middle Ages.

Along with these pious Jews came the radical political and socialist Jews, who believed that the only way to survive was through complete abandonment of religion. A third group who immigrated during this time represented the "middle-of-the-road" Jews, who were both religious and radical (Glazer, 1989).

It is important to understand the differences in religious behavior when caring for Jewish clients. All Jewish beliefs derive from the Torah (the five books of Moses) and the Talmud (the Rabbinic code). From the Torah come 613 commandments. The combination of the Torah and Talmud results in codes of law. Rather than referring to a body of doctrine, Judaism refers to a body of practices (Glazer, 1989).

As mentioned previously, four main religious Jewish groups exist today: Orthodox, Conservative, Reform, and Reconstructionist. The Orthodox Jew maintains a strict code of interpretation of the law, the Conservative

Jew maintains a less strict code of interpretation, and the Reform Jew follows a more liberal interpretation of the law. Reconstructionist Judaism is a little difficult to explain. Reconstructionists do not necessarily believe in God as a personified deity or that God chose the Jewish people. If they follow the laws of Judaism, they do so because of their cultural value. An example of the differences deals with the head coverings worn by men: the Orthodox Jew is obligated to keep his head covered at all times in reverence to God, the Conservative Jew keeps his head covered during times of worship, and the Reform and Reconstructionist Jews are not obligated to keep their heads covered.

The division between Jewish practices started in Germany in the nineteenth century, but it was not until Jews experienced the religious freedom of the United States that the Conservative and Reform movements thrived. The freedom experienced in the United States allowed the Jewish immigrant to question the narrow confines of orthodoxy and led to a desire to express religious beliefs and traditional practices in a less confining environment. The German Jews had begun to practice Reform Judaism. However, to the Eastern European Jew, Reform Judaism seemed empty (Howe, 1989). A movement known as "Conservatism," which had begun in nineteenth-century Germany, had a small beginning but appealed to the children of many Eastern European immigrants. According to Glazer (1989), Conservatism offered a compromise between the blind religious teachings of the Orthodox Jews and the scholarly endeavors of the Reform movement to break from tradition completely. Today, Reform temples are moving toward more traditional practices but maintain the belief that a person should be able to make choices based on knowledge of customs and their meanings.

In regard to religion, Jewish identity has changed through the generations. In the United States today, the sense of Jewish identity does not lie in the Old World religious observances. Most Jewish Americans do not observe the traditional Jewish Sabbath, nor are they active in their temple or synagogue. According to Sowell (1981), their identity lies not with the historical religious aspects of Judaism but with their ethnic or racial identity.

Changes in immigration laws have decreased the number of Jews entering the United States. However, since the time of the large immigration of Eastern European Jews, Jews from other countries have come to the United States under different circumstances. There are Jews who escaped or lived through the Holocaust, Jews who have emigrated from Communist Russia, Russian Jews who were able to leave after the collapse of the Communist party, and Jews who have arrived from many other countries of the world, including Ethiopia and Israel. Each group has added to the cultural diversity of the Jewish people. All have brought with them the culture of the land from which they emigrated. Because of the close ties that have developed between Jews of all nationalities, cultural traits have begun to blend. For example, descendants of Eastern European Jews talk about eating *falafel,* a food made from ground chickpeas, which originated in the Middle East.

A fear of many Jewish Americans is the effect of assimilation on their children. Jewish-American people do not want to appear different from other Americans because being different has led to thousands of years of persecution. However, many Jewish Americans do not want to lose the common thread that binds them to one another.

Although Jewish Americans make up only about 3% of the U.S. population, they are visible in many areas of U.S. culture. Today, an estimated 6,544,000 Jews reside in the United States (*Time Almanac,* 2011). Jewish Americans are distinguished members of the arts, academia, the sciences, medicine, law, and the political arena. Education is a large part of the Jewish culture, which has helped Jews in the United States succeed as they never could in other countries.

The desire to succeed, plus intermarriage, has caused some loss of Jewish identity. Some Jews today in the United States do not wish to be identified as Jewish for fear of discrimination in the workplace. Discrimination against Jews does exist in the United States, and many Jews are sensitive to anti-Semitism.

COMMUNICATION

Today the primary language of Jewish Americans is English. In the late 1800s the primary language of the Jews was Yiddish, which is a combination of German, Slavic, Old French, Old Italian, and Hebrew languages (Languages of the World, 2015; Rosten, 1999). The children of first-generation Jews, born to Eastern European parents, wanted to be accepted by the other children. Although Yiddish may have been spoken in the home, these children spoke English outside the home. Very few second-generation Jewish Americans understand Yiddish. However, almost all Jewish Americans know some Yiddish, and many Jewish conversations are sprinkled with Yiddish words. Some of these words have become a part of American English, such as *shtick* (or *shtück*) and *tush.*

Hebrew, which is the language of Israel, is rarely spoken by most Jews who do not live there. However, Hebrew is the language of the Torah, and many Jews can read it. An important part of Jewish religious education is the reading, speaking, and writing of Hebrew. *Shalom* is a Hebrew word that is commonly used by Jewish people to mean "peace," "hello," or "good-bye."

The Sephardic Jews have a language of their own, Ladino, which is similar to Old Spanish. It is not commonly spoken in the United States today.

Style

When communicating, Jewish people tend to be highly verbal and expressive, using hand gestures to punctuate their communication. They have a sharp sense of humor and usually prefer language that is direct and frank.

By changing the emphasis on certain words, the Jewish person changes the meaning of the message being conveyed (Languages of the World, 2015; Rosten, 1999). This change in emphasis is done easily in Yiddish and has been carried over into English. As an example, changing the emphasis on the words "Him you trust?" changes the meaning: "Him *trust*?" versus "*Him* you trust?" The first questions a person's judgment; the second implies that anyone who would trust the character of such a scoundrel must be an idiot.

Jewish humor may be viewed as sarcastic, and often the humor is directed at themselves. This self-directed humor has led to comments that Jewish humor comes out of self-hatred. Although Jewish humor may appear to be self-critical and sometimes self-deprecating, it does not stem from a form of Jewish masochism. One of the most popular beliefs is that Jewish humor arose as a way for Jews to cope with the hostility they found around them, sometimes using that hostility against themselves. It appears as if a Jewish person is telling enemies, "You don't have to attack us. We can do that ourselves—and even better" (Novak & Waldoks, 1981).

Jews today are sensitive to humor from "outside" sources. Jokes that are not appreciated when told by non-Jews include "JAP" (Jewish American Princess) jokes and those about "Jewing people down" (referring to Jews being cheap or unmerciful at bartering).

As Jews become more acculturated with each generation, the communication styles change. Jewish people who are third- or fourth-generation Americans are more likely to demonstrate the same communication style as their neighbors rather than that of their parents, grandparents, or great-grandparents. This type of acculturation is part of the history of Jews all over the world (Patai & Wing, 1989).

Touch

The use of touch varies among Jewish people; however, the use or nonuse of touch can be a critical issue with Orthodox Jews and must be carefully considered by the nurse. Because of Jewish laws regarding personal space and touching others of the opposite sex, it is important to ascertain to which religious group the client belongs. If the client is Orthodox, he or she will be very modest. Overexposure of

or touching the parts of the body associated with sexual activities can cause a great deal of distress. When caring for strict Orthodox Jewish clients of the opposite sex, the nurse should use touch only for hands-on care. To touch the client at any other time could be offensive because of the sexual connotations attached to casual touch. It is also important to note that, according to Jewish law, religious observances are not to be followed if doing so will endanger the person's health.

Implications for Nursing Care

Because older Jewish clients may be very verbal about what and how they are feeling, they may appear to be chronic complainers. Although it is difficult to remain nonjudgmental with a client who is considered a chronic complainer, it is important to remember that letting others know feelings is part of the Jewish culture. It may be difficult to assess pain levels of Jewish clients because they are very emotional when expressing their discomfort, and it may take persistence and patience to pinpoint the problem and its extent. Younger Jewish clients may be more articulate and may also complain less than their parents or grandparents as a result of acculturation.

Jewish communication style may lead to analytical sparring. Because of this tendency, teaching may be best accomplished using a question-and-answer style and open discussion.

SPACE

The Orthodox Jew is keenly aware of religious dictates regarding personal space that may or may not be invaded by members of the opposite sex. Many Orthodox Jewish men and women will not shake hands with a member of the opposite sex. This practice stems from the ruling in the Code of Jewish Law that forbids a man to smell the scent of a strange woman, to look upon her hair, or even to gaze upon her little finger (Kolatch, 1985; Rozovsky, 2015). An ultra-Orthodox Jewish man will not usually touch his wife in public.

Traditionally, Jewish people have also had practices about personal and social space. In times of sickness and during their elderly years, Jewish individuals have an acute desire to have members of their family and other Jews around them. This desire has been illustrated in studies of the elderly that indicate that elderly Jewish people in nursing homes adjust better if they have other Jews around them (Kaplan, 1970; Rozovsky, 2015).

Implications for Nursing Care

Judaic laws can lead to some misinterpretation by nurses and other health care providers. For example, during childbirth, if an ultra-Orthodox Jewish husband decides to participate in the delivery, his participation will be only verbal. He will not touch his wife during labor. This practice is associated with the laws of separation that dictate that avoidance is necessary during the time a woman has any vaginal bleeding. He will not view the birth because he is not permitted to view his wife's genital area. After the birth, he may lean over his wife (being careful not to touch her), smile, and say, *Mazel tov* (good luck, congratulations) (Bash, 1980; Lutwak, Ney, & White, 1988; Rozovsky, 2015). Some ultra-Orthodox husbands elect to participate only spiritually. If this is the case, they will sit with their prayer book and recite from the Book of Psalms. It is important to remember that this practice does not mean the man loves his wife any less than the man who actively participates.

Among the Orthodox Jews there are different groups. The "modern" Orthodox Jew cannot be distinguished by his or her dress, although some traditional Orthodox Jews are often recognizable by their appearance. The men usually have long earlocks and beards and wear a yarmulke (skull cap) or large black hats and long black frock coats. The women are modestly dressed in long-sleeved dresses and have wigs or scarves covering their heads.

With the increase of male nurses, the question arises regarding the assignment of a male nurse to a female Orthodox Jewish client. The Code of Jewish Law (Ganzfried, 1963) states that "a male is not permitted to attend to a woman who is suffering with a belly ache . . . but a woman may attend to a male who is so suffering. . . ." This passage may be interpreted to mean that a male nurse should not be assigned to care for a female client. If, however, only male nurses are available, this law would probably be waived because all laws are suspended in the case of severe illness. A law that addresses attendance of a male physician with a female client states that a physician is permitted to let blood and to feel the pulse or any other place of a woman, even if she is married, even the pudenda (external genital organs), as is customary with physicians, because he is merely following his profession (Ganzfried, 1963; Periara, 2015).

The nurse should be aware that since elderly Jewish clients in non-Jewish hospitals or nursing homes may adjust better with other Jews around them, it may be advantageous to have Jewish clients room together or at least be in proximity. This closeness will allow for increased comfort and offer the Jewish client the chance to interact with someone who "understands" him or her.

SOCIAL ORGANIZATION

The foundation of the Jewish culture is the nuclear family and the greater Jewish community. Controversy exists as to whether the Jewish community or the Jewish family has had the bigger influence on maintaining the Jewish faith and the Jews as a people (McDonald, 2001; Schneider, 1985).

Jewish families tend to be close-knit and child oriented (McDonald, 2001; Schlesinger, 1971). Jewish parents tend to "want better" for their children than they had themselves. It is not unusual to hear parents say that they have given up something they really wanted for the "sake of the children."

Family life of the Jewish Americans has changed through the years. The earlier Jewish family was male dominated, and the father made the major decisions. The mother's job was to care for the home, the children, and her husband. Today the delineation of duties is more obscure. Usually both parents work, often at jobs of equal financial and professional status.

The Jewish family structure is seen as protective. The Eastern European mother of the past got the reputation of being overbearing and overprotective. In the shtetls of Europe, the mother was the cohesive force in the home. This is still the case today, although younger women are not considered as overbearing or overprotective as their mothers and ancestors were.

In the Jewish family the child is seen as the means of maintaining Jewish existence. Therefore, education of the child in the Jewish faith and traditions is often seen as the most important thing a community, as well as the family, can do. In small Jewish communities, even communities too small for a rabbi, religious education of the children is seen as a priority. The fear of assimilation and annihilation increases the importance to the community of "sticking together" and educating the children.

Among the commandments that Jews are expected to follow are those that dictate the social relationships of family and community. These commandments dictate expected behavior toward parents and people within the community, such as the poor, teachers, rabbis, neighbors, ill people, the dying, and the dead.

Social orientation has helped maintain the Jewish people. When the Eastern European immigrants arrived in the United States, they were an embarrassment for the German Jews. However, commandments that control social behaviors dictated that the German Jews reach out to help the newcomers. This sense of kinship was so strong that Jews felt obliged to help one another, both in the United States and abroad. Today, this dictate is seen in the assistance offered Russian Jews, as well as other smaller groups of Jews from other countries, who immigrate to the United States.

Eastern European Jews brought with them a strong sense of community, which arose from their restricted lives within the shtetls. Furthermore, they were often held responsible for political events that occurred outside the Jewish quarters. Even though each Jew developed his or her own individuality, there was an intense feeling of "groupness," an identification with a common cultural heritage (Kolatch, 1985).

When the immigration laws of the 1920s resulted in decreased numbers of Eastern European Jews entering the United States, increased assimilation began to occur. Several significant events have helped slow the rate of Jewish American assimilation. The event that seems to have had the largest effect was the rise of Nazi anti-Semitism and its American counterparts. The Holocaust caused all Jews to realize that they were indeed brothers (Janowsky, 1964), and the memory of the Holocaust continues to have this effect on Jewish people. Other events that have had an effect on Jewish identification were related to the development of the state of Israel and the struggle of Israel to continue to exist despite a hostile environment. When Israel won the Six-Day War in 1967, the feeling of pride in the Jewish state was almost tangible. There seemed to be a stronger sense of "Jewishness" and an increased willingness to admit to being Jewish. Today, the tension in the Middle East continues to unite Jews.

Today, the Jewish American community is much more mobile than it was in the past. It is not unusual for the children to move away when they leave for college or marry. When a Jewish individual moves, often one of the first things he or she may look for is a Jewish affiliation. A Jew may not join a synagogue until the children are ready for religious school, but often he or she desires the company of other Jews despite the inability to join a synagogue until that time.

Implications for Nursing Care

When a Jewish person becomes ill, family and community resources are mobilized to assist the client. The Jewish faith contains a commandment to visit the sick. Therefore, friends, relatives, and neighbors will visit an ill Jewish client. If the client is very ill, the visitors will act as client advocates. It is important for the nurse to recognize the cultural implications of these visitors and to expect them to ask about the client.

Because of the protective attitudes of Jewish parents, they will often make arrangements to have someone with their child at all times if the child is hospitalized. Jewish parents may appear demanding and aggressive if they believe their child is not getting the care he or she "deserves." Handling the concerns of the parents may take patience on the part of the nurse. The nurse needs to remember that this cultural group highly prizes their children and sees the survival of the Jewish people as a responsibility of the next generation. This view places a large responsibility on the child to get well and on the parents to see that the child does get well.

TIME

The best way to classify Jewish people in relation to time orientation is to say that they are past, present, and future oriented. Jews are aware of their past—all 5000-plus years of it. They are also concerned about the present and are very involved with current social concerns, both Jewish and non-Jewish. One of the main precepts is *tikkun olam,* or repairing the world. They also look toward the future by insisting that their children be educated, religiously and secularly, and by participating in philanthropic activities to help the future of Israel.

The Jewish concern with the past is very obvious in American society, especially in relation to the Holocaust. Every Jewish person believes that this kind of atrocity should never happen again. By continuing to remind the world of the horrors that happened, not only to Jews but also to people of all faiths and ethnic origins, the Jewish people hope the world will never again let that type of event occur.

During happy occasions, such as a wedding, there is always something to remind Jews of their past. As an example, at the end of the wedding ceremony, the groom breaks a glass. One reason for this custom is to symbolize the destruction of the Jewish temple during the Roman invasion.

Past orientation is also seen following the death of a loved one (such as a parent, sibling, or spouse). On the anniversary of the death each year, a candle is lit and a prayer, the *kaddish* (meaning "holy"), is recited in honor of that person. In addition, the *kaddish* is recited at special times during the year for a loved one. In some congregations the *kaddish* is recited by the whole congregation in memory of those who have recently died or those who have no one to say the prayer for them. In relation to present-time orientation, Jews tend to be very social minded and are often involved in social movements. In many communities, Jewish congregations help run soup kitchens. In one southwestern city a rabbi was involved with the sanctuary movement.

From the Talmud comes the requirement that Jews care for all who are in need whether they are Jewish or non-Jewish. Because the concepts of charity and righteousness are so intertwined, the Hebrew word for "righteousness" (justice), *tzedaka,* has become the Hebrew word for "charity" (Kolatch, 1985). This concept has had an influence on the social system in New York City (Howe, 1989).

Another way that Jewish present-time orientation is apparent is in relation to an afterlife. Although Jews may believe that the spirit continues to live or reside with God after death, they are not concerned about an afterlife. What is considered important is doing good deeds on earth. During an interview regarding the belief in a soul, one woman summed up what has been written by other authors when she stated that it is the memory of one's good deeds that causes one to be immortalized (Schwartz, 1984).

Future-time orientation is apparent in issues concerning the education of children. Establishing schools, supporting schools, and furthering education are top priorities. Throughout the ages, education of the children in the Torah has been regarded as a duty. Originally it was the duty of the parents; eventually it became the duty of the community (Janowsky, 1964). Today, not only religious but also secular education is seen as important. In most Jewish households the children hear, from the time they are very young, that someday they will go to college. Education is highly prized as a way of securing the future for the child as well as for the Jewish community as a whole.

Another way that future-time orientation is apparent relates to concerns during illness. Jewish people not only want immediate relief but also worry about what the future implications of their illness will be. They worry about the effect of their illness on the future of their family members, their jobs, and their lives. According to Zborowski (1969), the intensity of their concern is greater than that of other Americans.

Many Jews tend to be punctual when it comes to appointments and become very upset when they arrive on time and have to wait for their appointment to begin. However, some Jewish people also talk about "Jewish standard time," which is at least 10 to 15 minutes later than regular time. Although there are many Jews who are very punctual (especially when it comes to appointments), general Jewish functions, such as weddings or bar mitzvahs, often begin late.

Implications for Nursing Care

Because Jewish people are past, present, and future oriented as well as emotionally expressive, they appear to feel joy, sorrow, illness, and so on with great intensity. They become very anxious when they do not feel well and may appear to be impatient about finding a cure. Jewish people have a tendency to worry about what the illness means in the present as well as the implications it has for the future.

Patience and honesty are necessary qualities for a nurse to display when dealing with Jewish clients. Demonstrating interest and concern will convey the message that the nurse cares about the ill person and may help decrease the amount of anxiety the client is feeling. Until a diagnosis is made, trying to help the anxious Jewish client put events into proper perspective may not work because the client reasons that the nurse cannot know what the future will hold if the physician does not know what is wrong.

It is important to understand that the high degree of outward anxiety the Jewish person may feel is probably more apparent in the older generation of Jews than in the younger generation because assimilation has caused them to exhibit more "acceptable" behavior patterns.

ENVIRONMENTAL CONTROL

Many Jewish people tend to be fatalistic about life. They may believe that they do have some control over their health, but God has the final say. This belief is apparent during Rosh Hashanah and Yom Kippur (the New Year and the Day of Atonement), when Jews pray to be written in the Book of Life for another year.

Health Care Beliefs

Jewish people have a religious requirement to maintain the health of the body as well as the soul. The origin of Jewish health care beliefs dates back to the Torah. Many of the 613 biblical commandments appear to be hygienic in intent. Several chapters in the Book of Leviticus (12–14), as well as other books in the Bible, are devoted to the control of disease (Kolatch, 1985; Washofsky, 2015). The Talmud continues to stress this concern for health. There are passages that deal with proper exercise, getting enough sleep, eating breakfast, and eating the proper diet.

Physicians are held in high esteem by people in the Jewish culture (Feldman, 1986; Washofsky, 2015). In biblical times the priests were physicians. When a Jewish person is ill, it is a duty to go to a physician, and it is the duty of the family to make sure the individual goes. The importance of health care is so great in this culture that Talmudic scholars stated that a person should not settle in a city without a physician (Feldman, 1986; Washofsky, 2015).

Some researchers contend that Jewish and Arab health locus of control discovered that Jewish people had a higher internal locus of health care control than Arab participants in the study (Cohen & Azaiza, 2007; Radwan, 2015). Jewish people believe physicians cannot heal without the participation of the client. They are also likely to question the physician if the client believes the physician is wrong about a diagnosis or treatment (Feldman, 1986; Radwan, 2015; Zborowski, 1969), and the Jewish client may decide not to follow the physician's orders. However, if the client chooses not to listen to the physician or does not agree with the physician, this individual is expected to seek the knowledge of another physician (Feldman, 1986; Radwan, 2015).

Seeking the best medical care, even obtaining a second opinion, is a religious dictate.

Health is one of the most frequent topics of conversation among Jewish people. With some Jewish people, especially older ones, good health is seen as an exception rather than the rule. The older individual may become preoccupied with the issue of good health because life may be viewed as a temporary lapse between one illness and another (Radwan, 2015; Zborowski, 1969).

The Jewish person believes that prevention of illness is important. Each family member tries to protect and warn the other members of dangers that may cause illnesses, which can make client teaching easier for the nurse. It is important to remember that client teaching in the Jewish family requires the cooperation of all the immediate family members.

There is an increased interest among Jewish adults in alternative or collaborative health care. It is not unusual to hear a group of Jews discussing the issues of fat content in food or the use of herbs to maintain health. In recent years, two healing centers that address prayer and healing have been developed in San Francisco and New York City. Healing services are held periodically in temples throughout the United States.

Illness Behaviors

When a member of a Jewish family is ill, the whole family suffers with the person. Each individual is expected to become a part of the process of helping the ill person feel better.

Complaining about discomforts is expected and accepted, especially in the older generation. Complaining fulfills several important functions: it gives relief through its cathartic function, it is a means of communication, it mobilizes the assistance of the environment, and it reaffirms family solidarity (Radwan, 2015; Zborowski, 1969).

When Jewish clients are admitted to the hospital, they may continue to behave as though they were at home. The Jewish client may attempt to mobilize the attention and sympathy of those in the new environment by using the same methods that worked in the home, so that what the nurse encounters may be a client who complains, cries, moans, and groans. When this behavior does not result in the reactions that would be received from the family, the client may attempt to temper reactions so that feelings of acceptance and being cared for are experienced.

If the client does not verbalize pain, another member of the family will usually do so. The reasoning is that the client may be too ill to tell the physician or nurse and that it is the family member's responsibility to communicate to obtain the attention the family member believes the loved one should have.

Zborowski's classic study (1969) of first-generation Jewish Americans in pain noted that these clients responded to questions with details that sometimes seemed to relate only marginally to the topic. In the study a simple question released a flow of responses that led to information about pain, illness, anxieties, intrafamily relationships, and so on. Probing was necessary to pinpoint specific information rather than to elicit a fuller answer to a question.

Second-, third-, and fourth-generation Jewish Americans seem to be a little less expressive about their pain. However, they do consider it wrong not to express their feelings. The expressive behavior of Jews seems to indicate that Jewish people believe that one cannot get help unless a complaint is made.

If oral complaining does not result in the type of behavior the client wishes to elicit from those around him or her, crying may be used. Crying, with many first-generation Jewish Americans, is acceptable behavior and is seen as an expression of frustration or pain and often results in the attention desired (Zborowski, 1969).

With increased American acculturation, each succeeding Jewish-American generation appears to be less expressive when in pain. The women may cry easily, but the men have adopted the American view that crying is not proper behavior for men. Second-generation Jewish American male clients tend to be less verbal about their pain than their fathers (Zborowski, 1969). For some Jewish people, however, the meaning of pain does not change, just the outward signs. For a Jewish person, pain, discomfort, and change in the state of good health are seen as a warning that something is wrong and that the professional health care system needs to be utilized.

Jews have been noted to have higher physician utilization rates than other groups, as well as having a heightened concern for maintaining health (Jacobs & Giarelli, 2001). Utilization of the health care system may involve getting the opinions of several physicians. The Jewish client recognizes that the physician is only another human, with the possibility of being incorrect. By getting at least one other opinion, the client can decide if the physician was correct or not. Before choosing the physician to see for a second opinion, the Jewish person will most likely ask a number of people who might have connections in the medical community for recommendations. Not only is a Jewish client likely to get a second or third opinion, but also this client may check the medical literature and search the Web for information about his or her condition and prescribed regimen. Schiller and Levine (1988) and Zborowski (1969) have noted that some of these activities seem to be based on a feeling that the client is the final judge and authority in matters pertaining to his or her health. In this case the physician is seen in the role of consultant and advisor.

Once the Jewish client accepts the physician's opinion, the client will also accept the prescribed treatment. The cultural belief is that to get well, one must cooperate with all therapeutic measures. Although the Jewish client will follow the prescribed regimen, the client expects the medication regimen to be individualized because illness is viewed as being individualized. Jewish patients today take a more active role in health care decisions.

In many cases, the client will want to know all about the prescribed treatment: what is expected of the client, what the side effects are, and, if a drug is being prescribed, the name of the drug. The client is unlikely to be content with, "It's good for you."

The Jewish client tends to observe carefully the effects of the drug or treatment on the system. Since many Jews believe that they are the ultimate judge of their condition, they may change the time they take a drug, increase or decrease the number of drugs taken, or reject the drug completely if they decide it is not helping or is harmful. Many times these decisions are made without consulting the physician. Careful, thorough explanations about the drug, its purpose, side effects, and why it was ordered are essential.

The future-oriented Jewish client may become hesitant to take analgesics because most drugs are viewed as "dope" and Jewish persons often fear addiction. This fear increases the problem for the client in pain who wants to receive pain relief but is afraid of addiction (Zborowski, 1969).

Wellness Behaviors

Jewish-American people tend to be more educated than most other American ethnic groups (Sowell, 1981), and the thirst for knowledge is apparent in their wellness behaviors. They tend to be well read on issues of health, and it is not unusual to hear Jews discussing the latest information on maintaining healthy diets, preventing disease, or following health-oriented regimens.

In years past, it was rare to see Jewish children involved in physical activities. Eastern European Jews tended to de-emphasize physical activity in favor of more intellectual activities that kept the children closer to home. This practice may have stemmed from the fears of child abduction that they brought with them from the "old country" (Sowell, 1981). However, this trend seems to be changing. Jewish children are now involved with soccer teams, baseball teams, and other physical activities. Their parents are also more involved in physical exercise. Jogging, tennis, racquetball, and aerobics are some of the activities that are attracting more Jewish participants as the importance of physical exercise is discussed in the media.

Maintaining certain laws is included in the wellness behaviors seen in Orthodox Jewish people. Many of these laws have been incorporated into the everyday habits of most Jewish Americans because they are good hygiene or they have been proved to be medically prudent. The following are examples of these laws taken from the Code of Jewish Law (Ganzfried, 1963):

1. The hands must be washed on awakening from sleep, after elimination of bodily wastes, after hair cutting, after touching a vermin, and after being in proximity to a dead human body.
2. The proper way of washing oneself is to take a bath regularly every week.
3. It is advisable for one to accustom himself to having breakfast in the morning.
4. One is forbidden to eat or drink out of unclean vessels, and the individual should not eat with hands that are not clean.

There is a belief, although there is no empirical evidence to support it, that the custom requiring washing hands before meals has contributed to lower morbidity and mortality rates. Plus, because of better hygiene, infant and child mortality rates have been lower in Jewish than in non-Jewish populations (Jacobs & Giarelli, 2001).

Kosher Diet, Religious Holidays, and Illness. Maintaining a kosher (*kasher*, "fit, proper") diet may pose a problem for some Jewish clients. As mentioned in Chapter 7, kosher meat is usually salted to help drain all the blood. This process presents a problem for a client on a low-salt diet unless the meat is soaked in water to remove as much of the salt as possible.

It is important for the nurse to consider what can be done for the Jewish client following a kosher diet if the hospital does not have a kosher supplier nearby. In this case it is possible to serve any fish that meets the dietary requirements of having fins and scales. It is also possible to serve dairy products as long as they are not contraindicated on the person's diet. These meals should be served on paper plates with plastic utensils because meat and milk products or dishes prepared with milk products should not be mixed.

If, because of medical dietary restrictions and the unavailability of kosher food, maintaining a kosher diet is impossible, the client must decide to waive the dietary restrictions. All commandments are suspended whenever a life is in danger, no matter how remote the likelihood of death (Feldman, 1986). Food is essential to maintain life; therefore, the client would be directed by the rabbi to eat whatever the hospital could provide that would help sustain life.

Yom Kippur (the Day of Atonement) and Passover (based on Hebrew *pesah*, "passing over") are two holidays that require special consideration. On Yom Kippur, Jewish people are required to fast for 24 hours. If this fast is considered physically or medically dangerous, however, the individual is required by law to put aside the law and eat. Passover requires that special foods be served. Passover, which falls in or near the spring of the year, is an 8-day holiday that celebrates the freedom of the Jews from Egypt. During these 8 days, certain foods must be "kosher for Passover" (*kasher le-pesah*). In addition, there are other foods that are forbidden, including any foods with leavening (bread, cakes made with baking soda or baking powder) or foods made with even a small amount of a grain product or by-product that is not specifically prepared for Passover. This prohibition includes many drugs and medications, such as those containing starch or grain alcohol. These drugs may be refused by the client unless they cannot be replaced and are urgently needed by the client.

Procreation

The use or nonuse of contraceptives is dictated by Jewish law, which requires one to "be fruitful and multiply." This can cause special problems for the woman who is unable to conceive or the woman who may have physical problems, making conception dangerous. There is a lengthy discussion of this issue in the *Mishnah* (a part of the Talmud containing the oral law). The final analysis is that the man is commanded to procreate, but the woman is not, because, it is believed, God would not impose on the "children of Israel" a burden "too difficult for a person to bear" (Gold, 1988). Since childbirth is painful and may be physically dangerous, it would be unfair for the Torah to impose the commandment for procreation on the woman.

When Jewish men were allowed two wives, this commandment was not a problem. Today, because monogamy is the rule in the Jewish community, procreation is seen as the couple's obligation. However, outside of the very Orthodox community, Jewish couples today decide on how many children they want, and most practice some form of birth control. Within the very Orthodox community, the use of birth control is discouraged unless pregnancy or delivery would be dangerous for the woman.

Couples who have a problem with fertility are encouraged to seek medical help. For the very Orthodox Jewish man, however, a problem arises in the collection of semen. Rabbis have declared that masturbation and the use of male contraceptives such as condoms are not permitted because the Talmud outlaws the spilling of seed. For this reason, the woman is usually tested first, and then, if no problem can be detected, the man may be tested. The very Orthodox Jewish husband will have to consult his rabbi before he consents to a sperm count. Since masturbation is considered taboo, it may be emotionally difficult for the man to collect his semen. This is not a problem for most non-Orthodox couples.

It is interesting to note that the role of companionship is given an equal place with procreation in the purpose of a Jewish marriage (Gold, 1988). To add to this idea of companionship, rabbis have also addressed the idea of sexual satisfaction being the right of both men and women within the bonds of marriage (Lutwak et al., 1988).

Organ Transplants

According to Jewish law, all body parts should be buried with the body after death (Jakobovits, 1975; Silberberg, 2015). However, if an organ transplant would save the life of another human being, it is permissible to donate the organ (Feldman, 1986; Silberberg, 2015). Even removal of the heart for transplantation is allowed so long as the dying person has experienced total brain death (Feldman, 1986; Kolatch, 1985).

Life-Support Measures

According to Jewish law, nothing may be done to hasten death; a client must be given every chance for life. However, if the use of mechanical systems would delay death rather than prolong life, they should not be used. If mechanical systems have been connected and they are not helping to prolong life but are delaying death, they may be removed (Feldman, 1986; Goffe, 2011).

The Dying Jewish Client

As there are commandments that control living for the Jew, there are also commandments that control dying. These commandments are usually followed strictly only by Orthodox Jews, but some of the behaviors that the nurse may see in other Jews are a result of the cultural knowledge that these commandments have created.

According to Jewish law, a person who is very ill and considered to be dying should not be left alone. One reason for this law is that the spirit is believed to depart from the body at the time of death, and if no one were present, the soul would feel alone and desolate (End of Life, n.d.; Some Modern Views, n.d.; Sperling, 1968). To satisfy this commandment, family members will often take turns sitting with the critically or terminally ill client. Asking family members to leave may cause family distress.

Jewish law also dictates that a client should be informed that death is near. However, because of two controversial passages in the Torah, some rabbis believe it is important to inform a dying individual about serious illness but not that death is near. Informing a person about a serious illness allows the individual time to put worldly affairs in order, as Isaac and Jacob did when they were told they would die (End of Life, n.d.; Heller, 1986; Some Modern

Views, n.d.). However, to tell a person that death is imminent removes all hope, and some Jewish people fear that this information may hasten death.

Judaism teaches that it is important to lead a good, decent, and helping life on earth. Since good deeds must be done on earth, the law requires a Jew to ask God to forgive those deeds that may have been against God or not in keeping with God's commandments. To fulfill this commandment, the dying person is encouraged to recite the confessional. If the individual is too sick to say the whole confessional, the individual is encouraged to recite the affirmation of faith, the *Shma*. If the dying person cannot repeat any of the confessional, the law says that it is up to the family or friends who are with the person to recite it. The recitation of the confessional is usually seen only with observant Jews.

Once death has been established, the eyes and mouth are closed by the son or nearest relative. In some Orthodox Jewish families, it is customary to remove the body from the bed and place it on a straw mat on the floor, with the person's feet toward the door through which the body will be taken. A candle is placed at the person's head to symbolize the "light," or joy and love the departed brought to others while alive (End of Life, n.d.; Some Modern Views, n.d.; Trepp, 1980). A sheet is placed over the person's face because it is disrespectful to the dead to permit others to see the ravages of death on the face (Sperling, 1968; Staff, 2015). The dead body is viewed as being contaminated by Orthodox Jews and is placed on the floor because the bed is viewed as being defiled by contact with the dead body; however, the ground is not considered defiled by contact (Sperling, 1968; Staff, 2015). It is important to understand that this behavior is rarely seen in most hospitals or nursing homes today.

Autopsy is not allowed by Orthodox Jews unless (1) it is required by governmental regulations, (2) the person had a hereditary disease and an autopsy may help safeguard the health of survivors, or (3) another known person is suffering from a similar deadly disease and an autopsy may yield information vital to that person's health (Jakobovits, 1975; Staff, 2015). If an autopsy is performed, all parts that are removed must be buried with the body. Autopsy does not pose a religious problem for the non-Orthodox Jew.

AIDS

It has been stated that acquired immunodeficiency syndrome (AIDS) "will cause psychological and social reactions that may change the character of human social life" (Edelheit, 1989; Farbiarz, 2010). In the Jewish community, AIDS poses a psychological, social, and religious problem. The problem lies in the traditional belief system of the

Jewish people: according to the Torah, homosexuality is an abomination, and premarital sexual activity is not permitted by the traditional rabbinate. This belief system is a potential cause of distress for Jewish homosexuals, or for any Jews who test positive for human immunodeficiency virus. They have to live not only with their disease but also with being an outcast of their culture.

Patient education in an Orthodox Jewish environment may be very difficult, and rabbis in all the religious groups are still trying to decide how to handle this situation. Some of them are addressing it and trying to teach about the disease and safe sex. It appears that Orthodox rabbis are handling the issue of "safe sex" by going to the law that states that methods to destroy or block the passage of the seed are not permitted. Rabbi Yonassan Gershom (personal communication, 1998) noted that the issue of safe sex should not be a problem for Orthodox Jews because sex outside of marriage is not permitted. When asked about issues of finger sticks or blood transfusions, Rabbi Gershom responded that each case would be considered on an individual basis. Homosexuality among Reform Jewish rabbis is recognized and accepted. There are Reform synagogues that have predominantly homosexual congregations. In 1997, the Reform Jewish movement agreed to ordain openly homosexual Jewish rabbis.

AIDS and the Jewish client is an area requiring great sensitivity for the nurse. The most important thing that the nurse can do for the Jewish AIDS client is to be there for support. These clients need to deal not only with a terminal illness and rejection by the general society but also with possible cultural and religious ostracism.

Circumcision

According to Jewish teaching, God made a covenant with Abraham in which God promised to bless Abraham and make him prosper if Abraham would be loyal to God. This covenant was entered into and sealed by the act of circumcision. Jewish people honor this covenant by having a *brit* (which means "sign of the Covenant," *bĕ rith*) on the eighth day of the baby's life. If the child is ill or was born prematurely, the *brit* is postponed until the infant is in good health. The circumcision is usually done by a *mohel*, who is trained to do circumcisions. This is a time of celebration, and usually the entire family and friends gather at the home of the baby's parents for this important occasion. Since the circumcision is performed in the home, the nurse should review the principles of circumcision care with the mother before discharge. The postcircumcision care is usually managed by the *mohel*. L'Archevesque and Goldstein-Lohman (1996) noted the importance of offering parents information about the different methods of circumcision, types of pain-control measures, and symptoms of possible complications. Parents should be educated about the expected amount of bloody staining and what would be excessive bleeding, as well as signs and symptoms of infection.

Implications for Nursing Care

Caring for Jewish clients may be viewed as difficult by the nurse. Jewish clients tend to be vocal about feelings, anxieties, and pain, but they may not be direct about what is bothering them. This type of verbalization can be difficult for health care providers who expect the client to be compliant, noncomplaining, and direct about needs. Nurses with judgmental attitudes may label the Jewish client as childish, which leads to treating the client as a child or ignoring the client as much as possible. It is important for the nurse to remember that for the Jewish client, this behavior may be part of the culture. The nurse must be patient and let the client know that the nurse cares about needs because this will lead to feelings of trust and may decrease what is seen as demanding behavior.

Demanding behavior is less likely to occur in second-, third-, or fourth-generation Jewish Americans, who are more aware of what is considered acceptable behavior by the general American culture. This awareness does not mean that they feel pain or anxieties any less.

Illness is often viewed by Jews as a family affair. Because the whole family is involved with the ill person's suffering, the whole family wants to know what is happening with or to the client. The family members often do not appear to trust the word of another family member and instead want to get the information directly from the physician or the nurse. To assist the family and decrease the amount of time numerous explanations may take, it may help to have a family conference. However, not all the members may show up at the same time, and the nurse may need to repeat the information. The most important message to convey to the family of a Jewish client is that of caring, not only about the client but also about each family member and the pain they are going through.

Assisting the client who is dying, as well as the family, requires knowledge of Jewish cultural practices and beliefs. The nurse needs to remain sensitive to the need for a confessional if death is imminent and the client is Orthodox. Studies have shown that following cultural practices helps decrease the amount of distress and disorganization felt by loved ones during the death and dying period (Dempsey, 1977; Ross, 1981). Therefore, it is the duty of the nurse to assist families in following customs related to death and dying. When an Orthodox Jew dies, the body must not be touched by a person of the opposite sex. One nurse recounted the story of a young Chassidic boy who died and was washed by the nurses on the floor before the father arrived. The father became so upset that a female had touched his son's body that he told the nurses not to touch him, left the hospital, and returned a few minutes later with some dirt and a bag. He covered the boy's body with the dirt, put him in the bag, and carried him out of the hospital. He did this because the body was considered contaminated. When an Orthodox patient dies, all clothing and dressing material with the patient's blood on it must be left with the patient (Sommer, 1995).

Jewish people are interested in illness prevention and may ask in-depth questions to clarify what is being said. They may ask many questions to weigh information for personal effect, and these questions should not be misconstrued to indicate mistrust of the health care professional.

When caring for a Jewish client, it is helpful for the nurse to know what form of religious practice is adhered to because the Orthodox Jewish client will follow religious practices more strictly than any other group. Unless the nurse works in an area that has a large number of Orthodox Jews, most Jewish clients cared for will be non-Orthodox and may not be affiliated with any group.

BIOLOGICAL VARIATIONS

Some people believe that a Jewish person can be recognized by physical appearance, and the "Semitic appearance" is occasionally related to cultural patterns (Goodman, 1979; Weiss, 2013). However, Jews differ greatly in physical appearance, depending on what part of the world they migrated to when forced out of Israel. Jews are not uniformly the same as far as height, hair and eye color, body structure, or shape of the nose is concerned. European Jews are White, Falashas (Ethiopian Jews) are Black, and Chinese Jews have Asian features. The differences among Jews from different parts of the world are the results of biological adaptation to the area of the world resided in, intermarriage with non-Jews, and conversion to Judaism (Goodman, 1979; Mourant, Kopec, & Domaniewsks-Sobczak, 1978; Weiss, 2013).

For determination of the extent of genetic similarity among Jews as opposed to non-Jews, studies of blood phenotypes have been done (Goodman, 1979; Mourant et al., 1978). As opposed to outward appearances, blood characteristics are unaffected by the environment.

Enzymatic and Genetic Variations

Although skin color, body size, and body structure vary, depending on the part of the world resided in, fingerprint patterns indicate a relatedness among Jews from Germany, Turkey, Morocco, and Yemen. The patterns of fingerprint whorls, loops, and arches are similar to those of non-Jews living in the Mediterranean area. This seems to indicate that the Jewish people, although appearing to be diversified genetically, still maintain a remnant of the Mediterranean gene pool.

To classify genetic differences of peoples, polymorphic blood groups, serum and cell proteins, and enzyme variants that have altered catalytic activity, kinetic properties, stability, or electrophoretic mobility are used. Since anthropological structures and simple genetic traits of Jews are difficult to define, Jewish genetic studies have concentrated on the genetic polymorphisms (Bray et al., 2010; Rothschild & Chapman, 1981). Data from these studies have concluded that (1) Jewish groups from different parts of the world are very different genetically, (2) Jews of a certain area tend to resemble the surrounding non-Jews more than they resemble Jews from other parts of the world, and (3) European Jews have a residue of non-European genes that resemble Mediterranean genes (Bray et al., 2010; Patai & Wing, 1989).

A classic study by Stevenson, Schanfield, and Sandler (1985) on immunoglobulin allotypes had interesting results. The multivariate analyses indicated that the Jewish populations may be derived from a common gene pool. When the results were plotted, all the Jews, except the Yemenite group, were genetically similar to each other. The European Jewish cluster is the most closely knit in similarity, and the Asian and North African Jewish clusters are closer to Middle Eastern groups than to European non-Jews.

In relation to genetic disorders, the Jewish population is divided into Sephardic Jews, Asian Jews, and Ashkenazi Jews. Since the largest number of Jews in the United States are Ashkenazi Jews (European), the rest of this discussion involves genetic disorders most prevalent in this group.

Of all the genetic disorders that occur most frequently in Eastern European Jews, the one receiving the most publicity is Tay-Sachs disease. This disease is recessively inherited and is characterized by the absence of an enzyme involved in fat metabolism, resulting in the accumulation of fatty substances in the brain and leading to gradual neural and mental degeneration, with death occurring around 3 or 4 years of age. Couples in which both partners are Jews of Eastern European descent should be counseled to have genetic screening done to prevent the possibility of having a child with this deadly disease.

In January 2001, the genetic mutation for another disorder common to Ashkenazi Jews was discovered (Jaffe-Gill, 2002; Jorde, Carey, Bamshad, & White, 2010; National Library of Medicine, 2015). This disorder, familial dysautonomia, is a deadly disease affecting children and often causing death before the age of 30. It is characterized by pain; wild fluctuations in blood pressure and body tem-

perature; and impaired chewing, swallowing, and digestion.

Although Gaucher disease is rare, it has a frequency of about 1 in 500 in Ashkenazi Jews (Mamopoulos, Hughes, Tuck, & Mehta, 2009; National Library of Medicine, 2015). The most common allele attributable to Gaucher disease is thought to be produced by an A to G mutation resulting in a single amino acid substitution (Jorde et al., 2010; National Library of Medicine, 2015). Gaucher disease is characterized by enlarged visceral organs, multiorgan failure, and a debilitating skeletal disease. The DNA tests available today are capable of detecting 97% of the mutations among the five most common Gaucher alleles in the Ashkenazi Jewish population (Jorde et al., 2010; Mamopoulos et al., 2009; National Library of Medicine, 2015).

Glucose-6-PD (G-6-PD) deficiency has been linked to severe jaundice that leads to kernicterus or even death in newborns (Kaplan et al., 1997; National Library of Medicine, 2015). Kaplan et al. (1997) conducted a classic study to determine whether the TA repeat promoter in the gene for uridinediphosphoglucuronate glucuronosyltransferase (EC1.1.1.49; UDPGT1) was associated with benign jaundice noted in adults (Gilbert syndrome) or to determine if this mutation could increase the incidence of neonatal hyperbilirubinemia in G-6-PD deficiency. Findings from this study suggested that neither G-6-PD deficiency nor the variant UDPGT1 promoter, by themselves, increased the incidence of hyperbilirubinemia. Findings from this study, however, suggested that UDPGT1 promoter, when coupled with G-6-PD deficiency, did ultimately increase the incidence of hyperbilirubinemia (Kaplan et al., 1997; National Library of Medicine, 2015).

Susceptibility to Disease

Susceptibility to disease for Jewish people depends on geographical origin. Some beliefs about Jewish susceptibility have no real scientific basis, such as the belief that Jews are more likely than others to have diabetes mellitus. Some studies have shown that Jews are no more susceptible to this disease than non-Jews from the same area of the world, as had been originally believed (Goodman, 1979).

Cancer. Certain cancers are more frequent in certain groups of Jews than in others. Stomach cancer is more prevalent among Jews from Europe and the United States. Colon and prostate cancer is prevalent in Jews of Eastern European descent. Breast cancer, the most frequent type of cancer for all Jewish female groups except those from Iran (Brandt-Rauf, Raveis, Drummond, Conte, & Rothman, 2006; Patai & Wing, 1989), has been found to be more common in Jewish women from Europe and the United

States than in those from Asia. Cancer of the ovary is generally higher in Jews from Europe than in those from Asia or Africa. Brandt-Rauf et al. (2006) and Darwish et al. (2002) conducted a study on subjects residing in the same geographical location. The primary purpose of the study was to evaluate and compare differences in molecular genetics among high-risk (Ashkenazi), intermediate-risk (Sephardic), and low-risk (Palestinian) people for colorectal cancer. Findings from this study suggested that Ashkenazi Jews have the highest rate of colorectal cancer and are generally diagnosed earlier than Sephardic Jews.

Studies indicate that 1% to 2% of American Ashkenazi Jewish women have a high incidence of specific mutations of *BRCA1* and *BRCA2* (Brandt-Rauf et al., 2006; Gene mutation, 1995; Jacobs & Giarelli, 2001). These changes have been associated with an increase in ovarian cancer and with a higher risk in breast cancer. A specific alteration (185delAG) appears to be found in Ashkenazi Jews and is considered to be ethnic specific (Brandt-Rauf et al., 2006; Key, 1997). While the *BRCA1* and *BRCA2* founder mutations have been clearly delineated among Ashkenazi Jewish women, this knowledge alone has not led to increased testing among this vulnerable population (Brandt-Rauf et al., 2006; Schwartz et al., 2002). Schwartz et al. (2002) conducted a study to determine whether a brief educational booklet regarding *BRCA1* and *BRCA2* could influence knowledge and attitudes and generate interest in testing among Ashkenazi women. Findings from this study suggested that, relative to breast cancer education, the genetic testing materials did lead to increased knowledge among these women, increased the perceptions of the risks and the limitations of the testing, and yet decreased the interest of these women in obtaining a *BRCA1/BRCA2* mutation test. Nonetheless, these researchers concluded that educational print material is an innovative way to educate high-risk individuals about *BRCA1/BRCA2* genetic testing (Schwartz et al., 2002).

Historically, rates of cancer of the cervix have been lower in Jewish women than in non-Jews (Brandt-Rauf et al., 2006; Patai & Wing, 1989). However, as Jews become more acculturated and the incidence of multiple sexual partners, as well as partners who are not circumcised, increases, so does the incidence of cervical cancer. Cervical cancer is an area of concern for some Jewish individuals and an area where client teaching is helpful.

HPC1/RNASEL was identified as a candidate gene for hereditary prostate cancer (Rennert et al., 2002). Rennert and associates (2002) identified a novel founder frameshift mutation *RNASEL*, 47delAAAG, in Ashkenazi Jews. In fact, when these researchers estimated the mutation frequency in this Ashkenazi population, they were able to determine that the frequency among 159 healthy young males was 4%

(95% confidence interval). However, among Ashkenazi Jews, the mutation frequency was significantly higher in subjects with prostate cancer as compared with a control group consisting of elderly males. It was interesting to note that 47delAAAG was not detected in 134 non-Ashkenazi subjects with prostate cancer. Findings from this study also suggest that the 47delAAAG null mutation is associated with prostate cancer in Ashkenazi Jewish men (Rennert et al., 2002).

Heart Disease. Data from a classic 1952 study of serum cholesterol levels in New York indicated a higher frequency of elevated serum cholesterol levels among Jews than among non-Jews. It is believed that elevated serum cholesterol levels may be caused by a single gene (Patai & Wing, 1989; Weisglass-Volkov & Pajukanta, 2010). If this is true, Ashkenazi Jews may have a higher frequency of the gene than Asian Jews, who seem to have a relatively low rate of elevated serum cholesterol levels.

It is commonly believed that Ashkenazi Jews are more prone to coronary disease than other Jewish ethnic groups or non-Jews are. In international comparisons of the rate of first-time myocardial infarctions among men, Israel ranks among the highest in the world if all types of infarcts (including clinically unrecognized infarcts) are included (Mourant et al., 1978). Although there is a relatively high incidence of infarcts in Israel, there is a low mortality rate. After numerous studies, the conclusion regarding heart disease in the Jewish population is that further studies need to be done to determine the frequency of the disease among Jews as well as the interplay between heredity and environment (Mourant et al., 1978).

Polycythemia Vera. Evidence indicates that polycythemia vera is more common in Ashkenazi Jews than in other ethnic groups (Prchal & Samuelson, 2009). In addition, there seems to be a higher prevalence of polycythemia vera in Jewish men than in Jewish women (Mourant et al., 1978).

Diabetes Mellitus. Diabetes has been referred to as the "Jewish disease" in Germany. Through ethnic Jewish studies done in Israel, an interesting phenomenon has been noted. A slightly higher percentage of Ashkenazi Jews than Sephardic Jews have diabetes. Also, in Yemenite and Kurdish newcomers to Israel, there are almost no cases of diabetes. However, in Yemenite and Kurdish settlers who have lived in Israel for more than 25 years, the same frequency of diabetes as with Ashkenazi Jews has been identified (Mourant et al., 1978; Patai & Wing, 1989). The results of this study indicate that dietary habits have an influence on the development of diabetes. The main dietary change in the older settlers as compared with the new arrivals has been an increased intake of sugar.

Although the incidence of diabetes in Jewish people has been indicated as being higher than in the general population, there has been no study to confirm this belief. Most of the studies on diabetes among Jews have been done in Israel. For a truer assessment of the prevalence of diabetes in the Jewish community, further studies outside Israel need to be conducted (Mourant et al., 1978).

Crohn's Disease. Studies indicate that Crohn's disease occurs in Jewish males more often than in Jewish females and in Jews more often than in any other White ethnic group (Mourant et al., 1978). Although the number of young people diagnosed as having this disease has been increased (Thompson, McFarland, Hirsch, et al., 1989), it is unknown if the increase is a result of a better awareness of the disease and improved diagnostic techniques or if there is an actual increase in the number of cases.

Ulcerative Colitis. Ulcerative colitis is seen more frequently in Ashkenazi Jews than in non-Jews or in any other Jewish ethnic groups. It has many similarities to Crohn's disease and may even be seen with Crohn's disease. The cause of ulcerative colitis is unknown, but familial tendencies have been noted; it occurs 10% to 15% more often in families of clients with ulcerative colitis than in families of control clients without the disease (Mourant et al., 1978).

Myopia. Jews seem to have a higher incidence of myopia than the general population, and it occurs more often in boys than in girls. It is important to understand that myopia is not caused by close bookwork, as was believed many years ago, but by a prevalence of low hypermetropia and factors that allow for a greater or longer development of the length of the eye. Vision screening is an important part of a physical examination for Jewish people, particularly Jewish children.

Nutritional Preferences and Deficiencies

Jewish people tend to eat a lot of dairy products, which becomes a concern in patients with a history of lactose intolerance. Lactose intolerance has been identified among some Jewish ethnic groups, and a study done in Israel identified approximately two thirds of the Jewish population in Israel as being lactase deficient. However, the researchers also noted that most of these clients were not aware of their milk intolerance, leading to the conclusion that the condition was relatively benign and asymptomatic in the Jews studied (Mourant et al., 1978). Any Jewish client with a history of diarrhea, nonspecific lower gastrointestinal symptoms, and abdominal pain should have a good dietary history taken to check for a history of milk intolerance. The nurse needs to determine any family tendency toward lactose intolerance, as well as the relationship between foods and the onset of abdominal symptoms.

It is important for the nurse to remember that not all Jews maintain a kosher diet and that some Jews are stricter about their diet than others. If the nurse is caring for an Orthodox Jewish client who is not eating properly because of the conflict between maintaining a kosher diet and eating institutional food, the nurse should consult with the family about bringing food from home. If the family cannot help with this situation, the client's rabbi may be consulted.

Psychological Characteristics

Jews have been labeled with certain personality traits for over 3000 years. According to the Bible, the Children of Israel, following their exodus from Egypt, were "stiff necked," quarrelsome, disobedient, and rebellious. In Talmudic literature the Jews are described as the "merciful sons of a merciful father." Greek and Roman authors, who were usually anti-Semitic, made derogatory comments on the Jewish character.

It was not until the 1930s that studies began to explore Jewish personality characteristics (Patai & Wing, 1989). All these studies involved Jewish Americans, and most involved college students. The conclusions derived from these studies are as follows (Patai & Wing, 1989):

1. Studies indicate that Jews are superior in intelligence to comparable groups of non-Jews, especially in verbal intelligence. It is questionable whether Jews are genetically more intelligent than non-Jews; the apparent superiority in intelligence may be attributable to the pressures from the Gentile world for Jews to rely on their brains in order to survive.

2. In scholarly, intellectual, literary, and artistic pursuits, Jews seem to be proportionately overrepresented. Whether this phenomenon is proof of special Jewish talent or the result of extraneous circumstances that attracted Jews to concentrate on certain areas is open for debate.

3. As far as character traits are concerned, it is difficult to pinpoint differences between Jews and non-Jews. Character traits seem to be formed more by personal experiences in the immediate environment than by historical conditioning. As an example, Jewish Americans have been characterized as being aggressive, and this aggressiveness may be attributable to the pressure placed on Jewish children by their parents to "have a better life" than they did.

Anti-Semitism is a concern for Jewish people. Within the Jewish community, mention is often made of Jewish fear in regard to anti-Semitism. Although the relative freedom experienced in the United States has led to a decrease in the practice of many Jewish rituals and possibly to the increased numbers of nonpracticing Jews, there are constant reminders that Jews are different and not always accepted by the general public. Today, in addition to constant reminders of the Holocaust, some Jewish people are also concerned about events in Israel.

Mental Health. The older medical literature indicates that the rate of occurrence of a variety of mental illnesses in Jews is high. In discussing this issue with numerous psychiatrists and leaders in the mental health field, Mourant et al. (1978) concluded at that time that necessary data are lacking to confirm that the old medical literature is correct.

One concern among psychiatrists and mental health workers in Orthodox Jewish sections is the apparent need for but lack of use of mental health facilities. To determine what discourages Orthodox Jews from seeking psychiatric professional help, a study was conducted with 20 Orthodox Jewish mental health outpatients; it revealed that Orthodox Jews attach a stigma to mental health treatment and to Jews who avail themselves of it. This stigma is partly the result of an association of mental health treatment with insanity and partly because of the fear that this knowledge will have a negative effect on matrimonial prospects (Wikler, 1986).

It is important for the nurse to remember that Orthodox Jews do not enter mental health treatment easily. In the case of an Orthodox Jew who may need psychiatric counseling, there may be resistance to overcome before treatment can be started. The prospective client may display a real concern about confidentiality that may be seen as paranoia. This paranoia needs to be understood within the context of the social risk involved.

Orthodox Jews who do seek mental health care usually choose the agency or therapist based on reputation. One agency that opened its office in the Williamsburg section of Brooklyn, New York, in the heart of the Chassidic and Orthodox Jewish sections, was picketed and threatened. Today, however, this center has earned the "grudging" respect of the community (Meer, 1987).

Alcoholism. The literature reports that Jews have had a low incidence of alcoholism in the past (Mourant et al., 1978). This assumption is questionable, and the incidence of cross-addiction, to both alcohol and another substance, may be higher among Jews than among non-Jews (Steinhardt, 1988). Lieberman (1987) has noted that Jews do not acknowledge a problem with alcohol because of their perception of what an alcoholic is. Many Jews view the alcoholic as a skid row bum, not a person who gets drunk and acts silly at a wedding or maybe drinks too much when celebrating a holiday or festival, even if this behavior occurs on a regular basis.

All the behaviors that characterize the alcoholic in general—denial, isolation, ignorance of the disease, and guilt—seem to be intensified in the Jewish alcoholic because of the myth of Jewish sobriety. Orthodox Jews seem to suffer the greatest from these symptoms (Steinhardt, 1988).

Studies done in the United States indicate that drinking disorders tend to increase in Jews as religious affiliation shifts from Orthodox, to Conservative, to Reform, to secular (Mourant et al., 1978). Some sociologists have suggested that alcoholism among Jews may increase as acculturation increases.

Of greatest concern to the Jewish community and to health care workers is the increasing alcohol and drug abuse among Jewish youth. It is important to educate the Jewish community on the facts that alcoholics are not just skid row, homeless people and that the ceremonial and social drinking of the Jewish community can increase the potential for alcoholism if it is not tempered.

Holocaust Survivors. Although the Holocaust has had a profound effect on Jewish feelings regarding "Jewishness" and persecution, the Holocaust survivors have had very little effect on the Jewish culture in the United States as a whole. The reason for this is that a relatively small number of Jewish Americans are Holocaust survivors. According to the Jewish Federation of North America (Ain, 2003), half the American survivors of the Holocaust (55,000 people) live in New York. Many studies have been done on the effects of the Holocaust on survivors (Kren & Rappoport, 1980; Rose & Garske, 1987). These studies have helped the medical profession, especially the psychiatric medical profession, to determine the effects of war atrocities on survivors.

Since the 1990s, there has been an increase in studies of adults who are child survivors of the Holocaust. The studies indicate that child survivors show an increased level of post-traumatic symptomatology; see the world as more negative, although more controllable and meaningful; and have a high vulnerability to stress (Cohen, Brom, & Dasberg, 2001). Although many of these studies were done in Israel, it is expected that all child Holocaust survivors will have similar symptoms.

Many Jews have a difficult time discussing the effects of the Holocaust and its devastation on Jewish families and communities. Jewish individuals sometimes leave the room when the Holocaust is mentioned or joke to relieve their distress or feelings of anger and bewilderment at how this type of event could occur in modern times in a country that was supposed to be "civilized."

The effects of the Holocaust on the survivors and their children are still being studied. From the literature comes evidence of anger, depression, withdrawal, and anxiety in the survivors (Krystal & Niederland, 1971; Steinitz & Szonyi, 1979). Bearing children was seen as a means for the survivors to replace their loved ones who were lost during "the War," and the children were seen as a source of new hope and meaning. Because of this transference, the children of the survivors were usually overprotected and had unrealistic expectations placed on them (Nadler, Kav-Venaki, & Gleitman, 1985).

Numerous studies have been done on children of Holocaust survivors. The results of these studies indicate that, on the whole, this population is well adjusted, with few significant psychopathological problems (Nadler et al., 1985; Rose & Garske, 1987; Steinitz & Szonyi, 1979). The biggest problems for these children seem to be related to the pressures they feel to protect their parents from any further physical or psychological pain and the desire to fulfill their parents' unrealistic need to have the child compensate for what has been lost. These pressures lead to feelings of guilt when the children attempt to become emancipated from their parents.

Personality characteristics that most studies have discovered in Holocaust survivors are repressed anger, feelings of guilt, depression, fears of abandonment, worries of personal injury, feelings of being different, strong feelings of Jewishness (even if they are nonpracticing Jews), concern for Jewish survival (often more intense than in non–Holocaust survivors), and desires to maintain Jewish traditions that may border on obsession (Nadler et al., 1985; Rose & Garske, 1987; Sorscher, 1994; Steinitz & Szonyi, 1979). Daughters of survivors have been found to be more susceptible to Holocaust-related symptoms than sons, and daughters whose parents did not talk about their experience had more problems than those whose parents talked about the experience (Sorscher, 1994).

Some Jewish people believe that it is important that the memory of the Holocaust never die and that no event like this should ever happen again. These same people believe there should never be mass destruction of any people. Perhaps protecting the memory of the Holocaust is one plausible explanation for the vast amount of literature that has been published regarding the Holocaust and its effect on the survivors. Some Jewish people believe that the Holocaust was just one more act of persecution against a people who have endured thousands of years of being victims of ignorance and misunderstanding.

Implications for Nursing Care

The nurse caring for a Jewish-American client should get a careful history of the client's eating habits. Many ethnic Jewish foods are high in animal and saturated fats. Since these are known to influence the amount of cholesterol in the body and since high cholesterol is known to be a factor in heart disease, dietary education is important in this cultural group. In addition, many prepared kosher foods are made with eggs as well as palm or coconut oil. Jewish clients who maintain a kosher diet must be cautioned to read labels carefully on all prepared kosher foods.

Because of the use of dairy products by this cultural group, as well as the high incidence of Crohn's disease and ulcerative colitis, a history regarding bowel habits and abdominal problems should be carefully obtained. The nurse needs to remain alert for any symptoms that may indicate lactose intolerance. In addition, the nurse needs to remain alert for signs of drug or alcohol abuse. Since alcohol consumption is considered permissible at religious and secular functions, excessive drinking on a routine basis may not be viewed as a problem by the individual or the family. Cultural beliefs and taboos may make educating the client about the potential for alcohol abuse difficult.

Assisting Orthodox Jewish clients in areas of psychological needs takes patience and understanding on the part of the nurse. Not only may clients have concerns about personal acceptance by peers but they may also worry that knowledge of psychiatric problems in the family will lead to potential problems in finding a suitable mate for themselves or future children. Going to counseling is equated with being "crazy," and being "crazy" is seen as a hereditary problem. Further education on psychiatric and emotional problems is needed to change negative attitudes about treatment.

SUMMARY

It is crucial that the nurse remember that not all Jewish clients are alike. Although some Jewish patients are Orthodox and follow the commandments strictly, other Jewish people, with each successive generation, have become more acculturated to the behavior of the people around them.

Caring for the Jewish-American client can be a challenge. Although nursing education traditionally has prepared nurses to view health from a singular professional perspective, health must also be understood from a cultural perspective when care is being provided to clients whose cultural background differs from that of the nurse (Leininger, 1985). Many educational programs are seeking to address this issue by providing transcultural experiences for student nurses. Other health care facilities are offering educational programs to new nurses and to nurses already in practice. One such experience related to the Jewish client is at Baycrest Centre for Geriatric Care in Toronto, Canada (Gorrie, 1989; Gould-Stuart, 1986; Rose, 1981). This program provides a transcultural experience for nurses in orientation and for selected nurses on a continuing care unit of the hospital. During this experience, differences between the Jewish culture and the secular culture are examined. Such educational programs can assist nurses in developing an increased understanding of the universality of various cultural attributes and the importance of culture to all individuals.

CASE STUDY

Esther Rosenbloom was admitted to a nursing home after a fall that resulted in a fractured hip. Esther, age 87, emigrated from Russia with her family in 1929, at 4 years of age. She was brought to the nursing home by her son-in-law, Nat, and her daughter, Bernice. Esther was admitted for physical therapy and is expecting to be discharged to her home after she learns to walk with a walker. Her home is a block away from her daughter and son-in-law's home.

Esther was raised in an Orthodox Jewish home in Brooklyn, New York, but joined the Conservative movement when she married at 24 years of age. Bernice, age 61, informs the nurse that although Esther follows Conservative Jewish thought, she maintains a kosher diet. The nursing home she is admitted to has very few Jewish clients and is unfamiliar with kosher diets. Bernice also mentions that her mother has abdominal difficulties if she ingests too much cheese or milk. Esther appears worried, is moaning, and is complaining of pain in her hip. Bernice's eyes appear red, as if she has been crying. Bernice

is wringing her hands and mentions that her mother has been uncomfortable and that she hopes the nurses at the nursing home will be able to keep Esther comfortable.

When the nurse asks Esther how she is feeling, she states in a whining tone of voice, "My hip hurts, and I want to go home. How are you going to feed me here? What do you know about kosher foods?"

When moving Esther from wheelchair to bed, the nurse notes that Esther does not seem to want to assist, despite the fact that the transfer sheet notes that Esther can move from wheelchair to bed with minimal assistance. When asked why she did not help, Esther replies, "I'm just too tired."

Esther is usually self-sufficient and very busy with her volunteer activities, despite decreased visual acuity, for which she wears glasses. Although Bernice mentions that her mother always worries about her bowels, Esther does not have a history of constipation. She is continent of urine and stool.

CARE PLAN

Nursing Diagnosis: Pain related to fractured hip and anxiety. Supportive data: complains of pain, appears upset and tense, has difficulty transferring from chair to bed

Client Outcome	Nursing Interventions
Pain will decrease.	1. Medicate as ordered. 2. Use comfort measures (such as relaxation techniques, diversional activities) to promote relaxation. 3. Assist client to a comfortable position. 4. Spend at least 10 minutes per shift, while client is awake, to allow for expression of feelings.

Nursing Diagnosis: Nutrition, altered, less than body requirements, related to religious and cultural dietary restrictions, plus possible lactose intolerance

Client Outcome	Nursing Interventions
Client will maintain weight within normal limits.	1. Determine client's likes and dislikes in foods that the institution can provide that meet with client's religious restrictions. 2. Request that family bring ethnic foods from home that client would enjoy. 3. Serve foods on paper plates with plastic utensils to avoid serving impermissible foods and non-kosher foods on same set of dishes. 4. Offer cheese or milk products in small amounts until tolerance can be determined. 5. If milk products are ingested, assess for abdominal cramps and diarrhea.

CARE PLAN—cont'd

Nursing Diagnosis: Anxiety related to situational crisis

Client Outcome	Nursing Interventions
Client will adjust to new living arrangements with minimal difficulty.	1. Spend time with client to allow verbalization of fears, discomforts. 2. Find activities client is interested in, and attempt to have client participate in facility activities. 3. Encourage independence. 4. Include client in decisions related to her care whenever feasible. 5. Allow family to spend as much time as desired with client. 6. Give client clear, concise explanations of anything that is about to occur. 7. Introduce client to other Jewish clients, and encourage them to visit with each other. 8. Remain nonjudgmental toward family and client. 9. Contact rabbi and ask him to visit if client wishes.

Nursing Diagnosis: Anxiety related to maturational crisis

Client Outcome	Nursing Interventions
Client will identify potential and actual sources of anxiety.	1. Encourage client to identify stressful life events experienced within the past year. 2. Spend specific amount of uninterrupted time with client to listen to her concerns. 3. Allow family to spend as much time with client as desired. 4. Involve family in client's care if desired. 5. Assist client in identifying sources of fear or tension. 6. Assist client in identifying activities that help decrease anxiety and encourage the use of these activities.

Nursing Diagnosis: Mobility, impaired physical, related to discomfort, fractured hip, and possible fear

Client Outcome	Nursing Interventions
Client will be able to transfer easily by self from bed to chair and ambulate with walker with minimal assistance.	1. Provide physical therapy daily. 2. Reinforce what client is learning in physical therapy. 3. Observe client's functional ability daily. 4. Encourage and compliment client liberally. 5. Encourage verbalization of fears and feelings regarding altered state of mobility. 6. Remain nonjudgmental when client is unwilling to perform to her ability. 7. Provide comfort measures, such as medication as ordered and padding of extremities where they may be prone to skin breakdown. 8. Do range-of-motion exercises to increase strength; instruct family in these exercises, and encourage them to encourage client. 9. Promote progressive ambulation. 10. Discuss use of distraction and other nonpharmacological pain relief. 11. Explain necessity of moving, even when in pain, to prevent arthritic conditions or contractions and increased stiffness.

Continued

◎ CARE PLAN—cont'd

Nursing Diagnosis: Injury, risk for, related to impaired mobility, decreased visual acuity, and new environment

Client Outcome	Nursing Interventions
Client will sustain no injury.	1. Encourage use of a walker, with assistance. 2. Assist client when she is getting short of breath, getting out of chair, or walking. 3. Be sure floor is dry and furniture and litter are out of the way when client is engaging in activities that may cause falls. 4. Instruct client and family regarding safety practices when client is using walker or transferring. 5. Keep side rails up when client is in bed. 6. Maintain bed in low position.

Nursing Diagnosis: Constipation related to decreased mobility

Client Outcome	Nursing Interventions
Client will not develop constipation.	1. Monitor frequency and characteristics of stools; record. 2. Recognize that client may have concerns about bowels because of age and culture. 3. Ask client if she has a specific routine at home, such as a normal time for defecation or use of prune juice (a favorite "remedy" for Eastern European Jews). 4. Encourage fluid intake of 2000 mL per day.

Nursing Diagnosis: Spiritual distress (risk for) related to separation from religious and cultural ties

Client Outcome	Nursing Interventions
Client will not express feelings of spiritual distress.	1. Listen for cues that client may be having spiritual distress (such as, "Why did God do this to me?"). 2. Remain nonjudgmental. 3. Acknowledge spiritual concerns and encourage expression of thoughts and feelings. 4. Find ways to help client maintain kosher diet. 5. Encourage client to continue her religious practices during hospitalization, and do whatever is necessary to help facilitate this. 6. Ask client if she desires rabbi to visit, and contact synagogue if necessary. 7. Introduce client to and help foster friendships with other Jewish clients. 8. If client can have a pass, and family and client desire it, make arrangements for client to attend Friday night or Saturday services.

CLINICAL DECISION MAKING

1. List ways that a kosher diet can be maintained while a client is in the hospital.
2. List religious needs a Jewish client may have while being hospitalized with which nursing staff can assist.
3. Identify three communication barriers that a nurse may encounter when giving care to a Jewish-American client.
4. List biological variations a Jewish client may have that will affect care given by a nurse.
5. Explain relationship characteristics that families of Jewish clients usually display toward a hospitalized relative.
6. Explain how Jewish people may react toward the impending death of a relative.

REVIEW QUESTIONS

1. When providing care for an Orthodox Jewish client, the nurse should do which of the following?
   a. Introduce self and shake hands.
   b. Use touch as a manner to show caring.
   c. Avoid touching the client on the head.
   d. Touch the client for "hands-on" care only.
2. To assist a hospitalized Jewish client following a kosher diet, the nurse should attend to which of the following?
   a. Serve seafood instead of meat.
   b. Suggest the client waive the dietary restriction.
   c. Serve meals on paper plates with plastic utensils.
   d. Serve different food on a different tray.
3. The nurse overheard two nursing assistants talking about a Jewish-American client whom they consider to be a chronic complainer. The best way for the nurse to handle the situation is to do which?
   a. Explain that letting others know feelings is a part of the Jewish culture.
   b. Agree with the staff and develop a plan to decrease complaints.
   c. Explain that being a perfectionist is a part of the Jewish culture.
   d. Avoid discussing the situation and do not assign them to care for the client.

REFERENCES

Ain, S. (2003). One-fourth of Holocaust survivors in US live below the poverty level. *The Jewish Federation of America*. Available at <http://www.jewishfederations.org/page.aspx?id=51886> Retrieved October 3, 2010.

Bash, D. M. (1980). Jewish religious practices related to childbearing. *Journal of Nurse-Midwifery, 25*, 5.

Brandt-Rauf, S. I., Raveis, V. H., Drummond, N. F., Conte, J. A., & Rothman, S. M. (2006). Ashkenazi Jews and breast cancer: the consequences of linking ethnic identity to genetic disease. *American Journal of Public Health, 96*(11), 1979–1988.

Bray, S. M., Mulle, J. G., Dodd, A. F., Pulver, A. E., Wooding, S., & Warren, S. T. (2010). Signatures of founder effects, admixture, and selection in the Ashkenazi Jewish population. *Proceeding of the National Academy of Sciences, 107*(37), 16222–16227.

Cohen, M., & Azaiza, F. (2007). Health-promoting behaviors and health locus of control from a multicultural perspective. *Ethnicity & Disease, 17*, 637–642.

Cohen, M., Brom, D., & Dasberg, H. (2001). Child survivors of the Holocaust: symptoms and coping after fifty years. *Israel Journal of Psychiatry, 38*(1), 3–12.

Darwish, H., et al. (2002). Fighting colorectal cancer: molecular epidemiology differences between Ashkenazi and Sephardic Hews and Palestinians. *Annals of Oncology, 13*(9), 1497–1501.

Dempsey, D. (1977). *The way we die.* New York: McGraw-Hill.

Edelheit, J. (1989). The rabbi and the abyss of AIDS. *Tikkun, 4*(4), 67–69.

End of life issues: a Jewish perspective. (n.d.). *My Jewish learning.* Available at <http://www.myjewishlearning.com/article/end-of-life-issues-a-jewish-perspective/> Retrieved April 25, 2015.

Farbiarz, R. (2010), The Jewish response to HIV/AIDS. *Jewish World Service.* Available at <https://ajws.org/what_we_do/education/resources/the_jewish_response_to_hiv_aids.pdf> Retrieved April 25, 2015.

Feldman, D. M. (1986). *Health and medicine in the Jewish tradition.* New York: Crossroad.

Ganzfried, S. (1963). *Code of Jewish law: a compilation of Jewish laws and customs.* New York: Hebrew Publishing.

Gene mutation in Jewish women. (1995). *Harvard Women's Health Watch, 3*(3), 7.

Glazer, N. (1989). *American Judaism* (2nd revised ed.). Chicago: University of Chicago Press.

Goffe, W. S. (2011). An estate planner's roadmap to the valley of the shadow of death: health care directives from religious perspectives. *Fear no evil.* Available at: <http://ssrn.com/abstract=1954212> Retrieve, April 25, 2015.

Gold, M. (1988). *And Hannah wept: infertility, adoption and the Jewish couple.* Philadelphia: Jewish Publication Society.

Goodman, R. (1979). *Genetic disorders among the Jewish people.* Baltimore: Johns Hopkins University Press.

Gorrie, M. (1989). Reaching clients through cross cultural education. *Journal of Gerontological Nursing, 15*(10), 29–31.

Gould-Stuart, J. (1986). Bridging the cultural gap between residents and staff. *Geriatric Nursing, 7*, 319–321.

Heller, Z. (1986). The Jewish view of death: guidelines for dying. In E. Kubler-Ross (Ed.), *Death: the final stage of growth.* New York: Simon & Schuster.

Howe, I. (1989). *World of our fathers.* New York: Shocken Books.

Jacobs, L. A., & Giarelli, E. (2001). Jewish culture, health belief systems, and genetic risk for cancer. *Nursing Forum, 36*(2), 5–13.

Jaffe-Gill, E. (2002). The next Tay-Sachs? *Moment (New York, N.Y.), 24.*

Jakobovits, I. (1975). *Jewish medical ethics.* New York: Bloch.

Janowsky, O. (1964). *The American Jew: a reappraisal.* Philadelphia: Jewish Publication Society.

Jorde, L., Carey, J., Bamshad, M., & White, R. (2010). *Medical genetics.* St. Louis: Mosby.

Kaplan, R. (1970). *An experience with residual populations in Detroit.* Paper presented at the annual meeting of the National Conference of Jewish Communal Service, Boston.

Kaplan, M., Renbaum, P., Levy-Lahad, E., Hammerman, C., Lahad, A., & Beutler, E. (1997). Gilbert syndrome and glucose-6-phosphate dehydrogenase deficiency: a dose-dependent genetic interaction crucial to neonatal hyperbilirubinemia. *Proceedings of the National Academy of Science of the United States of America, 94*(22), 12128–12132.

Kertzer, M. (1993). *What is a Jew?* New York: Collier Books.

Key, S. W. (1997). Three breast cancer gene alterations in Jewish community carry increased cancer. *Cancer Weekly Plus,* 14–17.

Kolatch, A. J. (1985). *The second Jewish book of why.* Middle Village, NY: J. David Publishers.

Kren, G. M., & Rappoport, L. (1980). *The Holocaust and the crisis of human behavior.* New York: Holmes & Meier.

Krystal, H., & Niederland, W. G. (1971). *Psychic traumatization: aftereffects in individuals and communities.* Boston: Little, Brown.

L'Archevesque, C. I., & Goldstein-Lohman, H. (1996). Ritual circumcision: educating parents. *Pediatric Nursing, 22*(3), 228, 230–244.

Leininger, M. (1985). Transcultural nursing: an essential knowledge and practice field for today. *Canadian Nurse, 80*(11), 41–45.

Lieberman, L. (1987). Jewish alcoholics and the disease concept. *Journal of Psychology and Judaism, 13*(3), 165–179.

Lutwak, R., Ney, A. M., & White, J. E. (1988). Maternity nursing and Jewish law. *Maternal and Child Health, 13,* 3.

Mamopoulos, A. M., Hughes, D. A., Tuck, S. M., & Mehta, A. B. (2009). Gaucher disease and pregnancy. *Journal of Obstetrics and Gynaecology, 29*(3), 240–251.

MacDonald, K. (2001). *The culture of critique: An evolutionary analysis of Jewish involvement in twentieth-century intellectual and political movements.* Westport, CT: Praeger Publislers.

Meer, J. (1987). An open door. *Psychology Today, 17.*

Mourant, A. E., Kopec, A. C., & Domaniewsks-Sobczak, K. (1978). *The genetics of the Jews.* New York: Clarendon Press.

Nadler, A., Kav-Venaki, S., & Gleitman, B. (1985). Transgenerational effects of the Holocaust: externalization of aggression in second generation of Holocaust survivors. *Journal of Consulting and Clinical Psychology, 53*(3), 365–369.

National Library of Medicine. (2015). *Genetics home reference. Familial dysautonomia (2015).* Available at <http://ghr.nlm.nih.gov/condition/familial-dysautonomia> Retrieved April 25, 2015.

Novak, W., & Waldoks, M. (1981). *The big book of Jewish humor.* Philadelphia: Harper & Row.

Patai, R., & Wing, J. P. (1989). *The myth of the Jewish race* (revised ed.). Detroit: Wayne University Press.

Popenoe, D. (2000). *Sociology* (11th ed.). Upper Saddle River, NJ: Prentice Hall.

Prchal, J. T., & Samuelson, S. J. (2009). *Polycythemia vera.* Available at <http://emedicine.medscape.com/article/957470-overview> Retrieved September 23, 2010.

Radwan, M. F. (2015). *Religion and locus of control.* Available at <http://www.2knowmyself.com/miscellaneous/locus_of_control_religion> Retrieved April 25, 2015.

Rennert, H., et al. (2002). A novel founder mutation in the RNASEL gene, 47delAAAG, is associated with prostate cancer in Ashkenazi Jews. *American Journal of Human Genetics, 71*(4), 981–984.

Rose, A. (1981). The Jewish elderly: behind the myths. In M. Weinfield, W. Whaffer, & I. Cotler (Eds.), *The Canadian Jewish mosaic* (pp. 199–200). New York: John Wiley & Sons.

Rose, S. L., & Garske, J. (1987). Family environment, adjustment, and coping among children of Holocaust survivors: a comparative investigation. *American Journal of Orthopsychiatrics, 57*(3), 332–342.

Ross, H. M. (1981). Societal/cultural views regarding death and dying. *Topics in Clinical Nursing, 3*(3), 1–16.

Rosten, L. (1999). *The joys of Yiddish.* New York: Galahad Books.

Rothschild, H., & Chapman, C. F. (Eds.), (1981). *Biocultural aspects of disease.* New York: Academic Press.

Rozovsky, L. (2015). *May I shake the lady's hand?* Available at <http://www.chabad.org/library/article_cdo/aid/1051760/jewish/May-I-Shake-the-Ladys-Hand> Retrieved April 25, 2015.

Sachar, A. L. (1965). *A history of the Jews* (5th ed.). New York: Knopf.

Schlesinger, B. (1971). *The Jewish family: a survey and annotated bibliography.* Toronto: University of Toronto Press.

Schneider, S. (1985). The non-Orthodox Jewish perspective of dying and death (Unpublished master's thesis). University of Arizona, Tucson.

Schwartz, E. (1984). The non-Orthodox Jewish perspective on dying and death (Unpublished master's thesis). University of Arizona, Tucson.

Schwartz, M., Benkendorf, J., Lerman, C., Isaacs, C., Ryan-Robertson, A., & Johnson, L. (2002). Impact of educational print materials on knowledge, attitudes, and interest in BRCA1 and BRCA2 testing among Ashkenazi Jewish women. *Cancer, 92*(4), 932–940.

Silberberg, N. (2015). *Why does Jewish law forbid cremation?* Available at <https://www.chabad.org/library/article_cdo/aid/510874/jewish/Why-Does-Jewish-Law-Forb> Retrieved April 25, 2015.

Some modern views on euthanasia. (2015). *My Jewish learning.* Available at <http://www.myjewishlearning.com/article/some-modern-views-on-euthanasia/> Retrieved April 25, 2015.

Sommer, B. (1995). Special consideration for Orthodox Jewish patients in the emergency department. *Journal of Emergency Nursing, 21*(6), 569–570.

Sorscher, N. (1994). Children of Holocaust survivors may inherit their parents' trauma symptoms. *The Psychology Letter, 6*(5).

Sowell, T. (1981). *Ethnic America*. New York: Basic Books.

Sperling, A. (1968). *Reasons for Jewish customs and traditions*. New York: Bloch.

Steinhardt, D. (1988). Alcoholism: the myth of Jewish immunity. *Psychology Today, 10*.

Steinitz, L. Y., & Szonyi, D. M. (Eds.), (1979). *Living after the Holocaust: reflections by children of survivors in America*. New York: Bloch.

Stevenson, J. C., Schanfield, M. S., & Sandler, S. G. (1985). Immunoglobulin allotypes in Jewish populations living in Israel and the United States. *American Journal of Physical Anthropology, 67*(3), 195–207.

Thompson, J. M., McFarland, G. K., Hirsch, J. E., et al. (1989). *Mosby's manual of clinical nursing* (2nd ed.). St. Louis: Mosby.

Time Almanac. (2011). New York: The Penguin Group.

Trepp, L. (1980). *The complete book of Jewish observances*. New York: Summit Books.

Washofsky, M. (2015). *Jewish living: a guide to contemporary reform practice* (rev. ed.). New York: UAHC Press.

Weiss, P. (2013). *The "genetic truth" of Jesus's "classically Semitic appearance," as revealed by Jeffrey Goldberg*. Available at <http://mondoweiss.net/2013/12/classically-appearance -revealed> Retrieved April 25, 2015.

Weissglass-Volkov, D., & Pajukanta, P. (2010). Genetic causes of high and low serum HDL-cholesterol. *Journal of Lipid Research, 51*(8), 2031–2057.

Wikler, M. (1986). Pathways to treatment: how Orthodox Jews enter therapy. *Social Casework: The Journal of Contemporary Social Work*, 113–118.

Zborowski, M. (1969). *People in pain*. San Francisco: Jossey-Bass.

Korean Americans

Jai Bun K. Earp

BEHAVIORAL OBJECTIVES

After reading this chapter, the nurse will be able to:

1. Describe the communication patterns of Korean Americans and the difficulties encountered when communicating in an English-speaking society.
2. Identify patterns of spatial behavior found among Korean Americans.
3. Relate family and social values commonly held by Korean Americans.
4. Describe the effect of cultural perspectives on time on the behavior of Korean Americans.
5. Relate the significance of Oriental herbal medicine for the health care of Korean Americans in the United States.
6. Describe the biological variations that affect health care for Korean Americans.

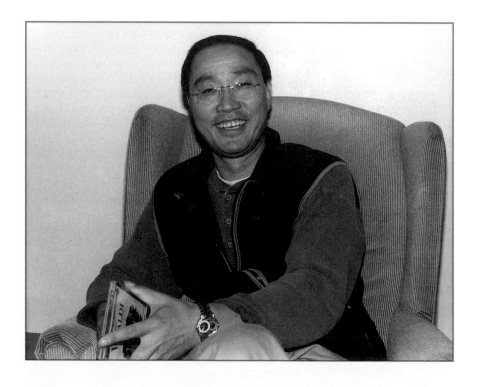

OVERVIEW OF KOREA

Often referred to as the "Land of the Morning Calm" (in Japanese, *Chōsen*) because of its spectacular mornings, Korea is a nation with one of the richest and most original cultures in East Asia and is one of the world's leading economic powers (Buzzle.com, 2010). A peninsula in the East Sea (Sea of Japan), Korea is bordered by thousands of islands, with China and Russia to the north and neighboring Japan to the east. The peninsula is 125 miles wide at its narrowest point and extends 625 miles from north to south.

Korean history dates back to 2333 B.C., with the founding of the state of Ancient Choson by Tan-Gun (Buzzle .com, 2010). Korea was united as a kingdom under the Silla Dynasty, 668 A.D. At times Korea was associated with the Chinese empire. A treaty that concluded the Sino-Japanese war of 1895 recognized Korea's complete independence. However, in 1910 Korea was forcibly annexed by Japan. Following World War II, Korea was occupied by the Soviet Union in the north and the United States in the south, with the thirty-eighth parallel designated as the line dividing the areas of occupation. North Korea became totalitarian like the Soviet Union and Communist China. South Korea became a free society like the United States; both aspired to erase the boundary and reunite Korea into a single state. These attitudes burst into flames on June 25, 1950, when the armed forces of North Korea invaded the Republic of Korea (Blumeson, 2010). In 1953, following 4 years of battle between the North and the South in the Korean War, an armistice was declared. Today the country remains one of the few nations in the world still affected by the Cold War. About 40,000 U.S. troops continue to guard South Korea at the thirty-eighth parallel demilitarized zone against another Communist invasion. In 2006, North Korea began a proliferation of missile testing. While this situation appeared to put the world at large in an extremely vulnerable position, in July 2007, the United Nations verified that North Korea had closed all five of its major nuclear facilities, which was a milestone in the efforts expended to get the country to give up its nuclear weapons program (CNN, 2007). Since that time, North Korea has reconstituted its nuclear programs, tested nuclear weapons and defied the free world's demands to cease nuclear armament. This situation remains unresolved. In 2010, a North Korean submarine torpedoed a South Korean naval vessel (verified), raising tension to new levels. North Korea continues to threaten South Korea and allied nations.

The South Korean landmass is only 38,486 square miles, slightly larger than Indiana. In contrast, the North Korean landmass is 46,541 square miles, slightly smaller than Pennsylvania. The population of North Korea is 22,912,177. In contrast, the population of South Korea is 48,636,068, which approximates the populations of California and Florida combined (Central Intelligence Agency [CIA], 2011; *Time Almanac*, 2011). If South Korea and North Korea were reunited, the country would be about the same size as Iceland or Portugal.

North Korea was ruled by Kim Jong Il from 1994 until his death in December of 2011. Kim Jong Il succeeded to this leadership position at the death of his father, Kim Il Sung. He was not only the head of state for North Korea, but also chairman of the National Defense Commission, a position accorded to the nation's highest administrative authority. As this text goes to press, speculation suggests that North Korea may move to a collective leadership model, with experienced advisors sharing power with designated successor Kim Jung Eun, son of Kim Jong Il. However, the ultimate political leadership of this tightly ruled Communist country is unclear at this time (Harlan, 2011). Similarly, the president of the Presidium of the Supreme People's Assembly, Kim Yong-nam, serves as the nominal head of state. Since June 7, 2010, the premier is CHOE Yong Rim (CIA, 2011). In North Korea, the labor force is 36% agricultural, with many dependent on the scarce farmland (14% arable land) for a basic subsistence. The per capita income is $1700 (CIA, 2011; *World Almanac*, 2011).

The president of South Korea, at this writing, is Lee Myung-bak (2008–) and the Prime Minister is Chung Un-Chan (2009–). In contrast to North Korea, South Korea has made great strides in developing its potential as one of the Far Eastern powers by blending nationalism, administrative efficiency, and semiauthoritarian rule (*Time Almanac*, 2011). The war left South Korea with virtually no natural resources (Kaltsounis & Shin, 1988). However, South Korea's export successes have been the result of the labor and skills of its people, with 67.7% of the labor force involved with services, 25.1% in industry, and 7.2% in agriculture (CIA, 2011). South Korea has made a remarkable economic transformation in the past several decades, with its per capita gross national product increasing from $87 in 1962 to $23,000 in 1987 (Park, 1988) to $28,000 in 2009 (*World Almanac*, 2011). Today, South Korea enjoys a hitherto undreamed of standard of living and is the sixth largest trading partner of the United States. The United States is the second largest export recipient of Korean goods, with major exports including electronic products, machinery, and passenger cars (*World Almanac*, 2011). Sponsorships of the Twenty-Third World Olympics in 1988, the International Council of Nurses Nineteenth Congress in Seoul in 1989, and the World Cup soccer matches in 2002, as well as winning gold medals in the 2008 Beijing Olympics represent a few examples of the economic confidence of the people of South Korea.

Unification of the peninsula is a hope held very close to the hearts of most Korean people (Lee, 1988). South Koreans have not forgotten the United Nations' commitment of the 1950s (Korean Conflict) and continue to partner with the ideals and democratic philosophy of the United States, a staunch economic, political, and military ally. In recent years, there have been unification demonstrations in South Korea by those who did not experience the previous aggression of the North. At an unprecedented summit meeting in Pyongyang in 2000, South Korean President Kim Dae Jung and North Korean leader Kim Jong Il agreed to work at reconciliation and reunification of their two countries. Kim Dae Jung was named winner of the 2000 Nobel Peace Prize for his efforts (*World Almanac,* 2011). In 2007, a second North/South summit took place between South Korean president Roh Moo-Hyun and the North Korean leader. However, unwillingness by the North to engage new President Lee Myung-Bak following his 2008 election left inter-Korean relations strained (CIA, 2011).

Mountains, valleys, and streams dominate the terrain of both North and South Korea. North Korea is almost completely covered by a series of north–south mountain ranges that are separated by narrow valleys. In North Korea, the Yalu River forms a part of the northern border with Manchuria (*Time Almanac,* 2011). South Korea is approximately 70% mountainous. In the north and east of South Korea, more than 10% of the land is 3000 feet above sea level. In South Korea, narrow plains and hills between the mountains provide the major land area for agriculture and other economic activities. Approximately 16.58% of the land is arable and is cultivated for rice, root crops, barley, soybeans, and vegetables (CIA, 2011).

South Korea has a clear delineation of four seasons, and its climate is characterized by cold winters and hot summers. The average temperature in the coldest winter month is below 28° F and in the warmest month is over 86° F. A humid summer monsoon from the Pacific lasts about 6 weeks in June and July. South Korean weather has been described by many as similar to that in Virginia.

The population density in South Korea is 501 people per square kilometer, with 81% of the people living in cities (*World Almanac,* 2011). The population of Seoul, the capital (the term *Seoul* also means "capital city"), is 10,287,847, and Pusan (*Cauldron-mountain*) has 3,504,900 inhabitants (Infoplease.com, 2010). In North Korea, the majority of the population is urban (61.1%), with the capital city of Pyongyang having the largest population of 3,228,000 (*World Almanac,* 2011).

OVERVIEW OF KOREAN AMERICANS

Although Korean immigration to the United States dates back to 1885, when three Korean men claimed to be political refugees, it was not until after the Korean War when sustained immigration started. Early immigrants during this time principally came to Hawaii to work as laborers in the sugar plantations solely for the purpose of making money and with the intention to return home. They had a "sojourner" mentality, never fully participating in American life.

The Immigration Act of 1965, the rapidly rising population level in Korea, and Korea's urbanization and rapid industrialization led to a dramatic increase in Korean immigration to the United States. In addition, the connection through the political-military alliance with the United States and the stationing of large numbers of U.S. military personnel allowed more female immigrants to the United States. These Koreans were largely well-educated professionals and students who wanted more freedom to live in a democratic society and who had no intention of going back (Jo, 1999). This created a "brain drain" phenomenon. However, dramatic improvements in economic and living standards in South Korea and the establishment of a civilian-controlled government in the 1990s caused a drop in immigration rates. Even some people who had immigrated to the United States earlier returned home during this period. It is interesting to note that the emergence of a favorable political, economic, and social climate in South Korea had an immediate effect on Koreans' decisions to immigrate.

LIFE IN THE UNITED STATES TODAY

According to the U.S. Bureau of the Census (2009), 1,754,354 Korean Americans reside in the United States, representing 0.4% of the total U.S. population and 9.5% of the Asian-American population. The growth rate for Korean Americans has slowed from 134.8% between 1980 and 1990 to 35.1% between 1990 and 2009 (U.S. Department of Commerce, Bureau of the Census, *American Community Survey,* 2015). Koreans are the fifth largest ethnic group among Asian Americans, following the Chinese, Filipinos, Indians, and Vietnamese (Ameredia, 2010). Of all Korean Americans residing in the United States, 44% live on the West Coast, 23% in the Northeast, 19% in the South, and 14% in the Midwest, which is a typical historical settlement pattern for Asian Americans (Ameredia, 2010). More than 75% of Korean Americans live in just 10 states: California, New York, New Jersey, Illinois, Washington, Texas, Virginia, Maryland, Pennsylvania, and Georgia (U.S. Department of Commerce, Bureau of the Census, *American Community Survey,* 2015; Ameredia, 2010).

Of the Korean Americans who resided in the United States between 1975 and 1979, 15.3% were foreign-born; between 1980 and 1990, 41.0% were foreign-born; between 1990 and 2000, 60% were foreign-born, and from 2000 to the present, 29.2% were foreign-born (U.S. Department of Commerce, Bureau of the Census, *American Community Survey*, 2015). Immigration has obviously contributed immensely to the growth of the Korean-American population over the past four decades. However, the percentage of Korean Americans who are foreign born differs considerably across time periods.

The median age of Korean Americans is 36.3 years, compared with 35.4 for other Asian Americans, and the national median age of 36.8 years for the general U.S. population. In addition, only 9.3% of Korean Americans are 65 years of age or older, compared with 12.7% of the general U.S. population (U.S. Department of Commerce, Bureau of the Census, *American Community Survey*, 2013).

Korean Americans maintain one of the highest levels of ethnic attachment of any Asian ethnic group. An extremely high percentage of Korean immigrants speak Korean, eat Korean food, and practice Korean customs a majority of the time. Further, a larger population of Korean Americans belong to ethnic associations (75%) than Filipino (50%) or Chinese (19%) do (Asian and Pacific Islander American Health Forum, 2010).

There are three major reasons Korean Americans maintain high levels of ethnic attachment. First, Korea is a small, homogeneous country with one language (Min, 1995). Second, most Korean Americans (55%) were affiliated with Korean ethnic churches prior to immigration, and 75% affiliate with Korean churches after settling in the United States, probably for practical and social reasons (Min, 2006). Third, Korean Americans tend to concentrate in small businesses, which strengthens Korean ethnicity. Many Koreans who do not operate small businesses are employed in these enterprises. This ties many Korean Americans together socially and culturally.

Although the ethnic bonds within the Korean-American communities provide a high level of nationalistic satisfaction, the same ethnic bonds have hindered Korean-American assimilation into the American society. American-born Korean Americans assimilate proportionately according to length of residence and education. Older immigrants cling to Korean food, language, customs, and newspapers, thus slowing assimilation compared with other Asian immigrant groups (Chang, 1999; Hurh & Kim, 1990). Korean Americans who have the opportunity to move through the American educational system, including universities, enhance the rate of assimilation while retaining pride of heritage.

Korean Americans are noted for high educational standards. In 2009, 61.1% of Korean-American males and 46.5% of their female counterparts had completed 4 or more years of university-level studies. Similarly, among Korean-American males, 91.5% as compared with 95.8% of their female counterparts 25 years of age or older held a high school diploma.

Children excel in school, particularly in math and science (Clark, 2000; U.S. Department of Commerce, Bureau of the Census, *The Asian Population*, 20013), which can be related to the struggle to achieve economic development after the Korean Conflict and the importance of education, which was emphasized in the home. Each year, over 99% of Korean students move from elementary school into middle school, and about 95% graduate from high school (U.S. Department of State, 2010). Korean children go to school more than 220 days a year for 5.5 days per week (Clark, 2000). Stress and competition to go to the top-rated schools have created some problems, such as loneliness (Simmons, Klopf, & Park, 1991), depression (Crittenden, Fugita, Bae, Lamug, & Un, 1992), and suicide.

Many Korean Americans view entering the workforce after college graduation as a serious lifetime commitment. Because of limited job opportunities, some Korean Americans do not look favorably at moving from job to job. In addition, some Korean Americans believe that attendance at the right school plays a major role in landing a prestigious position because many elite companies scout only capable people from the top-rated schools. Korean Americans, like other Asian Americans, are more likely to participate in the U.S. labor force than the U.S. population as a whole. Of the number of Korean Americans in the United States, 60.2% participate in the workforce. In general, 52.8% of Korean-American women participate in the labor force compared with 59.5% of all other women (U.S. Department of Commerce, Bureau of the Census, *American Community Survey*, 2015). Korean Americans are represented in various work occupations such as in management, professional, or related occupations (6.2%); service occupations (14.2%); sales or office occupations (27.7%); farming, fishing, or forestry occupations (0.1%); construction, extraction, maintenance, or repair occupations (3.6%); and production, transportation, or material moving occupations (U.S. Department of Commerce, Bureau of the Census, *American Community Survey*, 2013. In 2009, the median family earnings for Korean Americans was $64,142, compared with $62,367 for the rest of the general U.S. population (U.S. Department of Commerce, Bureau of the Census, *American Community Survey*, 2013). Korean Americans fare better than their counterparts regarding median individual income. In 2009, the median per capita income for Korean-American women was

$38,791, as compared with women in the rest of the general U.S. population at $35,299. Likewise, the median per capita income for Korean-American men was $50,659, as compared with $45,320 for men in the rest of the general U.S. population (U.S. Department of Commerce, Bureau of the Census, *American Community Survey,* 2013). Among Korean Americans, 11.4% live below the federally defined poverty level as compared with the 14.0% of the general U.S. population (U.S. Department of Commerce, Bureau of the Census, *American Community Survey,* 2013).

One major issue that prompted Korean adults to immigrate to the United States was consideration for their children's future. However, many elderly Koreans came over without a thorough awareness of their future or a plan (Messaris & Woo, 1991). Many Koreans found difficulty in leaving behind old cultural and social norms and adjusting to new ones (Moon & Pearl, 1991). Many of these individuals faced problems, including financial struggles, poor health, poor care practices, difficulty with social interactions, and mental problems such as *Hwa-byung,* which is a Korean culture-bound syndrome of suppressed anger and depression (Lin, 1983; Pang, 1990). Another major issue involves Korean-American men who suffer from loss of control and a sense of not belonging (Hurh & Kim, 1990). Many men followed their spouses who were nurses or physicians (it was easier for females to immigrate because of their professions) without adequate preparation for their own professional future and "equalization" of the male–female relationship.

COMMUNICATION

Language and Culture

Koreans use their own unique language, Hangeul. Hangeul is spoken by more than 78 million people in 31 different countries, including large groups in the former Soviet Union, Australia, United States, Canada, Brazil, and Japan (CIA, 2011). Hangeul is related to the Mongolian and Japanese languages and a large number of Chinese cognates (around 1300) exist in the Korean language (Buzzle.com, 2010). The Korean language is entirely different and capable of standing on its own (14 consonants and 10 vowels), and the language and literature have been greatly influenced by the Chinese (Chang, 1999). As noted, more than half of the words now used in Korean are of Chinese origin. With continued emphasis on learning Chinese because of the ruling Neo-Confucian philosophy of the earlier Chosun Dynasty, Chinese characters and Chinese words still occupy more than 50% of the text of Korean newspapers, magazines, and books today. Nevertheless, the Hangeul language was created in 1446 during the Joseon Dynasty to give the Korean people an alphabet that was learnable and usable

by all (Korean Cultural Service, 2006). The unique simplicity of Hangeul is reinforced by the fact that illiteracy is almost non-existent in Korea. Most Korean children have mastered their language by the time they reach school age (Korean Cultural Service, 2006).

The forced annexation of Korea by Japan from 1910 to 1945 prohibited the public use of the Korean language and forced Koreans to learn Japanese (Lee, 1988). Thus, many words used in Korean also have a Japanese origin (many of which are also from Chinese). However, the Korean language has a well-developed and extensive vocabulary, and Hangeul has been at the root of the Korean culture, helping to preserve its national identity and independence. Because of the simplicity and accessibility of the Korean alphabet, Hangeul is easy to learn, which has resulted in 100% literacy in Korea. Scientific design makes it easy to mechanize for computer utilization (Korean Overseas Informational Service, 1997). During the Japanese occupation, many Korean scholars worked to preserve the national language, which was critical in forging a strong national identity (Korean Cultural Service, 2006). The Japanese occupation, historical Chinese influence, and other foreign contacts have led to the integration of many indigenous words and loan words into the Korean language, mostly technological and scientific terms (Korean Cultural Service, 2006).

Dialect and Style

The usual commentary on dialect, style, emotional context, and kinesics does not apply to Hangeul as spoken by Koreans. Breadth of full language use and preciseness of pronunciation are most often the discriminators that identify and delineate higher-class (educated) from lower-class (less-educated) Koreans.

Verbal Communication

When abroad, a Korean being introduced to other Koreans, whether socially or professionally, will listen quite attentively before deciding to interact. This reserved behavior is related to the Korean equation of "reserved familiarity" until the individual has mastered the language and learned to know the individual. During conversation with an unfamiliar person, if there is a match between individuals, the individual is "in" and conversation will ensue. Of the Korean Americans residing in the United States, 79.2% speak only Korean at home, 46.7% do not speak English well, and 20.6% speak only English (U.S. Department of Commerce, Bureau of the Census, *American Community Survey,* 2009).

Use of Eye Contact and Kinesics

In public situations, Koreans are a "noncontact" group. In this sense, some Koreans have difficulty making eye contact or engaging in physical contact on streets, at markets, on subways, and in the workplace. However, in one-on-one and "acquaintance" situations, Koreans are very similar to Americans in interactions. With a familiar acquaintance, some Korean Americans will engage in eye contact. When conversing with familiar individuals, they will speak in the first person. Some Korean Americans are comfortable in face-to-face situations. However, some Koreans are still offended if, for instance, the sole of a shoe or foot is directed at them. Most Koreans who subscribe to this belief are willing to forgive "lack of knowledge" on the part of some Westerners in this regard. Basic courtesy, when sincerely exhibited by all parties, is a good-faith gesture that overcomes traditional Korean mores.

Confucian philosophy forms the basis for behavior and position within the social hierarchy (Van Decar, 1988). Etiquette is very important to Koreans, and it is a mistake to appear too familiar or informal. First names are used only within a family or a circle of close friends. For some Korean Americans, addressing or referring to people by name is considered a lack of proper respect and is believed to invoke evil spirits and lead to ill fortune.

Social Rank and Language

The idea of filial piety (*Hyo*: eternal indebtedness to the parents who gave children life) is so pervasive in Korean culture that the language itself is structured to reflect the junior–senior relationship of the parties in any given conversation (Clark, 2000). Different vocabulary and verb endings are used according to whether the person being addressed is of higher, equal, or lower rank or socioeconomic status than the speaker. Koreans accept filial obligations as part of life; these obligations set the patterns for getting along with other people and make it easier to know how to act in daily situations. Parents have a duty to their own ancestors to be wise, and it is children's duty to obey their parents and to repay them with loyalty and sincere effort (Clark, 2000).

Relationships outside the family are also modeled by filial piety. People understand how to behave toward others who are above or below them on the social scale (Clark, 2000). Many Korean Americans are very sensitive regarding the feelings of others. In most instances, Korean Americans are generous and agreeable and rarely say no to even an "impossible" request to prevent overt conflict and a breakdown of relationships (Fisher, 1996; Van Decar, 1988).

Implications for Nursing Care

More than 60% of Korean Americans were not able to speak English prior to immigration (Mangiafico, 1988). Many elderly Korean Americans who immigrated late in life may be quite intelligent and trilingual (Korean, Chinese, and Japanese), but they may not be able to communicate with health care professionals. Some elderly Korean Americans may have an attitude of "giving up on learning English." It is essential for the nurse to assess the linguistic abilities of the client. When translators are needed and Korean interpreters are not available, sometimes a Japanese or Chinese interpreter may be used to communicate with the client. If the client speaks and understands only Korean, a Japanese or Chinese interpreter might not be helpful. In these instances, the nurse may seek the assistance of a family member who speaks English to serve as a translator. However, children should not be used as translators, because this may create a reversal in the parent–child relationship and cause conflict. When communicating with a Korean-American client who has some knowledge of English, it is essential that the nurse speak slowly because this aids understanding. However, it is not necessary to speak loudly. Understanding and applying filial piety are of utmost importance during interaction with Korean Americans, be it polite body posture showing respect to elders or a sincere appearance of attentive listening.

SPACE

Distal spacing—between elderly and young, seniors and juniors, bosses and subordinates—is very subtle but quite distinct within the Korean community. If this spacing is ignored through ignorance or "cockiness," the person is considered a "black sheep" and will not be accepted socially.

Korean Americans, like some other Asian Americans (Chinese Americans, Japanese Americans), have a high tolerance for crowding in public spaces. For Korean Americans who immigrated from Korea, the ability to tolerate crowding probably developed in Korea as a result of the density of the population. South Korea is so crowded that its 47 million people live with 501 people per square kilometer (Infoplease.com, 2010).

Although Korean Americans can tolerate crowding, some avoid physical contact if possible. These individuals are uncomfortable in situations where physical contact is likely to occur. In addition, although some Korean Americans can tolerate higher degrees of crowding, they do not necessarily desire to engage in eye contact with unfamiliar persons.

Implications for Nursing Care

Because Korean Americans are basically a "noncontact" cultural group, until a relationship has been established, the nurse should attempt to establish an environment of trust and caring. Korean Americans are often perceived as extremely practical and thus, when confronted with sincerity, will respond in a manner of "Let's get the job done."

When interacting with an elderly Korean who does not speak the language, an interpreter who can convey sincerity should be used. It is essential for the nurse to remember that, although some Korean Americans are reported to have a higher tolerance for crowding, physical contact may not be acceptable, despite the closeness to the individual.

SOCIAL ORGANIZATION

Family

The average family size for Korean Americans is 3.6 people. The percentage of Asian-American families maintained by a husband and wife is 82%, which is slightly higher than the national average of 79%. Of the number of Korean-American families, only 12% are female-headed households, compared with the national average of 17%. A watershed percentage of women in the workforce has both enhanced tradition and extended opportunity to family unit members, especially females (U.S. Department of Commerce, Bureau of the Census, *Background Note, 2000*).

Historically, the Korean-American family has been the cornerstone of the culture. In most cases, father and sons have enjoyed preeminence as the leaders and undisputed decision makers (Van Decar, 1988). The traditional Korean family has been fixated on the need for a male heir, who is needed to guarantee the family line and lead the family in rituals that pay homage to ancestors, both in the home and at burial sites. The firstborn son inherits the mantle of family leadership and a greater property inheritance. Other sons receive lesser portions. Daughters receive very little, if any, inheritance. However, Pritham and Sammons (1993) investigated women receiving prenatal care in Korea and noted that only 35% felt having a male son was "important."

In Korea, marriages of daughters have been traditionally arranged, and elders have been respected and cared for. Gender biases may be held by some Korean Americans. However, since the Republic of Korea has leaped into the forefront of industrial export and partnership with the Western world, there has been a demand for qualified citizens with bachelor's, master's, and doctoral degrees, regardless of gender. This surge of national output and pride saw the competitive Korean educational system pushing those with potential to the top, regardless of gender. The movement toward equality in rights for women has threatened tradition both domestically and internationally. Although pure tradition is still found in the larger Korean rural society, the profound effect of this change is clearly visible in the matriculation picture at Korean universities. Essentially, modern mobility has strengthened relationships between couples and immediate family and has weakened traditional extended family obligations.

For some Korean-American families, problems have arisen when the wife has experienced professional upward mobility and the educationally prepared husband has not been able to find employment. Some Korean-American males have not been able to accept this situation and as a result have experienced enormous stress and anxiety. Some Korean-American males have discouraged their partners from continuing in competitive job tracks. This reaction appears to be adjusting with time because Koreans not only are rooted in tradition but also are very pragmatic and realistic.

Koreans as a whole are determined to increase their stock as an international economic partner. Korean Americans are an impressive example of how people can both assimilate and remain true to national heritage and family values. Korean-American communities have both become a part of the greater American society and begun to internalize to ensure homogeneity. Almost every major Korean community in the United States (that is, Los Angeles, San Francisco, New York, Baltimore, and Atlanta) and almost every city with a major university have organized local Korean schools to ensure that the culture, history, language, and tradition are not lost. Korean Americans today strive to balance American opportunity with knowledge and pride of heritage.

In a study on perceptions of elder abuse, elderly Korean-American women were substantially less likely to perceive a situation with an elder as abusive as were African-Americans or Caucasian Americans (Moon & Williams, 1993). Korean-American elderly were more likely to define abuse in a narrow context and were significantly less likely to seek help than the other groups.

Religion and Social Values

The social values of modern Korea reflect a blend of both old and new religious viewpoints. Shamanism, Taoism, Buddhism, and Confucianism were practiced in Korea long before Christianity (Clark, 2000; Min, 1995).

Although Buddhism is not the dominant influence in Korean life that it once was, it is still the biggest single religion, with 22.9 million (47%) adherents (*World Almanac*, 2011). Buddhism was originally not a religion but rather a doctrine of self-enlightenment, attainment of which would result in a deep understanding of one's own nature and place in the universe. This, in turn, engendered a way of "being-in-the-world" in which suffering would cease to exist and a timeless peace would be enjoyed.

Confucianism, entering Korea four centuries after Buddhism, was not so much a religion as a social ideology, exacting subordination of the son to the father, of the younger to the elder, of the wife to the husband, and of the subject to the throne. It inculcated filial piety, reverence for ancestors, and loyalty to friends, with strong emphasis on decorum, rites, and ceremony. With Japanese rule in 1910, the Confucian system disappeared. However, its basic values and premises lived on and continue to serve as the moral backbone of Korea (Korean Overseas Informational Service, 1996).

Christianity in Korea, although more recent, has been accentuated by the presence of 40,000 to 60,000 Westerners for more than 40 years. With the Westerners have come missionaries, astutely armed with modern learning, which isolated and withdrawn Korea badly needed. They had a powerful appeal to Koreans. As a result, approximately 20% of Koreans are church-going Christians. In addition, even more are influenced by the "Christian way." Unlike many Buddhists, Korea's Christians are fervent and devout to a point where they would probably feel quite out of place in a Western congregation (Korean Overseas Informational Service, 1996).

Many Koreans honor and practice a blend of traditional and modern religion, since Korea does not have one national religious creed. Although certain conflicts are recognized—that is, Confucianism versus Christianity—Korean Americans are able to harmonize the "best of both worlds." Korean Americans are generally more oriented to the future than to the ancient past and will adopt consistent, provable change, whether religious or political. Today, approximately half of the Korean population is affiliated with Buddhism or Christianity, while essentially the whole population is profoundly influenced by Confucian thought (Korean Overseas Informational Service, 1993).

Implications for Nursing Care

Although contemporary changes in traditional family customs have weakened the kinship and family structure, there is no question that Korean Americans are family oriented. Hospitalization of one becomes an entire family concern. The increasing importance of conjugal family relationships rather than the son–parent relationship has put sons and daughters-in-law at risk of great guilt if the parents become ill. Some Korean Americans may blame the illness of the father or mother on inadequate attention and care on the part of the child.

Although Koreans are exposed to many religions, it is important to note that Confucianism became the philosophical basis of family life as well as government and society. Respect for authority, balanced by affection and a sense of obligation toward one's subordinates, is central to the Korean way of life (Korean Overseas Informational Service, 1993). This may affect health care decision making for Korean Americans: for example, if an elder family member believes a medical procedure is necessary, the client will usually accede. Of course, the reverse may also

be true. If culturally appropriate care is to be rendered, it is essential to remember that the family is a primary social unit and family members must be included in the plan of care. In some instances, the client and the family may need counseling services to ensure proper intervention with the family.

TIME

According to Dodd (1987), time is an element of culture that belongs to a unique category in a nonverbal communication system. The organization of time is essential for some cultural groups. In other words, perceptions of time are culturally determined and are not culturally free (Dodd, 1987). Some Korean Americans believe that a person is in this world for only a brief time. For persons subscribing to this belief, life and living are viewed as a harmonious relationship between nature and the human being. Some Korean Americans, like some other Asian Americans, believe that every individual needs to learn to use time wisely. Thus, they are likely to believe that time should be used for activities such as performance of service for another person (Dodd, 1987).

Many Korean Americans are future oriented, which is derived from a Confucian belief in reincarnation. In this sense, many individuals who subscribe to this belief are likely to believe that it is essential to finish a task before beginning another one.

By virtue of culture, individuals can be either polychronic or monochronic in the organization of time. Hall (1966) described the time orientation of Asians as polychronic in contrast to the monochronic orientation of Westerners. Monochronically oriented individuals believe that it is essential to do one thing at a time. Persons who are monochronically oriented believe that accomplishments should be achieved during each task (Dodd, 1987). These individuals have an increased need for closure (finishing a task, ending a relationship). Monochronically oriented individuals generally think in a linear fashion. People who think in a linear fashion tend to internally process information in a sequential, segmented, orderly fashion (Dodd, 1987). For example, these individuals would sequence a meeting in this order: arrival, meeting, conclusion, action. They are likely to cycle through this sequence all day (Dodd, 1987). In contrast, polychronic individuals tend to think about and attempt to do many things at one time (Dodd, 1987). Persons who are polychronic can experience a high degree of information overload because they are trying to process so many things at one time. These individuals may also procrastinate because of information overload (Dodd, 1987). They may also tend to struggle harder to articulate abstractions without visualizations. Dodd (1987) concludes that polychronic individuals are very visually oriented. This orientation appears to be in concert with some research that indicates that these individuals may have either a right-brain or left-brain orientation. Right brain–dominant people tend to think more creatively, visually, and artistically than left brain–dominated individuals do, whereas left brain–dominant people tend to think more mathematically and linearly (Dodd, 1987). Because Korean Americans tend to be polychronically oriented and appear to be visually oriented, they are very likely to be right-brain dominant.

For some Korean Americans, having children is an essential life task. Sacrifice to bring up children in the best possible environment is an indescribable quest. For example, parents may be maintaining their living at the fish market, but they may send their children to the best private institution possible.

Many Koreans believe that people are reincarnated. They believe that those who perform good deeds and provide mercy for others in this world will be reborn as another human being, and that those who are bad in this world will be punished and be reborn as some sort of animal. Because of this belief, an intact body is necessary. Organ donation and transplantation are not seen as a virtue but as a threat to reincarnation.

Westerners tend to prioritize and schedule their lives. Compartmentalization of time occurs even in clinical settings such as the hospital. For example, in the hospital, rounds are made, temperatures taken, meals served, medicines dispensed—all on schedule.

Implications for Nursing Care

Time as viewed by Koreans is obviously a concept not held by Westerners in general. Nurses can expect cooperation in matters involving time, but when the client is suffering from anxiety and stress, the nurse must take time to communicate with the client to determine the client's needs.

ENVIRONMENTAL CONTROL

Illness and Wellness Behaviors

Several theories can explain the perceptions of illness by Korean people. One predominant health–illness theory governing Korean people is the equilibrium system, which emphasizes harmony and balance. Health derives from the harmonious relationship among elements of the universe, the human environment, and the supernatural world. Health also derives from the balance of the two major forces: *eum* (cold/dark, Chinese *yin*) and *yang* (hot/bright, Chinese *yang*). Disruption in the harmony of nature and imbalance between the two forces causes illness.

Dominance of *eum* creates problems related to cold, which makes a person depressive, hypoactive, and hypothermic. Examples of diseases from this dominance of *eum* are abdominal cramps, indigestion, and vaginal discharge. In contrast, dominance of *yang* causes a person to be hyperactive, hyperthermic, and irritable. Febrile seizures, stroke, and pimples are some examples of conditions related to *yang* dominance. Treatment for a person with dominant *eum* includes its replacement with *yang* to achieve balance, which includes providing hot food such as onions, peppers, ginger, and scallion roots. Giving cold food such as ice water, myung bean curd, cold noodles, and crab are some of the treatment modalities for those who have dominant *yang* problems (Hwang, 2000; Manderson, 1987).

Elderly Korean Americans consider drawing blood for laboratory work a very unfortunate event and may refuse. This idea stems from the fact that blood is considered life and removing blood from the body is considered as removing *ki* (Chinese *ch'i*), which is the very essence of life energy (Kim, 1992).

Oriental Herbal Medicine

The use of herbal medicines (*Han-yak*, "Chinese medicines") dates back to ancient Chinese practices. However, traditional Korean medicine has developed with its own characteristics (Pang, 1989). There are 396 distinct herbs and spices commercially available that are used either singly or in blended mixtures such as herbal decoctions (Hwang, 2000).

Today the power and influence of herbal medicine are evident in every city with a large Korean community, where many wholesale and retail herbal medicine shops may be found (*Korean American Journal*, 2002; *Korean Times*, 2002). Oriental herbal medicine doctors practice their trade by four common treatment methods: herbal medicine shops, acupuncture, moxibustion, and cupping. They may use one method singly or several in combination to treat clients.

Oriental medicine is based on the visual observation of behavior, physical properties of the body such as build, illness history, verbal responses, and radial pulses. After assessment, symptoms of disease are interpreted, and the treatment plan is devised on the basis of the metaphysical and cosmological philosophy of the concepts of *eum* and *yang* (Hwang, 2000; Pang, 1989, 1990).

If properly trained, Oriental medicine doctors have completed at least 6 years of education, with 2 years of premedical school and 4 years of Oriental Medical School. To practice in Korea, they also must pass a national licensing examination. Because of the popularity of holistic and alternative forms of health care, not only Oriental people are seeking herbal medicinal treatment in the United States, but also many Americans are seeking to have their health monitored by "herbal doctors" (Pang, 1989).

Oriental medicine doctors who have been assimilated into the American culture may incorporate biomedical technologies in making diagnoses. They may explain and make an analogy of their Oriental treatment in biomedical terms. It is likely that the number of Oriental medical doctors will increase as Korean communities become larger. In Atlanta alone, at least 20 Oriental medicine doctors are in official practice (*Korean American Journal*, 2002).

Because of the popularity and consumer demand, schools of acupuncture and Oriental medicine are increasing all over the United States, mainly in large metropolitan cities, and enrollment in these schools is expanding. Currently in the United States, these schools are 3 years in length for those who possess prior degrees. The curriculum includes at least 240 credits of theory and 1400 supervised clinical hours. Upon completing the curriculum, students must take national certification examinations to apply for state license to practice as a Licensed Acupuncturist (LAc), Acupuncture Physician (AP), or Doctor of Oriental Medicine (OMD or DAOM). The National Certification Commission on Acupuncture and Oriental Medicine administers the examinations, and the eligible candidates must pass the entire four-part examination, consisting of Biomedicine, Foundations of Chinese Medicine, Acupuncture, and Chinese Herbology. Some states (e.g., California) have their own licensing examination.

Nationally, the National Institutes of Health (NIH) established a National Center for Complementary and Alternative Medicine (NCCAM) to provide research funding related to complementary and alternative medicine, which includes herbs and acupuncture. The NCCAM is one of 27 centers within the NIH with a 2011 budget of $132 million. This sends a powerful message that the influence of Oriental herbal medicine in the American health care system is no longer minor and that insurance coverage for these services is quite probable in the near future.

Pregnancy and Postpartum Practices

Tae-kyo (prenatal training) is commonly practiced among some Korean-American women during pregnancy (Choi, 1986). Using *tae-kyo*, women are supposed to think only about good things in life and to maintain a calm attitude to ensure having a healthy baby. Pregnant Korean-American women are taught to eat only the right food in the right form, for example, an apple without nicks or spots (Pritham & Sammons, 1993). Pritham and Sammons (1993) note that in an investigation of Korean women receiving prenatal care at a U.S. military facility, the women reported that they had followed traditional beliefs in *tae mong*, a conception dream, and *tae-kyo* rituals for safe childbirth, as well as food taboos, including protein sources. The responses included positive maternal and paternal perceptions of pregnancy.

The nurse should appreciate that the possibility of not having a husband for support during delivery can cause anxiety, particularly when the husband can serve as translator. Limited language ability has been an obstacle for health care for Korean women, which can be enhanced by assistance from a more English-fluent husband (Park & Peterson, 1991).

During the postpartum period, women were instructed to have 21 days of bed rest with lots of seaweed soup for cleansing the body and providing fluid for adequate lactation (Giger, Davidhizar, & Wieczorek, 1993). However, this practice may be a dysfunctional health care practice because after delivery, a woman is in a hypercoagulable state (Giger, Davidhizar, & Wieczorek, 1993). However, many women nowadays go back to work and, because of the dangers of immobility, they do not stay on bed rest for long periods.

General Preventive Health Practices

Koreans have many general preventive health patterns. For example, during the hot summers in Korea, individuals tend to sweat more. Too much sweating is considered a loss of energy (*ki*) and negative to good health. Eating dog meat soup just before summer is believed to build stamina and strength by decreasing sweating (Hwang, 2000). Restaurants specializing in dog meat soup are abundant and busy in Korea.

Sex is regarded as a high energy consumer; therefore, sex drains *ki* from the body. Traditionally, both Korean men and women have been highly considerate of their partner's state of health; if one's health was not at its best or if one was "weak," sex might be abstained from in consideration of the situation.

The influence of Oriental herbal medicine on preventive health is very strong. Many Koreans take *bo yak* (an Oriental herbal medicine that tonifies the body and raises stamina and general health status) regularly at the beginning of spring for the purpose of enjoying health for the rest of the year. It is common for sons to present *bo yak* as their gesture of filial piety to their elderly parents each spring. Frequently, if daughters-in-law do not appear to be as vibrant, energetic, and obedient as they used to be soon after marriage into the family, it is the mother-in-law who suggests that the daughter-in-law take some *bo yak*. These rituals are often practiced in mostly well-to-do families, since *bo yak* is expensive and considered a luxury to many struggling families, although they know and appreciate the power of *bo yak*.

Another preventive health measure many Korean Americans practice is to visit fortune tellers, who may, in turn, forecast a person's health for the year. Visiting various religious shrines brings inner comfort and serenity and therefore is a positive health measure for the supplicant.

In general, Korean Americans have transformed from a culture of family-oriented caregiving and treatment to a culture of outreach to those who need to seek medical attention in which prevention is emphasized. Studies have shown that among Korean Americans, those who are more proficient in English, are more highly educated, and have health insurance are more likely to seek out available community health resources (Juon, Kim, Shankar, & Han, 2004). Culturally appropriate educational programs reaching out to the older, less-educated, less-English-proficient Korean-American populations should be developed. Nurses involved in community-focused interventions and outreach can play a significant role in acceptance of available services by Korean Americans.

Death and Dying

Many Korean Americans also believe that illness or death is fated and that they have no control over nature (Tien-Hyatt, 1987). Many Korean Americans equate admission to a hospital with a death sentence and may refuse to be admitted. This refusal may occur particularly with elderly Korean Americans, which, in turn, delays treatment. Among many Korean Americans, a do-not-resuscitate order is common because prolonging life might be viewed as unacceptable. In stark contrast, discussing a terminal illness with Korean Americans might be resisted by both the client and the family. Even today, some Korean Americans view the donation of organs and transplantations as a disturbance in the body. Health care professionals must broach such subjects with care (Kwon, 2006).

Many Korean Americans believe that dying should occur at home (Kwon, 2006). This concept is considered to be a "good death" among many Korean Americans. When a Korean or Korean American is dying, it is essential to bring that individual to the warmest part of the bedroom. Next, it is the obligation of the children, or *Imjong*, to watch at the deathbed of their parents. Often, a piece of cotton *sokkweng* will be placed on the dying person's mouth as this helps to check the last breath of the person (Kwon, 2006). In the past, it was the practice of some Koreans and Korean Americans to take a white shirt of the deceased out into the garden and, if possible, climb up to the roof and repeat the word *bok* ("return") three times. The purpose of this traditional ceremony, which is called *kobok,* refers to its literal translation: "calling back the spirit of the dead." Today, the *kobok* ceremony is not practiced as much as it once was (Kwon, 2006).

In Korea, the practice of embalming is not observed (Kwon, 2006). Because embalming is required in the United States, and a certified affidavit from five licensed embalmers is required for shipment of the body to any foreign country, this may cause concerns for a Korean American who is attempting to ship the body of a loved one to Korea (Kwon, 2006). Even today, the most important rites in the traditional funeral remain the *sup* (washing of the body) and the *yom* (binding). In a traditional Korean ritual with the body of the deceased, the body is washed with a piece of cloth or cotton that has been soaked in warm water. After washing, the body is bound with a long cloth known as a *yom* (Kwon, 2006).

Implications for Nursing Care

Many Korean Americans embrace more than one belief about their health–illness systems. As a result of these multiple beliefs, a variety of health care practices may be encountered by nurses. Persons who believe that sickness is from the action of a supernatural being may delay seeking health care until it is too late. They also may project a guilty conscience about their past behavior and act as though they have given up on recovering from the present illness. Nurses must be very authoritative in carrying out treatment plans for Koreans who exhibit such attitudes. Healing practices used by Korean clients should not be rejected automatically. Careful assessment is essential to provide culturally appropriate care.

It is essential for the nurse to recognize that many Korean Americans who are admitted to acute care or other health care facilities may be using both modern and herbal remedies simultaneously (Pourat, Lubben, Wallace, & Moon, 1999). This creates a problem of allergic and synergistic effects. Several specific cases of herbal-use conflicts have been reported (Lamba, 1993). Some herbal decoctions contain mistletoe, shave grass, horsetail, or sassafras and are certainly unsafe. Mistletoe contains viscotoxin, a mixture of toxic proteins that can produce anemia, hepatic and intestinal hemorrhage, and fatty degeneration of the thymus in experimental animals (Lamba, 1993). Most of these ingredients are crude complex mixtures that are neither uniformly prepared nor assayed for purity. Many contain a variety of unidentified allergens that may cause many potentially adverse effects. Some of the known allergenic materials include pollen (particularly from flower herbs), insect parts, and mold spores. Nurses must monitor the clients closely for potential side effects as well as synergistic effects of medicines in case they are dual users.

Health care practices that are based on the client's cultural beliefs must be honored when possible to ensure client compliance. If a client desires and truly believes in herbal medicine, some sort of collaborative health supervision may be the best solution for the client. Open discussion to enhance rapport and trust is a key ingredient for successful client-oriented care. One of the herbal medicine ingredients that is gaining tremendous popularity in the United States is ginseng (*Panax quinquefolius* and *P. ginseng*). Ginseng is used to raise stamina and power of thoughts, improve the tone of body organs, and increase longevity. The long-term properties of ginseng have been poorly researched. It is postulated, however, that long-term abuse of ginseng can cause hypertension. Other, but less frequently seen, side effects of ginseng include nervousness, sleeplessness, skin eruptions, morning diarrhea, and edema (Siegal, 1979). Nonetheless, despite the many hazards that have been alluded to, it should be understood that the majority of herbal products on the U.S. market are safe when properly used (Lamba, 1993).

In assessing the predictive factors of social context and ethnicity on childhood hepatitis B immunization status among Korean-American children in an urban area, Kim and Telleen (2001) found that the mother's history of adequate prenatal care was significantly related to immunization status. They found that major perceived barriers in accessing preventive health care were burdens of cost, language barrier, and difficulty in remembering the immunization schedule. Preventive health care providers must look beyond the mother's health beliefs and include beliefs and knowledge of the mother's social network.

BIOLOGICAL VARIATIONS

Body Size and Structure

Generally speaking, Korean Americans are shorter than other Americans. A direct correlation exists between age and height among Korean Americans: the older they are, the shorter they are (Molnar, 2006). This correlation exists because in the old days in Korea, meager living and lack of food prevented people from consuming enough nutritious food for growth (Overfield, 1995). Children born since the industrialization of Korea are considerably taller, although they are not as tall as children in the United States. Korean Americans have longer trunks and shorter lower extremities in general (Overfield, 1995). This may be attributable in part to genetic factors, but also from cultural habits. Koreans do not wear shoes in the house. They sit on *ondol* (hypocaust) floors that are generally heated from beneath by coal, called *yun-tan* (briquettes). Long years of sitting on the floor in a "Buddha" position prevents vertical blood circulation into the legs, which in turn prevents the legs from stretching and achieving adequate growth. Sitting also contributes to aches and weakening of the legs in many elderly Korean people because of the habitual stretching of thigh muscles above the knees (Overfield, 1995).

Adipose tissue deposition is less in Koreans than in Americans, which is largely a result of less fatty-food consumption. Shoulder-to-hip width is about the same in most Koreans (Overfield, 1995). For Korean-American women, breast-to-hip size is also about equal. Because of their small structure and body size, it is unusual for Korean-American women to wear large sizes of clothes.

Some Korean Americans tend to have less body hair than other Americans (Overfield, 1995). In fact, some Korean-American women do not have to shave their legs. Usually, hair that does appear on Korean Americans is not shaved because of the Confucian belief that such hair means good luck and that shaving it would be bad luck (Eshleman, 1992).

Skin Color

Koreans have a golden-brown skin tone as a result of a higher melanin composition in their skin (Molnar, 2006; Overfield, 1995). However, Korean Americans have a wide range of skin tones, mostly attributed to the degree of exposure to the sun. The majority of Korean and Korean-American infants have mongolian spots, which are dark pigmentations seen primarily in the posterior iliac crest and buttock areas (Overfield, 1995).

Enzymatic and Genetic Variations

A majority of Korean Americans have lactose intolerance because of a lack of lactase in the body. Thus, the Korean-American diet may not necessarily include milk. After consuming dairy products such as milk, cheese, or ice cream, some Korean Americans experience a feeling of bloating, frequent burping, abdominal cramping, diarrhea, and vomiting. Lactose intolerance is a relatively common condition and is found in approximately 90% of Orientals (Overfield, 1995).

Bone density among Korean Americans is lower than that in other Americans, creating a higher risk for osteoporosis (Ott, 1991). This low bone density is a result of both hereditary and dietary factors. Some of the risk factors for osteoporosis in Korean-American women include a thin, small bone frame and calcium intake of about half that of Western women (National Institutes of Health, 2002). Anemia is common among Koreans because of their predominantly vegetarian diet (Ott, 1991).

Koreans and Korean Americans tend to have a higher prevalence of insulin autoimmune syndrome (Uchigata et al., 1992). Insulin autoimmune syndrome is characterized by spontaneous hypoglycemia without evidence of exogenous insulin administration. High serum concentrations of total immunoactive insulin and presence of insulin autoantibodies in high titer are found (Uchigata et al., 1992).

Hantavirus disease, which is characterized by fever, headache, hemorrhagic manifestations, shock, and renal failure, can trace its origin to Korea (Levins et al., 1993) and is synonymous with Korean hemorrhagic fever with its high mortality. Although found in other parts of the world, this disease in Korea is much more severe. Treatment consists mainly in the use of careful fluid balance and circulatory support to prevent shock (Levins et al., 1993).

Diet

The Korean and Korean-American diets are known for high fiber content and spicy seasoning (Kim, Yu, Liu, Kim, & Kohrs, 1993). Two foods that have become synonymous with Korea are *kimchi* and *bulgogi* (Korea.net, 2007). *Kimchi* is a staple dish, eaten with every meal. A typical Korean meal consists of rice, soup, vegetables, meat or fish, and *kimchi*. *Kimchi* is a pungent, fermented dish consisting of salt-seasoned cabbage or turnips with garlic, green onions, ginger, red pepper, and shellfish (Korea.net, 2007). It is very nutritious and rich in vitamins, is an excellent source of fiber, and contains many of the nutrients and naturally occurring chemicals that can help combat certain forms of cancer. The combination of cabbage, garlic, and red chili peppers fermented with the other ingredients creates an ideal health food. To most Koreans, at home or abroad, a meal without *kimchi* is unthinkable (Korea.net, 2007). *Kimchi* is now found, increasingly, on supermarket shelves internationally.

Bulgogi, a marinated meat dish commonly known as "Korean barbecue," is extremely popular with Koreans and non-Koreans alike. *Bulgogi* is marinated in soy sauce, sesame, minced garlic, and other seasonings and cooked over a dome-shaped pan, often at the table. The grilled beef is eaten as is or wrapped in lettuce with garlic, green pepper, soybean, or red pepper paste. Chicken, lamb, squid, or octopus can also be cooked in this style, known as *bulgogi* barbecue. *Bulgogi* is tasty, healthy, and versatile (Korea.net, 2007). It can serve as a main course, hors d'oeuvre, or picnic item.

Koreans eat a great variety of vegetables and wild herbs, seasoned with various spices and aromatic herbs. Garlic, ginger, soy paste, soy sauce, and red pepper are favorite seasonings, and a liberal use of red pepper is what makes Korean food distinctively hot. Koreans eat only moderate amounts of protein and sugar, and fat intake is lower than in the typical American diet. Obesity is rare among Koreans.

Drug Interactions and Metabolism

Korean Americans, like other Asian Americans, metabolize alcohol by aldehyde dehydrogenase (Kudzma, 1992). This is in stark contrast to White Americans, who metabolize alcohol by the liver enzyme alcohol dehydrogenase. Since

Korean Americans tend to metabolize alcohol by aldehyde dehydrogenase, alcohol tends to work faster, causing circulatory and unpleasant effects, such as facial flushing and heart palpitations (Kudzma, 1992). Facial flushing occurs in 45% to 85% of Asian Americans after alcohol consumption (Kudzma, 1992).

Susceptibility to Disease

Because Korean Americans have a tendency to consume high amounts of carbohydrates, including vegetables and high-roughage foods, health alterations such as diverticulosis or inflammatory bowel diseases are uncommon (Song et al., 2010). Hypertension is the leading cardiovascular risk factor among elderly Korean Americans (Kim, Juon, Hill, Post, & Kim, 2001). Peptic ulcer disease is also common, which is due to the Korean-American's frequent consumption of spicy and salty food such as soybean mash sauce (*dwen jang*), soy sauce (*gan jang*), and hot pepper sauce (*ko choo jang*). Consumption of salty food traces back to earlier days, when refrigeration was unavailable and people were concerned about storing food for long times. Peppers were traditionally used for quick energy for the backbreaking labor of rice farming.

Cardiovascular Disease. Relatively few studies have been done regarding the cardiovascular risk factors among Asian Americans (Kim et al., 2001). Asian Americans are often excluded from clinical trials on various cardiovascular conditions because of the assumption that they do not have cardiovascular risk factors because of their body weight and tendency to follow diets of low animal fat. However, available data suggest more cardiovascular risk factors among Asian Americans than once thought, as a result of Koreans' lifestyle changes after coming to the United States (Lauderdale & Rathouz, 2000).

Klatsky and Armstrong (1991) examined 13,031 Asian people to determine if biological markers for cardiovascular risk factors existed. Findings from this study are suggestive that significant ethnic differences in risk factors exist and that health care professionals must target their public health efforts to reduce obesity, hypercholesterolemia, and hypertension among all Asian Americans. Findings from the study also suggest that smoking cessation among Asian-American women is imperative to reduce the potential for cardiovascular conditions (Klatsky & Armstrong, 1991).

Smoking. Smoking by men in Korea is a common thread in their social world and a prime component of Korean men's gender identity (Kim, Son, & Nam, 2005). Compared with their counterparts in Korea, Korean-American men show significantly decreased rates of both smoking and drinking. Increasingly, however, acculturated

Korean-American women are more likely to smoke and drink (Song et al., 2004). These reports of smoking changes among genders are very likely due in part to the stigmatization of smoking in the workplace (men) and the freedom of Korean-American women to smoke by choice without traditional family pressure to abstain.

Body Weight. It is true that Korean Americans do have lower body weight than Americans. However, there is a strong association between birthplace and years since immigration, which means that higher levels of body mass index were found in those U.S.-born and those who have been in the United States for a number of years (Lauderdale & Rathouz, 2000). Researchers (Klatsky & Armstrong, 1991; Yano et al., 1988) asserted that regardless of how low the blood cholesterol was, within 2 years of living in the United States, the blood cholesterol level of Asian Americans will go up to 200 mg/dL unless they continue to follow a diet similar to what they ate in their native land. Younger Korean Americans who have been living in the United States for at least 2 years and who are continuously exposed to diets high in animal fat must be checked for cardiovascular risk factors. Elderly Korean Americans who are set in their ways may be more prone to have salty vegetarian diets and must be monitored closely for cerebrovascular risk factors. When providing health teaching, health care professionals must remember that Korean Americans who were born in the United States may have the same risk factors as the rest of the U.S. population.

Korean Americans who are more acculturated consume more American food and less Korean food. American foods are adapted more at breakfast and Korean foods continue to dominate the dinner meal (Lee, Sobal, & Frongillo, 1999). Compared with their diets in Korea, Korean Americans generally increase their consumption of beef, dairy products, coffee, soft drinks, and bread, while decreasing their intake of fish, rice, and grains. However, the balance between carbohydrates and fat did not indicate dietary problems except for decreased intake of fiber and calcium.

Dietary factors contribute to the risk of developing metabolic syndrome. A study by Shin, Lim, Sung, Shin, and Kim (2009) indicated that those who consume more seaweed and oily food, as well as those whose eating habits include eating faster and frequent overeating, are associated with the risk of metabolic syndrome. There is a definite trend for the more acculturated Korean Americans to consume more Western food than the less acculturated Korean Americans. More acculturated Korean Americans tend to dine out more frequently and prepare less traditional Korean food at home (Park, Paik, Skinner, Ok, & Spindler, 2003).

HIV/AIDS. The number of Koreans being diagnosed with human immunodeficiency virus (HIV) infections and acquired immunodeficiency syndrome (AIDS)-related lymphoma is on the rise (Kim et al., 2008; Lee et al., 2010), but more than 90% of them are men; thus, Korean HIV/AIDS studies reflect the male population (Lee et al., 2009) and women are at high risk for heterosexual transmission of HIV. Korean women describe high levels of knowledge about HIV and AIDS risk factors, although they have less knowledge about transmission of the virus (Chang & Hill, 1996). Because the majority of HIV-infected women in Korea were infected by male sexual partners, early and active detection of HIV-positive men will facilitate earlier detection and prevention in women. In addition, HIV infection in Korea is primarily detected by voluntary testing with identification in public health centers. It is critical that the health care providers encourage voluntary testing for early detection to decrease the prevalence of HIV infection and AIDS progression (Lee et al., 2010). The level of HIV/AIDS knowledge among Korean adolescents is moderate (Yoo, Lee, Kwon, Chung, & Kim, 2005). Attitudes toward persons with HIV/AIDS are negative among both adolescents and women.

Communicable Disease. There are many communicable diseases such as malaria, dengue, filariasis, Japanese encephalitis, leishmaniasis, and plague, carried by various insects (Centers for Disease Control and Prevention [CDC], 2002). The reemergence of *Plasmodium vivax* malaria in South Korea in 1993, which peaked in 2000, put travelers on alert for a time (CDC, 2002). However, control programs, including early case detection and treatment, mass chemoprophylaxis of soldiers, and international financial aid to North Korea for malaria control, have been successful, and the situation is remarkably improved (Han et al., 2006).

Psychological Characteristics

Influenced by Confucian and Buddhist philosophy, Korean Americans are a very proud and independent people. Generally they do not ask for handouts in either the material or psychological realms. Korean Americans generally view psychological or psychiatric illness as shameful and do not usually reveal such afflictions to the public. In South Korea, mental patients may be locked in their rooms at home or left uncared for during the day when family members have gone to work (Kim, 1998). A number of mentally ill patients live alone when family members are unable to cope with the conflicts at home. In Korea there is a strong conflict between the preference for institutional care and an inability to address the volume of the need.

Hwa-byung (an ailment caused by pent-up resentment) is common among Korean Americans, particularly among elderly Korean females, and is categorized as a Korean culture-bound syndrome (Pang, 1990; Park, Kim, Kang, & Kim, 2001). *Hwa-byung* is believed to be caused by *han*—a bitter feeling, an unsatisfied desire, or a discontent caused by life's problems (Kudzma, 1992; Pang, 1990). Since Lee (1977) first studied *Hwa-byung* in 1977, studies related to this illness have increased. However, studies have usually focused on persons in psychiatric departments or clinics. These studies have revealed that *Hwa-byung* prevails in middle-aged, married women of lower socioeconomic status and lower educational background and in up to 11.9% of the population (Chi, Kim, Whang, & Cho, 1997; Moon, Kim, & Wang, 1988; Park, Min, & Lee, 1997). In a study by Park et al. (2001) in seven metropolitan areas and six provinces of Korea, 4.9% of women designated themselves as having had *Hwa-byung*. These researchers found rates of *Hwa-byung* were higher among women of low socioeconomic status, those living in rural areas, divorced or separated women, smokers, and drinkers. It is important that health care professionals appreciate the cultural lifeways in the pathogenesis of this illness and respond in a culturally sensitive manner (Park et al., 2001).

Kim (1995) notes that depression is higher among Korean Americans than in other ethnic groups and that problems associated with depression, such as family violence, substance abuse, and suicide, have sharply increased among Korean Americans during the immigration and acculturation process. Kim (1995) also suggests that lack of research on the cultural context of health behavior among Korean Americans has obstructed health care professionals from understanding mental health needs and has resulted in lack of culturally appropriate care.

Moon and Williams (1993) studied perceptions of elder abuse and help-seeking patterns among Korean American elderly women and noted that Korean Americans were substantially less likely to perceive a given situation as abusive than the African-American and Caucasian women studied. These subjects also differed significantly in intended use of formal and informal sources of help in the case of elder abuse.

Mental Health. Koreans have traditionally viewed mental illness as a family shame and stigma. Rather than actively seeking outside mental health treatment or resources, family members have cared for and protected their relatives suffering from a variety of mental health issues. Korean Americans, however, find themselves in an environment in which mental health is readily addressed through both individual and group approaches. Culturally relevant psychoeducational intervention has been found to be a useful treatment modality for mentally ill children of Korean Americans (Kim, Shin, & Carey, 1999). Family education

and community-based treatment programs can encourage Korean Americans to seek treatment for mental health challenges. Today's nurses can further acceptance of mental health treatment by Korean Americans by developing culturally relevant programs to achieve treatment needs (Donnelly, 2005).

Implications for Nursing Care

Korean-American clients may have food brought in by family members and friends while hospitalized. Some Korean Americans consider American food "too mushy," and many believe it has too many blended tastes. Knowledge of usual Korean diets will allow health care professionals to make informed choices about diet exchanges appropriate to the client's prescribed diet. For example, Korean clients on a bland or full liquid diet will gladly take, instead of orange juice and Jell-O, a rice soup and corn decoction, which complements the prescribed diet. Instead of strictly enforcing the prescribed diet and creating potential conflicts, mutual understanding can promote client cooperation with satisfactory outcomes.

Health care professionals must also remember that Koreans talk very little during mealtime because of the Confucian belief that the quality of the food should be appreciated in silence by concentrating on eating. Providing a quiet mealtime without interruption is vital and will enhance the client's nutritional intake.

Nursing caregivers should be aware that Korean Americans experience various levels of eating behavior changes as a result of cultural assimilation. Korean American dietary behavior will, however, differ by acculturation stage, and interventions should be tailored appropriately.

Nurses who attempt to develop a cultural appreciation of the Korean psyche can bring about more successful client outcomes, enhance family and institutional economics, and improve public attitudes toward our health care system. The nurse's alertness to indicators—some obvious, some subtle—can transcend Asian-Western cultural differences and create opportunities for more desirable physical and psychological results.

If a health-restoration regimen requires Korean American clients to consume milk or any other dairy products, lactose-free milk should be given. Comparable lactose-free food (such as tofu) can be substituted for dairy products.

Korean women tend to avoid sunlight to prevent their faces from becoming darker. They use parasols (*yang-san*) to avoid the sun and often use cosmetics to look lighter than their actual skin color. Most Korean women are sensitive about their skin color and allowing them in the medical setting to "fix" their faces to their satisfaction will ensure more positive client attitudes.

Because the development of insulin autoimmune syndrome is associated with a strong genetic predisposition, those Koreans who have insulin autoimmune syndrome should be instructed to carry sugar packs, chewing gum, or gumdrops with them at all times.

Calcium intake during childhood has long been related to bone density. Korean-American female clients of childbearing age should be encouraged to take calcium supplements to increase bone density. Compliance with their drug regimen must be monitored because Korean Americans have a tendency not to take prescribed medicines, if they do not have any obvious symptoms. Iron supplements should also be encouraged to prevent anemia.

For those with psychological or psychiatric problems, the best approach is to establish a relationship of trust with the client. Since Korean Americans are reluctant to reveal their feelings, time should be provided for them to sort through their problems. A consistent and caring approach will eventually cause the clients to open up and allow the health professionals to help them. If this approach is unsuccessful, they should be referred to appropriate psychiatric services. For the elderly, visits by a Korean of the same age group and background will often be the key to cooperation and problem solving. Mental health interventions should be approached with insight, empathy, and patience because of the long-standing negative attitude by Korean people toward mental illness (Kim, 1998).

SUMMARY

Korean Americans, like other Asian Americans, vary in their degree of acculturation. The nurse should recognize this diversity and remember that as much diversity is present as within any cultural group across racial, ethnic, and cultural lines. Some Korean Americans have developed cultural behaviors that are integral to their past and complementary to their present. Therefore, the nurse must develop a respect for the uniqueness of the individual. When the client is Korean American, illness or wellness behaviors should be considered from a cultural perspective so that culturally appropriate and competent care can be rendered.

CASE STUDY

A young Korean woman emigrated to the United States to pursue work and educational opportunities. A college graduate and nurse, she was granted a "green card" and had a job at the hospital in a major metropolitan area waiting for her. The now Korean-American nurse began assimilation upon arrival, making friends with American colleagues, buying a condo in a neighborhood, purchasing a car, and traveling when she could. She did not choose to live in the local "Koreatown" and associate socially with predominantly Koreans and retain a traditional diet. She acknowledged that since she chose to emigrate to the United States, she felt her future success would rely upon becoming a part of the United States' business and social environment and being accepted as "one of them."

Several years later, the young Korean woman, having risen in the nursing profession, having earned a doctorate, and having became a naturalized citizen, brought her 79-year-old widowed mother from Korea to live with her in the United States. The mother, an intelligent but shy woman, obviously was not thrilled with the cultural changes she was experiencing. Although fluent in Korean, Chinese, and Japanese, she had no interest in learning English, saying she was "too old." In spite of having her own bedroom and bath in her daughter's condo, she was quite isolated when the daughter was at work. The language barrier prevented her (or she prevented herself) from visiting local shops and parks or using public transportation. Depression became a factor and although her health was failing, she wanted to "go home." This was not an option because the Korean-American daughter was an only child and there was no one to go to in Korea. A Korean senior citizens group was located in a predominantly Korean part of the city and arrangements were made for transportation to two-per-week meetings of mostly older Korean ladies, who talked, cooked (Korean food), and did crafts for hours at a time. This, for a time, alleviated the mother's distress. However, medical problems began to demand her entry into the health care system.

The mother's first contact with health care began when the State's Department of Health demanded she travel to a clinic in another town for a tuberculosis tine test. She was reluctantly taken, processed, and seen by staff with no Korean-speaking capability and was literally pulled, poked, and prodded throughout the ordeal. This fertilized an already negative mindset concerning U.S. health care delivery. When hospitalization loomed, she dug in her heels, because culturally she viewed hospitalization as a one-way trip. The daughter, realizing all of the potential problems, met with hospital administrators and nursing management prior to admission to apprise them of the cultural situation and communication challenge. Upon

CASE STUDY—cont'd

arrival, a Korean-American clinical specialist met the mother and daughter, established rapport with the mother and accompanied her through processing and settling in. Her calm, respectful demeanor and language ability turned a potentially stressful situation into a calming, attitude-adjusting experience and garnered the mother's full cooperation. Nursing staff made small diet adjustments recommended by the daughter and courtesy flowed both ways. Dispensing of medicines was done calmly and accepting meds was tempered by the new accepting attitude. Doctors' conversations with the mother were usually accomplished with the daughter or a Korean-American staffer present. The cultural abyss was bridged through prior planning, communication, professional and courteous staff attitudes, and a caring atmosphere, which adjusted the Korean client's outlook from reluctance and stress to one of trust and compliance. Cultural perspective appropriately applied contributes immensely to positive outcomes.

◎ CARE PLAN

Nursing Diagnosis: Communication, impaired verbal, related to inability to speak dominant language

Client Outcome	Nursing Interventions
Effective communication between provider and family will be established.	1. Establish rapport with family members. 2. Assess family members' understanding of client's condition. 3. Encourage expression of feelings. 4. Support attempts to improve communication. 5. Assist in correction of faulty perceptions. 6. Speak slowly and in an unhurried manner. 7. Use translators to facilitate communication.

Nursing Diagnosis: Coping, ineffective individual, related to situational crisis, guilt, and faulty perceptions

Client Outcomes	Nursing Interventions
1. Client will verbalize need for more information or clearer understanding relating to the situation. 2. Client will demonstrate understanding of health status and verbalize any concerns.	1. Involve other family members in care of client as much as possible. 2. Clarify misconceptions. 3. Expand social networks. 4. Seek to understand client's perspective of situation. 5. Encourage expression of fear of information given.

CLINICAL DECISION MAKING

1. What are the two cultural values, beliefs, and practices unique to Korean Americans that affect health care?
2. Of which biological variations among Korean Americans should the nurse be aware?
3. How does culture affect illness and wellness behaviors exhibited by some Korean-American clients?
4. How can the nurse transcend a language barrier when a Korean-American client does not speak English?

REVIEW QUESTIONS

1. In meeting the dietary needs of Korean-American clients who practice the Confucian belief related to the appreciation of food quality, the nurse should attend to which of the following?
   a. Provide a quiet mealtime without interruption.
   b. Provide a well-balanced diet.
   c. Permit food brought in by family member.
   d. Provide for including rice in various forms.
2. The nurse is developing a plan of care to increase bone density for a Korean-American client, which should include a diet that contains which of the following?
   a. High in vitamin D
   b. High in vitamin C
   c. With milk and other dairy products
   d. With lactose-free milk and foods
3. When communicating with a Korean-American client, it is important for the nurse to apply filial piety, which includes which of the following?
   a. The nurse speaking slowly
   b. The nurse speaking loudly
   c. The nurse using a sincere appearance of attentive listening
   d. The nurse using hand gestures to emphasize the topic

REFERENCES

Ameredia (2010). *Korean American demographics.* Available at <http://www.ameredia.com/resources/demographics/korean.html> Retrieved September 23, 2010.

Asian and Pacific Islander American Health Forum (2010). *Ethnic health assessment for Asian Americans, Native Hawaiians, and Pacific Islanders in California.* Available at <http://www.jabsom.hawaii.edu/native/docs/publications/2010/Ethnic_Health_Assessment_for_Asian_Americans,_NHs,_&_PIs_in_California_8-10.pdf> Retrieved September 25, 2011.

Buzzle.com (2010). *Facts about South Korea.* Available at <http://www.buzzle.com/articles/facts-about-south-korea.html> Retrieved September 21, 2010.

Blumeson, M. (2010). Lessons learned: reviewing the Korean War. *ARMY: Association of United States Army Magazine, 60*(7), 59–64.

Centers for Disease Control and Prevention (CDC) (2002). *Malaria information for travelers to East Asia.* Available at <http://www.cdc.gov/travel/regionalmalaria/eastasia.htm> Retrieved June 17, 2002.

Central Intelligence Agency (CIA) (2011). *World factbook.* New York: Skyhorse.

Chang, K. (1999). Chinese Americans. In J. Giger & R. Davidhizar (Eds.), *Transcultural nursing: assessment and intervention.* St. Louis: Mosby.

Chang, S., & Hill, M. (1996). HIV/AIDS related knowledge, attitudes and preventive behavior of pregnant Korean women. *Image, 28*(4), 321–324.

Chi, S., Kim, J., Whang, W., & Cho, H. (1997). The study of the clinical aspects of Hwa-byung patients. *Journal of Oriental Neuropsychiatry, 8*(2), 63–84.

Choi, E. (1986). Unique aspects of Korean-American mothers. *Journal of Obstetric, Gynecologic, and Neonatal Nursing, 15*(5), 394–400.

Clark, D. N. (2000). *Culture and customs of Korea.* Westport, CT: Greenwood.

CNN.com (2007). Available at <http://www.cnn.com/2007/WORLD/asiacf/07/18/north.korea.inspectors.reut/index.html?iref=newsresearch> Retrieved August 14, 2007.

Crittenden, K., Fugita, S., Bae, H., Lamug, C. B., & Un, C. (1992). A cross-cultural study of self-report depressive symptoms among college students. *Journal of Cross-Cultural Psychology, 23*(2), 163–178.

Dodd, C. (1987). *Dynamics of intercultural communication* (2nd ed.). New York: W. C. Brown.

Donnelly, P. L. (2005). Mental health beliefs and help seeking behaviors of Korean American parents of adult children with schizophrenia. *Journal of Multicultural Nursing & Health,* 43–53.

Eshleman, J. (1992). Death with dignity: significance of religious beliefs and practices in Hinduism, Buddhism, and Islam. *Today's OR Nurse,* 19–20.

Fisher, N. E. (1996). *Cultural and ethnic diversity: a guide for genetics professionals.* Baltimore: Johns Hopkins University Press.

Giger, J., Davidhizar, R., & Wieczorek, S. (1993). In I. Bobak & M. Jensen (Eds.), *Maternity and gynecological care* (5th ed., pp. 43–67). St. Louis: Mosby.

Hall, E. T. (1966). *The silent language.* New York: Doubleday.

Han, E. T., et al. (2006). Reemerging vivax malaria: changing patterns of annual incidence and control programs in the Republic of Korea. *The Korean Journal of Parasitology, 44*(4), 285–294.

Harlan, C. (2011). North Korea likely to use collective leadership. *Washington Post,* December 21, 2011.

Hurh, W., & Kim, K. (1990). Adaptation and mental health of Korean male immigrants. *International Migration Review, 24*(3), 456–470.

Hwang, I. (2000). *Bang Yak Hap Pyun.* Seoul: Yam Lim.

Infoplease.com (2010). Available at <http://www.Infoplease.com/Ipa/A0107690.html> Retrieved September 12, 2011.

Jo, M. H. (1999). *Korean immigrants and the challenge of adjustment*. Westport, CT: Greenwood.

Juon, H. S., Kim, M., Shankar, S., & Han, W. (2004). Predictors of adherence to screening mammography among Korean American women. *Preventive Medicine*, 39(3), 474–481.

Kaltsounis, T., & Shin, S. (1988). South Korea: a country on the move. *Social Studies*, 79(4), 137–139.

Kim, S. K. (1992). Korean elderly women in America: everyday life, health, and illness. *Journal of Asian Studies*, 402–404.

Kim, M. (1995). Cultural influences on depression in Korean Americans. *Journal of Psychosocial Nursing*, 33(2), 13–18.

Kim, S. (1998). Out of darkness. *Reflections/Sigma Theta Tau*, 3, 7–9.

Kim, M. T., Juon, H. S., Hill, M. N., Post, W., & Kim, K. B. (2001). Cardiovascular disease risk factors in Korean American elderly. *Western Journal of Nursing Research*, 23(3), 269–282.

Kim, J. S., et al. (2008). Report of AIDS-related lymphoma in South Korea. *Japanese Journal of Clinical Oncology*, 38(2), 134–139.

Kim, Y., Shin, J., & Carey, M. P. (1999). Comparison of Korean-American adoptees and biological children of their adoptive parents: a pilot study. *Child Psychiatry and Human Development*, 29(3), 221–228.

Kim, S. S., Son, H., & Nam, K. A. (2005). The sociocultural context of Korean American men's smoking behavior. *Western Journal of Nursing Research*, 27(5), 604–623, comment 624–627.

Kim, Y., & Telleen, S. (2001). Predictors of hepatitis B immunization status in Korean American children. *Journal of Immigrant Health*, 3(4), 181–192.

Kim, K., Yu, E., Liu, W., Kim, J., & Kohrs, M. B. (1993). Nutritional status of Chinese, Korean, and Japanese American elderly. *Journal of American Dietetic Association*, 1416–1422.

Klatsky, A., & Armstrong, M. (1991). Cardiovascular risk factors among Asian Americans living in Northern California. *American Journal of Public Health*, 81(11), 1423–1428.

Korean American Journal (2002). News on Korean Americans. FL: Valrico, C3.

Korean Cultural Service (2006). *New York*. Available at <http://www.koreanculture.org/> Retrieved July 26, 2007.

Korea.net (2007). *Exploring Korea*. Available at <http://korea.net/exploring.do> Retrieved September 24, 2011.

Korean Overseas Informational Service (1993). *The Koreans*. Seoul: Jung Min SaMun Hwa Co.

Korean Overseas Informational Service (1996). *Korea: its history and culture*. Seoul: Jung Min SaMun Hwa Co.

Korean Overseas Informational Service (1997). *Korean cultural heritage*. Seoul: Jung Min SaMun Hwa Co.

Korean Times, Florida (2002). Altamonte Springs, FL: Update on Korean Americans, C2.

Kudzma, E. (1992). Drug interactions: all bodies are not created equal. *American Journal of Nursing*, 92, 48–50.

Kwon, S. Y. (2006). Grief ministry as homecoming: framing death from a Korean-American perspective. *Pastoral Psychology*, s11089–s12005.

Lamba, S. (1993). Be careful with herbal medicines. *Tallahassee Democrat*, D4.

Lauderdale, D. S., & Rathouz, P. J. (2000). Body mass index in a US national sample of Asian Americans: effects of nativity, years since immigration and socioeconomic status. *International Journal of Obesity and Related Metabolic Disorders: Journal of the International Association for the Study of Obesity*, 24(9), 1188–1194.

Lee, S. (1977). A study of the Hwa-byung (anger syndrome). *Journal of Korea General Hospital*, 1(1), 63–69.

Lee, J. H. (1988). Features of Korean history. *Social Studies*, 79(4), 147–152.

Lee, J. H., et al. (2010). Increasing late diagnosis in HIV infection in South Korea: 2000–2007. *BMC Public Health*, 10, 411.

Lee, J. H., Lee, E. J., Kim, S. S., Nam, J. G., Whang, J., & Kee, M. K. (2009). Epidemiological characteristics of HIV-infected women in the Republic of Korea: a low HIV prevalence country. *Journal of Public Health Policy*, 30(3), 342–355.

Lee, S., Sobal, J., & Frongillo, E. (1999). Acculturation and dietary practices among Korean Americans. *Journal of the American Dietetic Association*, 99(9), 1084–1089.

Levins, R., Epstein, P. R., Wilson, M. E., Morse, S. S., Slooff, R., & Eckardt, I. (1993). Hantavirus disease emerging. *Lancet*, 342(8802), 1292.

Lin, K. (1983). Hwa-byung: a Korean cultural bound syndrome? *American Journal of Psychiatry*, 140, 105–107.

Manderson, L. (1987). Hot-cold food and medical theories: overview and introduction. *Social Science and Medicine*, 25(4), 329–330.

Mangiafico, L. (1988). *Contemporary American immigrants: patterns of Filipino, Korean, and Chinese settlement in the United States*. Westport, CT: Praeger.

Messaris, P., & Woo, J. S. (1991). Image vs. reality in Korean Americans' responses to mass-mediated depictions of the United States. *Critical Studies in Mass Communication*, 8, 74–90.

Min, P. G. (1995). *Asian Americans: contemporary trends and issues*. Thousand Oaks, CA: Sage.

Min, P. G. (2006). *Asian Americans: contemporary trends and issues* (2nd ed.). Thousand Oaks, CA: Pine Forge Press.

Molnar, S. C. (2006). *Human variations: races, types, and ethnic groups* (2nd ed.). Englewood Cliffs, NJ: Prentice Hall.

Moon, A., & Williams, O. (1993). Perceptions of elder abuse and help-seeking patterns among African-American, Caucasian American, and Korean-American elderly women. *The Gerontologist*, 33(3), 386–395.

Moon, C., Kim, J., & Wang, W. (1988). The bibliographical study on stress and Hwa. *Journal of Korean Oriental Internal Medicine*, 9(1), 153–159.

Moon, S., & Pearl, J. (1991). Alienation of elderly Korean American immigrants as related to place of residence, age, years of education, time in U.S., living with or without children, living with or without a spouse. *International Journal of Aging and Human Development, 32*(2), 115–124.

National Institute of Health Osteoporosis and Related Bone Disease, National Resources Center (NIH-ORBD-NRC) (2002). Washington, DC: U.S. Government Printing Office.

Ott, S. M. (1991). Bone density in adolescents. *New England Journal of Medicine, 325*(23), 1646–1647.

Overfield, T. (1995). *Biological variations in health and illness: race, age, and sex differences* (7th ed.). New York: CRC.

Pang, K. Y. (1989). The practice of traditional Korean medicine in Washington, D.C. *Social Science and Medicine, 28*(8), 875–884.

Pang, K. Y. (1990). Hwa-byung: the construction of a Korean popular illness among Korean elderly immigrant women in the United States. *Culture, Medicine and Psychiatry, 14*, 495–512.

Park, Y. (1988). The geography of Korea. *Social Studies, 79*(4), 141–145.

Park, Y., Kim, H., Kang, H., & Kim, J. (2001). A survey of Hwa-byung in middle-age Korean women. *Journal of Transcultural Nursing, 12*(2), 115–122.

Park, J., Min, S., & Lee, M. (1997). A study on the diagnosis of Hwa-byung. *Journal of Korean Neuropsychiatry Association, 36*(3), 496–502.

Park, S., Paik, H., Skinner, J., Ok, S. W., & Spindler, A. A. (2003). Mothers' acculturation and eating behaviors of Korean families in California. *Journal of Nutrition Education and Behavior, 35*(3), 142–147.

Park, K., & Peterson, L. (1991). Beliefs, practices, and experiences of Korean women in relation to childbirth. *Health Care for Women International, 12*, 261–269.

Pourat, N., Lubben, J., Wallace, S., & Moon, A. (1999). Predictors of use of traditional Korean healers among elderly Koreans in Los Angeles. *The Gerontologist, 39*(6), 711–719.

Pritham, U., & Sammons, L. (1993). Korean women's attitudes toward pregnancy and prenatal care. *Health Care for Women International, 14*, 145–153.

Shin, A., Lim, S. Y., Sung, J., Shin, H. R., & Kim, J. (2009). Dietary intake, eating habits, and metabolic syndrome in Korean men. *Journal of the American Dietetic Association, 109*(4), 633–640.

Siegal, R. K. (1979). Ginseng abuse syndrome: problems with the pancreas. *Journal of the American Medical Association, 24*(15), 614.

Simmons, C., Klopf, D., & Park, M. (1991). Loneliness among Korean and American university students. *Psychological Reports, 68*(3), 754.

Song, Y. S., et al. (2004). Acculturation and health risk behaviors among Californians of Korean descent. *Preventive Medicine, 39*(1), 147–156.

Song, J. H., et al. (2010). Clinical characteristics of colonic diverticulitis in Korea. A prospective study. *Korean Journal Internal Medicine, June 25*(2), 140–146.

Tien-Hyatt, T. L. (1987). Keying in on the unique care needs of Asian clients. *Nursing and Health Care, 8*(5), 268–271.

Time Almanac (2011). Boston: Information Please, Inc.

Uchigata, Y., et al. (1992). Strong association of insulin autoimmune syndrome with HLA-DR4. *Lancet, 339*, 393–394.

U.S. Department of Commerce, Bureau of the Census (2000). *The Asian population 2000.* Washington, DC: U.S. Government Printing Office.

U.S. Department of Commerce, Bureau of the Census (2009). *American community survey, Koreans.* Washington, DC: U.S. Government Printing Office.

U.S. Department of Commerce, Bureau of the Census (2013). *American community survey.* Washington, DC: U.S. Government Printing Office.

U.S. Department of Commerce, Bureau of the Census (2015). *American community survey.* Washington, DC: U.S. Government Printing Office.

U.S. Department of State (2010). *Background note: South Korea.* Available at <http://www.state.gov/r/pa/ei/bgn/2800.htm> Retrieved September 20, 2010.

Van Decar, P. (1988). Teaching about Korea in secondary school. *Social Studies, 79*(4), 177–193.

World Almanac. (2011). New York: World Almanac Books.

Yano, K., et al. (1988). A comparison of the 12-year mortality and predictive factors of coronary heart disease among Japanese men in Japan and Hawaii. *American Journal of Epidemiology, 127*, 476–487.

Yoo, H., Lee, S. H., Kwon, B. E., Chung, S., & Kim, S. (2005). HIV/AIDS knowledge, attitudes, related behaviors and sources of information among Korean adolescents. *The Journal of School Health, 75*(10), 393–399.

23

French Canadians of Québec Origin

Mary Reidy

BEHAVIORAL OBJECTIVES

After reading this chapter, the nurse will be able to:

1. Understand the communication patterns and the dialectal variations of the French-Canadian people of Québec.
2. Describe the spatial needs, distance, and intimacy behaviors of the French-Canadian people of Québec.
3. Describe the time orientation and effects on treatment regimens of the French-Canadian people of Québec.
4. Describe the social organization of family systems among the French-Canadian people of Québec.
5. Identify the illness, wellness, and health-seeking behaviors of the French Canadians of Québec.
6. Identify beliefs, practices, and healers unique to the health value systems of the French Canadians of Québec.
7. Identify susceptibility of the French-Canadian people of Québec to specific disease or illness conditions.

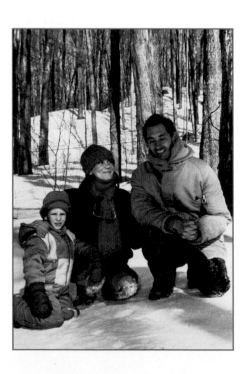

OVERVIEW OF QUÉBECERS

The people of Québec represent a rich cultural heritage of French settlers, native Canadians, as well as Scottish, Irish, English, and other immigrants from around the world. Québec (English /kwuh-bek'/, French /kay-bek'/, from the Micmac *kepek*, "narrows") is the only society in North America with a preponderance of French speakers (francophones). The early French settlers referred to themselves first as *Canadians* and later as *French Canadians* in order to differentiate themselves from British and other immigrants, who also began referring to themselves as Canadians. Today, the descendants of these French colonists call themselves "Québécois" (Québecer), and the term *French Canadian* has been largely replaced by *Québécois de souche*, designating "old-stock" Québecer (Québec Government Portal: Society, 2002a). The Québecers' social identity is the result of their cultural and geographic history, its congruence with personal history, contiguity with other Québecers, a common language, and the sentiment of the right to exist as an entity—an essential factor in the planning and providing of culturally appropriate care (Davidhizar & Giger, 2000; Gohier & Schleifer, 1993).

PROVINCE OF QUÉBEC

Québec, the largest of the 10 Canadian provinces, encompasses about one sixth of the Canadian landmass and is so vast that it could accommodate the United Kingdom five times over. Reaching almost to the Arctic Circle, it takes in the territory north of the Ottawa and St. Lawrence rivers. To the south of the St. Lawrence, it takes in the lowlands as far as the U.S. border, as well as the Gaspé Peninsula projecting into the Gulf of St. Lawrence. The borders are with Labrador, Newfoundland, and New Brunswick in the east; the American states of Vermont and New York in the south; and Ontario and Hudson Bay in the west. The province's lifeline, the St. Lawrence River, approaching 750 miles in length, together with the St. Lawrence Seaway, forms a direct link between the Atlantic Ocean and the Great Lakes. Because of this geographical location, Québec possesses three climate zones: humid continental in the central southern areas (warm summers, cold winters), subarctic farther to the north, and arctic in the far northern regions (long, cold winters; short, cool summers) (*World Almanac*, 2015).

The estimated population of Canada in 2011 was 33,476,688; the population of Québec was reported as 8.18 million with an annual mean growth rate of 4.7% (Institut de la statistique de Québec, 2013a); the median age of the population was 41.9 years; and by 2013 the immigrant population was estimated at 12.5% of the population

(Santé et Services sociaux de Québec, 2013). The province is home to some 73,000 native people, including 64,000 Canadian Indians from 11 aboriginal nations and 9000 Inuit people (Québec Government Portal: Society, 2002b). The total number of people residing in Quebec is 7,903,001.

The People and Culture of French Québec

While New France was claimed by Jacques Cartier in 1534, the actual settlement began in 1604. Québec traces its cultural origins to the Catholic colonists who came from Normandy and west central France and to the French explorers and traders who soon penetrated beyond the Great Lakes to the prairies (McGovern, 2002). Conflict between England and France, climaxing in the Seven Years' War (1756–1763), ended with a conquest by England. The colonists of New France formed bonds with the indigenous Huron and developed ties with the arriving Scottish traders, farmers, and merchants. In the years that followed, an agricultural-, family-, and church-oriented culture evolved that had a high degree of homogeneity and rapidly became differentiated from the French culture (Québec Government Portal: Society, 2002b; Rioux, 1974).

With power in the hands of England and extensive British immigration, the urban centers of Montréal and Québec City became predominantly English speaking. While the language of commerce was English and the British controlled business and trade until the mid-nineteenth century, agriculture, law, and medicine proved to be the primary professions of the French in the province. Large-scale Scottish migration in the eighteenth and nineteenth centuries contributed literate and skilled immigrants to the growing population (Herman, 2001). Further, a poor potato crop in Ireland, causing a widespread famine, prompted another wave of immigrants. A cholera epidemic at the peak of the immigration took numerous lives, resulting in many Irish children arriving as orphans. Although they were assimilated through adoption by French-speaking families, they often kept their own names, which explains names such as McNeill and Ryan among today's French-speaking population. More recent waves of immigration have added a further dimension of sociocultural complexity (Labrie, 1990; Tétu de Labsade, 1990).

In 2011, Québec welcomed 49,490 immigrants, more than half between the ages of 25 and 44 and with university education (Institut de la statistique de Québec, 2013). These included professionals, entrepreneurs, or workers; some were rejoining family members, and others (about 20%) were refugees. While most came from French-speaking countries like France, Morocco, Algeria, Congo, and Haiti, others were from China, the former Soviet republics, Romania, Sri Lanka, India, Pakistan, the former Yugoslavia, and Libya. Only about 15% of these immigrants chose to reside outside the Montréal area. Although overt and organized racism or extreme marginalization of Québec's ethnic minorities is rare, certain social, cultural, and racial barriers on one side, and resistance to total integration on the other, slow complete integration (McAndrew & Potvin, 1996). While Québec feels the duty to accommodate new immigrants, the "niqab" has become a flash point in the debate about the price such accommodation will cost society, as well as the focal point of a policy of the Québec Human Rights Commission restricting its use where identification is required (Scott, 2010).

POLITICAL DEVELOPMENT

After the English conquest, the political system of Canada took on the form of a parliamentary democracy, with the Crown as head of state. In 1867, the British North America Act established Canada as a federal state, with strong central powers. The federal government shares legal, fiscal, and social powers with the provinces. Criminal and international law are under federal jurisdiction in conformity with the British common law tradition. The provinces retain the power to enact civil legislation affecting private property, social welfare, and health. The Québec civil code, recently revised in detail rather than in spirit, is unique as it was inspired by French legal tradition.

Quiet Revolution

In the years after World War II, Québec underwent a rapid transition from a rural to an urban technological society. Starting in the 1950s, the control of political institutions and business enterprises shifted into the hands of French-speaking Québecers (Bouchard, 1992). However, well into the 1960s, Québecers were oriented to family and to the church. The latter, in Catholic Québec, not only dictated mores and behavior and served as the major social and health resource but also participated actively in political affairs. The so-called Quiet Revolution resulted in social, political, and behavioral transformations as extensive as any produced by violent revolution. Secularization resulted in changes in structure and power rather than in function or values. The state assumed control of schools, health care, and welfare programs.

Moreover, the Quiet Revolution stimulated feelings of nationalism and led to legislation to protect language and culture. The movement in favor of the political independence of Québec from Canada was also fueled, contributing to a charged emotional climate between those "for" and those "against" separatism and augmenting tensions between provincial and federal governments. Separatist sentiments peaked in the referendum on secession in October 1995, which rejected separatism by a narrow margin. Although the issue has remained on the political agenda, many Québecers feel that it is time to make the best of the current constitutional status and to redirect concerns to economic, health, and education priorities (CBC, 2010). However, 50 years after the Quiet Revolution, young English-speaking Québecers want to learn French and to live and work in Québec (Johnston, 2010).

Economy

The profound change in the politico-economy was associated with more families needing two sources of income to maintain living standards, women with higher education pursuing careers, a decline in the birthrate, and an increase in the number of the elderly (Lanthier & Rousseau, 1992). By 2010 in Québec, while there was no significant change in the number of women in traditionally female jobs (e.g., nursing), women were beginning to make inroads into male-dominated professions (e.g., medicine). In the greater Montréal area, more than half the jobs in the financial and business sector were filled by women, with a decline in women in senior management over a 10-year period (O'Donnell et al., 2006).

The Québec Employers Council on Prosperity reports that Québec currently faces an economic challenge (in terms of gross domestic product as compared with 34 other provinces and countries, Québec ranked twentieth). It is well positioned concerning university graduation, taxation on investments, spending on research, and the development of sustainable natural resources such as hydroelectric power, but it was rated less strongly in relation to certain areas such as economic integration of immigrants and public debt (Centre for Sustainable Living Standards, 2015; Dorval, 2010). However, since 2004, inflation has ranged annually between 0.6% and 2.3%. With a mean annual increase in the consumer price index of 1.6%, Québec knows greater price stability than 155 of the 160 countries for which the statistic was available (Centre for Sustainable Living Standards, 2015; Institut de la statistique de Québec, 2013).

Health Care

Catholic religious orders brought health care and hospitals to New France and were responsible for training many generations of nurses. Protestant religious groups and Scottish-trained physicians provided for the health of the English-speaking populace. The latter were influential in the development of scientific medicine and hospital organization in Québec and throughout the rest of Canada. In 1969, the province put into place a medical insurance program, followed in 1970 by the development of a network of social services (Anctil & Bluteau, 1986). By law, health care is offered by public access to hospitals, local community health centers, and affiliated community agencies, as well as to centers for residential and extended care, child and youth protection, and rehabilitation. In addition, a public insurance program for prescribed medications is in place for Québecers without private coverage (Québec Government Portal: Health, 2002a). Moreover, private care providers (e.g., medical imaging clinics) thrive in various urban centers (Derfel, 2005). Currently practicing in the province, there are 2.13 doctors per 1000 inhabitants, of whom approximately half are general practitioners (Institut de la statistique de Québec, 2013). However, the 10th Annual Canadian Medical Association Poll reports that, although the system delivers values for the financial investment, Québecers feel a certain dissatisfaction with overall quality of care that could be ameliorated by greater availability of family doctors, and that many fear that the demographic bulge of the ageing baby boomers requires reorganization of the system if it is to provide the health care wanted and needed (Fidelman, 2010).

Ordre des infirmières et infirmiers du Québec (OIIQ) supervises schools of nursing and professional practice, registers nurses, and carries out inspections of nursing practice in hospitals and community health centers. According to this association, 68,754 nurses (mean age: 42.3 years) are registered in Québec, 84% of whom report permanent employment and approximately two thirds of these working full time (OIIQ, 2010b). Intense movement is under way to ensure the baccalaureate degree as entry into practice, and currently 44.7% have university preparation; the others for the most part come from a collegial system, with hospital schools of nursing having been closed for many years (OIIQ, 2010c).

During the past years, the province has been involved in health care reform and a shift to ambulatory care, with the concurrent problems of high costs and shortages of staff and hospital beds. However, such reforms have increased professionalization in nursing practice and more autonomous roles in patient/family education (Reidy, 2005). Given current health care requirements, additional spaces have been opened in basic nursing programs, and the Ministry of Health has offered both substantial bursaries to augment advance nursing practice preparation in the universities and has announced the opening of 500 positions for advanced nurse practitioners within the health system (McCallum, 2010a; OIIQ, 2010b).

The OIIQ is also a leader in the promotion of a contemporary vision of nursing care that is professional, clinical, and evolving (e.g., in the development of new roles for an increased number of nurse practitioners and clinical specialists, in redefining the nurse role augmented by shared medical acts, or participating in team care) (Allard

& Durand, 2006; Laflame, 2010; OIIQ, 2009, 2010a, 2010b). A number of recent studies have also contributed to the development and validation of advanced nursing practice. These include a study by Murray, Reidy, and Carnevale (2010), which examined the process of conceptualization by future stakeholders of a new nurse practitioner's role in a pediatric emergency setting; they saw it having an essential clinical focus and themselves as active participants in both its development and implementation. Another such study performed by Dias, Chambers-Evans, and Reidy (2010) focused on how the consultation role of the clinical specialist emerged in an active care setting; it also included managing crises situations, ensuring continuity of care, and supporting other professionals, but it required constant clarification in the context of the clinical situation and the evolution of the system.

Education

During the nineteenth and most of the twentieth centuries, free schooling was provided to the eighth grade, and high schools and colleges were private, maintained for the most part by Catholic or Protestant religious groups. In 1943, attendance became compulsory in the Canadian school system. In 1960 and 1961, a series of laws was enacted that provided free universal education through the eleventh grade and compulsory education to 15 years of age (Audet & Gauthier, 1967). System restructuring led to a network of free postsecondary junior colleges; universities provided 3-year undergraduate programs, as well as graduate and professional education. School boards were originally organized according to religion, with Catholic and Protestant boards operating schools in both French and English. In 1993, the Supreme Court of Canada upheld the constitutionality of a 1988 law that reformed governance of school boards along linguistic rather than religious lines. By 2004 such reorganization had been completed throughout the province. Today, private schools, which may be religious or secular, coexist with the public system. Organizational school reform has centered on devolution of powers based on a philosophy of school-based autonomy, accountability, and parental involvement. Although concomitant curriculum reform focuses on competencies to enable students to acquire skills and adjust to a fast-changing world, the effects of the such efforts, as well as those directed to the integration of "at-risk" groups (such as non–French-speaking immigrants or children with learning needs) are still being determined (Branswell, 2010). However, level of schooling continues to improve; the number of Québecers with a university diploma rose from 12% in 1990 to 23% in 2009, and the proportion of those without a high school diploma dropped from 38% to 16% (Santé et Services sociaux de

Québec, 2013). More specifically, by proportion of the population, 7.8% held an advanced university degree; 18.1% held a bachelor's degree; 3.5% held a university certificate below the bachelor's level; 20.2% held a certificate or diploma college or CEGEP; 17.4% held a certificate or diploma of a trade school; 19.5% held a high school diploma; and 13.5% had no diploma (Institut de la statistique de Québec, 2013).

COMMUNICATION

Language and Culture

The French-Canadian people of Québec are a linguistic minority in North America and, as such, fear the eventual loss of their cultural identity. Despite their ongoing efforts to preserve the distinct nature of the French-speaking culture, they are bombarded by pervasive American political and cultural influences exerted through various media, including film, radio, television, magazines, and recordings (Labrie, 1990; Lamonde, 1991). The use of the Internet poses a particular dilemma in the reconciliation of international science and business with the protection of linguistic identity (MSNBC, 2000).

A charter (*Charte des Droits et des Lois*), which established French as Québec's official language, was established to protect Québec's language, culture, and identity (McKenzie, 2002). These laws have enabled the French language to prosper and promoted the use of French among newly arrived immigrants and within commercial enterprises and public institutions. Several organizations have been created to monitor and encourage the use of French—for example, the Commission for the Protection of the French Language, which handles complaints concerning the unavailability of health or social services by French-speaking clients, and the Office of the French Language, which is charged with maintaining the quality of the French language and administering French competency tests to individuals entering the health (and other) professions (Gouvernement de Québec, 2002).

French

French is the everyday language of most of the people of Québec and the foundation of their cultural identity. The language brought from the old country was shaped and refined for two centuries from an amalgam of accents and expressions of various regions of France, with the assimilation of American Indian words designating places, lakes, flora, and fauna. In speaking this language, the *r*s can be rolled, and long vowels, *t*s and *d*s can slide into certain front vowels with a postconsonantal *s* sound (Tétu de Labsade, 1990).

With the migration of rural populations to the cities and the common use of English in the workplace, a popular level of language often referred to as *joual* (literally, "stock of an anchor") was created. This type of speech, reserved for oral communication, incorporates English words into a syntax and grammatical system that is essentially French (Tétu de Labsade, 1990). The resulting speech patterns are, at times, quite remote from the standard French used by intellectuals, writers, and those in the media. In 2013, French was the native language of 99.3% of the population of Québec as compared with 21.1% in the rest of Canada (Institut de la statistique de Québec, 2013). Some 30% of the urban population is bilingual, speaking both French and English. Another 35 languages are spoken in the province, including Italian, Greek, Chinese, Native Indian dialects, Inuit, Slavic, Spanish, Chinese, Vietnamese, Persian, and Tamil (STATS Canada, 2015). Immigrants usually learn French as a second language and frequently learn English as a third language. However, the more than 50% non–French-speaking immigrants arriving yearly tax the process of integration into the French-speaking society (McKenzie, 2002).

Communication Behavior

As the French language evolved, so did the behavioral patterns of its speakers. For example, there is a tendency to use the familiar pronoun *tu* (you) soon after a first meeting or being introduced to someone—a habit frowned on in France (Tétu de Labsade, 1990). Québecers are warm-hearted people who express their thoughts and opinions openly, are expressive, and use their hands for emphasis when speaking. However, they do not use as many nonverbal movements as the Italians, Spaniards, or the continental French. They enjoy the interaction of social gatherings, celebrate important dates, have a quick sense of humor, and enjoy conversation and discourse. When these individuals are married with young children, they tend to associate with others in similar life situations. They express themselves in the performance, visual, and written arts; cinematography and television production flourish, along with theater, dance, and music; and events such as the yearly jazz festival have become international. Local artists not only are influenced by cultures from all over the world but also are becoming appreciated internationally.

Conversation on subjects having to do with community, day-to-day life, and children, composed of modern multimedia sources exist where people of both sexes discuss celebrities, politics, art, or world events. Modern media allows such virtual communication as, for example, real-time viewing of Montréal's city council meetings (Mennie, 2010) or use of an interactive Web site devoted to parenting (Boone, 2010). Women are not only aware of feminist concerns but are increasingly vocal concerning issues of status, needed services, and treatment by various government agencies (e.g., Montréal women have marched on the capital to sensitize law makers about women's rights [La Press Canadienne, 2010]).

Implications for Nursing Care

In Québec, as elsewhere, the nurse must respect the client's choice of language, not only to ensure clear communication but also to meet the requirements of Québec law. The Québec nurse realizes the centrality of good communication to patient/family care and education (Reidy, 2005). Most nurses and doctors are bilingual, and whether they work in traditionally anglophone (English-speaking) or francophone (French-speaking) health settings, they care for patients and families whose mother tongue may be French, English, or a host of other languages (Derfel, 2002). The ethnic mosaic that exists requires that the nurse be sensitive to the style, mode, and context of the communication patterns, not only of Québécois of different backgrounds and education but also of diverse ethnic groups in different stages of social and linguistic integration into the province (Vissandjée & Dupéré, 2000).

The nurse must be familiar with the popular Québec expressions used to designate parts of the body (such as *passage* for "vagina") or certain infections (such as *chaude pisse* for "gonorrhea") or health and illness. Those who are older or with a rural background might say that a person able to resist illness is as "strong as an ox" or "able as a bear," or when ill that the sufferer has a "weak constitution" (Dulong & Bergeron, 1980). When interacting with the older generation, the nurse should avoid using the familiar *tu* form because such usage is considered to show lack of respect.

SPACE

Conceptualization of Space

The representation of space in Québec's consciousness is process-oriented, related to urban-rural tensions and historical and social-political evolution, as well as to place-based identity (Chapman, 2000). This representation may be seen in three (interrelated rather than sequential) attitudinal themes: (1) spatial possession, depending on the underlying premise that specific groups can own, name, and control space; (2) spatial oppression, or domination or oppression by military force, patriarchy, class system, economy, or capitalism; and (3) spatial mobility, the tension between mobility and stasis, whether physical movement or identified with gender and ethnicity. The frame of reference consists of reterritorializing maps of power, domination, and marginalization.

Interpersonal Space

In public, Québecers tend to avoid physical contact and maintain a certain physical space. At work they may be in closer contact than in public, but individuals generally attempt to maintain a distance of 18 to 30 inches between themselves and others (Hall, 1990). Among friends and close relations, greater intimacy is permitted. Men may pat each other on the back or shake hands when they meet but seldom embrace or kiss. Women embrace or kiss cheeks but seldom walk arm in arm. Normally, physical contact in public is limited to young lovers, between adults and young children, or between adults at emotional or difficult moments when they require support.

Physical Space

Families generally live in apartments, condominiums, or single-family dwellings in the cities and suburbs, or in single-family dwellings in rural areas. Housing, particularly low-cost and public housing, is available chiefly in the larger cities, but there are homeless among the young, the addicted, and the chronically mentally ill (Desrochers, 2002). Despite immense territory, some 80% of the population is concentrated in the southern part of the province. Most people reside in the larger cities, such as Québec City (the capital), Montréal, Sherbrooke, Trois Rivières, or Laval. Montreal has been deemed the second happiest place in the world by a well-known travel guide (McCallum, 2010a); the first place went to a South Pacific island nation. Montréal is home to innumerable festivals (e.g., jazz, film, Haitian, fringe, fantasia, circus) during the summer, and for the past 180 years, without exception, it has hosted one of the world's largest St. Patrick's Day parades, turning the city completely green for the day (no matter one's ethnic background).

Implications for Nursing Care

An understanding of cultural geography can help nurses realize that space meanings are subtly constructed through a reworking of the past. Québecers are jealous and protective of their usually ample physical and personal space. In caring, the nurse avoids overly familiar attitudes, maintains distance when conversing, respects the privacy needs of patients and families, and recognizes the patient's sense of modesty when receiving intimate care.

SOCIAL ORGANIZATION

Family and Church

In early colonial days, families were large and stable, and family members felt a sense of belonging, not only to their land but also to the "Holy Mother the Church," accepting its dominance in health care, education, and population management (Fahmy-Eid & Dumont, 1983). During the period preceding the world wars, rural families often had 8 to 14 children, in order to provide additional help with farm work and out of respect for the teachings of the church. With the advent of the Quiet Revolution of the 1960s, the state assumed responsibility for the family through health and social services. By the late 1970s, changes in social attitudes and legislation permitted divorce, contraception, and abortion (Lazure, 1990).

Evolution of the Family

In the past, family roles were well defined: the father was head of the family and responsible for its material well-being, and the mother had specific household and possibly farm duties and was caregiver and religious educator. The family was seen in Québec as a group of parents and children united by multiple and varied ties, favoring the development of person and society, for mutual support during life (Gouvernement du Québec, 1985). Family roles remained relatively unchanged until women, under socio-economic pressures, began to join the workforce in greater numbers and became the heads of single-parent families. With the transition to the new generation of families, men and women began to reevaluate their familial roles; however, family functioning has not evolved without some difficulties (Valentine, 2001). Often the mother has maintained a double burden, still encumbered with her former tasks while assuming the obligations of outside employment. However, amid social change, the mother has remained the principal health care giver in the Québec family, instilling and supervising the practice of healthy habits within the family (Lazure, 1990; Thibaudeau & Reidy, 1985).

Québec suffered a major decrease in the birth rate in the 1960s and although the number of births had dropped to 76,100 by the year 2005, it had risen to 87,600 in 2008; however, abortions had risen from 1.4 in 1971 per 100 live births to 38.1 in 1999 (Institut de la statistique de Québec, 2013). By 2011, the birth rate was 9.9. Whereas the fertility rate was 1.69 children per woman in 2011, Britain's fertility rate was 1.7 and that of the United States was 2.1 (Institut de la statistique de Québec, 2013). In 2006, the mean number of children per family was 1.02; 83.4% of families were biparental, and, of these, 14.2% were reconstituted; 77.9% of single-parent families were headed by women (Institut de la statistique de Québec, 2010b). In 2006, 13% of Québec's children were growing up in low-income families (Santé et Services sociaux de Québec, 2013). Currently, about 32% of the adult population is not married (single, divorced, etc.); 38% are legally married and 20% live in common-law marriages (Institut de la statistique de Québec, 2010b). In Canada, more than 340,000 children

are growing up in mixed-race families, through inter-racial adoptions or in a growing number of ethno-cultural conjugal unions, composing 5.1% of Canadian couples who are mostly found in urban centers such as Vancouver, Toronto, or Montréal (Milan, Maheux, & Chul, 2010).

The two-parent family remains the ideal, the fathers of young children play a larger role in the care of children and their home environment, and the reconstituted family unit has become an accepted social phenomenon (Lacourse, 1999). However, a province-wide study of the health of families with children concluded that single-parent and reconstituted families seem more at risk than two-parent families. Whereas the regular use of alcohol varied little with type of family, smoking ranges from 28% in two-parent families, to 49% in single-parent families, to 54% in reconstituted families. Elevated psychological distress was reported in 18% of two-parent families but in 32% of the single-parent families and in 29% of the reconstituted families (Létourneau, Bernier, Marchand, & Trudel, 2000).

New Models of Interdependence

Québec society has evolved in such a way that diluted traditional networks of support built around family and relatives, the neighborhood, and various religious institutions (Lazure, 1990). However, changing cultural mores and options, emerging lifestyles, or shared problems over the past few years have stimulated the creation of new models of interdependence, individualization, and actualization for women, as well as legalization of gay and lesbian unions and adoptions (Fitterman, 2002; Lacourse, 1999). Regrouping of individuals into new networks of mutual aid or self-help is particularly significant. Community and volunteer organizations that have assumed many social and health functions for a variety of individuals are often inspired by needs no longer met by traditional means or by emerging social and health needs, such as persons living with acquired immunodeficiency syndrome (AIDS) (Stewart et al., 2001).

Aging of the Population

Demographic changes in the past 30 years have left Québec with a growing percentage of older citizens. The number of persons over 65 years is projected to grow from 1.2 million in 2011 to 2.3 million in the following 20 years; this group will then represent 25% of the population as compared with 9% in 1981 and 16% in 2011. There was also an increase in disabilities such as pain and decreased mobility with age: the rates were 8% in the 15–64 age group, 22.5% in those 64–74 years, and 46% in those over 75 years (Santé et Services sociaux de Québec, 2013). This general aging of the population includes an increase in the number of elderly women in relation to men, a proportion of about 3:2, and an increase in the number of the very old (i.e., over 80 years).

Youth

In 2010 in Québec, children, youths, and young adults composed 28.4% of the population (0–4 years, 5.3%; 5–9 years, 4.9%; 10–14 years, 5.5%; 15–19 years, 6.5%; 20–24 years, 6.2%) (Institut de la statistique du Québec, 2010b). Socioeducational problems are present (e.g., children with learning needs, homelessness, teenage pregnancy, drug addiction, street gangs), and whereas the general unemployment rate in Québec is about 9%, it is over 14% for youths 15 to 24 years of age (Institut de la statistique du Québec, 2010b). However, child and youth welfare is a priority for the province: there are provincial programs in pre- and postpartum care, scholastic adaptation for children with learning disabilities, recreation, and job training for youth and young adults.

Religion

Even with the British military conquest, the Catholic Church remained a social and political force in French Canada, defending faith, language, and culture (Orr, 1992). The church was actively involved in financial, educational, and health affairs. In the 1960s, however, the Quiet Revolution brought about greater separation of church and state. At that time, attendance at church declined greatly, and religious affiliations became more diversified (Orr, 1992). However, despite the decline in Catholicism's influence and practice, more than 6 million Québecers consider themselves to be Catholic. Many individuals conform to a model whereby one calls oneself "Catholic" and marks certain important life events in life by a church ceremony (baptism, marriage, funeral, and so forth) and continues to support a school system organized on religious groups (Laperrière, 1992). Today, Québec is noted for a growing interest in spirituality, a search for values, and diversification of beliefs and religious affiliations, including Protestantism, Judaism, Buddhism, Islam, Sikhism, Hinduism, and Seventh-Day Adventism (Québec Government Portal: Society, 2002c).

Implications for Nursing Care

The integration of extreme diversification of ethnic, cultural, and age groups in Québec presents a challenge for the nurse. By assessing the cultural attitudes of the client and family caregivers toward health, human reproduction, illness, and health care, the nurse takes the first step in assuring clients' enabling and empowerment. An investigation of community nurses in Montréal found that family participation was one of the most important facilitators to care, and that patient/family participation in care objectives was one of the most important nursing strategies (Reidy, 2005). Nevertheless, despite Québec's evolving social complexity, the social canvas of the province is still, in many ways, held together by the influence by the older generation, a sense of family, and sharing and mutual aid between generations. In working with single-parent families or those with limited financial means, the nurse may work with families whose members suffer from a variety of health and social problems. With feelings of powerlessness, whatever the family's status, self-confidence is undermined. The nurse can help family members understand their situation, participate in the care process, and deal with the health system. Within any family, efforts can be made to improve functioning in health matters, whether by improving competencies, direct support, information, and advice or by arranging access to resources. The nurse can also become an advocate for families so that they may obtain the social and health services to which they are entitled (Thibaudeau & Reidy, 1985; Thibaudeau, Reidy, d'Amours, & Frappier, 1984).

An aging population and a diminishing national health budget require that more community services be available to enable elderly people, with functional limits, to remain in their own homes. Day hospitals and centers staffed by multidisciplinary teams that offer various social services are increasing in number. Cossette, Lévesque, and Laurin (1995) note that both gender and kinship should be considered with respect to support when assisting French-speaking primary caregivers in providing care for aging and disabled relatives in the home.

TIME

Past and Present

The development and diffusion of time sense (the way we see and live time) is a phenomenon for the people of Québec that is related to the consciousness of time in the context of the value and rhythm of human life of a Catholic and rural society; the preciousness of time and calculation of time within the modernity of the educational system, urban industrialization, and the evolution of a city-based mechanized society; and the importance accorded to time in an era of developing communications (Watelet, 1999). French Québecers tend to attach primary importance to day-to-day affairs and to living in the present. Pleasure and sorrow are generally accepted as they occur, with an attitude that life goes on from one day to the next (Paquet, 1989). However, climatic and historic conditions have prompted planning to survive long and cold winters and a context of stability that provides structure for these values and attitudes. For older Québecers, time is intimately associated with religion. They envision the future with the hope of life after death. Anniversaries of the death of family members are often commemorated by a Mass. However, many of the young and urban, being less influenced by religion, tend not to follow such traditions. For women in modern Québec society, time has taken on a new meaning as working women assume a variety of roles (wife, mother, professional person).

Although time is determined by the flow of the successive seasons for rural populations, urban life is characterized by variations in the distribution of time as reported by study participants in a study by Laroche (2000); more than half expressed preference for engaging in free or leisure time activities, about 17% preferred time devoted to family and domestic responsibilities, and about 7% favored work time. In 1998, productive time for Québecers (work and domestic responsibilities) averaged 7.8 hours per day in households without children and 9 hours in those with at least one child (Laroche & Gauthier, 2002); however, living with children is associated with a negative impact on physical activities (Bacon, 2010). Time accorded to leisure activities (media, social, cultural, physical activities, and sports) totaled about 6 hours a week (Québec Government Portal: Society, 2002d). The most popular cultural activities were recreational games, dancing, audiovisual entertainment, plastic arts, and literary activities. Outdoor activities and sports accounted for time spent by people of all ages: more than 40% cycled; about one third camped, fished, or skied; and about 15% golfed, canoed, or rode snowmobiles.

Implications for Nursing Care

The nurse must consider the present-time orientation, often demonstrated by the importance attributed to practical goals, when interacting with families and individuals, as well as in the approach and content of health education. A verbal "contract" between the nurse and patient and family, of prioritized collaborative objectives including a time frame, often proves advantageous in enabling and in supporting self-care within the context of health promotion and therapeutic regimens.

ENVIRONMENTAL CONTROL

Attitudes toward Health

In intellectual circles in Québec, health is perceived as being in complete possession of one's physical and mental capacities and as a way of improving one's status, professional or otherwise (Paquet, 1989). For financially secure families, health is seen as an ideal state in which illness is absent, whereas illness is seen as a slow and insidious degradation of health that occurs over time. In lower socioeconomic groups, health is defined as the ability to work, to be self-sufficient, and to satisfy primary needs. The

disadvantaged often attach less value to a general state of good health, often seeking resolution of immediate problems without follow-up of long-term goals. Illness is seen as a stroke of bad luck, causing a momentary rupture in one's normal state of health.

More than 90% of Québecers over the age of 12 considered themselves to be healthy but reported visiting a health professional within the previous 12 months (Institut de la Statistique du Québec, 2010b). However, Lavasseur (2000) previously found that those from 45 to 64 evaluated their health more negatively than did the youth; the poorer and less educated rated their health less favorably, and persons employed saw themselves to be in better health than those who were unemployed. Factors associated with an unfavorable self-evaluation of health included problems with weight, limits on activities, consultations with health professionals, and psychological distress. The practice of medicine has always held a place of prestige and political power in Québec.

Published yearly by a local newspaper, a "barometer of the professions" including 30 professions/occupations indicates that Québecers sustain a level confidence of 97% in firefighters, 96% in nurses, and 91% in doctors, as compared with 40% in priests, 29% in lawyers, and 6% in the proverbial used car salesmen (Leger, 2010). However, with the advent of consumerism, the people of Québec began to participate more directly in health care decision making, and the ideology of the powerful medical establishment is now being questioned by both ordinary people and other health professionals. Various "alternative medicine" and spiritual approaches to health have become more popular, apparently in answer to a need for therapies that are global and allow greater personal control (Laforest, 1985). Furthermore, in a recent poll, three fourths of Québecers were found to be in favor of a special tax on energizing and sweetened drinks with the revenues being invested in health prevention (Lévesque, 2010).

Social Environment of Health

Because of the strong interrelationship between an individual's social environment and health and the value placed on families, Québec's health and welfare policy is directed to reinforcing family and social networks. A survey of 1014 people across the province asked, "What is the most important thing in life for you?" The answer was emotional life and support (43%) before more time, work, or money (Le Devoir, 1999). Further, a surrounding family was seen as essential, and the emotional and psychological affinity was viewed (61%) as most important to a successful life as a couple. In their study of the health and social support of Québecers, Julien, Julien, and Lafontaine (2000) concluded that men; persons widowed, separated, or divorced; and persons between the ages of 25 and 64 were comparatively more dissatisfied with their level of social interaction and social support. Men were more dissatisfied with living alone, and women in general had better social support. One person in four with a spouse, whether cohabiting or not, reported difficulties in the relationship. Further, in 2008, 12% of youths (3–14 years) experienced moderate or severe socioemotive difficulties, relational troubles being the most frequent and boys being more susceptible than girls (Santé et Services sociaux de Québec, 2013).

However, even though 65% of the population considered spiritual life to be very important, 64% seldom or never frequented a place of worship (Carkson, Pica, & Lacombe, 2000). Generally, it was those persons who considered themselves to be in a poor state of health or who were limited in their activities who most valued spiritual life and attendance at religious worship. Those persons who most frequently attended religious services were less likely to report a high level of psychological distress or suicidal ideas.

The work environment in Québec has been found to affect health; 3% of workers reported violence and 18% intimidation, and 8% of women and 2% of men were subjected to unwanted words or gestures of a sexual nature constraints at work (such as combined low level of work autonomy with a high level of psychological demand) were found to be associated not only with psychological distress but also with perceptions of poorer mental and general health. Certain work conditions (e.g., working nights, exposure to solvents or vibrations), as well as certain characteristics of the work environments (such as size of the company, work organization, age of workers), were found to be associated with a high risk of accidents (Arcand et al., 2000).

Physical Environment

Problems of pollution and waste management constitute a serious challenge to the environment in terms of costs, contamination, and health. A water-purification program, in Québec since 1981, involves water-processing plants and greater control of industrial waste (Thibault, 1989). Public awareness has intensified and public programs have been created concerning reducing atmospheric pollutants, recycling, composting, using natural products, disposing of dangerous household wastes, and cleaning up lakes and rivers. With collaboration between the province and its inhabitants, there has been a reduction from 28 to 7 (from 2007 to 2009) restrictions in the use of lakes because of blue-green algae (Santé et Services sociaux de Québec, 2013). Further, pesticides, which are linked to cancer and diseases affecting children, have been banned from use on private lawns and gardens, as well as on the grounds of schools and other provincially owned green spaces (Dougherty, 2002).

Determinants of health and well-being include physical activity and exercise, vaccinations, control of body weight, the practice of behavior proper to women's health, and the practice of safe sex. There has been an increase from 45% in 2003 to 54% in 2009 in the rate of Québecers who report being active, rather than sedentary, during their leisure time; however, in adolescence (12–17 years), girls are less physically active than boys (53%) (Santé et Services sociaux de Québec, 2010b). Although the rate of obesity is lower in Québec than in the rest of Canada, the number of obese children has almost tripled since 1981. Further, obesity related to health risk has also increased, with 32.7% of the province's adults now overweight and 15.5% obese (Institut de la statistique de Québec, 2010b); and obesity-related illnesses cost the Québec health care system more than half a billion dollars annually, or 5% of total direct health care costs in the province (Institut de la Statistique de Québec, 2010b).

In the mass inoculation of 2009, 57% of the population were vaccinated against the flu (H1N1); by the 2008–2009 school year, 90% of students in grade 4 were vaccinated against hepatitis B and 80% of girls in the third year of high school were vaccinated against human papillomavirus (Santé et Services sociaux de Québec, 2013). Moreover, in a study by Chénard, Daveluy, and Émond (2000), about 27% of women over age 15 practiced self-examination of their breasts, and 50% indicated that they had a medical examination of their breasts, 49% had a mammogram, and 44% had a Pap test within the past year. Oral contraceptives were used by more than 50% of women ages 18 to 24, and by about 7% of those over age 35, for a total of 57% of the female population.

Fournier and Piché (2000) noted that health professionals, other than physicians, are assuming increasing importance in the health care system. While health problems, incapacity, and psychological distress prompt consultation with a health professional, the most important factor in seeking health care is perception of one's state of health. Persons without a health problem were more likely to consult another professional rather than a physician. Infosanté (Info-Health), a telephone service in which nurses give information and advice on health and social matters, is available 24 hours a day, 7 days a week (Dunnigan, 2000). Seventy-five percent of the population knew of the availability of telephone service, and 32% of those used it.

Papillon, Laurier, Barnard, and Baril (2000) reported that in the 2 days prior to their study, half of their respondents had consumed at least one prescription or nonprescription medication. The proportion of women who consume medication is greater than that of men, although it should be noted that this use includes contraceptives and hormone replacements. Use increased with age, and non-prescription use increased with revenue and education. Trahan, Bégin, and Piché (2000) indicated that 6% of Québecers had been hospitalized and 4.2% had been treated in day surgery during the previous year. Persons living alone, the chronically ill, aged, and new single-parent mothers were the most likely to receive home care. Families, in partnership with home-care nurses from local community centers, were the principal source of help and care at home, following hospitalization or during long-term illnesses (Reidy, 2005). Further, 20% of Québecers 15 years or older cared for an aged person without remuneration (Santé et Services sociaux de Québec, 2010a).

Rituals Related to Death and Dying

Functionality, aging, spousal death, and dying are interrelated as the older Québecer "downsizes" from the family home to a smaller apartment or care environment and to a smaller set of "things." In Québec, such a move, often accompanied by a compulsion to divest themselves of many of their belongings, is called *casser la maison* (literally, "breaking the house"). An ethnographic study, realized in Montréal by Marcoux (2001) and seen as descriptive of the social organization of death across Québec, reveals that to *casser la maison* is not a means of merely separating from one's belongings; more essentially it is a ritualized form of ancestralizing oneself by placing those possessions with kin or other recipients, guaranteeing one's survival in memory. Marcoux argues that *casser la maison* begins with a compulsion toward detachment but evolves into the appropriation of the event in the reconstruction of self: the acceptance of the loss of status through the acceding to the higher status of ancestor.

For earlier generations in Québec, death was formalized and dealt with by adherence to the symbols and ceremonies of the Catholic Church, usually in the context of the family, and by a strong belief in an afterlife. Death and anniversaries of the death of family members are often commemorated by a Mass. Although in the 1950s cremation was unacceptable to Québec's Roman Catholics, with increased secularization and urbanization, it is now requested twice as often as body burials (Johnston, 1996).

Today, the final agony of death and all the emotions it provokes are frequently concealed from public view, since death usually occurs in an institution. Death is often perceived as the ultimate failure, by both family and health professionals, since it cannot be mastered or controlled by technology. However, the attitudes, values, and outlooks concerning the ethical problems of death, assisted suicide and euthanasia, treatment and cessation of treatment, and the accompaniment of the terminally ill are considered worthy of continued scientific study and philosophical discourse (Volant, 2004). A recent poll in Québec that indicated strong support for assisted death in end-of-life situations also reflected confusion between ceasing unusual measures to prolong life and euthanasia (Fedio, 2010).

Implications for Nursing Care

In a multicultural society like Québec, health and illness are, in part, determined by the degree of an individual's integration into a society and the social support supplied by the community. Social support has a preventive value if it is associated with networks that are stable, homogeneous, and dense and that provide a variety of links between individuals (Bozzini & Tessier, 1985). Health care planning must be sensitive to such diversity to be effective. A public-centered approach is at the heart of health and social service reform in Québec (Battaglini & Gravel, 2000). It is essential that the nurse be integrated into the interdisciplinary team in effective decision making about health and social services (Trudel, 1995).

Three differentiating factors contribute to health care assessment in a multicultural setting. First, nurses should note the meaning of *health* and *illness* in terms of the underlying significance of these concepts in the cultural group. Second, descriptions of symptoms, compliance with treatment, and reaction to pain will differ according to social level and ethnic origin. Third, the client's gender influences how individuals view their bodies and the adoption of dependent or independent behavior patterns with regard to health (Dorvil, 1985). These factors influence one's representation of illness, the way the client's illness is explained, the assumption of responsibility for personal health through self-care, and participation in the treatment regimen. Because women are ordinarily the principal health agents in the family, nursing interventions can be directed toward encouraging their collaboration in fostering healthful living habits.

In the larger cities, polluted air is associated with such problems as asthma, bronchitis, and allergies affecting the skin, eyes, and respiratory tract. Families could be advised to minimize use of possible allergy-producing substances found in rugs, bedding, and humidifiers in homes with young children, older people, persons suffering from asthma, or individuals with symptoms of acquired immunodeficiency. Prevention of symptoms caused by stagnant air in large buildings or factories also falls within the domain of the nurse concerned with the work environment and the reduction of worker absenteeism.

Since hunting and fishing are popular activities in Québec, it is of concern that certain pollutants may be present in fresh water and soil. Therefore, pregnant women should be advised against consuming freshwater fish or game during pregnancy. Even when women are not pregnant, the federal government recommends that fish from contaminated lakes be consumed no more than once a week to prevent accumulation of polychlorinated biphenyls in body tissues. The nurse's role includes participation in awareness campaigns, in short- and long-term preventive measures, and in research to determine possible interrelations between such factors as pollution, health, lifestyle, and heredity.

With the aging of the population and the subsequent increase in the incidence of chronic illnesses has come intensification in the use of various drugs and medicines in the community. It is the nurse's responsibility to help clients maintain their medical regimen and to inform them about the dangers of uncontrolled and irrational use of prescription or nonprescription drugs, of accidental or intentional intoxication, of teratogenic and iatrogenic effects, and of physical and psychological dependency.

BIOLOGICAL VARIATIONS

Genetic Factors

The various social, economic, and cultural practices of a given population influence the eventual formation of a genetic pool that determines the biological characteristics of a community and contribute to reducing or increasing the frequency of certain genes in the population (Bouchard & DeBraekeleer, 1991a). Such phenomena as migrations, successive waves of immigration, family inbreeding, and concentration of certain groups in specific areas are of particular consequence. Québecers of French origin have a specific genotype inherited from the original group of 5000 colonists (Bouchard & DeBraekeleer, 1991b). For example, the genetic abnormalities found in the populations of the Saguenay and Charlevoix regions of Québec represent an important public health problem in these areas. The most striking example is that of muscular dystrophy, a disorder of genetic origin characterized by a progressive increase in muscular debility (Bouchard, 1991). Its worldwide frequency is approximately 1 in 25,000 individuals. In the Saguenay region, the frequency is estimated to be 1 in 514 (DeBraekeleer, 1991). Familial hypercholesterolemia has a worldwide frequency of 1 in 500 in the general population; in the eastern part of the province, its frequency is estimated to be 1 in 15. Familial hypercholesterolemia has probably been the most carefully studied of the dominant chromosome abnormalities. The principal complication of this disease is coronary thrombosis in the young adult, which is often fatal (Bouchard & DeBraekeleer, 1991b). Cystic fibrosis is the most common fatal hereditary illness among Québecers. Its frequency of 1 in 895 births in the Saguenay region is higher than that in most

other populations. Tay-Sachs disease also seems to occur frequently in Québec. No treatment has been discovered for this condition, which occurs in infants from birth to 6 months of age (DeBraekeleer, 1991).

Life Expectancy

In 2008, life expectancy of Québecers reached 78 years for men and 83 years for women—a gain of about 6 years since 1981 (Santé et Services sociaux de Québec, 2013). However, it should be noted that the "disability-free" expectancy, which includes staying mobile and living outside a hospital or nursing home, is just over 70 years. Rural and northern Québec residents live shorter lives than the average Canadian; for example, the average life expectancy in Nunavik was only 66.7 years in 2005 (STATS Canada, 2015). However, from 1961 to 2008, the province showed a continuing reduction in peri-mortality (from 11.5 to 6.8 per 1000 live births) and in infantile mortality (from 31.5 to 4.0 per 1000 live births) (Santé et Services sociaux de Québec, 2013).

The leading causes of death in Québecers are cancer (33.2%) and heart disease (26.5%), with rates at about 175 per 100,000. Trauma and accidents (about 27 per 100,000) and suicide (12 per 100,000) are the major causes of death for persons under 20 years of age (Santé et Services sociaux de Québec, 2013).

Susceptibility to Disease

In 2009, the highest number of new cancer diagnoses among men were lung and prostate cancers and, among women, cancer of the breast. Approximately two out of three Québecers report at least one health problem that has imposed limits or required consultation with a health professional including allergies (25%), back problems (18%), hypertension (17%), arthritis or rheumatism (11%), migraines (9%), asthma (7%), thyroid problems (7%), and diabetes (6%). There was an increase in the incidence of diabetes from 5% in 1999–2000 to 8% in 2006–2007, with a rate of 21% in those over 65 years of age. An analysis of health problems by age indicates that allergies, asthma, and other respiratory afflictions are the most important problem for children and adults under age 24 and remain significant throughout the life span. Further in 2008, 9% of children in Québec were diagnosed with attention deficit disorder with or without hyperactivity; among these 58% were prescribed medication (Santé et Services sociaux de Québec, 2013).

Sexually and Intravenously Transmitted Diseases. Diseases transmitted sexually and through the bloodstream constitute a serious public health problem in Québec. About 75% of heterosexuals reported having only one sexual partner during the previous year. However, 1 in 10 of the sexually active had more than one partner, and 60% of these reported the at-risk behavior of not systematically using a condom. Further, nearly one half of sexually active teenagers (15–19 years) reported having failed to use a condom during any of their sexual relations during the previous year (Santé et Services sociaux de Québec, 2013)

Chlamydiosis is the most frequently reported sexually transmitted disease, rising from 8404 reported cases in 2000 to 15,869 in 2009. Reported cases of gonorrhea also increased; there were 381 cases in 2000 and 1883 cases in 2009. However, the incidence of hepatitis B has declined 17% since 2004, with 965 cases in 2009, and the incidence of syphilis is fairly low, with 370 cases in 2009 (Santé et Services sociaux de Québec, 2013).

Although Québec has the second highest number of cases of AIDS among Canadian provinces, the number of new diagnoses has stabilized per year from 2004 to 2009 (−18%) (Santé et Services sociaux de Québec, 2013). Bisexual and homosexual men under 40 years of age and intravenous drug users account for most cases of AIDS. However, whereas women infected with human immunodeficiency virus (HIV) constitute a significant group, the number of children infected by vertical transmission is small because of early treatment of infected pregnant women. They are concentrated in the Montréal area, where the women have contracted the disease either from infected male sexual partners or through intravenous drug use. Québecers have, in general, a positive attitude toward those living with HIV and AIDS (Leaune & Adrien, 1998).

Nutritional Preferences and Habits

From early colonial times, because of the harsh climate, the diet of Québecers has been rich in starchy foods and fat. A considerable portion of the family budget has been devoted to food. Beginning in the 1960s, the practice of eating in restaurants became more frequent, and fast foods, rich in fat and salt and poor in fiber and vitamins, became widely popular. In 2000, Chénard, Daveluy, and Émond concluded that 85% of Québecers had a positive perception of their food habits. However, a poor nutritional state was associated with the perception of a poor state of health, an elevated level of psychological distress, and poor social support, particularly among the very poor, the unemployed, and single-parent families. To combat the problem of undernourishment and hunger in disadvantaged children, food and milk programs are subsidized by the province. Furthermore, there has been an increase in the daily consumption of fruit and vegetables, from 25% of the population in 2003 to 54% in 2009, with a rate of consumption of 58% in the group with the highest income and

46% in the lowest (Santé et Services sociaux de Québec, 2013).

Psychological Characteristics and Coping

Tobacco, Alcohol, and Drug Abuse. There has been a significant reduction in the proportion of smokers in Québec, from 34% in 1998 (the year smoking was banned in public buildings, bars, and restaurants) to 23% in 2009 (Santé et Services sociaux de Québec, 2013). However, although the proportion of 12- to 19-year-old cigarette smokers has decreased from 50% to 15% in the same period, the proportion of this group smoking cigars and cigarillos has risen to 18%. Moreover, a study by the Quebec Coalition for Tobacco Control concludes that smokers are costing Québec about $930 million each year as tobacco-related illnesses are taking their toll on the health care system. The results indicate that 32.6% of hospital beds in Québec are occupied by people who either smoke or smoked heavily at one time. Currently, the Health Ministry is not only preparing to file a multibillion-dollar class-action lawsuit against the tobacco industry but is also considering stronger antismoking legislation, including banning smoking in cars when children are present. Further findings from this study suggested that flavored cigars really do not measure up because people were mostly noncompliant 67–70% of the time (Québec Coalition, 2010).

Québec rates second among Canadian provinces in per capita sales of alcohol. Québecers buy less hard liquor and more beer; of all red wine sold in the country, 44% is sold in Québec (Kalbfuss, 2002). In terms of alcohol consumption, 40% of Québecers reported being abstainers, 45% were occasional drinkers, and 14% regular drinkers. Nearly 20% of the population reported drinking to excess at least once a month during the previous year, and 13% used illicit drugs, usually marijuana. Moreover, during this same period, the proportion of high school students using drugs increased from 8% to 47%; however, of young people who reported not having used drugs in the past year, there was an increase from 57% in 2000 to 72% in 2008 (Santé et Services sociaux de Québec, 2013).

Mental Health. In 2008–2009, while 77% of the population 15 years or older declared themselves to be in very good or excellent mental health, 6% suffered from quite intensive stress in their everyday lives, and one worker in three experienced elevated stress at work daily. The most common mental health problems were major episodes of depression (5%), social phobias (2%), eating disorders (2%), and panic attacks (1.4%). Distress was experienced more frequently by women, youth under 24 years, the unemployed, and persons with low income (Santé et Services sociaux de

Québec, 2013). About 5300 Québecers were hospitalized for psychiatric problems; the most common diagnoses included affective and other psychoses, alcoholic psychosis, and schizophrenia (STATS Canada, 2002). In 2007–2008, the health system devoted 0.44 beds per 1000 inhabitants to psychiatric care.

The rate of suicide in Québec is among the highest both in Canada and in other industrialized countries. In the year 2008, 3% of the population over 15 years of age experienced suicidal ideation or attempted suicide. However, since the year 2000, there has been a reduction in the mortality rate attributable to suicide from 32 per 100,000 population in 1999 to 23 per 100,000 in 2008. In 2008, 77% of the deaths by suicide were by men, and the highest rate according to age was among people between the ages 40 and 49 (Santé et Services sociaux de Québec, 2013).

Implications for Nursing Care

The particular mortality and morbidity curves occurring in the Québec population, combined with severe budget limitations placed on health services, call for the creation of approaches targeting populations such as those who suffer from chronic illnesses, cancer and cardiac conditions, asthma, and diabetes. The evolution of these latter illnesses follows a pattern in which brief hospitalizations occur episodically, followed by long periods of time when the patient and family must learn to function at home within the limits imposed by the condition. As length of allowed hospitalizations becomes shorter, the nurse must develop educational interventions and home care approaches in order to facilitate the participation of the patient and the family caregiver, as well as enabling self-care and maintaining quality of life.

Health care and counseling in parallel with preventive and health programs, for Québecers exposed to venereal disease, also fall within the scope of nursing practice. Intervention should be designed to educate the public concerning the dangers of sexually transmitted diseases, especially AIDS, and the part played by intravenous drug use in the transmission of the latter. Moreover, nurses need to maintain open, nonjudgmental attitudes in their interactions with clients suffering from AIDS (Taggart, Reidy, & Grenier, 1992).

A "language of food" indicates not only how society views eating but also how a culture designates foods as normal and healthy. It also includes the personal adaptation that an individual or group makes concerning eating habits. Although socioeconomic and cultural factors influence the way these two concepts function, both must be considered when attempts are made to improve living habits. The perceived social requirement of staying slim, coupled with the burdens of motherhood and outside employment, causes many women to be undernourished or overweight. Given the importance of the relationship between nutrition, the health of newborns and adolescents, and osteoporosis in older women, much remains to be accomplished in the area of proper diets for women and children. The nurse's role includes participating in setting up and maintaining programs designed to reduce malnutrition in schools serving underprivileged children. School nurses are in a good position to assess needs and seek ways to foster healthful living habits among children and to act as a liaison between parents and teachers.

SUMMARY

The ethnic identity of French Canadians of Québec is witnessed in the attitudes and values common to them and in the knowledge they have of what it means to be a Québecois. They share a common background of the culture and ways of life of their ancestors, but one must accept that their ethnic identity varies in terms of content and degree relative to disparities such as age, education, and socioeconomic situation (Gohier & Schleifer, 1993). It is essential, however, for the nurse to remember that the people of Québec now live within an evolving multicultural society. To understand the significance of health and social behaviors of *les Québecois* (Québecers), it is essential that the nurse develop cultural competence and sensitivity to the unique culture of the people of Québec, as well as to the diverse ethnic and racial groups who blend to make up the larger heterogeneous, pluralistic society.

CASE STUDY

Marguerite Tremblay (born McNeill) married in 1939 at 16 years of age. Her husband, Théophile Tremblay, worked at a farm in the Laurentians. They were for the most part self-sufficient, with cows, a few sheep, and a market garden. They traded for certain goods and had a small cash crop. Life was hard, with workdays beginning before dawn and continuing until bedtime.

In 1970, at the death of Théophile, the eldest son, Étienne, took over running the family farm, where he continued to live with his wife, Estelle, and their children. Several years later, the land was expropriated to make room for a highway. The family, now composed of Mrs. Tremblay, Rose (her unmarried daughter), and Étienne and his children, moved to a small farm property in Ste-Rose. Mrs. Tremblay, with the help of Rose, raised Étienne's children after their mother died in childbirth.

Mrs. Tremblay, a good Catholic and farm wife, had 14 children between 1940 and 1966, 8 of whom survived to maturity (see Tremblay Family Tree, Figure 23-1). One of these children was born dead, one died after a premature birth, one died of meningitis, one died of polio, and one did not survive a hard winter. One son died in an automobile accident, when drunk, at 18 years of age.

The life situation of the surviving family members demonstrates how the family structure and religious practices have changed within the life span of one family.

Mrs. Tremblay has remained active and involved in the lives of her children and grandchildren. At 80 years of age, she suffered a cerebrovascular accident that left her with a left-sided hemiplegia. She has made only a moderate recovery. She requires help with transfers but can stand with a walker. She also requires help with many activities of daily living and spends much of her time in a wheelchair. She speaks slowly but is lucid, if somewhat anxious.

Mrs. Tremblay has been admitted to a long-term care unit because of her physical limitations and her immediate family's inability to care for her at home. She alternates between understanding the need for long-term care and fear that her family no longer needs her. Her family, particularly her eldest son and daughter, with whom she lived, feel guilty and fear that they are not doing their "duty," despite their own health problems and physical limitations.

Rose

Age 71; unmarried; lives with mother; suffers from obesity, diabetes, and osteoporosis; attends church and receives the sacraments regularly.

Étienne

Age 70; widower; farmer and truck driver; father of seven children, five of whom survived to maturity, all of whom have left home; suffers from severe arthritis.

Philippe

Age 66; notary; father of six children, five of whom lived to maturity; smoker; suffers from hypertension and hypercholesterolemia; wife has recovered from breast cancer.

Line

Age 63; married a farmer; worked as a volunteer for the parish church; mother of four children, all of whom survived to maturity.

Victor

Age 62; missionary in Africa; smoker; suffers from certain chronic parasitical infections.

Marie-Madeleine

Age 51; was a nun in a nursing order; after leaving the convent, has worked with adolescents with drug problems; does not practice her religion.

Catherine

Age 48; former teacher; divorced from a doctor; mother of two children; suffers from chronic anxiety and mild abuse of tranquilizers; has become a Christian Scientist.

Denise

Age 45; former commercial artist; unmarried; mother of one child whose father, an actor, died of AIDS; mother and child HIV positive; activist in AIDS self-help group; very interested in spiritual renewal but refuses her mother's pleas to return to the church.

CASE STUDY—cont'd

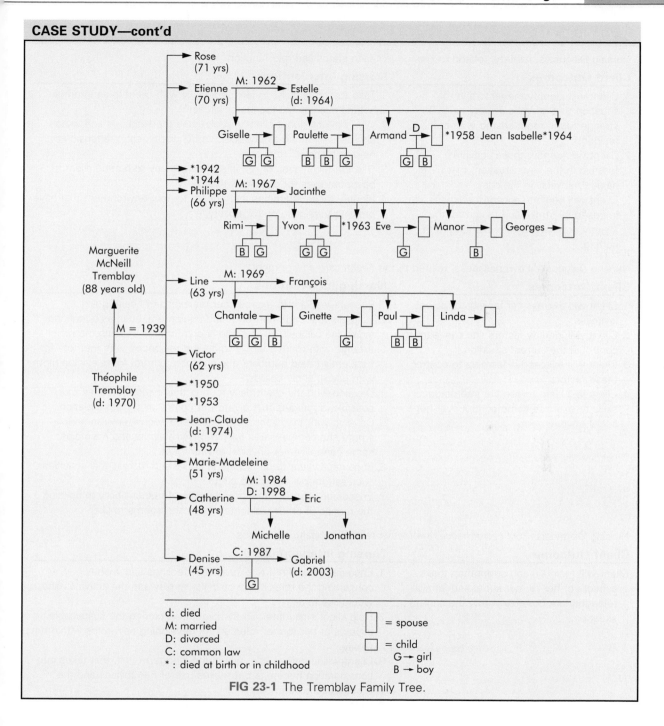

FIG 23-1 The Tremblay Family Tree.

◎ **CARE PLAN**

Nursing Diagnosis: Anxiety, related to change in health status and role function

Client Outcomes	**Nursing Interventions**
1. Client will identify the factors in the situation that provoke anxiety (such as strange room, room shared with other resident). 2. Client will identify those activities, feasible in the new situation, that have helped her relax in the past. 3. Client will begin to accept the limits imposed by stroke and to control the anxiety provoked by life in a long-term setting.	1. Take the time, daily, to talk personally with client in an informal setting such as the lounge or kitchen. 2. When talking about client's stroke, use the language and words she uses as much as possible. Verify client's comprehension of new or technical language. 3. Use the techniques of reminiscence therapy to remind client of past strategies for dealing with anxiety. 4. Identify those strategies appropriate to new environment that have previously helped control anxiety.

Nursing Diagnosis: Powerlessness, related to the health care environment

Client Outcomes	**Nursing Interventions**
1. Client will express her feelings of powerlessness. 2. Client will identify factors she can learn to control in the current situation. 3. Client will succeed in learning to control these factors. 4. Client will learn to use her interpersonal skills to exercise some control over her social environment.	1. Encourage client to express her feelings and health goals. 2. Help client arrange her room and equipment, such as telephone, radio, and call bell, so that she is comfortable in using them. 3. Arrange with client's family to have a telephone with memory for frequently called numbers and a remote control for television (both with user-friendly boards). 4. Develop with the client daily routine that incorporates, as much as possible, strategies that give client control in current situation. 5. Develop with the client a prosthetic and secure environment where she compensates for her physical limits and maintains some control of her physical environment. 6. Encourage client to participate in social and recreational activities such as group singing and bingo. 7. Encourage client's interest and sense of responsibility in building the morale of other residents whom she seems to like.

Nursing Diagnosis: Role performance, ineffective related to health alterations

Client Outcome	**Nursing Interventions**
Client will maintain and strengthen those aspects of her former social and familiar roles that are possible within the current situation.	1. Encourage the client to express her feelings and wishes concerning the roles she would like to play and the activities she would like to do. 2. Help client's daughter aid the client in exploring the sustainable aspects of her former roles and in developing new roles within the family. 3. Client will identify a role, within the long-term unit, that takes into consideration her limits but makes use of her abilities and the prosthetic environment. 4. Help the client understand and play her role in maintaining effective interrelationships between the generations of her family. 5. Develop a "caring" relationship with the client and explore with her the relationships she can develop and the roles she can play in interacting with other staff members, volunteers, and other residents.

CARE PLAN—cont'd

Nursing Diagnosis: Self-esteem (situational) low, functional impairment (left-sided hemiplegia) related to dependence on health care team within long-term care unit

Client Outcomes	Nursing Interventions
1. Client will express opinions and her preferences to both staff and family. 2. Client will participate in the various aspects of her care process (such as decision making, physical care, assessment). 3. Client will experience and express, through her body language, an increase in self-esteem.	1. Address the client by her name, Madame Tremblay, and never by "Mama" ("Maman") or other diminutives. 2. Respect the client's privacy and her physical space, and go slowly in manifesting a physical display of affection. Permit client to set the parameters of her social space. 3. Listen to the client, encourage her to use "I" in her conversation, respect her opinion, encourage her to make decisions, and respect those decisions. 4. Encourage the family to help client maintain her personal appearance by providing clothes that fit and are attractive, personal grooming equipment, and the like. 5. Compliment her on any improvements in appearance. 6. Work with occupational and physical therapy personnel to develop appropriate but practical and worthwhile projects (such as weaving, food preparation).

Nursing Diagnosis: Disturbed sensory perception (kinesthetic), related to sensory reception, transmission, and integration

Client Outcomes	Nursing Interventions
1. Client will begin to compensate for inability to identify position of body parts by developing other senses (sight, sensations of unaffected members, and so on). 2. Client will learn to master prosthetic aids to compensate for diminished motor coordination. 3. Client will understand the importance of practicing preventive and safety measures (such as skin care and proper shoes).	1. Validate with the client that she understands the effect of the stroke on her ability to function and that she realizes that certain false perceptions can occur because of this condition. 2. Work with the client so that she learns to use her "good" hand routinely and to use visual inspection to verify the position and location of her affected limbs. 3. Develop with the client compensatory routines such as turning her head to improve her visual field or repositioning items in her physical environment. 4. Show the client how to inspect her skin for pressure points, and help her develop a routine for turning and relieving these pressure points.

Nursing Diagnosis: Compromised family coping related to disabling progression that exhausts supportive capacity of significant persons

Client Outcomes	Nursing Interventions
1. Family will develop appropriate involvement of all family members in the client's current situation (such as involvement that encourages both affiliation and autonomy). 2. Family will mutually accept new roles of the client and the principal caregiver in the family. (Adapted from Ackley & Ludwig, 2002)	1. Clarify with the daughter, in terms of her limits and abilities, her new role as principal health caregiver in the family, emphasizing the essential nature of this new role. 2. Clarify with family members (especially the eldest son) the importance of visits and family celebrations, development of relationships with grandchildren, and keeping client informed of family events. 3. Include the daughter in the planning of the client's care. 4. Encourage family members to develop joint family projects such as a family photo album.

CLINICAL DECISION MAKING

1. How is public access to health care authorized in Canada, and what group of citizens are included under the authorization?
2. Describe how the work environment in Québec affects the health care of workers in Québec.
3. Describe the most commonly occurring genetic conditions found among French Canadians in Québec.
4. Describe the life expectancy by gender of French Canadians in Québec.
5. Describe the commonly occurring conditions to which French Canadians living in Québec are most susceptible.

REVIEW QUESTIONS

1. In promoting self-care for a client from Québec, the nurse needs to be sure to do which of the following?
   a. Include a spiritual plan of care.
   b. Include touch in the plan of care.
   c. Include the family in health teaching.
   d. Include a time frame with collaborative objectives.
2. In providing nursing care in Québec, the nurse realizes that the space meanings are implemented by which of the following?
   a. Standing close when communicating with a client
   b. Standing close when discussing familiar attitudes
   c. Maintaining distance when conversing with a client
   d. Shaking hands with the client before providing care
3. A nurse in Québec is doing dietary teaching for a pregnant woman. Because of environmental factors, the nurse should advise the client to do which of the following?
   a. Consume fish no more than once a week.
   b. Avoid consuming freshwater fish.
   c. Consume a vegetarian diet from a variety of sources.
   d. Avoid eating beef that is imported from England.

REFERENCES

Ackley, B. J., & Ludwig, G. (2002). *Nursing diagnosis handbook* (5th ed.). St. Louis: Mosby.

Allard, M., & Durand, S. (2006). L'infirmiere practicienne specialisee: un nouveur role. [Clinical nurse specialist: a new role]. *Perspective Infirmiere*, 3(5), 10–15.

Anctil, H., & Bluteau, M. A. (1986). *La santé et l'assistance publique au Québec, 1886–1986 [Québec health and social welfare, 1886–1986]*. Québec: Ministère de la Santé et des Services sociaux, Direction des Communications.

Arcand, R., Labrèche, F., Stock, S., et al. (2000). *Travail et santé [Work and health]. Enquête sociale et de santé [Health and social inquiry]* (pp. 525–570). Québec: Institut de la Statistique du Québec.

Audet, L. P., & Gauthier, A. (1967). *Le système scolaire du Québec: organisation et fonctionnement [Québec educational system: structure and function]*. Montréal: Librairie Beauchemin Limitée.

Bacon, S. L. (2010). *Children have a negative impact on physical activity among individuals with heart disease.* Press release Université de Montréal. Available at <http://www.eurekalert.org/pub_releases/2010-07/uom-cha072010.php> Retrieved on September 14, 2011.

Battaglini, A., & Gravel, S. (2000). *Diversité culturelle et planification de la santé. [Cultural diversity and health planning]. Dans culture, santé et ethnicité-vers une santé publique pluraliste [Culture, health and ethnicity—toward a pluralist public health]. Régie Régionale de Montréal-Centre et des Service Sociaux.* Montréal: Direction de la Santé Publique.

Boone, M. (2010). Creating a site relevant to parents. *Montreal Gazette*, A3.

Bouchard, G. (1991). Pour une approche historique et sociale du génome québécois [Historical and social approach to the Québec genome]. In G. Bouchard & M. DeBraekeleer (Eds.), *Histoire d'un génome: population et génétique dans l'est du Québec [History of a genome: population and genetics in eastern Québec]* (pp. 3–18). Québec: Les Presses de l'Université de Québec.

Bouchard, G. (1992). Sur les perspectives de la culture québécoise comme francophonie nord-américaine [On the perspectives of Québec culture as a French-speaking community in North America]. In P. Lanthier & G. Rousseau (Eds.), *La culture inventée, stratégies culturelles aux XIXe et XXe siècles [Cultural tendencies and cultural strategies of the nineteenth and twentieth centuries]* (pp. 319–328). Québec: Les Presses de l'Université de Québec.

Bouchard, G., & DeBraekeleer, M. (Eds.), (1991a). *Histoire d'un génome: population et génétique dans l'est du Québec [History of a genome: population and genetics in eastern Québec].* Québec: Les Presses de l'Université du Québec.

Bouchard, G., & DeBraekeleer, M. (1991b). Mouvements migratoires, effets fondateurs et homogénéisation génétique [Migratory shifts, founders effects and genetic homogenization]. In G. Bouchard & M. DeBraekeleer (Eds.), *Histoire d'un génome: population et génétique dans l'est du Québec [History of a genome: population and genetics in eastern Québec]* (pp. 281–321). Québec: Les Presses de l'Université du Québec.

Bozzini, L., & Tessier, R. (1985). Support social et santé [Social support and health]. In J. Dufresne, F. Dumont, & Y. Martin (Eds.), *Traité d'anthropologie médicale [Medical anthropology treatise]* (pp. 905–939). Québec: Les Presses de l'Université du Québec.

Branswell, B. (2010). Report card on educational reform. *Montreal Gazette*, A3.

Carkson, M., Pica, L., & Lacombe, H. (2000). *Spiritualité, religion et santé: une analyse exploratoire. [Spirituality, religion and health: an exploratory analysis]. Enquête sociale et de santé [Health and social inquiry]* (pp. 603–623). Québec: Institut de la Statistique du Québec.

CBC News. (2010). Bouchard calls the PQ too radical. *CBC News.* Available at <http://www.cbc.ca/news/canada/montreal/story/2010/02/18/lucien-bouchard-blasts-partiquebecois.html>.

Chapman, R. (2000). *Siting the Québec novel.* New York: P. Lang.

Chénard, L., Daveluy, C., & Émond, A. (2000). Conclusions général [General conclusions]. In *Enquête sociale et de santé [Health and social inquiry]* (pp. 628–643). Québec: Government of Québec.

Cossette, S., Lévesque, L., & Laurin, L. (1995). Informal and formal support for caregivers of a demented relative: do gender and kinship make a difference? *Research in Nursing and Health, 18*(5), 437–451.

Davidhizar, R., & Giger, J. (2000). Cultural competency matters. *International Journal of Health Care Quality Assurance, 13*(16/7), viii–xi.

DeBraekeleer, M. (1991). Les gènes délétères [Deleterious genes]. In G. Bouchard & M. DeBraekeleer (Eds.), *Histoire d'un génome: population et génétique dans l'est du Québec [History of a genome: population and genetics in eastern Québec]* (pp. 343–363). Québec: Les Presses de l'Université de Québec.

Derfel, A. (2002). Health care system is bearing up well. (Montréal). *The Gazette,* A1–A7.

Derfel, A. (2005). Medical-imaging clinics thrive. (Montréal). *The Gazette,* A1–A7.

Desrochers, P. (2002). Shattering shelter myths. (Montréal). *The Gazette,* B7.

Dias, M. H., Chambers-Evans, J., & Reidy, M. (2010). Le volet consultation du rôle d'infirmière spécialisée [The consultation role of the clinical nurse specialist]. *Canadian Journal of Nursing Research, 42*(2), 92–104.

Dorval, Y. T. (2010). Let's meet the challenge of prosperity in Quebec. *Montreal Gazette.*

Dorvil, H. (1985). Types de sociétés et representations [Types of societies and representations]. In J. Dufresne, F. Dumont, & Y. Martin (Eds.), *Traité d'anthropologie médicale [Medical anthropology treatise].* Québec: Presses de l'Université du Québec.

Dougherty, K. (2002). Keep off the grass: Québec bans pesticides linked to diseases (Montréal). *The Gazette,* A1–A2.

Dulong, G., & Bergeron, G. (1980). *Le parler populaire du Québec et de ses régions voisines: atlas.* Linguistique de l'Est du Canada. (10 volumes). Québec City: Office de la langue française (Éditeur officiel).

Dunnigan, L. (2000). *Recours au service téléphonique Infosanté CLSC. [Recourse to Info-health telephone service]. Enquête sociale et de santé [Health and social inquiry]* (pp. 429–443). Québec: Institut de la Statistique de Québec.

Fahmy-Eid, N., & Dumont, M. (1983). *Maîtresses de maison, maîtresses d'écoles: femmes, familles et education dans l'histoire du Québec [Housewives, school mistresses: women, families, and education in Québec history].* Montréal: Boréal Express.

Fedio, C. (2010). Most Quebecers ready to support euthanasia. *Montreal Gazette.*

Fidelman, J. (2010). *MD's nurses blame Quebec government for ER crisis.* Available at <http://www.montrealgazette.com/story_print.html?id=3279083&sponsor=>.

Fitterman, L. (2002). Married ... with controversy. (Montréal). *The Montréal Gazette.*

Fournier, M.-A., & Piché, J. (2000). *Recours aux services des professionnels de la santé et des services sociaux [Recourse to the services of health and welfare professionals]. Enquête sociale et de santé [Health and social inquiry]* (pp. 388–407). Québec: Institut de la Statistique du Québec.

Gohier, C., & Schleifer, M. (1993). *La question de l'identité: Qui suis-je? Qui est l'autre? [The question of identity: Who am I? Who are the others?].* Montreal: Les Éditions Logiques.

Gouvernement du Québec (1985). *Livre vert: pour les familles Québécoises [Green book: for Québec families].* Québec: Ministre du Conseil exécutif, Secrétariat à la politique familiale.

Gouvernement du Québec (2002). *La situation démographique au Québec: bukab 2002 [The demographic situation in Québec: Outline 2002].* Québec: Ministre du Conseil executive, Secrétartiat á la politique familial.

Hall, E. T. (1990). *The hidden dimension.* New York: Anchor Books.

Herman, A. (2001). *How the Scots invented the modern world.* New York: Crown.

Institut de la statistique de Québec (2010b). *Le Québec chiffres en main.* Gouvernement de Québec. Available at <http://www.stat.gouv.qc.ca/>.

Institut de la statistique de Québec, 2013 <http://www.stat.gouv.qc.ca/page404_an.htm>.

Johnston, D. (1996). Aging boomers put a spin on funeral industry. (Montréal). *The Gazette,* A1.

Johnston, D. (2010). Unending (r)evolution. *Montreal Gazette,* 41.

Julien, M., Julien, D., & Lafontaine, P. (2000). *Environnement de soutien [Support environment]. Enquête sociale et de santé [Health and social inquiry]* (pp. 499–522). Québec: Institut de la Statistique du Québec.

Kalbfuss, K. (2002). Québec drinkers in the red. (Montréal). *The Gazette,* 1–12.

Labrie, N. (1990). La question linguistique et les communautés culturelles au Québec [Québec linguistic issue and cultural communities]. In L. Guilbert (Ed.), *Identité ethnique et interculturalité: état de la recherche en ethnologie et en socio-linguistique [Ethnic identity and interculturalism: state of research in ethnology and in sociolinguistics]* (pp. 33–46). Sainte-Foy: CELAT (Centre d'Études sur la Langue, les Arts, et les Traditions populaires des Francophones en Amérique du Nord), Université de Laval.

Lacourse, M. T. (1999). *Famille et société [Family and society]* (2nd ed.). Montreal: Chenelière.

Laflame, F. (2010). La contribution des infirmières . . . au sein des équipes multidisciplinaires de première ligne [The contribution of front line nurses within multi-disciplinary teams]. *Perspective Infirmière.*

Laforest, L. (1985). Pratiques médicales et évolution sociale [Medical practices and social evolution]. In J. Dufresne, F. Dumont, & Y. Martin (Eds.), *Traité d'anthropologie médicale [Medical anthropology treatise]* (pp. 267–280). Québec: Les Presses de l'Université du Québec.

Lamonde, Y. (1991). *Territoires de la culture québécoise [Québec cultural territories].* Québec: Les Presses de l'Université de Laval.

Lanthier, P., & Rousseau, G. (1992). *La culture inventée, stratégies culturelles aux XIXe et XXe siècles [Cultural tendencies and cultural strategies of the nineteenth and twentieth centuries].* Québec: Institut québécois de Recherche sur la Culture.

Laperrière, G. (1992). La place du catholicisme [The place of Catholicism]. Dossier: Catholicisme et société distincte [Catholicism and distinct society]. *Présence, 2*(5), 21–23.

La Press Canadienne. (2010). Des femmes marchent à Montréal pour sensibliser Ottawa et Québec (Women march from Montreal to sensitize Ottawa and Quebec). *Yahoo News.* Available at <http://qc.news.yahoo.com/s/capress/10037/nationales/femmes_marche_montreal&printer=1> Accessed September 14, 2011.

Laroche, D. (2000). Indicateurs pour des activités quotidienne [Indicators of daily activities]. *Donnée sociodémographique en bref* [Sociodemographic data in brief] *4*(6), 5–6.

Laroche, D., & Gauthier, H. (2002). Quelque résultats sur l'emploi du temps [Some results about the use of time]. *Donnée sociodémographique en bref,* [Sociodemographic data in brief], *6*(2), 1.

Lavasseur, M. (2000). *Perception de l'état de santé [Perception of health status]. Enquête sociale et de santé [Health and social inquiry]* (pp. 259–269). Québec: Institut de la Statistique du Québec.

Lazure, J. (1990). Mouvance des générations. Condition féminine et masculine [Generational sphere of influence. Female and male status]. In F. Dumont (Ed.), *La Société québécoise après 30 ans de changements [Québec society after 30 years of change]* (pp. 27–40). Québec: Institut québécois de Recherche sur la Culture.

Leaune, V., & Adrien, A. (1998). *Les Québécois face au sida: Attitudes envers les personnes vivant avec le VIH et gestions des risques [Québecers in regards to AIDS: attitudes toward persons living with HIV and the management of risks].* Montréal: Direction de la santé publique, Régie régional de la santé et de services sociaux de Montréal-Centre.

Le Devoir, L. F. (1999). *Une grande enquête Sondagem—Le Devoir sur les priorités et les aspirations des Québécois.* Montreal: [A Great survey—Le Devoir on the priorities and the aspirations of the people of Quebec].

Leger, J.-M. (2010). Le baromèter des professions [The barometer of the professions]. *Journal de Montreal.* Available at <http://fr.canoe.ca/cig-bin/imprimer.cgi?id=609261> Retrieved September 14, 2011.

Létourneau, E., Bernier, B., Marchand, P., & Trudel, G. (2000). Familles et santé [Families and health]. In *Enquête sociale et de santé [Health and social inquiry]* (pp. 271–293). Québec: Institut de la Statistique du Québec.

Lévesque, L. (2010). Les Québécois favorables à une taxe sur les boissons sucrées et de la prévention [Quebecers favor a tax on sweetened and energizing drinks and on prevention]. *Yahoo! Santé Québec.* Available at <http://qc.sante.yahoo.ca/health_news_popup.asp?channel_id=36&news_id=3064&section_name=channel_health_news&section_name_value=cardiovasculaire> Retrieved September 14, 2011.

Marcoux, J. S. (2001). The "casier maison" ritual. *Journal of Material Culture, 6*(2), 213–235.

McAndrew, M., & Potvin, M. (1996). *Racisme au Québec: éléments d'un diagnostique [Racism in Québec: elements of a diagnosis].* Québec: Ministère des Affaires internationales de l'immigration et des Communications du Québec.

McCallum, J. (2010a). *Quebec to introduce 500 front line nurses into system, up from 25.* Available at http://www.montrealgazette.com/story_print.html?id=3279083&sponsor=.

McGovern, S. (2002). 66,000 jobs, jobs, jobs. (Montréal). *The Gazette,* A1–A2.

McKenzie, R. (2002). Vivre l'immigration français [Long live French immigration]. (Montréal). *The Gazette,* B1–B4.

Mennie, J. (2010). Life from Montreal, its city council. *Montreal Gazette,* A7.

Milan, A., Maheux, H., & Chul, T. (2010). *A portrait of couples in mixed unions. Statistics Canada.* Government of Canada.

MSNBC. (2000). *Web-threat to French in Québec: "le combat" over the web.*

Murray, L., Reidy, M., & Carnevale, F. A. (2010). Stakeholders' conceptualization the nurse practitioner's role in a pediatric emergency department. *Nursing Leadership, 22*(4), 88–100.

O'Donnell, V., Almey, M., Lindsay, C., et al. (2006). *Women in Canada: a gender-based statistical report. Statistics Canada.* Government of Canada.

Ordre des infirmières et infirmiers du Québec (2009). *Les infirmières praticiennes spécialisées: un rôle à propulser, une intégration à accélérer [Nurse practitioners: a role to promote, and integration to accelerate].* Montréal: Ordre des infirmières et infirmiers du Québec.

Ordre des infirmières et infirmiers du Québec. (2010a). Programme d'inspection professionnelle de l'exercice infirmier [Professional inspection program for the practice of nursing]. *Le Journal, 7*(3), 5.

Ordre des infirmières et infirmiers du Québec. (2010b). Les infirmières partage deux nouvelles activités avec les médecines [Nurses share two new activities with doctors]. *Le Journal, 7*(2), 1, 5.

Ordre des infirmières et infirmiers du Québec (2010c). *Évolution de l'effectif de la profession infirmière au Québec—Données au 31 mars 2006 [Evolution of the workforce of the professional nurse in Québec—data from March 31 2006].* Montréal: Ordre des infirmières et infirmiers du Québec.

Orr, R. (1992). Notre héritage Catholique [Our Catholic heritage]. Translated by Serge Gagnon. Dossier: Catholicisme et société distincte [Catholicism and distinct society]. *Présence, 1*(5), 11–13.

Papillon, M.-J., Laurier, C., Barnard, L., & Baril, J. (2000). *Consommation de médicaments [Consumption of medications]. Enquête sociale et de santé [Health and social inquiry]* (pp. 245–267). Québec: Institut de la Statistique du Québec.

Paquet, G. (1989). *Santé et inégalité sociales: un problème de distance culturelle [Health and social inequality: cultural gap].* Québec: Les Presses de l'Université de Québec.

Québec Coalition for Tobacco Control. (2010). *Smokers occupy one-third of hospital beds.* Commissioned by Québec Coalition for Tobacco Control. Retrieved November 8, 2011 from <http://www.cbc.ca/news/health/story/2010/08/16/montreal-study-smokers-health-care-system.html>.

Québec Government Portal. (2002a) *Health.* Available at <http://www.gouv.qc/Vision>.

Québec Government Portal. (2002b). *Society.* Available at <http://www.gouv.qc/Vision/Societe/ProtraitDemographique_en.html>.

Québec Government Portal. (2002c). *Society.* Available at <http://www.gouv.qc/Vision/Societe/ProtraitHistorique_en.html>.

Québec Government Portal. (2002d). *Society.* Available at <http://www.gouv.qc/Vision/Societe/ProtraitsDistinctives_en.html>.

Reidy, M. (2005). The educational role of the nurse in the context of the shift to ambulatory care (Unpublished dissertation). Universite de Québec a Montréal.

Rioux, M. (1974). *Les Québécois [The Québecers].* Paris: Seuil.

Santé et Services sociaux de Québec (2013). *État de santé de la population québécoise–quelques repères [State of health of the Quebec population–a number of tables of information].* Québec: Gouvernement de Québec.

Scott, M. (2010). Niqab: The new flash point. *Montreal Gazette,* B1.

STATS Canada. (2002). Available at <http://www.statcan.ca> Retrieved on June 28, 2007.

Stats Canada (2015). Retrieve from <http://www.statcan.gc.ca/start-debut-eng.html> February 1, 2015.

Stewart, M. J., Hart, G., Mann, K., Jackson, S., Langille, L., & Reidy, M. (2001). Telephone support group: intervention for persons with haemophilia and HIV/AIDS and family caregivers. *International Journal of Nursing Studies, 38*(2), 209–225.

Taggart, M. E., Reidy, M., & Grenier, D. (1992). Attitudes d'infirmières francophones face au sida [French-speaking nurses' attitudes toward AIDS]. *Infirmière canadienne/Canadian Nurse, 88*(1), 48–52.

Tétu de Labsade, F. (1990). *Le Québec: un pays, une culture [Québec: a country, a culture].* Montréal: Boréal.

Thibaudeau, M. F., & Reidy, M. (1985). A nursing care model for the disadvantaged family. In M. Stewart (Ed.), *Community health nursing in Canada* (pp. 269–286). Toronto: Gage.

Thibaudeau, M. F., Reidy, M., d'Amours, F., & Frappier, G. (1984). *La santé de la famille défavorisée: évaluation de l'application d'un modèle de soins infirmiers auprès de familles défavorisées qui utilisent les services du CLSC [Health of the disadvantaged family: assessment of the application of a nursing care model in disadvantaged families using community health clinics].* Montréal: Faculté des Sciences infirmières, Université de Montréal.

Thibault, M. T. (1989). Environnement [Environment]. In R. Asselin (Ed.), *Le Québec statistique 1989 [1989 Québec statistics]* (59th ed., pp. 261–291). Québec: Les Publications du Québec.

Trahan, L., Bégin, P., & Piché, J. (2000). *Recours à l'hospitalisation, à la chirurgie d'un jour et au services post-hospitaliers [Recourse to hospitalization, day surgery and post-hospital services]. Enquête sociale et de santé [Health and social inquiry]* (pp. 409–428). Québec: Institut de la Statistique de Québec.

Trudel, A. (1995). Nurses as members of administrative boards. *Canadian Nurse, 91*(5), 37–40.

Valentine, H. (2001). The increasingly assertive ladies of Québec. *Le Québécois Libre,* 92. Available at <http://www.quebecoislibre.org/011110–8.htm> Retrieved June 28, 2007.

Vissandjée, B., & Dupéré, S. (2000). La communication interculturelle en contexte clinique: une question de artenariat [Intercultural communication in a clinical context: a question of partnership]. *In Revue canadienne de recherche en sciences infirmières [Canadian Review of Nursing Research], 32*(1), 99–113.

Volant, E. (2004). L'accompagnement des mourants: aux limites du sens—une ethique du seuil [The companionship of the dying: at the end of life—an ethic of the threshold]. *Frontieres, 17*(1), 83–86.

Watelet, H. (1999). *Temps et culture [Time and culture]. Quatre essais sur temps et culture [Four essays on time and culture]* (pp. 5–8). Montréal: Centre interuniversitaire d'études québécois & Institut d'études canadiennes.

World Almanac. (2015). New York: World Almanac Books.

24

Puerto Rican Americans

Sherrica Miller

BEHAVIORAL OBJECTIVES

After reading this chapter the nurse will be able to:

1. Describe methods a nurse can use to enhance communication with a Puerto Rican.
2. Explain the importance of personal space to some Puerto Rican women.
3. Describe the importance of family relationships for Puerto Ricans.
4. Discuss the effect of time orientation on health promotion activities for Puerto Ricans.
5. Identify the role of folk and spiritual healers for some Puerto Ricans.
6. Discuss biological variations that may be found in Puerto Ricans.

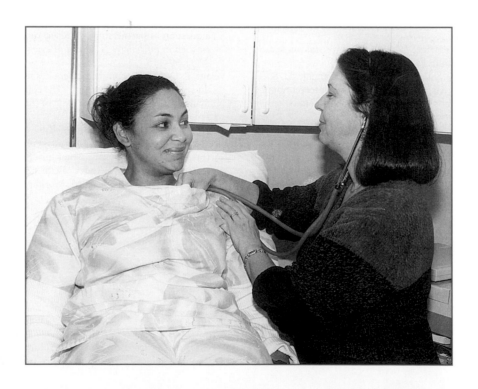

OVERVIEW OF PUERTO RICO

The commonwealth of Puerto Rico is located in the Caribbean Sea about 1000 miles east-southeast of Miami. Puerto Rico is to the east of Haiti and the Dominican Republic (La Hispaniola) and to the west of the Virgin Islands. With a land area of 3425 square miles, Puerto Rico is approximately three times the size of Rhode Island (Central Intelligence Agency [CIA], 2015). Its territory includes the islands of Culebra, Vieques, Descecheo, and Mona. Puerto Rico has a high central mountain range, dry and fertile northern coastal plains, low eastern mountains, and the El Yunque rain forest (CultureGrams, 2002).

In the fifteenth century, some 50,000 indigenous Taino Indians inhabited the territory and called the island *Boriken* or *Borinquen,* which means "the great land of the valiant and noble Lord" or "land of the great lords" (Welcome to Puerto Rico: History, 2015). This word is still used to designate the people and island of Puerto Rico. When Christopher Columbus arrived in 1493 and claimed the island for Spain, the Taino Indians lived in small villages, organized in clans, and were led by a chief. The Taino lived off the tropical crops, including pineapples, cassava, and sweet potatoes, supplemented by seafood. Spanish colonizers who arrived in 1508 were welcomed by the Taino, who offered these colonizers gold nuggets they picked out of the river. The seaside port, which later was named San Juan and today is the capital, quickly became Spain's most important military outpost in the Caribbean. The Spaniards constructed a wall around San Juan. A massive fort on the harbor, San Felipe del Morro Castel, was erected to protect the city with garrisoned troops. The Spaniards also established gold-mining operations, which lasted until 1570, when the gold stores were depleted.

Under the rule of Juan Ponce de León, the governor appointed by the Spanish crown, the first *repartimiento* (colonial forced labor system) of Puerto Rico was established. Indians were offered to officials and colonists as wage-free, forced labor. When several priests protested the treatment of the Indians, the Spanish crown instituted the *encomienda,* which required the Indians be taught the Catholic religion and be paid for their labor. However, the Indians continued to be treated as slaves, and those who resisted were killed, which resulted in the annihilation of much of the male population. Only a few Indians escaped into the remote mountains of the island. Many of the remaining women were taken by the Spanish settlers for mates, and their offspring become known as *jibaros.* With industrialization and migration to the cities, few *jibaros* remain today (Welcome to Puerto Rico: People, 2015). African slaves were brought to the island as sugarcane was introduced, with slavery continuing until 1873

(CultureGrams, 2002). The slaves imported from Africa came from Sudan, Congo, Senegal, Guinea, Sierra Leone, the Ivory Coast, and the Gold Coast, adding further diversity to the island's racial mix. Furthermore, some French families from both Louisiana and Haiti, Scottish and Irish farmers escaping depressed economies, Italians, Germans, and even Lebanese people moved to Puerto Rico and contributed to the cultural and racial mix that makes the Puerto Rican culture unlike any other. This historic intermingling has resulted in an island where racial problems are minimal (Welcome to Puerto Rico: Puerto Rican Culture, 2015).

Over the centuries, the Spaniards fought off attempts by the French, Dutch, and British to capture control of the island. Nevertheless, after the Spanish-American War, in 1898, the Treaty of Paris ceded Puerto Rico to the United States, thus adding American influence to the culture. In 1917 Puerto Ricans were given U.S. citizenship.

In 1952 the people voted in favor of commonwealth status. As a commonwealth, Puerto Rico is a self-governing part of the United States. Puerto Rico's executive power resides in the governor and a bicameral legislature made up of a Chamber of Representatives of 53 members and a Senate of 27 members, who have control over the internal affairs of Puerto Rico. Puerto Rico is divided into 78 municipalities, each of which has an elected mayor and municipal assembly (Welcome to Puerto Rico: Government, 2015). Puerto Rico has one resident commissioner with a voice but no vote in the Congress of the United States. As U.S. citizens, Puerto Ricans are subject to military service and most federal laws, and they have free movement in and out of the United States. However, as residents of the commonwealth, they pay no federal income tax on locally generated earnings, nor can electoral votes be cast by Puerto Rico in the U.S. presidential elections.

Currently, Puerto Ricans are divided over whether to request the United States for statehood or to remain a commonwealth (CultureGrams, 2002). A view of the Internet version of the *Puerto Rico Herald* (http://www.puertorico-herald.org) indicates numerous articles related to the political future of Puerto Rico, including one titled, "What should the U.S. Congress do about Puerto Rico's political status?"

Puerto Rico is a strategic location for the U.S. military in the Caribbean. This setting gives the U.S. military access to North, Central, and South America, and Puerto Rico is a center for U.S. military training, surveillance, and weapons testing (Welcome to Puerto Rico: Government, 2015). Since the closure of U.S. bases in Panama in 1999, Puerto Rico has provided the home for military forces in Latin America and for the U.S. Army South.

With a population of 3,620,897 (July 2014 estimate) and density of 1057.5 people per square mile (2014 estimate),

Puerto Rico is one of the most densely populated islands in the world and is more densely populated than any of the other states (CIA, 2015; U.S. Department of Commerce, Bureau of the Census, 2013). Some 71% of the population lives in urban areas. Approximately one third of the population is concentrated in the San Juan-Carolina-Bayamon metropolitan area; 75.8% are White, 12.4% are Black, 0.4% Amerindian, 0.2% Asian, and 10.8% are mixed and other (CIA, 2015; Welcome to Puerto Rico: People, 2015). A total of 98.8% of the population considers themselves Hispanic (*World Almanac,* 2015). According to 2014 estimates, the birthrate is 10.90 per 1000 live births, the average annual rate of growth is 0.65%, the infant mortality rate is 7.73 per 1000 live births, and the life expectancy at birth is 79.09 years (75.46 years for males and 82.80 years for females) (CIA, 2015; Welcome to Puerto Rico: People, 2015; *World Almanac,* 2015).

Puerto Rico is a major hub of Caribbean commerce and tourism, boasting a diversity of attractions in an unvarying climate that ranges year round from 75° to 85° F (Porter & Prince, 2000). San Juan provides one of the world's busiest cruise ship ports and is among the most dynamic cities in the West Indies (Porter & Prince, 2000). Romantic resorts, private villas, and remote offshore islands offer attractive honeymoon destinations. The chief crops of Puerto Rico include coffee, plantains, pineapples, tomatoes, sugarcane, bananas, mangos, and ornamental plants. Chief industries are pharmaceuticals, manufacturing of electronics and apparel, and tourism. Some 19% of the labor force is employed by the government. In spite of marked success in Puerto Rico's developmental efforts, the per capita median income (2009 estimate) of $14,905 is low by U.S. standards, but high by the World Bank estimates that considers high-income countries as having a gross national income per capita of $16,300 (2014 estimate) (Welcome to Puerto Rico: Government, 2015). The unemployment rate of 16% (2015) means some persons live off public assistance (CIA, 2015). The median family income is $27,017 (U.S.) compared with the rest of the general U.S. population at $52,029 (U.S. Department of Commerce, Bureau of the Census, *American Community Survey,* 2013). In 2008, it was estimated that some 48.8% of the total population of people in Puerto Rico lived below the poverty level, which is defined by Health and Human Services for a family of three at $15,670 per year and for a family of four at $18,240 (Welcome to Puerto Rico: People, 2015).

IMMIGRATION TO THE UNITED STATES

The open borders allow migration of Puerto Ricans to the United States. As American citizens, they are neither immigrants nor aliens (Spector, 2004). Initial settlements of Puerto Ricans were in New York. In the 1950s, an average of 40,000 Puerto Ricans migrated yearly, so that by 1970 more than 1.4 million Puerto Ricans lived in regions across the United States. When the economy in the United States declined in the 1970s, thousands returned to Puerto Rico. When the Puerto Rican economy declined, social programs from the U.S. government were provided.

In mainland United States, Puerto Ricans make up the second largest Hispanic subgroup in the United States and represent 9.7% of the country's Hispanic population (U.S. Department of Commerce, Bureau of the Census, *American Community Survey,* 2013; U.S. Department of Commerce, Bureau of the Census, *Hispanic Briefs,* 2013). Today, nearly 4.6 million Puerto Ricans reside in mainland United States, predominantly in the Northeast, with large numbers in New York and metropolitan New Jersey (CIA, 2015; U.S. Department of Commerce, Bureau of the Census, *American Community Survey,* 2013).

As citizens, Puerto Ricans do not require a work visa to live or work in the United States, significantly simplifying travel back and forth. However, while travel can be done without difficulty, problems with the English language, lack of financial resources, and health problems present significant acculturation problems that require assistance from culturally competent professionals (Cohen, 1972). Among the Puerto Rican population in the United States, 25.7% live in poverty, compared with 14.3% of the total population (U.S. Department of Commerce, Bureau of the Census, *American Community Survey,* 2013). As an ethnic group and minority, Puerto Ricans in the mainland United States may encounter prejudice not experienced on an island where racial diversity is the norm.

COMMUNICATION

For many years Spanish and English were both designated as the official languages of Puerto Rico. Even though few Puerto Ricans spoke English, English was the official language of instruction, and children were forced to learn English in school (Juarbe, 2005). In 1991, in response to pleas from the people, the Puerto Rican legislature passed a bill that made Spanish the island's official language. However, in 1993 the governor restored equal status to Spanish and English (Welcome to Puerto Rico: Description, 2015). Today, Spanish tends to be used at home and in schools, the mass media, and business, whereas English is used for all federal matters, is spoken in all major tourist areas, and in most schools is taught as the second language. Puerto Ricans from large cities are most likely to be able to read, understand, and speak at least some English (Juarbe, 2005).

It is important for the nurse to appreciate that the Spanish spoken by Puerto Ricans may differ significantly from the Spanish spoken by individuals from other Hispanic cultures. An example of this is found in the use of *Escala de Inteligencia para Ninos,* which is a translation of the Wechsler Intelligence Scale for Children developed in Puerto Rico but used widely for testing with many Spanish-speaking children. When Christine Miracle (1981) tried to use this test with Aymara children in Bolivia who were bilingual in Spanish and Aymara, a number of overt and covert problems were identified. The language presented overt problems, and differences in cultural heritage between the two groups taking the test presented covert problems. When a word was taken from American English to Puerto Rican Spanish to Bolivian Spanish and from White middle-class children in the United States to Puerto Rico to the poor rural American Indian children in Bolivia, both the word and the meaning changed.

Puerto Ricans are sensitive people and are quick to express feelings of love and affection, or *carinosos.* They are known for their hospitality and desire warm and smooth interpersonal relationships, or *simpaticos* (Juarbe, 2005). Gratitude and respect are often expressed to others, including health care providers, by gifts of homemade food. Since showing respect properly is highly valued in the culture, rejection of a gift can be interpreted as an insult.

Puerto Ricans are fond of fiestas (celebrations) and celebrate not only U.S. federal holidays but also many holidays unique to Puerto Rico, including Three Kings Day (January 6), the Discovery of Puerto Rico Day (November 19), and Constitution Day (July 25). Tourists can easily find festivals and carnivals to add to their holiday itinerary when visiting Puerto Rico (Porter & Prince, 2000). Many Puerto Ricans living in the United States continue to celebrate Puerto Rican holidays.

Tone of voice is important in communication for Puerto Ricans; their tone is typically melodic and peaceable (Juarbe, 2005). A Puerto Rican may misinterpret the nurse's use of high pitch and voice inflection as confrontational when this is not intended.

Puerto Ricans are generally accustomed to shaking hands when greeting people. Close friends may grasp shoulders and kiss each other on the cheek. While women may kiss women or men in this way, men do not greet other men with a kiss. However, a man may embrace a good friend or relative (*compadre*) with a hug after a long absence. It is common for females to touch each other with their hands during communication. In greeting, more traditional Puerto Ricans may avoid eye contact as a sign of respect. Avoidance of eye contact may also be practiced when greeting the elderly as a sign of respect.

For most Puerto Ricans, self-respect is communicated by pride in personal appearance, particularly by what is worn in public. In Puerto Rico, parties and social gatherings are occasions where formal dress is expected, with shirts and ties for men and dresses or skirts and blouses for women. Sloppy, overly casual, or revealing dress is not considered appropriate. The traditional clothing once associated with Puerto Rico is no longer worn, but *Espiritistas* or faith healers may wear white outfits, hats, and handkerchiefs on selected days.

When addressing others in formal situations, Puerto Ricans may use titles to show respect. A Puerto Rican may use a title recognizing the person's profession alone or in combination with a surname. It is most respectful to address an older person by combining the title with the person's first name.

Implications for Nursing Care

Lack of ability to speak English has been related to lack of adequate treatment for Puerto Ricans in the United States. While Spanish literature for teaching may be available, the literacy level of the patient may not allow the literature to be understood. When a Spanish-speaking translator is available, the dialect of the translator may be so different that the Puerto Rican patient does not clearly understand what is being explained. Rogler (1999) noted that translators can make many errors in translating a language even when they are familiar with that language. When a translator lacks the cultural and linguistic background to recognize words in a language that may change meaning from one culture to the next, the translation can lack accuracy (Bonder, Martin, & Miracle, 2002).

When interpreters are used, it is important to consider the topic to be discussed and the gender of the interpreter. If the topic carries a stigma such as acquired immunodeficiency syndrome, tuberculosis, or sexual behavior, a patient may be more likely to express concerns to an interpreter than to a family member and to express concerns to the interpreter that they do not want this information disclosed to the health care provider. Thus, it is necessary to convey to the patient that no information should be communicated to the interpreter that the patient does not want the health care provider to know. For some topics related to sexual matters, same-sex family members will be more effective translators than an interpreter of the opposite sex.

Ruiz (1983) noted that when dealing with Puerto Rican patients who have come from an agrarian society, even if the care provider or interpreter speaks Spanish, the patient may have difficulty with good control of the Spanish language. Additionally, in contrast with other Hispanic persons, it is essential to understand the nonverbal communication and symbolism that Puerto Ricans convey with hand gestures and facial expressions, which are critical to understanding the patient's communication.

It is important for the nurse to appreciate that a Puerto Rican patient may be very hesitant to use a bedside commode or bedpan and may refrain from having a bowel movement during hospitalization because of embarrassment. The nurse may be able to provide adequate privacy that enables a patient on bed rest to use a bedpan by being aware of the stress this causes the patient. Even when a Puerto Rican is sick, self-care for personal needs or care by a family member of the same sex may be preferred over having care provided by medical care providers. The nurse should be flexible and adapt care to be culturally appropriate.

The nurse must appreciate the value that Puerto Ricans place on saving face. For example, a patient who has limited grasp of the English language may be hesitant to ask a nurse to slow down or repeat what is said. The importance of respect in verbal and nonverbal communications should be recognized and accepted with cultural understanding, for example, accepting a patient's gift of homemade food to show appreciation and respect. Because Puerto Ricans are particularly sensitive to feeling slighted, the nurse should be attentive to actions that may be interpreted as rejection (CultureGrams, 2002).

SPACE

Puerto Ricans are accustomed to standing close together when talking. A Puerto Rican may feel insulted if the other individual in a social or professional interaction moves away even slightly during the conversation (CultureGrams, 2002). On the other hand, personal space can be a significant issue for some Puerto Rican women, who are conscious of maintaining a reasonable distance with persons of the opposite sex. Younger Puerto Ricans may relate distance to being stereotyped as nonassertive.

Implications for Nursing Care

Since spacial needs and interpretations vary, it is important to assess each individual in relation to spacial needs. Spatial needs will vary with sex, age, and position.

SOCIAL ORGANIZATION

The family, including both nuclear and extended members, is highly valued in the Puerto Rican culture. In fact, in most Puerto Rican families all activities, decisions, and social and cultural standards occur in the context of the family (Juarbe, 2005).

In Puerto Rico, the total fertility rate is 1.64 (2014 estimate), and 70% of Puerto Rican women report use of contraception to control family size. The average family size in Puerto Rico is 3.6 people. The marriage rate is 9.2 per 1000 persons, with a divorce rate of 4.47 per 1000 (CIA, 2015; Welcome to Puerto Rico: People, 2015). Older Puerto Ricans are often rejecting of nonheterosexual preferences, and subsequently gay and lesbian choices may not be revealed to older family members (Juarbe, 2005).

Puerto Ricans tend to rely on older adults and elder family when making decisions. In some families, the oldest son or daughter is the one with final decision-making authority over health matters (Juarbe, 2005). When a health-related decision is to be made, a wife will typically consult her husband. Even in an emergency situation, the nurse should be sure to ask a Puerto Rican woman if her husband needs to be consulted regarding consent for treatment of a Puerto Rican male. This may be also the case if another family member is to be included in the decision-making process. In some situations, an older woman in the family will have authority and a respected role in decision making. For younger families it will usually be the man who takes responsibility for decisions. Since generational differences may exist as well as differences related to generation of migration to the United States, the nurse must be sensitive and assess each patient for decision-making responsibility within the family. Sick individuals are expected to assume a passive role in terms of care responsibilities and allow themselves to be taken care of by a family member. Family members generally prefer to provide support for individuals needing care in the home themselves rather than involving home care or home-making services; for example, an elder daughter or son may assume care responsibilities for an elderly parent and a wife for the husband rather than involving an outside caregiver.

It is important to avoid stereotyping individuals who are Hispanic since many differences exist between Hispanic cultures. For example, Sokol-Katz and Ulbrich (1992) investigated family structure in relation to alcohol and drug use among Mexican, Puerto Rican, and Cuban-American adolescents. Whereas Mexican-American adolescents in female-headed households had higher rates of drinking, drug use, and overall risk-taking behavior, Puerto Rican adolescents in female-headed households had higher rates of overall risk-taking behaviors, and Cuban-American adolescents' behavior did not show any relationship to family structure. Thus, relationships and influences within the family structure vary among different Hispanic groups.

Children are highly valued members of the Puerto Rican culture and represent a significant portion of the population: 18.1% of the population of Puerto Rico is 0 to 14 years of age, while 65.4% is 15 to 64 years of age and 12.2% is 65 years and over (Welcome to Puerto

Rico: People, 2015). Mothers assume the greater role in physical care of children, and a father's role is for financial needs. The socioeconomic environment of some Puerto Rican families places children at higher risk for health problems. Wasserman, Brunnelli, Rauh, and Alvarado (1994) reported that high rates of poverty, poor housing, violence, and high rates of mental illness in adults place children in Puerto Rican families at higher risk for both health problems and acquired disability, such as head trauma, lead poisoning, and spinal injury. Research has provided data that suggest values of Puerto Rican parents may hamper optimal functioning of children with disabilities. Gannotti, Handwerker, Groce, and Cruz (2001) investigated sociocultural influences on disability status in Puerto Rican children. These investigators conclude that Puerto Rican values of interdependence, *anonar* (pampering or nurturing behaviors), and *sobre* protective (overprotectiveness) influence parental expectations for the capacity of children with disabilities and need to be taken into account when evaluating scores on the Pediatric Evaluation of Disability Inventory and in establishing plans of care.

When a family member is sick, it is expected that close and distant family members, as well as neighbors and friends, will visit to provide support. The nurse should attempt to accommodate the need of some Puerto Rican families to have someone with a hospitalized patient on an ongoing basis.

Attitude toward victims of child sexual abuse varies among cultures and has been found to be more positive in Puerto Rican families. Rodriguez-Strednicki and Twaite (1999) found that Puerto Rican adults evaluated victims more positively than did Cuban-American adults and thus are less likely to stigmatize the child.

Pregnancy is a time for indulgence for many Puerto Rican women. Men are supportive and tolerant of pregnant women. Although most Puerto Rican women follow a diet, exercise is viewed as inappropriate. Therefore, it is helpful for the nurse to encourage exercise and good nutrition in order to avoid excessive weight gain. During labor, fathers generally assume a passive supportive role, and many prefer not to be in attendance at the delivery. Vaginal delivery is preferred since there is some stigma that a cesarean section suggests a "weak woman" (Juarbe, 2005). Many women from rural areas prefer breastfeeding; women who work may combine breastfeeding with formula. A tradition for the first meal after delivery for some Puerto Ricans is homemade fresh chicken soup. Some Puerto Rican women's birth recuperation includes avoiding housework and hair washing for 40 days. Male babies are traditionally circumcised at birth.

Researchers conducted a study to investigate the cultural differences in the relationship between maternal sensitivity, emotional expression, and control strategies during the first year of life, comparing middle-class island Puerto Rican and mainland Anglo mother–infant pairs. All mothers were interviewed in their homes by ethnically matched interviewers in their native language. According to the researchers, the Puerto Rican mothers used physical control in a meaningful and predictable manner in their interactions with their infants. The Puerto Rican mothers persistently and actively structured interactions with their infants in a manner consistent with their long-term socialization goal, teaching infants to be attentive, calm, and well-behaved, compared with teaching infants to be assertive and self-confident. The researchers concluded that their findings supported the need to explore the role of culture in early relationship formation and to define culturally specific definitions of sensitive caregiving (Carlson & Harwood, 2003).

In a small city in the northeastern United States, research was conducted to explore the experience of fatherhood among young Puerto Rican fathers whose sexual partners were teenagers when their first child was born. The setting was selected because of the persistently high adolescent birth rates in this urban environment. Of the 40% Hispanic population in the city, 90% are Puerto Rican. The 30 fathers participating in the study were Puerto Rican, ranging in age from 14 to 24 when their first child was born, and had an income below the federal poverty guidelines. Two findings were unanticipated by the researchers: (1) ten (33%) of the fathers interviewed reported that they had planned pregnancy with their partner for at least a year and (2) children challenged the fathers to act more responsibly in the world on behalf of their children. The fathers acknowledged concern about how their children perceived them and that children made them aware of their mortality. The unexpected findings, although not generalizable, emphasize the importance for nurses to recognize that reproductive health behaviors occur beyond stereotypical assumptions. The positive and affirming component of identity helps to explain the persistence of adolescent pregnancy, in spite of health promotion messages to avoid it (Foster, 2004).

Since 85% of Puerto Ricans are members of the Roman Catholic Church, beliefs related to Roman Catholicism are a significant influencing factor for many Puerto Ricans. For example, when a new store opens in San Juan, the owner often invites a priest to bless the business. When individuals plan a meeting, one may say *Si Dois quierre,* or "If God will" (Kent, 1992). The other 15% are Protestants (8%), nonreligious (2.3%), and others (3%) (Welcome to Puerto Rico: People, 2015). There is a separation of church and state; however, because of the high numbers of Catholics, Catholic traditions and customs prevail among the people.

Puerto Ricans consider themselves a religious people and often attribute good fortune to the deity. However, although most Puerto Ricans and Puerto Rican Americans are Christians, many also practice *espiritismo,* or spiritualism, a blend of Indian, African, and Catholic beliefs. The belief that good and evil spirits are present and can be encouraged or warded off with the proper herbs and rituals is often still present among Puerto Ricans who live in the United States. Even if Puerto Ricans in the United States do not actively practice spiritualism, many respect the beliefs (Kent, 1992).

The literacy rate in Puerto Rico is 94.1% (Welcome to Puerto Rico: People, 2015). Puerto Ricans value education, and families encourage children to not only finish high school but also attend college. This importance is underscored by the fact that a teacher's salary in Puerto Rico in 1997 was $1500 a month, far above the mean income. Puerto Rico has 50 institutions of higher education and rates sixth in the world for college education rates. Some 56% of college-age persons are attending institutions of higher learning (Welcome to Puerto Rico: People, 2015).

Implications for Nursing Care

The nurse should be aware that Puerto Ricans have a strong need for family support and that decision making usually occurs in a family context. The nurse should also be aware that Puerto Ricans in the United States are also likely to be strongly loyal to their country and to feel a strong sense of nationalism. Rather than calling themselves *Americanos,* many Puerto Ricans prefer to call themselves *Puertorrique-nos* or *Boricuas.* When referring to "my country," the reference is usually to Puerto Rico rather than the United States. Some Puerto Rican descendants born in America refer to themselves as Puerto Ricans, saying, "I am Puerto Rican, but I wasn't born there." When the nurse is able to speak knowledgeably about Puerto Rican culture or has visited the country, even if only to get off a cruise ship at San Juan for a few hours to visit Fort San Cristobal or the El Yunque rain forest, this familiarity will facilitate a bond with the patient (Zbar, 2001). Puerto Ricans in the United States are generally eager to talk about their plans to return and visit their homeland (Welcome to Puerto Rico: People, 2015). Thousands of Internet sites are available to keep Puerto Ricans in the United States in touch with what is happening in Puerto Rico and to provide opportunities to share thoughts and feelings. *The Puerto Rico Herald* is available in both English and Spanish online.

It is important for the nurse to consider that appropriateness of maternal responses and reproductive health behaviors is based in part on cultural factors. Assessment of mother–child interactions must be understood in terms of cultural beliefs about parenting and child development

(Carlson & Harwood, 2003). The power of gender relations in adolescent health behavior must be considered an integral part of the solution to unintended pregnancy among teenagers. Male partners must be included in a comprehensive approach to contraceptive counseling and preparation for parenting (Foster, 2004). Health behaviors, as well as personal development, occur in a context of cultural values.

TIME

The Puerto Rican concept of time is generally relaxed and more social than clock oriented. In other words, the social interaction occurring at the moment is considered more important than scheduled appointments. If a friend, relative, or business associate drops by unexpectedly, a Puerto Rican will often stop what is being done in order to visit, regardless of other commitments.

Implications for Nursing Care

The social orientation to time often sometimes serves as a barrier to punctuality with scheduled health care appointments. It is important to emphasize to the patient that the office schedule is often not flexible and arriving late may mean that the appointment will have to be rescheduled.

ENVIRONMENTAL CONTROL

Puerto Ricans tend to have a serene rather than fatalistic view of life. Most Puerto Ricans feel that destiny, a deity, spirits, or spiritual forces control events that occur, health, and death (Juarbe, 2005). Illness may be attributed to heredity, sin, lack of personal attention to health, an evil spirit, or a disharmony of environmental forces within the individual. A person under the control of an evil spirit or forces will seek a spiritualist to perform an intervention. A disharmony of environmental forces can be treated by foods, medicines, and herbs, all of which, the Puerto Ricans believe, will restore a positive internal environment.

Some Puerto Ricans believe in *Santeria,* a belief that originated among the Yoruba people in Nigeria and was brought to Puerto Rico with the importation of the Yoruba slaves. In order to be compliant with the demand to practice the Catholic religion, the Yoruba identified their gods (*Orishas*) with names of Catholic saints (Gonzalez-Wippler, 1992). Certain saints were attributed with curative powers for various health conditions. The *Santeria* belief system is practiced by *santeros,* who are sought out by many Puerto Ricans for treatment of symptoms that are described by Western medicine as symptoms of mental illness. Mumford (1973) reported that of Puerto Rican patients seen in an outpatient mental health clinic in New

York, 73% had already sought out a *santero*. Ruiz (1983) reported that in the early 1970s, 85% of the Puerto Ricans seen with mental problems went to both Catholic church on Sunday and spiritualistic centers during the week. In fact, Puerto Ricans, who seek Western medical treatment for mental illness, may fear being rejected by their community for this action. Puerto Ricans have traditionally placed great faith in the power of the *santero* to listen and to perform an appropriate treatment that makes the person feel "special" and thus restores damaged self-esteem. *Santeria* can be practiced in any location—for example, the individual's home, a storefront, or a college dormitory (Spector, 2004). A *santero* may wear a white robe and beaded bracelet as a sign of identity and when ceremonies are performed.

Wearing amulets is a traditional healing practice that some Puerto Ricans still practice. A small black fist (*azabache*) or small black rabbit foot may be tied on a child to protect him or her from evil. Removal of the object may be thought to produce illness, misfortune, or even death, so it should not automatically be done by the nurse in the process of giving care. It is important to ask for permission before removing such objects and to be aware that in time of crisis amulets may provide hope and reassurance (Juarbe, 2005). For some families, a priest's benediction may be requested before removal of an amulet. The nurse should also ask permission before removing rosary beads from a patient's neck. The family or patient may agree to allow the rosary beads to be moved to the patient's hand if they interfere with care. The family or patient may also desire to have other items of religious significance near the patient, including candles, pictures or statues of saints, or holy water. The family may want to use aromatic oils and lotions to rub the body as a way to ward off evil spirits.

Whereas many Hispanics believe in hot and cold diseases, Puerto Ricans have further classified remedies (food and medications) as hot (*caliente*), cold (*frio*), and cool (*fresco*). Treatment of a hot disease is with a cold or cool remedy, whereas treatment of a cold disease is with a hot remedy (Spector, 2004). An example of a hot illness is constipation; an example of a cool medicine that can be used to treat this problem is milk of magnesia. Another hot illness is diarrhea, which may be treated with the corresponding cold treatment, bicarbonate of soda (Schilling & Brannon, 1986). Ear disorders or aches, which are considered cold illnesses, can be treated with olive oil, which is a hot treatment (Juarbe, 2005). Since many Puerto Ricans classify penicillin as a hot remedy cure, they should be instructed that this drug should not be used to treat the hot conditions of diarrhea and constipation (Harwood, 1971). If a baby is being given infant formula containing evaporated milk, which is classified as hot, use of whole milk should be avoided because it is classified as cool. In other words, hot and cold food and medications should not be combined (Harwood, 1971).

In a review of the literature on barriers to health care access for Latino children, the authors identify that children account for more than 39% of the major subpopulations of Latinos (Mexican American, Puerto Rican, and Cuban American) in the United States. Because children are a large, rapidly expanding population that are disproportionately likely to be poor, to be uninsured, and to have parents with limited educational attainment, they are at greater risk for poor health and underutilization of health services. The authors report that folk medicine practices may lead to delay or complication of conventional health care. The potential for folk practices to act as barriers to health care is described by an example reported from an inner-city Puerto Rican community in Connecticut: 64% of the children had experienced *empacho* (a gastrointestinal illness); 77% of the parents reported that they took their child to a *santiguadora* (a folk healer in the Puerto Rican community) for treatment; 58% used home remedies; and 37% visited a physician. While visiting a physician was the initial choice for only 9% of the parents, 85% sought another form of treatment afterward, primarily *santiguadora* (Flores & Vega, 1998).

Spector (2004) lists folk diseases described by Puerto Ricans, including (1) *susto*, a sudden fright causing shock; (2) fatigue, with asthma-like symptoms; (3) *empacho*, which is pain and stomach cramps caused by lack of food digestion; (4) *mal ojo*, a sudden, unexplained illness; and (5) *atoque*, falling to the ground with wild movements of arms and legs and screaming. Folk illnesses may be treated with folk medicine, by a relative or friend, or in some cases by Western-style medicine and health care providers.

Rituals Related to Death and Dying

Puerto Rican families can be expected to maintain cultural death rituals. Enabling Puerto Rican families to grieve and honor the dead in a culturally appropriate manner is essential to the delivery of culturally competent care (Munet-Vilaro, 1998). In some Hispanic families, there is a code of silence in which the dying individual is not informed of the impending death (Rivera-Andino & Lopez, 2000). If a family member is dying, the family may want to keep constant vigil in a waiting area. The spiritual leader is expected to be with the patient when death occurs. When death has occurred, the person who serves as a family spokesperson should be the one to receive this information. The family may want to kiss and touch the body to say goodbye. After a death, a private area should be available for discussion with and by the family and to allow for expressions of emotion, including crying, feeling faith, being nauseated, or vomiting (Juarbe, 2005). Puerto Ricans usually support organ donation since this is a way to help others. Nevertheless, the nurse should be sensitive to which family members in the family structure should provide authorization. Autopsies are generally viewed as a violation of the body. If an autopsy is necessary, it is essential that the requirement is explained and that the family spokesperson has given consent (Juarbe, 2005).

Since a large proportion of Puerto Ricans are Catholic, death rituals are described as heavily influenced by Catholic beliefs, wherein spirituality is important and there is a continuing relationship between the living and the deceased through prayer and visits to the gravesite (Lobar, Youngblut, & Brooten, 2006).

Implications for Nursing Care

The importance of family must be recognized by the nurse. Strong family ties and high levels of instrumental and affective support are characteristic in Hispanic subgroups (Talamantes, Gomez, & Braun, 2000). The potential for parental belief systems to act as an access barrier is an important consideration. It is important, when responding to the concerns of Puerto Rican patients and their families, to explore what types of treatment interventions have already been attempted to relieve symptoms. Through respect and acceptance, alternative practices to treatment can be discussed and integrated into conventional management of childhood illness (Flores & Vega, 1998). In many cases, because of beliefs about the causes of illness, it is essential to combine both home remedies and other beliefs with use of Western medicine to obtain an optimal outcome.

When providing health teaching about health promotion activities, it is important to explain how the relationship works between health prevention activities and future health. When Puerto Rican patients believe they have control over future events, taking action will be more likely. The nurse should be aware that being underweight and thin tends to be associated with ill health, whereas being overweight is associated with health. It is important to realize that teaching about the need for regular exercise may contradict the value placed on being overweight, an indication of economic advantage.

On matters of end-of-life decision making, the nurse must be aware that collectivist rather that individualist decision making is supported by the values of *familismo* and *espiritismo*. When end-of-life care planning is considered, levels of acculturation, literacy, linguistic isolation, and values must be taken into account to promote open communication, mutual understanding, and cultural accommodation (Talamantes, Gomez, & Braun, 2000).

BIOLOGICAL VARIATIONS

Body Size and Structure

People in different racial groups vary according to body size and structure. Some examples of research involving Puerto Ricans will be noted. Cephalometric radiography is an important aspect of treatment for orthodontic deviations. Evanko, Freeman, and Cisneros (1997) noted that when norms for White European Americans and Black Americans of African descent were compared with those for Puerto Ricans, there were significant differences between ethnic groups in the dentoalveolar region. Similarities were noted in the upper face height and the anterior cranial base length. The purpose of this study was to facilitate the treatment of Puerto Ricans by means of the development of a standard mesh diagram.

Bermudez, Becker, and Tucker (1999) report the development of sex-specific equations for estimating stature of elderly Puerto Rican and other Hispanic persons by using knee-height equations. Previously published equations significantly overestimated stature of Hispanic subjects. Estimated stature of frail elderly is influenced by socioeconomic status as well as ethnicity. Mott et al. (1999) investigated the relationship of age and body fat in four ethnic groups to test the hypothesis that body fat is lower in the elderly than in middle-aged persons. Whereas Asians, Blacks, and Whites showed a highly significant curvilinear relationship between age and body fat, Puerto Rican men did not. Lauderdale et al. (1998) concluded that elderly Puerto Ricans are at less risk for hip fracture than Whites, Blacks, and other Hispanic populations studied.

Genetic Deviations

Santiago-Borrero and Valcarcel (1994) reported that Puerto Rican infants are at higher risk for congenital malformation, particularly neural tube defects, and for genetic diseases such as hypothyroidism and abnormal hemoglobins compared with other Hispanic babies because of low birth weight.

Susceptibility to Disease

Major causes of death per 100,000 population in Puerto Rico (2014) included the following (National Center for Health Statistics, Health, United States, 2014; Welcome to Puerto Rico: People, 2015):

- 142.6 Heart and cardiovascular disease
- 95.4 Cancers
- 55.1 Diabetes
- 38.0 Cerebrovascular disease
- 29.2 Pneumonia and influenza

Asthma. The 1982–1984 Hispanic Health and Nutrition Examination Survey reported high rates of asthma among Puerto Rican children in the Northeast when compared with Mexican and Cuban children (Carter-Pokras & Gergen, 1993). Crain et al. (1994) reported high rates of asthma among Puerto Rican children in an inner-city study. Ledogar, Penchaszadeh, Garden, and Acosta (2000) reported that in a study of Puerto Ricans and other Latinos in a New York metropolitan area, Puerto Ricans were more likely than other Latinos to have asthma. These researchers supported the suggestion of other researchers that gene–environment interactions may well play a part in asthma prevalence among Puerto Ricans (Colb, Pappas, Moran, & Lieberman, 1993). Other researchers have observed that the reasons for the significantly higher prevalence of active asthma for the Puerto Rican children may be key to improved understanding of asthma pathophysiology, prevention, treatment, and correlated social and environmental factors (Flores et al., 2002).

Asthma prevalence among U.S. adults was analyzed by specific variables, including age, gender, race, and ethnicity. Lifetime asthma was found to be significantly higher among Puerto Ricans (17%) than among any other racial/ethnic group. In an analysis where race/ethnicity were considered together with geographic region, Puerto Ricans in all regions of the United States had high rates of asthma. These researchers also concluded that further study of gene–environment interactions among Puerto Ricans is needed to explore the susceptibility to asthma-triggering responses (Rose, Mannino, & Lederer, 2006).

Wright and Giger (2010) conducted a study to profile California's Hispanic children, which included Puerto Ricans with asthma ranging from 1 to 5 years of age, addressing their demographics, their health care access, their asthma severity, their disability caused by asthma, and their health care utilization patterns. A sample of 149 Hispanic children was used who had a medical doctor's diagnosis of asthma. A secondary analysis of parental reports of their children's asthma was done using the California Health Interview Survey (CHIS) (2001). Findings from this study suggested that within the past 12 months, young Hispanic children with asthma had increased emergency department use because of their asthma (58.5%) as compared with visits to their regular care provider, increased hospitalizations (77.1%), and daily asthma control medication (53.4%). Most children had mild asthma severity (43.6%) and sometimes had their physical activity limited (26.8%) because of asthma. Further analysis suggested that California's young, Hispanic children with asthma have high utilization of health care services caused by asthma.

Visual Impairments. In a study by Lee, Gomez-Marin, Lam, Ma, and Vilar (2000), Puerto Rican children and adolescents in New York City were found to have a significantly higher prevalence of usual-corrected visual acuity impairment than Cuban Americans, Mexican Americans, and non-Hispanic Whites in samples drawn from Miami and five southwestern states. The findings suggest that compared with their counterparts, the Puerto Rican children and adolescents may not be receiving similar corrective refractive care, may have more severe ocular diseases, or both. Awareness of visual impairment is important since it has been related to poor school performance, learning disabilities, and juvenile delinquency (Evans, 1968; Flax, 1970; Snow, 1983). In another study related to visual acuity, Lee, Gomez-Marin, and Lam (2000) investigated the relationship between lifetime history of depression and visual acuity in Hispanic adults. The data indicated that although there was a higher relationship between impaired acuity and Mexican Americans and Cuban Americans and incidence of depression, no significant relationship was found in Puerto Ricans.

Obesity. Childhood obesity has been described as a major health problem in the United States, affecting nearly 25% of American children. In a longitudinal health survey, it was found that among Hispanic adolescents aged 12 to 18 years, obesity patterns were greater among Puerto Ricans than among other Hispanic subpopulations. Childhood obesity has important health consequences for children, is a major precursor of adult obesity, and is an important risk factor for hypertension. Additionally, an acculturation and assimilation effect was identified by the researchers, indicating the significant effect that second- and third-generation Hispanics are more likely to be obese. The researchers remarked that during adolescence, constraints linked to the family may be overridden by peer and other effects in situations where shifts in diet and physical activity that promote obesity are influenced by acculturation and assimilation (Popkin & Udry, 1998).

Obesity is a risk factor for diabetes, cardiovascular disease, and some cancers. Obesity rates for Puerto Rican women are high, at 28% to 39%. Dietary factors, including high intake of animal fat, may be associated with the increased risk (Glanz, Croyle, Chollette, & Pinn, 2003).

Wright (2011) conducted a community-based participatory research study to profile Hispanic children in Los Angeles, California, which included Puerto Ricans ranging from 7 to 12 years of age, addressing their demographics, weight status, and physical activity behaviors. A sample of 140 Hispanic children ($n = 140$) from Los Angeles–based elementary schools was used. In addition, a secondary analysis of parental reports of their children's asthma was done using the CHIS (2001). Findings from this study suggested that many urban, Hispanic children (39.0%) had a body mass index (BMI) greater than the 85th percentile for gender and age, girls (31.7%) had lower levels of weekly physical education class attendance, and girls (28.8%) and monolingual Spanish-speaking students (24.5%) had lower participation in team sports. Children with a BMI greater than the 85th percentile for gender and age had lower levels of weekly physical activity and team sports participation (13.1%). Further findings from this study suggested that Hispanic children in this sample (Los Angeles) have higher BMIs and have lower physical activity behaviors compared with other children in the same cohort.

Diabetes. Type 2 diabetes mellitus, previously known as *non–insulin-dependent diabetes,* is a major health problem among Latinos. In a study involving Puerto Ricans in the United States and Mexican Americans with type 2 diabetes, Lipton et al. (1996) found while most patients spoke only or mostly Spanish, 14% had received instruction in English alone. Most have a basic understanding of the disease, and more than half reported positive health behaviors in the past year, but 54% of the Puerto Rican Americans and 26% of the Mexican Americans had been admitted to the hospital or had used the emergency room for diabetes-related conditions. Tucker, Bermudez, and Castaneda (2000) investigated the prevalence of type 2 diabetes among Hispanic elders of Caribbean origin. The investigators found that prevalence was higher among Puerto Rican elders and noted that ethnicity was more strongly associated with diabetes status and control than were socioeconomic or measured health behavior variables.

The attitude of health professionals also affects treatment. For example, Lipton, Losey, Giachello, Mendez, and Girotti (1998) investigated attitudes and issues in treating Puerto Ricans in the United States with type 2 diabetes. The practitioners agreed that communication with patients was hindered by low reading levels, lack of proficiency in English, and an excessive respect for physicians. These emotional barriers to adequate treatment were often more important than financial concerns even among low-income patients. In this study, fear of insulin therapy was also a factor that contributed to use of folk remedies to treat diabetes. An additional cultural complication was that since many Puerto Rican individuals considered family needs to be more important than individual needs, adhering to a treatment regimen can be viewed as self-indulgence and thus not compatible with family values. This research illustrates the necessity of considering a variety of factors that may influence the delivery of culturally competent care, including communication, family values, and environmental control.

Overall, Latino subgroups (e.g., Puerto Ricans, Cubans, and Mexicans) have been described in recent studies as exhibiting differences in sociodemographic characteristics, health status, and use of health services that are often greater than differences among ethnic groups. The health disparities experienced by many Latino subgroups result from complex interrelated factors. In addition to being one of the most rapidly growing populations, the Latino population in the mainland is one of the youngest, with 36% under the age of 18 years. Barriers to health promotion and disease prevention can be reduced by addressing inadequate access to care related to a disproportionate poverty rate and level of uninsurance, as well as a shortage of Spanish-speaking health care workers. It is imperative to understand the issues related to access to health promotion and disease prevention for this vulnerable population in order to improve the quality of health care delivered and to help eliminate the racial and ethnic disparities (Betancourt, Carrillo, Green, & Maina, 2004).

Cancer. The burden of cancer is not distributed equally; many racial and ethnic minorities suffer disproportionately from cancer. Cancer-related health disparities are related to risk factors and early detection strategies. The most common cancers among Puerto Rican women from 1992 to 1998 were cancers of the breast and lung and non-Hodgkin's lymphoma. According to the National Cancer Institute (2006), rates of mammography have increased since the 1980s among Puerto Rican women—just under half of Puerto Rican women report having had a mammogram within 3 years—but Hispanic women in general are substantially less likely than their non-Hispanic counterparts to have had a recent Pap test. Higher smoking rates were found among Puerto Rican women (30.3%) on the mainland, more than most Hispanics and other ethnic groups, but studies suggest that women in Puerto Rico smoke less than on the mainland (Glanz, Croyle, Chollette, & Pinn, 2003; National Cancer Institute, 2006).

Implications for Nursing Care

It is important for the nurse to be aware that health and quality of life for Puerto Ricans are affected by a multifaceted combination of biological variations and demographic and socioeconomic factors. In a study conducted between 1996 and 2000 in Puerto Rico, lower income was positively correlated with self-reported decreased quality of life and increased mental and physical illness. Persons with higher income have fewer unhealthy days regardless of sex, whereas persons of low income have more unhealthy days. Older women, persons with less education, persons unable to work, and those who were overweight or who had diabetes or high blood pressure reported more days when they were physically or mentally unhealthy (Centers for Disease Control and Prevention [CDC], 2002). Nurses must respect the traditional beliefs and cultural contexts of illness and health-seeking behaviors. They must also understand the skepticism and distrust based on experience with discrimination and exclusion that minority groups may experience. Multidisciplinary and collaborative approaches with ethnic minority communities are important to develop relevant health improvement initiatives.

SUMMARY

The Puerto Rican population totals almost 4 million, with approximately 47% living in Puerto Rico and the remaining 53% living in the mainland United States. With an open border between Puerto Rico and the United States, Puerto Ricans are increasingly traveling back and forth. The nurse should be prepared for differences that may challenge the nurse in the delivery of culturally competent care.

CASE STUDY

Maria, a 24-year-old Puerto Rican, came to America with her husband 2 years ago. They both communicate in English and are employed at the local community college. Maria is expecting their first child. Maria's mother recently came to live with them so that she can "pamper" Maria and help when the baby is born.

Maria is 5 feet tall and weighs 110 lb at her first visit to the clinic. The nurse determines that Maria is in the second trimester at about 20 weeks' gestation. Maria states that she has not been eating very much lately because she is afraid she will get "too fat" like her older sisters did when they had babies. Her mother has told her about the cool and cold foods that she should eat during pregnancy and the hot foods that she should eat after the baby is born. Her mother has warned her not to mix hot and cold remedies. Maria wants to do what her mother tells her out of respect and feels guilty when she eats the wrong things.

Maria voices concern that her husband may want to be with other women now that she is getting a bigger "belly." She states that she has seen other Puerto Rican men do this. She also wants her husband to be with her during labor and delivery.

CARE PLAN

Nursing Diagnosis: Altered nutrition, less than body requirements related to concern about weight gain and following traditional dietary requirements of culture of origin

Client Outcomes	Nursing Interventions
1. Client will gain approximately 1 lb per week for the remainder of her pregnancy.	1. Take a diet history. Ask Maria to recall what she had to eat at meals and as snacks in the past 24 hours. Determine if this is a usual pattern. Give Maria a food intake record to list what she eats in the next 2 days. Have Maria complete a food frequency questionnaire and bring it to her next prenatal visit.
2. Client will maintain a hemoglobin level about 10.5 g/dL throughout her pregnancy.	2. Use a U.S. Department of Agriculture MyPlate graphic to explain the recommended foods and serving sizes during the last weeks of her pregnancy and after the baby is born. Emphasize that it is possible to follow the traditions of her Puerto Rican heritage and still keep her figure after delivery. Encourage her to ask her mother to put in the names of foods to eat during pregnancy. Give her another MyPlate graphic for her mother to note the foods to eat after the baby is born.
	3. Explain the importance of keeping her appointments, having the lab work done, and eating foods rich in nutrients. These things are all important for the health of her developing baby, as well as for Maria's health during and following delivery.
	4. Point out specific foods that she prefers to eat that are especially healthy for her and her baby. For example, corn tortillas and cheese are good sources of calcium, meat (beef, pork, chicken, fish) is rich in protein, and vegetables and fruits (chili peppers, tomatoes, beets, cabbage, chayotes, bell peppers, string beans, avocado, bananas, coconut, lima beans, white beans, barley water, raisins, watercress, onions, peas, kidney beans) are excellent sources of vitamins and minerals.

Continued

CARE PLAN—cont'd

Nursing Diagnosis: Risk for altered health maintenance related to nonassertive communication patterns of family members, as evidenced by Maria's comments about her husband's sexual behavior in the last part of her pregnancy and her guilt when not eating what her mother says she should eat

Client Outcomes	Nursing Interventions
1. During the first clinic visit, client will verbalize her plan for regular prenatal visits and explain the benefits of visiting the clinic regularly. 2. The client and family members will express concerns with the nurse and with each other.	1. Encourage Maria and her husband to talk about their concerns about Maria's pregnancy by using broad opening statements, such as "Many couples have concerns about continuing sexual intercourse during pregnancy...." 2. Explain what will be done at the following prenatal visits and how these activities are important to the health of the baby and Maria. 3. Offer explanations for all aspects of the prenatal visit. Explain the size and development of the growing baby. 4. Explain how sexual activities between husband and wife can change during the pregnancy so that it is comfortable. Reassure them that it will not harm the baby. 5. Explain the dangers of unprotected sex with multiple partners for all members of the family. Sexually transmitted diseases can cause long-term illness and even death. Human immunodeficiency virus is life-threatening for the father. It can be transmitted to Maria via sexual intercourse and then to the developing fetus through the placenta. Other diseases may be mild in adults but catastrophic for the developing fetus and the newborn, such as cytomegalovirus, rubella, herpes, and hepatitis B. Specific medications are used to treat sexually transmitted diseases, such as syphilis, gonorrhea, chlamydial infection, and trichomoniasis. If untreated, these diseases are also life-threatening for the developing baby. 6. Encourage Maria and her husband to write down their concerns, call the office any time, and talk about their feelings to each other. 7. Before leaving the room, ask Maria and her husband to state what their plan is in regard to future clinic visits. 8. Explain how they can be involved with childbirth classes and provide a tour of the hospital prior to delivery.

CLINICAL DECISION MAKING

1. Describe the culturally based explanations of why some pregnant Puerto Rican women may be extremely concerned about their weight gain during pregnancy.
2. Explain possible correlations between cold and hot foods and diet during pregnancy discussed by Puerto Rican women.
3. List questions that may facilitate discussion between a Puerto Rican husband and wife and the nurse related to beliefs about sexual activities during pregnancy.
4. Relate the effect of beliefs related to environmental control and preventive health care for some Puerto Rican clients.
5. Explain the individuals, by family role assignments, who may be involved in decision making concerning child and infant care among some Puerto Rican families.
6. Describe the values and beliefs about pregnancy and children commonly held by Puerto Ricans.
7. Describe how stereotyping Puerto Ricans as similar to other Hispanic Americans can lead the nurse to errors in patient care.
8. Describe how a health care provider's approach to the patient by the health care provider can be individually and uniquely focused while still utilizing knowledge about common behaviors and beliefs held by some Puerto Ricans.

REVIEW QUESTIONS

1. A pregnant Puerto Rican client comes to the clinic. Because of the cultural implications, the nurse needs to consider which of the following for this client?
   a. Service lifestyle
   b. Inclusion of the extended family
   c. Diet and exercise
   d. Prayers and rituals

2. A Puerto Rican client is being scheduled for a follow-up visit to the clinic. For this client it is important for the nurse to do which of the following?
   a. Emphasize to the client to be prompt as the office schedule often is inflexible.
   b. Emphasize the importance of coming for the appointment that day.
   c. Inform the client of the appointment in writing.
   d. Emphasize the importance of bringing the father to the next visit.

3. When using an interpreter for a Puerto Rican client, it is important for the nurse to do which of the following?
   a. Convey to the client that no information should be communicated to the interpreter that the client does not want the nurse to know.
   b. Use a same-sex family member as the interpreter.
   c. Use a translator who is familiar with the language.
   d. Provide the interpreter with available Spanish literature for teaching.

REFERENCES

Bermudez, O., Becker, E., & Tucker, K. (1999). Development of sex-specific equations for estimating stature of frail elderly Hispanics living in the northeastern United States. *American Journal of Clinical Nutrition, 69*(5), 992–998.

Betancourt, J. R., Carrillo, J. E., Green, A. R., & Maina, A. (2004). Barriers to health promotion and disease prevention in the Latino population. *Clinical Cornerstone, 6*(3), 16–29.

Bonder, B., Martin, L., & Miracle, A. (2002). *Culture in clinical care.* Thorofare, NJ: Slack.

California Health Interview Survey (CHIS). (2001). *UCLA Center for Health Policy Research.* Available at <www.chis.ucla.edu>.

Carlson, V. J., & Harwood, R. L. (2003). Attachment, culture, and the caregiving system: the cultural patterning of everyday experiences among Anglo and Puerto Rican mother-infant pairs. *Infant Mental Health Journal, 24*(1), 53–73.

Carter-Pokras, O., & Gergen, P. (1993). Reported asthma among Puerto Rican, Mexican-American, and Cuban children, 1982 through 1984. *American Journal of Public Health, 83,* 580–582.

Centers for Disease Control and Prevention (CDC). (2002). Health related quality of life—Puerto Rico, 1996–2000. *Morbidity and Mortality Weekly Report, 51*(8), 166.

Central Intelligence Agency (CIA). (2015). *The world factbook.* Chicago: Skyhorse.

Cohen, R. (1972). Principles of preventive mental health programs for ethnic minority populations: the acculturation of Puerto Ricans to the United States. *American Journal of Psychiatry, 128*(12), 79.

Colb, C., Pappas, J., Moran, E., & Lieberman, J. (1993). Variants of alpha 1-antitrypsin in Puerto Rican children with asthma. *Chest, 103,* 812–815.

Crain, E., Weiss, K., Bijur, P., Hersh, M., Westbrook, L., & Stein, R. E. (1994). An estimate of the prevalence of asthma and wheezing among inner-city children. *Pediatrics, 94,* 356–362.

CultureGrams. (2002). *Culture grams standard edition* (Vol. 1). Salt Lake City, UT: Brigham Young University.

Evanko, A., Freeman, K., & Cisneros, G. (1997). Mesh diagram analysis: developing a norm for Puerto Rican Americans. *Angle Orthodontist, 67*(5), 381–388.

Evans, J. (1968). Relationships between visual skills and behavioral disorders. *Journal of the American Optometry Association, 39,* 623–640.

Flax, N. (1970). The contribution of visual problems to learning disability. *Journal of the American Optometry Association, 41,* 841–845.

Flores, G., et al. (2002). The health of Latino children: urgent priorities, unanswered questions, and a research agenda. *Journal of the American Medical Association, 288*(1), 82–90.

Flores, G., & Vega, L. R. (1998). Barriers to health care access for Latino children: a review. *Family Medicine, 30*(3), 196–205.

Foster, J. (2004). Fatherhood and the meaning of children: an ethnographic study among Puerto Rican partners of adolescent mothers. *Journal of Midwifery & Women's Health, 49*(2), 118–125.

Gannotti, M., Handwerker, W., Groce, N., & Cruz, C. (2001). Sociocultural influences on disability status in Puerto Rican children. *Physical Therapy, 81,* 1512–1523.

Glanz, K., Croyle, R. T., Chollette, V. Y., & Pinn, V. W. (2003). Cancer-related health disparities in women. *American Journal of Public Health, 93*(2), 292–298.

Gonzalez-Wippler, M. (1992). *Santeria-African magic in Latin America* (2nd rev. ed.). New York: Julian Press.

Harwood, A. (1971). The hot-cold theory of disease: implications for treatment of Puerto Rican patients. *Journal of the American Medical Association, 216,* 1154–1155.

Juarbe, T. (2005). Puerto Ricans. In J. Lipson, S. Dibble, & P. Minarik (Eds.), *Culture and nursing care.* San Francisco: UCSF Nursing Press.

Kent, D. (1992). *America the beautiful. Puerto Rico.* Chicago: Children's Press.

Lauderdale, D. S., Jacobsen, S. J., Furner, S. E., Levy, P. S., Brody, J. A., & Goldberg, J. (1998). Hip fracture incidence among elderly Hispanics. *American Journal of Public Health, 88*(8), 1245–1247.

Ledogar, R., Penchaszadeh, C., Garden, C., & Acosta, L. (2000). Asthma and Latino cultures: different prevalence reported among groups sharing the same environment. *American Journal of Public Health, 90*(6), 929–935.

Lee, D., Gomez-Marin, Q., & Lam, B. (2000). Current depression, lifetime history of depression, and visual acuity in Hispanic adults. *Journal of Visual Impairment and Blindness, 94*(2), 85–96.

Lee, D., Gomez-Marin, Q., Lam, B., Ma, F., & Vilar, N. F. (2000). Prevalence of usual-corrected distance visual acuity impairment in Hispanic and non-Hispanic children and adolescents. *Pediatric and Perinatal Epidemiology, 14*(4), 357.

Lipton, R., Losey, L., Giachello, A., Corral, M., Girotti, M. H., & Mendez, J. J. (1996). Factors affecting diabetes treatment and patient education among Latinos: results of a preliminary study in Chicago. *Journal of Medical Systems, 20*(5), 267–276.

Lipton, R., Losey, L., Giachello, A., Mendez, J., & Girotti, M. H. (1998). Attitudes and issues in treating Latino patients with type 2 diabetes: views of healthcare providers. *Diabetes Educator, 24*(1), 67–71.

Lobar, S. L., Youngblut, J. M., & Brooten, D. (2006). Cross-cultural beliefs, ceremonies, and rituals surrounding death of a loved one. *Pediatric Nursing, 32*(1), 44–49.

Miracle, C. (1981). Intelligence testing and the Aymara. In M. J. Hardman (Ed.), *The Aymara language in its social and cultural context* (pp. 240–247). Gainesville, FL: University Presses of Florida.

Mott, J. W., Wang, J., Thornton, J. C., Allison, D. B., Heymsfield, S. B., & Pierson, R. N., Jr. (1999). Relation between body fat and age in 4 ethnic groups. *American Journal of Clinical Nutrition, 69*(5), 1007–1013.

Mumford, E. (1973). Puerto Rican perspectives on mental illness. *Mount Sinai Journal of Medicine, 6*(40), 771–773.

Munet-Vilaro, F. (1998). Grieving and death rituals of Latinos. *Oncology Nursing Forum, 25*(10), 1761–1763.

National Cancer Institute. (2006). *Cancer control and population sciences: cancer in Puerto Rican women.* Available at <http://dccps.nci.nih.gov/womenofcolor/puerto.html> Retrieved May 25, 2006.

Popkin, B. M., & Udry, J. R. (1998). Adolescent obesity increases significantly in second and third generation U.S. immigrants: the national longitudinal study of adolescent health. *Journal of Nutrition, 128*, 701–706.

Porter, D., & Prince, D. (2000). *Frommer's Puerto Rico.* Chicago: IDG Books World Wide.

Rivera-Andino, J., & Lopez, L. (2000). When culture complicates care. *RN, 63*(7), 47–48.

Rodriguez-Strednicki, O., & Twaite, J. (1999). Attitudes toward victims of child sexual abuse among adults from four ethnic/cultural groups. *Journal of Child Sexual Abuse, 8*(3), 1–24.

Rogler, L. (1999). Methodological sources of cultural insensitivity in mental health research. *American Psychologist, 54*, 424–433.

Rose, D., Mannino, D. M., & Lederer, B. P. (2006). Asthma prevalence among US adults, 1998–2000: role of Puerto Rican ethnicity and behavioral and geographic factors. *American Journal of Public Health, 96*(5), 1–9.

Ruiz, P. (1983). Cultural factors in diagnosis and treatment: transcript of the panel discussion. *ACP Psychiatric Update, 3*(2), 2–6.

Santiago-Borrero, P., & Valcarcel, M. (1994). Maternal and child health and health care in Puerto Rico. In G. Lamberty & D. Coll Garcia (Eds.), *Puerto Rican women and children: issues in health, growth, and development* (pp. 39–54). New York: Plenum Press.

Schilling, B., & Brannon, E. (1986). *Health related dietary practices. Cross-cultural counseling: a guide for nutrition and health counselors.* Alexandria, VA: U.S. Department of Agriculture and U.S. Department of Health and Human Services, Nutrition and Technical Services Division.

Snow, R. (1983). The relationship between visual and juvenile delinquency. *Journal of the American Optometry Association, 54*, 509–511.

Sokol-Katz, J., & Ulbrich, P. (1992). Family structure and adolescent risk-taking behavior: a comparison of Mexican, Cuban, and Puerto Rican Americans. *International Journal of the Addictions, 27*(10), 1197–1209.

Spector, R. (2004). *Cultural diversity in health and illness* (6th ed.). Upper Saddle River, NJ: Pearson Prentice Hall.

Talamantes, M. A., Gomez, C., & Braun, K. L. (2000). Advance directives and end-of-life care: the Hispanic perspective. In K. L. Braun, J. H. Pietsch, & P. L. Blanchette (Eds.), *Cultural issues in end-of-life decision making* (pp. 83–100). Thousand Oaks, CA: Sage.

Tucker, K., Bermudez, O., & Castaneda, C. (2000). Type 2 diabetes is prevalent and poorly controlled among Hispanic elders of Caribbean origin. *American Journal of Public Health, 90*(7), 1288–1293.

U.S. Department of Commerce, Bureau of the Census. (2013). *American community survey: Puerto Ricans.* Hyattsville, MD: U.S. Government Printing Office.

U.S. Department of Commerce, Bureau of the Census. (2013). *Hispanic Briefs, Population Reports.* Hyattsville, MD: U.S. Government Printing Office.

Wasserman, G., Brunnelli, S., Rauh, V., & Alvarado, L. (1994). The cultural context of adolescent childrearing in three groups of urban minority mothers. In G. Lamberty & C. Coll Garcia (Eds.), *Puerto Rican women and children: issues in health, growth, and development* (pp. 137–160). New York: Plenum Press.

Welcome to Puerto Rico. Description. (2015). Available at <http://welcome.topuertorico.org/descrip.shtml> Retrieved March 21, 2011.

Welcome to Puerto Rico. Government. (2015). Available at <http://welcome.topuertorico.org/government.shtml> Retrieved March 21, 2011.

Welcome to Puerto Rico. History. (2015). Available at <http://welcome.topuertorico.org/history.shtml> Retrieved March 21, 2011.

Welcome to Puerto Rico. People. (2015). Available at <http://welcome.topuertorico.org/people.shtml> Retrieved March 21, 2011.

Welcome to Puerto Rico. Puerto Rican Culture. (2015). Available at <http://www.welcome.topuertorico.org/culture> Retrieved March 21, 2011.

World Almanac. (2015). New York: World Almanac Books.

Wright, K. N. (2011). Influence of body mass index, gender, and Hispanic ethnicity on physical activity in urban children. *Journal for Specialists in Pediatric Nursing, 16*(2), 90–104.

Wright, K., & Giger, J. N. (2010). California's young Hispanic children with asthma: disparities in health care access and utilization of health care services. *Hispanic Health Care International, 8*(3), 155–164.

Zbar, J. (2001). *Explorer of the seas.* Miami, FL: Royal Caribbean International.

25

Nigerian Americans

Cordelia Chinwe Nnedu

BEHAVIORAL OBJECTIVES

After reading this chapter, the nurse will be able to:

1. Integrate an understanding of patterns of communication behaviors that may be found among Nigerian Americans to nurse–client interactions.
2. Describe spatial behavior and beliefs that may be found among Nigerian Americans.
3. Determine the impact of the sociocultural and spiritual beliefs of Nigerian Americans to the health care system and acceptance of health care services.
4. Describe modifications in care that may be necessary for a client on African time.
5. Describe the interrelatedness of problem solving, cultural demands, and crisis intervention among Nigerian Americans.
6. Develop a culturally appropriate plan of care for a Nigerian-American woman with malaria.

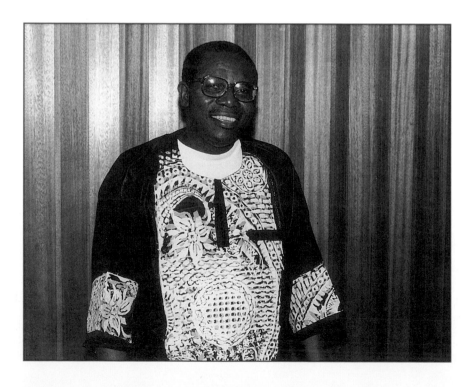

OVERVIEW OF NIGERIA

Nigeria lies within latitudes 4°1′ and 13°0′ North and longitudes 2°2′ and 14°30′ East and is bordered in the North by the Niger Republic, in the East by the Republic of Chad and Cameroun, in the West by the Republic of Benin, and in the South by the Atlantic Ocean. The country occupies a total surface area of approximately 656,425 square miles (923,768 square kilometers), comparatively more than twice the size of the state of California; it has 800 km of coastline and ranks as one of the largest countries in the world (Kalu, 2014; Nigeria Global AIDS Response Progress Report [GARPR], 2014).

In the coastal and southeast portions of Nigeria, the rainy season usually begins in February or March as moist Atlantic air, known as the *southeast monsoon,* invades the country. By April or early May in most years, the rainy season is under way throughout most of the area south of the Niger and Benue river valleys. Farther north, the rain does not usually start until June or July. The peak of the rainy season occurs through most of northern Nigeria in August, when air from the Atlantic covers the entire country. In southern regions, this period marks the August dip in precipitation. Although rarely completely dry, this dip in rainfall, which is especially marked in the southwest, can be useful agriculturally, because it allows a brief dry period for grain harvesting.

Most of Nigeria's inhabitants are Black Africans who live in rural areas in homes made of grass, dried mud, or wood. A group of related families often lives in a compound. Nigeria also has large, crowded cities, which include Lagos, the former capital, leading port, and center of finance and commerce, and Abuja, which is the present capital of the country (Kalu, 2014). Overcrowding in cities, where people often go in search of jobs, has contributed to slums of mud huts that line unpaved streets.

Nigeria is ethnically diverse, with more than 250 ethnic and cultural groups. The languages include English (official), Hausa, Yoruba, Igbo, and over 500 other indigenous languages (Nigeria GARPR, 2014). The Hausa have lived in the northern area for more than a thousand years. The Hausa live in many cities and move around as traders and itinerant workers. During the 1200s, the Fulani began to settle in the Hausa territory and in the 1800s with the Islamic revolution took control of the region. The two peoples intermixed and today are sometimes called the *Hausa-Fulani* (Central Intelligence Agency [CIA], 2015). The Yoruba live mainly in southwestern Nigeria and constitute the second largest group. Many Yoruba live in cities and farm the surrounding countryside. The Igbo form a majority of the individuals living in southeastern Nigeria, with a small proportion of the Igbo (Western Igbo) living

close to the Edo in the southwest. The Tiv and Nupe live in Central Nigeria; the Edo, Urhobo, and Itsekiri live in the Edo and Delta states; the Ijaw live in the Rivers state; the Efik and Ibibio live in the Cross River state, and the Kanuri live in northeastern Nigeria. The groups have varying customs, cultural behaviors, and political organizations.

The life expectancy in Nigeria is 54.1 years for females and 52.3 for men, with more than 41.2% of the population age 14 or younger. The birthrate is 36.07 per 1000, with an infant mortality rate of 72.97 deaths per 1000 live births in 2013. The death rate is five deaths per 1000 population (Nigeria GARPR, 2014). The Nigerian population is growing at an annual rate of 1.966% (CIA, 2015). The per capita gross national product was listed at $5353.38 in 2014, while the literacy rate (2005–2010) was 61% (Human Development Report, 2014). In 2014, Nigeria's gross domestic product (GDP) became the largest in Africa, worth more than $500 billion, and overtook South Africa to become the world's twenty-sixth largest economy. By 2050, Nigeria is expected to become one of the world's top 20 economies (Kalu, 2014). Nigeria ranks 176th among all nations for health expenditure per capita and 184th for overall health attainment (CIA, 2015).

The majority of Nigerians earn their livelihood by farming, fishing, or herding. Nigeria ranks among the world's leading producers of cocoa, peanuts, palm oil and palm kernels, and rubber. Other important crops include beans, cassava, corn, cotton, millet, rice, sorghum, and yams. Nigerian farmers also raise goats, poultry, and sheep. Nigerian fishing crews catch shrimp and other seafood, whereas herders in the north raise cattle. Although only 15% of the country's total area is used for growing crops, more than half of Nigeria's land is suitable for farming and grazing. Forests cover about one third of the land, and rivers, lakes, and streams provide an abundance of fish (CIA, 2015).

Since the 1960s, the oil industry has brought new wealth to the nation. The wealth that Nigeria gained from oil exports in the 1970s attracted many people from neighboring lands searching for work. However, in the early 1980s declining oil prices began to hurt the economy of Nigeria, and beginning in 1983 the government ordered foreigners living in Nigeria illegally to leave. Nevertheless, the wealth brought by the oil industry has allowed Nigeria to develop industries, improve the educational system, and modernize agricultural practices. In addition to oil, there are deposits of tin and columbite, gas, coal, iron ore, lead, limestone, natural gas, and zinc (Nigeria GARPR, 2014).

Nigeria is rich in the variety and quality of its art. Traditional African sculpture influenced Pablo Picasso and other modern Western artists (Onwudiwe, 2002). Terracotta (clay) figures created by the Nok civilization in central

Nigeria date back to 500 B.C. Other famous art media include the traditional sculptures of bronze and brass figures of Ife and Benin; wood carvings from the Yoruba people; wooden masks from forest areas; and paintings on sculptures, on textiles, and as body decoration. Nigerian music features drums, xylophones, and various string and wind instruments and is often part of dance and dramatic performances that are popular forms of entertainment and cultural expression. The Nigerian culture has been passed on in oral stories rather than written, with popular forms including chants, folk stories, proverbs, and riddles. Since the mid-1900s, Nigerian authors have begun to record stories in English as well as in local languages. In 1986, Wole Soyinka, a Nigerian playwright, poet, and novelist, became the first African writer to win the Nobel Prize for literature (CIA, 2015).

In addition, Nigeria continues to experience long-standing ethnic and religious tensions. Nigeria is now experiencing its longest period of civilian rule since independence. The general elections of April 2007 marked the first civilian-to-civilian transfer of power in the country's history. In January 2010, Nigeria assumed a nonpermanent seat on the United Nation's Security Council for the 2010–2011 term.

HISTORY

Early History

People have lived in what is now Nigeria for thousands of years (Eluwa, Ukagwu, Nwachukwu, & Nwaubani, 1988). In fact, archeologists have dated tools they found to 40,000 years ago (CIA, 2015). Human skeletons, rock paintings, and prehistoric settlements provide documentation of the early civilizations. Agriculture or the domestication of plants and animals served as the main occupation of the earlier inhabitants. In 500 B.C., iron civilization emerged with one major center at Nok. Clay figures of animals and people produced by the Nok civilization are among the oldest known examples of African sculpture (CIA, 2015). In the east, Igbo Ukwu bronzes reveal a society in existence by 900 A.D. Not only do the artifacts show impressive artwork, but they also yield information about trade with neighbors and with communities as far away as the Sahara and Venice (Falola, 2001). Like agriculture, iron technology brought significant changes in people's lives. Iron tools and weapons were more effective than stone, bone, or wooden ones. Technology was altered, with great consequences on farming, urbanization, and settlements.

The development of kingdoms can be dated to the kingdom of Karem in about 700 A.D. in the area now known as *Chad*. Islam was adopted as early as the 1000s as the religion in Karem, and it expanded as a dominant religion. In the early 1800s, a Muslim religious leader turned almost all of the northern region into a Muslim empire (Eluwa, Ukagwu, Nwachukwu, & Nwaubani, 1988; Falola, 2001; Uwazie, Albert, & Uzoigwe, 1999).

The Coming of the Europeans

The Portuguese were the first Europeans to reach Nigeria. In the late 1400s, a trade center near Benin was established, and a trade in slaves with the African leaders was begun (CIA, 2015). The first kingdom to receive Christianity was Benin, as European missionaries arrived. Dutch, British, and other European traders competed for the control of the slave trade. By the 1700s, the slave trade was led by the British. However, in 1807 the British government outlawed the slave trade, and ships carrying slaves were captured, with the slaves returned to the mainland. Slave trade was replaced by trade in palm oil and other agricultural products (CIA, 2015). British missionaries converted many freed slaves to Christianity, which then spread along the coastal areas and in the southwest. Christianity was accepted in Nigeria in 1842. It is interesting to note that prior to the introduction of religions, Nigerians believed and worshipped only God. They believed in deities, which originated from the traditional conception of the universe.

British Rule

During the late 1800s, the British established protectorates in parts of southern Nigeria. Throughout Nigeria, there were unsuccessful battles against the establishment of British rule (CIA, 2015). In 1900, the charter granted to the Royal Niger Company was revoked, paving the way for the creation of the Protectorate of Northern Nigeria. By 1906, all of southern Nigeria had become the Colony and Protectorate of Southern Nigeria. Finally, in 1914, the British protectorates in both south and north were merged to create modern Nigeria, named after the River Niger and under the control of a governor based in Lagos (Aminu, 2002).

To govern the local communities and to ensure that various ethnic units were differently managed, the British government introduced a system of indirect rule, or divide and rule. The first high commissioner of northern Nigeria and the first governor-general of Nigeria was the architect of indirect rule (Falola, 2001). The effort to reject the political and cultural domination of British rule gave birth to nationalism. The western and eastern regions obtained internal self-government in 1957, and the north did so 2 years later. The north feared the domination of federal power by the southern elites; the south feared that the north would use its vast size to advantage; and the minorities in all the regions were afraid of domination by the

Hausa, Igbo, and Yoruba. Thus, on one hand, there was joy at the impending end of British rule (Falola, 2001). On the other hand, there was fear that regionalism and ethnic differences would tear the country apart. The United Kingdom granted Nigeria independence on October 1, 1960.

The Republic of Nigeria and Military Rule

In 1963 Nigeria became the Federal Republic of Nigeria, with a federal constitution and a parliamentary system based on that of the United Kingdom. However, the next 16 years were marked by repeated coups and failed governments. In 1979, the British form of government was discarded, the U.S. style of government was adopted, and a president was installed. Unfortunately, the new president failed to pay attention to declining oil revenues, poverty, and falling living standards, and in 1983 a successful coup placed the military in power (Ogbu, 1999). From 1984 to 1999, Nigeria endured the most turbulent years of its modern history under three successive ineffective military regimes (Falola, 2001).

Following an April 2014 statistical "rebasing" exercise, Nigeria has emerged as Africa's largest economy, with 2013 GDP estimated at US$ 502 billion. Oil has been a dominant source of government revenues since the 1970s. Regulatory constraints and security risks have limited new investment in oil and natural gas, and Nigeria's oil production contracted in 2012 and 2013. Nevertheless, the Nigerian economy has continued to grow at a rapid 6% to 8% per annum (pre-rebasing), driven by growth in agriculture, telecommunications, and services, and the medium-term outlook for Nigeria is good, assuming oil output stabilizes and oil prices remain strong. Fiscal authorities pursued countercyclical policies in 2011–2013, significantly reducing the budget deficit. Monetary policy has also been responsive and effective. Following the 2008–2009 global financial crises, the banking sector was effectively recapitalized and regulation enhanced. Despite its strong fundamentals, oil-rich Nigeria has been hobbled by inadequate power supply, lack of infrastructure, delays in the passage of legislative reforms, an inefficient property registration system, restrictive trade policies, an inconsistent regulatory environment, a slow and ineffective judicial system, unreliable dispute resolution mechanisms, insecurity, and pervasive corruption.

Economic diversification and strong growth have not translated into a significant decline in poverty levels—over 62% of Nigeria's 170 million people live in extreme poverty. President Muhammadu Buhari has established an economic team that includes experienced and reputable members and has announced plans to increase transparency, continue to diversify production, and further improve fiscal management. The government is working to develop stronger public–private partnerships for roads, agriculture, and power (CIA, 2015).

IMMIGRATION TO THE UNITED STATES

The African diaspora, the forced migration of West Africans between the sixteenth and nineteenth centuries, was the starting point for the arrival of Nigerians in the United States. European slave traders purchased or captured an estimated 10 million people on the west coast of Africa and transported them to the Caribbean and the Americas. Today, however, Nigerians leave by choice. Although education is said to be free and compulsory in Nigeria, some children and youths are too busy trying to help earn a living for their families to receive an education (CIA, 2015). Opportunities for higher education are limited. Thus, many Nigerians have come to the United States for the primary purpose of obtaining an education and on student visas that limit work.

However, with the initiation of visa lotteries, Nigerians from all walks of life have been allowed and are eager to enter the United States (Washington Visa Center, 2014, http://www.nigeriaembassyusa.org/index.php?page=visas). Whereas the hardships encountered in Nigeria make it seem impossible for most families to make ends meet, the United States has been seen as the land of opportunity. The high cost of living, lack of jobs, lack of medical staff and medicine, and political dissent are strong motivators for Nigerians—particularly men trying to meet the needs of a family—to leave the country. Others who are single leave in hopes of bettering themselves. While at one time Nigerians considered it shameful to complete one's education abroad and remain abroad, today it is more acceptable to leave the country with no intention of returning to live there permanently. Leaving with the opportunity to send money home for the family is seen as a noble goal.

By 2014, the U.S. Census reported that 221,000 Nigerians were residing in the United States (Gambino, Trevelyan, & Fitzwater, 2014; U.S. Department of Commerce, Bureau of the Census, *American Community Survey*, 2014). Because many Nigerians entered America during the slave trade era and are undoubtedly not included among Americans reporting Nigerian origin, it should be noted that many more Black Americans have ethnic origins from this African country than those listed on the census.

COMMUNICATION

The official language of Nigeria is English, which is taught in schools throughout the country (CIA, 2015). Since many schools were established by the British, it is British English that is taught and understood. However, English is not the country's most commonly used language, since each of the more than 250 ethnic groups has its own distinct language. The most widely used languages are those of the three largest ethnic groups: the Igbo of the southeast speak Igbo, the Yoruba of the southwest speak Yoruba, and the northerners speak Hausa. Ethnic languages are spoken at home and outside. The majority of rural dwellers speak their ethnic language and do not comprehend English (Ikezuagu, personal communication, 2002).

Pidgin English, however, is the predominant language of communication, with only educated individuals using British English. Pidgin language became a necessary way to communicate. Because of diversity in ethnicity, Pidgin became a way for these mixed groups to comprehend each other. Pidgin English is regarded by many as "broken English." Some rural dwellers do not speak or comprehend Pidgin English but are limited to their ethnic dialect (Ikezuagu, personal communication, 2002).

The majority of Nigerians speak more than one language. They may use their ethnic language on most occasions and speak English or another language at other times. In addition, the 50% of Nigerians who are Muslims may use Arabic while taking part in various religious activities (CIA, 2015).

Since Nigerians who have immigrated tend to be educated or in school after they arrive, most Nigerian Americans speak the English language fluently. The 2000 census noted that only 9.5% of Nigerian Americans did not have a good command of the English language. It was noted that 53.1% spoke a language other than English (U.S. Department of Commerce, Bureau of the Census, *Population Profiles*, 2015).

Mannerisms vary during communication, which may be construed as disrespectful by outsiders. For example, it is not a sign of dishonesty, but of respect, for a younger person not to make eye contact with an elder or a person in authority when the elder or authority figure is talking. People of rank or age dominate discussion.

Nigerian Americans are less likely to engage in intimate behavior, such as touching, kissing, or hugging in public. A traditional Nigerian couple in love may not go to the movies, hold hands, or kiss one another in public places. Even married Nigerians are less likely to show intimate behavior in public or even in health care settings. For example, if the Nigerian-American husband is present during labor, the nurse should not expect intimate touching behavior. Failure to express intimate emotion, even to a sick person or one receiving medical treatment, should not be misinterpreted as lack of caring (Falola, 2001).

In addressing an older person, a younger person uses socially accepted words before his or her name, for example, Sister-Joyce, Aunti-Joyce, and Ndaa Joyce. Respect can also

be shown by the manner of greeting (for example, bowing), the forms of address (honorifics), and other expressions approved by the culture. For many Nigerian Americans, it is not proper to address elders and senior people by their first names. Greetings in the morning are considered mandatory for proper etiquette by some Nigerian Americans, and it is proper to first inquire about the state of health. The younger person is expected to greet the elder first out of respect for age. The freedom to use first names is allowed only to seniors and superiors. Some Nigerian Americans consider it an insult to call elder siblings by their first name (Falola, 2001).

Nigerians are very proud of traditional titles, and it is not uncommon to address people with their occupation before their names, such as Engineer Ngozi Nnedu (instead of Ms. Ngozi Nnedu). Those who have done the pilgrimage to Mecca are addressed as Alhaji (for men) and Alhaja (for women). One of the most sought-after titles in Nigeria is *Chief,* which is considered more important than a doctoral degree. Those who hold traditional titles, such as *Chief, Emir, Oba,* or *Eze,* enjoy higher status in the community. Some of these titles are inherited, but wealthy individuals may receive titles as a result of their achievements. A Nigerian American who has such a title is likely to continue to value it and to desire this title to be used by others as a form of respect (Falola, 2001).

Implications for Nursing Care

It is important for the nurse and other health care professionals to assess the comprehension level of the Nigerian-American client and family since an immigrant's common language may be an ethnic language or Pidgin English rather than English. Even if the client and family speak English, the nurse should be aware that words have different meanings and may be stated with different implications. Nurses, who tend to speak fast, should talk more slowly until the comprehension level is clearly evaluated. If necessary, a translator may be used to ensure clear communication, particularly of medical terms and procedures that require more complex understanding. When new immigrants or relatives visiting from Nigeria, who are less versed in English, enter the health care system, a family member fluent in English will commonly accompany the individual to provide linguistic and other forms of support.

It is frightening for the newly immigrated Nigerian American or the Nigerian visiting America to be sick and in unfamiliar surroundings and not to be able to comprehend the language of the health care professionals. The nurse should always begin the assessment phase by establishing rapport. Part of this initial encounter involves finding out how to address the client because titles are important and preferences may vary. If the phrase "your age mate" is used in response to a first-name approach, this can indicate lack of acceptance of the first-name approach or indication of seniority in age (Amadi, personal communication, 2002). Addressing the client appropriately is a stepping stone toward acceptance and meaningful health care delivery.

In general, the nurse's approach and way of speaking to the Nigerian client will set the tone for how the client reacts to health care professionals. The nurse should be aware that hurrying behaviors may annoy the Nigerian American. The Nigerian-American client may feel this conveys a lack of concern and lack of time to give adequate care. It may be interpreted as not being good enough for the nurse. A hurried approach can also result in the client not asking for help in order to not disturb the nurse.

Cooperation with treatment and care routines will be fostered through communication with and involvement of the family. It is important to include the spouse or other family where possible in planning and giving care. Culturally competent nurses gain credibility because they do not exclude or ridicule traditional beliefs but rather incorporate them in the total plan of care. Often the nurse may have to negotiate with the client or family to carry out the essential medical treatments as well as include cultural practices. For example, some obstetricians in this country are now prescribing cabbage leaves as an adjunct in lactation suppression. Leaves have been used for decades in medical treatments throughout Nigeria.

The ability to use proverbs, analogies, and stories to support a case is highly valued and will enhance communication with Nigerian Americans. Pictures and models are also useful when explaining medical procedures to an individual whose English may be limited.

The nurse may be surprised to find that a newly immigrated Nigerian is fascinated with the opportunity to see a television and listen to the radio. It is more easily understood when the number of televisions (61 per 1000) and radios (197 per 1000) in Nigeria is known (CIA, 2015). Even a newspaper may seem surprising to an immigrant Nigerian since the daily newspaper circulation in Nigeria is 24 per 1000. Patient teaching in the form of cartoons and videos may be particularly fascinating to the Nigerian-American adult or child.

Nurses interacting with a Nigerian American should follow these guidelines adapted by Haq (1998) for communicating in a culturally competent manner:
1. Establish primary language first and assess need for qualified interpreters.
2. Be aware of importance of body language—by both the nurses and the clients.
3. Establish the need for a family member or religious leader to be present.
4. Be aware of appropriate eye and touch contact.
5. Allow enough time for storytelling and long histories.
6. Adapt the physical examination to meet privacy and modesty needs.
7. Avoid a hurried, impatient, or distracted demeanor.

SPACE

Personal space includes the area that surrounds a person's body and the objects within that space. Although spatial requirements vary from individual to individual, within a cultural group individuals tend to behave similarly (LaMar, 2013). Space is an important concept for Nigerian Americans. In general, African-Americans are more comfortable with a much closer personal space, whether in the home or in the health care agency (Sue, 2003). Activities that occur in spaces in the home generally involve many members of the family. Within a home setting, Nigerian Americans may have multiple families residing together. In Nigeria, where polygamy may have been practiced, multiple wives may live in one home and share a small space with other wives and their children.

For Nigerian Americans, the nature of any conversation determines the distance and sound intensity between the participants in the conversation. Confidential information tends to be shared in low voices and in very close proximity. Other information may be shared with loud voices without consideration for proximity (Amadi, personal communication, 2002).

Implications for Nursing Care of the Childbearing Family

Pregnancy and childbirth are the fundamental part of marriage, and births tend to be celebrated by the family with parties. A married couple is expected to have a child within 9 months of marriage. Failure to do this will often result in gossip. Most of the time, the female will be blamed. If the couple is unable to conceive, the man's family will often blame the woman. The woman will be the first to seek infertility treatment. Acquaintances will wonder about her past life. The question is often "What did she do in her youth to warrant this predicament?" People will wonder how many abortions she committed in the past to make it impossible to conceive a child. All these agonizing statements are made before a visit to a clinic. Even after a visit is made to the clinic and the woman is cleared of any reproductive problems, there is always doubt concerning the tests performed at the clinic. Most of the men will seek medical care for infertility without the knowledge of the wives. Nurses should respect their need for privacy while at the same time encouraging communication with their spouses. It is important to inform clients about the relationship among stress, pregnancy, and treatment outcome.

The nurse working with the family during the delivery process should be aware of beliefs that Nigerian Americans may have related to childbirth. The exception to wanting the whole family in close proximity is the childbirth situation. In labor and delivery, it will not be unusual for older Nigerians to shy away, especially during active labor. The maternity nurse needs to recognize that staying away from labor and delivery is not a sign of lack of love but of respect. The presence of the husband during childbirth varies for Nigerian Americans, who may be used to traditional birth attendants assisting with the delivery (Spector, 2004). It will not be unlikely for the husband to stay out of the childbirth unit the majority of the time. Some men comment that they will not do what their fathers did not do, signaling that this behavior is not the Nigerian way of life and that their fathers were not present when their mothers were giving birth.

The nurse should be aware that during childbirth, the Nigerian-American woman may receive a lot of visitors. Most visitors will bring food to the hospital, and many people will volunteer to do things for the woman. Nurses can use family and friends as an important resource. They can assist in care; in fact, the client may expect them to do so.

The nurse should be aware that pain is perceived differently across cultures and for Nigerians, particularly at childbirth (Davitz, Sameshima, & Davitz, 1976). Nigerians newly arriving in the United States may not favor certain pain management regimens used in labor and delivery (for example, epidural anesthesia). Cesarean section is seen as a failure in fulfilling this particular female role. The couple will wait to the very end to agree to a cesarean section, regardless of the pain the woman may be experiencing or the condition of the fetus.

In a study by Onah (2002) with 279 infertile women in southeastern Nigeria, 69% were unwilling to adopt, stating it was psychologically unacceptable and that adoption was not a solution to their infertility problem. Only 21% actually knew how to adopt, and only 27% knew the correct meaning of adoption. Thus, while motherhood was highly valued, adoption was not commonly seen as an option for a woman who could not bear children. It is not unusual for the adopted child to be ridiculed and discriminated against by the kinsmen.

Nigerian culture includes many myths, rituals, and the use of herbs in attempts to regulate women's fertility. A culturally competent practitioner will incorporate some of the traditional beliefs while providing care to Nigerians. It is advisable to discuss personal beliefs and practices with clients and to plan care with the client and husband.

In Nigeria, some customs frown at premarital sex, and others advocate spacing children 2.5 to 3 years following childbirth.

Implications for Nursing Care

In the health care setting and in relation to situations of illness, birth, or death, Nigerian Americans tend to be more comfortable when distances are narrowed. This may involve distance between the client and family or between the health care professional and the client and family. Nigerian Americans tend to feel that the narrower the space between individuals, the greater the acceptance level.

In general, Nigerians tend to have a more permissive style where space is concerned. In fact, some Nigerians like crowds—the more the better. Thus, the nurse should not be surprised to find a number of family members crowded into the client's room in a health care setting. The nurse should be aware that family is very important to persons of Nigerian origin and attempt to accommodate the client's need for the presence of family whenever possible. When appropriate, the nurse should give the client the option to decide who should be allowed to be present when health care is provided.

Social Organization

Family.   The family is a biological and social unit for Nigerian Americans. Most Nigerian-American families are patrilineal, and rights of inheritance are traced through the male members of the family. In a patrilineal system, men have inheritance rights, and women may receive only a small share or nothing. Also in such a patrilineal system, when a woman marries, she becomes a permanent member of the husband's lineage. All children, irrespective of gender, belong to the father's kinship group. The children will treat their father's cousins as brothers and sisters and refer to them as such (Falola, 2001; Kayongo-Male & Onyango, 1984).

As the patriarch, the Nigerian-American man seeks resources to support his usually large family and many dependents. Polygamy (the practice of having multiple wives) is still practiced in many parts of Nigeria and contributes to increased numbers of dependents. The man's ability to be responsible for the needs of many people is interpreted as a measure of success. The typical Nigerian-American husband does not have household duties.

In many Nigerian families, whether in the United States or in Nigeria, the role of the woman is related to the family. In most families, women carry out all the household tasks, sometimes with the help of relatives or servants. In a study by Tomkiewicz and Adeyemi-Bello (1996), data suggested that American and Nigerian female management aspirants are likely to experience barriers to advancement in Nigeria because of attitudes by both Nigerians and Americans toward women as managers. Nigerian males, especially, were found to have a negative view of women as managers. If women are placed in positions of authority by expanding multinational organizations, the attitudes of the Nigerian males were predicted to impede opportunities offered women (both native and expatriate) and the goals of equality in American corporations.

Extended families, in which parents, children, their spouses, grandchildren, and other relatives live under one roof, are common in rural areas. Family relationships are guided by a strict system of seniority. Although the extended family system is changing, a tradition of mutual caring and responsibility is very strong in Nigerian family life.

The common dress of many family members living in cities in Nigeria is Western-style clothing. However, other city dwellers and most people in rural areas wear traditional clothing. For men and women in Nigeria, traditional garments include long, loose robes made of white or brightly colored fabrics. Men may wear short, full jackets with shorts or trousers. Small round caps are popular head coverings for men, while Nigerian women may wear scarves tied like turbans. Nigerian Americans usually wear Western-style clothes but often have traditional garments for special occasions.

Migration, new occupations, Western education, and foreign religions have had significant consequences on gender roles, marriage, customs, and family life for Nigerian Americans. The more educated tend to favor small, monogamous nuclear families. Nevertheless, most Nigerian Americans continue to cherish children, have men as the head of the households, and tend to have large families. The 2000 census found that household size for 19.8% of Nigerian Americans was five or more persons, for 15.2% was four persons, and for 16.4% was three persons (U.S. Bureau of Commerce, Bureau of the Census, *Population Profiles*, 2012).

Marriage

The Nigerian institution of marriage is unconventional by Western standards. The traditional and Islamic systems of polygamy flourish within every social class. Women expect very little from men in terms of companionship, personal care, and fidelity. Their relationships exist without the emotional elements (Qualls, 2010). Polygamy is a crucial component of many women's lives. Marriage is the unification of two families, not merely of the couple alone. It unites the couple's lineages and clans. Family role is reflected in the choice of partners, the religious ceremonies that accompany marriages, the bride's wealth, and the intervention of members of the lineage to resolve marital

problems. When a couple wants to divorce, the two people involved tend to consider the feelings and roles of other lineage members (Falola, 2001).

Practices such as child marriage are disappearing among Nigerians, although girls are still encouraged to marry early. Arranged marriages are becoming less common. Even when the choice is made by the partners themselves, the families still become involved in information gathering to ensure that the other family has a good reputation and an acceptable medical history. If a certain disease is thought to be hereditary, a family in which such a disease appears is avoided in order to prevent possible contamination. Most parents still prefer that their children marry a member of the same ethnic group as themselves. This may be difficult in the United States, where the number of persons of the same ethnic group may be limited.

Whether traditional or modern, a marriage requires the exchange of bride's wealth and religious ceremonies, both of which involve many people as participants in an important social institution and contract. The customs are also designed to ensure the survival and stability of the relationship. In Islamic, Christian, and court marriages, other ceremonies will follow to legalize the marriage (Falola, 2001). In the traditional wedding, the gods and ancestors are invoked to bless the marriage. Ceremonies take different forms from one area to another. Among the Ibibio in the southeast, part of the marriage preparation is for women to go to a fattening house, where they eat large quantities of food to gain weight. Weight gain is seen as a sign of beauty. At the same time they receive training in cooking, childrearing, and managing a home (Falola, 2001).

Married couples place emphasis on responsibility and respect for one another, attention to the moral upbringing of children, attention to the education of the children, fidelity in monogamous couples, and caring for the needs of the extended families. These values have persisted for most Nigerian immigrants to the United States.

Religion

Christianity and Islam are the two dominant religions in Nigeria. Muslims represent about 50% of the population and are concentrated in the north and southwest (Nigerian GARPR, 2014; Spector, 2004). Christians make up 40% of the population and are found predominantly in the south and the middle belt. The remaining 10% practice indigenous beliefs native to Africa. For some Nigerians, elements and practices of Islam, Christianity, and the indigenous religions coexist. Islamic law is practiced in a dozen northern Nigerian states. This has presented problems, especially for females. In 2002, amid an international outcry, death sentences were handed down to two Nigerian Muslim women convicted of adultery under Islamic law.

The women were pregnant and unmarried. This law discriminates between men and women since men can be convicted of adultery only on the testimony of four witnesses (Minchakpu, 2002).

For many Nigerians, ancient indigenous practices such as masquerades, priesthood practices, and secret societies coexist with Muslim and Christian traditions. In the majority of cases, the type of education students are exposed to is directly related to their religion. For example, northern Muslims are likely to attend a Koranic school, while the southern Christians are likely to attend a European-style school. For many Nigerian Americans, beliefs about religion play an important role in personal behavior. For example, their attitude toward death is affected by religious beliefs. It may be important for a Catholic Nigerian American, even one who has not been an active church member, to see a priest when death is imminent (Enang, 2000; Wilkinson & Treas, 2011).

Regardless of the present religious beliefs of the Nigerian American, personal behavior may be affected by the deep-rooted religious beliefs of their ancestors, for example, traditional beliefs about the conception of the universe. In Nigeria, in the Igboland, ancestors conceived the universe as being made of this visible world, namely, the firmaments (*Igwe*) and earth (*Ala*) (Ogbu, 1999). Human beings, animals, and plants live on the earth. The earth gives food to sustain life. It is in the earth that persons are buried when they die. Consequently, the earth is very much revered, culminating in a ritual known as *Ime Ala,* meaning to celebrate the earth. Early Nigerians believed that within the universe there exist certain inexplicable forces that intrude in the lives of the people. These metaphysical forces—for example, the earth and the firmaments—control the days and nights from which the Nigerian market days, *Eke, Orie, Afo,* and *Nkwo,* derive their names. The same forces control the seasons and the lunar year. The metaphysical forces are neither human beings nor dead ancestors, even though they have the attribute of human beings. Dead ancestors, sometimes referred to as *mmuo* or *ndimmuo,* are consistently remembered because they, too, are believed to form part of the universe. These beliefs are the basis for the concept of bad spirits and good spirits held by many Nigerian Americans. Bad spirits are those who lived bad lives and were referred to as the *devil's angels.* The good spirits, or God's angels, lived good lives while on earth. Heaven and hell are where the good or the bad go after death. Some Nigerian Americans believe there are men and women who have the power to interpret and to arrest the evil machinations of the devil's angels that intrude into their lives. These men and women are consulted when the need arises. Sacrifices are offered to the good spirits by these men and women to invoke their aid

in preserving and perpetuating the lineage and in stopping the forces of the evil spirits that intrude into an individual's life (Ogbu, 1999).

In the traditional belief, the Supreme Being known as *God* stands above metaphysical forces and is recognized by all as the creator of everything in the universe, including all the metaphysical forces already mentioned. The term *god* with the small letter *g* was coined by the early colonial masters with their Christian missionary agents to discredit traditional religious practices, which they described as worshiping false gods (Ogbu, 1999).

Implications for Nursing Care

When caring for the Nigerian American, the nurse should appreciate that ethnic background influences health practices and responses to illness. Ethnicity is a stimulus in a person's response to pain and disease. The nurse should be knowledgeable about the impact of family, religion, and ethnicity on the Nigerian-American client to provide culturally competent care and to gain a working relationship with the client in order to meet health care needs.

In 1996, a Nigerian grandmother was arrested in Brooklyn, New York. She had allowed her 6-year-old grandson to be slashed on the face with African tribal marks (Egyir, 1996). It is important for the nurse to appreciate that ethnic practices and values may continue regardless of the location of the person of Nigerian ethnic origin. Even though this incident was assessed as abuse in New York City, the grandparents and mother were not being abusive according to generations-old Yoruba beliefs and customs. Another ethnic practice that has existed for years in some parts of Nigeria is female genital mutilation (FGM).

The national prevalence rate of FGM is 41% among adult women. Evidence abounds that the prevalence of FGM is declining. The ongoing drive to eradicate FGM is tackled by the World Health Organization (WHO), the United Nations International Children's Emergency Fund, the Federation of International Obstetrics and Gynecology, the African Union, the economic commission for Africa, and many women's organizations. However, there is no federal law banning FGM in Nigeria. There is need to eradicate FGM in Nigeria. Education of the general public at all levels with emphasis on the dangers and undesirability of FGM is paramount (Okeke, Anyaehie, & Ezenyeaku, 2012).

In the summer of 2002, the Nigerian legislature considered passing a law banning FGM and imposing a 2-year jail term for offenders (Lagos, 2002). The legislation is controversial and has yet to be passed. Thus, a nurse may encounter adult Nigerian-American females who were born in Nigeria and may be victims of this traditional practice.

Moodley (2000) found that research on the structure of illness perceptions consistently suggests the five following dimensions: (1) identity, the label placed on the illness and its symptoms; (2) causes, ideas about how one gets the illness; (3) consequences, the expected outcome; (4) timeline, ideas about the duration of the illness; and (5) controllability/cure, belief about the extent to which the illness can be cured or controlled.

Asuni (cited in Moodley, 2000) compared African traditional healing methods with the European model and suggested that the "why" questioning and interpreting of conflict and illness are given more emphasis than the "how" model used by Western health care professionals. Western methods divide illness into different categories of somatic, psychological, and psychosomatic, but the majority of Nigerians do not. They do not split themselves into good and bad parts but express their distress as "when part of me is ill, the whole of me is ill, irrespective of what the illness is" (Moodley, 2000, p. 4).

TIME

The concept of time indicates the focus of the culture as well as providing a method of marking the past, present, and future events. Nigerian-American children are socialized to accept the values and practices in relation to time as aspects of culture that should not be challenged or questioned. Parents inculcate in the children that they stand in the circle of history, where their ancestors represent the past, their parents represent the present, and they represent the future. Thus, children are trained to cherish the past, respect the present, and work so their own future will be successful. Children may see their grandparents and accept the reality that they will be obliged to take care of their own parents at an old age (Amadi, personal communication, 2002; Falola, 2001; Ogbu, 1999).

In Nigeria, the use of time varies from exact dates and events to so-called African time, known in the United States as "colored people time" (Umegeh, personal communication, 2002). For example, a Nigerian woman is most likely to state that her last menstrual period occurred 2 days before or after Christmas. Also, those who were born prior to birth registration in a particular area will state their date of birth in relation to an event. For example, Ms. Ezenwa (Igbo) may state her date of birth as the year in which "two nights occurred in one day," meaning the solar eclipse. This is the eclipse of the sun, which occurred in 1948. Ms. Nwankwo may state her date of birth to be the year when there was a salt scarcity in Nigeria. Nigeria experienced a scarcity of salt in the early 1940s as a result of world war. *African time* refers to lack of punctuality. An 8 A.M. appointment may mean 12 noon.

Implications for Nursing Care

In working with Nigerians whose birth dates predated birth registration, the nurse should ask for events happening during the client's birth time in order to come up with an estimated date of birth. If certain medication must be taken at a certain time, the nurse must stress the importance of taking the medication on time. It will also help if other family members are included in this decision. In planning care with the client, the implication(s) of taking medication on time or late must be stressed. Nigerians like examples, stories, and what will happen if the regimen is not followed, in order to be compliant. Some believe that once they begin to feel better, the need for medication is no longer present. As a result, they may not complete the prescription for an antibiotic or malaria treatment. A story or education in terms of the implications of not completing antibiotic therapy can be a helpful way to communicate the importance of compliance.

For those Nigerian Americans who maintain African time, the nurse should emphasize that this time orientation is not helpful for medications on a required routine and that haphazard usage could be detrimental to health. The nurse should be aware that some Nigerian Americans are unlikely to take prescribed medications whether a set time is required or not. The nurse must stress the importance of the medications and the consequences of nonadherence. It may be helpful to have the teaching done by a Nigerian nurse if one is available since the Nigerian client will be more likely to believe the Nigerian nurse. If one is not available, it is also important to appreciate that a client will be more likely to be compliant when the nurse who gives the instructions takes time with the teaching and acts in a caring manner.

ENVIRONMENTAL CONTROL

Most Nigerians believe that illness is a natural occurrence resulting from disharmony and conflict in some area of a person's life. Since the majority of Nigerians believe strongly in extended family relations, an illness in one individual is perceived as a crisis in the whole family. Depending on the type of illness, family members will join together to discuss the best plan of care for this one person. Also, depending on the age of this person, the ill person may not participate in this discussion. There is also the notion that illness is a result of forces in the environment, such as witchcraft or voodoo. For persons with these beliefs, it is usually felt that Western medicine has no effect on witchcraft or voodoo. As a result, the individual's family may seek the help of a traditional healer for treatment (Amadi, personal communication, 2002; Falola, 2001; Ogbu, 1999; Umegeh, personal communication, 2002).

According to Roy and Andrews (2008), changes in environmental setting can have a pronounced effect on the person's state of adaptation. These changes tend to affect the individual's senses and include such stimuli as temperature changes, different noise levels, or unusual diet. The presence of unfamiliar people or absence of familiar ones may be an external environmental change that affects health. Drugs, alcohol, and tobacco, which can influence the person's internal environment, are also factors related to environmental control.

Health Care Practices

Health care practices in Nigeria range from home remedies to spiritual healers to, as a last resort, clinics or hospitals. Thus, Nigerian Americans may tend to see clinics or hospitals as the final treatment of choice rather than the first. Home remedies and spiritual healers may be considered cultural practices. Cultural health practices utilized by Nigerian Americans can be categorized as efficacious (beneficial), neutral, or dysfunctional (Kalu, 2014). Efficacious cultural health practices are those practices that are viewed as beneficial to the client's health status, although they can differ vastly from modern scientific practices; for example, certain family planning practices are deemed efficacious. Many Nigerian-American couples use rituals, herbal approaches, and similar practices to regulate fertility for cultural, economic, or personal reasons. Some of these beliefs and practices are not effective birth control measures. A number of research studies support the health care practices used in Nigeria. For example, Oyelami, Agbakwuru, Adeyemi, and Adedeji (2005) reported the positive effect of grapefruit seeds in treating urinary tract infections. Okeniyi, Olubanjo, Oguniest, and Oyelami (2005) reported the benefits of honey in healing incisions of abscessed wounds.

Neutral cultural health practices have no effect on the health status of an individual. Although some health care practitioners may consider neutral health practices irrelevant, the nurse must remember that such practices may be extremely important because they may be linked to beliefs that are closely integrated with an individual's behavior, for example, drinking tea made from various harmless roots and weeds and jumping up and down or sneezing after intercourse to dislodge the sperm (Delano, 1996; Keller, 1996; Pillsbury, 1982).

Dysfunctional cultural health practices may be dangerous or counterproductive and should be discouraged. The Nigerian belief that sex during menstruation will turn people into albinos is not harmful (Keller, 1996). In actuality, intercourse during menstruation will have less likelihood of resulting in pregnancy, so in this respect it could be said to be efficacious in terms of the risk of pregnancy.

In some African countries, some women douche with hot water, salt, vinegar, lemon, or even potassium after sex to abate pregnancy. Nurses must stress the consequences of these dysfunctional practices.

Other potentially harmful pregnancy prevention traditions include eating arsenic and castor oil seeds and soaking cotton wool in pepper and inserting it into the vagina as a barrier method (Keller, 1996). It is also believed in some circles that participating in vigorous exercise will result in spontaneous abortion. Some unwed mothers have tried this practice, and some claim it was successful in causing an abortion (Delano, 1996).

Folk Medicine

Folk medicine is one of people's earliest uses of the natural environment to promote their own well-being and involves the use of herbs, plants, minerals, and animal substances to prevent and treat illnesses (Spector, 2004). Folk medicine existed in Nigeria before the introduction of Western medicine. It is believed that herbal medicine goes back to ancient civilizations that studied and made observations of the various plants growing around them. Fellow inhabitants were treated by use of medicinal plants (Mudzafar, 1999). Christianity has tended to sway people away from folk medicine. However, most ethnic groups in Nigeria still practice folk medicine, and many brought these practices with them as they immigrated to the United States (Falola, 2001).

There are different kinds of folk medicines, including cures of sicknesses caused by natural or unnatural events. Natural sicknesses are believed to be caused by forces in nature as a result of the wear and tear of life or by exposure to some natural contaminants. On the other hand, unnatural sicknesses are caused by fellow human beings who are jealous of the person or as a result of evil doings by the person, referred to as *karma*. There is no formal education for the practice of folk medicine. Old medicine women or men pass down their knowledge of the curative properties of plants to an heir or to selected individuals who become the recipients of such powers (Spector, 2004).

The classification of the sickness will determine where treatment is sought. The majority of rural dwellers will seek the help of traditional or folk medicine practitioners first. In South Africa, for instance, 60% of the population still relies on traditional plant-based medicine. Indigenous peoples and Indians of the Amazon rainforest have for centuries used their knowledge of medicinal plants. In fact, some entire communities and indigenous tribes of the rainforest earn a living by collecting medicinal plants from the wild.

There are different kinds of medicine men or herbalists. The good ones provide concoctions to promote adaptation and wellness. The bad ones provide concoctions that are detrimental to health and are believed to cause death. The latter kinds are responsible for magic, voodoo, and witchcraft. They are very cheap. The good native doctors are very expensive; they scare their clients and their family members enough to cough out any amount of money in order to be safe. They often provide their clients with charms to wear or oils to rub as prophylaxis (Amadi, personal communication, 2002).

Persons who can afford Western medicine, primarily city dwellers, will seek the services of a trained medical doctor first. However, for persons without financial resources, the more reasonable cost of folk medicine may cause this to be the treatment of choice. Other factors contributing to the popularity of folk medicine include the long-standing cultural belief that the treatment will work and the lack of availability of medical doctors, even if resources to pay were available. Unlike medical doctors, the traditional healers and practitioners of folk medicine are available in every village. Therefore, Nigerians often seek medicine men and women who use plant-based medicine in most of their treatments of aches, pains, and infertility. Traditional Nigerian healers and practitioners of folk medicine can also be found in America through use of Nigeria Infonet, a premier search engine for Nigeria and Nigerian Americans.

Folk medicine treatments range from drinking the water from selected leaves after boiling to cure malaria and certain fevers, to the wearing of beads or ornaments to ward off evil spirits. It is a general belief that the leaves talk to traditional healers, telling the healer what the leaves will cure. Certain roots are soaked in homemade hot drinks and are dispensed as specified by the traditional healers, who are also known as *native doctors.*

Traditional healers treat measles by drawing lines all over the body with liquid from a certain seed. The lines turn black after several hours and remain in place for several days. The lines are believed to prevent the worsening and side effects of the disease. Placing a traditional necklace with charms around a child's neck can prevent convulsions. Most illnesses, especially those that result in complications, are believed to be caused by one's enemies or those who do not want one to progress. One's closest relative, the mother-in-law being at the top of the list, causes almost all the infertility cases.

Medicinal plants deserve attention because they are of great value to most Nigerians. The Zulu, said to have known the medicinal uses of some 700 plants, used the fever-leaf to treat malaria cases all over Africa. In some parts of Africa, the bark of the willow (*Salix capensis*) is used in treating rheumatism complaints. This plant comes from a family known for salicylic acid, which is the active ingredient in aspirin (Mudzafar, 1999). In Nigeria, certain herbal preparations are made to treat skin infections. Herbal preparations have antibacterial activity against gram-positive bacteria, which cause skin infections.

Mudzafar (1999) noted that in 1952 a distinguished Nigerian in England was suffering from severe psychotic episodes and was not responsive to the treatment given by the English doctors. To help him, a traditional Nigerian doctor was called. By using the rauwolfia root, he managed to relieve the patient of psychosis. Rauwolfia comes from a family of plants used for the modern-day reserpine, which was first used to treat psychosis and today is used to help control blood pressure.

Customs and Rituals Related to Death and Dying

Death is revered by Nigerians. Traditional Nigerians believe that family members owe the deceased rites and burial customs, which will assist on the journey to join the ancestors. If rites are violated, the deceased will torment any member of the family by inflicting some ailment that defies medical explanation. The spirit is left wandering between the living and dead and cannot be fully integrated with the ancestors. According to Nnedu (personal communication, 2006), the family must do everything possible, even if it necessitates borrowing funds for burial money. In the Akpulu community of eastern Nigeria, a family that has more than one death must complete burial rites for the first family member before proceeding to rites for the next.

An individual's mode of living, religious affiliations, profession, and class dictate the type of burial rite to be performed. For example, the burial rite for a title holder is different from that for a non–title holder. Likewise, the burial rite for women is different from that for men. Lastly, the burial rite for a married man is different from that for a single man.

The burial ceremony of an Ozo titled man in Igboland is mainly performed in three stages. The first stage is the interment. When an Ozo title holder dies, the relations must be quickly informed. Each title holder has to perform some ritual of killing a cock to disengage himself from any further cultural ties with the deceased. A cock may be substituted with a fowl's egg. The individual holds the egg in his hand, makes a circle over his head with the hand raised, and finally throws the egg away while muttering the words of disengagement in the process. A further ritual of stripping the deceased of his title is performed. The significance of this ritual is the belief that the title holder came to this world naked and without a title and must return in a similar way. The relative of the deceased will bathe and dress the remains for viewing. The bathing or cleansing is to ensure purity and qualification of admittance into the home of the ancestors (Olajubu, 2003). While traveling to visit the bereaved, individuals may act happy and joke. However, as soon as they are in close proximity, the emotional tone may change dramatically. The viewing of the dressed-up corpse evokes strong emotion, resulting in the cries of women and deep sighs from the men. The corpse is laid to rest on a spot in the family compound amidst booming guns. Cemeteries are very seldom used. The burial brings the first stage to a close.

The second stage is the showcase stage, which is referred to as *Igba Okwukwu* in some parts of the Igboland. Because of the expense involved, family members do not hurry into this stage, which is also called *wealth demonstration*. The ceremony starts in the evening of Orie Market day and is known as *Ura Ozu* (night vigil for the corpse) (Ogbu, 1999). During this time, native musical instruments are at work, with people dancing and chanting. The guns known as *nkponala,* which are stuck to the ground at an interval of a foot or two from each other and filled with gunpowder, are fired at regular intervals (Ogbu, 1999). The gunshots signify the departure of a great man. A set of songs provided by women reminds the widow of her new status, and its attending implications are rendered by women (Olajubu, 2003). At dawn of a market day, guns boom. The talking drums call out the names of dignitaries as they arrive. The drummers are rewarded with cash gifts. In appreciation for the gifts, the donor is given heroic names reminiscent of the deeds of the ancient warriors as if the donor were one of the heroes (Okparaeke, personal communication, 2006).

Each of the deceased man's sons-in-law must bring with him the traditional dish known as *oku-akwu.* This is a large basin overstuffed with large pieces of yams boiled in palm oil with a large cooked leg of a goat placed on top of it, or a large boiled fish (Ogbu, 1999). This dish is accompanied with a gallon or two of palm wine. The food is for the female relatives of the deceased, who leave their marital homes to spend several days in the home of the deceased. It is not unusual for the sons-in-law to try to outdo each other by presenting additional gifts, such as a goat, ram, or cow. Each in-law is usually accompanied by a cultural dancing group or entertainers or masquerade to grace the occasion. The ceremony lasts for about 8 days, with friends and well-wishers coming from far and near to pay tribute. The crowd thins down each succeeding day until the last stage is reached.

The final stage is the celebration in the market square and is known as *iku ozu* (Ogbu, 1999). This takes place on the fourth or eighth day of the ceremony described previously according to the status of the deceased. During this stage, a gun is fired to appease the dead, which marks the end of the ceremony and indicates that the daughters of the deceased may return to their marital homes.

The widowhood rites are also complex. The widow is expected to be in mourning and to remain behind closed doors for a specified period of time. The woman is not allowed to apply makeup or attend to her hair. She may wear only black attire to signify grief. She is exempt from her activities as part of her grief process. Her late husband's family may shave off all her hair as a sign of respect to her late husband. It is of note to mention that husbands mourn for their wives differently.

When a married woman dies or is about to die, her close relations are notified without delay. Her relatives are responsible for cleansing her with water and soap and for dressing her for viewing. The deceased woman's male relations will return to their respective homes while the females remain with the corpse. The women engage in singing and dancing while the eldest son and the eldest daughter, accompanied by a few relations of the husband, visit the home of their mother to solicit the male relatives to come and bury her. This visit is usually accompanied with gifts. The burial of a woman can be as elaborate as those of men depending on the wealth of her children. Observers are there for different reasons. Some are there for sympathy; some are there because of the good foods that are served to all in attendance; and some are there for criticism, watching how many livestock animals were slaughtered, the type of burial casket, and the jewelry of the deceased.

Implications for Nursing Care

Problems in health care occur when the needs of certain individuals are not considered (LaMar, 2013). Lack of respect for cultural diversity can cause physical, emotional, and spiritual distress if care that is provided is not meaningful to the client. When a health care professional demonstrates respect for culture, it is more likely that health care resources will be used by the people who need them. People from different cultures, races, religions, and backgrounds should be made to feel welcome and respected for their unique health beliefs. Personal cultural beliefs should be considered when developing the plan of care (Geissler, 1998; Spector, 2004).

Nurses need not hold the same views as their Nigerian-American clients but must respect their cultural, spiritual, and religious beliefs. Nurses demonstrate cultural competency when they allow their client's beliefs to mold and direct the care they provide, within accepted standards of practice.

Delano (1996) advised health care professionals to take advantage of nonharmful rituals to promote the acceptance of modern family planning. An existing Nigerian ritual, placing an object made of red feathers (called a *teso*) on the floor, is believed to make it impossible for any man to have sexual intercourse with an adolescent girl until the spell is removed. Other rituals practiced that are not harmful include ineffective notions that pregnancy can be prevented when women avoid the sun or moon at certain times or wear charms, including dead spiders, children's teeth, or leopard skin bracelets. Leopards are believed to scare away unwanted pregnancy (Delano, 1996).

Practices that are not harmful, such as rituals or story-telling, may offer innovative ways to teach the physiology of menstruation and Western contraceptive practices or to encourage correct and consistent use. According to Delano (1996), health care professionals gain credibility for teaching family planning in ways that do not exclude or ridicule traditional beliefs.

BIOLOGICAL VARIATIONS

It is well accepted that people differ culturally and socio-economically. Less is known about how people differ biologically, although knowledge of this area is significantly expanding with research on biological differences (LaMar, 2013).

When giving care to Nigerian Americans, nurses should appreciate that because a significant diversity exists within this vast group, it is critical to conduct an individual health assessment and base care on data collected rather than on stereotypical assumptions concerning Nigerian or Black individuals. In addition to having differing behaviors and beliefs, Nigerians also differ biologically, both within groups of Nigerians and from other groups. For example, Nigerians experience different processes of development and aging and may manifest illness differently from other groups (for example, White Americans or South Africans). The data concerning biological variations among Nigerians are limited and present a challenging area of opportunity for the nurse researcher. Data available in the literature will be discussed.

Birth Weight

It is the dream of every Nigerian to have a neonate whose weight is average to above average. Some see it as a sign of wealth or being able to take care of one's wife financially. Northern Nigerian men are usually taller than the southerners, and southern women are on average heavier than northern women. This difference can be attributed to diet and lifestyle. It is a well-known fact that southerners consume a lot of carbohydrates, whereas northerners consume a lot of meat and milk products from animals that accompany them in their nomadic lifestyle (Falola, 2001).

Skin Color

Skin color, or pigmentation, is determined by the amount of melanin. Melanin is a water-insoluble polymer of various compounds derived from the amino acid tyrosine. It is one of two pigments found in human skin and hair and adds brown to skin color. The various hues and degrees of pigmentation found in the skin of human beings are directly related to the number, size, and distribution of melanosomes within the melanocytes and other cells. Besides its role in pigmentation, melanin absorbs ultraviolet light and therefore plays a protective role when skin is exposed to the damaging rays of the sun. Dark-skinned individuals are not immune to sunburn but may not burn as easily as Whites do (LaMar, 2013). Hence, the dark skin color may be nature's way to protect sub-Saharan residents.

The skin color of Nigerians varies from very light tan to very black. The skin color is attributed to the geographic location in Nigeria, as well as from mixed ancestries. The surface of the body is determined by climate (Ogbu, 1999). New Guinea highlanders and sub-Saharan Africans are about as different from each other genetically as any human beings on earth. Yet they have physical similarities because of where they live, including dark skin to protect against the rays of the sun.

Susceptibility to Disease

Hypertension. Scientists have known for some time that the rate of hypertension in rural West Africa is lower than in any other place in the world, except for some parts of the Amazon basin and the South Pacific (Cooper, Rotimi, & Ward, 2002). People of African descent in the United States and the United Kingdom have among the highest rates of hypertension in the world. Cooper, Rotimi, and Ward (2002) stated that the shift suggests that something about the environment and lifestyle of European and American Blacks, rather than a genetic factor, is the fundamental cause of the altered susceptibility to high blood pressure. These researchers established facilities in communities in Nigeria, Cameroon, Zimbabwe, St. Lucia, Barbados, Jamaica, and the United States. Later on in the research, the focus was only on Nigeria, the United States, and Jamaica. The Nigerian community used in this study is a rural one in the district of Igbo-Ora. The residents of Igbo-Ora are typically lean, engage in physically demanding subsistence farming, and eat the traditional Nigerian diet of rice, tubers, and fruit. Nations in sub-Saharan Africa, of which Nigeria is among the largest, do not keep formal records on mortality and life expectancy, but based on local studies, the researchers assumed that infections, especially malaria, are the major killer. The research revealed that adults in Igbo-Ora have an annual mortality risk of 1% to 2%. Cooper, Rotimi, and Ward (2002) noted that those who survive to older ages tend to be quite healthy, and blood pressure was not found to rise with age. Thus, it is important for nurses to educate Nigerians to continue some of the lifestyle patterns taught by the ancestors and to caution clients about the implications of adopting the Western way of life in entirety.

Yeh et al. (1996) studied 397 civil servants in Nigeria to assess the role of socioeconomic status and serum fatty acids for the relationship between intake of animal food and cardiovascular risk factors. Civil servants were selected for the study since they provided persons of differing socioeconomic status for the study. Those with more resources were noted to consume more meat, milk, and eggs. The researchers concluded that fatty acids in absolute weight concentration reflected the amount of fat intake. The level of total fatty acids was directly related to cardiovascular risk factors in the Nigerians studied. They noted that follow-up of such populations in cultural transition can facilitate the understanding of the true roles of animal fat intake in the early evolution of atherosclerosis.

Cancer. Based on the WHO's worldwide cancer data, West African men have much lower prostate cancer incidence and mortality compared with African-American men. Specifically, Nigerian men are 10 times less likely to develop prostate cancer and 3.5 times less likely to die from the disease than African-American men (Odedina, Ogunbiyi, & Ukoli, 2006).

Lactose Intolerance. Lactose intolerance exists among Nigerian Americans. Thus, the nurse should avoid automatically teaching every Nigerian to drink milk. Calcium can be obtained in other ways—for example, from seafood and leafy vegetables or by adding vinegar to the water when cooking a soup bone for homemade soup to decalcify the bone. Also, lactose-free dairy products can be suggested to this group.

Alzheimer's Disease. Hall et al. (2006) investigated cholesterol, *APOE* genotype, and Alzheimer's disease (AD). They noted that increased levels of cholesterol and low-density lipoprotein cholesterol were associated with increased risk of AD in individuals without the *APOE4* allele, but not those with this allele. There was a significant interaction between cholesterol, *APOE4,* and the risk of AD in the Yoruba, a population with lower cholesterol levels and lower incidence rates of AD than African-Americans.

Malaria. Malaria is a common health problem in Nigeria. When a Nigerian enters the health care system with fever of unknown origin, she or he must be tested for malaria. Malaria is an infectious parasitic disease that can be acute or chronic and is frequently recurrent. Four kinds of malaria can infect humans, categorized by the causative organism: *Plasmodium falciparum, P. vivax, P. ovale,* and *P. malariae* (Centers for Disease Control and Prevention [CDC], 2014). Malaria is not endemic to Nigeria but occurs in more than 100 countries. According to the Centers for Disease Control and Prevention, more than 40% of the people in the world are at risk.

The WHO estimates that there are 300 to 500 million new cases of malaria each year, culminating in 1.5 to 2.7 million deaths annually worldwide. About 1200 cases of malaria are diagnosed in the United States each year. The WHO noted that most cases in the United States are in immigrants and travelers returning from malaria-risk areas, mostly from sub-Saharan Africa and the Indian subcontinent (CDC, 2014). Humans get malaria from the bite of a malaria-infected mosquito.

Pathophysiology of Malaria. When a mosquito bites an infected person, it ingests microscopic malaria parasites found in the victim's blood. These parasites begin multiplication. The multiplication may last for about a week or more before infection can be passed to another person. At the end of the multiplication period, if this mosquito bites another individual, the parasites travel from the mosquito's mouth into the person's bloodstream and then to the person's liver. While in the liver, they continue to grow and multiply. This is the incubation period; the individual will not exhibit any signs and symptoms of the disease.

The parasites live in the liver and reenter the bloodstream into the red blood cells (RBCs). The incubation period can last from 8 days to several months (CDC, 2014). As the RBCs continue to grow, they will eventually burst, freeing the parasites to attack other RBCs. As the RBCs burst, toxins are also released. It is the toxin that is responsible for the signs and symptoms seen in clients suffering from malaria. If a mosquito bites this person during this time, it will ingest the tiny parasites, and the cycle of malaria infestation is repeated. Other modes of transmission of the malaria parasites are through blood transfusions and from mother to fetus across the placental barrier.

Measures to Combat Malaria. Malaria is a difficult disease to control largely due to the highly adaptable nature of the vector and parasites involved. While effective tools have been and will continue to be developed to combat malaria, inevitably, over time the parasites and mosquitoes will evolve means to circumvent those tools if used in isolation or used ineffectively. To achieve sustainable control over malaria, health care professionals will need a combination of new approaches and tools, and research will play a critical role in development of those next-generation strategies (U.S. Department of Health and Human Services National Institutes of Health, 2014). According to Alalu and Ojeme (2002), the Nigerian government is determined to fight malaria. The Nigerian Ministry of Health planned to launch a three-pronged campaign targeted at promoting awareness of the use of insecticide-treated nets (ITNs), prepacked antimalarial drugs, and intermittent presumptive treatment for pregnant women (Alalu & Ojeme, 2002). Shulman et al. (1999) demonstrated that intermittent treatment with sulfadoxine-pyrimethamine during the second and third trimesters decreased the risk of severe anemia in primigravidas living in areas with a high prevalence of malaria infection. The sample for this study included 1264 primigravida women who attended the prenatal clinic with a viable singleton pregnancy. At the time of recruitment, the women were at 16 to 30 weeks' gestation. Women with a hemoglobin level below 6 g/dL, severe preeclampsia, or a clinical diagnosis of malaria were excluded. The authors also concluded that the mechanisms underlying the adverse effects of malaria in pregnancy are not well understood. The vision is "a malaria-free Nigeria." The goal is to halve malaria-associated mortality by 2015 and again by the end of 2016. According to Lambo (2014), the Federal Ministry of Health, National Malaria Control Programme published a five-year strategic plan: 2006–2010 for the control of malaria in Nigeria. There are a set of core interventions and cross-cutting interventions that form the framework of the strategic plan. The objectives are related to achieving ITN distribution to a minimum of 80% of the country by 2010. The publication also indicated that there would be indoor residual spraying in urban areas with poor access to health care services. Lambo continued that strategies to prevent malaria during pregnancy include strengthening the malaria component of focused antenatal care, supporting the national roll-out of focused antenatal care with intermittent preventive treatment and sulfadoxine/pyrimethamine during pregnancy. Also encouraging pregnant women to attend prenatal care at least twice during their pregnancy is important. The recommendation is to treat uncomplicated and severe malaria with artemisinin-based combination therapies.

The problems facing the strategic plan include an increase in the resistance of malaria parasites to drugs, the nonavailability of the very effective antimalarial commodities such as artemisinin-based combination therapies, and access to care for those residing in the rural villages (Lambo, 2014).

Travel Hints for Malaria Prophylaxis

- Visit health care provider 4 to 6 weeks before foreign travel for any necessary vaccinations and a prescription for an antimalarial drug.
- Take antimalarial drug exactly on schedule without missing doses.
- Prevent mosquito and other insect bites. Use *N,N*-diethyl-meta-toluamide (DEET) insecticide on exposed skin and flying-insect spray in the room where you sleep.
- Wear long pants and long-sleeved shirts, especially from dusk to dawn. This is the time when mosquitoes that spread malaria bite.
- Sleep under a mosquito bed net that has been dipped in permethrin insecticide if you are not living in screened or air-conditioned housing (CDC, 2014).

AIDS (HIV) Risk

The first case of acquired immunodeficiency syndrome (AIDS) in Nigeria was reported in 1986. Consequently, and in line with guidelines from the WHO, the government adopted antenatal clinic sentinel surveillance as the system for assessing the epidemic. Sentinel survey data showed that the human immunodeficiency virus (HIV) prevalence increased from 1.2% in 1991 to 5.8% in 2001. After 2003, the prevalence declined to 4.4% in 2005 before slightly increasing to 4.6% in 2008. Results from the latest round of sentinel survey data shows that the national prevalence was 4.1% in 2010 (Federal Ministry of Health [FMOH], 2014) Trend analysis of HIV prevalence from sentinel surveillance in Nigeria indicates that the epidemic has halted and is showing signs of stabilizing at about 4% from 2005 to the present.

Similarly, based on projected HIV estimates of 2013, about 3,229,757 people now live with HIV while it is estimated that 220,394 new HIV infections occurred in 2013. A total of 210,031 died from AIDS-related cases. It is also estimated that a total of 1,476,741 required antiretroviral drugs in 2013. Although the most-at-risk populations contribute to the spread of HIV, heterosexual sex, particularly of the low-risk type, still makes up about 80% of transmissions. Mother-to-child transmission and transfusion of infected blood and blood products, on the other hand, account for the other notable modes of transmission.

In 2013, Nigeria continued a commitment toward meeting the vision of Millennium Development Goal to halt and reverse the HIV/AIDS epidemic in the country and promote the achievement of universal access to HIV/AIDS prevention, treatment, care, and support in line with global commitments. With the valuable support of local and international partners, the country has seen the epidemic profile change significantly from HIV prevalence of 5.8% in 2001 to 4.1% in 2010. Attaining the status of a country with a stable HIV epidemic among adults 15–49 years old between 2001 and 2011 is a significant achievement, though there are still gaps and challenges with access to HIV/AIDS service by eligible persons. Reviews of the national response further helped to identify some other key challenges that revolve around limited domestic financing of the response, weak coordination at national and state

BOX 25-1   Estimated Number of People Living with HIV/AIDS in Nigeria

People Living with HIV/AIDS	Adult (15–49) Rate (%)	Women with HIV/AIDS	Children with HIV/AIDS	AIDS Deaths	Orphans Due to AIDS
3,400,000	3.1	1,700,000	430,000	240,000	2,200,000

n = 2.6 million, 2007 estimate.
Data obtained from UNAIDS/WHO (2013); HIV and AIDS in Nigeria (2014).

levels, inadequate state government contribution to resourcing for the response, challenges with human resources for health, weak supply-chain management systems, and limited service delivery capacity and access to HIV services.

The 2014 Nigeria GARPR report highlights the progress in the national response and the collective efforts stakeholders have made in Nigeria in the year 2013 while providing evidence that will further strengthen the need to do more toward ensuring that we reach our country goals, objectives, and targets for HIV response (Nigeria GARPR, 2014). At the end of 2013, the data in Box 25-1 were available from UNAIDS and the World Bank (2014).

Chemical Abuse. Drug abuse is defined as excessive or inappropriate use of a substance by a person, such use being considered or judged to be illegal by the culture and resulting in harm to the person or society (Asuni & Pela, 1986; Odejide, 2006). The situation in Nigeria and the lifestyles of Nigerians have dramatically changed over past years under the influence of industrial and urban development. Development has in turn changed the way in which some Nigerians relax.

Until the recent past, information on drug abuse among Nigerians was minimal and largely based on studies on in-school populations and small populations in the urban areas. The focus of the Nigerian Drug Law Enforcement Agency (NDLEA) is on drug couriers, rather than on leaders of drug-trafficking groups. Based on the assessment by NDLEA (2014), the general picture emerging is one of widespread use and an estimated lifetime consumption of cannabis (10.8%), followed by psychotropic substances (mainly the benzodiazepines and amphetamine-type stimulants) (10.6%), and to a lesser degree heroin (1.6%) and cocaine (1.4%) in both urban and rural areas. The use of volatile organic solvents (0.053%) is reportedly becoming popular, especially among street children, in-school youth, and women.

This study reported abuse of various local plants among youth and the unemployed. Abuse included smoking of paw paw (papaya) leaves and the seeds of zakami, which grows widely in most of the northwestern and north-central regions of Nigeria. The study findings, including the age of first use and pattern of abuse, confirm that the 10- to 29-year-old age group is the most vulnerable group for drug abuse in Nigeria. In addition, a high usage rate of cannabis, cocaine, and heroin was found among prostitutes, commercial drivers, motor park touts, and law enforcement agents.

Reasons cited for abusing drugs include sociocultural displacement of the young people through rapid urbanization and modernization; general poverty levels that increase the vulnerability of children to street or peer pressure for survival; and beliefs among prostitutes, commercial drivers, and law enforcement agents that narcotics increase their energy for tedious and long hours of work. The easy availability of narcotics and psychotropic drugs in the country increases the exposure of the vulnerable and facilitates subsequent use.

According to Murray and Zentner (2008), therapy is usually entered into as a result of family pressure, often in the form of threatened financial loss, such as the withdrawal of inheritance, or a crisis event, such as attempted suicide or arrest. The behavior and illness of the drug abuser can control the entire family, yet in Nigeria there are limited treatment opportunities, which often cost money that is not available. The outlook for treatment is bleak. Since some Nigerian Americans may have been drug users before immigration, an understanding of drug use in Nigeria is important for the nurse to respond knowledgeably when the client enters the health care system in America.

Alcohol use is forbidden to individuals adhering to Islamic law. Beer and a wine that is made from the sap of palm trees are popular beverages in Nigeria for persons not adhering to Islamic law who do not live in the states in the north; in those states, Islamic law is applied to both civil and criminal cases (CIA, 2015).

Epilepsy. Danesi and Adetunji (1994) studied 265 epileptic patients in Lagos, Nigeria. Clients used alternative treatments before seeking hospital treatment. This study noted that only 14.6% of the clients who had previously used African traditional medicine continued with such treatment after initiation of hospital treatment. Two thirds of the clients who had used spiritual healing continued with that treatment, suggesting that many of the clients perceived some continued benefit from the alternative treatments. The researchers concluded that alternative medicine, especially spiritual healing, cannot be considered irrelevant in the management of epilepsy in Africa.

Ebola. Ebola is a rare and deadly disease caused by infection with a strain of Ebola virus. The 2014 Ebola epidemic is the largest in history, affecting multiple countries in West Africa including Nigeria. It is spread through direct contact with blood and body fluids of a person already showing symptoms of Ebola. It is not spread through the air, water, food, or mosquitoes. The symptoms may appear anywhere from 2 to 21 days after exposure to Ebola virus (CDC, 2015). On July 20, 2014, the Ebola virus was introduced into Nigeria via Lagos by a Liberian passenger. The world stood still in anticipation of impending doom in Nigeria, but the response was quick and decisive (Dung, 2014). The WHO reported that 20 people were infected and 8 of them succumbed to the virus (a 60% success rate). At publication, the WHO has declared Nigeria Ebola free. Nigeria responded promptly and aggressively to a single case of Ebola.

Psychological Characteristics

Nigerian-American families have close ties to one another. Stressful events are discussed among family members and close friends. According to Lazarus and Folkman (2012), psychological stress is a particular relationship between the person and the environment that is appraised by the person as taxing and/or exceeding his or her resources and endangering his or her well-being. There are universal stressors that would affect most people—for example, illness, accidents, and catastrophic events. However, because of individual interpretations of events, stressors are frequently person-specific (Carson, 2000). For most Nigerian Americans, when universal stressors are present, the family attempts to be supportive, and the recipient of the stressors is not left alone. Nigerians take turns staying with the afflicted person or family.

Nurses need to be aware that Nigerian Americans may attempt to hide certain illnesses from other family members. For example, psychiatric illness is often known only to the husband if the wife has the problem or vice versa. It is a taboo to admit that one's family member is a psychiatric patient. Mental illness is a shameful stigma in the Nigerian culture. There are reasons for this denial. The patient's children may find it difficult to get a Nigerian spouse because Nigerians believe that such illnesses are hereditary. They fear that their children might inherit it.

The nurse should also be aware that Nigerians with a psychological illness such as depression may not share their symptoms with a health care professional because of the negative connotation that goes with depression. A person's behavior during illness is culturally defined in terms of how she or he should act and what illness means for the person. Understanding this situation and seeking reasons for behavior help avoid stereotyping and labeling a person as uncooperative and resistant just because the behavior is different. People from different cultural backgrounds classify health problems differently and have certain expectations about how they should be helped. If cultural differences are ignored, the nurse's ability to assess and help the clients and their ability to progress toward a personally and culturally defined health status may be hampered. Murray and Zentner (2008) advise that nurses should be able to translate their knowledge of the health care system into terms that match the concepts of their clients.

Sometimes psychological stress felt by Nigerian Americans is related to their vision to succeed in the United States. Nigerians have typically come to the United States with a vision, often to acquire an education and return home to move mountains. Sometimes the road to realizing this dream is twisted or curved in many directions that place the individual in a dilemma. There is the feeling of failure with its accompanying stress. Nigerians believe in survival. Even when Nigerians obtain an education and cannot find jobs suitable for their educational qualifications, they will often engage in other activities, for example, taxi driving, to survive. There is a saying among Nigerians: "I did not cross the Atlantic to make a fool of myself" (Nnedu, personal communication, May 27, 2002). Nevertheless, it may be important for the nurse working with the Nigerian-American client to help the client identify goals and how these goals can be achieved in order to reduce psychological stressors.

BIOLOGICAL VARIATIONS

Implications for Nursing Care

Because Nigerians tend to have dark skin, assessment of skin color is an important aspect of the nurse's health assessment. The nurse should be knowledgeable of differences in skin assessment for persons with dark skin as opposed to light skin. Pallor represents vasoconstriction. A brown-skinned person appears yellow-brown, and a black-skinned person appears ashen gray; mucous membranes, lips, and nail beds are pale or gray. Erythema and inflammation are assessed by palpating for increased warmth of skin, edema, tightness, or induration of skin. Streaking and redness are difficult to assess in black-skinned individuals. Cyanosis is tissue hypoxia. For the assessment of cyanosis in Nigerians, evaluate the color of the lips, tongue, conjunctiva, palms, and soles of feet to either confirm or rule out a pale or ashen gray color. Nurses should apply light pressure to create pallor; in cyanotic tissue, color returns slowly by spreading from the periphery to the center. Ecchymosis occurs when deoxygenated blood seeps from broken blood vessels into subcutaneous tissue. In assessing Nigerians or people of color, the nurse should observe the oral mucous membrane or conjunctiva for color changes, which can range from purple-blue to yellow-green to yellow. Petechiae represent intradermal or submucosal bleeding. In black-skinned clients, oral mucosa or conjunctiva will show purplish-red spots. Jaundice is the accumulation of bilirubin in the tissues. In dark-skinned clients, the nurse should observe the sclerae of their eyes, oral mucous membrane, palms of the hands, and soles of the feet for yellow discoloration (Murray & Zentner, 2008). Other characteristics that can be seen on the skin of Nigerians are birthmarks, which are believed to be God's special mark of identification. The birthmark is darker than one's skin color and can be seen on different parts of the body. Also, there are tribal marks, with various patterns, that can be seen on the faces of some Nigerians.

There is a paucity of information on Nigerians who abuse chemicals in the United States. Also, there is limited information on the number of Nigerians with HIV/AIDS in the United States. The majority of Nigerians received the bacille Calmette-Guérin (BCG) vaccine against tuberculosis (Spector, 2004). Nurses should ask their Nigerian clients whether they received BCG vaccine as part of their childhood immunization prior to engaging them in tuberculin skin testings. BCG tends to interfere with the result of the purified protein derivative test, and a false-positive result may occur. Therefore, before instituting drug therapy, the results should be confirmed with a chest x-ray.

It is important for the nurse to realize that in helping countries that are underdeveloped to meet health care needs, environmental degradation that leads to droughts, soil erosion, famine, malnutrition, and related diseases must be addressed. A country cannot advance with military activities that contribute to the devastation of the environment and increase the vulnerability of the economically disadvantaged. Equality in health care can become a worldwide vision for health if there is progress toward a holistic approach, health improvements in socioeconomic development, community participation with emphasis on self-reliance and self-determination, and the concept that health is not delivered by a few but must be nurtured and cared for by all (Kaseje, 1995). Nurses need to be world leaders in improving the health of persons not only in the United States but also in underdeveloped countries like Nigeria that have such dire health care needs.

SUMMARY

As a result of visa lotteries, Nigerians from all socioeconomic levels have entered the United States and may enter the health care delivery system seeking care. Some persons entering the United States through the lottery may have no understanding of English. The needs of a client who cannot speak English can be met by using an interpreter or a family member who accompanies the client. When an interpreter is used, the nurse must allow ample time for interactions since use of an interpreter will slow the conveyance of information.

Some Nigerian Americans may adhere closely to traditional practice, whereas others may not. Therefore, the nurse must not base care on the assumption that all Nigerians can be treated similarly. Some Nigerians practice Western medicine, others combine traditional practices and Western practice, and still others believe that Western medicine is not an appropriate remedy for some illnesses. The nurse must assess the client for belief practices and integrate traditional practices and Western practices when appropriate into a culturally sensitive plan of care. Cultural differences should be anticipated not only for refugees, immigrants, and first-generation immigrants but also for persons even further removed in time from their country of origin and for persons from other regions within any country.

For many immigrant Nigerians, the United States is seen as the land of opportunity for education, jobs, and possible advancement. The nurse should appreciate that as Nigerians have immigrated to America, many have struggled to improve the standard of living they experienced in Nigeria. For some, the socioeconomic status of their family of origin has been an influencing factor to work hard and be successful. For others, commitments to family and knowledge of family living in Nigeria in an impoverished situation have motivated them to succeed in order to save money to send home. Some Nigerian Americans want to stay involved with Nigeria. The nurse can suggest the Internet as a way to access associations and organizations that allow Nigerian Americans to unite and provide support to each other and to family and friends in Nigeria (Nigeria Infonet, 2014 http://www.nigeriainfonet.com). Unfortunately, caution should be used in responding to unknown persons since the Internet has recently been used for scams that have resulted in staggering losses to individuals (from $52,000 to more than $5 million). Persons have been asked to help in transferring money out of Nigeria into the victim's country with a percentage in cash for an administrative fee. While starting small, the con artist asks for more and more money. There have been more than 30 arrests between 1999 and 2001 for cross-border telemarketing schemes. The new government of Nigeria and the Central Bank of Nigeria have assisted in fighting this fraud (Munroe, 2001).

CASE STUDY

Mrs. Ngozi Iweka is a 32-year-old in her twenty-eighth week of gestation with her eighth pregnancy. She has had six full-term pregnancies, no preterm births, and one abortion. The sixth pregnancy resulted in spontaneous abortion at 10 weeks of gestation. She has four daughters and a son. Mrs. Iweka arrives at the emergency department with the complaint of bouts of chills and sudden fever for 2 days, general malaise, joint pain, loss of appetite, and headache. She states that she has not eaten in 2 days. Mrs. Iweka returned from Nigeria following a 6-week vacation.

Physical examination yields the following: temperature, 103.7° F (39.8° C), (tympanic) pulse, 128; respirations, 28 and labored; and SPO₂, 98% on room air. Her skin was warm, dry to touch, and flushed, and moderate splenomegaly and tender hepatomegaly were noted. Fundal height was appropriate for gestational age, and the fetal heart rate was 180 beats/min. Blood work showed leukopenia, increased indirect serum bilirubin, and a platelet count less than 50,000/mm³.

◎ CARE PLAN

Nursing Diagnosis: Hyperthermia related to the disease process

Client Outcome	Nursing Interventions
The patient will maintain normal body temperature, carry pregnancy to term, have good skin turgor, and maintain laboratory values and urinary output within normal limits.	1. Keep client comfortable. Advise her to cover herself lightly with blankets when hot and to replace wet linens if sweating. 2. Instruct client to take antimalarial drug as ordered. 3. Administer acetaminophen (Tylenol) every 3–4 hours for temperature above 101° F (38.3° C). 4. Instruct client to take oral fluid of choice. 5. Assess vital signs every 4 hours. Take temperature by oral or tympanic method. 6. Give sponge bath using tepid or cool water if temperature is 102° F (38.5° C). 7. Encourage rest and energy conservation. 8. Assess the skin for color, temperature, and gooseflesh. 9. Take fetal heart rate every 4 hours until temperature returns to normal. 10. Perform daily nonstress test. 11. Monitor laboratory values.

Nursing Diagnosis: Knowledge deficit related to a lack of understanding of the effects of malaria on pregnancy outcome

Client Outcomes	Nursing Interventions
1. Client and family are able to explain the process of malaria and its implications for her unborn child. 2. Client is able to explain the importance of antimalarial drugs and cooperates with the recommended dosage schedule. 3. Client gives birth to healthy neonate. 4. If complications develop for the fetus, they are detected quickly and therapy is instituted without delay.	1. Discuss the complications of malaria with client and family. 2. Instruct client and family on the importance of taking the prescribed antimalarial drugs as ordered by the doctor. 3. Instruct client on the importance of monitoring fetal well-being with daily movement count. 4. Instruct client to call her physician immediately if abnormal findings occur.

Continued

◎ CARE PLAN—cont'd

Nursing Diagnosis: Ineffective family coping related to depression resulting from the risk on fetus with exposure to malaria infection

Client Outcomes	Nursing Interventions
1. Signs of potential problem are detected quickly and intervention instituted. 2. Client will seek prompt medical attention when signs of problems occur. 3. A healthy neonate is born at term.	1. Discuss symptoms of potential problem. 2. Stress importance of taking medications as directed, and inform the physician promptly when changes are noticed (such as decreased fetal movement). 3. Instruct family members of need for prompt attention to any problems. 4. Encourage client to verbalize feelings and concerns about pregnancy; ask what is the most worrisome aspect; be supportive of all her responses.

Nursing Diagnosis: Risk for altered health maintenance related to lack of knowledge about ways in which malaria is contracted

Client Outcomes	Nursing Interventions
1. Client is able to discuss malaria, its methods of transmission, the implications for her fetus, and measures she can take to avoid future exposure to malaria parasites. 2. Healthy neonate is delivered. 3. Client will implement health measures to avoid contracting malaria in the future.	1. Discuss how malaria is transmitted by the *Anopheles* mosquito. 2. Educate client on malaria prophylaxis. 3. Inform client of the side effects of some of the antimalarial drugs; for example, quinine has oxytocic properties that can cause uterine contractions and premature labor. 4. Go over signs and symptoms of preterm labor, and advise the client to call the health care provider without delay should any occur.

Nursing Diagnoses—Definitions and Classifications 2012–2014. Copyright © 2012, 1994–2012 by NANDA International. Used by arrangement with Wiley-Blackwell Publishing, a company of John Wiley and Sons, Inc. In order to make safe and effective judgments using NANDA-I nursing diagnoses it is essential that nurses refer to the definitions and defining characteristics of the diagnoses listed in the work.

CLINICAL DECISION MAKING

1. State three strategies that may help health care workers to communicate effectively with their Nigerian clients.
2. Discuss the pathophysiology of malaria infection.
3. Discuss the effects of malaria on the growing fetus and its treatment.
4. Compare and contrast the similarities and differences in family structure between Nigerians and Americans.
5. What are the nurse's roles in the management of a pregnancy complicated with fever resulting from malaria infection?
6. Prepare an educational pamphlet on malaria prevention to be given to Nigerian clients.

REVIEW QUESTIONS

1. A 25-year-old Nigerian client has just delivered her first baby. Based on the nurse's past experience with a Nigerian family, the nurse assumes that family members will gather to care for the mother and infant. This is an example of which of the following?
   a. Discrimination
   b. Ethnocentrism
   c. Racism
   d. Stereotyping
2. A nurse's ability to use proverbs, analogies, and stories to support a case is highly valued and will enhance communication with Nigerian Americans. Which of the following is correct about this statement?
   a. True
   b. False
   c. Not applicable
   d. Neutral
3. An illness in a Nigerian individual is considered to be which of the following?
   a. A personal, individual problem
   b. A crisis in the individual's whole family
   c. A societal problem
   d. Unrelated to voodoo or witchcraft

REFERENCES

Alalu, C., & Ojeme, V. (2002). *Health ministry distributes 4000 nets*. Nigerian Health Ministry: VanGuard.

Aminu, J. (2002). *About Nigeria*. Available at <http://www.mapsofworld.com/nigeria/about.html> Retrieved September 24, 2011.

Asuni, T., & Pela, O. (1986). Drug abuse in Africa. *Bull Nar, 38*, 55–64.

Carson, V. B. (2000). *Mental health nursing, the nurse-patient journey* (2nd ed.). Philadelphia: Saunders.

Centers for Disease Control and Prevention (CDC). (2014). *Malaria: general information*. Available at <http://www.cdc.gov> Retrieved December 28, 2014.

Centers for Disease Control and Prevention (CDC). (2014). Available at <http://wwwnc.cdc.gov/travel/yellowbook/2012/chapter-3-infectious-diseases-related-to-travel/malaria.htm> Retrieved December 21, 2014.

Centers for Disease Control and Prevention (CDC). (2015). *Ebola (Ebola virus disease)*. Accessed at <http://www.cdc.gov/vhf/ebola/>.

Central Intelligence Agency (CIA) (2015). *The CIA world factbook, 2015*. New York: Skyhorse Publishing.

Cooper, R. S., Rotimi, C. N., & Ward, R. (2002). *The puzzle of hypertension in African-Americans*. Available at <http://www.scientificamerican.com/> Retrieved August 29, 2014.

Danesi, M., & Adetunji, J. (1994). Use of alternative medicine by patients with epilepsy: a survey of 265 patients in a developing country. *Epilepsy, 35*(2), 344–351.

Davitz, L., Sameshima, Y., & Davitz, J. (1976). Suffering as viewed in six different cultures. *American Journal of Nursing, 76*, 1296–1297.

Delano, G. (1996). *Guide to family planning* (2nd ed.). Ibadan, Nigeria: Spectrum Books.

Dung, E. J. (2014). *The place of Nigeria in the world economy*. A speech delivered at Nigeria's 54th independence day celebration, organized by the Nigerian American Association (NAC) of south central Alabama, Montgomery, Alabama.

Egyir, W. (1996). Grandma arrested, grandpa sought in tribal slashing. *New York Amsterdam News, 87*(28), 17.

Eluwa, G. I. C., Ukagwu, M. O., Nwachukwu, J. U. N., & Nwaubani, A. C. N. (1988). *A history of Nigeria for schools and colleges*. Singapore: FEP International.

Enang, K. (2000). *Nigerian Catholics and the independent churches: a call to authentic faith*. Immensee, Switzerland: Neue Zeitschirigt for Missionswissenchaft.

Falola, T. (Ed.), (2001). *Culture and custom of Nigeria*. Westport, CT: Greenwood.

Federal Ministry of Health (FMOH) in Global AIDS response, country response, Nigeria GARPR 2014. Available at <http://www.unaids.org/sites/default/files/country/documents/NGA_narrative_report_2014.pdf>.

Gambino, C. P., Trevelyan, E. N., & Fitzwater, J. T. (2014). *The foreign-born population from Africa*. Available at <http://www.census.gov/content/dam/Census/library/publications/2014/acs/acsbr12-16.pdf>.

Geissler, E. M. (1998). *Pocket guide to cultural assessment* (2nd ed.). St. Louis: Mosby.

Hall, K., et al. (2006). Cholesterol, APOE genotype, and Alzheimer disease: an epidemiologic study of Nigerian Yoruba. *Neurology, 66*(2), 223–227.

Haq, M. B. (1998). Cultural competency in nursing. In J. M. Leahy & P. E. Kizilay (Eds.), *Foundations of nursing practice: a nursing process approach* (pp. 81–100). Philadelphia: Saunders.

Human Development Report. (2014). Available at hdr.undp.org/en/2014-report.

Kalu, N. K. (2014). Brief history of Nigeria. *The Nigeria-American Community, South Central Alabama, Inc., 1*(1), 10–16.

Kaseje, D. (1995). Africa: the role of nursing in health care in the context of unjust social, economic, and political structures and systems. *Nursing and Health Care, 16*(4), 209–214.

Kayongo-Male, D., & Onyango, P. (1984). *The sociology of the African family*. New York: Longman.

Keller, S. (1996). Traditional beliefs, part of people's lives. *Family Health International, 17*(1), 1–6.

Lagos, A. (2002). BMJ.com news roundup. *British Medical Journal, 324*(7345), 1056.

LaMar, J. (2013). Culture and ethnicity. In P. A. Potter, A. G. Perry, P. Stockert, & A. M. Hall (Eds.), *Fundamentals of nursing* (8th ed., pp. 101–115). St. Louis: Mosby.

Lambo, E. (2014). *In Nigeria 5-year strategic plan: 2006–2010 roll back malaria*. Available at <http://www.ncbi.nlm.nih.gov/pmc/articles/PMC3751122/>.

Lazarus, R., & Folkman, S. (2012). *Stress appraisal and coping*. New York: Springer.

Minchakpu, O. (2002). Where adultery means death. *Christianity Today, 46*(6), 34.

Moodley, R. (2000). Representation of subjective distress in black and ethnic minority patients: constructing a research agenda. *Counselling Psychology Quarterly*, 159–174.

Mudzafar, J. (1999). *Herbal medicine: nature's very own pharmacy*. Available at <http://www.sibexlink.com> Retrieved November 25, 2014.

Munroe, S. (2001). *Arrests in Nigerian letter scam*. Available at <http://canadaonline.about.com/library/weekly/aa071401a.htm> Retrieved December 6, 2014.

Murray, R. B., & Zentner, J. P. (2008). *Health assessment and promotion strategies through the life span* (8th ed.). Stamford, CT: Appleton & Lange.

National Agency for the Control of AIDS (NACA). Global AIDS response, country progress report. National Center for Health Statistics. (2014). *Health, United States 2014*. Hyattsville, MD: U.S. Government Printing Office.

Nigeria Global AIDS Response Progress Report (GARPR), 2014. Available at <http://www.unaids.org/.../documents/NGA_narrative_report_2014.pdf> Retrieved December 18, 2014.

Nigerian Drug Law Enforcement Agency (NDLEA). (2014). *Nigeria country profile*. Available at <http://www.ndlea.gov.ng> Retrieved December 13, 2014.

Odedina, F., Ogunbiyi, J., & Ukoli, F. (2006). Roots of prostate cancer in African-American men. *Journal of the National Medical Association, 98*(4), 539–543.

Odejide, A. (2006). Status of drug use/abuse in Africa: a review. *International Journal of Mental Health and Addiction, 4,* 87–102.

Ogbu, C. N. (1999). *A brief history of Akpulu: from the earliest times to 1980.* Enugu, Nigeria: Unik Oriental Press.

Okeke, T. C., Anyaehie, U. S. B., & Ezenyeaku, C. C. K. (2012). An overview of female genital mutilation in Nigeria. *Annals of Medical and Health Sciences Research, 2*(1), 70–73.

Okeniyi, J., Olubanjo, O., Oguniest, T., & Oyelami, D. (2005). Comparison of healing of infected abscessed wounds with wild honey and eusol dressing. *Contemporary Medicine, 11*(3), 511–523.

Onah, H. (2002). The knowledge, attitude and practice of child adoption among infertile Nigerian women. *Journal of Obstetrics and Gynaecology, 22*(2), 211.

Olajubu, O. (2003). *Women in the Yoruba religious sphere.* New York: State University of New York Press.

Onwudiwe, E. (2002). *Nigeria. World book online, Americas edition.* Available at <http://www.aolsvc.worldbook.aol.com/wbol/wbPage/na/ar/co/391300> Retrieved June 24, 2010.

Oyelami, O., Agbakwuru, O., Adeyemi, L., & Adedeji, G. (2005). Effectiveness of grapefruit seeds in treating urinary tract infections. *Journal of Alternative and Complementary Medicine, 11*(2), 369–371.

Pillsbury, B. (1982). Doing the month: confinement and convalescence of Chinese women after childbirth. In M. Kay (Ed.), *Anthropology of human birth.* Philadelphia: F. A. Davis.

Qualls, A. (2010). *Women in Nigeria today.* Available at <http://www.postcolonialweb.org/nigeria/contwomen.html> Retrieved August 31, 2014.

Roy, C., & Andrews, H. (2008). *The Roy adaptation model: the definitive statement.* Norfolk, CT: Appleton & Lange.

Shulman, C. E., et al. (1999). Intermittent sulphadoxine-pyrimethamine to prevent severe anemia secondary to malaria in pregnancy: a randomized placebo-controlled trial. *Lancet, 353,* 632–636.

Spector, R. E. (2004). *Cultural diversity in health and illness* (6th ed.). Upper Saddle River, NJ: Prentice Hall.

Sue, D. (2003). *Counseling the culturally different: theory and practice* (4th ed.). New York: John Wiley & Sons.

Tomkiewicz, J., & Adeyemi-Bello, T. (1996). Briefly noted. *Communication Abstracts, 19*(3), 423.

UNAIDS. (2014). *National Agency for the Control of AIDS (NACA) Federal Republic of Nigeria global AIDS response country progress report Nigeria (GARPR), 2014.* Retrieved from <http://www.unaids.org/sites/default/files/country/documents/NGA_narrative_report_2014.pdf>.

U.S. Department of Commerce, Bureau of the Census (2012). *Population profiles by age, sex, race, and Hispanic origin, Summary File 3.* Washington, DC: U.S. Government Printing Office.

U.S. Department of Health and Human Services. National Institutes of Health. (2014). *Prevention and control of malaria.* Retrieved from: <http://www.niaid.nih.gov/topics/Malaria/research/Pages/control.aspx>.

U.S. Department of Commerce, Bureau of the Census, (2015). *American Community Survey,* Washington, DC: U.S. Government Printing Office.

Uwazie, E. I., Albert, I. O., & Uzoigwe, G. N. (Eds.), (1999). *Inter-ethnic and religious conflict resolution in Nigeria.* New York: Lexington Books.

Wilkinson, J. M., & Treas, L. S. (2011). *Fundamentals of nursing* (2nd ed.). Philadelphia: F. A. Davis.

Yeh, L. L., Kuller, L. H., Bunker, C. H., Ukoli, F. A., Huston, S. L., & Terrell, D. F. (1996). The role of socioeconomic status and serum fatty acids in the relationship between intake of animal foods and cardiovascular risk factors. *Annals of Epidemiology, 6*(4), 290–300.

Ugandan Americans

Anita Hunter

BEHAVIORAL OBJECTIVES

After reading this chapter, the nurse will be able to:

1. Discuss sociocultural influences in Uganda that differentiate Ugandan culture from American culture and affect assimilation of Ugandan Americans.
2. Discuss the hierarchical patterns of communication that may be utilized by Ugandan Americans.
3. Explain Ugandan customs related to space.
4. Discuss barriers Ugandan Americans may face when seeking health care or health information.
5. Name Ugandan practices surrounding childbearing and dying.
6. Explain tropical diseases and genetic diseases or impairments that may be observed in a Ugandan after arrival in the United States.
7. Identify nursing measures that can be taken to provide culturally competent, effective care to Ugandan Americans.

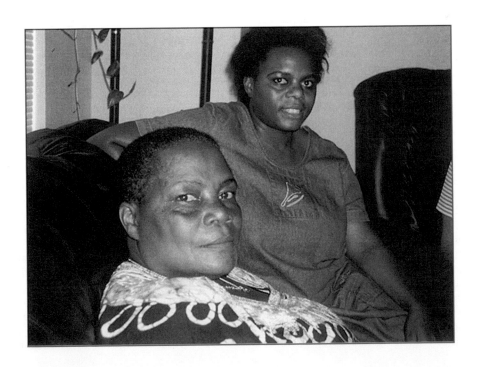

OVERVIEW OF UGANDA

Uganda is located in East Africa, along with Kenya and Tanzania. Named the "Pearl of Africa" by Winston Churchill for its lush green beauty, Uganda encompasses 91,135 square miles—approximately twice the size of Pennsylvania. Although it straddles the equator, its altitude of over 2037 feet at the lowest point above sea level moderates its temperature to an average range between 72° and 92° F, with variations related to location and season (Central Intelligence Agency [CIA], 2014; Facts about Uganda, 2013). There are two rainy seasons, approximately March to July and September and October. There are three main areas: swampy lowlands, fertile plateaus, and desert regions. Lake Victoria, once the largest lake in the world, forms part of the southern border. The Nile, which begins at Jinja, meanders northwest across the country before continuing northward to the Mediterranean Sea. Five large national parks provide protection for large animals, such as elephants, hippos, giraffes, chimpanzees, and the endangered gorillas. Landlocked, Uganda borders the Democratic Republic of Congo on the west, Rwanda and Tanzania on the south, Sudan on the north, and Kenya on the east (Facts about Uganda, 2013).

Historically, the kingdom of Buganda was well established by the eleventh century, with an army and well-defined administration. When Uganda's borders were drawn, the country included this and other kingdoms, plus many independent organizations. Missionaries arrived from Europe in the late nineteenth century, winning converts for the Protestant church (Britain) and for the Catholic Church (France), leading to religious skirmishes. When the British claimed Uganda as a protectorate, the British government set up a replica of the British system, and Protestantism spread. Today the religious denominations are Roman Catholic (42%), Protestant (42%), Muslim (12%), other (3%), and none (1%) (Facts about Uganda, 2013).

In 1962, independence was granted, with Milton Obote as prime minister and the Kabaka Mutesa II (King of Buganda) as president. Since then, Obote, Idi Amin, and Obote again have had dictator rule until 1986 when General Yoweri Museveni assumed power and formed the National Resistance Movement government. Museveni's "non-party" democracy has brought sufficient improvement and stability to the country despite the uprising of the Lord's Resistance Army (LRA). The LRA, supported by Sudan, conducted violent abduction of children at night, turning them into boy soldiers or sex slaves. The LRA killing raids have led to displacement of thousands into internal camps and have sent over 250,000 to flee to neighboring countries (Facts about Uganda, 2013). The LRA is

no longer in Uganda but does operate on the borders of the Congo. After the new constitution of 1995 authorized elections, Museveni was elected president in 1996 and has remained in power ever since (Facts about Uganda, 2013).

Representatives to Parliament are elected from every county, with seats reserved for a woman from each district, disabled, youth, and workers (CIA, 2014). Amin abolished the kingdoms, but in 1994 Museveni allowed the kingdoms to exist publicly, giving them little authority except to promote their respective cultural practices. In spite of efforts to stamp out bribery and corruption, government and other institutions are still heavily affected by these problems.

The economy is based on agriculture, providing income to 80% of the workforce; women perform most of this work. The primary cash crops are coffee, tea, tobacco, and cotton, but government efforts to diversify have led to increasing exports of tilapia, soybeans, spices, flowers, and other produce. Uganda is blessed with fertile soil and abundant rainfall, engaging the poor and illiterate in subsistence farming (CIA, 2014). Economic recovery has taken remarkable strides under President Museveni. Reduction of poverty is the chief goal of the government. The population living in poverty declined in 2009 from 56% to 24%; however, 84% of the population live in poor rural areas and within that population, the poverty rate is between 40% and 60% (Rural Poverty in Uganda). Privatization of hotels and businesses formerly owned by the state has been a boon to economic stability. Transport is readily available in the capital city of Kampala, in the main towns, and on paved highways, but the rural areas suffer from a lack of public transport (Facts about Uganda, 2013).

Almost 84% of the population is rural, with the majority of urban dwellers inhabiting Kampala. Uganda is a melting pot of 48 distinct ethnic groups representing three different linguistic groups: Bantu, Nilo-Hamites, and Nilotic (Facts about Uganda, 2013). All of these groups were merged into the country of Uganda during the colonial period, setting the stage for later ethnic rivalries, armed conflict, and human rights abuses (Facts about Uganda, 2013). Buganda is the largest of the Bantu groups, making up 17% of the population and living in the southern part of the country (locals call it the "central" region). Colonialists curried favor with the people of Buganda and rewarded them with leadership positions. Thus, the seat of government developed in the central region. Some citizens of Asian descent reside in Uganda. The citizens who were deported by Amin in 1972 began returning to their businesses after a formal invitation from President Museveni in 1991 (Facts about Uganda, 2013). In addition, Uganda has hosted refugees from across its borders, especially Sudan, the Democratic Republic of Congo, and Rwanda.

The family is the most important center of life for Ugandans. Families tend to be very large, live in close-knit groups, and include extended family that both give and receive support—financial or otherwise—as needed. Although outlawed in Uganda, polygamy is culturally acceptable, providing the husband has the means to support more than one wife and the numerous children that are likely to follow (Uganda, 2015). In very rural communities, marrying the deceased brother's wife, girls marrying at age 13, sex with children, and child sacrifices may still be practiced (Hunter, unpublished data, 2015). Children are indoctrinated into the roles and mores of their group, and the eldest provides for aging parents (Facts about Uganda, 2013). The couple's parents have been known to negotiate marriage, usually after the couple have chosen to marry one another and often after they have one or more children. The groom's family agrees upon the bride's price, which is likely to include a number of cows but may also include goats, a dress for the bride's mother, and money. An educated bride brings a higher bride's price. Marriage means the husband has "ownership" of the wife, making divorce difficult, and spousal rape and abuses are accepted practices (Uganda, 2015).

By 2012, children composed up to approximately 56% of Uganda's population. There are 2.7 million orphans in Uganda, of whom 1.2 million have been orphaned by acquired immunodeficiency syndrome (AIDS); one in seven children will die before he or she reaches the age of 5 years (African Network for the Prevention and Protection of Children Against Child Abuse and Neglect [ANPPCAN], 2013). A son is favored over a daughter because of the expectation that he has more potential for earning a good living. Therefore, he is more likely to receive education and health care according to the father's preferences. Though the report by the ANPPCAN indicates that only 20% of children in Uganda are malnourished, those figures don't match this author's findings, which indicate that 80% of the 440 children assessed had body mass indexes of 13 and were short for age as measured by World Health Organization (WHO) standards; 50% were microcephalic (Hunter, unpublished data, 2015).

The youth literacy rate in 2010 was 85.67%, with young men at 89% and young females at 64%; the overall adult literacy rate was only 73% (United Nations Educational, Scientific, and Cultural Organization (UNESCO), 2015). Such literacy ability means the individual can, with understanding, read and write a short, simple statement on his or her everyday life. This makes teaching and learning about child and adult health somewhat problematic as terminology and written instructions are not understood or followed.

The gender equity campaign at the government level with Museveni's support of women in politics still has a long way to go in changing mindsets of people outside of Kampala, as poverty, gender norms, and cultural traditions still dictate the future of girls in Uganda. SALVE International (2015a) reports that 12% of girls are married by age 15, with 48% married by 18. Women's reproduction rate is 6.14 children/woman, which places Uganda fourth in the world for average birthrates. Given the decimation of their population from AIDS, it is understood why reproduction is encouraged; however, many of these women are poor, malnourished, cannot sustain a healthy full-term pregnancy or adequately breastfeed a newborn as they still have several toddlers suckling. The deaths of women during childbirth, though lower than previous reports, is still reported at 6000 per year, and 1 in 13 women are at high risk for dying while giving birth. Traditional practitioners deliver 41% to 43% of births at home or in a clinic setting, not by a trained health professional. One in 7 children do not reach adolescence. Women with higher education have decreased rates of child mortality because they have fewer children, better nutrition, better access to health care, and jobs. Unfortunately, higher education does not protect these women from domestic violence. Domestic violence is the norm, with more than 60% of women experiencing such violence in their lifetime. Personal communication with various professionals in Uganda since 2007 has found that much of the violence is related to alcohol consumption and the women who are able to obtain jobs although there are no jobs for the men (SALVE, International, 2015a). Women are gaining their political voice because they constitute 25% of the legislators and 27% of government ministers (Facts about Uganda, 2013).

In 1996, universal primary education was passed into law, paving the way for all primary children to attend government-sponsored schools for free. However, parents must supply the uniforms, books, and pens. Attendance is not compulsory, but enrollment of primary age children is 100% (Facts about Uganda, 2013). The demand for free education is high, and there are not enough classrooms and supplies to handle the requests. It is not uncommon for classes to have well over 100 students, with very little in the way of facilities, with overworked teachers heading them. This means that for most of the population, especially those who want a higher quality education, the only other option is private school. In Uganda, private schools vary enormously in fees and quality. Paying school fees is beyond many families, especially when they have a lot of children. Depending on relatives to help with the finances or donations from foreigners interested in helping means that many children will go without an education, thereby limiting their future potential to support themselves or a family.

Only 12% of females and 18% of males between ages 13 and 19 years are enrolled in secondary schools, and only 3% of the relevant age group is enrolled at the tertiary level (SALVE International, 2015b). Makerere University is the oldest and largest university of the seven in the country, with a growing student body and a wide range of programs, including public health, medicine, and nursing (Facts about Uganda, 2013).

Currently 7.2 % of the population is living with human immunodeficiency virus (HIV), with an estimated 1.4 million people that includes 190,000 children. Sixty-two thousand people died from AIDS in 2011, and the incidence in adolescents and young adults is rising, which is attributed to the same phenomenon that is occurring globally: young people believe that AIDS can be cured because of the drugs that are now available (Avert, 2013). Despite these facts, with the increasing access to health care and treatment for HIV/AIDS, current estimates find the population is now 35,918,915, with a growth rate of 3.24%, birth-rate at 44.17 per 1000, infant mortality at 60.82 per 1000, and an increasing life expectancy at 54.46 years (Facts about Uganda, 2013).

In 2014 the median per capita income of Ugandans was $1375 (World Bank, 2014, http://www.worldbank.org/en/about/annual-report. Retrieved on September 24, 2015). This income must feed, house, clothe, educate, and obtain health care for the family members. On $3.76 or less a day, such costs are not possible. Construction appears to be the primary growth area. Agriculture is the highest employer of personnel but is unlikely to achieve high rates of growth because of supply-side constraints such as lack of infrastructure, irrigation, and modern machinery (Table 26-1).

The health of Ugandans is precarious because health care is expensive. There is minimal primary health care, and few can afford to pay for the management and stabilization of chronic health problems. Public and environmental health has not been a top priority, and many Ugandans use traditional healers, often delaying entry into the medical center until it is too late. Many do not have adequate sanitation facilities, 56% do not have access to improved drinking water sources, and many are malnourished, especially the women and children (particularly lacking protein and essential vitamins and minerals). This puts them at risk for severe anemias, foodborne and waterborne tropical diseases such as malaria, typhoid fever, schistosomiasis, bacterial diarrhea, and hepatitis A. Malaria is still the leading cause of morbidity and mortality in Uganda, with the world's highest malaria incidence (rate of 478 cases per 1000 population per year). Uganda has the third largest malaria burden in Africa and the sixth largest in the world. Malaria is responsible for up to 40% of all outpatient visits, 25% of all hospital admissions, and 14% of all hospital deaths. Child deaths due to malaria are between 70,000 and 100,000 every year, a death toll that far exceeds that of HIV/AIDS. Additionally, malaria affects maternal morbidity and mortality and is attributed as a direct or indirect cause of 65% of maternal mortality and 60% of spontaneous abortion. Additionally, 15% of life years lost to premature death are due to malaria, and families spend 25% of their income on this disease (Bauer, 2014).

Unfortunately, chronic hypoxia from the decreased oxygen-carrying capacity evident with decreased red blood cells (RBCs) and the destruction of RBCs that occurs with malaria has resulted in such sequelae in children as developmental delays, microcephaly, cognitive impairment, short stature, and impaired fertility (Bangirana et al., 2011). This further exacerbates the precarious health state of many Ugandans.

UGANDAN AMERICANS

Ugandans are latecomers as immigrants to America. From 1989 to 2000, the average intake of immigrants had been 423 per year, but from 2001 through 2004, that average rose to 553. In addition, between 2000 and 2004, the yearly

TABLE 26-1   Average Monthly Income by Region and Residence (UGX)

Region	2005–2006			2009–2010			
	Urban	Rural	Total	Urban	Rural	Total	USD
Kampala	347,900	—	347,900	959,400	—	959,400	$362.00
Central	320,200	192,600	209,300	603,800	336,800	389,600	$147.00
Eastern	261,700	144,100	155,500	361,000	151,400	171,500	$64.72
Northern	209,000	76,200	93,400	361,200	117,200	141,400	$53.36
Western	313,100	144,200	159,100	479,000	282,300	303,200	$114.42
Uganda	306,200	142,700	170,800	660,000	222,600	303,700	$114.60

Uganda National Household Surveys Report 2009/2010, Uganda Bureau of Statistics. Available at http://www.ubos.org/UNHS0910/chapter7.Average%20Monthly%20Household%20Income.html.

average of Ugandans naturalized was 331, the yearly average granted asylum was 104, and the yearly average of refugees and asylees granted lawful permanent resident status was 50. A total of 5587 nonimmigrant Ugandans were admitted in fiscal year 2004 as students, workers, businessmen, tourists, or relatives of U.S. citizens (McCabe, 2011; Uganda, 2015). At one time, refugees from the civil war were given scholarships to North American colleges. Many of those students continued in university education and became U.S. citizens. More recently, nonimmigrant visitors have joined students in seeking political asylum, often to escape persecution or rebel activity.

The cultural differences between Ugandan Americans and Black Americans are immense, especially considering that both cultures share similar origins and skin color. Ugandans, arriving from a country where they predominate culturally, perceive themselves to be more like Whites in the United States yet are dismayed to find themselves feeling like "cultural impostors" and assigned to low social status in a country where institutional racism prevails (Otengho, n.d.).

Western civilization has traditionally viewed Ugandans as passive people. Their willing servitude and nonaggressive behavior often are the results of tribal structure that discouraged individual self-promotion. The culture of the Baganda was authoritarian, and obedience to the king was crucial. The tradition of giving all power to a village chief, the era of colonialism, and the repressiveness of men like Obote and Amin had taught them obedience, even servitude, and survival.

English is Uganda's official language. Refugees who lived in rural areas, however, find American culture is very different from what they left behind. American life poses challenges for those who have not seen escalators, refrigerators, traffic lights, and scan-your-own grocery checkouts. Many Ugandans immigrate for better educational opportunities. Unfortunately many immigrants not enrolled in a university are unable to work at the same position or in the same field in the United States without further study to meet American standards. A highly educated and skilled group of immigrants, Ugandan immigrants hold one of the highest proportions of postschool qualifications of any ethnic group and were the ethnic group with the highest proportion of qualified people who were unemployed (14%). More than 93% had completed secondary school in the United Kingdom, "O level," and 46.2% were educated to diploma or degree level. Women's educational levels lagged significantly behind men's (Uganda, 2015). Ugandan immigrants experience discrimination from Blacks and Whites, not only on the basis of color but also because they are African immigrants (personal communication with American Ugandans, 2014).

Ugandan Americans tend to establish single-family homes where children learn reverence for God and their family and prefer to join family members already in the United States. Ugandan immigrants take part in community and school events in much the same way as other Americans. The children of Ugandan Americans assimilate into American culture. Immigrants with professional employment are geographically scattered, although significant communities have developed in metropolitan areas such as Atlanta, Sacramento, Dallas, and St. Petersburg (Uganda, 2015).

COMMUNICATION

Ugandan culture is a mixture of various traditions and practices. In Uganda, people may break into song and dance, even in the streets, when they hear good news. If you are invited to someone's home, it is polite, but not required, to bring a gift for your host or hostess. Wives are automatically included in invitations unless it is specified otherwise. In conversation, most topics can be discussed freely, and national and world affairs and the arts are the most popular topics. There are also many native languages. Luganda is probably the most widely known because it is the language of the largest group, the people of Buganda, and because it is widely spoken in the capital city. Native speakers of several other languages can readily understand it because of the similarities. English is spoken as a second language by nearly all people because they were born into a family that spoke a tribal language. Ugandan English diction and idioms strongly follow British English in vocabulary and pronunciation (Uganda, 2015).

Ugandan upbringing incorporates a strict code of conduct, including etiquette. To convey respect when meeting a friend or colleague, one must inquire about the other's welfare using "madam" or "sir." Then it is polite to make other inquiries about the person's family, work, or sleep. One should stand to greet an elder or person of high status (Facts about Uganda, 2013). Taboos prevent children from speaking when adults are holding a conversation and younger people from expressing anger or their opinions to elders. Parents prefer to visit their children in person rather than by letter writing. Speaking softly is the norm, especially when showing deference. A person who raises his or her voice volume is considered to be rude and angry and is said to be "shouting." Shaking hands upon meeting a friend or acquaintance is far more common than hugging and is expected. Shaking hands on departure is also appropriate. To express one's pleasure at the meeting, a person will hold the right wrist with the left hand. Hugging is reserved for greeting special friends and relatives or visitors not seen for a long time. It is more prevalent in western

Uganda. In public, no hand holding, embracing, stroking, or sexually suggestive touching is acceptable between the sexes, not even from sweethearts or spouses. Sometimes men will walk hand in hand with other men. Touch is acceptable as necessary for rendering health care, but unwanted touch causes emotional discomfort (Uganda, 2015).

Two nonverbal communication behaviors are significant because they demonstrate the hierarchical nature of the culture. It is considered impolite to make direct eye contact with a superior in age or status, so people direct their gaze downward while bowing the head slightly to convey respect. Traditionally in Buganda, a woman must kneel to the floor in respect when greeting a man; likewise, a child must kneel when greeting an adult. Any time a person uses both hands for giving or receiving a gift, intense appreciation is conveyed. Gestures may be used when talking. Sighing or stretching while visiting is considered rude, crossed arms are considered belligerent, and a woman crossing her legs when seated ignores this taboo (Facts about Uganda, 2013). Ugandans in pain have been acculturated to bear it in silence. Neither facial expression nor writhing nor moaning communicates that one is in pain (personal communication with health professional at Holy Innocents Children's Hospital in Mbarara, Uganda, January 2015).

Ugandans guard their privacy about interpersonal relations and communication, extending to a lack of openness at times even with their children. In business dealings and friendships, they are very tactful and indirect when discussing sensitive issues in order to avoid embarrassment. Criticism is considered rude. Euphemisms are plentiful and masterfully used. For example, rather than say the word "intercourse" even in health care assessment or teaching, they will use terms such as "when the wife serves the husband" or "when the husband meets his wife" (personal communication with the health professionals and religious professionals in Mbarara, Uganda, 2015). They are not averse to discussing information of an intimate nature but are diplomatic in their approach. Uganda was one of the earliest countries to launch an educational campaign for AIDS prevention that has proved successful because of the ability to publicly discuss specific prevention methods (Facts about Uganda, 2013).

Implications for Nursing Care

The style of speaking may be the first clue to many nurses that they are caring for an African immigrant rather than an American-born Black. Expressing interest in learning about them personally or their culture is likely to encourage trust and understanding. The nurse should listen carefully to their concerns and preferences, as well as any family members who may have information related to the patient. Preferences may include a care provider of the same sex.

The first introduction to the patient should be formal, using a title or both names, but friendly and solicitous about the patient and the family. Professional nursing was begun in Uganda in 1993, so current immigrants are not likely to appreciate the contribution that professional nurses can make to their health care. To build trust, take time with the introduction and then explain your nurse role in order to gain permission for your intended nursing actions. Because Ugandans have experience with being promptly treated for their symptoms, they may lack patience for a long history or for being asked similar questions at every visit, which American health professionals find necessary for making a diagnosis.

Maintaining a calm, conversational, low-volume tone will prevent offense to the patient. Nurses should also speak clearly and distinctly in a formal way, rather than use slang or colloquialisms, in order to avoid misunderstanding and repetition. Keep in mind that some American English vocabulary and medical terminology may be difficult for the Ugandan immigrant to grasp and understand fully (personal communication with a Ugandan trained as a nurse in the United States, 2013). Avoidance of joking, teasing, and sarcasm can prevent the misinterpretation that is more likely to occur in cross-cultural exchanges. Because euphemisms are commonly used, they may facilitate communication regarding matters of a delicate nature. Analogies may help in providing health education. However, evaluation of the effectiveness of the communication when using any method is essential. Ugandans, who note even small details, readily absorb visual illustrations, but use of illustrations is enhanced if any humans in the illustration bear some resemblance to people of their own ethnicity. Encouraging their personal and cultural character strengths of acceptance, determination, and optimism can support them in health-seeking behaviors while showing respect (Hunter, unpublished data, 2015).

Ugandan patients appreciate a handshake upon meeting and parting. It is essential to remember that for some Ugandan Americans, patting, stroking of the back or arms, or hand holding may be uncomfortable because touch, especially with strangers, is unacceptable. The provider should gain permission for touch necessary for health assessment or treatment. The family provides all personal care, including bathing, toileting, bed making, and feeding, whether in a Ugandan hospital or at home. Therefore, Ugandan patients are likely to feel more comfortable when female family members provide these services. They may also find comfort in having a family member nearby when their condition or treatment is discussed with them by the health professional.

Nurses must assess Ugandan patients carefully regarding the presence and extent of their pain. A master's thesis completed at Mulago Hospital in Kampala, Uganda, found that the almost half the nurses lacked knowledge on key pain assessment principles and 44% did not always agree with patients' statements about pain (Kizza, 2012). Some of this can be explained by the cultural traditions of not expressing pain and the belief that if one does complain, one is not seen as "strong" but as weak and therefore needs to "toughen up." Nurses should offer pain control even though the patient demonstrates no signs of being in pain.

Ugandans may avoid eye contact with health care professionals as a sign of deference for their status and expertise. Maintaining eye contact is considered rude, much as in the Asian culture. Thus health professionals should learn to use eye contact appropriately to indicate they are listening and absorbing without appearing aggressive and disrespectful.

SPACE

In Uganda, a spatial distance of about 3 to 4 feet is maintained face-to-face between men and women in public, with the same distance applied shoulder-to-shoulder in many instances. However, in public buses, churches, waiting rooms, or schools with space constraints, people sit very close together, with bodies, stools, or chairs touching each other.

Some Ugandan families do not allow the children to enter the bedroom of the parents or babies to sleep in the parents' bed (personal communication with parents in Uganda, 2013). Other territorial proscriptions include not using the cup, eating utensils, or clothing belonging to elders or esteemed persons. Chairs are reserved for adults. Children must sit on mats on the ground or floor. In most households, guests leave their shoes at the door and will be offered the best chair in the house (Facts about Uganda, 2013).

Fathers seldom accompany their pregnant wives to the hospital for delivery and never accompany them during delivery. In the large teaching hospital in Uganda, fathers are not yet allowed in the labor ward. A baby is tied on the mother's back at all times until the child can walk, and thereafter as necessary until a newborn sibling fills that space. Close physical contact allows breastfeeding to continue up to around 2 years (Facts about Uganda, 2013).

Implications for Nursing Care

While most conversation is conducted in Ugandans' personal space, they are not insulted by invasion of their intimate space when nursing or health care dictates the necessity of it. Every effort should be made to avoid exposing the patient unnecessarily, especially from the waist to the knees. Some Ugandans feel embarrassed when they must accept care from a health care provider of the opposite sex; however, during this author's experience in Uganda at the Children's Hospital and in community outreach health assessments, no such embarrassment was noted. Patients were pleased they were being attended to regardless of gender.

Couples may need instruction about the value of husbands accompanying their wives into labor and delivery. Husbands may need additional information about specific behaviors they should demonstrate in relation to their wives and newborns in the various stages of childbirth and the postpartum period.

Breastfeeding for 2 years is the cultural norm for immigrants of African descent, with premature cessation considered a social stigma. In the West, breastfeeding is encouraged, but infant feeding remains the mother's choice. The first-generation immigrant feels strong cultural and economic pressures to breastfeed. The challenge for nurses is to support Ugandan Americans in continuing this prevailing tradition and to teach them how to be socially appropriate in a country where exposed breasts in public has a different connotation from their traditional ethnic values, and where advance planning is required to continue breastfeeding when socioeconomic pressures demand early return to work.

SOCIAL ORGANIZATION

Ugandan families are patriarchal, with urban families commonly residing under one roof. However, the patriarchal family may also include a second wife or as many as seven or more wives (usually in rural areas). In these cases, it is the prerogative of the husband to select another wife and move her into his compound, where he generally builds a separate dwelling for her and her offspring. The term *wife* refers to a woman with whom he lives, not necessarily a woman to whom he is married by law because Ugandan law now precludes polygamy. A *girlfriend* usually means a person with whom one is intimate. A woman has few rights and very seldom owns property; cultural practice prevents her from inheriting property when her husband dies (Facts about Uganda, 2013). Consequently, women are at high risk for domestic violence for any perceived disobedience to males and when unwanted pregnancy or induced abortion occur. Homosexuality is "illegal" in Uganda; thus, such family units are unknown (CIA, 2014).

All families belong to a clan that is most akin to a very large extended family. Each clan has a totem or symbol of honor. If the totem is a fish, for example, those clan members refrain from eating fish to ensure good luck. Marriages between members of the same clan are taboo. The individual, or the self, is interdependent on the community or group (Uganda, 2015). Ugandans maintain community in the United States by means of telephone, email, conventions, goat roasts, and other social gatherings.

Roles of various family members are clearly taught and understood. Men must take the financial and moral responsibility of head of the household. Their tasks include protecting the family, paying educational and health care expenses, buying clothing, clearing the bush, building shelter (except in certain areas where this is a woman's duty), and conducting barter trading or business transactions. They do not help with childcare, cooking, or any household chores. Women have responsibility for management of their households, looking after their husband, providing food for the household (usually by first tilling the soil and harvesting the vegetables or crops), caring for the sick and elderly, and maintaining the health of their children and family. Sometimes they sell produce in the market. Educated and urban women are pursuing careers and trying to merge the responsibilities of a home and a vocation (Facts about Uganda, 2013; Uganda, 2015).

Children's roles are also well defined. They are expected to remain silent when adults are conversing unless spoken to. Children are taught that boys play with boys and girls with girls. The birth of a boy is celebrated more than the birth of a girl. Boys are groomed for their roles as men. Their fathers teach them to tend livestock, hunt, trade, farm, and perform any specialized skills held by the father, such as ironworking, pottery, or bark-cloth making. A particular clan specializes in a particular skill. In eastern Uganda, a few groups circumcise boys as a rite of passage. Girls are started early to care for the household and children by learning cooking, basketry, pottery, laundry, and childcare. Although the practice is outlawed in Uganda, a few groups in northeastern Uganda still clandestinely practice female circumcision as a rite of passage on 9- to 13-year-old girls. Children legally belong to the father and his family regardless of the death or divorce of the mother (Facts about Uganda, 2013). Young men, although trained in the work and role of men and expected to stay out of the kitchen, insist they are able to cook and manage their households when single and unmarried because they learned it by watching their mothers. Single immigrant men are forced to learn to cook and clean because of the absence of female relatives.

Male immigrants from Uganda have a greater problem of acculturation than females because American women have more rights and more fluid role assignments, and they expect assistance with household duties—concepts that strike at the very heart of Ugandan men's identity. Female immigrants delight in their increased rights, opportunities for greater independence, and sense of freedom (personal communication with female immigrants to the United States, 2013). Fathers send their children to the best schools they can afford because that was their role in Uganda, and good schools also mainstream their children into American culture.

About two thirds of the Ugandan population is said to be Christian; the remaining one third follows Islam. While Ugandan Americans are likely to practice the same religion as they did in Uganda, most are reported to be Christian. Religion is a major coping resource and in Uganda a major educational resource for health, healthy living, and similar issues (Hunter, unpublished data, 2015). First-generation immigrants may miss the assistance of babysitting, finances, and emotional support from grandparents and extended family. They may move to other geographical areas for economic opportunities that do not allow them to maintain close ties with other Ugandan immigrants. Families might experience an "assimilation gap" when second-generation young people acculturate quickly while the parents or first generation lags in adapting to the new culture; however, adolescent immigrants and second-generation adolescents encounter different stressors from those their parents faced—a concept known as cultural marginality, or "passive betweenness" (Wade, 2013). To which culture do they belong when they are treated in public as African-Americans without that history and at home being treated as Ugandan without having lived very long, if at all, in Uganda?

Implications for Nursing Care

Nurses are in the habit of assessing patients regarding their family relationships because of their importance for home caregiving, exposure to infectious illnesses, or genetic influences. Tracing the ancestry of any one Ugandan can be difficult because all their names are given them at birth or soon after. Very little record keeping outside the hospital occurs in relation to births, or deaths, but lineage is conveyed in oral history. However, in the United States, wives (and children) take the husband's name, often adding it to their other names.

The mother is customarily the decision maker in regard to health care for their children while the father pays the bills. The nurse should consult with the mother regarding the issues involved, and she will consult with the father as necessary. If extended family is in the vicinity, they may be expected to assist with the health care giving or financial obligations of the family. Adults will make their own decisions about health care. They are most likely to turn to a health professional for advice when making their decisions (Uganda, 2015). Education and belief in religion are linked to Ugandans' preference for Western health care over traditional healers (personal communication with Ugandan Americans, 2014).

A family member is present at all times with a hospitalized patient and should be instructed about how he or she may be of assistance with such tasks as bathing, feeding, medication administration, and safety issues (for example, related to side rails, bed height, ambulation, toileting, and call signals) because they come from a country where these matters are not applicable or very different. Spiritual insight and religious beliefs and practices will guide the person and family in a time of illness. Therefore, it is important for the nurse to assess how those religious beliefs and practices can reinforce this and aid in healing (Uganda, 2015).

It is essential to remember that Ugandan Americans may need assistance to learn new role behaviors as necessitated by illness in the family. Explanations that capitalize on their traditional standards, such as providing well for their families or seeing their children successfully through school, are likely to be the best motivators for positive change. In addition, referral to social service agencies, especially those that cater to African immigrants, can be a valuable aid. In a study by Muwanguzi and Musambira (2009), Ugandan Americans found that many Americans did not make them feel welcomed as demonstrated by the lack of American understanding of what the Ugandan was saying because of accent differences, the attitude of superiority and discrimination presented by the American, attitude of disrespect and rudeness. It is important that American professionals practice cultural respect and sensitivity so as not to perpetuate this sense of unwelcomeness.

TIME

Time tends to be future oriented for young Ugandans who are setting educational and career goals while planning how those goals can be achieved and working diligently to reach them. The young people say that their elders are more past-time oriented, as they prize former days of glory and significance while resisting new ways of living because they cannot imagine the future as better than the past. The young also feel that experiences in the past help them plan for the future. Time orientation may vary between tribal groups, as well as by age.

Young, educated Ugandans are usually quite conscious of "keeping time," as they say, or being "on time," whereas rural Ugandans have no concept of punctuality. On the other hand, some of the young people do not seem concerned if they are tardy. If tardy, they may apologize without necessarily changing their behavior or suffering any unpleasant consequences for their lateness. Many Ugandans do not make appointments to visit friends, clinics, or business offices; they just make their way to the office and are seen on a first-come, first-served basis (personal communication with Ugandans around the country, 2015; Uganda, 2015).

In Uganda, it is expected that a wife will bear a child within the first year of marriage. Other time periods related to childbearing are clearly understood. The mother is expected to breastfeed for about 2 years, to stay in her house for the first 2 weeks after the child's birth, and to resume sexual relations after 2 to 3 months. In the past, family planning has not been widely accepted because a large family was considered to be a sign of wealth and would guarantee that one was well cared for in old age. Traditional men do not want their wives to use family planning methods. Now family planning is more acceptable as "child spacing," with four children spaced two or more years apart considered the ideal family. Family planning makes it possible for the father to provide education for all his children and possibly university education as well. Ugandan immigrants to Britain and the United States average two children per family (personal communication with Ugandans in Mbarara and Kampala, 2015).

Immigrants to the United States are shocked by the speed of Americans' conversation and everyday work, and that people would be so rude as to eat "on the way" (while walking or driving). They eventually realize that Americans value time and want to make the most of it in order to make a decent living. They hope their children will learn to balance the speed of life in the United States with important Ugandan values like stopping to visit with friends.

Implications for Nursing Care

Ugandan Americans can be expected to attend to ill family members in a timely fashion. They have a high regard for the American health care system and the skills of American health care professionals. However, they are inclined to self-treat first before seeking the care of a health care professional. Self-care is likely to consist of over-the-counter drugs, tea, herbs, or special foods if the condition is not believed to be serious. A pharmacist is considered an authority on treating illnesses in Uganda and is likely to be consulted. Frustration may occur in the United States because pharmacists cannot give antibiotics or controlled substances without a prescription. Although commonly used in rural Uganda, traditional healers and the herbal remedies they apply are not available in the United States.

The nurse should take responsibility for initiating discussion with Ugandan women of childbearing age about family planning methods, using the term *child spacing*. Condoms should be encouraged as a preventive measure against HIV for sexually active adults, accompanied by appropriate teaching regarding testing and other preventive methods.

Ugandan Americans find they must wait longer for health care than in Uganda and exercise some degree of patience while the practitioner makes a diagnosis and then offers treatment. On the basis of their previous experience in Uganda, where treatment is based on the symptoms and the limited supply of drugs available for treatment, they tend to expect the expert to identify their problem as soon as they have related the symptoms. A brief explanation about the range of possibilities and the diagnostic process may be of some assistance.

ENVIRONMENTAL CONTROL

Ugandan culture is steeped in external locus of control, with social, fatalistic, or supernatural explanations related to health and illness. Most people believe that a Supreme Being is in control of the natural order of the universe and accept a harmonious linkage of sacred and secular realities. The most significant explanations of the cause of AIDS, illness, or death are beliefs in curses (witchcraft) invoked by other people, God's will or punishment, or retribution by ancestral spirits (Kaliba et al., 2011). Problem solving is now taught in school and church; parents teach the behaviors necessary for certain roles. At higher education levels, the emphasis is on learning facts, with little attention given to practical application. At the worksite, the worker's job is to perform certain tasks in a prescribed sequence with a lack of emphasis on assessment of the situation, priority setting, or customer satisfaction (Ssekajugo, 2012). There is a national movement toward preparing college graduates in Uganda to achieve the workplace expectations required of others in the United States and Europe, but overcoming traditional behaviors related to time and the lack of understanding about immediacy and timeliness of project completion as well as the social responsibilities of the young to their elders or those they consider the "big man" will make such movement a slow process.

Regardless of their belief that they are different, Ugandan women are subject to the same triple jeopardy by Americans as other Black women: sexism, racism, and classism. In addition, they may suffer discrimination as immigrants and as Africans. Consequently, low socioeconomic status and poverty, especially if they are single, may put them at risk for poor nutritional status, lack of access to health care, and inadequate prenatal care. Lack of education and low income are known risk factors for disease and death in Black people.

A large percentage of Ugandan men have earned higher degrees, some of them in Uganda. However, their high academic achievement has not translated into well-paid responsible positions suited to their abilities. Ugandan education is not deemed equivalent to American education, but just how those with an American higher degree can be so poorly rewarded remains a mystery. A study of African-Americans, Caribbeans, and African immigrants confirms that not only do they earn at the lowest level of these three groups but also that the higher their education, the more they accept mismatched job placement (Docquier & Rapoport, 2012).

Financial hardship is a significant stressor affecting assimilation of Ugandan immigrants. In addition to the economic stress, discrimination, and frustration in upward career mobility, Ugandans named their loneliness from loss of close relationships and their lack of cultural knowledge in adapting to new unfamiliar norms as barriers to assimilation.

Numerous cultural beliefs and practices are related to both preventive health and treatment. Some have demonstrated effectiveness, such as the hybrid *Artemisia annua anamed* designed to be grown in the tropics for tea as a treatment for malaria and an herbal treatment for pain relief of herpes zoster in HIV-infected patients. Other traditional practices in Uganda are documented, but modern educated immigrants prefer Western medicine and deny using traditional treatments except tea or readily available herbs for mild symptoms (Namuddu et al., 2011).

Death and Dying Issues

In Uganda, dying patients are cared for at home by the women of the family. Hospice care has been available to aid in pain control in some areas of the country. It is not uncommon for terminal patients to be taken to the hospital as a last resort.

Most Ugandans face illness or death with quiet acceptance. However, participating in the death rituals and looking after daily needs and other family members carry them forward (Dean, 2011). Death rituals in particular are clear for each ethnic group. HIV/AIDS survivors were found to face their adversity with constructive living, thereby demonstrating resilience, resourcefulness, and hope, and an absence of self-pity and resentment.

At the time of death, wailing is spontaneous and recurs at the burial (funeral). In some ethnic groups, the family together washes the dead body. The family retrieves the body for burial. The body is returned to the home or the hometown where the person originated, and a funeral is organized the next day if possible. An all-night vigil takes place, with singing of hymns as necessary to stay awake. If out-of-town relatives are expected to arrive, the funeral might be put off for up to 4 days. Embalming does not take place, and postmortem examinations, organ donations, and autopsies are rare out of respect for the deceased.

Because Ugandans do not embalm, this may create a problem when bodies are shipped back to Uganda from the United States—embalming is required in the United States. In fact, a certified affidavit from five licensed embalmers is required for shipment of the body to any foreign country (African Religions, 2015). During the period of waiting for the funeral, none of the grieving family does any work, goes to school, or serves others for 2 to 4 days. Leave of absence for a family funeral can be as long as a week (personal communication with Holy Innocents Children's Hospital CEO). A ceremony referred to as "last funeral rites" or "second burial" is held either immediately after the burial or up to a year later. A delay allows time to prepare a feast and to put legal affairs in order. The ceremony may contain speeches, singing, dancing, prayer, or reading of a will, plus the naming of an heir to take over the responsibilities of the person who died. Hindus practice cremation in Uganda, but other people are buried in their family's banana plantation or garden near the house. The funeral, grave digging, burial, and cementing over of the grave may all take place on the same day. After a person dies, he is called "the late [former name]" in order to respectfully allow his spirit to rest (Dean, 2011).

Implications for Nursing Care

A goal of health teaching should include developing internal controls in patients to enhance their health. Assessment of health knowledge should be the first step in every teaching situation. Nurses can teach problem solving and making appropriate choices in relation to health care issues. Health teaching that provides guidelines for wellness and illness allows Ugandan Americans to accept responsibility for their own health. Education is an important influence on Ugandans' choice of conventional health care rather than alternative health care. Nurses should be alert to possible misconceptions related to health care and present correct information gently in a style that informs but is not condescending or critical. All procedures and medical terminology should be explained fully and repeated, along with the rationale for the procedure.

Immigrants report that they have been thwarted in carrying out their usual rituals when death occurs. At the time of death, health care providers can negotiate with family caregivers about traditional rituals they may wish to perform, and privacy should be afforded for the ritual or for mourning within legal limitations. They may wish to return the body to its home in Uganda, but the price for following this practice is usually prohibitive. They vow to return the bones to Uganda some day. They negotiate with cemetery superintendents to have the deceased buried while they are still present at the gravesite. Many attend churches in the United States and will, no doubt, find comfort in the ministry of their respective religion and religious leader.

BIOLOGICAL VARIATIONS

Nutritional Preferences and Deficiencies

Nutritional preferences correspond to the leading crops in Uganda. Plantains or green bananas called *matoke* are the preferred food in central Uganda and might be considered the national dish. Cassava, maize, and millet are grown in some areas and can be cooked into a salt-free porridge. Sweet potatoes, Irish potatoes, cabbage, pumpkin, tomatoes, onions, carrots, and avocadoes are popular. Rice is grown in the country. Various types of spinach and sweet potato vines provide green vegetables. Red beans and groundnuts (peanuts) are popular and provide a source of protein. Unfortunately, schoolchildren are often served only red beans and posho (cornmeal) everyday. Pineapples, papayas, mangoes, bananas, and passion fruits are plentiful. Ugandans generally eschew sweets, using bland cakes for special occasions only. Although goats are plentiful, Ugandans seldom drink goat milk and prefer cow's milk. Beef and freshwater fish are available, but few people can afford to purchase this food. Muslims avoid pork (Hunter, unpublished data, 2015).

Ugandans eat fresh, unprocessed food daily and are therefore unhappy with American food offerings when they relocate. They find American food too salty, too sweet, too greasy, and too processed with unknown and possibly dangerous chemical additives. They experience difficulty in finding their preferred foods, and knowing how to cook new vegetables using ovens and ranges rather than the wood or charcoal they had previously used. Initially they find difficulty eating any American food, and coupled with the lack of exercise they get in the United States after walking miles every day for work or fetching water or harvesting crops, may experience digestive problems, bowel changes, and obesity and its sequelae.

Enzymatic and Genetic Variations

Ugandans exhibit a range of skin pigmentation from medium brown to very black, depending upon genetic influences. A range of body builds and heights can also depend on racial origins, clan or family lines, or the region in the country in which they are born. Many of the tallest are Acholi from the north. In the central and southwest regions, body build is more typically Bantu or round. In the past, an overweight person signified wealth. With more education and an expanding worldview, younger Ugandans are becoming more weight conscious. Diabetes mellitus and cardiac disease are quite common among overweight adults. In a country where vegetables are bountiful and sweets spurned, teeth are usually in good condition. Most men and many women choose to wear their hair quite short. This facilitates neatness and grooming. Contemporary plaiting is becoming popular as women find the money to pay for this service (Uganda, 2015).

Susceptibility to Disease

Hypertension, Diabetes, Asthma, and Strokes. Hypertension is known have a much higher incidence in African-American and immigrant Africans than in Whites. Diabetes is 60% more common; they are two and a half times more likely to suffer a limb amputation and five and a half times more likely to suffer kidney disease than other people with diabetes; they are three times more likely to die of asthma than White Americans; strokes will kill four times more 35- to 54-year-old Black Americans than White Americans; and they develop high blood pressure earlier in life, with nearly 42% of Black men and more than 45% of Black women aged 20 and older having high blood pressure (DeNoon, 2015).

Sickle Cell Anemia. Ugandans are subject to the genetically inherited disorder sickle cell anemia, in which sickle-shaped erythrocytes clump together and hemolyze, thus preventing oxygen from reaching the cells and causing anemia, ischemia, and infarction with attendant joint pain. For some time it has been believed that a person with sickle cell anemia is not subject to malaria, but this is incorrect.

Chronic Obstructive Pulmonary Disease. Chronic obstructive pulmonary disease had affected only a small number of Ugandans because cigarette smoking and air pollution had been minimal; however, over the past decade pollution has significantly increased because of the increased industrialization and deforestation (Facts about Uganda, 2013). In rural villages and urban communities, cooking is still performed indoors with little if any ventilation outside so women and children are having an increased amount of respiratory problems (personal observation in Uganda over past 7 years).

Substance Abuse. According to United Nations (UN) statistics, 37,000 people in Africa die annually from diseases associated with the consumption of illegal drugs. The UN estimates there are 28 million drug users in Africa; the figure for the United States and Canada is 32 million. Young people in consumption countries were identified as the most vulnerable section of the population, especially those who were unable to resist peer pressure and start experimenting with drugs (Ndinda, 2013). This author, across the 7 years of working in Uganda, has noted increasing drug use among adolescents and young adults in the larger cities in Uganda where the environment is much like our own major cities (full of people with hopes for a better future but who have lost that hope because of lack of eligibility for meaningful work or general lack of open job positions).

According to a WHO comparison of per-capita consumption in liters of pure alcohol, Ugandans—at 19.47 liters per year—out-drink all other nations (Rufus, 2010). There is a 20% rise in alcohol abuse, especially in young people ages 13 to 21 and an increase in the use of drugs like cocaine, heroin, cannabis, and tobacco. Unfortunately, the outcome of such abuse can be HIV, cardiovascular disease, liver disease, and mental health problems. Experts attribute many mental health problems of women to habitual alcohol use among men, which leads to domestic abuse, stress, and, eventually, mental illness (Uganda Harm Reduction Network, 2013).

Mental Diseases. In Uganda, currently 35% of the population—about 11.5 million people—suffer from some form of mental illness, with depression being one of the most common (Kavuma, 2010). Many Ugandans still blame mental health problems on witchcraft or other supernatural causes. Treating people with mental health conditions is problematic because of the lack of drugs, the costs of medical interventions, and the lack of trained specialists (there are only 28 psychiatrists for a population of 33 million people) (Kiwawulo, 2010). Post-traumatic stress disorder (PTSD), the most common mental ailment in northern Uganda, is a result of rebel activity, abductions, political clashes, and various types of violence (Kiwawulo, 2010). PTSD may be even worse for Ugandans seeking political asylum in the United States because they face the relocation stressors mentioned before in addition to the memories or nightmares of fear or torture they experienced in Uganda (Kiwawulo, 2010).

Cancer. Malinga (2010) has reported that the incidence of cancer is on the rise in Uganda related to lifestyle changes like consumption of fatty foods, alcohol, heavy smoking, and decreased exercise, especially by those who are more affluent. In February 2010, Sankaranaryanan et al. reported that only 13% of the people diagnosed with cancer survive (except for breast cancer, with a survival rate of 46%). Cervical and breast cancers are the biggest killers among women in Uganda, while prostate, liver, lung, penile, urinary bladder, and esophageal cancers and Kaposi's sarcoma (common among HIV/AIDS patients) are common among men.

In general, the prognosis of cancer patients in Uganda is very poor. For example, 5-year relative survival is 8.3% for colorectal cancer and 17.7% for cervical cancer in

Uganda, compared with 54.2% and 63.9%, respectively, for Black-American patients. Such poor prognoses are most likely due to the lack of access and affordability of early diagnosis and treatment options in the country (DeNoon, 2015).

Tropical Diseases. Malaria is the leading cause of morbidity and mortality in Uganda, caused most often by the protozoa species, *Plasmodium falciparum,* which is transmitted by mosquito bite, transfusion, shared needles, or vertically (mother to fetus). An average of 320 Ugandans die every day, mostly pregnant women and children below 5 years (the most vulnerable victims), causing between 70,000 and 110,000 deaths per year (Yeka et al., 2012). With its complex cycle through the liver and blood, malaria may have an insidious onset or erupt suddenly after the victim is in the United States for several years when the immune system becomes compromised, because the virus can remain dormant in the liver for several years. American health professionals may not suspect malaria in infected patients with fever and alternating chills and sweating, or may lack diagnostic or treatment expertise. The disease causes severe anemia and hepatosplenomegaly and can be rapidly life-threatening. Fortunately, the infection is easily identified from a blood smear or rapid diagnostic test on a pinprick specimen, and drug treatment can be effective. Artemether-lumefantrine is the current national first-line regimen for uncomplicated malaria (Yeka et al., 2012).

A 2014 report by the CDC stated that approximately 1500 to 2000 cases of malaria are reported every year in the United States and in 2011 reached a high of 1925 cases. Such cases are usually present in immigrants from malaria-endemic countries returning to their homeland to visit families but not protecting themselves against the disease. Only 63 cases of locally transmitted mosquito-borne malaria have occurred since 1957; however, 97 cases of transfusion-transmitted malaria have been reported in the United States.

In addition to malaria, Ugandan immigrants are troubled with positive tuberculin tests, necessitating 6 months of antitubercular treatment. Immigrants may have received bacillus Calmette-Guérin (BCG) immunizations against tuberculosis, ensuring that their tuberculin skin test will always be positive. In fact, BCG and the oral polio vaccine (OPV) are now given to all children at birth or first contact. The OPV is given again, along with the diphtheria, tetanus, and pertussis, *Haemophilus influenzae* type B, and hepatitis vaccines, through 14 weeks; the measles vaccine is given at 9 months; and vitamin A is given every 6 months, up to 10 doses (Zaramba, 2011).

Other tropical diseases that should be considered in Ugandan immigrants of less than 1 year's residence include visceral leishmaniasis, human African trypanosomiasis, trachoma, Buruli ulcer, soil-transmitted helminths, schistosomiasis, lymphatic filariasis, brucellosis, ascariasis (roundworms), and onchocerciasis (Gautret et al., 2012). Some tropical diseases have long incubation periods and can therefore be transported when the traveler is symptom free, and some diseases are prone to relapse. A hemorrhagic fever such as Ebola may have a long incubation period but rapidly erupts into severe illness, progressing to disseminated intravascular coagulation and death. The Ebola virus is easily passed from human to human in body fluids, and barrier precautions need to be immediately implemented. Ebola had a mortality rate of 50% for health care workers (CDC, *Ebola virus,* 2014). The infection carried so much stigma that the workers were often reluctant to remain on duty, especially when barrier supplies were inadequate, and they were shunned by colleagues and their own families if they stayed (CDC, *Ebola virus,* 2014).

Hepatitis. Hepatitis A, B, C, and D are also prevalent conditions divided into acute disorders (hepatitis A, E, G) and those with acute and chronic states (hepatitis B, C, D). They are spread by the fecal–oral route, perinatally, percutaneously, through blood or blood products, or by unprotected intercourse. Treatment is mostly supportive, although several medications are available, depending on the individual disorder. Prevention is through proper sanitary conditions, vaccination, and education on risk factors (Teshale et al., 2010). If untreated, these conditions contribute to liver cancer and liver transplants.

Implications for Nursing Care

In the first year of migration, immigrants can benefit from a thorough assessment of their dietary intake, gastrointestinal system, and exercise regimen. Until they can locate and learn how to prepare their preferred foods in American kitchens, Ugandans are seriously distressed by American food offerings and the choices they must make in regard to food. One reported that he failed to eat anything for 2 months after arrival, and another reported an early visit to the emergency department with severe constipation (personal communication with recent Ugandan immigrant, 2015). Immigrants should be encouraged to exercise and take an adequate fluid intake, and be informed that tap water is potable. Parasites are often found in East African immigrants, even those without noticeable symptoms. Several studies point to the need to screen all immigrants within 3 months of arrival and up to 1 year with a stool specimen for microscopy and blood tests for serology and complete blood count in order to identify infectious organisms and anemia (CDC, Medical Screening, 2014).

It is imperative for nurses assessing a patient to identify the country of origin or country recently visited. Whenever the Ugandan patient seeks treatment, a thorough history of previous infection with tropical diseases and previous living environment in Uganda should be taken to rule out a possible tropical disease. If the patient exhibits symptoms suggestive of an infection, thorough examination of body fluids and stool or sputum should be implemented. The nurse should ensure the safety of other patients, staff, and him- or herself with standard precautions, barrier precautions if a hemorrhagic fever is suspected, or a mask appropriate to TB prevention.

Malaria commonly relapses when a person has experienced unusual stress or is immunocompromised. The lack of knowledge about malaria on the part of American health care personnel is a source of frustration to sufferers of this unpleasant illness. Nurses should familiarize themselves with the symptoms and the chemotherapy suitable for treating this disease. Nurses need to listen carefully to patients' ideas about what illness they might have and what treatment has been effective in the past.

In Uganda, use of the word *fever* means "malaria." Nurses should be alert to this meaning in using this word with African immigrants. Ugandans use the term *flu* to refer to upper respiratory viral symptoms similar to the common cold or sore throat. They do not use the term *cold*.

Physiological assessment of black skin may be difficult for some nurses. For best results, it should be conducted in indirect sunlight. Mucous membranes, lips, and nail beds are the best places to observe for pallor that appears ashen gray. Palpation must be used to check for erythema. The area will be warmer, tight, and edematous, while the underlying tissues will be hard. When assessing for cyanosis, close inspection of the lips, tongue, conjunctiva, palms of the hands, and soles of the feet again will demonstrate an ashen gray color, and a blood return to the palms of more than 1 second after being pressed is a positive sign. History of trauma, along with swelling of the surface, indicates ecchymosis. Observe the sclerae for yellow discoloration when assessing jaundice, but this may be misleading if carotene deposits cause the discoloration. Also check the buccal mucosa, palms of the hands, and soles of the feet for yellowish coloration.

There have been many studies about the differences between black and white patients on the pharmacotherapeutic responses to treatment for cardiac disease and asthma. It is important for nurses to understand the ethnic and racial differences to drug therapies regardless of race.

The possibility that lactose intolerance may affect the patient should be considered, especially when assisting with meal planning or feeding. Family caregivers for inpatients should be encouraged to bring preferred foods from home after conferring with the dietitian, if dietary restrictions have been ordered.

Immigrants suffering from PTSD and depression, which often occur together, may demonstrate somatization, such as gastrointestinal disorders; "re-experiencing phenomena," such as nightmares and flashbacks; "avoidance of stimuli associated with being tortured," which may mean avoidance of other Ugandans or people in uniform; and "physiologic symptoms of increased arousal and reactivity of the sympathetic nervous system" (WHO, 2012), such as hypertension, sleep disturbances, and exaggerated startle response. Because of the stigma associated with mental illness by Ugandans, *stress* would be a more acceptable term to use for these diagnoses.

SUMMARY

Ugandan Americans want quality conventional health care, and they expect to receive it in the American health care system. In comparison to their experiences in Uganda in earlier times, they appreciate the use of advanced technology; the cleanliness and quality of health care facilities; the education and expertise of health care providers; and the fair, polite, caring treatment they receive in America. However, they may delay treatment for economic reasons, especially if they do not have access to adequate insurance. Poor, single women are most likely to find the cost of health care to be a barrier. First-generation immigrants cope with health care barriers by using their character strengths of acceptance, determination, and optimism, along with survival instincts learned in Uganda and their spiritual faith or well-being. Encourage discussion about their beliefs regarding food, healing and health, child spacing, infant care, family relations, or medications in order to reinforce positive beliefs and behaviors that optimize their health and coping or to dispel any misconceptions. Keep in mind that the terminology used may be different from American English and American medical terminology, and the nurse may need to carefully and discreetly define some aspects of health teaching. Euphemisms for sensitive issues, analogies, and illustration with pictures, models, or gestures are teaching techniques that can be effective with Ugandan Americans.

Ugandans value politeness, modesty, and respect, and any effort by the nurse to try to understand the culture of patients, to value their ethnic loyalty, to include family members, to respectfully personalize care, to preserve their modesty, or to support the patient in self-care will be rewarded with gracious appreciation, as well as learning for both the nurse and the patient.

CASE STUDY

Mrs. Josephine Tumusiime, 36, arrives at the emergency department accompanied by her 14-year-old daughter, Justine. Mrs. Tumusiime's temperature is 102.6° F. She reports being very weak and dizzy, with joint aches of 3 days' duration, headache, chills, and "sweats." She has been unable to eat because of nausea since the aching started and has taken only tea several times a day. She says she has had "fever" many times when she lived in Uganda. There her mother knew which roots to use for treatment. Her mucous membranes are dry, so intravenous fluids are started.

Some history is elicited from Justine, who said the patient has been in this city since the family arrived from Uganda 3 years ago. The father sought political asylum and brought her mother and a sibling a few years later. Although the patient is a teacher, having received a certificate from a teacher's institute, she is not qualified to teach in the United States. She is working nights cleaning offices and taking education courses at the university during the day. About 2 weeks ago, some items were missing from her place of work, and she has been questioned repeatedly and accused of theft, causing her a great deal of stress. In addition, her final examinations are scheduled for next week. Justine appears tense and frightened after divulging this information. The patient says her husband is away at a conference in another state, but she isn't able to name the hotel or city where he is staying.

After the physician verifies the presence of malarial parasites in a blood smear, he orders intravenous antimalarial drugs, an antipyretic, and an analgesic. The patient's low erythrocytes and hemoglobin are treated with a hematinic. When her temperature returns to normal, she is discharged from the hospital with an oral antimalarial drug and instructions to complete the entire course of treatment.

CARE PLAN

Nursing Diagnosis: Hyperthermia related to relapse of malaria

Client Outcome	Nursing Interventions
The patient maintains temperature below 100° F.	1. Monitor temperature every 2 hours until within normal range. 2. Offer oral fluids every hour while awake. 3. Administer antimalarials as ordered. 4. Instruct patient how to take antimalarial on discharge, along with the rationale for completing the entire course of treatment.

Nursing Diagnosis: Altered tissue perfusion (peripheral) related to anemia

Client Outcomes	Nursing Interventions
1. The patient demonstrates increased tissue perfusion with pink, dry skin and strong peripheral pulses and is alert and oriented. 2. The patient's vital signs are within normal limits.	1. Assess patient for cyanosis, capillary refill, and skin condition. 2. Assess vital signs and level of consciousness at least every 4 hours. 3. Review laboratory values for improved RBC count and hemoglobin concentration. 4. Administer oxygen as needed. 5. Administer hematinic as ordered. 6. Teach patient about foods high in iron, as well as rationale for increasing iron in the diet at this time.

Nursing Diagnosis: Pain related to joint aches and headache from hemolysis of erythrocytes and toxins in blood

Client Outcome	Nursing Interventions
The patient will verbalize reduction in pain following administration of pain relief measures.	1. Ask patient about the presence of pain, and have her rank it using a scale. 2. Offer analgesic at reasonable intervals. 3. Encourage patient to request analgesic as needed. 4. Teach patient to use nonmedicinal pain relief measures, such as listening to music or prayer.

Continued

◎ CARE PLAN—cont'd

Nursing Diagnosis: Impaired verbal communication related to fatigue and to cultural differences in English dialect, leading to misinterpretation by health personnel and the patient and family

Client Outcomes	Nursing Interventions
1. The patient will express satisfaction that health professionals have understood her. 2. The patient will verbalize understanding of health teaching.	1. Greet patient and family member with respect, using correct titles. 2. Speak slowly, distinctly, formally, and softly. 3. Inquire about the patient and family welfare when greeting the patient in order to develop rapport. 4. Listen carefully to the message conveyed and the intended meaning, clarifying as necessary. 5. Direct communication to supporting family member until energy level returns. 6. Provide brief explanations prior to each nursing measure, especially if it is necessary to invade intimate space in order to gain permission. 7. Assess patient and family for misconceptions regarding the illness and treatment, and provide correct information. 8. Accompany verbal health teaching with written directions or diagrams.

Nursing Diagnosis: Ineffective family coping: compromised related to absence of spouse and extended family available for support and needs

Client Outcomes	Nursing Interventions
1. Family members will identify internal strengths and individual and family coping skills. 2. Family members will identify need(s) for support. 3. Patient will verbalize person or agency she will contact for assistance to meet identified need(s).	1. Commend daughter Justine for taking responsibility for assisting mother. 2. Assess and reinforce internal sources of strength. 3. Explain to Justine how she can help her mother in the hospital while maintaining the safety of all involved. 4. Refer to social services, university counseling office, or community agencies catering to women and immigrants to assist with identified needs.

Nursing Diagnosis: Spiritual distress related to belief in supernatural as possible cause of illness and feeling isolated in a culturally foreign setting

Client Outcomes	Nursing Interventions
1. Patient and daughter will name community sources of spiritual support. 2. Patient will name a plan of action to cope with stress.	1. Encourage verbalization of concerns and discomfort by using therapeutic techniques. 2. Acknowledge awareness of concern, validating feelings as appropriate. 3. Assess religious–spiritual orientation. 4. Offer referral to chaplain or clergyperson, if desired. 5. Educate patient on the relationship of stress to physical illness. 6. Explore with patient and daughter organizations in the community that can provide the needed spiritual support. 7. Assist patient to identify appropriate stress relief methods for her situation.

CLINICAL DECISION MAKING

1. How should this patient be greeted upon her arrival at the facility?
2. How is it possible for Mrs. Tumusiime to become infected with malaria in the United States?
3. Does Mrs. Tumusiime's stress on the job have any relationship to her relapse of malaria?
4. What is the danger in untreated malaria?
5. Why might Justine have misgivings about the background information she has given the nurse about her family?
6. In what ways might this family typify Ugandan-American immigrants?
7. How is Mrs. Tumusiime's anemia related to her malaria?

REVIEW QUESTIONS

1. Because of their skin color, geographical location of Uganda, and the tendency of some Ugandans to contract malaria, what condition is said to be a condition of adaptation for Ugandans and Ugandan Americans?
   a. Sickle cell anemia
   b. Glucose-6-phosphate dehydrogenase (G-6-PD)
   c. Dumping syndrome
   d. Metabolic syndrome
2. Mr. Akello has been admitted to your unit. He was diagnosed with a myocardial infarction. When you assess Mr. Akello, you note that he appears to be wincing and to be in obvious pain. However, when you ask Mr. Akello if he is in pain, he denies pain. Based on your cultural assessment of a Ugandan American, you recognize that some Ugandan Americans may do which of the following?
   a. Bear pain stoically, so offer him pain medication.
   b. Verbalize extensively about pain, so do not worry.
   c. Tend to bring herbal remedies from home, so the pain has been relieved.
   d. Tend to meditate and thus are able to relieve their pain.
3. As you talk with Mr. Akello, you learn that the primary structure of the Ugandan family is likely to be organized in which of the following ways?
   a. Nuclear
   b. Extended
   c. Clan
   d. Tribes

REFERENCES

African Network for the Prevention and Protection of Children against Child Abuse and Neglect (ANPPCAN). (2013). *The current situation for children in Uganda*. Available at <http://www.anppcanug.org/wp-content/uploads/press_kits/The_Sit_of_Child_in_Ug.pdf>.

African Religions. (2015). *Encyclopedia of death and dying*. Available at <http://www.deathreference.com/A-Bi/African-Religions.html>.

Avert. (2013). *HIV and AIDS in Uganda*. Available at <http://www.avert.org/hiv-aids-uganda.htm>.

Bauer, R. (2014). *Malaria in Uganda*. Available at <www.jbpub.com/.../skolnik/.../Malaria%20in%20Uganda,%20Bauer.doc>.

Bangirana, P., et al. (2011). *Malaria with neurological involvement in Ugandan children. Effect on cognitive ability, academic achievement, and behavior*. Available at <http://www.malariajournal.com/content/10/1/334> Retrieved February 4, 2015.

Centers for Disease Control and Prevention (CDC). (2014). *Ebola virus information*. Available at <http://www.cdc.gov/vhf/ebola>.

Centers for Disease Control and Prevention (CDC). (2014). *Medical screening of US-bound refugees*. Available at <http://www.cdc.gov/immigrantrefugeehealth/profiles/congolese/medicalscreening/index.html>.

Central Intelligence Agency. (CIA). (2014). *The world factbook: the CIA*. New York: Skyhorse. Available at <https://www.cia.gov/library/publications/the-world-factbook/>.

Dean, K. (2011). *Ugandan death traditions*. Available at <https://mysendoff.com/2011/06/uganda-death-traditions/> Retrieved January 29, 2015.

DeNoon, D. J. (2015). Why 7 deadly disease strike blacks most: health care disparities heighten disease differences between African-American and white Americans. *WebMD*. Available at <http://www.webmd.com/hypertension-high-blood-pressure/features/why7-deadly-diseases-strike-blacks-most> Retrieved February 6, 2015.

Docquier, F., & Rapoport, H. (2012). Globalization, brain drain, and development. *Journal of Economic Literature, 50*(30), 681–730.

Facts about Uganda. (2013). Available at <http://www.factmonster.com/country/uganda.html> Retrieved January 27, 2015.

Gautret, P., et al. (2012). Infectious diseases among travellers and migrants in Europe. *Surveillance and Outbreak Report, Eurosurveillance, 17*(26). Available at <http://www.eurosurveillance.org/ViewArticle.aspx?ArticleId=20205> Retrieved February 2, 2015.

Kaliba, A. R., et al. (2011). Locus of control and readiness to conjure and believe in mystical powers among small business operators in Entebbe, Uganda: a multilevel Rasch rating scale model analysis. *African Journal of Business Management, 5*(17), 7258–7271. doi:10.5897/AJBM10.983; ISSN 1993-8233.

Kavuma, R. M. (2010). Changing perceptions of mental health in Uganda. *The Monitor*.

Kizza, I. B. (2012). *Nurses' knowledge and practices related to pain assessment in critically ill patients at Mulago Hospital, Uganda* (Master's thesis). Muhimbili University of Health and Allied

Sciences. Available from Health Digital Library. <http://ihi.eprints.org/1598/>.

Kiwawulo, C. (2010). *Uganda: mental health—over 11.5 million countrymen suffer disorders*. The New Vision.

Malinga, J. (2010). Should Uganda be tackling cancer? *The Guardian*. Retrieved from: <http://www.theguardian.com/katine/katine-chronicles-blog/2010/mar/23/health-news> September 24, 2015.

McCabe, K. (2011). *African immigrants in the U.S.: Migration Policy Institute*. Available at <http://www.migrationpolicy.org/article/african-immigrants-united-states> Retrieved February 4, 2015.

Muwanguzi, S., & Musambira, G. W. (2009). The transformation of East Africa's economy using mobile phone money transfer services: a comparative analysis of Kenya and Uganda's experiences. *Journal of Creative Communications*, 4(2), 131–146.

Namuddu, B., et al. (2011). Prevalence and factors associated with traditional herbal medicine use among patients on highly active antiretroviral therapy in Uganda. *BMC Public Health*, 11, 855. Available at <http://www.biomedcentral.com/1471-2458/11/855/> Retrieved February 5, 2015.

Ndinda, L. (2013). *Illegal drug use on the rise in Africa*. Available at <http://www.dw.de/illegal-drug-use-on-the-rise-in-africa/a-16614023> Retrieved January 30, 2015.

Rufus, A. (2010). Who drinks the most alcohol? *The Daily Beast*. Available at <http://www.thedailybeast.com/articles/2010/12/29/drinking-stats-who-drinks-the-most-alcohol.html> Retrieved January 30, 2015.

Rural Poverty in Uganda. (n.d.). *Rural poverty portal*. Available at <http://www.ruralpovertyportal.org/country/home/tags/Uganda>.

Sankaranaryanan, R., et al. (2010). Cancer survival in Africa, Asia, and Central America: a population-based study. *Lancet Oncology*, 11(2), 165–173.

SALVE International. (2015a). *Being a woman in Uganda*. Available at <http://www.salveinternational.org/salve-explained/being-a-woman-in-uganda/>.

SALVE. (2015b). *Education in Uganda*. Available at <http://www.salveinternational.org/salve-explained/education-in-uganda/>.

Ssekajugo, D. (2012). Workplace environment in selected multinational companies in Kampala, Uganda. *International Journal of Business and Management Tomorrow*, 2(12). Available at <http://dx.doi.org/10/1257/JEL.50.3.681> Retrieved February 2, 2015.

Teshale, E. H., et al. (2010). Hepatitis E epidemic, Uganda. *Emerging infectious disease*. Available at <http://wwwnc.cdc.gov/eid/article/16/1/09-0764_article>.

Uganda. (2015). *Countries and their cultures*. Available at <www.everyculture.com/To-Z/Uganda.html>.

Uganda Harm Reduction Network Justification (UHRNJ). (2013). Available at <https://ugandaharmreduction.wordpress.com/2013/09/> Retrieved February 3, 2015.

United Nations Educational, Scientific, and Cultural Organization (UNESCO) Institute for Statistics. Retrieved from: <http://www.uis.unesco.org/Pages/default.aspx>. 9-23-2015.

Wade, L. (2013). Assimilation among 1st and 2nd generation immigrants. *Sociological Images*. Available at <http://thesocietypages.org/socimages/2013/04/13/assimilation-among-1st-and-2nd-generation-immigrants/> Retrieved February 1, 2015.

The World Bank. (2014). *Uganda overview*. Available at <http://www.worldbank.org/en/country/uganda/overview>.

World Health Organization (WHO). (2012). *Mental Health Policy and Service Development Department of Mental Health and Substance Abuse World Health Organization: Uganda*. Available at <http://www.who.int/mental_health/policy/country/uganda_country_summary_2012.pdf> Retrieved February 5, 2015.

Yeka, A., et al. (2012). Malaria in Uganda: challenges to control on the long road to elimination: epidemiology and current control efforts. *Acta Tropica*, 121(3), 184–195. doi:10.1016/j.actatropica.2011.03.004; [Epub 2011 Mar 21].

Zaramba, S. (2011). *Uganda National Expanded Programme on Immunization Multiyear Plan 2010–2014*. Available at <file:///C:/Users/anita/Downloads/UgandaComprehensive%20multi-year%20plan%20for%202010-2014%20-%20Year%202011.pdf> Retrieved February 6, 2015.

27

Jordanian Americans

Najood G. Azar, Linda G. Haddad, and Mary Grace Umlauf

BEHAVIORAL OBJECTIVES

After reading this chapter, the nurse will be able to:

1. Describe the political, historical, and religious influences that have shaped modern Jordan and influenced migration of Jordanians to the United States.
2. Describe how advances in communications and travel influence acculturation of Jordanian immigrants now and in the future.
3. Explain the cultural values related to space among traditional Jordanian Americans.
4. Identify social customs related to social interactions among family members and between unrelated men and women commonly observed among Jordanian Americans.
5. Explain the importance of the past to traditional Jordanian Americans.
6. Recognize the influence of Islamic values on the acceptability of various infertility treatments and of genetic screening for heritable conditions.
7. Identify hereditary diseases that are prevalent among Jordanians and describe how culture has contributed to incidence.
8. Describe the effects of Western lifestyle practices on health outcomes among Jordanians and Jordanian Americans.

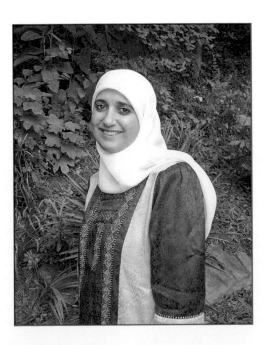

OVERVIEW OF JORDAN

The Hashemite Kingdom of Jordan is a developing country in the Middle East, bound by Israel and the Palestinian lands on the west, Syria on the north, Iraq on the east, and Saudi Arabia on the east and south. In land area, Jordan is slightly smaller than Indiana. In 2007, the population was estimated at 6,407,085 people (*World Almanac*, 2015), with 33% of the population residing in the capital city of Amman (Central Intelligence Agency [CIA], 2015). In 2013, the gross domestic product was U.S. $40.02 billion, which yields a $6100 per capita rate (CIA, 2015). The average number of persons per family is 5.1, and the fertility rate is 3.8. The birth rate (per 1000 population) is 25.23 with an average birth interval of 31 months (CIA, 2015; Department of Statistics, 2010). Unlike some countries in the region, Jordan has no oil or gas reserves. Thus, it has been said that the most valuable export has been their human capital, university-educated professionals such as engineers and health care workers, including nurses. Many of these professionals immigrate to the West because of their technical expertise and because their English skills are strong. English is taught in elementary schools in Jordan, and the universities teach the sciences in English using textbooks from Great Britain and the United States.

Several hundred years ago, the collective area of Jordan, Palestine, and Syria was a single administrative entity, a *vilayet*, of the Turkish Ottoman Empire. At the conclusion of World War I, the Western powers divided the remains of the Ottoman holdings. Under the League of Nations mandate, the area east of the Jordan River was given over to the British and was called *Transjordan*. In 1946 the mandate ceased, and the country became fully independent, with its own constitution under the reign of a member of the Arabian Hashemite dynasty, King Abdullah ibn Hussein. At this juncture, the formal name was changed to the Hashemite Kingdom of Jordan. After the assassination of King Abdullah in 1951, he was succeeded by his grandson, King Hussein bin Talal, in 1952. For nearly 50 years, King Hussein ruled Jordan as a constitutional monarchy with a bicameral legislature. During his reign, significant advances were made in education, public health, modernization, and infrastructure development (*Time Almanac,* 2011). King Abdullah bin al-Hussein assumed power following the death of his father, King Hussein, in 1999 and has maintained the existing policies of a constitutional monarchy with a bicameral parliament.

As a result of policies that promoted education, health, and public welfare, there is evidence of consistent improvement in quality of life in Jordan. For example, in 2009 the population of Jordan was 6.4 million, which is twice the number counted in 1988 and four times that of 1970 (CIA, 2015; World Bank, 2013). This dramatic increase in population has been attributed to a high population growth rate, plus dramatic improvements in life expectancy and reduced infant mortality. For example, life expectancy at birth increased from 46.9 years in 1960, to 62.6 years in 1980, to 70.6 years in 2000, to 72.7 in 2008, and to 74 in the year 2012 (World Bank, 2013). Although fertility levels have declined from a high of 8 children born per woman in 1964 to a low 3.3 in 2013, improved childhood survival rates have increased the numbers of young people who will soon enter marriageable age. According to the CIA 2015 report, 35.8% of the population was under age 15 years, whereas only 5.1% of the total population was over the age of 65 (CIA, 2015). However, Jordan's centralized regional location and political stability during the reign of King Hussein and his son King Abdullah have been affected by periodic waves of refugees from the West Bank, the Gaza Strip, Lebanon, and Iraq. Although persons of Palestinian descent make up more than half the total population, the number of registered Palestinian refugees and the recent influx of Iraqi and Syrian refugees is estimated at 1.7 million persons (CIA, 2015).

Jordan is often referred to as a labor-exporting country, this by virtue of a well-educated and skilled labor force (Embassy of Jordan, 2012; *World Almanac*, 2015). College education is free at public universities for those who qualify, and unemployment is a significant problem in the country for almost all graduates. Thus, entire graduating classes of engineers, physicians, and pharmacists look for work elsewhere in the Middle East, in Great Britain, and in the United States. The nursing shortage is a consistent finding worldwide, but Jordanian nurses often seek work outside of Jordan because of better salaries and opportunities to work in hospitals with better technological infrastructures. Even when labor migration is permanent, the practice of remittance of a portion of the worker's salary to family members in Jordan is common. This practice continues today in the United States and is an indication of continuing ties and identity between an immigrant and the family of origin.

Although there has been an influx of Palestinians into Jordan over the past century, they have retained their tribal identity. Thus, Jordan has two main tribal groups: (1) Jordanians whose ancestors were Bedouins and (2) Palestinians. Both groups include Muslims and a small minority of Christians, about 2.2% of the total population of Jordan (CIA, 2015; *World Almanac*, 2015). Like other Arabs, Palestinians have maintained their ethnic identity and may make this evident by displaying or wearing their tribal *kaffiyeh,* the traditional Arab man's scarf head covering. The Palestinian design is distinctive, an open black basket weave pattern on a predominantly white fabric, compared with the Jordanian design, which is a denser network design of bright red embroidery on a white background. The scarf may be worn in the traditional fashion as a head covering by men, along with a special woven rope crown, an *egal*. When there is an escalation in conflict in the West Bank in Israel, wearing the Palestinian *kaffiyeh* in the United States is likely to convey political solidarity for families who are endangered by the conflict. On these occasions, both men and women in the United States may wear clothing with the Palestinian design or prominently display the *kaffiyeh* in their shops and businesses.

OVERVIEW OF JORDANIAN AMERICANS AS AN ETHNIC GROUP

Between 2006 and 2010, there were 60,056 resident Jordanian Americans (U.S. Department of Commerce, Bureau of the Census, *American Community Survey,* 2013). Arab Americans live throughout the United States, and about one third of Arabs are concentrated in California (Los Angeles County), Michigan (Wayne and Oakland counties), and New York (Brooklyn). Another third reside in Illinois, Maryland, Massachusetts, New Jersey, Ohio, Texas, and Virginia. On the average, Arab Americans are better educated than other Americans. Likewise, college attendance is also higher than average, and the percentage of those earning degrees is double. As a group, Arab Americans are more likely to be self-employed, entrepreneurs, or in sales. About 60% of those employed do so as executives, professionals, and office and sales staff. As with other workers, types of employment are also related to area of residence. For example, there are more Arab-American executives in Washington, DC, and Anaheim, California; more sales workers in Cleveland, Ohio, and Anaheim; and more manufacturing workers in Detroit, Michigan. Nationally, Arab Americans have incomes that are higher than average, although incomes are below average in certain locations, such as in Detroit and Anaheim (100 Questions, 2001; U.S. Department of Commerce, Bureau of the Census, *American Community Survey,* 2013).

IMMIGRATION OF JORDANIANS TO THE UNITED STATES

Large waves of Arab immigration to the United States can be traced to as early as 1875 and continued until about 1920. Most of these early immigrants were Christian. This early period was a reflection of economic depression in Lebanon and Syria resulting from Japanese competition in the silk market and a plant epidemic that affected vineyard production. A second wave of immigration began in the 1940s as a result of the Arab–Israeli conflict and civil war.

This second wave of immigration included many more asylum seekers, students, persons who were financially secure, and Muslims (100 Questions, 2001; U.S. Department of Commerce, Bureau of the Census, *American Community Survey,* 2013).

The electronic age has provided immigrants ready access to news and contact with their home country and family of origin. As a result, the process of acculturation for the current generation of immigrants has changed substantially. The information age has provided real-time access to happenings in almost any city in the world. The Internet, Web cameras, social networking programs (e.g., Facebook, Twitter), Internet-based phone services (e.g., Skype), and satellite communications have created affordable access to native-language newspapers, live video, contemporary music and films, and local television programming from places on the other side of the globe. International telephone service is more reliable and affordable than ever before, which allows immigrants to communicate with families and communities much more easily and much more often. The proliferation of ethnic specialty stores in the United States has made it easier for immigrants to maintain native food patterns and to furnish their homes in the same style as relatives at home. The growth of ethnic communities in the United States has also facilitated the building of mosques and churches, which provide religious services in the native style and language. As a result of these technological innovations and changes in U.S. communities, Jordanian Americans and other ethnic groups will be able to maintain or re-establish their cultural identity and cultural preferences much more easily than previous generations. Thus, it is important for nurses to be informed about cultural differences to provide culturally sensitive and culturally specific care to patients, based on their individual ethnic background and country of origin.

COMMUNICATION

Arabic is a Semitic language derived from Aramaic, Hebrew, various Ethiopian languages, and others. It is the official language of Jordan and dates back to pre-Islamic Saudi Arabia. Arabic is also the language of the Qur'an, the holy book of Islam. However, there is a small minority of people who have another native language (such as Circassians and Armenians). In addition, English is currently taught as a second language at the elementary school level. Jordanian university programs also teach engineering and the sciences in English, using U.S. and British textbooks. Arabic has a formal written and spoken form, Modern Standard Arabic, which is used in books and newspapers, as well as in diplomatic settings and on television news. In colloquial use, Jordanians are said to employ the Levantine dialect of

Arabic (100 Questions, 2001; U.S. Department of Commerce, Bureau of the Census, *American Community Survey*, 2013).

Social custom dictates that greetings between persons are ritualized with greetings such as "Welcome" and "How is your health?" and responded in kind with "Welcome to you" and "My health is good, thanks be to God." Among friends and family, these exchanges can be very animated between persons of the same sex or between older persons and much younger persons. These verbal greetings among friends and family are often observed, along with a handshake and a kiss on both cheeks (right cheek to right cheek first, and then left to left). In formal or business settings, greetings are more likely to be limited to a more formal verbal exchange and handshaking alone. Muslim women, particularly those who are covered, usually refrain from touching or shaking hands with men other than family members. These women often lift the right hand and place it flat on the upper chest just below the left clavicle. This gives visual acknowledgment of the other person's intention to shake hands but avoids physical contact. A proper response to this gesture is a slight bow or nod of the head or the same hand motion and placement. Some covered women may actually shake hands with a man but only after quickly pulling her long sleeve over her hand to prevent actual skin-to-skin contact.

Jordanians often raise their voices when trying to convey important information or to make a particular point. Children may complain loudly about a minor need or in defense of their behavior. In health care settings, they may exaggerate physical symptoms of pain (Zahr & Hattar-Pollara, 1998). In business and family settings, both men and women speak loudly and quickly over each other to clarify their vantage point in the discussion. No offense is taken or given in these verbal exchanges, which might be taken as offensive or hostile by the average American.

Public display of affection between men and women is highly discouraged, and touching is very limited between unrelated men and women in Jordan. This prohibition is related to the importance of family honor, *sharaf el 'aar.* Loss of honor primarily results from the loss of virginity or the promiscuity (actual or perceived) of women in the family. A breach in family honor is an important family concern and a significant source of stress among mothers of female teenagers in newly immigrated families (Hattar-Pollara & Meleis, 1995). Jordanian social custom supports behaviors that visibly separate women from men outside of the family group. Avoidance of touch in social settings may be more pronounced, particularly among covered Muslim women. For example, a covered woman will avoid sitting directly next to a man on public transportation. She will seek out seating next to another woman or child first

or avoid sitting if at all possible. Taking a child, particularly a boy child, along on grocery shopping excursions also provides a social and physical barrier to having too much contact with unrelated men. Thus, Jordanians may appear to go to extreme means to cloister females to guard against even the perception of impropriety.

However, there is a great deal of touching permitted by persons of the same sex without an assumption of homosexual behavior. Although it is more common to see men holding hands or women holding hands as they walk down the street in Jordan, this behavior is less likely to be observed in the United States because of the greater sensitivity to homosexual behavior in the United States. In contrast, within the family, Jordanians are very affectionate with their children. Hugging and touching are also fairly common between children and are frequently focused on the smallest child in any family group.

In formal settings, communication is measured but is hospitable and very gracious. Among friends and family, a great deal of collective energy and focus is invested in communication. In greetings, negotiations, or disagreements, voices are often raised and speech is very rapid. Disapproval, such as when a child misbehaves, is often expressed in a minimal fashion by shaking the head "no" or by making a clicking noise with the tongue. It is very uncommon to observe physical violence or spanking in this culture.

Along with a propensity to speak loudly, Jordanians also use their hands for emphasis while speaking. Commonly, the hands are kept close to the body while gesturing. Just as with the prohibitions against touching between sexes, eye contact in public between unrelated men and women is generally avoided.

Implications for Nursing Care

Because there are different communication behaviors expected of men and women in the Jordanian culture, nurses must be prepared to conform to gender-based expectations as well. Male nurses may be limited in trying to interact with Muslim girls and women but conversely find that the men are more than ingratiating. Female nurses will find fewer barriers to entering the home and working with mothers and children, while Jordanian-American men may seem more distant or too aggressive. In addition, recently immigrated women who do not work outside the home may have poor English-language skills and not know what to expect from health care providers in the United States. Children may be called upon to act as translators, which may limit the nurse's ability to conduct detailed health histories or to inquire about sensitive family issues, such as family violence, abuse, or infertility.

SPACE

Although there are few limits to same-sex touch and contact, proximity takes on a negative connotation between the sexes outside of the family group. Jordanians are highly affiliative and value close proximity within the extended family group. Close proximity is reserved for families, and children have close physical contact with all adult members. Nonfamily may also be welcomed into the family circle, but this interaction will be much more limited if the parties are not of the same religion, either Christian or Muslim. Visitors who are women will be expected to interact more with the women of the family, and male visitors will be expected to interact more with the male members of the household.

In traditional home settings, there will often be one or two large sitting rooms with multiple stuffed chairs and couches, plus many small end tables. These rooms are furnished to accommodate large family gatherings while allowing for the men to congregate in one room and the women in the other. If there is only one sitting room, women may congregate in the kitchen area, or men will congregate outside if weather permits.

Implications for Nursing Care

It is essential to remember that close proximity is reserved for family and that all children have close contact with adult family members. Therefore, the astute nurse should remember that because Jordanians are highly affiliative and tend to value close proximity within the extended family group, it is important to respect distance in the relationship between the nurse and client. In addition, it may be necessary to include the entire extended family in the plan of care for the Jordanian client.

SOCIAL ORGANIZATION

Regardless of religion, social life and identity are centered on the family and family roles. The extended family and patrilineal family ties to clans and tribes persist in modern-day Jordan. For example, after marriage both Christian and Muslim women may keep their family name, and the children take the name of the father. Gender and age affect roles in the family, with home life being a focus of women and higher social status afforded to older members of the family. Children are highly valued in the Arab culture, and infertility is viewed as a significant problem in the family context and for the couple, especially the woman. Traditionally, women were expected to have children very soon after marriage, and the birth of a son was an important milestone of achievement for the woman and for the individual nuclear family. However, in Jordan, violence against

women may occur when family "honor" is threatened. The most extreme form of violence against women is an "honor killing." Human Rights Watch continues to publicly object to Jordanian law where murder of a relative believed to be engaged in extramarital sex carries a reduced sentence as a function of protecting the family's honor (Human Rights Watch, 2009). Thus an intentional or unintentional violation (e.g., rape or even suspicion of sexual activity) can bring dishonor. Thus, the family, not just the spouse or father, may perceive the social injury and feel compelled to act on it. Therefore, in situations where cultural ties are still strong, the family may condone and contribute to domestic violence against women by male family members (including siblings and uncles).

As with other immigrant populations, the degree of acculturation will depend upon the time since immigration, proximity to communities of similar ethnic background, and how closely the migrated family maintains contacts with the family of origin. Jordan has enjoyed a positive political relationship with the United States for many years (U.S. Department of State, 2014). As a result, short-term visas for entry into the United States have always been available under certain conditions. Conversely, visas to enter Jordan have few limitations. Owing to the emphasis on family connections, even those who are U.S. born are readily welcomed back into the family group with few reservations. Many families also sponsor the immigration of other family members into the United States. As a result, a given family may be able to maintain a strong Jordanian identity some generations after immigration.

Even today, it is not uncommon for a Jordanian-American man to travel to Jordan just to find a suitable spouse. Although these marriages are not arranged in the strict sense, the family plays an important part in finding and approving the final choice. Family background is extremely relevant to the suitability of a prospective bride or groom. This is but one reason why spouses are often selected from within the extended family. However, culturally preferred consanguinity poses significant risks; as a result, mandatory premarital genetic testing for β–thalassemia carriers began in 2004 (Hamamy, Al-Hait, Alwan, & Ajlouni, 2007).

Religion

Although many Americans view Arabs as Muslim, the social and political history of Jordan includes both the Christian and Muslim religions. Because Christian Arabs immigrated to the United States much earlier than most Muslims, this subpopulation may not be as readily visible as more recent Muslim arrivals. For example, the churches in Jordan are almost exclusively Orthodox Catholic but include others, such as Seventh Day Adventist and Baptist churches. In the United States, there are numerous Maronite Catholic churches that provide services in Arabic. Thus, Arab Americans can maintain religious and language traditions long after immigrating.

On the other hand, the growth of Islam in America is much more recent. However, mosques also provide instruction in Arabic because their holy book is in Arabic. Their tradition states that the meaning of the text is purer in Arabic and that translation dilutes the intended meaning. As a result, Jordanian-American children can receive ongoing religious and language instruction that reinforces the traditional values and ethnic identity of the family. The number of mosques in the United States has grown significantly, with 1583 mosques counted in 2006 (The Pluralism Project, 2006), up from 1209 in 2001 and 962 in 1994. In 2001, 32% of mosques were started in the 1980s, and 30% were established in the 1990s. About 80% are located in metropolitan neighborhoods, with fewer in the West than in other regions of the country. Mosque membership is diverse, but the average percentage of Arab Americans is 25% nationally. Of the general membership, 75% are men, 81% have high school diplomas, 48% are college graduates, 47% are age 35 or younger, 11% are over age 60, and 24% have household incomes below $20,000, compared with the U.S. median household income of $41,000 (Bagby, Perl, & Froehle, 2001).

In general, Jordanians are Sunni Muslims who are characterized as more moderate in their practices than, for example, the Shiites of Iran. Islam has some important rubrics and practices that should inform health care delivery and nursing practice. The duties of Muslims for the five pillars of Islamic faith are *shahada,* affirmation of the faith; *salat,* daily prayer; *sakat,* almsgiving; *sawm,* fasting during the month of Ramadan; and *hajj,* pilgrimage to Mecca (Metz, 1989). In addition, abstinence from alcohol, abstaining from sex outside of marriage, and dietary restriction against pork or pork products are important prohibitions. Islam encourages women (and girls after the onset of menses) to be devout by being modest in dress and action. This includes not drawing attention to themselves by speaking loudly or displaying their beauty, particularly their hair, in the presence of men outside the immediate family. Among Sunni Muslims, the choice and degree of "covering" is the choice of the individual woman and is not supposed to be coerced by spouse or family. Some women choose to cover themselves from head to toe by wearing a headscarf, veil, gloves, and a floor-length skirt, all in black. However, this practice is not common among Jordanian women. More often, Jordanian-Muslim women do not cover their faces and will wear head scarves that compliment their long coatlike dresses that cover their usual clothing (e.g., slacks and blouses).

Religion, either the tradition of Christianity or Islam, is woven into the fabric of family history and identity. Thus, Jordanian-American families may have very strong feelings against marriage outside the faith. In particular, women may suffer family expulsion for dating a man who is not of the same faith. Further, interfaith marriages are likely to suffer from forced isolation and will lose access to important family supports. This can have a long-term impact on both parties, such that the woman may lose the support of her mother, sisters, and aunts for her maternal role and the man may lose financial and occupational contacts for employment or business.

Implications for Nursing Care

Because of the emphasis on confidentiality in health care, it may seem awkward when the families of Jordanian patients offer little privacy during encounters with health care providers. In order to balance the imperatives of patient confidentiality and the cultural norms of the patient, it is always advisable to ask permission from the patient before discussing their health matters in front of family members who may be present. This may be particularly important if the nurse suspects rape, abuse, or suspicious accidents. Also, nurses should be aware that the virginity status of unmarried woman of any age is an extremely sensitive and serious issue. Although this may become a standard practice in many settings, it is better for the nurse to err on the side of protecting the privacy and safety of all patients. This may include taking immediate action when protective services are indicated (e.g., a women's shelter or protective custody of a minor).

Dietary issues, fasting during Ramadan, and limited cross-gender contact present important challenges for direct nursing care. Nursing staff must be attentive to provide food that does not violate religious or cultural preferences. That is, patients and families will need assurance that meals provided will be *halal* (kosher) or they may not eat at all. Likewise, nurses must be aware of the practice of fasting from food and water over daylight hours during the month of Ramadan. Although the seriously ill are exempt from this religious requirement, nurses will need to assess and counsel diabetic patients about their individual risks before Ramadan begins. Safe adjustments can be made in medication dosing based on having only early morning and late night meals, but patients need careful anticipatory education to avoid complications (Al-Arouj et al., 2005). In addition, adult Muslim patients may refuse care by health care providers of the opposite sex, even in emergency settings, particularly if care involves intimate contact (Padela, Schneider, He, Ali, & Richardson, 2010). Thus, nursing staff should anticipate this sensitivity about cross-gender interaction with Muslim patients to avoid mis-communication that can interfere with delivering quality nursing care.

Given the increasing number of Arab and Middle-Eastern immigrants to the United States, it is important to recognize the role of religion in the lives of these special groups. In addition, we all need to be aware of prevalent stereotypes that infer that every Arab or every person wearing a black-and-white Palestinian scarf is a Muslim, which is not true. Even so, the increasing religious diversity of the population simply means that nurses need a working understanding of related practices and how they may affect patient behavior and nursing practice. When the objective is providing better care for patients, community and religious leaders can also serve a key role in providing contacts and access to hard-to-reach groups in their midst. For example, the recent innovation of "parish nursing" can be extrapolated to offering services for women and children at a local mosque. Thus, nurses and local health care agencies can capitalize on how religious tradition brings these immigrant communities together to improve access to care overall.

TIME

Because of the importance of family history, honor, and continuity, Arabs tend to value the past as an important part of identity. Right living and moral behavior in the present are viewed as contributing to maintaining the family, the most important construct in Islamic society, and to the good of the greater community. The common belief of Muslims and Christians in an afterlife, heaven and hell, and the eternal nature of the soul also conveys the importance of present behavior on the future.

Like people in many developing countries, Jordanians are not dependent on the clock, and attention to timekeeping is likely an index of acculturation to the American way of life. Because social networks play such an important part in daily life, Jordanian Americans may expect allowances in regard to arriving late or early for appointments. If there is some perceived urgency or special circumstance involved, Jordanians are likely to press time limits and are willing to request favors from personal contacts or to argue their case with strangers.

Because new immigrants may be unfamiliar with the limits of scheduling systems, it would be appropriate to explain the limits of clinic and laboratory hours in out-patient settings. It would also be reasonable to carefully outline how to obtain urgent care services after hours and on weekends, particularly for young mothers and for families with small children. Given the intrinsic value of children, families are more than willing to comply

with complicated treatment plans if the behaviors or expectations are congruent with their belief systems and within their economic and physical ability to achieve them.

Health care providers can reinforce compliance with treatment strategies and care plans by emphasizing the importance of regular immunizations and well-baby checkups on health and development. The primary health care model is not unfamiliar to recent immigrants from Jordan, and their culture reinforces the value of personal efforts to generate positive health outcomes.

Implications for Nursing Care

Recognizing that an immigrant family may not have ready access to transportation or that the number of small children in a household complicates even short excursions for clinic visits is an important aspect of care planning. Social service programs and home health visits may be needed in communities where there are income and language barriers among newly immigrated families. In these settings, it would be most appropriate for local agencies to create alliances with local mosques and Islamic centers to develop a collaborative referral system or social service programs for their members. One report, *The Mosque in America*, by Bagby et al. (2001), describes many programs offered at mosques that can be used as models for new programs in collaboration with existing community agencies.

ENVIRONMENTAL CONTROL

In Islamic countries, there is a saying central to the culture that has two meanings: "God willing" or "if God wills it" (إنْ شاءَ الله pronounced "in sha'allah"). In the strictest sense, the phrase asserts and confirms the absolute dependence of humankind on the beneficence of a higher power. Islam is built upon this premise, and the Islamic view of life is constructed around it. Both good and bad events are attributed to God's will. As a result, members of this culture may accept illness with resignation and fatalism. Although this belief may be an underlying tenet, it has not kept Islamic societies from adopting and using primary health care models or from Westernizing health care delivery systems. Like many new immigrant groups, for Jordanian Americans barriers to obtaining health care services are usually related to language, transportation, economic status, number of dependents in the home, and/or the severity and chronicity of diseases of family members. Without the ability to communicate and sufficient resources to access necessary health care services, families may be overwhelmed by the apparent hopelessness of their circumstances and thereby seek psychological and emotional solace in accepting "God's will." However, this is a normal adaptive response to extremes of stress, which can be refocused with the help of the nurse. To illustrate this point, it is common practice in the Arab culture to withhold informing seriously ill patients that they have a cancer diagnosis. Between family and patients, it becomes the classic "Don't ask, don't tell" situation. The intent on both sides is to protect the other from being upset. However, when King Hussein was diagnosed with and treated for cancer in the early 1990s, his diagnosis was made public. As a result of this cultural breakthrough, private citizens funded the first cancer hospital in the Middle East, El Amal Hospital in Amman (الأمل). The name of the hospital translated in English is "hope." This also illustrates the second meaning of "in sha'allah"—the speaker acknowledges that, with effort and some degree of good fortune, the desired outcome will be achieved. This additional meaning conveys recognition that a given individual may do all that is expected, but other circumstances may have a greater impact on the outcome. So when the nurse instructs a family member on a regimen of care for a patient, the reply may be "in sha'allah," which means "I will try." The health care provider who recommends a treatment that does not have a 100% cure rate could also use this phrase. This would affirm hope for the best results, even though a total cure cannot be guaranteed.

Folk Beliefs and Folk Practices

Jordan is no longer a developing country and has progressed to having a nationalized health care system. Public and private health care services and pharmacies are becoming more numerous every year, and the use of folk medicine is becoming less common. However, there are some traditions that persist or that may be seen among immigrants. As observed in many other cultures, the "evil eye" is a negative force, and small children are most vulnerable (Zahr & Hattar-Pollara, 1998). A blue glass amulet resembling an eye configured in the palm of an upraised hand is a common symbol in the culture. It is not unusual to see toddlers with a small blue eye amulet pinned to their clothing to ward off evil and protect the child from harm. In addition, among Muslims there is a folk belief that fear or being frightened can induce sudden fever, sleeplessness, and malaise among children as well as adults. The treatment for this condition is to use a special bowl with inscriptions from the Qur'an. Water is placed in the bowl and left overnight. In the morning the ill person drinks the water from the bowl while the prayers inscribed on the rim of the bowl are read. However, these practices have more significance among older or less educated persons and may not be encountered among immigrants, who are likely to be better educated.

Illness and Wellness Behaviors

Westernization of lifestyle and diet is emerging as an important health problem in Jordan. In studies of health-promoting lifestyles, many Jordanians, particularly women, demonstrate the erosion of healthy behaviors by modernization (Haddad, Shoater, Al-Zyoud, & Umlauf, 2010; Kofahi & Haddad, 2005; Madanat, Brown, & Hawks, 2007). The aggressive marketing of high-fat fast food products in the Middle East has also compounded the negative effect of a Westernized lifestyle on health outcomes. Diseases that have been common in Western countries for many years—obesity, diabetes, and hypertension (HTN)—have increased in Jordan as lifestyle and diet have become more Westernized (Madanat, Troutman, & Al-Madi, 2008). For example, a recent epidemiological survey in Jordan (n = 1121) reported an increase in the age-standardized prevalence for obesity in northern Jordan (28.1% men, 53.1% women) (Khader, Batieha, Ajlouni, El-Khateeb, & Ajlouni, 2008). This notable difference between men and women was irrespective of age or measure used. In addition, body mass index–defined obesity and high waist circumference were significantly associated with impaired fasting glycemia, diabetes mellitus, HTN, low HDL-cholesterol and hypertriglyceridemia.

In addition, smoking in Jordan is an important health risk, and the prevalence has always been very high (44% men; 5% women). Likewise, smoking is also common among adolescents aged 12 to 18 years (32% males; 11% females) and among college students (50% males; 6.5% females) (Corrao, Guindon, Sharma, & Shokoohi, 2000; Haddad & Malak, 2002). Women and youths are more likely to smoke in private and in their homes (Warren et al., 2000). This pattern of behavior contributes to passive smoke exposure of children throughout the day, not just when the men are home. Because of the strong influence of culture and marketing in the United States and Jordan, smoking cessation may be particularly difficult for Jordanian Americans. Thus, culturally specific and culturally sensitive antismoking programs should be developed to reach this high-risk and traditionally insulated segment of the population.

Cumulatively, many studies show the potent negative impact of adopting a Westernized lifestyle (a high-fat diet, high sodium intake, exercise avoidance, and stress) in lieu of maintaining the healthy aspects of a native culture. Metabolic syndrome is becoming more common in Jordan (Khader, Batieha, El-Khateeb, Al-Shaikh, & Ajlouni, 2007) and obesity is significantly associated with high blood pressure, high cholesterol, and asthma (Zindah, Belbeisi, Walke, & Mokdad, 2008). Nurses and other health care providers would do well to encourage maintenance of the traditional Mediterranean diet, exercise, and health-promoting behaviors that were indigenous in the culture traditionally.

Death Rituals or Customs

Islamic cultures have burial traditions that reflect practices of people who lived in hot climates. One important difference is that burial is expected to occur soon after death, the same day or no later than the afternoon of the next. Among Muslims, the body is prepared for burial by washing it and wrapping it in white linens. Christians, on the other hand, dress the body for burial in good clothing, more like the American custom. However, embalming is not customary in Jordan, and the notion of autopsy is very distasteful to Arabs in general. In contrast, organ donation is viewed as a positive gesture when indicated.

Implications for Nursing Care

Without a basic understanding of the distinct culture of modern Jordan, the unique health needs of Jordanian-American families might be overlooked. For example, smoking is already endemic in Arab populations, and the adoption of the poor eating habits of our indigenous population (high-fat fast foods) through acculturation is an alarming trend. Thus, programs designed to address health initiatives may need to be adapted to make them acceptable and effective among Jordanian Americans.

BIOLOGICAL VARIATIONS

Given that Jordan is located in the Eastern Mediterranean, the people of the area typically have olive or medium dark complexions, smaller stature, brown eyes, and dark straight or curly hair. In recent history, military occupation by the British, Turks, and others have added to the gene pool blue eyes, taller stature, fair complexions, and lighter hair coloring. Arabs are also known for having large noses and skin that tans easily. This may be an adaptive physiological mutation associated with the desert climate of the area.

Nutritional Preferences and Deficiencies

The traditional diet of Jordanians is described as the Mediterranean diet, which primarily includes fresh fruits and vegetables, bread, olive oil, nuts, and legumes (beans and lentils). This diet has been described as one of the most healthful in terms of preventing cardiovascular disease and cancer (Willett et al., 1995). Although Jordanian-American youth are susceptible to adopting Western eating habits in order to be accepted by peers, persons of all ages in the United States are at nutritional risk. However, the Westernization of lifestyle and dietary practices in Jordan has resulted in the same chronic metabolic and cardiovascular diseases found in the United States.

Genetic Variations

Cultural and religious pressures to maintain coherent family groups has contributed to the prevalence of consanguineous marriage in Jordan and many Middle Eastern countries. According to the March of Dimes *Global Report on Birth Defects* (Christianson, Howson, & Modell, 2006), the rate of birth defects in Jordan is one of the highest in the world (73.3 per 1000 live births). Other countries in the Middle East share similar high rankings for congenital birth defects because of the cultural preference for consanguinity. For example, a study of 3269 new mothers in northern Jordan found that 49% had consanguineous marriages (Obeidat, Khader, Aarin, Kassawneh, & Al Omari, 2010). In this sample, the rates of low birth weight (13.9% vs. 10.1%), preterm delivery (19.9% vs. 12.3%), and births with congenital anomalies (4.1% vs. 0.8%) were greater in consanguineous families. Further, the odds ratios (ORs) for preterm delivery (OR = 1.5, 95% confidence interval [CI] 1.2, 1.9) and congenital malformations (OR = 6.5, 95% CI 2.8, 15.3) were significantly associated with consanguinity.

Numerous genetic conditions commonly found in Jordan are likely to be found among Jordanian Americans. These include Bardet Biedl and Meckel syndromes, phenylketonuria (Teebi, 1994), congenital nephrotic syndrome (Hamed & Shomaf, 2001), thrombophilia (Awidi et al., 1993), cystic fibrosis (Rawashdeh & Manal, 2000), glucose-6-phosphate dehydrogenase deficiency (Karadsheh, Moses, Ismail, Devaney, & Hoffman, 2005), and muscular dystrophy (Al-Din et al., 1995; Al-Qudah & Tarawneh, 1998; Najim Al-Din et al., 1996). The most common inherited conditions are familial Mediterranean fever (FMF) and various types of hemoglobinopathies, which are otherwise uncommon in the United States.

Familial Mediterranean fever or familial paroxysmal peritonitis is characterized by recurrent high fever and peritonitis with infrequent symptoms of pleuritis, arthritis, skin lesions, and pericarditis. This disease is chronically episodic, with a usual onset between ages 5 and 15 years. The severity and frequency of attacks are variable and tend to decrease with age, during pregnancy, or when resulting in amyloidosis. This condition is sporadic, and no laboratory tests are diagnostic. Early manifestation of the disease may be mistaken for appendicitis or perforated bowel and result in unnecessary surgical intervention. As a result, diagnosis depends upon clinical findings and presentation, including ethnicity; positive family history; recurrent, self-limited peritonitis; and excellent health otherwise (Beers & Berkow, 1999). FMF is an autosomal recessive trait that apparently demonstrates a diverse number of genetic mutations in the Jordanian population (Hamamy, Al-Hait, Alwan, & Ajlouni, 2007; Medlej-Hashim et al., 2000).

Thalassemia is an autosomal-dominant microcytic anemia that is particularly common in Jordanians and persons of Mediterranean ancestry. Thalassemia (Mediterranean anemia, thalassemia major or minor) describes a heterogeneous group of hereditary disorders that involve defective hemoglobin synthesis and ineffective erythropoiesis (Beers & Berkow, 1999). It is broadly classified into two types of disorders according to the affected hemoglobin chain synthesis: alpha (associated with a reduced or absent alpha-chain synthesis) and beta (associated with a reduced or absent beta-chain synthesis). In beta-thalassemia, persons with a single gene are carriers and have asymptomatic mild to moderate microcytic anemia (thalassemia minor), which seldom requires treatment. Persons with two genes have a severe, potentially life-threatening anemia (thalassemia major, Cooley's anemia) with hemoglobin values under 6 g/dL. Inheritance of both sickle cell and thalassemia genes is also a common finding in Jordan. Thus, because Jordanian Americans may still follow the cultural preference for consanguineous marriages, these relatively unusual disorders may appear more frequently in the United States than in the past.

Implications for Nursing Care

When providing genetic and reproductive counseling for Muslim families, the nurse should be aware of how Islam views various forms of assisted reproduction and contraception. First, there are no prohibitions in Islam against contraception as long as it is temporary in nature. Because large families are viewed as desirable, contraception is an important aspect of helping women with birth spacing. However, sterilization is not supported in Islam unless the health of the mother would be endangered by pregnancy or when there are already children in the home with serious inherited disorders (Albar, 1999).

Further, infertility and genetic problems are serious family situations. For example, in Jordan Islamic law recognizes infertility as sufficient grounds for divorce. Options for increasing family size that Americans take for granted are not necessarily viable options in Jordanian families. For example, adoption of foundlings or children from outside the family group is a rare and unusual circumstance in Jordan or in Islamic societies. Even then, the adoption is acceptable only as long as the child retains his or her original family name. The importance of family lineage in Muslim cultures is so strong that changing the child's name is viewed as unacceptable.

In addition, fertility options involving surrogacy or donated sperm, eggs, or pre-embryos are not acceptable in Islam because procreation is limited to participation by husband and wife alone. Various forms of diagnostic screening of congenital malformations are also acceptable during pregnancy. That is, genetic diagnosis, in vitro fertilization, and implantation of blastulae free of defects are acceptable practices to Muslims. According to Islamic law, abortion is acceptable under certain specific conditions:

1. A committee of specialized physicians has determined that the fetus is grossly malformed and that its life would be a calamity for both the family and itself.
2. The malformation must be untreatable, unmanageable, and very serious.
3. The abortion may only be carried out prior to day 120 after conception (Albar, 1999).

Islamic law, however, does not provide guidance for conditions such as Down syndrome, phenylketonuria, or thalassemia, which fall in a gray ethical area. In the end, nurses must acknowledge that couples may choose to follow or reject these guidelines based on individual circumstances. The cultural value of children and family life may ultimately outweigh religious prohibitions against treatment options that are readily available in the United States.

SUMMARY

Although many Jordanian Americans have lived in the United States for many years, they seldom relinquish their identity as Arabs or their religious heritage. Like waves of immigrants over the past centuries, these groups will establish new roots in the United States while retaining many of the traditions of their homelands. Our own history shows that these transplanted groups maintain a unique identity for long periods in spite of great distances. However, with advances in electronic communication and the ease of travel, immigrants may retain their original cultural identities longer than ever before. In any case, nurses must be prepared to provide care that is culturally sensitive, culturally adapted, and translated into Arabic, if necessary. One of the hallmarks of nursing is that the best nurses are always learning and growing professionally. Thus, learning about new cultures is not just an added burden but adds to the diversity of the practice of nursing itself.

CASE STUDY

Mr. Ali Hamad has brought his 67-year-old father, Issa, to the primary care clinic. Ali is a computer engineer who immigrated to the United States 8 years ago, but his recently widowed father has only been in the States for about 2 months. The son has brought his father to the clinic because he has run out of the blood pressure medications that he brought from Jordan. The son can only provide a limited health history for his father who speaks only Arabic. "My father tells me that he takes blood pressure medicine but cannot tell me the name of it. But I have noticed that he gets up several times at night to use the toilet to urinate and his clothing is getting tighter through the middle." The patient's vital signs are as follows: temperature, 97.5° F; pulse, 76; respirations, 24; blood pressure 140/95, height, 5′ 3″; weight, 177 lb; BMI, 31.4. The cardiovascular exam findings include the following: heart sounds are regular rate and rhythm, apical and radial pulses are equal, pulses are equal bilaterally, no carotid or abdominal bruits, but positive for edema of feet and ankles. The patient appears to be in no acute distress and is dressed appropriately. With the son providing translation of instructions, a clean catch urine specimen was obtained (nitrites: negative; glucose: positive). During the exam, the nurse inquires about relevant cultural or religious health practices. The patient's son reports that his father will insist on fasting during Ramadan, which is about 2 months away. After consulting with the physician about findings of metabolic syndrome, the nurse orders a complete metabolic profile, CBC, EKG, CXR, and a consultation with the clinic diabetic education specialist who is knowledgeable about the implications of fasting during Ramadan.

◎ CARE PLAN

Nursing Diagnosis: Communication, impaired verbal, related to cultural differences

Client Outcome	Nursing Interventions
Client will use alternate methods of communication effectively.	1. Communicate with the patient (Issa) through his son (Ali). 2. Obtain translator, if necessary, for communicating technical medical explanations and dietary plans. 3. Inquire if the family has additional support available to assist with meal planning. 4. Accept communication style of Jordanians, who raise their voices when excited. 5. Use visual aids and written pamphlets when explaining medical and nutritional interventions. Provide educational materials and dietary planning materials in Arabic.

Nursing Diagnosis: Ineffective therapeutic regimen management

Client Outcome	Nursing Interventions
Client's family will reduce illness symptoms of family members.	1. Teach family about necessity of monitoring blood sugar multiple times each day and the importance of meal planning and caloric management. 2. Teach family about the roles of the diabetic educator and the clinic staff in supporting patients with newly diagnosed type 2 diabetes. 3. Have lab work drawn by an individual who is the same sex as client (male draws male, female draws female). 4. Explain limits of clinic and laboratory hours. 5. Explain how the patient can obtain urgent care services when the clinic is closed. 6. Explain importance of follow-up care for Issa at the clinic and with the diabetic educator to keep him healthy. Type 2 diabetes requires long-term management rather than a one-time treatment or cure. 7. Identify potential support groups within Muslim community for others with diabetes who are planning to fast during Ramadan. 8. Give written instructions and explanations regarding all of this information. Provide materials in Arabic.

Nursing Diagnoses—Definitions and Classifications 2012–2014. Copyright © 2012, 1994–2012 by NANDA International. Used by arrangement with Wiley-Blackwell Publishing, a company of John Wiley and Sons, Inc. In order to make safe and effective judgments using NANDA-I nursing diagnoses it is essential that nurses refer to the definitions and defining characteristics of the diagnoses listed in the work.

CLINICAL DECISION MAKING

1. Describe the geographical location of Jordan, and indicate how this region of the world and the political turmoil experienced by Jordanians may have a profound political impact on the health and well-being of recently immigrated Jordanian Americans.
2. Describe culturally competent techniques the nurse can use to facilitate communication with the Jordanian client who speaks some English but mostly Arabic.
3. Describe the five pillars of Islam, and relate these pillars to the care of the Jordanian-American client.
4. Describe the role of women in traditional Muslim society and relate how this role assignment might affect rendering culturally competent care.
5. Describe how the observance of Ramadan may affect the rendering of culturally competent care and identify ways to effectively alter care plans to accommodate the client and the family during this period of extended fasting.
6. Relate how the culturally competent nurse who is from a different cultural and religious orientation can learn to appreciate the differences between personal religious values and those of the Islamic client.
7. Describe the Islamic view or locus of control and how this may possibly affect the plan of care.
8. Describe the values, beliefs, and attitudes of some Jordanian Americans regarding infertility, artificial insemination, and adoption and how these variables may affect health care choices. Explain how the astute nurse may intervene in a culturally sensitive way to assist the client and family in efficacious decision-making.

REVIEW QUESTIONS

1. A female student nurse who is caring for a dying Jordanian patient who is Muslim is annoyed when the family rewashes him after she has already bathed him. The student's annoyance is most likely a sign of which of the following?
   a. Confusion associated with lack of adequate cultural knowledge
   b. Intolerance associated with immaturity
   c. Anxiety due to the student nurse's lack of organization
   d. Appropriate commitment to hospital procedures
2. When Muslims visit dying family members in a hospital setting, as a part of their culture they are obligated/required to do which of the following?
   a. Be accepting of visitor limitations
   b. Visit five times a day
   c. Visit 5 consecutive days with the sick family member
   d. Remain until death
3. An Islamic practice regarding death and burial for the Islamic is that practices centering on the dead must focus on which of the following?
   a. Buried facing the holy city of Mecca
   b. Buried only after an autopsy is performed
   c. Buried after embalming within 3 days
   d. Buried with no embalming the same day or no more than 24 hours after death

REFERENCES

100 questions and answers about Arab Americans. (2001). Accessed at <http://www.bintjbeil.com/E/news/100q/index.html> Retrieved November 16, 2014.

Al-Arouj, M., et al. (2005). Recommendations for management of diabetes during Ramadan. *Diabetes Care, 28*(9), 2305–2311.

Albar, M. A. (1999). Counseling about genetic disease: an Islamic perspective. *Eastern Mediterranean Health Journal, 5*(6), 1129–1133.

Al-Din, A. S., et al. (1995). Multiple sclerosis in Arabs in Jordan. *Journal of the Neurological Sciences, 131*(2), 144–149.

Al-Qudah, A. A., & Tarawneh, M. (1998). Congenital muscular dystrophy in Jordanian children. *Journal of Child Neurology, 13*(8), 383–386.

Awidi, A. S., et al. (1993). Hereditary thrombophilia among 217 consecutive patients with thromboembolic disease in Jordan. *American Journal of Hematology, 44*(2), 95–100.

Bagby, I., Perl, P. M., & Froehle, B. T. (2001). *The mosque in America: a national portrait*. Washington, DC: Council on American-Islamic Relations.

Beers, M. H., & Berkow, R. (Eds.), (1999). *Merck manual of diagnosis and treatment*. Whitehouse Station, NJ: Merck.

Central Intelligence Agency (CIA) (2015). *The world factbook*. Available at <https://www.cia.gov/library/publications/the-world-factbook/geos/jo.html> Retrieved November 16, 2014.

Christianson, A., Howson, C. P., & Modell, B. (2006). *Global report on birth defects*. White Plains, NY: March of Dimes Birth Defects Foundation.

Corrao, M. A., Guindon, G. E., Sharma, N., & Shokoohi, D. F. (Eds.), (2000). *Tobacco control country profiles*. Atlanta: American Cancer Society.

Department of Statistics (Hashemite Kingdom of Jordan) and Macro International Inc. (2010). *Jordan population and family health survey 2009*. Calverton, MD: Department of Statistics and Macro International Inc.

Embassy of Jordan (Hashemite Kingdom of Jordan) (2012). *Fact sheets, overview*. Available at <http://jordanembassyus.org/page/economy#> Retrieved November 16, 2014.

Haddad, L. G., & Malak, M. Z. (2002). Smoking habits and attitudes towards smoking among university students in

Jordan. *International Journal of Nursing Studies, 39*(8), 793–802.

Haddad, L., Shoater, A., Al-Zyoud, S., & Umlauf, M. G. (2010). Knowledge, attitudes and beliefs of Jordanian high school students about substance abuse. *Journal of Transcultural Nursing, 21*(2), 143–150.

Hamamy, H., Al-Hait, S., Alwan, A., & Ajlouni, K. (2007). Jordan: communities and community genetics. *Community Genetics, 10*, 52–60.

Hamed, R. M., & Shomaf, M. (2001). Congenital nephrotic syndrome: a clinico-pathologic study of thirty children. *Journal of Nephrology, 14*(2), 104–109.

Hattar-Pollara, M., & Meleis, A. I. (1995). Parenting their adolescents: the experiences of Jordanian immigrant women in California. *Health Care for Women International, 16*, 195–211.

Human Rights Watch (2009). *Jordan: tribunals no substitute for reforms on "honor killings" changes to penal code needed to help save women's lives.* Available at <http://www.hrw.org/news/2009/09/01/jordan-tribunals-no-substitute-reforms-honor-killings> Retrieved December 2, 2014.

Karadsheh, N. S., Moses, L., Ismail, S. I., Devaney, J. M., & Hoffman, E. (2005). Molecular heterogeneity of glucose-6-phosphate dehydrogenase deficiency in Jordan. *Haematologica, 90*, 1693–1694.

Khader, Y., Batieha, A., Ajlouni, H. M., El-Khateeb, M., & Ajlouni, K. (2008). Obesity in Jordan: prevalence, associated factors, comorbidities and change in prevalence over ten years. *Metabolic Syndrome and Related Disorders, 6*(2), 113–120.

Khader, Y., Batieha, A., El-Khateeb, M., Al-Shaikh, A., & Ajlouni, K. (2007). High prevalence of the metabolic syndrome among northern Jordanians. *Journal of Diabetes and Its Complications, 21*, 214–219.

Kofahi, M. M., & Haddad, L. G. (2005). Perceptions of lung cancer and smoking among college students in Jordan. *Journal of Transcultural Nursing, 16*(3), 245–254.

Madanat, H. N., Brown, R. B., & Hawks, S. R. (2007). The impact of body mass index and Western advertising and media on eating style, body image and nutrition transition among Jordanian women. *Public Health Nutrition, 10*(10), 1039–1046.

Madanat, H. N., Troutman, K. P., & Al-Madi, B. (2008). The nutrition transition in Jordan: the political, economic and food consumption contexts. *Promotion & Education, 15*(1), 6–10.

Medlej-Hashim, M., et al. (2000). Genetic screening of fourteen mutations in Jordanian familial Mediterranean fever patients. *Human Mutation, 15*(4), 384.

Metz, H. C. (Ed.). (1989). *Jordan: a country study.* Washington, DC: GPO for the Library of Congress.

Najim Al-Din, A. A., Kurdi, A., Mubaidin, A., El-Khateeb, M., Khalil, R. W., & Wriekat, A. L. (1996). Epidemiology of multiple sclerosis in Arabs in Jordan: a comparative study between Jordanians and Palestinians. *Journal of the Neurological Sciences, 135*(2), 162–167.

Obeidat, B. R., Khader, Y. S., Aarin, Z. O., Kassawneh, M., & Al Omari, M. (2010). Consanguinity and adverse pregnancy outcomes: the north of Jordan experience. *Maternal Child Health Journal, 14*, 283–289.

Padela, A. I., Schneider, S. M., He, H., Ali, Z., & Richardson, T. M. (2010). Patient choice of provider type in the emergency department: perceptions and factors relating to accommodation of requests for care providers. *Emergency Medical Journal, 27*(6), 465–469.

The Pluralism Project (2006). *The distribution of Muslim centers in the U.S.* Harvard University. Available at <http://www.pluralism.org/resources/statistics/distribution.php> Retrieved November 23, 2014.

Rawashdeh, M., & Manal, H. (2000). Cystic fibrosis in Arabs: a prototype from Jordan. *Annals of Tropical Paediatrics, 20*(4), 283–286.

Teebi, A. S. (1994). Autosomal recessive disorders among Arabs: an overview from Kuwait. *Journal of Medical Genetics, 31*(3), 224–233.

Time Almanac. (2011). *Time Almanac powered by Britannica.* Chicago: Encyclopedia Britannica.

U.S. Department of Commerce, Bureau of the Census (2013). *American Community Survey, Statistical portraits of the foreign-born.* Washington, DC: U.S. Government Printing Office. Available at: <http://www.census.gov/prod/2013pubs/acsbr10-20.pdf> Retrieved November 16, 2014.

U.S. Department of State (2014). Bureau of Near Eastern Affairs. *U.S. Relations with Jordan.* Available at <http://www.state.gov/r/pa/ei/bgn/3464.htm> Retrieved December 2, 2014.

Warren, C. W., et al. (2000). Tobacco use by youth: a surveillance report from the Global Youth Tobacco Survey project. *Bulletin of the World Health Organization, 78*(7), 868–876.

Willett, W. C., et al. (1995). Mediterranean diet pyramid: a cultural model for healthy eating. *American Journal of Clinical Nutrition, 61*(Suppl. 6), 1402S–1406S.

World Almanac. (2015). *Infobase Learning.* New York.

World Bank (2013). *World development indicators—Jordan.* Available at <http://data.worldbank.org/indicator/SP.POP.TOTL?cid=GPD_1> and <http://data.worldbank.org/topic/health?display=default> and <http://data.worldbank.org/indicator/SP.DYN.LE00.IN> Retrieved November 16, 2014.

Zahr, L. K., & Hattar-Pollara, M. (1998). Nursing care of Arab children: consideration of cultural factors. *Journal of Pediatric Nursing, 13*(6), 349–355.

Zindah, M., Belbeisi, A., Walke, H., & Mokdad, A. H. (2008). Obesity and diabetes in Jordan: findings from the Behavioral Risk Factor Surveillance System, 2004. *Preventing Chronic Disease, 5*(1), 1–8.

Cuban Americans

Thad Wilson and Miguel A. Franco

After reading this chapter, the nurse will be able to:

1. Describe verbal and nonverbal communication behaviors of persons of Cuban descent.
2. Have an awareness of Cuban Americans' spatial comfort zone.
3. Discuss family values that are commonly held by Cuban Americans.
4. Discuss the past-, present-, and future-time orientation that may be held by Cuban Americans, depending on generation of immigration.
5. Describe beliefs held by persons who espouse the cult of Santeria.
6. Discuss health problems that may be related to biological variations of persons of Cuban descent.

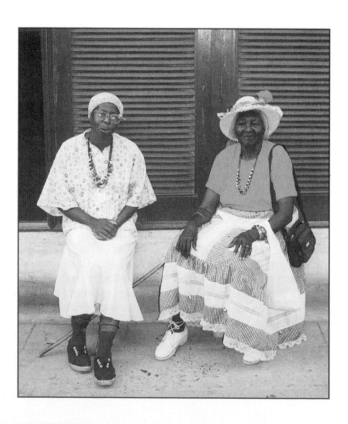

OVERVIEW OF CUBA

Cuba is located in the Caribbean on the westernmost part of the West Indies. To the north are Jamaica and the Bahamas, and to the south are the Cayman Islands and Haiti. Havana, on the northwest coast, is 90 miles from Florida's Key West, while the Pinar del Rio Province on the west coast is 130 miles from Mexico's Yucatan Peninsula. Cuba, an island of 42,803 square miles, is the largest island in the Caribbean and the fifteenth largest island in the world. Cuba also lays claim to a small island, Isla de la Juventud, and some 4200 coral cays and islets. Mountain ranges separate the country into three regions (*World Almanac, 2015*).

When Columbus reached Cuba in 1492, some 50,000 Indians, primarily fishermen and hunters, occupied the island. The island was conquered for the Spanish crown, and seven settlements were founded. In the early sixteenth century, the first Black slaves from Africa arrived in Cuba. These slaves were primarily Yoruba, from the southwestern part of Nigeria. The slaves brought aspects of their culture that are still present in food, music, and practices of spiritualism. Chinese workers were also brought to work in the sugarcane fields. Some of these workers were able to earn enough money to start their own businesses and married women from other ethnic groups, particularly *criollo* women (Spaniards born in the New World). Except for the British occupation of Havana in 1762–1763, Cuba remained under control of Spain until 1898. An economy driven by the slave-based sugar plantations was aided by mechanization of milling. Sugar continues to be the chief product and chief export to this day.

Despite numerous uprisings throughout the 1800s, Cuba remained under Spanish rule until José Martí, a Cuban national hero, championed a revolution in 1895. At that time the United States joined the international protest over Spain's treatment of Cuba. In 1898 the United States officially declared war on Spain in response to the sinking of the USS *Maine* in Havana. The Spanish–American War resulted in the defeat of Spain, and Cuba was granted its independence. During that period, an agreement was struck between the United States and Cuba that has had long-lasting effects in the minds of many exiled Cuban Americans. More specifically, according to the Platt Amendment to the Cuban constitution, the United States agreed to provide a military presence on the island to assist in maintaining the governmental stability initiated by the revolution. The U.S. peacekeepers remained in Cuba until 1934. However, a 99-year lease permits the United States to maintain a strategic naval base at Guantánamo Bay, on the southeast side of Cuba. To this day, many exiled Cuban Americans find comfort in knowing that the U.S. military

(whom many Cubans and Cuban Americans perceive as anti-Castro) still resides on the island.

In 1952, Fulgencio Batista seized control of the government, and a harsh dictatorship was established. However, Batista was overthrown in 1959, when Fidel Castro and a rebel band seized control. With Castro serving as the official head of state, sweeping economic and socialistic changes were initiated, and a system of cooperatives was instituted. Cattle, tobacco lands, banks, and other American interests were nationalized, with little provision for compensation to their former owners. Subsequently, relations with the United States were broken off, and a trade embargo, which remains in effect, was initiated. Poor sugar crops and the embargo further damaged the economy, and, in spite of aid from Communist countries, rationing practices were enacted. While civil unrest and various efforts to overthrow the regime occurred, Castro maintained control. In 1962, the United States discovered that the Soviet Union had brought nuclear missiles into Cuba. After a stern ultimatum from President John F. Kennedy on October 22, the missiles were removed. In 1967, in an overture to enhance relations, the United States and Cuba signed an agreement to exchange diplomats and to regulate offshore fishing. However, full ties were not restored, and some sanctions continued.

Throughout the 1970s and much of the 1980s, Cuba enjoyed the financial and political support of many Communist countries. Steady economic growth and advances were made in social security, public health, and education. However, the economy was severely hampered by the collapse of the Communist bloc in the late 1980s and the subsequent withdrawal of Soviet subsidies, worth $4 to $6 billion annually (Central Intelligence Agency [CIA], 2015). Increased trade sanctions by the United States also contributed to a deteriorating economic situation throughout the early 1990s. Trade sanctions were tightened even further in 1996, after two aircraft operated by an anti-Castro exile group based in Miami were shot down by Cuban Air Force pilots off the shores of Cuba. In an apparent humanitarian effort, Pope John Paul II visited Cuba in 1998 and called for an end to the U.S. economic sanctions. The pope urged Castro to release political prisoners and increase political and religious freedom. A softening of relations did occur, and sanctions were eased in 1999.

Cuba again made international news in 2000, when a Cuban child, Elián González, survived a capsized boat accident and was rescued off the Florida coast. After a 7-month legal battle, the U.S. government agreed, over the protestations of his relatives and the Cuban-American community in Miami, to return Elián to his father in Cuba (BBC News, 2000). This decision by the U.S. government led to subsequent changes. These included the passage of a bill allowing food and medicine sales to Cuba, somewhat relaxed travel regulations that allowed more Cuban Americans to visit Cuba, and Castro's decision to spend $120 million over a specified period to purchase food and agricultural products from key farm states. These actions energized pro-Cuba attitudes in the U.S. Congress, and the lifting of the trade embargo became a topic of debate (Kornbluh, 2002). The U.S. government tightened travel restrictions significantly in 2004 and again in 2006, allowing Cuban Americans to return to the island only once every 3 years instead of every year and restricting the amount of U.S. cash that can be spent there to $50 per day. In response, Cuba banned the use of dollars, which had been legal currency in the country for more than a decade (*Miami Herald*, 1999; *World Almanac*, 2015).

In 2006, Fidel Castro began transferring many powers over to his brother, Raul, because of personal illness. In February 2008, Fidel Castro formally resigned from office, ending an almost 50-year rule. Despite renewed U.S. economic interest in Cuba and some policy shifts under President Barack Obama (including legal travel to Cuba by students, churches, and cultural groups), experts agree that normalization of U.S.–Cuban relations was unlikely in the near future (Sweig, 2010). But when the Archbishop of Buenos Aires, Jorge Mario Bergoglio, was elected as Pope Francis in March 2013, he reached out to American President Barack Obama and Cuban leader Raul Castro in hopes of mending the diplomatic relations between the two countries. The Pope personally followed up and offered to mediate between the two countries as they held secret talks that spanned 18 months (Latza Nadeau, 2014). On December 17, 2014, Presidents Obama and Castro announced a deal to restore diplomatic relations and the liberalization of travel and remittances between their respective countries (White House, 2014).

Although the Obama administration would like to normalize relations with Cuba, there are still major hurdles to overcome. The president would like to lift the trade embargo, move Cuba toward democracy, and increase diplomatic presence in Cuba. But Congress is not likely to lift the embargo soon, and Cuba appears to have the goal of maintaining the status quo while maximizing the economic gain of the agreement and to be removed from the State Sponsors of Terrorism list (Robbins, 2015).

In 2014, Cuba had a population of 11,047,251 residents, representing ethnic groups that include mulatto and mestizo (26.6%), Black African (9.3%), and White (64.1%) (CIA, 2015; *World Almanac and Book of Facts*, 2015). The population was growing annually at a rate of 0.22% until 2008, when it began decreasing slightly (UN Data, 2014). Cuba has an aging population; 19.6% are over the age of 60 years, and this percentage is growing as the birthrate

remains low (UN Data, 2014). Havana has a population of 2.116 million people. Some 75% of the Cuban population is urban, with a population density of 262 per square mile (U.S. Department of State, 2015).

The island has 2500 miles of coastline. Low hills and fertile valleys cover more than half of the country, with 24% arable land. The chief crops include sugarcane, tobacco, rice, coffee, and citrus. There are 6000 plant species in Cuba, and land fauna includes crocodiles, lizards, and 15 species of snakes (CIA, 2015; *Lonely Planet World Guide*, 2010; *World Almanac*, 2015). Other resources include timber, cobalt, nickel, iron, copper, manganese, and salt. Pharmaceutical production is another source of Cuban development. More than 1000 people work at Cuba's Genetic Engineering and Biotechnological Center in Havana. Cuba's biotechnical products and technology currently reach markets in more than 40 countries and generate about $100 million annually (Evenson, 2007). The labor force of Cuba is 23% agricultural and 53% services. The gross domestic product is U.S. $72.3 billion, with a per capita gross domestic product of U.S. $10,200 (CIA, 2015). Major trading partners are Canada, China, Venezuela, the Netherlands, and Spain and a major shift away from Russia, China, Iran, and North Korea (CIA, 2015).

The tourism income is $1.846 billion (*World Almanac and Book of Facts*, 2015), and numerous travel guides outline opportunities in Cuba (e.g., Kindersley, 2011) as a vacation spot for cycling, travel, hiking, and swimming. Cuba is advertised as the Caribbean's largest and least commercialized island. The relative political isolation has prevented it from being overrun with tourists, a selling point used to promote Cuban travel in Canada and Europe (*Lonely Planet World Guide*, 2010). The peak tourist time is in the dry season from December to April, when planeloads of Canadians and Europeans arrive to enjoy the sun and beaches. Christmas, Easter, and the period around July 26 (the anniversary of the revolution) are also peak tourist times. The hotter wet season lasts from May to October and is also the time when hurricanes are most prevalent. The average annual temperature is 75° F.

Many Cuban citizens are experiencing an easing of political and religious restrictions. On the other hand, Cubans currently get by on an average monthly income in pesos equal to $8 to $20 a month, and state-rationing exacts a daily struggle (*Havana Guide*, 2010; UN Data, 2014). Cubans use their monthly income and ration cards for subsistence items in government peso stores in order to purchase rice, sugar, peas, cooking oil, tobacco, coffee, beans, and soap. Children under 7 may receive milk, some eggs, and meat, but otherwise meat and vegetables are not available at the government peso store. Other goods, including meat and more expensive items, are available at state-run stores. Many Cubans receive money from family members in other countries or a private income from pedaling bicycle rickshaws for tourists, running gypsy cabs, engaging in black market sales, opening small cafés in their homes, or renting rooms (*Havana Guide,* 2010). There is less poverty in Havana than in rural areas, since in Havana enterprising individuals can more easily supplement their peso income with personal and tourist-related enterprises.

Despite the U.S. embargo and the challenges faced after the fall of the Soviet Union, Cuba has produced better health outcomes than most Latin American countries (Drain & Barry, 2010; Hougendobler, 2014). In Cuba, the median age is 37.8 years; the life expectancy is 77.2 years for males and 81.2 years for females; and there are 11.02 births per 1000 and 7.29 deaths per 1000. The infant mortality rate is 4.5 per 1000. The number of persons in Cuba with human immunodeficiency virus (HIV) or acquired immunodeficiency virus (AIDS) is 3300 (>0.1%). There are 67.2 physicians per 10,000 inhabitants (CIA, 2015; Drain & Barry, 2010). Cuba spends 10.0% of the gross domestic product on health care, significantly less than the United States (17.9%) and most European countries. The positive health outcomes are probably more related to the focus on health and prevention of disease than on the amount of money spent (CIA, 2015; Drain & Barry, 2010).

IMMIGRATION TO THE UNITED STATES

Opportunities in the tobacco industry in Tampa and Miami between 1895 and 1905 resulted in the establishment of small, tight Cuban communities in these Florida cities (CIA, 2015; Varela, 2005). By settling within these communities, it became possible for these Cubans to retain a strong ethnic identity and maintain cultural values and practices. Another wave of immigrants came to the United States in the 1940s and 1950s for jobs related to military production and because increased trade and commerce between the United States and Cuba facilitated immigration.

When Castro assumed control in 1959, opponents were imprisoned or executed. Lack of promised liberties and the threat of Communist rule caused many middle- and upper-class individuals who had supported the Castro regime to immigrate to Miami, Tampa, and New York, thus expanding already existing Cuban settlements. It is estimated that, in the initial years of rule by Castro, some 700,000 Cubans emigrated, primarily to the United States (*World Almanac and Book of Facts,* 2015). It is significant to note that many of these individuals had grown accustomed to receiving high-quality health care as a result of their socioeconomic status prior to Castro's revolution. In contrast, some later immigrants who did not hold middle- and upper-class positions prior to the revolution were not accustomed to being benefactors of health care and did not come to the United States with the expectation of high-quality health care.

In 1978, as a result of pleas for liberation, Castro agreed to release political prisoners to the United States. Some 120,000 Cubans immigrated in 1980 in what was referred to as the *Mariel Boat Lift* (CIA, 2015; Varela, 2005). It was later determined that among these immigrants were mentally ill patients and criminals. Some of the criminals remained in jails in the United States until 1987, when Castro agreed to take back some 2500 Cuban prisoners. The 1987 agreement allowed 20,000 Cubans to immigrate to the United States each year. Many were relatives of those already in the United States. Cuban Americans represent one of the few minority groups in the United States who are predominantly refugees, not immigrants, many of them professionals and entrepreneurs.

In the 1990s, Cubans, desperate to get out of Cuba, increasingly tried to bypass the immigration regulations and make their way to Florida on small boats. Finally, in 1994, demonstrations against the Cuban government prompted loosening of the immigration restrictions, and a United States–Cuba accord was signed to end the illegal and dangerous exodus of "boat people." In 1995, U.S. policy shifted again with the announcement that 20,000 Cuban refugees held at the Guantánamo base would be admitted to the United States; however, any more boat people caught fleeing the island would be sent back to Cuba (*Miami Herald,* 1999). By 1999, it was estimated that 1550 Cubans had been repatriated under the immigration agreement (*Miami Herald,* 1999). Nevertheless, illicit migration to the United States using homemade rafts, alien smugglers, or falsified visas continues. In 2013, it was estimated that 14,251 Cubans crossed the straits to Florida and set foot on U.S. soil, with only 25% being deterred by the U.S. Coast Guard (CIA, 2015).

In 2010, 1.8 million people of Cuban descent were residing in the United States (Ennis, Ríos-Vargas, & Albert, 2011). The largest number of Hispanics in Florida are Cuban American (Ennis, Ríos-Vargas, & Albert, 2011). In a relatively short time, Cubans have been able to advance economically and obtain a higher standard of living in the United States than other Hispanic groups. Compared with other Hispanic groups, Cuban Americans have higher average educational attainment, larger family incomes, and lower poverty rates (U.S. Department of Commerce, Bureau of the Census, *American Community Survey,* 2015). For example, in 2011 the median annual individual income was $24,400, higher than the median earnings for all U.S. Hispanics ($20,000) but lower than the median earnings for the U.S. population ($29,000) (Brown & Patten, 2013).

Many Cuban Americans maintain the political stance of exiles waiting for Fidel Castro, and now his brother, to die or be overthrown (Anton & Hernandez, 2002). In fact, many identify themselves as "Cuban" despite having been born in the United States (Varela, 2005). Barlow, Taylor, and Lambert (2000) investigated "feelings of being American" among White-American, African-American, and Cuban-American women. In contrast to other groups, Cuban Americans reported neither feeling they were American nor believing that they were perceived as such by White Americans. However, feelings of inclusion increased with length of residence. The majority of the Cuban Americans in Miami-Dade County tend to be conservative, Republican, and anticommunist, though there may be a change away from the Republican party in the future (Moreno & Wyatt, 2013).

In spite of their exiled history, Cubans have tended to make the necessary adjustments to fit into the United States, preferring to use dialoguing, rather than resorting to violence, to address Cuba's problems. The retention of cultural values and practices from their Cuban heritage has not diminished and in some cases would appear to have enhanced success in the United States as musicians, poets, athletes (particularly in the sport of baseball), and business executives (Anton & Hernandez, 2002; Eckstein, 2006).

It is noteworthy that Cuban Americans have become successful in politics. Today, the Miami Cuban Americans are a powerful political force in the United States. Approximately 90% of Miami-Dade County Cuban Americans are registered to vote (Moreno & Wyatt, 2013). It has even been suggested that the impact of sending Elián González back to Cuba influenced the defeat of the Democratic party in the 2000 election in Florida since the presidential nominee, George W. Bush, opposed sending Gonzalez home and thus received strong support in Florida (Schneider, 2001).

COMMUNICATION

Spanish is the official language of Cuba, although Cubans often shorten words by dropping letters. The accent and some expressions are similar to the Spanish of Andalusia, although the accents tend to vary by the three main regions of Cuba (Bay, 2006; Ganon, 1998). Cuban Spanish has an African influence and also incorporates some words from the Taino Indians and some English words (Ganon, 1998). Today, English is a required course in secondary schools and is increasingly learned by persons interested in the tourist industry.

Eckstein (2006) identified that not speaking English is a significant problem for some first-generation Cubans in the United States. However, second-generation Cubans are more likely to speak both Spanish and English. However, unlike other non-English immigrant groups, Spanish is more likely to still be spoken in the home, within the Cuban community, and by elderly persons who do not have much reason to interact with an English-speaking community. Many Cuban Americans have incorporated English words into spoken Spanish (Ardilla, 2005).

A common greeting among Cuban men entails a firm handshake. Handshakes are often used when entering or leaving a home or greeting a group. On the other hand, women tend to kiss each other once on the cheek and offer a verbal greeting. Kissing on the cheek can be observed between younger members of the opposite sex. Elderly people are greeted with gestures indicative of respect.

Cubans commonly address others by first names. Among friends or co-workers, nicknames may be used. Strangers may address each other using the word *Companero/Companera* (Comrade), *Señor* (Mr.) or *Señora* (Mrs.). Common verbal greetings include "Buenos días!" (Good morning), "Buenas tardes!" (Good afternoon), and "Buenas noches!" (Good evening). "Buenas" (hello) is commonly used as a greeting when passing another on the street, while "Hasta luego!" (So long) is used in parting (Bay, 2006).

Nonverbal communication by Cubans includes use of hand gestures when talking to reinforce ideas and emotions. Conversation is lively and frequently loud and forceful. Most Cubans consider maintaining eye contact important, particularly in formal situations. Some Cuban individuals consider lack of eye contact a sign of insincerity or perhaps spite. Beckoning may occur by waving fingers inward with the palm down. Holding a palm up when beckoning is considered a hostile gesture (Bay, 2006). Silence can mean uncertainty or awkwardness.

Music has been an integral part of Cuban culture since the African slaves brought rhythms and ritual dances from the Santeria religion. Over time, rhythms and dances were blended with Spanish guitars and melodies. In the 1920s, much of the United States was enamored of rumba rhythms, which became fused with jazzy horn sections into big-band sounds. Cuban music is a combination of instruments including guitars, *tres* (a small Cuban stringed instrument with three pairs of strings), double bass, bongos, claves, maracas, and voice. Mambo, bolero, salsa, and cha-cha-cha music also have contributed to the popularity of Cuban music today (*Lonely Planet*, 2010).

Implications for Nursing Care

Although Cuban Americans tend to be educated, literate, and bilingual, it is important for the nurse to assess comprehension of the English language. The elderly Cuban American is more likely to speak only Spanish (Eckstein,

2006). The nurse should ascertain if it is easier for the patient to understand information, patient teaching, or consent materials in Spanish. It is important when materials are translated from English to Spanish to ascertain the reliability and validity of the translation, since research has shown direct translation from one language to another may change the meaning of a message (Xin, 2011).

When the patient does not speak English, a Spanish-speaking person (preferably a Cuban interpreter) who speaks the dialect of the patient should be used. The patient may prefer interpretation to be done by a family member. When issues related to a terminal prognosis or sexuality are involved, the patient may prefer to speak only with older members of the immediate family. However, if an HIV/AIDS diagnosis is to be discussed, the Cuban patient may not want this information discussed with another family member. In this situation, if a translator is needed, it is important to find a translator who is preferably a health provider outside the family. The nurse should be aware that Cubans often use a loud tone of voice in normal conversation and that commands or requests may seem to be direct and aggressive. The nurse should not interpret loudness as rudeness. It is also helpful to be aware that Cubans typically are spontaneous and outgoing. It is generally not considered impolite to interrupt others during conversation. The nurse should be aware that privacy is an important consideration. Highly sensitive or personal information may be withheld from the nurse.

The family may prefer that certain information regarding illness and prognosis be withheld from the patient. In some cases, it is important to discuss information with the family to determine what information should be shared with the patient and by whom. Whereas more acculturated patients will be more likely to want to be informed of serious information, less acculturated patients may prefer that information be given to family members who will share it as they see fit.

SPACE

Cubans tend to stand close to others when talking. Touching or tapping another person may be done to make a point. In the United States, Cubans have tended to choose to live in tight communities, close to other Cubans. This facilitates a high level of identity with Cuban culture. When persons in the family are sick or in need, when possible, other family members will physically appear as a means of support. Cubans may take advantage of the travel authorized by the U.S. Treasury Department's Office of Foreign Assets Control, which allows persons to travel to Cuba to visit close relatives (U.S. Department of State, 2015).

Implications for Nursing Care

The nurse should not be surprised when a Cuban American who learns of an ill family member feels a sense of urgency to be at that person's side. Physical presence of family members to provide support is highly valued, so hospital rooms filled with family and friends are common.

SOCIAL ORGANIZATION

Family Structure

Although Cuban Americans often feel strongly about a variety of social organizations, for most, the family is the most important social unit. Cubans share the Latino value of *familismo,* in which families are seen as an important source of support and identity. In addition, the cultural importance attached to *personalismo* indicates an emphasis on trust, respect and warmth in social relationships (Crockett, Brown, Iturbide, Russell, & Wilkinson-Lee, 2009). Traditionally, the Cuban family has been patriarchal, with a dominant male and a dependent female (Rivera et al., 2008). These roles have changed somewhat as a result of women entering the work force in larger numbers (UN Data, 2014). Although younger couples may develop more egalitarian relationships, traditional family roles and values persist. Women often take the role of emotional provider and mediator, which can be burdensome when combined with the other roles in the family (Rivera et al., 2008). Children tend to have strong relationships with parents and to be supported long after becoming adults. Whether in Cuba or in Miami, when a daughter becomes 15 years old, an extravagant birthday party announces arrival at the age of courting. Elderly people are offered respect by children and extended family. Elders assist in care of younger generations, and in turn when they need care, they are usually cared for within the home. Traditionally, nursing homes are used for the sick or elderly only if the family is unable to provide care.

In a classic study by Thomas and DeSantis (1995), feeding and weaning practices of Cuban and Haitian immigrant mothers in South Florida were assessed. Findings revealed that social, economic, and political factors in both Cuba and Florida affected beliefs and practices. Cuban mothers expected and encouraged weaning from the breast to the bottle and introduction of solid foods at an early age. These expectations, as well as prolonged bottle-feeding, relate to the common Cuban belief that a healthy child is a chubby child (Garcia, 2004). Often the overweight child, by medical standards, is seen as normal or even underweight (Garcia, 2004; Kaufman & Karpati, 2007). Another factor that contributes to early weaning is the Cuban concept of femininity and sexual attractiveness, which associates breastfeeding with deformity of the breast and therefore decreased female attractiveness to men (Garcia, 2004). An additional cultural value that promotes early and prolonged bottle-feeding is that crying is decreased because the bottle acts as a pacifier. Crying is considered an unacceptable behavior for infants and preschool children, with quietness being associated with happiness and contentment. Latina women associate crying by a child with the inability to meet a child's physical and psychoemotional needs (Kaufman & Karpati, 2007). Last, the impact of women entering the work force and the convenience of bottle-feeding cannot be overlooked (Faraz, 2009). It is important for the nurse to be aware of cultural beliefs that promote early weaning and prolonged use of the bottle for Cuban-American children. Patient teaching needs to address criteria for defining a "healthy" baby, the meaning of crying, and alternative ways to respond to crying.

Religion

Prior to Castro, 85% of the population was cited as Roman Catholic (*World Almanac and Book of Facts*, 2015). However, until recently the society was highly secularized, with most people showing little interest in organized religion. Until 1991, governmental policy excluded persons with religious beliefs from membership in the Communist party. Today, there exists a resurgence in religion, and there is growth in many congregations. Some 1800 churches and chapels are present on the island. The population is currently listed as 47% Catholic, 5% Protestant, and 22% nonreligious. Although Catholicism is the most prevalent faith group, many Cubans combine ideas of African voodoo origin to form beliefs known as *Santeria* into their customs and practices. The practice of Santeria combines practices from the worship of Orisha, with its associated rituals, animal sacrificing, wearing of amulets, incantations, magic, and spirit possession practiced by the Yoruba tribe of Nigeria, and the cult worship of Roman Catholic saints or *santos*. It has been estimated that approximately 5% of Cubans practice Santeria (*Time Almanac*, 2011).

Small numbers of people in Cuba practice spiritualism, which emphasizes communication with the dead, and *brujeria*, a form of witchcraft (Bay, 2006). Churches are required to register with the Cuban government and to adhere to rules of association. Religious beliefs are not discussed in school.

It is estimated that 85% of Cubans in South Florida are professing Catholics. However, Cuban Americans tend to practice a personalized religion, with many families having shrines at the entrance to their homes, yards, or place of business. Crucifixes, pictures, or statues of saints are common inside the home. The religious holidays of Christmas, Three Kings Day (*Los Tres Reyes Magos*), and the festivals of *La Caridad del Cobre* (September 8) and Santa Barbara (December 4) are occasions for celebration (Bay, 2006). Christmas Eve (*Noche Buena*) is also celebrated, with a pig cooked over charcoal and followed by attendance at midnight Mass. Some holidays that Cuban Americans recognize honor both a Catholic saint and an African god, such as St. Lazarus's Day (December 17). Cuban Americans may celebrate other Cuban holidays, including Liberation Day (January 1), Labor Day (May 1), the Anniversary of the Attack on the Moncada Garrison in Santiago de Cuba in 1953 (July 26), and the beginning of the War of Independence from Spain (October 10). Mother's Day is recognized on the second Sunday in May (Bay, 2006).

Education

Castro increasingly advanced education as a priority in Cuban society and as a way to promote Communist thinking (Menocal, 2001). Primary, secondary, technical, and higher education are provided to all citizens free of cost. Preschool is available in urban areas. Education is considered mandatory by the state for children between ages 5 and 12. Some 90% of children continue to secondary school, even if it means leaving a rural area to live at a boarding school. Graduates of secondary school may take college entrance exams or attend a technical training institute. Special schools are available for the mentally or physically challenged and for students gifted in the arts and sports. It is estimated that there is one teacher for every 45 inhabitants in Cuba (Bay, 2006). The literacy rate in Cuba is 95% (*World Almanac and Book of Facts*, 2015).

Students in secondary school are likely to live in a boarding school in a rural area, dividing their time between school and agricultural labor. However, even though most boarding schools are often combined with farm work, food may be limited and supplemented by parental gifts. While education is free, the lack of incentive of higher wages for professionals prompts some students in universities to drop out of school. While a doctor, engineer, or lawyer may earn twice as much as a laborer, a waiter or guide without much education may easily earn more money by obtaining "tips" (Menocal, 2001). In the United States, among Cuban-American males, 75% are high school graduates or higher, compared with 76.0% of Cuban-American females. Similarly, 24.6% of Cuban-American males held at least a bachelor's degree, compared with 25.0% of Cuban-American females (Ogunwole, Drewery, & Rios-Vargas, 2012).

Implications for Nursing Care

It is important for the nurse to appreciate that an immigrant from Cuba will have experienced a different level of care, depending on social class and time of immigration. More recently, Cubans have become accustomed to a system of primary health care and to the delivery of health care services to the community. However, the family is still central to health practices. Since Cuban families often care for the elderly in their homes, it is important for the nurse to use creative and culturally appropriate strategies to assist family members to be caregivers. Both professionals and caregivers reported that the "online discussion" was valuable and useful in facilitating the provision of care in the home setting.

Death is also an event that occurs in a community context. Tangible aid is offered to the family by providing assistance with doing household chores, making funeral arrangements, giving gifts of candles and floral wreaths, and providing hospitality for family and friends who have traveled from afar. Memories are kept alive by remembering the dead on birthdays, the anniversary of the death, and visits to the grave. The nurse should be aware that when death occurs, it is normal for Cuban Americans to express grief openly and with loud crying. Immediate female family members will usually wear black during mourning.

The nurse should be aware that Cubans and Cuban Americans may take opposite political positions about the present Cuban government and the position of the United States toward Cuba. Cuban Americans who supported Batista and who emigrated from Cuba may still be considered counterrevolutionary by the present supporters of Castro. Cubans in America may have opposite ideas on the best future for Cuba, with some thinking the United States should intervene with military force while others advocate for a more peaceful resolution to the conflict (Robbins, 2015). Thus, information available to the nurse about Cuba and from Cubans may appear irreconcilable. The nurse should be aware that a Cuban American may have family in Cuba that could receive retaliation for a position that does not support the prevailing government.

The nurse should be aware that Cuban Americans may belong to a variety of church groups. Since religious beliefs vary, the nurse should assess a Cuban patient for religious orientation and needs. The predominant religion of Cuban Americans continues to be Catholic. For Catholics, praying and reciting a rosary, worship of important saints, confession, and communion may be important practices to be included in the plan of care (Varela, 2005). The nurse should also appreciate and respect that Cuban Americans, much like many other Americans, may use an eclectic approach to health-seeking practices, combining Western medicine with folk medicine, home remedies, and use of *santeros* and spiritualists (Hockenberry & Wilson, 2013). Santeria and a *santero* priest may be used when Western medicine and the church fail to offer healing. While most ceremonies conducted by a *santero* are held in the home, if

the patient desires the ceremony to be conducted in the hospital, health care professionals should respect this choice. The nurse should not assume that a Cuban American will practice the Santeria religion. It is estimated that while Cuban Americans may be familiar with the Santeria religion, only a relatively small percentage (5% to 10%) of more recent immigrants in Miami may actually practice the Santeria religion.

It is important to note that as in any culture where slavery has been part of the nation's history, there is a likelihood of prejudice. Nurses need to be aware of the possibility of discriminatory racial dynamics, especially among the elderly of this community. Given that prior to the Castro revolution the "well-to-do" in Cuba were accustomed to having black servants, many elderly Cubans continue to harbor attitudes and values of a more antiquated period. However, those Cuban Americans who have become acculturated and have internalized mainstream values related to class and race are less likely to subscribe to such attitudes and discriminating behaviors.

TIME

Cubans tend to have a more casual view of time and to de-emphasize punctuality and schedules. The pleasure of the event takes on more importance than ending the event at a precise time (Bay, 2006). However, as Cubans have become more acculturated to the United States, social time orientation is often replaced with clock orientation and adhering to scheduled appointments (Bay, 2006). Elderly individuals or those who have recently arrived may be more likely to practice a social time orientation.

Elderly Cubans or persons who have been more recent arrivals may appear to have a past orientation and focus on return to Cuba. Many Cubans who have become acculturated to the United States and who have a strong desire to be financially successful are more future-oriented.

Implications for Nursing Care

The nurse should be aware of the need to assess for time orientation, which may vary with the level of acculturation, age, and profession. Patient teaching regarding follow-up with medical and nursing care, treatments, and medications should be altered in response to the patient's time orientation.

ENVIRONMENTAL CONTROL

Cuban Americans may combine beliefs of internal control with external control. Beliefs in internal control are evidenced in the activities of Cubans in Cuba to earn money to improve their lifestyle and control their environment in spite of the Communist society. This pattern of working for success has resulted in the financial success of many Cuban Americans.

Cubans may rely on family as their primary source of health information and practice home remedies that have a tradition of success. Older women are often sought out for advice on how to treat illness. Nevertheless, Cuba's health care system is a government priority, and even with the fall of the Soviet Union, Castro has been successful in implementing an organized national health system that includes 267 hospitals and more than 420 clinics throughout the country that promote primary as well as secondary health care (Bay, 2006; Nayeri & Lopez-Pardo, 2005; Wilson & Russell, 2004). Many childhood diseases have been eradicated by vaccinations. Family doctors are assigned to each community, and it is estimated that there are 6.7 physicians for every 1000 people, which is significantly higher than most other countries, including the United States (2.5 physicians/1000). There are 9.1 nurses per 1000 residents, which is similar to the United States (9.8) (World Bank, 2014). Nurses in Cuba include licensed practical nurses and diploma and degree nurses who are registered. Diploma nurses study for 3 years in polytechnic schools of health, while degree nurses study for 5 years at universities with health and medical facilities. If nurses are needed, more students are selected and streamed into a nursing program so Cubans do not suffer from a shortage of nurses (Havana Medical Sciences University, 2012). Level of education, income, access to care, the presence of insurance, and level of acculturation influence use of health services in the United States. While Cubans are increasingly exposed to Western medicine, use of folk practices still exist. In many Cuban American communities such as Little Havana in Miami, stores called *botanicas* sell herbs, ointments, oils, powders, incenses, and religious figurines, which are believed to break curses, drive away evil spirits, bring luck, or relieve physical ailments. *Botanicas* may also sell Santeria necklaces and animals for ritual sacrifice (Reeser & Cintrón-Moscoso, 2012). Medicinal plants may be used for teas, potions, salves, or poultices. Fruits and vegetables may be used for specific physical problems.

Rituals Related to Death and Dying

The death and dying process among Cuban Americans is juxtaposed by the immediate sadness and grief tied to the death of a loved one and the subsequent festive atmosphere at the wake. Although the majority of Cuban Americans does not actively practice their faith, religion plays a central role during the time of death. It is not unusual for a priest, rabbi, or other religious figure to provide some ceremonial ritual with the patient prior to his or her death. Moreover,

family members experience such an occurrence as a signal of imminent death as well as a rite of passage into heaven (O'Dea, personal communication, 2006).

When death is imminent, it is common for immediate family members and extended family members to convene in lobby areas and take turns being at the bedside of the dying patient. Expressions of grief are common at the bedside of the dying patient, yet these expressions do not usually reach boisterous levels. However, upon notification that the patient has died, it is not uncommon to find pronounced expressions of grief from those present at the hospital.

It is important to note that demographic variables influence many decisions upon the death of a parent of a Cuban American. Most Cuban Americans have witnessed both traditional U.S. (i.e., Americanized) death rituals as well as more traditional Cuban death rituals. Despite strong acculturation and adaptation of North American values and norms, at the time of a parent's death, the customs observed are almost exclusively Cuban.

The norm is for a wake service to be observed the day after the announcement of the death. Extreme care is taken to ensure that relatives and significant others are notified in person (via telephone if need be) to announce the death and to exchange information regarding where the wake will be held and where the funeral services will be observed.

Given the estrangement many Cubans feel as a result of becoming refugees, it can be considered an extension of Castro's victory if loved ones are not notified in a timely fashion that a loved one has died. For many, finding out "through the grapevine" after the funeral services concluded adds to a feeling of estrangement and defeat. Given the political upheaval that native Cubans experienced in the 1960s and 1970s, it is not uncommon for representatives of anti-Castro municipalities to pay their respect by attending these services.

Numerous factors dictate the dynamics of a Cuban American wake and funeral service. These include the religious identity of the deceased and/or the economic status of the family of the deceased. Catholics traditionally have a priest present at the wake who provides a short prayer service. It is customary for family members to spend the night at the site of the wake until the funeral the following day. The site of the wake usually allows for a gregarious and jovial social reunion (a celebration of the deceased person's life) the afternoon and eve of the wake and gradually turns more sullen as the funeral mass approaches. Note that it is very common for Cuban *bodegas* (corner stores) to be located near the site of the funeral home. This allows for the bereaved to provide Cuban coffee to one another. Hence, it is common to encounter a strong scent of coffee in the parlor where the deceased is at rest.

After the funeral Mass is held (at either a Catholic church close to the funeral home or the church where the deceased was a parishioner), a procession moves to the cemetery unless the deceased is cremated. Often, economic factors dictate whether the deceased is cremated (which is considerably less expensive) or whether there will be a burial at a cemetery. When there is a burial, the committal service concludes with prayers led by the priest who presided over the funeral Mass. Again, economic dynamics dictate whether or not there will be a reception after the committal service.

Whereas the majority of wake and funeral rituals has a strong Catholic presence, in nearly 10% of these Catholic ceremonies, Santeria rituals are also practiced. These rituals range from placing relics of saints at the feet of the deceased in the coffin to the breaking of pottery as the hearse leaves to take the deceased to his or her final resting place.

Less common are Jewish ceremonies. They too have different customs depending on whether the bereaved practiced Orthodox, Conservative, or Reform rituals. Whereas Orthodox Jews partake primarily in solemn and sullen expressions of grief for 7 days and bury their departed in a wooden coffin the day after the death, Conservative and Reform Jews partake in rituals that allow a more jovial expression of emotion and greater latitude in such matters as the attire the deceased wears and the style of the coffin (O'Dea, personal communication, 2006).

When anticipated, cultural norms will dictate who in the family should be informed first. Less acculturated Cubans will want the person performing the care to be told first, as well as the male head of the family or, if he is not available, the closest relative. Traditionally, the family contacted the clergy as well as telling the patient. Support by the extended family is highly valued, with notification of family members and subsequent visits to the dying or bereaved being the expected norm. If a patient is dying in the hospital, the family will expect to stay close to the patient, including staying overnight (Varela, 2005).

Death rituals are routinely performed according to the individual family's beliefs and by the religious official who is summoned (Catholic priest, Protestant minister, rabbi, or *santero*). If the *santero* is officiating, death rites may include chants, ceremonial gestures, and animal sacrifice. Most Cuban families will want measures taken to prolong life, as well as to make the patient comfortable. In most cases, in-hospital medical care is valued over dying at home. After the person's death, a funeral wake that may last for 2 or 3 days is usually held in the funeral parlor, where the immediate family is supported by friends and extended family members.

Implications for Nursing Care

The nurse should appreciate that some Cuban Americans may continue to use a variety of folk remedies and folk practices to prevent and treat illness. Health practices will vary with socioeconomic status, time of immigration, level of acculturation, education, and feelings of self-efficacy.

BIOLOGICAL VARIATIONS

A number of studies have compared the Hispanic ethnic groups. What is particularly noteworthy is that when Hispanic groups are studied by subgroup, conclusions consistently vary among groups. The infant mortality rate for Cubans (5.8 per 1000 births) and Mexican Americans (5.34 per 1000 births) is significantly less than Puerto Ricans (8.01 per 1000 births), which may be due to the large percentage of Cuban-American mothers who receive prenatal care in the first trimester (80.4%) compared with Puerto Rican mothers (68.1%) (Centers for Disease Control and Prevention [CDC], 2011; National Center for Health Statistics, 2014). Davis, Kreutzer, Lipsett, King, and Shaikh (2006) investigated asthma incidence among Mexican, Puerto Rican, and Cuban Americans. They noted the highest incidence among Cuban Americans (23.0%) followed by Puerto Rican Americans (22.8%) and Mexican Americans (13.2%). They proposed that the differences may be genetic or a relation of the time lived in the United States, because the longer a subgroup is in the United States, the higher the incidence of asthma.

Although Cubans vary in their ethnic origin, research involving Cuban Americans suggests some biological variations exist. Sevush, Peruyera, Crawford, and Mullan (2000) noted that in a comparison of Apo-Eε 4 frequencies for Cuban-American and White non-Hispanic persons with and without Alzheimer's disease, the Apo-Eε 4 allele conferred as large a risk for Alzheimer's disease in Cuban Americans as for White non-Hispanics. This finding differs from those for Hispanic subjects as a whole.

Espino and Franz (2002) assessed the effect of skin color of darker skinned Mexicans and Cubans on occupational ranking. This interesting study found that darker skinned Mexicans and Cubans face significantly lower occupational prestige than their lighter skinned counterparts, even after adjustment for factors that influence performance in the labor market. Conversely, no such conclusive evidence was found that skin-color differences impact occupational prestige scores for Puerto Ricans. This study confirmed earlier studies that dark-skinned Mexican Americans and Cuban Americans face higher levels of discrimination in the labor market, whereas dark-skinned Puerto Ricans do not.

Susceptibility to Disease

Vision Impairment. Kodjebacheva, Brown, Estrada, Yu, and Coleman (2011) found that 95% of Latino first graders with visual acuity problems lacked eyeglasses. Lam, Lee, and Gomez-Marin (2000) investigated eye care for adults and found Puerto Rican adults to have significantly higher prevalence of visual impairment and to be significantly less likely to become unimpaired with usual correction than Cuban Americans. The researchers concluded that of Hispanic groups studied, Cuban Americans may have less severe eye disease and/or may be receiving better eye care.

Diabetes. In the past 20 years the number of Hispanics in the United States has almost doubled, but the number of Hispanics with diabetes is almost fivefold (Aponte, 2009). The percentage of Hispanics diagnosed with diabetes is 12.8%, almost double that of non-Hispanic whites (7.6) (National Diabetes Surveillance System [NDSS], 2012). According to the Centers for Disease Control and Prevention (2011), other Hispanic-American groups have a higher age-adjusted prevalence of diabetes than Cuban Americans (13.8% for Puerto Ricans, 13.3% for Mexicans, and 7.6% for Cubans), yet Cuban Americans had the highest proportion of diabetes as the underlying cause of death (44%) as compared with Puerto Ricans (39%) and Mexican Americans (37%). Aponte (2009) similarly found that Cuban Americans with diabetes had higher systolic blood pressures, higher cholesterol, and higher creatinine levels than other Hispanic groups.

Huffman, Vaccaro, Nath, and Zarini (2009) found that Cuban Americans with type 2 diabetes given education on meal planning were statistically more likely to have an improved HA1c. Evaluation of environmental, personal, social, cultural and gender-specific barriers to following a meal plan and scheduling meals are warranted. For the development of a successful intervention for this population, culturally appropriate and relevant interventions with a refresher course 6 to 9 months following the intervention are recommended (Huffman, Vaccaro, Nath, & Zarini, 2009).

Mental Illness. Oquendo et al. (2001) investigated depression among ethnic groups. The 1-year prevalence rate among Cuban Americans was 2.5%, as compared with 3.6% among Whites, 2.8% among Mexican Americans, and 6.9% among Puerto Ricans. It is significant to note that the rate of depression was lowest among Cuban Americans. Alternatively, elder Cuban Americans are at greater risk of depressive symptoms than other ethnic groups and are not likely to access services due to the stigma of mental illness among their peers (Park, Jang, Lee, Ko, & Chiriboga, 2013; Rojas-Vilches, Negy, & Reig-Ferrer, 2011).

Substance Abuse. Investigators have also studied alcohol use among Hispanic populations. Use patterns differ significantly. Delva et al. (2005) noted that although Hispanic youth are overrepresented among students who use drugs, Cuban American males were less likely to use marijuana, cocaine or participate in heavy drinking compared to Mexican American, Puerto Rican, and other Latino American students. The authors also reported that Cuban Americans reported a relatively moderate alcohol consumption pattern that resembled that of non-Hispanic Whites, whereas women of Hispanic populations (Mexican American, Cuban American, and Puerto Rican) had a lower consumption rate, although it increased with level of acculturation.

Low Birth Weight. According to the most recent data, 7.6% of infants born to White parents with a high school education weigh less than 2500 grams at birth. The percentage of low-birth-weight children born to Hispanics or Latinos, as a collective group with similar education, is 7.0%. When divided by country of origin, differences appear: Mexican, 6.4%; Puerto Rican, 9.9%; Cuban, 8.2%; and Central and South American, 6.3% (National Center for Health Statistics, 2014).

Nutritional Preferences and Habits

In Cuba, dietary choices are often based on food that is grown locally and that is readily available. Cuban cuisine generally combines Spanish and African techniques. *Arroz con frijoles* (rice and beans) is the traditional meal. Rice is served at most meals, along with other dishes that may include potatoes, sweet potatoes, yucca (cassava), platanos (plantains), or tomatoes. When eggs are available, they may be boiled, fried, or prepared as an omelet (called a *tortilla*). Corn provides a basis for many foods including cornmeal. Dishes like *arroz con pollo* (chicken and rice) and *picadillo* (minced beef and rice) are common Cuban cuisine, as are soups made with plantains, chickpeas, or beans.

Roast pork is a luxury food eaten on special occasions or when funds are available. Lack of funds may also limit other meats in the diet. In coastal areas, seafood is popular. Tropical fruits are eaten in season. Sweets are eaten as desserts or snacks when available. Coffee is generally served sweet and strong. Cuban beer (*cerveza*) and Cuban cocktails are enjoyed by tourists, as well as by Cubans when funds permit (*Lonely Planet World Guide*, 2010).

As well as being served in Cuban homes in the United States, foods for Cuban tastes are increasingly being served in restaurants with a Cuban clientele. The McDonald's restaurants in Miami-Dade County in Florida serve products targeted at Cuban Americans. The breakfast menu's Latin McOmelet combines eggs with diced tomatoes, onions, ham, and spicy cheese and is served on a roll rather than on a biscuit, bagel, or English muffin. The Cuban Sandwich, available from lunchtime on, layers ham, pork, Swiss cheese, pickles, and mustard on toasted Cuban bread. Chicken McNuggets get a special mango-pineapple sauce. A special dessert is *dulce de leche,* a caramelized, milk-based confection much like a custard.

Implications for Nursing Care

It is important for the culturally competent nurse to be aware that persons included in the Hispanic culture must be assessed and evaluated individually. It is noteworthy that research that includes various Hispanic cultures frequently finds differences when the cultural groups are considered separately. According to National Center for Health Statistics (2014), the prevalence of persons under the age of 65 without health insurance for all Americans was 16.7% whereas for all Hispanic Americans it was 36.2% (Cuban, 22.0%; Puerto Rican, 17.7%; Mexican, 39.1%). In addition, Hispanics with diabetes, high blood pressure, or heart disease are less likely to receive clinical services monitoring these diseases than non-Hispanic Whites (Huffman, Vaccaro, Nath, & Zarini, 2009). Thus, national origin should be considered when providing care as well as social and economic factors.

The nurse should also be aware that in a patriarchal culture (such as the Cuban culture) the issues of HIV may become intertwined with homophobic values and attitudes held by some members of this culture. Therefore, the nurse practitioner must be especially attentive to confidentiality parameters when discussing and dealing with topics related to HIV.

SUMMARY

Cuban Americans have come to the United States in immigrant waves and thus have different levels of acculturation. The nurse must carefully assess the beliefs and values of each client in order to deliver culturally sensitive and appropriate care.

CASE STUDY

Recent Cuban immigrants, Maria, 22, and her 3-year-old son, Antonio, are being seen by the nurse practitioner at a community clinic in Miami, Florida. As the nurse interviews the mother, she notes that Antonio is given a bottle whenever he begins to fuss. When the bottle is empty, Maria opens a bag containing other bottles and provides him with another. The nurse observes Antonio to be "plump" and heavier than the standard weight for a child his age. When the nurse comments on Antonio's "baby fat," Maria beams and says, "I'm glad Antonio is fat. It's a sign he is in good health. He never cries and is such a good boy. But I wish I could get him to eat more. His cousins are all heavier than he is and it makes me feel bad. I don't want my family to think I am a bad mother."

CARE PLAN

Nursing Diagnosis: Health-seeking behaviors related to lack of knowledge regarding need for preventive health behaviors, as evidenced by Maria stating, "I'm glad Antonio is fat. It's a sign he is in good health."

Client Outcomes	Nursing Interventions
1. Antonio will maintain ideal weight according to standard weight for age and height.	1. Determine Antonio's weight and height. Compare results with standard weight for his age and height.
2. Maria will explain ways to provide other nutritious foods for Antonio now that he has teeth and different nutritional needs as a 3-year-old.	2. Inspect Antonio's skin, hair, nails, eyes, ears, nose, and throat, and praise Maria for raising such a healthy boy as you point out healthy findings.
3. Maria will state ways that identify Antonio's physical wellness and strength.	3. Discuss the advantages of maintaining ideal weight even in childhood, such as prevention of diabetes and cardiovascular disease.
	4. Teach Maria about proper nutrition, using a visual aid of the MyPlate diagram showing suggested proportions of various food groups for healthy eating.

Continued

5. Ask Maria which of the following foods her family eats: grains, vegetables, fruits, meat, poultry, fish, dry beans, eggs, nuts, milk, yogurt, and cheese.
6. Encourage her to include Antonio in family meals and to put various foods on his plate for him to feed himself.
7. Encourage Maria to offer water instead of a bottle of milk.
8. Explain that children who drink only milk become anemic (low in iron) and have increased dental caries.
9. Explain that Antonio has a need for fresh fruit, vegetables, and all the foods on the food pyramid, in order to be healthy with strong bones and for protection against infection and illness.
10. Assess Antonio's gross motor development and point out his skills:
    - Walks upstairs using alternate feet (3 years)
    - Walks downstairs using alternate feet (4 years)
    - Stands on one foot (3 years)
    - Rides tricycle (3 years)
    - Hops on one foot (4 years)
    - Jumps off one step (3 years)
11. Assess Antonio's fine motor development and discuss with Maria how this demonstrates intellectual and psychomotor skills:
    - Builds a tower of blocks (3 years)
    - Copies circles, may add facial features (3 years)
    - Handles scissors well (5 years)
12. Encourage Maria to praise Antonio for independent functions, such as putting on his socks, shoes, pants, and shirt.

Nursing Diagnosis: Ineffective health maintenance related to inability to make thoughtful judgments, as evidenced by Maria's statement, "He never cries and is such a good boy. Whenever he fusses, I give him a bottle of milk, and when the bottle is empty, I give him another one. I wish I could get him to eat more."

Client Outcomes	Nursing Interventions
1. Maria will follow a mutually agreed upon health care maintenance plan for Antonio.	1. Ask Maria how she might arrange her daily schedule in order to introduce solid healthy foods in Antonio's daily activities.
2. Maria will discuss her fears of implementing the changes in Antonio's health regimen.	2. Ask what Antonio does for fun.

CARE PLAN—cont'd

3. Suggest age-appropriate play and toys:
   - Things to help develop gross motor skills, such as a tricycle, wagon, sandbox, outside slide and swing, wading pool
   - Imitation play with trucks, cars, telephone, doctor or nurse kit, hats, tools, and the like
   - Toys and activities to foster fine motor skills, self-expression, and cognitive development: blocks, carpentry tools, illustrated books, puzzles, paints, crayons, clay, and bubble blowing
   - Television, when supervised, can be educational and provide a quiet activity
   - Imaginary playmates, which are common at this age and can help children deal with loneliness and fears
4. Ask Maria what her concerns are about giving water instead of milk in a bottle to Antonio when he fusses.
5. Suggest that these changes could be gradual, perhaps giving a bottle after each meal instead of any time he fusses.
6. Suggest that Maria use a play activity with Antonio when he fusses during the day instead of giving him a bottle of milk.
7. Encourage Maria to call or return in 2 weeks to discuss how things are going with the changes in Antonio's eating and play activities.
8. Rehearse with Maria what she will say to family members about her decision to not give a bottle of milk when Antonio fusses.
9. Rehearse with Maria how she will define a healthy 3-year-old when discussing Antonio's appearance with family members.

Nursing Diagnoses—Definitions and Classification 2012–2014. Copyright © 2012, 1994–2012 by NANDA International. Used by arrangement with Wiley-Blackwell Publishing, a company of John Wiley and Sons, Inc. In order to make safe and effective judgments using NANDA-I nursing diagnoses it is essential that nurses refer to the definitions and defining characteristics of the diagnoses listed in the work.

CLINICAL DECISION MAKING

1. What are two cultural values unique to Cuban Americans that affect health care?
2. Which two biological variations of Cuban Americans should the nurse be aware of?
3. What are differences that may affect Cuban Americans who immigrated at different times?
4. What folk beliefs are practiced by some Cuban Americans?

REVIEW QUESTIONS

1. The Cuban American considers making eye contact to be which of the following?
   a. Socially unacceptable
   b. Rude and aggressive
   c. Important, especially in formal situations
   d. Of no importance when communicating with another person
2. A nurse interacting with a recent immigrant from Cuba could expect that the individual is which of the following?
   a. Is literate
   b. Is illiterate
   c. Has no knowledge of the English language
   d. Has received very poor health care
3. Cuban Americans express grief in which of following ways?
   a. Only within the context of family
   b. With reserve and quiet
   c. Openly, with loud crying
   d. In the form of somatic complaints

REFERENCES

Anton, A., & Hernandez, R. (2002). *A vibrant history of a people in exile*. Philadelphia: Kensington.

Aponte, J. (2009). Diabetes-related risk factors across Hispanic subgroups in the Hispanic Health and Nutritional

Examination Survey (1982–84). *Public Health Nursing, 26*(1), 23–38.

Ardilla, A. (2005). Spanglish: an Anglicized Spanish dialect. *Hispanic Journal of Behavioral Sciences, 27*(1), 60–81.

Barlow, K., Taylor, D., & Lambert, W. (2000). Ethnicity in America and feeling "American." *Journal of Psychology, 134*(6), 581–600.

Bay, A. (2006). *Cuba. Culturegrams 2006.* Orem, UT: Millennial Star Network.

BBC News. (2000). *Cubans threaten Miami disruption.* Available at <http://news.bbc.co.uk/2/hi/americas/704943.stm> Retrieved on September 28, 2011.

Brown, A. & Patten, E. (2013). Hispanics of Cuban origin in the United States, 2011. *Pew Research Center.* Available at <http://www.pewhispanic.org/2013/06/19/hispanics-of-cuban-origin-in-the-united-states-2011/> Retrieved January 30, 2015.

Centers for Disease Control and Prevention (CDC). (2011). *National Diabetes Fact Sheet (2011).* Atlanta, GA: U.S. Department of Health and Human Services, Centers for Disease Control and Prevention.

Centers for Disease Control and Prevention (CDC). (2011). *CDC Health Disparities and Inequality Report—United States 2011. MMWR* Supp. 60.

Central Intelligence Agency (CIA). (2015). *The World Factbook.* Available at <https://www.cia.gov/library/publications/the-world-factbook/geos/cu.html> Retrieved January 30, 2015.

Crockett, L., Brown, J., Iturbide, M., Russell, S., & Wilkinson-Lee, A. (2009). Conceptions of good parent-adolescent relationships among Cuban American teenagers. *Sex Roles, 60*, 575–587.

Davis, A., Kreutzer, R., Lipsett, M., King, G., & Shaikh, N. (2006). Asthma prevalence in Hispanic and Asian American ethnic subgroups: results from the California Healthy Kids Survey. *Pediatrics, 118*, e363–e370.

Delva, J., Wallace, J. M., O'Malley, P. M., Bachman, J. G., Johnston, L. D., & Schulenberg, J. E. (2005). *American Journal of Public Health, 95*(9), 1494–1495. <http://doi.org/10.2105/AJPH.2005.070516>

Drain, P., & Barry, M. (2010). Fifty years of U.S. embargo: Cuba's health outcomes and lessons. *Science, 328*, 572–574.

Eckstein, S. (2006). Cuban emigres and the American dream. *Perspectives on Politics, 4*(2), 297–307.

Ennis, S., Ríos-Vargas, M., & Albert, N. (2011). The Hispanic population: 2010. *Census Briefs, C2010BR-04* U.S. Census Bureau.

Espino, R., & Franz, M. (2002). Latino phenotypic discrimination revisited: the impact of skin color on occupational status. *Social Science Quarterly, 83*(2), 612–624.

Evenson, D. (2007). Cuba's biotechnology revolution. *MEDICC Review, 9*(1), 1–10.

Faraz, A. (2009). Clinical recommendations for promoting breast feeding among Hispanic women. *Journal of the American Academy of Nurse Practitioners, 22*, 292–299.

Ganon, M. R. (1998). *Cuba. Peoples of the world.* Danbury, CT: Grolier.

Garcia, R. (2004). No come nada. *Health Affairs, 23*(2), 215–219.

Havana Guide. (2010). Available at <http://www.havana-guide.com/lifeinhavana.html> Retrieved January 25, 2011.

Havana Medical Sciences University. (2012). *Brief overview of the BSc in nursing curriculum.* Available at <http://instituciones.sld.cu/ucmh/files/2012/11/BSc-Nursing-overview.pdf> Accessed February 12, 2015.

Hockenberry, M., & Wilson, D. (Eds.). (2013). *Wong's essentials of pediatric nursing* (9th ed.). St. Louis: Mosby.

Hougendobler, D. (2014). *The public health implications of normalized U.S.-Cuba relations. O'Neill Institute for National and Global Health Law.* Available at <http://www.oneillinstituteblog.org/public-health-implications-normalized-u-s-cuba-relations/> Retrieved February 1, 2015.

Huffman, F., Vaccaro, J., Nath, S., & Zarini, G. (2009). Diabetes self management: are Cuban Americans receiving quality health care? *Journal of Health and Human Services Administration, 32*(3), 279–304.

Kaufman, L., & Karpati, A. (2007). Understanding the sociocultural roots of childhood obesity: food practices among Latino families in Bushwick, Brooklyn. *Social Science and Medicine, 64*, 2177–2188.

Kindersley, D. (2011). *DK eyewitness travel guide: Cuba.* London, England: Revaluation Books.

Kodjebacheva, G., Brown, R., Estrada, L., Yu, F., & Coleman, A. (2011). Uncorrected refractive error among first-grade students of different racial/ethnic groups in southern California: results a year after school-mandated vision screening. *Journal of Public Health Management and Practice, 17*(6), 499–505.

Kornbluh, P. (2002). Opening to Cuba. *Nation (New York, N.Y.: 1865), 275*(13), 6.

Lam, B., Lee, D., & Gomez-Marin, O. (2000). Prevalence of usual-corrected binocular distance visual acuity impairment in Hispanic and non-Hispanic adults. *Ophthalmic Epidemiology, 7*(1), 73–83.

Latza Nadeau, B. (2014). The Pope's diplomatic miracle: ending the U.S.-Cuba Cold War. *The Daily Beast.* Available at <http://www.thedailybeast.com/articles/2014/12/17/the-pope-s-diplomatic-miracle-ending-the-u-s-cuba-cold-war.html> Retrieved January 31, 2015.

Lonely Planet World Guide. (2010). *Cuba.* Available at <http://www.lonelyplanet.com/cuba> Retrieved November 10, 2010.

Menocal, A. (2001). *Cuba climbing. Survival in the museum of the revolution.* Website no longer available.

Miami Herald. (1999). *U.S. repatriates 20 Cubans.*

Moreno, D., & Wyatt, J. (2013). *Cuban-American partisanship: a secular realignment? Cuban Research Institute: School of International and Public Affairs.* Available at <https://cri.fiu.edu/research/commissioned-reports/> Retrieved February 1, 2015.

National Center for Health Statistics. (2010). *Health, United States, 2009: with special feature on medical technology.* Hyattsville, MD.

Nayeri, K., & Lopez-Pardo, C. (2005). Economic crisis and access to care: Cuba's health care system since the collapse of the

Soviet Union. *International Journal of Health Services, 35*(4), 797–816.

National Diabetes Surveillance System (NDSS). (2012). *Age-adjusted percentage of people aged 20 years or older with diagnosed diabetes, by race/ethnicity, United States, 2010–2012.* Available at <http://www.cdc.gov/diabetes/pdfs/data/2014-report-estimates-of-diabetes-and-its-burden-in-the-united-states.pdf> Accessed February 12, 2015.

Ogunwole, S., Drewery, M., & Rios-Vargas, M. (2012). The population with a bachelor's degree or higher by race and Hispanic origin: 2006–2010. *American Community Survey Briefs,* U.S. Bureau of the Census.

Oquendo, M., Ellis, S., Greenwald, S., Malone, K. M., Weissman, M. M., & Mann, J. J. (2001). Ethnic and sex differences in suicide rates relative to major depression in the United States. *American Journal of Psychiatry, 158*(10), 1652–1658.

Park, N. S., Jang, Y., Lee, B. S., Ko, J., & Chiriboga, D. (2013). The impact of social resources on depressive symptoms in racially and ethnically diverse older adults: variations by groups with differing health risks. *Research on Aging.* Available at <http://roa.sagepub.com/content/early/2013/05/06/0164027513486991> Accessed February 11, 2015.

Reeser, D., & Cintrón-Moscoso, F. (2012). Immigrant health care niches: exploring the role of botánicas in Tampa, FL. *Explorations in Anthropology, 20*(10), 1–17.

Rivera, F., Guarnaccia, P., Mulvaney-Day, N., Lin, J., Torres, M., & Alegria, M. (2008). Family cohesion and its relationship to psychological distress among Latino groups. *Hispanic Journal of Behavioral Sciences, 30*(3), 357–378.

Robbins, C. A. (2015). U.S.-Cuba relations: three things to know. *Council on Foreign Relations, January 30, 2015.* Available at <http://www.cfr.org/cuba/us-cuba-relations-three-things-know/p36063> Retrieved January 30, 2015.

Rojas-Vilches, A., Negy, C., & Reig-Ferrer, A. (2011). Puerto Rican and Cuban American young adults and their parents. *International Journal of Clinical and Health Psychology, 11*(2), 313–341.

Schneider, W. (2001). Elian Gonzalez defeated Al Gore. *National Journal, 33*(17), 1274.

Sevush, S., Peruyera, G., Crawford, F., & Mullan, M. (2000). Apolipoprotein-E epsilon 4 allele frequency and conferred risk for Cuban Americans with Alzheimer's disease. *American Journal of Geriatric Psychiatry, 8*(3), 254–256.

Sweig, J. (2010). *A reform moment in Cuba?* Available at <http://www.cfr.org/cuba/reform-moment-cuba/p22617> Retrieved January 31, 2011.

Thomas, J., & DeSantis, L. (1995). Feeding and weaning products of Cuban and Haitian immigrant mothers. *Journal of Transcultural Nursing, 6*(2), 34–42.

Time Almanac. (2011). Chicago: Encyclopedia Britannica.

UN Data. (2014). *Cuba.* Available at <http://data.un.org/CountryProfile.aspx?crName=cuba> Retrieved February 1, 2015.

U.S. Department of Commerce, Bureau of the Census. (2015). *American community survey.* Washington, DC: U.S. Government Printing Office.

U.S. Department of State. (2015). *Background note: Cuba.* Available at <http://www.treasury.gov/resource-center/sanctions/Programs/pages/cuba.aspx> Retrieved January 31, 2015.

Varela, L. (2005). Cubans. In J. Lipson & S. Dibble (Eds.), *Culture and clinical care.* San Francisco: UCSF Nursing Press.

White House. (2014). *Statement by the President on Cuba Policy Changes.* Available at <http://www.whitehouse.gov/the-press-office/2014/12/17/statement-president-cuba-policy-changes> Retrieved February 1, 2015.

Wilson, T., & Russell, J. (2004). Health care and nursing in Cuba. *Reflections in Nursing Leadership, 30*(4), 32–35.

World Almanac and Book of Facts. (2015). New York: World Almanac Books.

World Bank, (2014). <http://www.worldbank.org/en/about/annualreport> Retrieved September 24, 2015.

Xin, S. (2011). Translation as a key dimension of social life. *Theory and Practice in Language Studies, 1*(1), 119–121.

Amish Americans

Deborah R. Gillum

After reading this chapter, the nurse will be able to:

1. Describe patterns of communication used by Amish Americans.
2. Explain practices related to space that may influence interpersonal interactions between persons of Amish heritage and health care providers.
3. Relate the importance of family and religion to everyday practices of Amish Americans.
4. Explain the implications of the past-time orientation of the Amish in terms of health care practices.
5. Describe attitudes and beliefs of the Amish that influence health care.
6. Explain biological variations that may be found among the Amish.

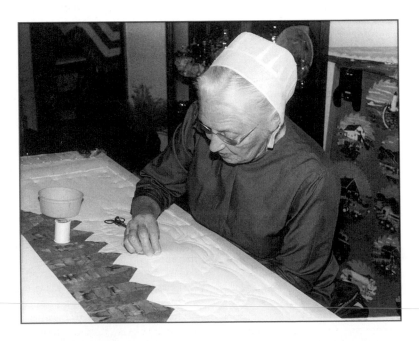

The author would like to thank Karon Schwartz and Mervin R. Helmuth for past contributions to this chapter. This chapter is also dedicated in memory to Karon Schwartz.

OVERVIEW OF THE AMISH

The Amish are direct descendants of the Anabaptists of sixteenth-century Europe. The Anabaptists originated in Switzerland in 1525, when a few individuals decided to separate from the Catholic Church. These reformers were named *Anabaptists,* or "rebaptizers," because they felt Scripture did not support infant baptism. There were also other issues, such as pacifism, separation of church and state, commitment to live peaceably with the world, and church discipline, that caused others to see this small group as "devil inspired, odd and antisocial" (Hostetler, 1993, p. 27). The Anabaptists became a persecuted group. Many were tortured or exiled and even put to death over the next century throughout Western Europe. Despite this, the group gave birth to three religious movements in existence yet today: the Mennonites (of Dutch origin), the Hutterites, and the Swiss Brethren (Hostetler, 1993). The Amish, named after their leader Jacob Ammann, are a branch of the Swiss Brethren (Gross, 1997).

Jacob Ammann was born in Switzerland and moved to the Alsace region of France in 1693, where he became an elder and spokesperson for the Anabaptists in that region. Ammann suggested changes, such as taking communion twice a year rather than once; always including foot washing as part of the communion service; and strictly enforcing the discipline of *meidung,* including ex-communication, with wrongdoers. He demanded unconditional answers from the area churches and succeeded in polarizing them, with neither side willing to compromise their beliefs. This dialogue continued throughout the middle 1690s, and gradually a division took place in the Swiss Brethren group (Roth & Springer, 2002). The followers of Ammann became known as *Amish,* although this name was not used until they left Europe.

The Amish came to North America from Germany's Palatinate region and the Alsace part of France, along with a large number of other religious groups, including the Mennonites, to escape war and religious persecution. The first wave of Amish came to North America between 1714 to 1770 (Nolt, 1992). Some came at the personal invitation of William Penn, who traveled in the Palatinate and proclaimed the religious freedoms in America. The Swiss Brethren, known as *Amish,* and the Mennonites, also from Switzerland, bought 10,000 acres from William Penn in what is now Lancaster County in Pennsylvania and are still thriving today. It is in this county that the oldest North American Amish community still exists. All of the groups that came from the Palatinate spoke a dialect that became known as *Pennsylvania Deitsch* (German) or more popularly as *Pennsylvania Dutch.* The European Brethren soon spread the word that the Amish in North America were

prospering and were not being confronted by wars and governments. The personal and religious freedom in the New World and the French Revolution of 1789–1799, as well as the Napoleonic Wars, precipitated a second wave of immigrants from 1815 until 1860. Many of this latter group settled in Ohio, Indiana, Illinois, and Iowa. There are no Amish in Europe today. Those who stayed lost their Amish identity and reunited with other Anabaptist groups.

The Amish immigrated to the United States and Canada and have gone through philosophical changes that led to divisions within this ethnoreligious culture. This is due in part to the fact that *Ordnung* (or rules) is unwritten and open for interpretation by church members and bishops. The term *Old Order Amish* is a nineteenth-century label that is used in America to describe groups that are more traditional (Hostetler, 1993). Some less traditional Amish are referred to as *New Order Amish* or *Conservative Amish Mennonites* (Randell-David, 1989; Wenger & Wenger, 2003). Some factional groups have been named after their leaders, for example, Egi and Beachy Amish. These more progressive groups stand between the parent group, the Mennonites, and the Old Order Amish (Hostetler, 1993). The term *Amish* is often used in a general sense to refer to anyone in this religious group, regardless of the order or the traditions and customs that are followed.

For the purposes of this chapter, the name *Amish* is used to describe the Old Order Amish, the most traditional of the Amish groups. Old Order Amish generally use the horse and buggy as a primary form of transportation, live off the land, do not have electricity or telephones in their homes, accept traditional biblical interpretations without question, and emphasize separation from the world (Randell-David, 1989). The Amish refusal to use electricity eliminates the possibility of mass media within the home and helps preserve traditional values (Kraybill, 2001). However, in some districts, diesel-powered generators are used to run indoor lights and refrigerators; other modern conveniences, such as the cell phone for the purpose of business, have been incorporated in some districts in recent years.

All Amish families living in a district belong to the same "church" and meet together in a member's home, shed, or barn for church services every other Sunday. When a district gets too large to be able to meet comfortably in a member's home, the district is divided into two churches (districts). This involves "choosing" and installing a bishop. Every church district has its own bishop and ministers who set the *Ordnung.* Hence, there are variations between individual districts in what members are allowed to do. The Amish do not want to interfere in the will of God, and they take special precautions to do this, for example, in the important matter of selection of a new preacher. Church members will process and finally suggest names of three or four men to be in the "lot." However, the choice of the "lot" is left to God by placing a piece of paper in a song book, mixing up the books, and letting each candidate pick one book. The person who picks the book with the piece of paper hidden inside is recognized as being called by God to be a minister for life.

The exact number of the Amish living in the United States is unknown. The Amish are organized in settlements that are made up of church districts. A settlement can have from 1 to 200 districts, with each district being made up of 25 to 40 families (Elizabethtown College, 2014). A 2014 census of settlements estimated there were 480 settlements in 30 states (Elizabethtown College, 2014). The Amish have an annual growth rate of 3% per year. The population is expected to double in 18 to 20 years (Elizabethtown College, 2014). The largest number of settlements were in four states: Ohio, Pennsylvania, Indiana, and Wisconsin (Elizabethtown College, 2014). Settlements are found as far south as Florida and as far west as Idaho (Elizabethtown College, 2014). The establishment of new settlements is the result of increased population along with a search for affordable farm land and a higher degree of government tolerance of their cultural distinctiveness.

The average Amish family has five or more children (Elizabethtown College, 2014). Amish women have a prolonged childbearing time, about age 20 to 45, and fertility rates can be extremely high. This capacity to double the population about every 18 to 20 years means new districts and even settlements must be developed continuously, which makes it difficult to keep accurate population counts (Elizabethtown College, 2014). Today, the total Amish population in the United States is greater than 290,000, with as many as 140,000 of these being children under 20 (Elizabethtown College, 2014).

Since the rules by which the Amish live vary between districts, it is difficult to make generalizations concerning the Amish as a whole. Health professionals who seek to provide culturally competent care to Amish in a given area should ask the individual about values, beliefs, and practices related to health care or particular aspects of health care as it applies to their local and current health situation. In 2006, some Amish beliefs and practices became well known when a milkman in an Amish community in Pennsylvania took students hostage in an Amish school and killed five girls. The nation watched in disbelief as the Amish community returned anger with love as they comforted the family of the killer (Death toll, 2006).

COMMUNICATION

Amish adults are bilingual, and many are trilingual (Beachy, Hershberger, Davidhizar, & Giger, 1997). The first language of virtually all Amish children is Pennsylvania Dutch, or more correctly, Pennsylvania German. Pennsylvania Dutch is a German dialect that in America has become a mixture of German and English. Sometimes an English word is simply given a German accent if a German word is not readily available. Pennsylvania Dutch could be called the Amish social language. It is often the only language children know until they start school. It is the language used by the family at home and for all Amish social events. The second language Amish learn is English. They start learning words at home, but the primary learning takes place when they start their formal schooling, whether in a public or Amish school. Most Amish, particularly adults, can speak English well. English may be considered the language for interaction with outsiders. English is the only written language Amish regularly use, both with each other and the outside world.

The third language of the Amish is German, often referred to by the Amish as *High German,* which is used primarily in church services. Many Amish who attend a church school learn to read German. Amish have difficulty holding a lengthy conversation in German because it is not commonly used in social dialogue. Even in church services, which used to be primarily in High German, more and more Pennsylvania Dutch words are used. The only time High German is used in the purest sense is for reading from the Bible or prayer book or for singing from the *Ausbund,* the original songbook of the Swiss Brethren prior to the Amish split.

Amish people tend to be quiet and are not likely to raise their voices in public places. An Amish person will avoid attracting attention in keeping with the desire of the Amish person to be humble. Quietness and use of nonverbal communication are considered appropriate in the Amish culture.

The Amish culture can be classified as a high-context culture (Leininger & McFarland, 2006; Wenger, 1988). Messages flow freely, have deep meaning, and have many levels, unlike the low-context cultures, where verbal communication is the primary means for sending messages. The Amish communicate with overt and explicit manifestations but also have covert and implicit communications, as well as gestures that outsiders may not note or understand (Hostetler, 1993). One author witnessed a physician explaining to an extended family why a particularly expensive procedure should be done for a child. The grandfather did not speak, but when the son looked at him, he lowered his head and bent it toward the side. The message of disapproval had been given, and the son understood his father's thoughts on the issue. This communication could have been missed by a health professional from a low-context culture unaware of the meaning of this nonverbal message.

Amish use a nonverbal screening process, particularly with outsiders. If the Amish person is not sure they can trust the outsider, certain topics are not discussed or are discussed with difficulty.

Outside of a good firm handshake and a Sunday greeting with a holy kiss of a person of the same gender, Amish adults do very little public touching; this also applies to husbands and wives. Even in the privacy of their homes, a husband and wife will not engage in physical holding and kissing, particularly in the presence of children. The lack of personal contact between newlyweds is evidenced in the traditional marriage ceremony. On the other hand, a lot of touching takes place with children as they interact with adults.

Implications for Nursing Care

Establishing trust is the cornerstone of the provider–patient relationship and the foundation of quality health care delivery and outcomes (Gamble, 2006). A health care provider working with the Amish patient and family should begin with a firm handshake, quietly provide an introduction and a greeting of name and purpose, and indicate that it is a pleasure to meet the individual or appreciation that the person has come. If the health care professional can speak a little German or Pennsylvania Dutch, a few words will facilitate the development of trust and provide a commonality around which to relate, especially when talking to children under the age of 5. For example, a nurse with Amish roots contracted with a government agency to draw blood from a group of preselected, multigravida Amish women in a cancer research project. The nurse obtained the blood from all but one woman. A few weeks later, the agency contacted the nurse and questioned the high rate of participation. The nurse explained that he introduced himself in Pennsylvania Dutch, spent 10 to 15 minutes explaining the blood test, and provided his personal background. After this brief discussion, which sometimes included eating popcorn together, the woman extended her arm and the blood was drawn.

Another example, on a pediatric unit where Amish children come for care, the Amish children are well behaved, sometimes stoic, and often shy. However, when the nurse spoke to the children in Pennsylvania Dutch, the response was dramatic. The children were less shy, less fearful, and even smiled. Parents, too, were more at ease, more willing to talk, and more trusting when they felt they had an advocate.

Strategies that can assist in developing trust with the Amish include:
1. Ask questions if unsure of cultural practices.
2. Approach with a handshake.
3. Speak slowly and softly.
4. Have knowledge of Amish customs.
5. Visit with the individual to get to know the person.
6. Explain about the cost before doing procedures.
7. Provide only care that the client desires.
8. Let family members stay with hospitalized patients.

Touch by health care professionals in the context of giving care is generally accepted. The health care professional should be aware that nonverbal expressions of familiarity, such as hugs in public by someone of the opposite sex, are generally not acceptable. Amish are reticent to talk about family problems, mental illness in the family, and sexual activity. If the health care provider needs to address these topics, they may be discussed more easily in a private conversation with the client or family member. If a relationship is present or can be established, this will facilitate conversation. Full disclosure may not come until trust has been developed between the Amish client and the health care provider.

Amish communicate love and concern by presence. Personal visits, particularly during illness or crisis, are common. In fact, there is almost an expectation to visit a sick family member, close friend, or neighbor. Since Amish do not live in town and hire a van to take them to visit a person in a hospital, they may ask other family or friends to go with them to share the expense. Therefore, Amish patients in a hospital often receive large numbers of visitors at one time. To some Amish patients, the number of visitors is a visible sign of being cared about. To provide culturally competent care for the Amish patient and family, it is important for hospital personnel to adjust rules on numbers of visitors. Visitors do not have to all be in the room at one time to be supportive. Some may go into the room, make their presence known, and withdraw to the hallway in order to allow others to fit into the room. Even having a large number standing in the room is usually not disruptive since volume is kept low. This is particularly true if the patient is gravely ill or near death. This is a time when family members want to be near their loved one. The Amish want to be present in the event that the dying person may have a deathbed message for them (Schwartz, personal communication, 2006).

SPACE

The Amish like space. The Amish find rural living or small villages and towns the most suitable setting for living with their family. Many have large houses, yards, and gardens. Rooms in the house tend to be large, particularly the living room, dining room, and kitchen, which are used frequently for hospitality and food preparation. The Amish enjoy inviting company. Meals for company may involve having 20 or more persons around the table. After dinner, sitting and visiting for extended periods of time are expected. Men sit and talk in the living room. All of the women help with the cleanup and may stay in the kitchen and talk or join the men in the living room. The large house is also useful for the one or two Sundays a year when the church service is held in the family home. These functional rooms are cleared of some furniture, and benches are placed in rows for the church service. The people sit in close proximity for the church service, which may last up to 4 hours. Men and women do not sit together at a church service but do so at other social events.

Amish maintain a cultural boundary between themselves and the outside world. They live among the "English" and participate in that world, yet they keep themselves separate. They constantly work at maintaining the appropriate boundary between themselves and the outside world, as they have for centuries. One may see a sign advertising farm produce at the end of a lane, inviting the outsiders to come and buy the produce. But one also sees and experiences the subtle hints of separation. The bottom of the sign will say "No Sunday Sales." Signs are common when Amish engage in entrepreneurial work. On some farms, buyers select their produce, make their own change from a money pot sitting beside the produce, leave their money, and never see an Amish person.

Implications for Nursing Care

The boundaries between the Amish persons and the outside world are more relaxed when responding to health care professionals. A professional caring for the Amish in the office or hospital can generally follow customary procedures of privacy and professionalism. However, the health care professional should be aware that the Amish may not be as free to show their bodies to their children or spouse. During personal care, the professional should offer the option of family members waiting in another location. Guardedness about personal privacy is relaxing somewhat among the younger generation in some settlements.

The health care professional should be aware that Amish family members care deeply about one another but that this affection is expressed in private, and it is unlikely to be seen in the health care setting. If a husband on a maternity unit appears aloof or even cool, this should not be interpreted as a lack of caring for his wife. Children on a pediatric unit are likely to be subdued and less demonstrative. This is a result of their training to respect adults and elders and to show restraint. In addition, there may be a language barrier, since most Amish children up to the age of 6 do not speak English.

SOCIAL ORGANIZATION

Family Systems and Family Roles

The Amish family is a nuclear family in the traditional sense. It consists of one man and one woman of the same ethnicity and religion who remain married for life. Most Amish get married in their early twenties and are expected to raise large families. An extended family with multiple generations may live in the same house or on the same farm. Grandparents may live in a *Dauddy Haus,* which may have an enclosed connection to the main house. Families that do not live on a farm will have extended family living next door or in the community. Amish live in a community, where children are expected to care for aging parents. Since aging parents have been part of the household and have helped with childrearing and gardening over the years, it is not difficult for Amish families to continue to care for them in their illness and death.

Amish families are paternal in structure, with the man taking on the roles of breadwinner, head of the family, and disciplinarian. Farming is the traditional occupation for the Amish man. However, with the increased cost of farmland and the high fertility rates, farming is an impossible goal for many. In some larger settlements, increasing numbers of Amish have moved to small farms that cannot support the family. Consequently, even though it is not an Amish value, many men work away from home in occupations such as carpentry, woodworking, construction, and other small industries in the "English" world. This work brings issues that conflict with the primary cultural values, such as the male role model not being at home during the day, not enough meaningful work for the children to do, and the male's exposure to modern worldly values at work.

Income of Amish families varies widely, not unlike the general population. The young Amish farmer with 5 to 10 children may struggle to provide for basic essentials and have little money for health care expenses. The Amish man working in a factory may receive a good income. Without needing to spend money on manufactured clothes, a car, insurance, education, or entertainment, income may be spent on a nicer home, traveling to visit family, or saved for future needs.

Amish women seldom work outside the home after marriage and having children but may sell quilts or baked goods to help with the family income. A woman is expected to bear children and care for her husband and family. She does her own sewing and preserves garden goods, most of which are grown on the farm or large garden. Some women will work outside the home prior to marriage or may continue to work outside the home if they remain single, which is considered undesirable by the Amish. Amish women see their role as wife and mother. Amish women define health as the ability to care for their husband and family and to participate in community activities without too many aches or pains (Schwartz, 2002).

Children are expected to assist with tasks at home at a very early age. By the age of 12 they will have many responsibilities, including caring for the garden and general farm work. Children learn very early that they are an important part of the community. They learn that the community expects them to take on responsibilities and to value and support what is good for the community. Amish children tend to be shy with outsiders.

Individualism is not a virtue in Amish culture. The Amish state that they want to be for others and not for self (Schwartz, 2002). A "good Amish person" tries to fit in and not stand out in the community. Pride is seen as a negative attitude. Pride is more often used to describe the opposite of humility, a characteristic God desires from individuals. This does not mean that Amish people cannot develop their gifts or skills but that their talents should be used to benefit the community and not violate the *Ordnung*. It is not uncommon to see women and girls do farm work. This is particularly true if the older children are girls. However, it is rare to find the Amish male doing housework on a regular basis.

Gender role conflicts, although not obvious to the outsider, may arise in the area of financial management. If the skill of financial management lies with the female, it may cause some internal conflict that will not be obvious to outsiders. The male is usually considered the financial manager, and even for minor medical expenses, the husband needs to be included in the discussion.

The Amish family is clearly defined in structure and roles. The Amish family teaches its values by living the expectations. Amish children are often dressed like their parents and, although they are not expected to be little adults, they are expected to participate in the life of the community as much as they can. A preschooler may be expected to help gather eggs or carry water to others in the field. Sunday is not a workday except for those activities that have to be done, like milking cows. No business is transacted on Sunday. Every other Sunday is church Sunday in the district, and everyone is expected to be present if they are not ill. The Sunday in between is a day of rest, and often the afternoon is used for visiting the ill or friends, or attending church services in another district.

Religious Principles

To understand the Amish culture, it is important to understand the basic Amish religious principles. The Amish strive to incarnate the teachings of Jesus into a voluntary social order (Hostetler, 1993). First and foremost, the Amish believe in separation from the world. The Amish believe they are to live in the world but not be conformed to the world (Romans 12:2). It is from this belief that they dress differently and conduct their daily lives with few amenities. This separation also means not marrying an outsider or "English" person and not developing business partnerships with outsiders (Brewer & Bonalumi, 1995). The Amish refuse to bear arms or to go to court to bring suit against someone for a wrong. Generally, they choose to move rather than "fight" the state over some issue that violates their religious principles. Obedience to God and humility constitute a pervasive theme in the community, and pride (*hochmut*) is abhorred (Hostetler, 1993). Although the Amish value being separated from the predominant society, they will work in it and relate to it. The Amish will not judge other persons, including being on a jury, believing instead that God is the only judge. The Amish will not try to convert outsiders to their ways, although they may try to suggest at times that another's behavior may not be biblical, as they understand it.

The process of helping its members to live and understand this separateness is found in the *Ordnung*, the rules and regulations developed by the community (Gross, 1997). These regulations are decided upon by a group of leaders who present them to the congregation for discussion and response twice a year, just prior to Communion Sunday. This is not a written document but an oral understanding of the beliefs and behaviors of the community. This concept is particularly important for the health care professional to understand because, while similar, not every church district has the same rules and regulations. If an Amish patient is hesitant or not compliant, one could ask if this is not allowed by the *Ordnung*. The *Ordnung* classifies what is worldly or sinful within the community and the world. Amish individuals voluntarily submit to the rules and regulations of the *Ordnung* and allow others to help them avoid emphasizing power, wealth, and status. The Amish try not to stand out or be different in their society but, rather, try to fit into the social order of love and brotherhood within the church district.

The church district is the home church for all members who live within its borders. The functions of the district, besides preaching, are baptisms, marriages, and funerals (Hostetler, 1993). Discipline of members is also carried out in the home district. Outside authority and other districts have no jurisdiction over a member. Likewise, a member has no recourse outside the home district. This pertains to church or community matters and not to state or legal matters. The Amish abide by the civil laws unless the law violates a basic principle of Amish belief.

Much of Amish life and behavior has a religious or biblical base. The most important part of Amish life is *Gelassenheit*, or submission to the will of God. It is based on the words of Jesus, "Not my will but thine be done." For the Amish, this translates into serving others and giving up individuality and selfishness. It is manifested in many aspects of Amish life, such as:

- Personality: reserved, modest, calm, quiet
- Values: submission, obedience, humility, simplicity
- Symbols: dress, horse, carriage, lantern
- Structure: small, informal, local, decentralized
- Ritual: kneeling, foot washing, confession, shunning (Kraybill, 2001, 2003)

Any technology or action that does not uphold the *Gelassenheit* principles is not allowed and may even be considered sinful. These unwritten decisions are part of the *Ordnung*. These rules help define what it means to be Amish. As technology changes, new rules may be added, or older ones may change, but the basic rules have stayed in place throughout the history of the Amish. The *Ordnung* will have many similarities in every church district, but each community will have its own variations on what will be accepted and what will not. The strictness of the rules and the method of enforcement depend on the bishop of each church district. Differences from one church to another may be confusing to outsiders. What is important for the health professional to know is that the *Ordnung* says very little about the use of modern medicine. The use of a particular medical technology may be discussed at a church meeting twice a year just prior to Communion, where leaders and members debate its ramifications as they understand them. The decision may have less to do with technology than with the rules of *Gelassenheit*. A bishop will consider a variety of aspects in making a decision. If the bishop decides a medical technology threatens the values or traditions of the Amish, it is banned. However, blood transfusion, organ donation, cardiac bypass surgery, and organ transplantation are generally accepted (Wenger & Wenger, 2003).

Education

Amish sought the freedom to educate their children in their own private schools. In 1972, there were seven districts in Wisconsin educating their children through eighth grade in their own schools with Amish teachers. Some of the teachers had only a general equivalency diploma. The State of Wisconsin attempted to force these children to attend public schools. Normally, the Amish resist repressive laws for a period of time and try to work things out with the state. However, the Old Order Amish do have a "Steering Committee" made up of bishops, deacons, and laymen that work to negotiate these types of situations with the state and federal government (Olshan, 2003). If the issue cannot be resolved, they have tended to move to a state more tolerant of their views. The Wisconsin situation caught the attention of several outside groups and lawyers, who finally forced a Supreme Court ruling (Mackaye, 1971). The Supreme Court ruled in 1972 that imposing mainstream cultural values on the Amish via the public schools would in essence destroy the culture and thus allowed them to maintain their own schools and educational system. In the next 25 years, the number of church districts in Wisconsin more than quadrupled. The number of Amish schools has increased in some settlements since the Supreme Court ruling.

The more conservative Amish districts build their own schools and have their own people teach with state oversight. The Amish are not against good basic education. Many Amish pupils test above the norm in their states (Lindholm, 1997). The mixed-grade, one-room schoolhouses, which are typical of pre-1945 rural America, are preferred because of the importance of transmitting Amish values and because they are more amenable to local control (Wenger & Wenger, 1998). Fisher and Stahl (1997) reported that in 1948 the Amish began looking at secular education and concluded that some of the curriculum was contrary to Amish beliefs. Materials that supported the Amish ways of life were selected. Many books used in many Amish schools have copyright dates of the 1960s and earlier; thus, up-to-date science and health information is not present. Rather, children are taught the importance of discipline, of helping each other, of obedience and truthfulness, and of the idea that what is good for the group is also good for the individual. Children are taught how to live and to prepare for death in the Amish tradition.

Public school education is perceived as a threat to the culture. The Amish are concerned about the time required to bus students out of their home communities and the subjects that are viewed as "unnecessary," such as advanced math and computer technology, which have little relevance to the Amish tradition (Meyers, 1994). They are concerned with the instruction in a value system that is antithetical to the Amish way of life in which individual achievement and competition are promoted (Meyers, 1994). They have a tendency to shun higher education because they know that those who complete high school leave the church and become "English." The emphasis is on practical education or education for the simpler life. Consequently, few Amish complete high school, and almost none has a college education.

In more heavily populated settlements, more Amish children attend public school. Most are taken out of school at age 16. Many public school districts that have a number of Amish children attempt to develop policies, course requirements, and student activities that the Amish will not find problematic.

Amish Youth

Amish youth are permitted to experience the world in their late teens; this is known as *Rumspringa* (Hostetler, 1993). Some allowances are made for dressing more "English," perhaps having a car (which some may park at an "English" neighbor's house rather than at home), or participating in typical activities experienced by "English" teenagers. The message is clear that such activities are in violation of community rules and sometimes even state law, but since the Amish youth are not baptized members yet, they are not told to stop the behavior or banned from the church. The Amish youth know that this way of life must be left behind when they decide to be baptized and join the church. Most Amish youth who participate in such activities know these are a violation of community values but have little intention or desire to leave the community. The Amish community and bishops accept this behavior as "sowing wild oats" and tend not to make a big issue out of it, because it allows these youth to put it away later and come back to the church. A health care professional should not be confused when caring for a youth who looks "English" but has Amish values and ideas associated with the traditional Amish. Considering the enticements of the culture around them, it is remarkable that 85% of Amish youth choose to join the church and to maintain the values they have been taught throughout adult life (Elizabethtown College, 2014; Wenger & Wenger, 1998).

The Amish and the State

The Amish are not a financial liability to the state (Lindholm, 2002). There is little or no unemployment, virtually no divorce, and very little delinquency among its youth. As a group they are trustworthy and hard workers, and they do not join unions, which makes them desirable as employees (Banks & Benchot, 2001; Blair & Hurst, 1997). The Amish are law abiding (unless a law violates the *Ordnung*), do not bring suit for personal gain against anyone, and are cooperative and compassionate, as an "English" neighbor discovered when the whole community showed up to help rebuild a barn that had burned (Kraybill, 2003).

Implications for Nursing Care

The health care professional should be aware that some health care decisions may be based on the *Ordnung*. Some health care professionals think that Amish do not believe in or approve of immunizations. There are a few districts where this is true; however, immunization rejection by an Amish person is more often based on ignorance, cost, or some other rationale. Thus, it would be appropriate for a health professional to discuss the pros and cons for rejecting a health treatment with an Amish person to see if it is based on the *Ordnung* or due to some other belief or

situation. Amish are aware of the religious waivers one can use to avoid immunizations and may use that route when their refusal may actually be an issue of cost. Husbands, who often accompany their wives and children when seeking health care, are the gatekeepers for the family's health care decisions (Schwartz, 2002).

Birth control is forbidden in most church districts. However, with increasing numbers of Amish moving out of farm settings, many Amish are starting to consider the number of children a family should have. Farms provided a natural environment to teach the work ethic that is not available in a nonfarm setting. Decisions or rationales related to birth control are not for public discussion. The methods used for birth control may include condoms, withdrawal, or abstinence. The Amish have also discovered the limitations of these methods, so some look to other options. One physician in northern Indiana reported to the author that he performed a number of vasectomies on Amish men on Friday afternoons. The physician felt the procedure was done without the sanction or knowledge of the Amish bishops because he was located out of the mainstream Amish community. The health care professional should approach the question of birth control with caution because Amish generally reject it. However, if the nurse senses that the Amish patient wants to discuss birth control, the advantages and disadvantages of options should be offered (Beachy et al., 1997).

Health care interventions need to be designed for the Amish in a culturally sensitive manner that considers the values and needs of the group. For example, the state health department asked a nurse to assist in an intervention in a settlement where several Amish children had died from pertussis. The state health department presenters gave explanations to the bishops on immunization theory and how it protects children by giving a controlled disease so the body could build its antibodies without causing major harm. The presenters stressed that children did not have to die from this disease if immunized. This was an important point because Amish desire children and see them as a gift from God. The death of a child is seen as a great loss. After a discussion time with the bishops over a full-course lunch, it became clear that the issue was not refusing to get immunizations because of *Ordnung* but more the cost of getting everyone in a family with 4 to 10 children immunized, since free immunizations were not available. A proposal finally emerged. The state would bring a team to their schoolhouse and charge a fair price for the vaccine, and the bishops would promote the event in the churches. Several weeks later, the immunizations took place.

It is important for the health care professional to appreciate the value of the Amish in placing others in the context of family, relatives, and community. In the hospital, it is not unusual for an Amish person to stop a person in the hall who is wearing distinctive Amish dress, shake hands with an Amish stranger, and ask in Pennsylvania Dutch, "Who are you?" Within minutes, they may discover that they are distant relatives or have a mutual acquaintance. At the same time health care professionals need to be aware of the privacy of the patient and not divulge patient information just because the inquirer is Amish. Amish women especially are very private and do not want private matters to become public even in the community in which they live (Schwartz, 2002).

The simple question "Who are you?" is a powerful networking tool that the "English" may not understand in dealing with the Amish. For example, a CEO of a hospital was to meet with an Amish leader to finalize an agreement to have the leader sign a contract or come to an understanding of how payment of a hospital bill would be handled if one of their members should use the CEO's facility. The CEO wanted to proceed as quickly and efficiently as possible, which is not an Amish value. When the CEO started pushing for some sort of an agreement, the Amish person pulled back and said, "I don't even know you." The CEO was stunned. This did not mean that the Amish man needed to know what degrees and credentials the CEO had, because those have little meaning to the Amish community. Rather the statement meant that the Amish person wanted to know about integrity in business dealings. An evaluation of trustworthiness will be established by determining "who you are." It is imperative for all health care workers to work on building trust by being open and honest with the Amish patient (Weyer et al., 2003).

Birthing centers have been established to respond to the needs of the Amish. Financing may be largely provided by the Amish community (Kreps & Kreps, 1997). The *Wall Street Journal* reported negotiations between hospitals and religious communities to reduce cost of health care to Amish and Mennonites (Millman, 2006).

The social support in the Amish community is evident in care of the elderly. Amish are seldom found in a nursing home. An Amish person may be sent home from a hospital sooner than other patients with like diagnoses and treatments because of the desire of the family to have the sick individual at home where care can be provided and because of the desire to lessen the expense of the hospital (McCollum, 1998). Most Amish persons will not have traditional insurance or Medicare unless they have worked in a factory. The health care professional may wonder how Amish can afford to pay large medical and hospital bills without private insurance. In some areas the Amish community has contracted with health care providers who will discount their bills by 20% or more since they know the bill will be

paid in a timely fashion. Several hospitals have developed a special rate for a normal delivery in obstetrics if the bill is paid prior to the hospitalization. Some Amish have what is called "Amish Aid," or a mutual insurance for large hospital bills or losses of any kind, although they do not call it "insurance." When a hospital bill is received that a family cannot pay, the church leaders in the district will take responsibility for starting the mutual insurance process. If it is not a large bill, the district may take care of it by asking members to contribute. If it is a larger bill, it is divided up among some or all the districts in a settlement or even several settlements. On a Sunday morning a leader of each district will announce each family's share of a certain hospital bill. Individuals will give this person cash, which he will put in his pocket to count when he gets home. If not enough money is collected for a district's share, it will be announced again at the next church meeting until the sum has been collected. These needs may also be announced in *The Budget* (an Amish newspaper) with a request to shower the person or family with cards or prayers (*The Budget,* 2015). Some church districts and settlements have gone to fund-raising activities such as auctions of donated items or meals (for example, a haystack supper) (see Box 29-1 for the recipe). The added benefit of these activities is that non-Amish family and friends can participate in the financial needs of a particular person. Some settlements are seeing that the high cost of health care is a major concern. Some settlements have started a hospital insurance fund that individuals can voluntarily join by paying a certain fee into the fund regularly, which makes them eligible to draw upon the fund in case of need (Greksa & Korbin, 1997). Some Amish groups are collaborating with local health care agencies to ensure lower health care costs.

TIME

As a culture the Amish are present- and past-oriented. Many aspects of living have changed very little since the 1600s, including dress, lifestyle, and religious services. The Amish value using time efficiently and productively. Since traveling to town with horses takes more time, trips are limited. While work is considered valuable, reserving time for visiting is important because relationships are highly valued. Women often make the clothes for the family. Traditionally they have used the old Singer treadle sewing machine. Today, more modern equipment, such as non-electric, battery-powered sewing machines, may be used for making clothes. Some items, such as underwear and men's shirts, may be purchased. The pocket must be removed from the shirt, but today the buttons, formerly removed, are generally left on men's shirts. Trousers will usually button or snap and have no outside pocket. In the

---

BOX 29-1 Amish Haystack Dinners

Submitted by June Yoder, a school nurse at Honeyville School in Goshen, the grand prize ($50,000) winner of Newman's Own in 1995.

2 lb ground beef
1 package taco seasoning mix (dry)
1 14-oz jar (or 1½ cups) tomato-based pasta sauce*
1½ cups shredded cheddar cheese†
2 cups crushed soda crackers or saltines
1 9-oz bag tortilla chips, crushed
2 cups cooked rice, prepared according to package directions
1 head iceberg lettuce, shredded
1 cups diced tomatoes
1 cup chopped onions
1 cup chopped carrots
1 cup sliced pitted ripe olives
1 cup diced green peppers
1 cup diced celery
1 cup crumbled cooked bacon
1 cup sunflower seeds
1 11-oz jar salsa*

Brown ground beef with taco seasoning in 12-inch skillet over medium-high heat; add pasta sauce. Simmer until meat is cooked through and liquid evaporates. Put all ingredients in individual bowls. Heat cheese sauce if used. Let diners serve themselves, layering as follows: lettuce, crushed chips, crackers, meat mixture, rice, the rest of the vegetables, and ending with cheese sauce, bacon, sunflower seeds, and salsa. Serves 12.

*Prize-winning recipe used Newman's Own.
†For a moister "haystack," use one 12-oz container of pasteurized process cheese sauce, heated through.

---

early Amish church, buttons were not allowed and only hooks and eyes were used, which rapidly became a symbol of the Amish people. A homemade shirt may still use the hook and eye instead of buttons. Women tend to have few if any buttons on their clothes; in particular, the Sunday dress is likely to be held together by the strategic placement of straight pins. Women wear a white organdy kapp (or head cap) in keeping with the Biblical teaching that a woman's hair is to be covered (1 Corinthians 11:5–6). The cap is worn day and night. A black bonnet may cover the white cap to protect the cap against the weather (Hostetler, 1993). Rules for dress are established within the districts and follow traditional plain clothes, with long sleeves for the women and a cape and apron. Men wear broad-fall pants with suspenders and black, broad-brim hats.

The Amish have learned to live in the present while still maintaining the boundaries of what is Amish and what is not. When the Amish work in factories, they have learned to use modern tools. Some Amish have their own workshops with modern tools that are run via the power of a large diesel engine. This is allowed for the exclusive use of the shop and the livelihood of the family. Persons whose income is not derived from farming frequently have more time and money to spend in the local economy. In areas of dense Amish population, local businesses, such as fast food restaurants and department stores, have often provided accommodations for Amish customers in the parking lots where they have placed hitching posts, horse shelters, and concrete pads for the horses (since concrete is cooler for the horses than blacktop). Despite their mode of travel, Amish are typically on time or early for appointments. It is common for many Amish to arrive at church services an hour early, preventing lateness, and allowing time for the important activity of visiting with the host family and other church members in attendance.

Implications for Nursing Care

With their past-time orientation, the Amish are excellent historians. Amish are likely to know what diseases or conditions run in the family and can often give this information for several generations. Although the medical terms may not be known, illnesses are described in general terms, such as "Uncle Sam died of liver problems." Because they are less present- and future-time oriented, Amish are less concerned with concepts of illness prevention. Since visits to a health professional are expensive, they are reserved for illnesses that cannot be cured with home and folk remedies (Sharpnak, Griffin, Benders, & Fitzpatrick, 2010). Thus the patient may be in more serious condition when finally arriving for medical treatment. This is gradually changing as they learn to trust the medical system.

When caring for hospitalized Amish women, the nurse should be aware of the desire for privacy and modesty. Requesting that a woman put on scrub pants for leg exercises after a knee replacement, for example, should not be done. In addition, the nurse needs to be cognizant of the need for prayer coverings. Some women may want to keep a prayer covering on at all times. This may be true even during surgery or other procedures. This request should be accommodated as much as possible in order to respect the woman's commitment to her religious roots and upbringing and to provide culturally congruent care.

ENVIRONMENTAL CONTROL

The Amish believe in an external locus of control. The overriding way of life is God's will in all things. The Amish believe that God acts in everyday situations and that events both positive and negative are under God's control and are His will. While this may appear to be fatalistic, they believe in using the knowledge God has given to care for self, family, and others.

The Amish view the body as the temple of God and believe they should do what they can to help the body to heal itself and that God will guide them in this effort, allowing that God's way is the natural way (Schwartz, 2002). This often includes taking a home remedy or a particular product recommended by a family member or friend. Patent medicines may be used for a number of complaints (Palmer, 1992). This is frequently the first step in their own health care and is referred to by Wenger (1995) as the folk aspect of Amish health care. The folk aspect includes taking herbs of various kinds, vitamins, or juices. Amish tend to believe that "natural" things are more helpful, which may open the door for quackery (Landmark series, 1984). For some, a practice called *Brauche,* or *pow-wowing,* is used. *Brauche* is a type of faith healing by a *Braucher,* who uses words, charms, and sometimes physical manipulation to heal common illnesses, such as colic in babies (Wenger, 1995). *Brauche* is thought to work best with babies since they cannot talk (Miller-Schlabach, 1992). Some Amish use *Brauche* because a *Braucher* tends to be readily available and accepts donations rather than charging fees for service (Palmer, 1992). While *Brauche* is generally considered an acceptable form of health care and a gift of God, some Amish communities are beginning to consider it questionable (Wenger, 1995).

Other alternative therapies that are popular with the Amish include chiropractic, reflexology, foot massage, and iridology. Miller-Schlabach (1992) reported that 100% of Amish persons surveyed used a chiropractor. *The Budget* advertises folk remedies or alternative health care providers (*The Budget,* 2015). Criteria for choosing options in health care include family tradition, proximity of the care provider, testimony of others, cost, and an attitude of respect by the care provider (Brewer & Bonalumi, 1995; Wenger, 1995). When the natural way does not take care of the symptoms, the Amish then seek "the medical way" (Schwartz, 2002). This may result in waiting too long for treatment or going to Mexico for treatment such as laetrile and other medicines that have not been approved by the Food and Drug Administration in the United States.

Since birthing is seen as a natural process, Amish women underutilize pregnancy care (Campanella, Korbin, & Acheson, 1993). While most Amish women see a doctor during the pregnancy, Adams and Leverland (1986) noted that 22% of women waited until the sixth month to seek prenatal care. Pregnancy care tends to be sought earlier for the first child but tends to be delayed in subsequent parities. Adams and Leverland (1986) found that 90% of the Amish women in a Pennsylvania study had their first child in the hospital but only 59% had their last child in the hospital. Many Amish women desire an alternate birthing experience, such as a birth at a birthing center or a home birth, rather than hospital care. Despite the low-tech approach to birthing used by the Amish, infant mortality is below the national average (Campanella et al., 1993).

Rituals Related to Death and Dying

When someone is critically injured in an accident, the decision not to use all the options to save life may be influenced by expense as well as by the will of God. This becomes more difficult when the person is young or a child, but, even then, the will of God is taken seriously. While death results in sorrow, there is still hope because the dead person has gone to a better place. To do everything to live a while longer can be viewed as lack of faith. The Amish view death as a part of life, and letting a natural death run its course is part of preparing to meet God. The Amish tend to be pragmatic about health care. If an alternative therapy is thought to work, they may try it rather than seeing a physician (Gillum et al., 2011). When an Amish person is near death, it is extremely useful to have the patient in a private room to allow as many visitors as can comfortably stand. The visitors may sing softly to the client to make the journey to their God more peaceful. Death is not feared but rather a solemn and profound event in the life of a person. Amish persons tend to prefer to die at home without the interference of institutional rules. When an Amish person faces death, it is important for the health care professional to be an advocate to ensure that personal needs and desires are met. For example, the family may need someone to explain how to say "no" to a doctor if they really do not want a procedure to continue. It is very difficult for persons in this high-context culture to say "no" to the rational reasoning of the health care system. When the health care professional hears "I'd rather not" in a quiet Amish voice, this may mean an emphatic "no!" The Amish will not refuse medical technology if there is a good prognosis, but they do not value the extension of life if it brings only more suffering. The patient may desire that the family or some other community members help decide how things should be done. Ultimately, the outcomes, regardless of intervention, are considered God's will, and the Amish are at peace with that (Gillum et al., 2011).

Implications for Nursing Care

The Amish recognize most health practices and practitioners as useful and will use them in an eclectic manner if they are trustworthy. Health care professionals, including physicians and nurse practitioners, are usually selected only after other options have been exhausted and at the recommendation of a friend or someone else in the community. It is important to gain the patient's trust and to elicit information about other remedies that have been tried. In recent years, getting information about other health practices among the Amish has been less of a problem, with alternative practices becoming more generally acceptable and understood. Historically, Amish would not divulge such information, knowing that it was not considered an approved treatment.

BIOLOGICAL VARIATIONS

Susceptibility to Illness

There are biological variations and consequently variations in susceptibility to illness between ethnic and cultural groups. Since the Amish do not have insurance for health care and are hesitant to participate in preventive treatments, the health professional could expect a higher incidence of preventable conditions among the Amish. For example, the health care professional could expect that use of well water and infrequent dental care would predispose this population to increased rates of dental disease and caries. An older study by Bagramian, Narendran, and Khazari (1988) found just the opposite. Amish children had only one third to one half the problems of non-Amish children. This difference was attributed to not snacking between meals, although desserts were part of a larger meal several times a day.

Obesity and High Blood Pressure. Both obesity and high blood pressure could be expected because of the Amish's Germanic background and diet, as well as not placing a high value on slimness and dieting. While no major difference in blood pressure from the general population was found, obesity is prevalent in the Amish community (Gillum, Staffileno, Schwartz, Coke, & Fogg, 2010). The propensity for the Amish female to be more obese starts after age 25; this may reflect the frequency and number of pregnancies in this age group. Obesity is also more tolerated by the Amish, with little stigma attached. Thus, Amish are less likely to diet or to exercise to lose weight. Exercise for the sake of exercise can be seen as wasting time or even as vanity. Incorporating exercise into the daily functional tasks would be a more appropriate intervention strategy for this population.

Communicable Diseases. The lack of immunizations in some communities can cause major outbreaks of illness. Amish tend to visit other Amish friends and relatives in other settlements rather than take a traditional vacation. The possibility of one individual from Ohio, who has been exposed to a communicable disease, traveling to a low-immunized settlement is real. The Centers for Disease Control and Prevention (CDC) became aware of this in 1979, when a number of polio cases in Amish communities in Pennsylvania, Wisconsin, and Canada all had social connections (CDC, 1979).

Cancer. In the largest Amish settlements in the world, cancer incidence rates are significantly lower than among the non-Amish (Westman et al., 2010). They also appear to have significantly lower cancer screening health practices (Katz et al., 2011). Of four religious sects, two of which were religious and genetic isolates (Amish and Hutterites) and two of which were not (Seventh Day Adventists and Mormons), Troyer (1988) showed a reduced rate of cancer among all four religious groups compared with the population as a whole, suggesting lifestyle as a factor. The Amish generally had the lowest rate of cancer overall, but the rates of breast cancer and juvenile leukemia were higher. The Amish are very aware of the deadly nature of cancer and would know who of their relatives died from cancer. For those and other reasons, many Amish are very open to participating in studies to find cures for such conditions.

Alzheimer's Disease and Diabetes. Two conditions becoming more prevalent in the Amish are Alzheimer's disease (AD) and type 2 diabetes mellitus. Both showed a low incidence in studies done in the Amish from Lancaster County, Pennsylvania. Holder and Warren (1998) studied 121 individuals older than age 65 and 74 persons older than age 60 and found only 5 individuals who met the criteria for AD. This was less than 50% of the expected rate and in line with what another study found in the northern Indiana and southern Michigan Amish settlements. Lifestyle was the only reasonable explanation for this decreased rate. Van der Walt et al.'s study (2005) of inherited mitochondrial haplogroups suggested that the lower incidence of AD may be nuclear genetic factors.

The prevalence of diabetes mellitus in the Amish is approximately half that of Caucasians. The heritability of diabetes-related traits is significant (Hsueh et al., 2000). The Amish are an ideal population to conduct genetic research. They are an isolated population that marry within the church, often within the same district, and almost never marry an "English." Because of this relatively closed gene pool, there is a much greater possibility for a genetic condition within the gene pool to manifest itself. The Amish keep excellent records of family trees for generations. The availability of a database has been a treasure trove for genetic research, which works from numerous pedigrees that are often referred to by numbers, such as *Amish Pedigree Number 110.*

Genetic Variations

Researchers have found the Amish generally quite willing to participate in genetic studies and to discuss the genetic conditions found in their families (Brensinger & Laxova, 1995). Where previously Amish were hesitant to agree to studies related to mental disorders, this resistance has appeared to relax. However, action as a result of research data is not always congruent with findings. Brensinger and Laxova (1995) found that having a child with a genetic condition did not deter subsequent reproduction, although some parents asked about natural family planning. They also found that most had not had genetic counseling and that the persons questioned indicated they would not agree to genetic testing. This is congruent with the strong belief of the Amish not to use birth control and to leave matters of this nature up to prayer and God. The Amish are quite aware of many of the genetic conditions within their families and settlements (Shachtman, 2006). This has not appeared to decrease the fertility rate.

Amish see a child born with a genetic condition as "special" as the result of God's will, and as much a child of God as any other child (Armstrong, 2005; Shachtman, 2006). They understand the extra care such a child may require, but there is often an acceptance of the child by the family and the community that amazes the "English" world. This acceptance allows the child to be incorporated into the daily activities of the Amish world in very healthy and helpful ways. Since the culture is geared more toward low technology, many of these "special" persons can be fairly productive in that society. The Amish can teach the modern world many lessons on how to accept and incorporate these children into the family and community.

Researchers have found certain types of genetic conditions within certain settlements of Amish. For example, in Lancaster County, Pennsylvania, glutaric aciduria is found more frequently and is the only known source for "Amish microcephaly" (Brensinger & Laxova, 1995; Rosenberg et al., 1999). Lancaster County also has a fairly large number of Amish with maple sugar urine disease (although this condition can be found in other settlements), as well as several extremely rare conditions, such as the liver disease Crigler-Najjar syndrome. The Holmes, Wayne County, Ohio, settlement has a high rate of hemophilia B, and there is a high incidence of limb-girdle muscular dystrophy in the settlement of Allen and Adams County, Indiana (McKusick, 1964).

Implications for Nursing Care

The health care professional must consider genetic aspects when working on pediatric and obstetrical units with an Amish population. Not only will such a closed gene pool highlight the known genetic conditions in the population, but occasionally, rare genetic conditions will be evident. An awareness of patterns of inbreeding among the Amish can cause the health professional to be more alert for the assessment and discovery of rare genetic conditions.

Amish are starting to acknowledge mental illness among themselves more openly. A big drawback for them is in-patient care, where they are required to mingle with the "English" for weeks, as well as being exposed to prolonged periods of television watching. To address some of these issues, an in-patient Amishlike home was built in Indiana for Amish persons receiving treatment. This was built and paid for by the Amish and is partially maintained and staffed by the Amish. This arrangement costs considerably less, has close proximity for therapy but maintains that desired separation, and keeps Amish values in its operation. Through creative care strategies of this type, health care professionals can assist the Amish in maintaining cultural values while at the same time receiving optimal care.

It is important for the health care professional to be aware that Amish tend to be stoic. Therefore, an assessment of pain requires more than a question about the presence of pain and needs to include a nonverbal assessment for indications of pain, as well as knowledge of the degree of pain that may be present in certain situations. The Amish may have difficulty with the 0–10 scale because they do not think in terms of degrees. Either they have pain or they do not have pain. A chiropractor said he quit asking the severity of the pain when the Amish patients said, "If I did not have pain I would not come." In addition, the "smiley face" pain scale may seem dichotomous to the Amish person—who can tell pain from a smile? The best way to assess is to ask if the person has some pain and then proceed to explain that pain medication will help the person sleep better and heal faster so that they may go home. Amish have no particular objection to taking pain medications, but, for some, to ask for medication or to admit to pain may be considered a sign of weakness. The Amish woman will be aware of the biblical directive that birthing will involve pain and thus expects pain and feels it should be accepted (Genesis 3:16).

▌ SUMMARY

The Amish are a branch of the Anabaptist religious movement, which started in Switzerland in 1525. They became a distinct group in the Alsace, France, region in 1697 through the strong leadership of Jacob Ammann. In the early 1700s, they began immigrating to the United States, where they became officially known as the *Amish*. The oldest settlement is in Lancaster County, Pennsylvania, but they have moved to many states, primarily east of the Mississippi. Unlike most cultures that have come to the United

States, the Amish have maintained many of the customs, beliefs, and dress of their ancestors. They live among the "English" but never in isolation from other Amish. They live in settlements, which are further divided into districts. Each district is a church group with its own ministers and bishop. The bishop sets the rules for the district. Most church districts will have many of the same rules, but each district will also have its own unique rules. Health care professionals need to understand that the general rules of each church district may be slightly different from another. It is essential to ask the patient and family about personal health care beliefs within the parameters of the church district to which the patient belongs. Amish are not averse to most modern health care and technology. They may choose not to use it because of cost and God's will. They are not against advanced technology; however, the low-tech or natural way is their first line of treatment for symptoms.

They are a humble people who try to live out their religion in everyday life. Death is a part of life and therefore the will of God. Thus, the Amish person may not choose every possible treatment to prolong life. The Amish use folk, alternative, and modern medicine in their own eclectic ways and see the value of one as much as the other. The community is very active in meeting the needs of its members and participates in helping individuals with losses or large hospital expenses. It is best if health care professionals take the time to get to know the person, do not push an agenda, and seek to understand the Amish ways of life and views on health. Do not seek to promote the medical model in health care; explain treatments and procedures until the Amish understand. Seek to develop the trust of the Amish people, and experience a deeper relationship with a unique culture that has stood the test of time in a fast-paced modern world.

CASE STUDY

Sarah Miller, an 85-year-old Amish woman, has had diabetes for 45 years. She was admitted to the hospital with extreme circulatory deficiency and evidence of early gangrene of the left foot. After discussion with some of her family members, she decided to go ahead with a below-the-knee amputation. Following surgery, she did quite well the first day, but when the nurse made her rounds the next morning, she found Sara mumbling and not being able to move her right arm and leg. The physician was notified, it was determined she had had a stroke, and the appropriate medications for dissolving a clot were ordered. As the day progressed, she got worse. By the next day, she did not try to speak but would squeeze the nurse's hand when spoken to.

Mrs. Miller was married when she was 18 to Sam, who became the district bishop when he was 47. He died of a coronary 5 years ago at the age of 82. They had eight children (four boys and four girls) 2 to 3 years apart, with the last one being born when Sarah was 40. The children were all married, and all but one lived as an Amish person in the local Amish settlement. Junior, the second male child, became "English" before marriage and continued to live in the area. Mrs. Miller has 42 grandchildren and 105 great-grandchildren.

Her children were asking questions about Sarah's prognosis, but no one was able to give them clear answers. Sarah had no living will—that would be left up to the family or the community to decide. After several days, she was not improving and may have gotten worse. She was having more difficulty with swallowing and was being maintained on IV fluids. The family had been coming daily to be with her. There were 20 visitors in the hallway and in her room. The family asked about the possibility of taking her home.

The medical staff agreed that going home with home health care visits was a possibility. The arrangements were started, but that evening the nurse found Sarah not responding with the hand squeeze and in an apparent coma. The family was notified that death may be imminent. The family gathered at the hospital that evening.

◎ CARE PLAN

Nursing Diagnosis: Communication, verbal, impaired related to alteration of central nervous system

Client Outcomes	Nursing Interventions
1. Client will communicate with family and friends by squeezing the hand for a yes or no. 2. Client will be pain-free as evidenced by nonverbal cues.	1. Explain her communication of a hand squeeze to visitors. 2. Determine the meaning of the nonverbal cue of a squeeze. 3. Have family or friends shake her hand and introduce themselves. 4. When speaking to her, use short sentences she can answer by a squeeze. 5. Encourage family and friends to visit even though she cannot speak. (This probably will not be a problem for this culture.) 6. Encourage just sitting in silence after introductions. 7. Encourage visitors to sing softly to her as a way of making her aware of their presence.

Nursing Diagnosis: Acute pain related to actual tissue damage (amputation)

Client Outcome	Nursing Interventions
Client will be pain-free, evidenced by nonverbal cues.	1. Be proactive in giving pain medications because of the stoic nature of the culture and the fear of doctors ordering too many pills. 2. Observe blood pressure and other physical nonverbal signs of pain. 3. Explain that you are giving some medication to make her more comfortable rather than using the word *pain*.

Nursing Diagnosis: Grieving, anticipatory

Client and Family Outcome	Nursing Interventions
Client and family will feel they have been allowed to practice cultural traditions as though the client were at home.	1. Include the family in caregiving activities. 2. Make an effort to have the client in a private room. 3. Encourage as many persons to be in the room as want to be. 4. Respect the need for privacy. 5. Introduce yourself with a handshake and express how glad the client must be to know the visitor is here. 6. Make it quite clear that no one needs to leave the room when the nurse comes in to do something unless you specifically need to have some or all of them leave. 7. Encourage them to sing softly to the client. 8. Accept the family values in a very nonjudgmental manner. 9. Be an advocate for the family and client. 10. Discuss the possibility of someone staying overnight in the room with the client. 11. Orient long-term family members to food sources and showers. 12. Spend a few minutes in the room being silent with the family. (Even sit and hold client's hand.) 13. If comfortable, say a short prayer for the client and family. (They normally do not do this themselves in public places but speak very kindly of nurses who have done that.) 14. As a primary caregiver of a client who has died, the family would be pleased if you came to the viewing at the family home.

CLINICAL DECISION MAKING

1. Why does one not see an Amish person living in a large city or an individual family living by themselves?
2. What values do Amish place on folk, alternative, and modern medicine, and how do they tend to use them?
3. Do Amish have any taboos toward using modern medicine?
4. What determines whether they choose to use a particular medical technology?
5. How do Amish pay for surgery and/or a hospital stay?
6. How can you begin to develop a trusting relationship with an Amish client?
7. What can a nurse do to make life in the hospital more culture-specific for an Amish client?
8. Why will one Amish person say he does not believe in doing some health care practice but another Amish person does not seem to have a problem with it?

REVIEW QUESTIONS

1. Which language is the first language of almost all Amish children?
   a. English
   b. German
   c. Pennsylvania Dutch
   d. Yiddish
2. Amish Americans tend to maintain boundaries between themselves and the outside world. When responding to health care professionals, these boundaries are generally expected to be which of following?
   a. Maintained
   b. Intensified
   c. Relaxed
   d. Forgotten
3. The Amish people have learned to live in the present. Culturally, their essential time orientation is to which of the following?
   a. Present
   b. Past
   c. Future
   d. Subjunctive

REFERENCES

Adams, C., & Leverland, M. (1986). The effects of religious beliefs on the health care practices of the Amish. *Nurse Practitioner, 11*(3), 58–63, 67.

Armstrong, P. (2005). Special children. *Journal of Midwifery & Women's Health, 3*(50), 241–242.

Bagramian, R., Narendran, S., & Khazari, A. (1988). Oral health status, knowledge, and practices in an Amish population. *Journal of Public Health Dentistry, 48*(3), 147–151.

Banks, M., & Benchot, R. (2001). Unique aspects of nursing care for Amish children. *The American Journal of Maternal/Child Nursing, 26*(4), 192–196.

Beachy, A., Hershberger, E., Davidhizar, R., & Giger, J. (1997). Cultural implications for nursing care of the Amish. *Journal of Cultural Diversity, 4*(4), 118–126.

Blair, R., & Hurst, C. (1997). Amish health care. *Journal of Multicultural Nursing and Health, 3*(2), 38–43.

Brensinger, J., & Laxova, R. (1995). The Amish: perceptions of genetic disorders and services. *Journal of Genetic Counseling, 4*(1), 27–47.

Brewer, J., & Bonalumi, N. (1995). Cultural diversity in the emergency department: health care beliefs and practices among the Pennsylvania Amish. *Journal of Emergency Nursing, 21*(6), 494–497.

The Budget. (2015). Sugar Creek, Ohio: The Budget.

Campanella, K., Korbin, J., & Acheson, L. (1993). Pregnancy and childbirth among the Amish. *Social Science and Medicine, 36*(3), 333–342.

Centers for Disease Control (CDC). (1979). Poliomyelitis: United States and Canada. *Morbidity and Mortality Weekly Report, 46*(50), 1194–1195.

Death toll at five from shooting. (2006). *The Goshen News,* 1.

Elizabethtown College. (2014). *The Young Center for Anabaptist and Pietist Studies: Amish Population by State.* Available at <www2.etown.edu/amishstudies/Index.asp> Retrieved April 1, 2015.

Fisher, S. E., & Stahl, R. K. (1997). *The Amish school.* Intercourse, PA: Good Books.

Gamble, V. N. (2006). Trust medical care and racial and ethnic minorities. In D. Satcher & R. Pamies (Eds.), *Multi-cultural medicine and health disparities* (pp. 437–448). New York: McGraw-Hill.

Gillum, D., Staffileno, B., Schwartz, K., Coke, L., & Fogg, L. (2010). The prevalence of cardiovascular disease and associated risk factors in the Old Order Amish of northern Indiana: a preliminary study. *Online Journal of Rural Nursing and Healthcare, 10*(2).

Gillum, D., Staffileno, B., Schwartz, K., Coke, L., Fogg, L., & Reiling, D. (2011). Cardiovascular disease in the Amish: an exploratory study of knowledge, beliefs, and healthcare practices. *Holistic Nursing Practice, 25*(6), 289–297.

Greksa, L., & Korbin, J. (1997). Influence of changing occupational patterns on the use of commercial health insurance by the Old Order Amish. *Journal of Multicultural Nursing and Health, 3*(2), 13–18.

Gross, L. (1997). *Background dynamics of the Amish movement: the Dutch Mennonites vis-à-vis the Swiss Brethren: pivotal individuals within the Swiss Brethren division of the 1690s, and the question of Reformed (Calvinist) influence.* Mennonite Historical Library, Goshen College, Goshen, Indiana. Available at <http://www.goshen.edu/mh/>.

Holder, J., & Warren, A. (1998). Prevalence of Alzheimer's disease and apolipoprotein E allele frequencies in the

Old Order Amish. *Journal of Neuropsychiatry, 10*(1), 100–102.

Hostetler, J. (1993). *Amish society* (4th ed.). Baltimore: Johns Hopkins University Press.

Hsueh, W. C., et al. (2000). Diabetes in the Old Order Amish: characterization and heritability analysis of the Amish Family Diabetes Study. *Diabetes Care, 23*(5), 595–601.

Katz, M. L., et al. (2011). Cancer screening practices among Amish and non-Amish adults living in Ohio Appalachia. *The Journal of Rural Health, 27,* 302–309.

Kraybill, D. (2001). *The riddle of the Amish culture* (revised ed.). Baltimore: Johns Hopkins University Press.

Kraybill, D. (Ed.), (2003). *The Amish and the state.* Baltimore: Johns Hopkins University Press.

Kreps, G., & Kreps, M. (1997). Astonishing "medical care." *Journal of Multicultural Nursing and Health, 3*(2), 44–47.

Landmark series on quackery aimed at Amish. (1984). *NCAHF Newsletter, 20*(1), 4–9.

Leininger, M., & McFarland, M. R. (2006). *Culture care diversity and universality: a worldwide nursing theory* (2nd ed.). Boston: Jones and Bartlett.

Lindholm, W. (1997). *U.S. Supreme Court case: is there religious freedom in America—for the Amish?* Available at <http://amishreligiousfreedom.org/case.htm> Retrieved April 1, 2015.

Lindholm, W. (2002). *Excerpts from the defense brief (Supreme Court ruling on Amish education)* (revised). Available at <http://amishreligiousfreedom.org/defense.htm> Retrieved April 1, 2015.

Mackaye, W. (1971). High court hears Amish school case. *Washington Post,* B7.

McCollum, M. (1998). The uninsured: uncovered—and unfazed. *Hospitals and Health Networks,* 38.

McKusick, V. A. (1964). Dwarfism in the Amish. *Transactions of the Association of American Physicians, 77,* 151–168.

Meyers, T. (1994). The Old Order Amish: to remain in the faith or to leave. *Mennonite Quarterly Review, 68*(3), 378.

Miller-Schlabach, N. (1992). Current health practices of old-order Amish (Unpublished master's thesis). University of South Florida, Tampa, FL.

Millman, J. (2006). How the Amish drive down medical costs. *Wall Street Journal, 247,* B1, B12.

Nolt, S. M. (1992). *A history of the Amish.* Intercourse, PA: Good Books.

Olshan, M. (2003). The National Amish Steering Committee. In D. Kraybill (Ed.), *The Amish and the state.* Baltimore: Johns Hopkins University Press.

Palmer, C. V. (1992). The health beliefs and practices of an Old Order Amish family. *Journal of the American Academy of Nurse Practitioners, 4*(3), 117–122.

Randell-David, E. (1989). *Strategies for working with culturally diverse communities and clients.* Washington, DC: U.S. Department of Health and Human Services.

Rosenberg, M., et al. (1999). Genetic mapping of a locus for Amish microcephaly. *American Journal of Human Genetics, 65*(Suppl. S), 2512.

Roth, J., & Springer, J. (Eds.), (2002). *Letters of the Amish division: a sourcebook.* Goshen, IN: Mennonite Historical Society.

Schwartz, K. (2002). Breast cancer and health care beliefs, values, and practices of Amish women. *Dissertation Abstracts International, 29*(1). (UMI No. 3047587.)

Shachtman, T. (2006). Medical sleuth. *Smithsonian, 11*(36), 23–30.

Sharpnak, P. A., Griffin, M. T., Benders, A. M., & Fitzpatrick, J. J. (2010). Spiritual and alternative healthcare practices of the Amish. *Holistic Nursing Practice, 24*(2), 64–72.

Troyer, H. (1988). Review of cancer among 4 religious sects: evidence that life-styles are distinctive sets of risk factors. *Social Science and Medicine, 26*(10), 1007–1017.

Van der Walt, J., et al. (2005). Maternal lineages of Alzheimer disease risk in the Old Order Amish. *Human Genetics, 118*(1), 115–122.

Wenger, A. (1988). The phenomenon of care in a high context culture: the Old Order Amish. *Dissertation Abstracts International, 29*(1). (UMI No. 8910384.)

Wenger, A. (1995). Classic article: cultural context, health, and health care decision making. *Journal of Transcultural Nursing, 7*(1), 3–14.

Wenger, A., & Wenger, M. (2003). The Amish. In L. Parnell & B. Paulenka (Eds.), *Transcultural healthcare* (2nd ed.). Philadelphia: F. A. Davis.

Westman, J. A., et al. (2010). Low cancer incidence rates in Ohio Amish. *Cancer Causes and Control, 21*(1), 69–75.

Weyer, S. M., et al. (2003). A look into the Amish culture: what should we learn? *Journal of Transcultural Nursing, 2*(14), 139–145.

Irish Americans

Cheryl M. Martin

BEHAVIORAL OBJECTIVES

After reading this chapter, the nurse will be able to:

1. Identify specific communication approaches for Irish Americans that influence health and wellness behaviors.
2. Explain the distance and intimacy behaviors of Irish Americans and their influence on health and wellness behaviors.
3. Describe the traditional roles of Irish-American family members.
4. Identify the Irish-American orientation to time and its influence on social and psychological behaviors.
5. Recognize cultural factors that affect the health-seeking behaviors of Irish Americans.
6. Recognize physical and biological variances that exist within and across Irish-American groups to provide culturally appropriate nursing care.

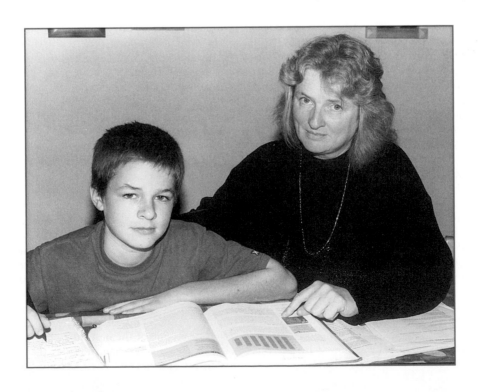

OVERVIEW OF IRELAND

The Republic of Ireland covers approximately 85% of the island known as *Ireland*. It comprises 26 counties that became the Irish Free State in 1921. In 1937 the Irish Free State was given the Gaelic name *Eire* by the constitution. Ireland is bordered on the northeast by Northern Ireland (Ulster), which today remains a part of the United Kingdom, and by the Atlantic Ocean to the west and south. St. George's Channel, the Irish Sea, and the North Channel separate Ireland from Great Britain by distances averaging at least 50 miles (80 kilometers).

The Republic of Ireland is primarily an agricultural country and is noted for the Irish potato. Industry is flourishing, and mining has become increasingly important because of recent discoveries of lead, silver, zinc, and copper deposits. Most of the countryside in Ireland is lowland situated less than 500 feet above sea level, and it is underlain by limestone rock. Most of the surface is covered by glacial drifts that are a legacy of the Pleistocene Ice Age. In some places in Ireland, the drifts have been shaped into distinctive landforms that form a continuous belt across the island.

Most of Ireland has a cool, maritime climate. For example, in July temperatures vary from 61° F in the south to 57° F in the north. Winters are extremely mild, with January temperatures varying from 44° F in the Valentia to 40° F in the northeast.

Ireland was colonized by settlers from Europe. For at least 5000 years, successive waves of settlers arrived from the island of Great Britain. Each group of settlers contributed to the heritage of the modern Irish nation. Even today, the Celtic influence remains dominant in Ireland. However, the eastern portion of Ireland has been particularly influenced by the Anglo-Normans, whose initial invasion in 1170 was followed by the subsequent immigration of settlers from England, Wales, and Scotland. The population of Ireland rapidly expanded during the eighteenth and early nineteenth centuries and reached a peak of 8.1 million people in 1841. However, the Great Potato Famine that began in 1845 brought a reversal of the population trend as a result of the many deaths and massive migration to the United States and Great Britain (Your Irish, 2015). This exodus continued over the next 100 years, and by 1921 the population of Ireland numbered little more than half of the original 1845 figure.

In the early , the Irish revolted against Britain in a battle for home rule. At the Easter Rebellion in Dublin in 1916, Irish nationalists unsuccessfully attempted to throw off British rule. In 1919, the rebels proclaimed Ireland as a republic. Unfortunately, this was followed by guerrilla warfare against the British until 1921, when a peace was negotiated by General Michael Collins (Your Irish, 2015). In 1922, the Irish Free State was established as a dominion and one of six northern counties constituting the United Kingdom. In 1948, Eamon de Valera, American-born leader of Sinn Fein (meaning "our own"; pronounced/shin fayn/), who had won establishment of the Free State in 1921 in negotiations with Britain's David Lloyd George, was defeated by John Costello, who demanded final independence from Britain. The Republic of Ireland was proclaimed in 1948 when it withdrew from the British Commonwealth (Your Irish, 2015). Nevertheless, in a claim not recognized by Ireland, the British government reasserted its claim to incorporate the six northeastern counties into the United Kingdom. In 1993, the Irish and British governments agreed on a plan to resolve the Northern Ireland issue, and in 1994 a cease-fire was announced by the Irish Republican Army (IRA). However, when peace talks lagged, the IRA returned to its terror campaign in 1996, which continued until 1997, when a new cease-fire was announced. In September 1997, Mary Robinson, the first woman president, resigned and Mary McAleese, the first northerner to hold the office, assumed the presidency. However, unrest continues to plague Northern Ireland, with periods of conflict following peace plans and a lagging hope of lasting peace in sight (Countries and Their Culture, 2015). Since Queen Elizabeth visited Ireland in 2014, relations between the countries have improved (Irish in Britain, 2014). Although discrimination is illegal in Britain, the ongoing conflict with the Irish has affected Irish who are working in Britain (Irish in Britain, 2014). It was noted in Irish in Britain (2014) that racial discrimination and prejudice against Irish nurses can be found in British health care facilities. This is not without deleterious effects. For example, it has been noted that there is a higher incidence of mental illness among Irish-born women in Britain (Leavey, Rozmovits, Ryan, & King, 2007).

Over the years, music has played an important role in Irish history. In the , Irish music, including spiritual music, Irish Catholic hymns, Irish songwriter and singer Mary Coughlan, and the Irish *céilí* (ceilidh, Gaelic for "party," especially one with dancing and music) bands, and the Chieftains received national recognition (Music, 2010; Warner, 2009). In 2001, the band U2 was the top band in Ireland, and several Irish singers had international musical hits (Newsline, 2001). Ensemble performance groups like Riverdance (since 1994) and Celtic Woman (since 2004) have received international acclaim presenting Irish song and dance programs around the world. James Galway is considered one of the best flute players in the world. Ireland's 99% literacy rate indicates that education is also valued (Countries and Their Culture, 2015).

Research concerning health care problems in Ireland is evident in the health care literature. For example, there has been a dramatic increase in the percentage of infants born to unmarried mothers in Ireland over the past decade. For the first 50 years of the 20th century, 2% of all registered births were to single mothers. In 1975 the figure had risen slightly to 3.7%. Within 10 years, it had risen to 8.5%, and in 1990 the figure stood at 14%. In 2010, it was reported that of 18,844 births, 6205 births were registered as outside of marriage, accounting for 32.9% of all births in Ireland (Central Statistics Office Ireland, 2010).

Another recent health problem in Ireland is a dramatically increasing suicide rate in all age ranges. Numerous meetings and websites document the governmental initiatives regarding this issue (Depression and Suicide, 2013). In contrast, the undetermined death rate has fallen off. This has implications both for improving measurement procedures and for suicide prevention (Bates, 2005; Department of Public Health, 2001; Irish Mental Health Coalition, 2007). Interestingly, there is little information in the Irish medical literature on smoking. However, a ban on smoking in workplaces and public spaces was enacted in May 2007 (Biege, 2010). Another health problem noted in the Irish medical literature relates to incontinence in the elderly. It was noted that only 33% of general practitioners studied were aware of the incontinence status of their clients over 75 years of age (Prosser & Dobbs, 1997). Research in Ireland has also suggested that self-neglect in later life, or Diogenes syndrome, may be a significant problem (Johnson & Adams, 1996). Samuels (2012) noted that older people in Ireland experience considerable ill health and social deprivation. Work by Manning, Curran, Kirby, Taylor, and Clancy (1997) indicated that there may be a prevalence of teenage asthma with associated allergic conditions in Ireland. Finally, alcoholism is historically an ongoing problem, with binge drinking being the norm (Your Irish, 2012).

Against a background of fundamental change in the Irish health care environment, MacDougall and Doran (1995) conducted a survey to determine the information needs of all health care practitioners. This survey revealed serious deficiencies in access, awareness, and availability of information for both staff and clients and recommended a comprehensive national health information strategy to coordinate the future development of health sciences information services. These changes have taken place, and nurses are expanding their roles to provide appropriate information and care across departments and health care (McIlfatrick, McKenna, Gray, & Hinds, 2002) is continuing to evolve (Heenan & Birrell, 2009). Irish nurses are recognized for their innovations; for example, Irish nurses are credited with making an important contribution in Calcutta (Development, 2015), for providing effective community public health partnerships for persons with mental health issues (Lakeman, 2012), for uniting with American nurses in the development of advanced cardiovascular life support training in Ireland (Irish Heart Foundation, 2015), and for developing better care for the elderly (McGee, Molloy, O'Hanlon, Layte, & Hickey, 2008).

The population of Ireland is approximately 4,553,000 World Almanac, 2015). Dublin, the largest city in Ireland with 1,018,500 inhabitants, is the capital (World Almanac, 2015). The life expectancy in Ireland of males is 75.76 years, while for females it is 81.24 years. The infant mortality rate is 5.31 per 1000 live births (CIA, 2011; World Almanac, 2015). Ireland's human immunodeficiency virus (HIV) and acquired immunodeficiency syndrome (AIDS) rate is 0.2% (2800) of the population (CIA, 2011). The per capita income is $31,900, with an unemployment rate of 4.3% (World Almanac, 2015). The economy has been growing (Countries and Their Cultures, 2015), and tourism to Ireland is increasingly promoted. Kiesnoski (2001) noted that the market history suggests that Irish Americans are the best target for promotional campaigns. Many visit family but while in Ireland are also consumers of tourism products, renting cars, and patronizing hotels and restaurants. Immigration to the United States continues to be an attractive alternative for many who are distressed by the political unrest that has so long prevailed in Ireland. However, once a country plagued with high unemployment, high inflation, slow growth, and a large public debt, Ireland has undergone an extraordinary economic transformation over the past 15 years. The "Celtic Tiger" has become a leader in high-tech industries, and recently the economy has grown as much as 10% (World Almanac, 2015). In fact, many European economists postulate that Ireland is continuing to distance itself wisely from the debt crisis experienced by other European countries such as Greece (Countries and Their Cultures, 2015). In 2010, the yield on 10-year Irish government bonds actually closed below 8% for the first time since the EU–International Monetary Fund bailout, but the yield is now back to levels seen in October 2010, suggesting that indeed Ireland is righting its financial course.

IMMIGRATION TO THE UNITED STATES

The large number of Catholic Irish immigrants of the famine years were not the first Irish people to immigrate to the United States. The famine immigrants were preceded by their Irish countrymen in the seventeenth and eighteenth centuries, although in smaller numbers. Many of the earlier immigrants, particularly during the seventeenth and eighteenth centuries, were Protestants from the northern county of Ulster and thus came to the United States under less dramatic circumstances than the later immigrants did. The early Ulster immigrants arrived in the United States just in time to help the Americans win independence from England. At that time many Irish-American immigrants regarded themselves as members of the Anglo-American society. This distinction was made not to deny their Irish origin but to embrace their new heritage. During the Civil War, more than 150,000 joined the Union army. Since much of the White population of the Confederate states was native-born, there was less of a drive in the Southern army to recognize heritage than there was in the Union forces, where, for example, the fabled Meagher's Irish brigade went into battle with an emerald green flag with a golden harp in its center (Unit History Project, 2014). Meagher led Irish Americans who were recruited from among common laborers in the Twenty-Eighth Massachusetts Regiment in a daring performance to "clear the way" for brother units. One of the best-known Irish nationalists in America, Meagher used his oratorical skills in Boston's Music Hall to whip up enthusiasm among the Irish for the effort (Unit History Project, 2014). By the mid-, Irish organizations were established in the major cities of the United States (Rapple, 2015). Today, Irish descendants regard their Irish extraction more as a point of historical interest than as an identification with social relevance for their lives. According to Lee and Casey (2006), Irish Americans, in the process of adapting to American life, began to think and behave like their American counterparts. Ethnic lines are blurred and it is difficult to tell differences between Irish and Americans (Rapple, 2015). Today, however, there are as many Americans descended from Irish Protestants as from Irish Catholics, so the tight-knit communities that kept the anti-British cause alive are fast disintegrating (Rapple, 2015). Irish Americans have become so assimilated into the mainstream of American society that today they are likely to be professionals or managers and less likely to be laborers, service workers, or factory workers (Countries and Their Cultures, 2015).

Approximately 40 million people of Irish descent reside in the United States (U.S. Department of Commerce, Bureau of the Census, *American Community Survey*, 2015). The Irish immigrant population has been steadily increasing since the early and increased dramatically in 1994, with 14.1 million between 1971 and 1980, 32.8 million from 1981 to 1990, 20.6 million from 1991 to 1993, and 17.3 million immigrants in 1994 alone (U.S. Department of Commerce, Bureau of the Census, *American Community Survey*, 2015). In addition, it was estimated that in 1992 there were 36,000 undocumented Irish immigrants (U.S. Department of Commerce, Bureau of the Census, *Statistical Abstract*, 2011). Irish ranks as the second largest ancestry group in the United States, outranked only by German. Irish is the largest ancestry group in five states in the Northwest and ranks third (after German and African-American) for having the largest ancestry group in a state (U.S. Department of Commerce, Bureau of the Census, *American Community Survey*, 2015). The number of Irish descendants has resulted in St. Patrick's Day being celebrated on March 17 each year in communities across the United States by Irish and non-Irish alike (Rapple, 2015; Your Irish, 2015).

COMMUNICATION

The official language of Ireland is Irish (Irish Gaelic). However, English is recognized as the second official language. English is universally spoken throughout Ireland, and approximately 27% of the population knows both Irish and English. Irish is more widely used in the west and is the first language of people in remote areas.

To understand the development of language in Ireland, it is essential to understand the historical significance of Celtic (usually pronounced /kel-tic/) languages. Because the Celts (/kelts/) developed a written language quite late, the people were forced to rely heavily on the oral transmission of laws, customs, religions, and philosophy; poetry became a useful mnemonic device for transmitting tradition. According to legend, the ancient heroes of the mythological cycle, which included Finn MacCool and Cuchulain, were clearly in love with the sound of their own voices. Modern-day Irish people are much like the ancient Celts; much wit and humor are part of communication (Kwintessential, 2014). Greeley (1993) suggested that, for Irish people, playing with the language provided not only a means of communication but also a portion of their enjoyment and pleasure. It should be noted that languages throughout the world that have survived from an earlier period have not only elaborate language structures but also more extensive vocabularies. The suggested reason is that spoken language needs to be more flexible and descriptive than written language.

For people in the western part of Ireland, the vocabulary is about one half as extensive as the vocabulary of the well-educated English speaker in London. It also has been noted that people who live in the *Gaeltacht* (/gail-tahht/) or the Irish-speaking regions in the west tend to have an extensive English-speaking vocabulary. Although a modern-day Irish language exists, the Irish language for all practical purposes was almost destroyed during the second half of the nineteenth century with the onslaught of the English language. Some phrases attributed to the Irish, such as "Top O' the Mornin'," are not commonly heard in Ireland, where Rapple, (2015) noted that "Hi," "Hiya," and "Howarya!" or, in rural areas, a polite "Hello," are the common terms. An effort has been made to increase the understanding and use of Gaelic through TV programs financed by the government, as well as schools using only Gaelic (Rapple, 2015).

Because many Irish persons arrived in the United States with knowledge of English, assimilation into the predominant culture was enhanced. However, despite the use of English words, some words have different meanings for the Irish. For example, the word *homely*, which is commonly used in the United States to describe someone who is plain and not attractive, is used by some Irish people as an endearing word to describe hospitality. An Irish guest after a dinner may hug the host or hostess and say, "Thank you for being so homely." In Ireland it is considered inappropriate to ask for a "ride" from a cab driver. Instead, the word *lift* or *drive* is used.

Nonverbal actions have special significance for the Irish. For example, holding up two fingers with the palm facing one's face is a hand gesture meant to be obscene (Lasky, 1996). In business or professional relationships, it is not considered proper to give gifts. Instead, tokens of appreciation with special significance, such as Vermont maple syrup or California wine, are appreciated (Kwintessential, 2014).

In Ireland, "Mac" before a family name describes the "son of," and "O" is used to mean "descended from." Gaelic names such as Brian, Maureen, Sheila, Sean, and Moria are popular first names for Irish-American children. Names are typically written with the surname. First names are commonly used in informal situations (Wilson, 2003).

The Irish tend to dress up rather than dress casually for business or professional events. The nurse should not be surprised if a newly immigrated Irish client comes to a health care agency very well dressed. Brightly colored traditional Irish costumes can still be seen in America by persons performing Irish dances and can be noted in Ireland at special holiday events (Rapple, 2015).

Implications for Transcultural Nursing Care

It is important for the nurse to understand that some Irish Americans who may be encountered in the health care system may not have an extensive vocabulary, but the words they speak may be used with exaggeration. Because language is a form of entertainment and power for some Irish people, the client may attempt to communicate needs through flowery and sometimes exaggerated words. On the other hand, some Irish tend to ignore pain and to provide no words of complaint. Therefore, it is essential for the nurse to carefully evaluate physical signs and symptoms of pain in addition to oral descriptions to accurately assess the need for nursing intervention. Because of this variety of responses, it is particularly important for the nurse to be careful to not stereotype Irish-American clients relative to pain response (Spector, 2004). The astute nurse must keep in mind that the Irish-American client may tend to be overly verbose in descriptions of conditions, but this does not imply that the client is not being objective or accurately descriptive about the nature of the condition. The nurse should use a combination of open- and closed-ended questions to solicit specific information from which culturally appropriate nursing care can be planned. When assessing the client, the nurse should be aware that some Irish Americans tend to avoid saying the word "no." Instead, phrases such as "I'll let you know" or "we'll see" or "perhaps" are used. It is important for the nurse to try to analyze context and demeanor to determine if the response is really negative (Rapple, 2015).

Zola (1966) compared Italian Americans and Irish Americans and their descriptive methods of presenting complaints. The findings of the study indicated that when Italian Americans and Irish Americans were asked, "Where does it hurt?" Irish-American respondents were more likely to locate chief problems in the eyes, ears, nose, or throat. In a similar question, the respondents were asked to identify the most important areas of the body. Again, for the Irish-American respondents, the emphasis was on the eyes, ears, nose, and throat. Another finding of the study was that the Irish Americans more often than the Italian Americans denied that pain was a part of their illness. When Irish-American respondents were asked about the presence of pain, some of them hedged their replies with qualifications such as "It is more a throbbing than a pain," or "It is not really a pain; it feels more like sand in my eye," or "It feels more like a pinprick than a pain." The conclusion of the study was that Irish Americans, through such comments, were reflecting something more than an objective reaction to their physical condition. Irish Americans were found to describe their chief problems in terms of specific dysfunctions. What appeared to emerge from the study was that Irish people limit and understate their physical difficulties, whereas Italians spread and generalize theirs.

With the increasing numbers of Irish clients, it is helpful to have health care materials translated into Irish. However, translating client-teaching materials and various assessment materials to the Irish has not always been completely successful. For example, Aroian, Patsdaughter, Levin, and Gianan (1995) attempted to utilize the Brief Symptoms Inventory to assess psychological distress among Polish, Filipino, and Irish immigrants by translating the form into the respective languages. It was found that the scale in its translated form was able to measure psychological distress with all three immigrant groups. However, problems with the psychoticism subscale occurred across all three immigrant groups, indicating that this subscale should be interpreted with caution when used with immigrants. Thus, although English translation to another language on written assessment materials is sometimes helpful, it cannot be assumed to be accurate.

SPACE

Space is an essential component in a cultural framework of nursing because from the beginning of modern time, philosophers, mathematicians, psychologists, and ethnologists have studied the phenomenon of space. *Territoriality, proximity,* and *personal space* are all terms that have been used to describe space. The word *territoriality* was initially used to describe the physical area that animals claim as their own and defend from predators, but in modern times the term has been extended to describe human behavior as well (Hall, 1981). Hall (1963) coined the term *proxemics* to describe the use of space as an elaboration of a culture. According to Hall (1990), individuals by virtue of their culture have four ways of perceiving distance: as intimate distance (from 6 to 8 inches), as personal distance (from 6 inches to 4 feet), as social distance (from 4 to 12 feet), and as public distance (from 12 to 25 feet). Hall (1990) concluded that the use of space explains communication in various cultures.

Space is a cultural phenomenon that is infrequently noted in the literature about the Irish. Greeley (1993) has noted, however, that Irish-American students often require more time to become articulate and self-confident in a high-powered academic environment and that this can be seen in the student's spatial relationships with others. The Irish-American student is more likely to sit off in a corner for several semesters, only to be "discovered" later as having produced brilliant work, for the most part in solitude (Griffin, 2001). Some authors (Griffin, 2001; Hoobler & Hoobler, 1995) have also noted that Irish individuals are less likely to be physically affectionate in both their interpersonal and their family relationships.

Implications for Nursing Care

The use of space, in its simplest terms, is a means of nonverbal communication (Stillman, 1978). How individuals feel about their own personal space determines how much intrusion by others is considered acceptable. Because health care often occurs in what is described as an *intimate zone,* spatial issues have important implications for the nurse.

The personal space of some Irish Americans is limited, and they are perceived as having a past-time–oriented culture that relies heavily on extended family ties (Kwintessential, 2014). They may be accustomed to having family members close by, increasing their need for proximity of family members during illness. However, according to

Countries and Their Cultures (2015), despite the closeness of the family unit, Irish-American families have a tendency to collapse the personal space inward, more so than in other cultures. It has been noted that Irish-American families have difficulty expressing love and affection. Some have more difficulty in expression with close family members than with more distant persons, creating an isolated and greatly expanded personal space. Others express feelings somewhat readily with a close group of intimates but not with persons more distant. The nurse should be cognizant of the possible effects of attitudes and values about space that may affect individuals from different cultures. One major objective for the nurse may be to assist the family in recognizing the need to convey warmth, feelings, and attitudes in order to create a supportive and nurturing spatial environment for the client that will promote recovery.

SOCIAL ORGANIZATION

Family

The famine years had a profound effect on the structure of the Irish-American family. As the famine progressed, the resulting experiences dramatically altered the family system in Ireland. Immigrants brought this altered family structure to the United States and formed their own ethnic societies. Most of those who immigrated to the United States from Ireland were between 15 and 35 years of age, since it was these able-bodied individuals who were most able to leave (Lee & Casey, 2006).

Ireland stands alone in losing such a large proportion of its population to emigration. Even in modern times, more Irish people live outside Ireland than in it, and most Irish families have at least some members living in the United States (Griffin, 2001). A wide range of disparity has been noted regarding the link between Irish Americans and the family in the homeland. For some Irish Americans, there appears to be an almost mystical link between the family in the United States and the roots in Ireland. These roots often lead to a particular farm that may still be inhabited by a remnant of that particular clan. For other Irish Americans, there is almost no link remaining, except the knowledge that an ancestor originated in Ireland. The family values and ethnic traits are often transmitted to the next generation unconsciously by imitation of the parental model.

Before the famine years, families in the southern and western parts of Ireland were traditionally Irish speaking, Catholic, and subsistence farmers. The typical couple married early, had many children, and on the father's death subdivided the land among the sons. The agricultural pattern of the prefamine years no doubt was instrumental in creating the almost total reliance of the Irish on the potato crop. However, this pattern of continuous subdividing of the land among family members also contributed to the close family bonds, as were evidenced by parental demands for respectful attention and obedience to marriages arranged by the parents. These family bonds continued even after immigration to the United States, as evidenced by the fact that it was the responsibility of many immigrants to send money back to Ireland to pay the passage for another family member to come to the United States (Lee & Casey, 2006).

Marriage

In the past, there was intense social pressure among Irish Americans to select mates from the Irish Catholic community. Therefore, the Irish neighborhoods in the United States often served as the social context for the meeting and pairing of the young immigrants (Wessel, 1931). For the early Irish settlers, marriage with non-Irish Catholics was a permissible alternative. However, these marriages generally followed a preferential hierarchy in which the early-arriving English or German Catholics were considered more suitable than the later-arriving Irish Catholics (Abramson, 1973). By the time of the third generation of immigrants, a tendency was noted for the socially aspiring Irish Catholic to marry a Protestant or even convert to Protestantism. These practices were generally disapproved of by other Irish-American Catholics. Even today in stable communities in the United States, intermarriage between Irish families remains one of the clearest distinctions of social acceptance and social equality in the Irish-American community.

Bachelorhood and spinsterhood are infrequent among Irish Americans (Countries and Their Cultures, 2015). The typical Irish-American Catholic woman marries at 22 years of age, and the typical Irish-American Catholic man marries at 24.5 years of age. Although this is a bit older than the American average, the practice in ancient Ireland was to delay marriage until the early 30s. The mean number of children for Irish-American families is 2.6, compared with the national mean of 2.4. As family planning becomes more progressive among Irish-American Catholics, the number of children is decreasing.

Role of Women. One traditional view of Irish women was that they were controlling matriarchs on whom sons and husbands were dependent (Rapple, 2015). A contrasting view held that male dominance began as a pattern in Ireland after the mass emigrations. Women were expected to be subservient in every way and assist their husbands with what was considered "men's work" in addition to completing their own traditionally female tasks. However, many women emigrated alone, accentuating the strength and resolve of women; today, many are involved in professional occupations (Rapple 2015).

Irish-American women are more likely than their Anglo-American counterparts to view the wife–mother role as the dominant one in marriage. The findings are also suggestive that Irish-American women view the mother's working as detrimental to children and see the role of the wife as a helper to her husband, although these views are changing to reflect more mainstream thought (Rapple, 2015).

Role of Men. Meagher (2005) has noted that although Irish men, particularly when intoxicated, may spin tall tales and recite romantic poetry about their true love, in intimate relationships they often become awkward and tongue-tied and may become clumsy, if not rough, in any attempts at intimacy. The male dominance that began in Ireland as a result of the change in family structure between 1840 and 1940 is paralleled even today among Irish Americans (Countries and Their Cultures, 2015).

Children and Adolescents

Haigh, Wang, Fung, Williams, and Mintz (1999) investigated pretend play interactions of Irish-American children, noting that compared with Chinese children studied, specific culture communities tend to create distinctive developmental pathways. In a study of adolescents in England and Ireland, Porteous (1985) noted that the Irish adolescents had a less mature pattern than their English counterparts; however, Irish adolescents in the study admitted to having more worries. The conclusion of the study was that cultural differences are specifically reflected in adolescent experiences.

Religion

In Ireland and in the United States, the primary cultural force and national unifier of Irish culture has been the Catholic church (Rapple, 2015). In fact, the parish rather than the neighborhood has traditionally defined the family's social context (Rapple, 2015). The Church of Ireland is an independent Anglican church found in both the Republic of Ireland and Northern Ireland, tracing its episcopal succession from the pre-Reformation church in Ireland. Christianity is believed to have existed in Ireland before the missionary activities of Patrick, the patron saint of Ireland, in the late fifth century. The early church in Ireland was monastic, without parochial or diocesan divisions or central government. If there was authority within the structure of the church, it rested with the abbot and the bishops.

In Ireland, the Catholic church has been faced with a dilemma because of the desire to preserve the Catholic moral tone. In this regard, the Catholic church has found it necessary to relegate the prevention of AIDS through the promotion of condoms and safe sexual practices to the government. Most Catholic churches advocate abstinence before marriage and avoidance of sexual behavior by some high-risk groups, such as homosexuals.

Political Influences

Immigrants from Ireland have contributed significantly to the development of the United States from its inception (Rapple, 2015). In fact, eight Irish individuals signed the Declaration of Independence, and five died in the Boston Massacre. About one third of the people in the United States can trace all or part of their lineage to Irish ancestry. It has been reported that three presidents, including Andrew Jackson, James Buchanan, and Chester Arthur, were sons of Irish immigrants. Irish individuals have been active in all walks of American life, including the formation and growth of trade unions and active service on police forces across the country, and have served admirably in the Army and in the Navy (Rapple, 2015).

Irish Americans have enjoyed a significant and spectacular rise in the political arena in this country, in part because of block voting in large cities, where they generally were the largest single group. This voting practice assured the Irish of political influence by the , particularly in Boston, where the first Irish-American mayors were elected. During this same period in New York, the Irish, including noted Irish-American political bosses John F. Fitzgerald, Richard J. Daley, "Big Tim" Sullivan, and James Michael Curley, controlled many political machines. The success of the Irish resulted partially from their strong sense of group solidarity, their fluency with the spoken word, and their personal charm. Historically, the Irish were known as the most successful enhancers of corrupt politics. Today, the voting patterns for Irish Americans remain about the same as that for other Americans. In addition, with the election of the first Irish-Catholic president in 1960 (John F. Kennedy), the issue of an Irish-Catholic president was resolved.

Implications for Nursing Care

The nurse must keep in mind that the one reemerging theme among Irish Americans is the significance of the family and family structure, which may be difficult for people from other cultures to perceive. Because Irish Americans are viewed as having a relational orientation that is lineal in nature (see later discussion), nursing interventions are likely to be successful only if family involvement in the care and treatment of the client is maximized.

Kluckhohn and Strodtbeck (1961) viewed relational orientation in families as having three subdivisions: lateral (collateral), lineal, and individualistic. For families with a lateral (collateral) mode of orientation, the goals and welfare of laterally extended groups, including siblings and peers, take on paramount importance. This type of family assumes responsibility for all of its members. Therefore, the goals of the individual family members become subordinate to those of the family group. When the lineal mode is present as the major focus in family groups, the goals and welfare of the group may also have primary importance because the family members view culture and kinship bonds as the primary basis for maintaining lineage.

It is important for the nurse to seek the family's advice and opinions on treatment for the client. In addition, since the family is perceived as being a source of anxiety and tension because of restricted family roles, it is important for the nurse to assist the family in identifying the boundaries and characteristics of each role. If the family determines that the boundaries are restricted and do not overlap, the nurse must accept this fact and recognize and appreciate that such families function with a hierarchical ranking of family roles. Therefore, lack of recognition on the part of a nurse may foster feelings of anxiety and tension on the part of those persons who are considered to be at the top of the hierarchical ranking, such as the father or the mother.

A contrasting mode held by some families is the individualistic mode of orientation. For families with this orientation, individual goals are viewed as being more important than specific lateral or lineal goals. In this type of family, each member is held responsible for personal behavior and is therefore judged according to personal accomplishments (Rapple, 2015).

Because Irish Americans tend to delineate roles and behaviors within the family structure on the basis of gender, it is important for the nurse not to minimize the significance of ranked ordering of behavior. For example, some Irish-American women may view their role as primary caretaker of the family. Therefore, when they are ill, their role function is greatly compromised. In this case, the client must be assisted to develop strategies to help the family meet its needs in the absence of the primary caretaker.

It also is important for the nurse to remember that for some Irish Americans, religion and religious views take on paramount importance in maintaining the social integrity of the individual. The astute nurse should solicit information on religious practices that are deemed essential to the optimal functioning of the Irish-American client. Lack of recognition of the significance of religious beliefs may augment problems and difficulties encountered with illness.

TIME

According to Kluckhohn and Strodtbeck (1961), the cultural interpretation of time has a three-point range of variability that consists of past, present, and future orientations. Based on this model, Irish Americans are viewed as having a past-oriented culture. Kluckhohn and Strodtbeck have noted that all cultures must deal with all three time orientations. Cultures differ regarding time perspective in the preferential ordering of the orientations, and a great deal about a society can be learned and predicted from this preferential ordering. For example, Irish Americans are perceived as members of a first-ordered, past-oriented society because some Irish Americans have a strong allegiance to the past, worship their ancestors, and have a strong family tradition. In addition, persons from cultures with past-oriented time perspectives may have the attitude that nothing new ever happens in the present or will ever happen in the future because it all happened in the distant past. For example, an Irish American who is shown a new invention may remark, "Our ancestors were making something similar to this 100 years ago." Persons in the dominant culture may find it difficult to understand the respect that Irish Americans have for tradition, and at the same time some Irish Americans do not appreciate the typical American disregard for tradition.

On the other hand, many Irish of today are present and future oriented, working hard to achieve a future objective. The Irish tend to maintain a hard work ethic and to have difficulty tearing themselves from a long day at the office to indulge in a social function (Rapple, 2015). Timing for business functions is considered very important, but the opposite is true of social gatherings, with fun-filled functions usually beginning 20 to 30 minutes late. Nevertheless, once a party has started, Irish Americans tend to indulge in light-hearted events enthusiastically and often late into the night.

Implications for Nursing Care

Since some past-oriented people are perceived as lacking an understanding of rhythmicity and periodicity, it is likely that they may also be perceived as being noncompliant regarding scheduled medical and therapeutic interventions. Some individuals with a past-time orientation view humanity as being subjugated to nature; therefore, there may be a tendency for a fatalistic orientation that affects the time orientation. In other words, some people with a past-time orientation believe that time and nature will alleviate the problem and tend to wait until the last possible moment to seek medical intervention for acute or chronic medical problems.

The astute nurse must recognize that noncompliance is not necessarily an inherent quality of the personality but may be related to a lack of understanding regarding the time perspective. For example, individuals with a past-oriented perspective view time as being elastic, and

therefore a moment in time has the possibility of being recaptured (Mbiti, 1990). The nurse should plan activities that encourage the client to adhere to the necessary aspects of the time perspective, as in the case of time-released insulin or heart medication. The client should be encouraged to relate adherence to a medical regimen to a business schedule that requires adherence to a fixed schedule (Lasky, 1996).

ENVIRONMENTAL CONTROL

Locus of Control

Kluckhohn and Strodtbeck (1961) developed a five-concept value-orientation framework that consists of (1) perceptions of human nature, (2) relationship of the human with nature, (3) time orientation, (4) activity orientation, and (5) relational orientation. In this model, Irish Americans are viewed as belonging to a past-oriented culture because some Irish Americans believe that humanity is basically evil and subjugated to nature, and so their family and social relationships are lineal in nature. Also, they tend to cling to a past-oriented value orientation regarding the family and family relationships and tend to consider past values and traditions of paramount importance to future growth and development. Irish Americans were more fatalistic, less authoritarian, less anxious, and more trusting than their Anglo-American counterparts. Because Irish Americans hold a value orientation that views man as being subjugated to nature, some Irish Americans are viewed as having an external locus of control.

Perception of Illness

According to the classic work of Zola (1966), every individual deals with problems in a way corresponding to his or her problem orientation. For Irish Americans, the worldview of life is expressed through fasts, which are symbolic of prior deprivations in their lives. Some Irish Americans have life patterns that have alternated between overindulgence and self-deprivation (Zola, 1966). Many psychologists believe that the expected and limited nature of these irregular, extreme cycles is correlated with alcohol use and that for some Irish Americans continued use of defense mechanisms to ignore or dispel previous conditions or symptoms is the norm rather than the exception. Some Irish Americans have a view of life that states that "life is black and long suffering and therefore the less said about life the better" (Zola, 1966). This statement best reflects the way in which some Irish Americans handle the concept of illness.

Although in some cultural groups ignoring bodily complaints is not normative, for some Irish Americans this appears to be a culturally prescribed and supported defense mechanism and the typical way of coping with psychological and physiological needs. For example, some Irish Americans will say, regarding an illness, "I ignore it as I do most other things." This point reemphasizes the fact that for some Irish Americans there is a tendency to understand the implications of the illness but, at the same time, to refrain from expressing illness-related complaints.

Illness and Wellness Behaviors

The consistency of the Irish illness behavior can also be perceived in two other contexts. First, for some Irish Americans, illness or the perception of illness helps perpetuate a self-fulfilling prophecy. Some people believe that the way in which Irish Americans communicate complaints, but do very little to make treatment easy, has assured them of continued suffering (Zola, 1966). Second, for some Irish Americans, illness behavior can be linked to sin and guilt ideology, which seems to pervade a major portion of Irish American society today. This is evidenced by the fact that in the Irish-American culture there is great restraint toward opening the door for constant temptation that must be denied. The perception held by some Irish Americans is that the flesh is weak and the individual is very likely to sin. This theme is reinforced even in the way symptoms are localized. According to Zola (1966), Irish Americans localize complaints in the eyes, ears, or throat, which might be a symbolic reflection of the more immediate source of sin and guilt. For example, it might be said that these three localized areas of complaints are congruent with what should have been seen, heard, or said.

Folk Medicine

Some Irish Americans subscribe to folk medicine beliefs that can be perceived as neutral health practices (neither having benefit nor producing harm), such as the "blessing of the throat" and the wearing of holy medals to prevent illnesses. Additional folk medicine beliefs that are considered neutral include the practices of tying a bag of camphor around the neck to prevent flu during the flu season, never looking in a mirror at night, closing closet doors to prevent evil spirits from entering the body, and above all maintaining a strong family with lots of love to prevent illnesses. Additional methods to prevent illness and protect health include not going to bed with wet hair, drinking nettle soup to clear the blood, and eating porridge at night before going to bed. Irish methods to restore health that are likely to have little effect include tying onions to wrists or dirty socks around the neck to cure a fever; curing a cold by eating a whole raw onion with a shot of whiskey; curing flatulence by placing one's bottom toward the fire; and wrapping hot bread, sugar, and soap in a linen cloth and placing it on an infection to cure boils and cuts (Rapple, 2015).

Other folk medicine beliefs practiced by some Irish Americans may be perceived as harmful, such as eating a lot of oily foods, cleansing the bowels every 8 days with senna, and seeing a doctor only in an emergency. For some Irish Americans, the first level of intervention is often home treatment because of the belief that a doctor should be seen only in an emergency, and this practice may create a reactive rather than a preventive model of treatment. For example, for a throat condition, the first level of intervention may be to paint the throat with iodine or kerosene or to soothe with honey and lemon. Another example of a practice that might be perceived as harmful is the home treatment of nausea and other stomach ailments that might have serious implications with such remedies as drinking hot tea, taking castor oil, or eating potatoes or gruel.

Some Irish Americans subscribe to folk medicine practices that may be perceived as beneficial, such as getting lots of rest and going to bed early, enjoying fresh air and sunshine, exercising outdoors, dressing warmly, and keeping the feet warm. Many also believe one must eat good food, take vitamins, and balance the diet. In addition, there seems to be an overriding belief that to stay healthy one must be goal oriented and nurture a strong religious faith. The combination of positive thinking along with these healthful practices can contribute to optimal wellness (Rapple, 2015).

Rituals and Customs for Death and Dying

Death is considered by the Irish as a part of life and a family affair. Because of the close ties to either the Catholic or Protestant church, that institution plays a significant role in death practices and rituals. Because of the close family unit, it is important that the nurse allow family and friends to remain with the dying to provide comfort for both.

When a person dies, the body is "laid out" in preparation for burial. Then friends and relatives assemble for a wake or time of vigil around the deceased. With the advent of funeral homes, the all-night wake is rarely observed now; however, the mourners are present at other times. The mourners pray for the soul of the departed, and, if the mourners and deceased are Catholic, the rosary is recited many times (Your Irish, 2015).

There are quantities of food available for friends and relatives, including alcoholic beverages. These continue to be consumed until after the morning funeral service when lunch is served (Rapple, 2015).

An old tradition, less observed today, is that of "keening." This consists of deep wailing over the body to help the soul make its way to the other world. Keening has to be timed just right so as not to wake the "devil's dogs" who might stop the soul. However, if keening waited too long, the soul had already gone on alone, which was to be avoided (Your Irish, 2012).

Implications for Nursing Care

The astute nurse must devise a teaching plan that emphasizes the importance of preventive techniques to maintain optimal wellness and prevent illness. The nurse should recognize the importance of assisting the client in developing a sensitivity and an understanding about wellness that will alleviate fatalistic beliefs about life in general and illness in particular. It is important for the nurse to understand that compliance with a health regimen is much more complex than the mere recognition and prescription of such a plan. The nurse must keep in mind that philosophical beliefs and attitudes play a major role not only in the perception of health and wellness but also in compliance behavior.

Because the first level of treatment for an illness for some Irish Americans may be home treatment, it is important for the nurse to ascertain for the client which of these practices are neutral or beneficial and thus may be incorporated into the plan of care and which of these practices are harmful. The nurse must devise teaching strategies that assist the client in developing an understanding about harmful folk medical practices in order for such practices to be eliminated from the typical health care regimen of the client. The nurse must realize that complete avoidance of harmful practices is initially difficult and that a reduction in such behaviors should be considered significant.

BIOLOGICAL VARIATIONS

Genetic Variations

It has been found that some Irish people have genetic susceptibility to certain biological variations. Some examples of research will be provided. However, it is important to note that within the Irish people are subgroups. North, Martin, and Crawford (2000) note variations found among the Travellers of Ireland, an itinerant population subdivision within the Irish people. The researchers noted that unique historical events influence population structure and affirmed a previously studied hypothesis concerning the distinctiveness of people in the midland counties.

Neural Tube Defects. Boyne Research Institute (2014) conducted research that indicates neural tube defects (NTDs) may result from a genetic susceptibility interacting with environmental exposures occurring early in pregnancy. A high-rate area of Ireland was compared with a low-rate area of Italy. The results of their study support the notion that geographic differences in occurrence of NTDs are attributable at least in part to differing prevalences of genetic susceptibility factors. Byrne and Carolan (2006) also noted the adverse reproductive outcomes among pregnancies of aunts and (spouses of) uncles in Irish families with NTDs. Yet another study by O'Leary et al. (2006) revealed reduced folate carrier polymorphisms and NTD risk in an Irish population.

Tay-Sachs Disease. Van Bael, Natowicz, Tomczak, Grebner, and Prence (1996) noted that non-Jewish Americans with an Irish background have a significantly increased frequency of heterozygosity at the *Hex A alpha* subunit gene locus. These data actually allow for a frequency estimate of deleterious alleles for Tay-Sachs disease among Irish Americans of 1 in 192 to 1 in 52, respectively. In contrast, non-Jewish Americans with ancestry from Great Britain do not differ from the general population for risk for Tay-Sachs disease. These distinctions have been confirmed more recently, and screening for the disease is being recommended for Irish Americans (McCullough, 2012).

Teeth. A study on bimaxillary dental protrusion was conducted with a sample of 20 Northern Irish people. On average, tooth size for the overall maxillary and mandibular dentition was 5.7% larger in the bimaxillary sample than in the control sample (McCann & Burden, 1996).

Sarcoidosis. Kay, Saffra, and Har-El (2002) noted that sarcoidosis, a systemic chronic granulomatous disease of unknown etiology, may affect persons of any race or ethnicity, but it more commonly affects African-Americans, Scandinavians, and the Irish.

Cystic Fibrosis. When mutations of chromosomes were studied in Northern Irish persons with cystic fibrosis (CF), it was determined that three major CF mutations are *delta F508*, *G551D*, and *R117H* (Hughes et al., 1996). Mutation *G551D* of exon 11 of the CF transmembrane conductance regulator gene is one of the most common mutations in clients of European origin (Cashman et al., 1995). Ireland continues to have one of the highest rates of CF in the world.

Abdominal Aortic Aneurysm. A high incidence of abdominal aortic aneurysm was identified among brothers of clients diagnosed with this illness. This study among an Irish population suggests the need to counsel siblings on their risk of aneurysm (Irish Heart Foundation).

Pain. Lipton and Marbach (1984) conducted a study to examine interethnic differences and similarities in reported pain experiences among African-Americans, Irish persons, Italians, Jewish persons, and Puerto Ricans and found that responses, attitudes, and descriptions of pain were relatively similar after controlling for variables shown by previous studies to influence reported pain experiences. These variables included symptom history; signs elicited on physical, radiographic, and laboratory examinations; and social, cultural, and psychological data. No significant intraethnic differences were noted regarding the clients' emotionality (that is, stoicism versus expressiveness) in regard to pain and the overall interference in daily functioning attributed to pain. The data suggest that the pain experiences reported by African-American, Italian, and Jewish clients were almost identical, whereas the pain experiences of Irish and Puerto Rican clients appeared to be relatively distinctive from those of the other groups and from those of each other. The variable that most influenced differences for Irish clients was social assimilation. The conclusion of the study was that intraethnic homogeneity is present for most aspects of the pain experience; however, intraethnic heterogeneity also exists for factors that influence the experience of pain.

HIV Risk

Of the number of reported cases of human immunodeficiency virus (HIV) in the United States among Irish Americans, there is a low incidence reported for homosexuals (Lewis, 1988). The number of reported cases of AIDS among Irish Americans appears to be predominantly related to intravenous drug use (Butler & Mayock, 2005). This is confirmation of previous research (Walsh, 1987), in which 11,640 persons in Ireland were tested for antibodies to HIV. Of this number, 626 were found to have antibodies to the virus, and 412 of these were identified as being intravenous drug users, including 28 infants born to mothers who were intravenous drug users (Lewis, 1988). The data would indicate that Irish people subscribe, in part or in full, to the doctrines of the Catholic church, which include monogamous relationships, no premarital intercourse, and no homosexual relationships. On the other hand, lack of sexual enhancement, failure to relieve aggressive tendencies, and characteristics of a dominant family lifestyle may be related to the incidence of HIV among Irish persons who are intravenous drug users (Lewis, 1988). MacHale and Newell (1997) studied the level of knowledge regarding sex education. Although the level of knowledge was found to be generally high, one third of sexually active respondent Irish schoolgoing teenagers were involved in high-risk behavior. For students who were sexually active, only 67% used condoms all the time, whereas 33% used them sometimes or never.

Psychological Characteristics

Christopher (2000) investigated 100 Irish immigrants for psychological well-being. Findings revealed that number of annual health care appointments, higher resilience, and greater life satisfaction were the strongest predictors of psychological well-being in a hierarchical regression analysis testing the association of psychological well-being with demographics, resilience, and life satisfaction.

Alcoholism. Among American ethnic groups, Irish Americans have been ranked the highest or near highest in terms of heavy alcohol intake, loss of control, and untoward social consequences (Rapple, 2015). Pubs are a popular and common venue for revelry in Ireland. Beer without ice and beer mixed with lemonade (a shandy) and served warm are favorite Irish drinks (Lasky, 1996). The Irish in Ireland have ranked among the highest groups internationally for the prevalence of alcohol-related problems (Lee & Casey, 2006). When compared with men in England and Wales, men in Ireland are more likely to drink at high-risk levels and are more likely to experience drinking problems than are their counterparts (Harrison, Carr-Hill, & Sutton, 1993).

Greeley (1972) concluded that the Irish often drink for reassurance, to escape from intolerable psychological burdens, and to repress sexuality and aggressiveness. Molyneux, Cryan, and Dooley (2006) discovered that 91% of persons identified as having an alcohol use disorder were binge drinkers. Greeley (1972) has further characterized the domination of the Irish-American mother as a causative factor in male alcoholism because she rules her family by strong will or by subtly manipulating the sympathies of her husband and children. Ablon and Cunningham (1981) have substantiated the possibility of female domination as an etiological factor in the development of alcoholism among Irish men. They found that problem drinking was positively linked most closely to the Irish and that in cases where a man's parents were both Irish, a serious alcohol problem was likely to be present. They also found that in cases where a man had an Irish mother but a father from another ethnic group, and if that father was characterized as a heavy drinker, even if not an alcoholic, the subject was likely to have a drinking problem. Farren and Dinan (1996) also noted that a significantly higher percentage of alcoholics studied had a positive family history of alcoholism. Johnson and Glassman (1999) investigated the moderating effects of gender and ethnicity on the relationship between effect expectancies and alcohol problems with Irish-American men and women in the New York metropolitan area. Both gender and ethnicity were found to moderate with links between aggressive and self-control expectancies and drinking problems.

Adolescents and Drinking Behavior. O'Connor (1978) noted that an expectation for enhanced sociability was directly related to drinking among Irish young adults. The respondents in this study had a prominent wish for a reduction in anxiety. Very little information is available regarding the drinking behavior of Irish adolescents. More information about adolescent Irish drinking would be helpful in addressing Irish adult drinking behavior.

Christiansen and Teahan (1987) studied the drinking behavior of Irish adolescents in two stages. The first stage compared the drinking behavior of Irish adolescents with the drinking behavior of American adolescents. During the second stage, the adolescents' expectations regarding the effects of alcohol were measured. In the study it was believed that adolescent expectancies might initially arise from social learning processes, including acculturation from parents who drink or are alcoholics. However, the data from the study are suggestive that Irish adolescents drink less and experience fewer alcohol-related problems than their American counterparts across all ethnic adolescent groups, including Irish Americans. The findings are not surprising because approximately 95% of the population in Ireland is Roman Catholic, and adolescents are prohibited from drinking as a religious decree at the time of confirmation and are expected to pledge abstinence until 21 years of age. Although Irish adolescents did not report as many alcohol-related problems as their American counterparts, when social drinking occurred among these adolescents, drinking-related problems were noted. A conclusion was that Irish adolescents had a lower expectation for sexual enhancement; however, they believed that alcohol would result in increased arousal and release of aggression.

The problems identified in Irish adolescents, such as lack of sexual enhancement and lack of ability to release aggression, have also been noted among adult Irish alcoholics. Although Irish adolescents are noted to drink less than their American peers and experience fewer alcohol-related problems, Ireland has one of the highest rates of alcoholism among the adult population.

Schizophrenia. Straub, MacLean, O'Neill, Walsh, and Kendler (1997) have presented some support for a possible schizophrenia vulnerability locus in region 5q22–31 in Irish families. Primm et al. (2005) also related the *Epsin 4* gene on chromosome 5q, which encodes the clathrin-associated protein enthoprotin, and is therefore involved in the genetic susceptibility to schizophrenia. This was the result of a genome scan for schizophrenia genes in 265 Irish individuals. It has been noted that allelic variation at the *DRD2* locus or other genes in the surrounding chromosomal region do not account for the genetic susceptibility

(Su et al., 1993). However, it has been noted in the British literature that since 1971 Irish-born people in Britain have the highest rates of first and subsequent admissions to psychiatric hospitals of any immigrant group (Doolin, 1994). They are three times more likely to be admitted to a mental institution than White British-born people and twice as likely to be admitted as a person of Afro-Caribbean origin, the next highest group (Cochrane, 1989). Numerous studies have indicated Irish have a consistently high vulnerability to a variety of mental disorders (Leavey et al., 2007; Schizophrenia, 2012). Doolin (1994) suggests that Irish men are more likely to be diagnosed as alcoholic than schizophrenic in Britain, suggesting a stereotypical and racist view of Irish people being drunks. Stopes-Roe and Cochrane (1980) also noted that ethnic group membership has been shown in England to be one of the sociodemographic variables that is related to overt or diagnosed level of psychopathology.

Bipolar Disorders. In a study, 92 Irish families with a total of 106 proband-parent trios were genotyped for three previously known polymorphisms within *hSERT* (*5-HTTLPR*, intron 2 *VNTR*, and *3'UTR B/T*). Data from two- and three-polymorphic marker haplotypes revealed a number of marker combinations with evidence of association (Mynett-Johnson et al., 2000). It is important to identify and treat affected persons (Kelly, 2013).

In a study of 92 families with a total of 10,638 illnesses, Kealey, Roche, Claffey, and McKeon (2005) also noted a linkage and candidate gene analysis of 14q22–24 in bipolar disorder, which support the *GGHI* as a novel susceptibility gene. Using a collection of Irish sibling-pair nuclear families, the authors found a modest evidence of linkage.

Implications for Nursing Care

The nurse should remember that for Irish Americans, alcoholism is influenced by a variety of factors, including patterns and characteristics of the family, social and economic conditions, and psychological orientation, rather than a biological variation per se. Because some Irish-American adults and adolescents drink for reassurance and to escape what is perceived as an intolerable burden, the nurse must develop strategies to teach such individuals more positive ways to alleviate stress and tension. Such individuals should be taught to verbally communicate feelings and anxiety rather than repressing or denying such feelings. The client must be taught the value of verbal expression to communicate needs. In addition, it is important to assist these clients in developing positive outlooks on life that may be perceived as positive coping strategies. The nurse also must remember the value of working not only with the client but also with the family because of the perception of family relationships as being paramount to a healthful existence.

The nurse might devise a family systems strategy that identifies perceived and actual roles within the family structure. After the roles are delineated, the nurse should assist the family in identifying undesirable behaviors manifested by persons in the particular roles. Changing behaviors that negatively affect the entire family system cannot be accomplished overnight. Such interventions will probably need repeated reinforcement. However, the nurse must remember that because some Irish Americans report that their drinking behavior is a result of their situation in life, it is important to consider the family's social and economic variables as a realistic beginning point in the initial intervention and treatment of such clients.

SUMMARY

Irish Americans have enjoyed extraordinary success in the United States. Although once faced with religious bigotry and economic hardship, they managed to cope with these problems and frequently turned them to their advantage. Irish descendants have become household names, including Robert Redford, Eugene O'Neill, Robert Kennedy, Andrew Jackson, John F. Kennedy, Henry Ford, and F. Scott Fitzgerald. Presidents Kennedy, Reagan, and Clinton each traveled to Ireland and claimed Irish ancestry, prompting pride by Irish Americans never felt before (Rapple, 2015).

The Internet offers intriguing and diverse information on Irish festivals, Irish heritage centers in states ranging from California to Illinois, Irish Americans telling their stories, and the role Irish Americans are playing in the United States.

Nurses should develop a sensitivity and understanding of individuals from a transcultural perspective to provide culturally appropriate nursing care. Nursing schools throughout the United States should incorporate transcultural courses and transcultural concepts into the nursing curriculum to foster the development of a transcultural understanding. One such institution that has developed a course to facilitate transcultural understanding is Vanderbilt University, which has a course titled "International Perspectives of Nursing and Health Care." This course was designed to offer graduate and undergraduate students an experiential learning opportunity for the development of a theoretical base in nursing and health care in countries other than the United States. During this experience, students spend time in Dublin, Edinburgh, and London. Macy and Morgan (1988) described the experiences of students in this course; for example, while in Dublin, students noted that 90% of the deliveries were attended by midwives, who were usually assisted by student midwives. Students were able to compare the differences in nursing and medical techniques found in other countries and to assess the need to modify care based on transcultural concepts.

CASE STUDY

Mr. Jonathon McMartin, a 46-year-old Catholic Irish American, is admitted to an inpatient alcoholic treatment center at a local hospital. Mr. McMartin came to the United States 10 years ago with his wife and his five children, who now range from 11 to 23 years of age. Of the five children, four still live at home. In addition, Mr. McMartin's mother and father live within five blocks of him. Mr. McMartin also has seven siblings; three of these siblings still reside in Ireland, and four live in the same city as Mr. McMartin. Mr. McMartin reports to the nurse therapist who admits him to the unit that his problem occurred because he feels isolated from his immediate family. He states that his wife is very cold and unaffectionate and appears to mobilize the children to her way of thinking. Mr. McMartin says his children appear very distant from him and closer to their mother. He also reports that as a child growing up he felt the same way about his mother and father: he felt close to his mother and very distant from his father. Mr. McMartin reveals to the nurse that he believes he can stop drinking any time he desires.

⊚ CARE PLAN

Nursing Diagnosis: Health maintenance, ineffective, related to unachieved developmental tasks

Client Outcomes	Nursing Interventions
1. Client and family will verbalize a desire to learn more about alcoholism and appropriate techniques to reduce symptoms. 2. Client and family will verbalize a willingness to comply with a psychiatric therapeutic regimen. 3. Client and family will verbalize an understanding of the need to comply with routine, scheduled follow-up visits to maintain an alcohol-free environment.	1. Identify with client and family sociocultural factors that influence health-seeking behaviors. 2. Determine with client and family their knowledge level about alcoholism and the severity of this illness. 3. Determine with client and family their willingness to adapt to an alternative lifestyle free of alcohol.

Nursing Diagnosis: Parenting, impaired risk for, related to lack of family cohesiveness

Client Outcomes	Nursing Interventions
1. Parents will display attentive, supportive parenting behavior. 2. Parents will develop realistic expectations of self, spouse, and children within the family system.	1. Assist parents in identifying present expectations of self, spouse, and children within the family system. 2. Assist family in developing and creating a positive learning environment for family growth. 3. Identify with family perceived areas of failure to meet expectations. 4. Provide family with opportunities to express feelings about unmet expectations. 5. Assist family in identifying major components within role identity that may create conflict within family system. 6. Encourage family to engage in closeness-related behavior, such as touching, to develop a more cohesive family system.

Nursing Diagnosis: Communication, impaired verbal, related to sociocultural variables creating interpersonal distance in family

Client Outcomes	Nursing Interventions
1. Family will be able to communicate with health care personnel about personal and family-related needs. 2. Family will be able to communicate feelings about interpersonal relationships and effects of alcohol on the family system.	1. Assist family in developing adequate communication techniques to communicate feelings and anxieties to one another. 2. Assist family in developing the ability to determine discrepancies in communicated verbal and nonverbal behavior. 3. Assist family in developing appropriate language skills and nonverbal perception to decrease the possibility of family perception.

Continued

CARE PLAN—cont'd

Nursing Diagnosis: Dysfunctional family processes: alcoholism related to lack of problem-solving skills

Client Outcomes	Nursing Interventions
1. Each family member will be able to send precise, understandable messages to one another through appropriate verbal and nonverbal communication. 2. Family will participate in care and maintenance of the alcoholic family member. 3. Family will assist nurse in assisting client to return to a high level of wellness. 4. Family will verbalize difficulties encountered in seeking appropriate external resources.	1. Determine family's understanding of client's condition. 2. Determine support systems available to family from external resources. 3. Determine with family supportive networks of friends and extended family members. 4. Involve family in care and management of client. 5. Encourage family to verbalize fears and anxieties.

Nursing Diagnosis: Social isolation related to inability to engage in satisfying personal relationships

Client Outcomes	Nursing Interventions
1. Client and family will verbalize positive and realistic feelings about self and the family system. 2. Client and family will make positive statements about self and the family system and display appropriate behavior accordingly. 3. Assist family in developing an understanding about the need for the client to engage in psychotherapy, whether as an individual or in a group. 4. Client and family will perceive self and family in a positive manner.	1. Design and implement client and family education to clarify values and beliefs that are perceived as negative influences. 2. Encourage client and family to engage in family therapy. 3. Client and family will set realistic goals for self and the family system and implement a plan to follow through on activities to achieve these goals. 4. Encourage family to seek and attend appropriate self-help groups.

Nursing Diagnoses—Definitions and Classifications 2012–2014. Copyright © 2012, 1994–2012 by NANDA International. Used by arrangement with Wiley-Blackwell Publishing, a company of John Wiley and Sons, Inc. In order to make safe and effective judgments using NANDA-I nursing diagnoses it is essential that nurses refer to the definitions and defining characteristics of the diagnoses listed in the work.

CLINICAL DECISION MAKING

1. List appropriate nursing interventions that can be implemented to facilitate communication within this family system.
2. Describe the family structure of some Irish-American families and the effect the family organization may have on health-seeking behaviors, and explain how this may affect nursing interventions when providing care for Mr. McMartin.
3. Identify how Mr. McMartin's behavior may be affected by time and space variables.
4. List at least two etiological reasons for the development of alcoholism within an Irish-American family.
5. Identify sociocultural variables within an Irish-American family that may facilitate perceived emotional distance.

REVIEW QUESTIONS

1. In Ireland and in the United States, the primary cultural force and national unifier of the Irish has been which of the following?
   a. The matriarchal family
   b. The Catholic Church
   c. The potato famine
   d. The work ethic
2. Alcoholism among Irish Americans is influenced by which of the following? (Mark all that apply.)
   a. Biological variation
   b. Patterns and characteristics of the family
   c. Economic conditions
   d. Psychological orientation
3. The Irish-American family expresses love and affection with which of the following mannerisms?

a. With difficulty
b. With great ease
c. With warmth and feeling
d. With discipline and rules

REFERENCES

Ablon, J., & Cunningham, W. (1981). Implications of cultural patterning for the delivery of alcoholism services. *Journal of Studies on Alcohol*, 42(Suppl. 9), 185–206.

Abramson, H. (1973). *Ethnic diversity in Catholic America*. New York: John Wiley & Sons.

Aroian, K., Patsdaughter, C., Levin, A., & Gianan, M. (1995). Use of the Brief Symptom Inventory to assess psychological distress in three immigrant groups. *International Journal of Social Psychiatry*, 41(1), 31–46.

Bates, T. (2005). Suicide in Ireland—everybody's problem. *Forum on Integration and Partnership Aras an Uachtarain*. Available at <http://www.hse.ie/eng/services/list/4/Mental_Health_Services/NOSP/Research/suicide2005.pdf> Retrieved October 15, 2011.

Biege, B. (2010). *No smoking in Ireland: the Irish smoking ban*. Available at <http://goireland.about.com/od/safetyinireland/qt/smoking_ban.htm?p=1> Retrieved August 18, 2010.

Boyne Research Institute. *Irish families with neural tube defects*. (2014). Available at <www.boyneresearch.ie/ntd.html>.

Butler, S., & Mayock, P. (2005). "An Irish solution to an Irish problem": harm reduction and ambiguity in the drug policy of the Republic of Ireland. *International Journal of Drug Policy*, 16(6), 415–422.

Byrne, J., & Carolan, S. (2006). Adverse reproductive outcomes among pregnancies of aunts and (spouses of) uncles in Irish families with neural tube defects. *American Journal of Medical Genetics*, 140(1), 52–61.

Cashman, S. M., et al. (1995). Identical intragenic microsatellite haplotype found in cystic fibrosis chromosomes bearing mutation G551D in Irish, English, Scottish, Breton and Czech patients. *Human Heredity*, 45(1), 6–12.

Central Intelligence Agency (CIA). (2011). *The world factbook*. Available at <https://www.cia.gov/library/publications/the-world-factbook/geos/ei.html> Retrieved April 18, 2011.

Central Statistics Office Ireland. (2010). *Births, deaths and marriages in quarter 2*, 2010. Available at <http://www.cso.ie/newsevents/pressrelease_vitalstatisticsquarter22010.htm>.

Christiansen, B., & Teahan, J. (1987). Cross-cultural comparisons of Irish and American adolescent drinking practices and beliefs. *Journal of Studies on Alcohol*, 48(6), 558–562.

Christopher, K. (2000). Determinants of psychological well-being in Irish immigrants. *Western Journal of Nursing Research*, 22(2), 123–140.

Cochrane, R. (1989). Mental hospital admission rates of immigrants to England: a comparison of 1971–1981. *Social Psychology*, 24, 2–11.

Countries and Their Cultures: Ireland. (2015). *Every culture*. Available at <http://www.everyculture.com/Ge-It/Ireland.html>.

Department of Public Health. (2001). *Suicide in Ireland: a national study*. Department of Public Health.

Depression and Suicide. (2013, December 1). *Irish Central*. Available at <www.irishcentral.com/news/depression-and-suicide>.

Development: across the gaping earth blasted by hatred: concern in Bangladesh. (2015). *History Ireland*. Available at <www.historyireland.com/20th-century-contemporary-history/development-across-the-gaping-earth-blasted-by-hatred-concern-in-bangladesh/>.

Doolin, N. (1994). The luck of the Irish? *Nursing Standard*, 8(46), 40–41.

Farren, C. K., & Dinan, T. G. (1996). Alcoholism and typology: findings in an Irish private hospital population. *Journal of Studies in Alcohol*, 57(3), 249–252.

Greeley, A. (1972). *That most distressful nation: the taming of the American Irish*. Chicago: Quadrangle Books.

Greeley, A. (1993). *The Irish Americans: the rise to money and power*. New York: Warner Books.

Griffin, W. (2001). *The Irish Americans: the immigrant experience*. Illinois: Beaux Arts Editions; Fairfield, CT: Rizzoli International Publications.

Haigh, W., Wang, W., Fung, H., Williams, K., & Mintz, J. (1999). Universal, developmental, and variable aspects of young children's play: a cross-cultural comparison of pretending at home. *Child Development*, 70(6), 1477–1488.

Hall, E. T. (1963). A system for the notation of proxemic behavior. *American Anthropologist*, 65(5), 1003–1026.

Hall, E. T. (1981). *The silent language*. New York: Fawcett.

Hall, E. T. (1990). *The hidden dimension*. New York: Doubleday.

Harrison, L., Carr-Hill, R., & Sutton, M. (1993). Consumption and harm: drinking patterns of the Irish, the English, and the Irish in England. *Alcohol*, 28(6), 715–726.

Heenan, D., & Birrell, D. (2009). Organizational integration in health and social care: some reflections on the Northern Ireland experience. *Journal of Integrated Care*, 17(5), 3–12.

Hoobler, D., & Hoobler, T. (1995). *The Irish American family album*. New York: Oxford University Press.

Hughes, D., Hill, A., Macek, M., Redmond, A. O., Nevin, N. C., & Graham, C. A. (1996). Mutation characterization of CFTR gene in 206 Northern Irish CF families: thirty mutations, including two novel, account for approximately 94% of CF chromosomes. *Human Mutations*, 8, 340–347.

Irish in Britain. (2014, April 7). *The silver voice*. Available at <https://thesilvervoice.wordpress.com/tag/irish-in-britain/>.

Irish Heart Foundation. (2015). Available at <www.irishheart.ie/iopen24/about-us-t-1.html>.

Irish Mental Health Coalition. (2007). *From neglect to respect: a 10-point agenda for action by the new Irish Government on mental health*. Dublin, Ireland: Irish Mental Health Coalition. Available at <http://www.sirl.ie/other/repository_docs/107.pdf> Retrieved October 14, 2011.

Johnson, J., & Adams, J. (1996). Self-neglect in later life. *Health and Social Care in the Community*, 4(4), 226–233.

Johnson, P., & Glassman, M. (1999). The moderating effects of gender and ethnicity on the relationship between effect expectancies and alcohol problems. *Journal of Studies on Alcohol, 60*(1), 64–69.

Kay, D., Saffra, N., & Har-El, G. (2002). Isolated sarcoidosis of the lacrimal sac without systemic manifestations. *American Journal of Otolaryngology, 23*(1), 533–535.

Kealey, C., Roche, S., Claffey, E., & McKeon, P. (2005). Linkage and candidate gene analysis of 14q22–24 in bipolar disorder: support for GCHI as a novel susceptibility gene. *American Journal of Medical Genetics, 136*(1), 75–80.

Kelly, P. (2013). Importance of hitting the bipolar nail on the head. *Irish Medical Times*, March 1. Available at <www.imt.ie/clinical/2013/03/importance-of-hitting-the-bipolar-nail-on-the-head.html>.

Kiesnoski, K. (2001). Eire's tourism board calls Irish-Americans home. *Travel Weekly, 60*(88), 6.

Kluckhohn, F., & Strodtbeck, F. (1961). *Variations in value orientation*. Evanston, IL: Row, Peterson.

Kwintessential. (2014). *Ireland—Language, culture, customs, and etiquette*. Available at <www.kwintessential.co.uk/resources/global-etiquette/ireland.html>.

Lakeman, R. (2012). What is good mental health nursing? A survey of Irish nurses. *Archives of Psychiatric Nursing, 26*(3), 225–231.

Lasky, J. (1996). Ireland: culture bytes. *Chronicle Features*, November 22, 1997.

Leavey, G., Rozmovits, L., Ryan, L., & King, M. (2007). Explanations of depression among Irish migrants in Britain. *Social Science and Medicine, 65*, 231–244.

Lee, J. J., & Casey, M. R. (2006). *Making the Irish American: history and heritage of the Irish in the United States*. New York: New York University Press.

Lewis, C. (1988). AIDS in Ireland. *Canadian Medical Association Journal, 138*, 553–555.

Lipton, J. A., & Marbach, J. J. (1984). Ethnicity and the pain experience. *Social Science and Medicine, 19*(12), 1279–1298.

MacDougall, J., & Doran, B. M. (1995). Health care information services in Ireland. *Topics in Health Information Management, 16*, 1–9.

MacHale, E., & Newell, J. (1997). Sexual behavior and sex education in Irish school-going teenagers. *International Journal of Studies in AIDS, 8*, 196–200.

Macy, J., & Morgan, S. (1988). Learning on the road: nursing in the British Isles and Ireland. *Nursing Outlook, 36*(1), 40–41.

Manning, P., Curran, K., Kirby, B., Taylor, M. R., & Clancy, L. (1997). Asthma, hay fever and eczema in Irish teenagers (ISAAC protocol). *Irish Medical Journal, 90*, 110–112.

Mbiti, J. (1990). *African religions and philosophies* (2nd ed.). Portsmouth, NH: Heinemann.

McCann, J., & Burden, D. (1996). An investigation of tooth size in Northern Irish people with bimaxillary dental protrusion. *Europe Journal of Orthodontics, 18*(6), 617–621.

McCullough, M. (Nov. 16, 2012). Tay-Sachs disease screening might become recommended for Irish Americans. *Philly.com*. Available at <http://articles.philly.com/2012-11-16/

news/35135852_1_tay-sachs-gene-tay-sachs-babies-jewish-genetic-disease>.

McGee, H. M., Molloy, G., O'Hanlon, A., Layte, R., & Hickey, A. (2008). Older people-recipients but also providers of informal care: an analysis among community samples in the Republic of Ireland and Northern Ireland. *Health and Social Care in the Community, 16*(5), 548–553.

McIlfatrick, S., McKenna, H., Gray, A., & Hinds, M. (2002). Health and social care futures in Ireland: the need for crossboundary work. *Journal of Clinical Nursing, 11*, 349–356.

Meagher, T. (2005). *The Columbia guide to Irish American history*. New York: Columbia University Press.

Molyneux, G. J., Cryan, E., & Dooley, E. (2006). The point-prevalence of alcohol use disorders and binge drinking in an Irish general hospital. *Irish Journal of Psychological Medicine, 23*(1), 17–20.

Music. (2010). *Celebrating St. Patrick and the Irish*. Available at <http://www.biography.com/st-patrick/irish-music.jsp> Retrieved August 18, 2010.

Mynett-Johnson, L., et al. (2000). Multimarker haplotypes within the serotonin transporter gene suggest evidence of an association with bipolar disorder. *American Journal of Medical Genetics, 96*(6), 845–849.

Newsline. (2001). *Billboard, 113*(14), 71.

North, K., Martin, L., & Crawford, M. (2000). The origins of the Irish Travellers and the genetic structure of Ireland. *Annals of Human Biology, 27*(5), 453–465.

O'Connor, J. (1978). *The young drinkers: a cross-national study of social and cultural influences*. London: Tavistock.

O'Leary, V. B., et al. (2006). Reduced folate carrier polymorphisms and neural tube defect risk. *Molecular Genetics and Metabolism, 87*, 364–369.

Porteous, M. A. (1985). Developmental aspects of adolescent problem disclosure in England and Ireland. *Journal of Child Psychology and Psychiatry, 26*(3), 465–478.

Primm, J., et al. (2005). The Epsin 4 gene on chromosome 5q, which encodes the clathrin-associated protein enthoprotin, is involved in the genetic susceptibility to schizophrenia. *American Journal of Human Genetics, 76*(5), 902–907.

Prosser, S., & Dobbs, F. (1997). Case-finding incontinence in the over-75. *British Journal of General Practice, 47*(421), 498–500.

Rapple, B. (2015), Irish Americans. *Encyclopedia.com*. Available at <http://www.encyuclopedia.com/topic/Irish_Americans.aspx>.

Samuels, T. (3/5/2012). Program inspired lonely death of elderly Irishman. *New York Daily News*. Available at <www.nydailynews.com/life-style/health/program-inspired-lonely-death-elderly-irishman-expands-older-irish-americans-citywide-article-1.1032107>.

Schizophrenia—its not just an Irish condition. (2012, August 18). *NAMA Wine Lake*. Available at <https://namawinelake.wordpress.com/2012/08/18/schizophrenia-its-not-just-an-irish-condition/>.

Spector, R. (2004). *Cultural diversity in health and illness* (6th ed.). Upper Saddle River, NJ: Prentice Hall Health.

Stillman, M. (1978). Territoriality and personal space. *American Journal of Nursing, 78*, 1671–1672.

Stopes-Roe, M., & Cochrane, R. (1980). Mental health and integration: a compromise of Indian, Pakistani, and Irish immigrants to English. *Ethnic and Racial Studies, 3*, 316–341.

Straub, R., MacLean, D., O'Neill, F., Walsh, D., & Kendler, K. S. (1997). Support for a possible schizophrenia vulnerability locus in region 5q22–31 in Irish families. *Molecular Psychiatry, 2*, 148–155.

Su, Y., et al. (1993). Exclusion of linkage between schizophrenia and the D$_2$ dopamine receptor gene region of chromosome 11q in 112 multiplex families. *Archives of General Psychiatry, 50*(3), 205–211.

Unit History Project: Meagher's Irish Brigade. (2014). Available at <dmna.ny.gov/historic/reghist/civil/brigades/meaghersBrigade.html>.

U.S. Department of Commerce, Bureau of the Census. (2009). *American Community Survey*. Washington, DC: U.S. Government Printing Office.

U.S. Department of Commerce, Bureau of the Census. (2015). *American Community Survey*. Washington, DC: U.S. Government Printing Office.

U.S. Department of Commerce, Bureau of the Census. (2011). *Statistical abstract of the United States*. Washington, DC: U.S. Government Printing Office.

Van Bael, M., Natowicz, M., Tomczak, J., Grebner, E. E., & Prence, E. M. (1996). Heterozygosity for Tay-Sachs disease in non-Jewish Americans with ancestry from Ireland or Great Britain. *Journal of Medical Genetics, 33*(10), 829–832.

Walsh, J. (1987). AIDS. *The Irish Times*, 8.

Warner, M. (2009). *The history of traditional Irish Music, eHow*. Available at <http://www.ehow.com/about_5349022_history-traditional-irish-music.html> Retrieved August 18, 2010.

Wessel, B. (1931). *An ethnic survey of Woonsocket, Rhode Island*. Chicago: University of Chicago Press.

Wilson, S. (2003). Irish-Americans. In L. Purnell & B. Paulanka (Eds.), *Transcultural health care* (2nd ed.). Philadelphia: F. A. Davis.

World Almanac. (2015). New York: World Almanac Books.

Your Irish. (2015). History. *Your Irish.com*. Available at <http://www.yourirish.com/history> Retrieved January 15, 2015.

Zola, I. (1966). Culture and symptoms: an analysis of patients' presenting complaints. *American Sociological Review, 31*, 615–630.

ANSWER KEY TO REVIEW QUESTIONS

CHAPTER 1

CHAPTER 2

1. Answer: A
   Cognitive Level: Comprehension
   Nursing Process: Assessment
2. Answer: D
   Cognitive Level: Application
   Nursing Process: Assessment
3. Answer: B
   Cognitive Level: Knowledge
   Nursing Process: Implementation

CHAPTER 3

1. Answer: B
   Cognitive Level: Application
   Nursing Process: Implementation
2. Answer: A
   Cognitive Level: Application
   Nursing Process: Assessment
3. Answer: A
   Cognitive Level: Knowledge
   Nursing Process: Assessment

CHAPTER 4

1. Answer: C
   Cognitive Level: Knowledge
   Nursing Process: Planning
2. Answer: C
   Cognitive Level: Knowledge
   Nursing Process: Assessment
3. Answer: D
   Cognitive Level: Application
   Nursing Process: Planning

CHAPTER 5

1. Answer: C
   Cognitive Level: Knowledge
   Nursing Process: Implementation
2. Answer: A
   Cognitive Level: Knowledge
   Nursing Process: Planning
3. Answer: A
   Cognitive Level: Knowledge
   Nursing Process: Implementation

CHAPTER 6

1. Answer: B
   Cognitive Level: Application
   Nursing Process: Assessment
2. Answer: A
   Cognitive Level: Application
   Nursing Process: Planning
3. Answer: A
   Cognitive Level: Knowledge
   Nursing Process: Planning

CHAPTER 7

1. Answer: D
   Cognitive Level: Knowledge
   Nursing Process: Assessment
2. Answer: A
   Cognitive Level: Application
   Nursing Process: Assessment
3. Answer: A, C, & D
   Cognitive Level: Knowledge
   Nursing Process: Assessment

CHAPTER 8

1. Answer: A
   Cognitive Level: Knowledge
   Nursing Process: Assessment
2. Answer: D
   Cognitive Level: Application
   Nursing Process: Implementation
3. Answer: A
   Cognitive Level: Application
   Nursing Process: Assessment

CHAPTER 9

1. Answer: C
   Cognitive Level: Knowledge
   Nursing Process: Implementation
2. Answer: B
   Cognitive Level: Knowledge
   Nursing Process: Implementation
3. Answer: B
   Cognitive Level: Knowledge
   Nursing Process: Planning

CHAPTER 10

1. Answer: C
   Cognitive Level: Knowledge
   Nursing Process: Assessment
2. Answer: D
   Cognitive Level: Knowledge
   Nursing Process: Assessment
3. Answer: B
   Cognitive Level: Knowledge
   Nursing Process: Planning

CHAPTER 11

1. Answer: C
   Cognitive Level: Knowledge
   Nursing Process: Assessment
2. Answer: B
   Cognitive Level: Application
   Nursing Process: Implementation
3. Answer: D
   Cognitive Level: Knowledge
   Nursing Process: Assessment

CHAPTER 12

1. Answer: A
   Cognitive Level: Application
   Nursing Process: Implementation
2. Answer: B
   Cognitive Level: Application
   Nursing Process: Assessment
3. Answer: D
   Cognitive Level: Knowledge
   Nursing Process: Assessment

CHAPTER 13

1. Answer: B
   Cognitive Level: Knowledge
   Nursing Process: Planning
2. Answer: A
   Cognitive Level: Knowledge
   Nursing Process: Assessment
3. Answer: D
   Cognitive Level: Knowledge
   Nursing Process: Assessment

CHAPTER 14

1. Answer: A
   Cognitive Level: Knowledge
   Nursing Process: Assessment
2. Answer: A
   Cognitive Level: Knowledge
   Nursing Process: Assessment
3. Answer: A
   Cognitive Level: Knowledge
   Nursing Process: Assessment

CHAPTER 15

1. Answer: A
   Cognitive Level: Knowledge
   Nursing Process: Implementation
2. Answer: B
   Cognitive Level: Knowledge
   Nursing Process: Implementation
3. Answer: D
   Cognitive Level: Application
   Nursing Process: Implementation

CHAPTER 16

1. Answer: A
   Cognitive Level: Knowledge
   Nursing Process: Assessment
2. Answer: C
   Cognitive Level: Knowledge
   Nursing Process: Assessment
3. Answer: B
   Cognitive Level: Knowledge
   Nursing Process: Assessment

CHAPTER 17

1. Answer: A
   Cognitive Level: Knowledge
   Nursing Process: Assessment
2. Answer: C
   Cognitive Level: Knowledge
   Nursing Process: Assessment
3. Answer: C
   Cognitive Level: Knowledge
   Nursing Process: Assessment

CHAPTER 18

1. Answer: A
   Cognitive Level: Knowledge
   Nursing Process: Planning
2. Answer: B
   Cognitive Level: Knowledge
   Nursing Process: Planning
3. Answer: D
   Cognitive Level: Knowledge
   Nursing Process: Evaluation

CHAPTER 19

1. Answer: B
   Cognitive Level: Application
   Nursing Process: Implementation
2. Answer: B
   Cognitive Level: Knowledge
   Nursing Process: Assessment
3. Answer: A
   Cognitive Level: Knowledge
   Nursing Process: Implementation

CHAPTER 20

1. Answer: D
   Cognitive Level: Application
   Nursing Process: Planning
2. Answer: B
   Cognitive Level: Application
   Nursing Process: Implementation
3. Answer: D
   Cognitive Level: Knowledge
   Nursing Process: Assessment

CHAPTER 21

1. Answer: D
   Cognitive Level: Application
   Nursing Process: Implementation
2. Answer: C
   Cognitive Level: Application
   Nursing Process: Implementation
3. Answer: A
   Cognitive Level: Application
   Nursing Process: Implementation

CHAPTER 22

1. Answer: A
   Cognitive Level: Application
   Nursing Process: Implementation
2. Answer: D
   Cognitive Level: Application
   Nursing Process: Planning
3. Answer: C
   Cognitive Level: Knowledge
   Nursing Process: Assessment

CHAPTER 23

1. Answer: D
   Cognitive Level: Application
   Nursing Process: Assessment
2. Answer: C
   Cognitive Level: Application
   Nursing Process: Assessment
3. Answer: B
   Cognitive Level: Knowledge
   Nursing Process: Implementation

CHAPTER 24

1. Answer: B
   Cognitive Level: Knowledge
   Nursing Process: Assessment
2. Answer: A
   Cognitive Level: Knowledge
   Nursing Process: Analysis
3. Answer: A
   Cognitive Level: Application
   Nursing Process: Assessment

CHAPTER 25

1. Answer: D
   Cognitive Level: Application
   Nursing Process: Assessment
2. Answer: A
   Cognitive Level: Application
   Nursing Process: Implementation
3. Answer: B
   Cognitive Level: Knowledge
   Nursing Process: Assessment

CHAPTER 26

1. Answer: A
   Cognitive Level: Knowledge
   Nursing Process: Assessment
2. Answer: A
   Cognitive Level: Knowledge
   Nursing Process: Assessment
3. Answer: C
   Cognitive Level: Knowledge
   Nursing Process: Assessment

CHAPTER 27

1. Answer: A
   Cognitive Level: Knowledge
   Nursing Process: Planning
2. Answer: D
   Cognitive Level: Knowledge
   Nursing Process: Planning
3. Answer: B
   Cognitive Level: Knowledge
   Nursing Process: Assessment

CHAPTER 28

1. Answer: C
   Cognitive Level: Knowledge
   Nursing Process: Assessment
2. Answer: A
   Cognitive Level: Analysis
   Nursing Process: Assessment
3. Answer: C
   Cognitive Level: Knowledge
   Nursing Process: Assessment

CHAPTER 29

1. Answer: C
   Cognitive Level: Knowledge
   Nursing Process: Assessment
2. Answer: C
   Cognitive Level: Comprehension
   Nursing Process: Assessment
3. Answer: B
   Cognitive Level: Knowledge
   Nursing Process: Assessment

CHAPTER 30

1. Answer: B
   Cognitive Level: Knowledge
   Nursing Process: Assessment
2. Answer: B, C, & D
   Cognitive Level: Comprehension
   Nursing Process: Assessment
3. Answer: A
   Cognitive Level: Knowledge
   Nursing Process: Assessment

INDEX

Page numbers followed by "*f*" indicate figures, "*b*" indicate boxes, and "*t*" indicate tables.